Drugs for the Treatment of Respiratory Diseases

Respiratory diseases affect millions of people each year and represent a major health burden around the world. This timely reference surveys and evaluates the drug treatments available for the main categories of lung diseases including asthma and chronic obstructive pulmonary disease, lung cancer, cystic fibrosis, pulmonary vascular disease, lung cancer, and respiratory infections. The recent increase in asthma in certain populations underlines the importance of finding effective new treatments for these diseases. This publication, a comprehensive reference, is one of the first to survey current and novel drug treatments for this group of diseases. It is certain to establish itself as an essential source of reference for respiratory physicians, clinicians and clinical pharmacologists.

Drugs for the Treatment of Respiratory Diseases

EDITED BY

Domenico Spina
The Sackler Institute of Pulmonary Pharmacology,
King's College London, UK

Clive P. Page
The Sackler Institute of Pulmonary Pharmacology,
King's College London, UK

William J. Metzger
National Jewish Medical and
Research Center, Denver, CO, USA

AND

Brian J. O'Connor
The Sackler Institute of Pulmonary Pharmacology,
King's College London, UK

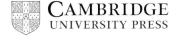

PUBLISHED BY THE PRESS SYNDICATE OF THE UNIVERSITY OF CAMBRIDGE
The Pitt Building, Trumpington Street, Cambridge, United Kingdom

CAMBRIDGE UNIVERSITY PRESS
The Edinburgh Building, Cambridge CB2 2RU, UK
40 West 20th Street, New York, NY 10011–4211, USA
477 Williamstown Road, Port Melbourne, VIC 3207, Australia
Ruiz de Alarcón 13, 28014 Madrid, Spain
Dock House, The Waterfront, Cape Town 8001, South Africa

http://www.cambridge.org

First published 2003

Printed in the United Kingdom at the University Press, Cambridge

Typeface Utopia 8½/12 pt.   *System* QuarkXPress®   [SE]

A catalogue record for this book is available from the British Library

Library of Congress Cataloguing in Publication data

Drugs for the treatment of respiratory diseases / edited by Domenico Spina . . . [et. al.].
      p. ; cm.
Includes bibliographical references and index.
ISBN 0 521 77321 0 (hardback)
1. Lungs – Diseases – Chemotherapy. 2. Respiratory agents. I. Spina, Domenico.
[DNLM: 1. Respiratory Tract Diseases – drug therapy. 2. Anti-Allergic Agents – therapeutic
use. 3. Respiratory System Agents – therapeutic use. WF 145 D7947 2002]
RC756 .D784 2002
616.2′4061–dc21   2002023390

ISBN 0 521 77321 0 hardback

Contents

Colour plate section between pp. 12 and 13.

Contributors

Editors

Domenico Spina
The Sackler Institute of Pulmonary Pharmacology
Department of Respiratory Medicine and Allergy
GKT School of Medicine
King's College London
Bessemer Road
London SE5 9PJ, UK

Clive P. Page
The Sackler Institute of Pulmonary Pharmacology
Division of Pharmacology and Therapeutics
GKT School of Biomedical Science
5th Floor Hodgkin Building
Guy's Campus
London SE1 1UL, UK

W.J. Metzger*
National Jewish Medical and Research Center
1400 Jackson Street, Denver, CO 80206, USA

Brian J. O'Connor
The Sackler Institute of Pulmonary Pharmacology
Department of Respiratory Medicine and Allergy
GKT School of Medicine
King's College London
Bessemer Road
London SE5 9PJ, UK

*now deceased

Contributors

Steven Abman
Division of Pulmonary Sciences and Critical Care Medicine
University of Colorado Health Sciences Center
4200 East Ninth Avenue, C272
Denver, CO 80262, USA

John J. Adcock
Pneumolabs (UK) Ltd
NPIMR, Y Block
Watford Road
Harrow, Middlesex HA1 3UJ, UK

Peter J. Barnes
Department of Thoracic Medicine
National Heart and Lung Institute
Imperial College School of Medicine
Dovehouse Street
London SW3 6LY, UK

Brydon L. Bennett
Signal Research Division
Celgene Corporation
5555 Oberlin Drive
San Diego, CA 92121, USA

Desmond N. Carney
Department of Medical Oncology
Mater Hospital
Dublin 7, Ireland

Mario Cazzola
Department of Respiratory Medicine
Division of Pneumology and Allergology
A. Cardarelli Hospital
Naples, Italy

Peter V. Dicpinigaitis
Department of Medicine
Albert Einstein College of Medicine
Bronx, New York, USA

Ahmed Z. El-Hashim
Department of Applied Therapeutics
Faculty of Pharmacy, Kuwait University
PO Box 249, Kuwait, SAFAT 13110

Lawrence G. Garland
Formerly at Acambis PLC
100 Fulbourn Road
Cambridge CB1 9PT, UK

Adi F. Gazdar
Hamon Center for Therapeutic Oncology Research
NB8.106, UT Southwestern Medical Center
5323 Harry Hines Blvd
Dallas, TX 75235-8593, USA

Pierangelo Geppetti
Department of Experimental and Clinical Medicine
Pharmacology Unit, University of Ferrara
Via Fossato di Mortara 19, 44100, Italy

Mark W. Geraci
Division of Pulmonary Sciences and Critical Care Medicine
University of Colorado Health Sciences Center
4200 East Ninth Avenue, C272
Denver, CO 80262, USA

Nicholas J. Gross
Building 1, Room A342, Hines VA Hospital
Roosevelt and 5th Avenues
Hines, IL 60141, USA

Masakazu Ichinose
Department of Respiratory and Infectious Diseases
Tohoku University School of Medicine
1-1 Seiryo-machi Aoba-ku
Sendai 980 8574, Japan

Peter K. Jeffery
Imperial College at the Royal Brompton Hospital,
National Heart and Lung Institute
Sydney Street
London SW3 6NP, UK

Neil A. Jones
The Sackler Institute of Pulmonary Pharmacology
Pharmacology and Therapeutics Division
GKT School of Biomedical Sciences
5th Floor Hodgkin Building
Guy's Campus, London SE1 1UL, UK

Michael Keane
Division of Pulmonary and Critical Care Medicine
Department of Internal Medicine
University of Michigan Medical Center
3916 Taubman Center, Box 0360
Ann Arbor, MI 48109-0360, USA

Alan G. Lamont
Catalyst Biomedica Ltd
183 Euston Road
London NW1 2BE, UK (formerly at Acambis PLC)

Alan J. Lewis
Signal Research Division
Celgene Corporation
5555 Oberlin Drive, San Diego, CA 92121, USA

Joseph P. Lynch III
Division of Pulmonary and Critical Care Medicine
Department of Internal Medicine
University of Michigan Medical Center
3916 Taubman Center, Box 0360
Ann Arbor, MI 48109-0360, USA

David G. McCormack
A.C. Burton Vascular Research Laboratory
Division of Respirology, London Health Services Centre
Departments of Medicine, Pharmacology and Toxicology
University of Western Ontario
London, Ontario, Canada

Maria G. Matera
Institute of Pharmacology and Toxicology
Medical School
Second Neapolitan University, Naples, Italy

Sanjay Mehta
A.C. Burton Vascular Research Laboratory,
Division of Respirology, London Health Services Center,
Departments of Medicine, Pharmacology and Toxicology
University of Western Ontario, London, Ontario, Canada

Paul M. O'Byrne
Firestone Regional Chest and Allergy Unit
St Joseph's Hospital, 50 Charlton Avenue East
Hamilton, Ontario L8N 4A6, Canada

Brian J. O'Connor
The Sackler Institute of Pulmonary Pharmacology
Department of Respiratory Medicine
King's College London
Bessemer Road, London SE5 9PJ, UK

Clive P. Page
The Sackler Institute of Pulmonary Pharmacology
Division of Pharmacology and Therapeutics
GKT School of Biomedical Science
5th Floor Hodgkin Building
Guy's Campus, London, SE1 1UL, UK

Andrew Peacock
Scottish Pulmonary Vascular Unit, Level 8, Western
Infirmary
Dumbarton Road, Glasgow G11 6NT, UK

John F. Price
Department of Child Health, King's College Hospital
Denmark Hill, London SE5 9RS, UK

R.G. Gary Ruiz
Department of Child Health, King's College Hospital
Denmark Hill, London SE5 9RS, UK

Tarek Saba
Scottish Pulmonary Vascular Unit, Level 8, Western
Infirmary
Dumbarton Road, Glasgow G11 6NT, UK

Yoshitaka Satoh
Signal Research Division
Celgene Corporation
5555 Oberlin Drive
San Diego, CA 92121, USA

Jeremy M. Segal
Departments of Medicine and Molecular Biochemistry
Stritch School of Medicine, Loyola University of Chicago, IL,
USA

Domenico Spina
The Sackler Institute of Pulmonary Pharmacology
Department of Respiratory Medicine and Allergy
King's College London
Bessemer Road, London SE5 9PJ, UK

Norbert F. Voelkel
Division of Pulmonary Sciences and Critical Care Medicine
University of Colorado Health Sciences Center
4200 East Ninth Avenue, C272
Denver, CO 80262, USA

Athol U. Wells
Interstitial Lung Disease Unit
Departments of Radiology, Pathology and Physiology
Royal Brompton Hospital
Sydney Street, London SW3 6NP, UK

Robert Wilson
Royal Brompton Hospital
Sydney Street, London SW3 6NP, UK

Ignacio I. Wistuba
Department of Pathology
Pontificia Universidad Catolica de Chile
PO Box 114-D, Santiago, Chile

Hilary H. Wyatt
Department of Child Health, King's College Hospital
Denmark Hill, London SE5 9RS, UK

Preface

In 1991, Jim Metzger and I edited a volume called *Drugs and the Lung*. A decade on, we thought that sufficient new information had been obtained to warrant a new book and this volume reflects the culmination of a considerable effort of many individuals including my new co-editors Dom Spina and Brian O'Connor, plus all the contributing authors. Lung diseases still represent a considerable burden to the healthcare system globally and have significant impact on the socio-economic situation in many countries around the world. The incidence of asthma continues to rise in many western countries with no cure in sight. Furthermore, tuberculosis, pulmonary infections and COPD are far from optimally controlled and not surprisingly therefore, there continues to be a considerable amount of interest in the development of novel therapies for a wider range of lung diseases. Perhaps, just as importantly, continual appraisal of optimal use of existing therapies continues with guidelines for the treatment of asthma and COPD now being commonplace in many western societies. This book represents a comprehensive collection of chapters regarding the current status of a wide range of drugs in use for the treatment of lung diseases, as well as providing an excellent overview of the many new drug classes under development. We have tried to ensure that, where possible, all chapters have a bias towards clinical information about drugs, but drawing on information from in vitro and animal studies where appropriate. We hope this book will be of interest to clinicians, scientists and students as a resource about drugs for the treatment of respiratory diseases.

Tragically, my colleague and friend Jim Metzger died half-way through this project. Jim was an excellent mentor to me along with fellow editors and was responsible for teaching me a lot about allergy and clinical immunology. I share his tragic loss with his devoted family and many friends. Jim had contributed enormously to the field of lung diseases and we hope this book will help provide a lasting memory of him.

Clive P. Page
on behalf of all the editors
March 2002

Part I

Asthma and COPD

Pathology of asthma and COPD : inflammation and structure

Peter K Jeffery

Imperial College at the Royal Brompton Hospital, London, UK

Introduction

It is widely recognized that neither asthma nor COPD are disease entities but rather each is a complex of inflammatory conditions that have in common airflow limitation (syn. obstruction) whose reversibility varies (Fig. 1.1). The characteristics and distinctions between mild stable asthma and COPD have been reviewed[1,2]. However, these differences become less clear when the conditions become severe or there are exacerbations due to infection or other cause. An understanding of whether or not there are fundamental differences of inflammation and airway/lung structure between these two conditions is relevant to clinical decisions regarding both initiation and long-term treatment and to patient management during exacerbations. In the longer term it is of value to the design of specific therapy for asthma and COPD and to their prevention. Whilst the definitions of asthma and COPD highlight the differing degrees of airflow variability and reversibility[3,4], there is a prevailing clinical impression that, with age, there is often overlap and a progression from the reversible airflow obstruction of the young asthmatic to the more irreversible or 'fixed' obstruction of the older patient with COPD. The Dutch hypothesis encompasses the idea that both conditions are extreme ends of a single condition[5]. In the author's opinion it may, in the future, be less relevant to be concerned with the clinical labels of 'asthma' or 'COPD' and more important to ascertain and target treatment to the predominant pattern of inflammation and structural change that prevails in each patient.

Asthma may be divided into extrinsic (also called allergic or atopic), intrinsic (late onset or non-atopic) and occupational forms. At this time the pathologist cannot distinguish between these distinct clinical forms of asthma: there are alterations that appear to be common to all forms. COPD is associated, usually, with the smoking habit as the relationship between cigarette smoking and COPD is a strong one statistically. Three conditions can contribute, the degree varying in each patient, to the clinical expression of COPD: chronic bronchitis (syn. mucus hypersecretion), chronic bronchiolitis (syn. small airways disease) and emphysema, inflammatory conditions broadly affecting bronchi (airways with cartilage in their wall), bronchioli (membranous or non-cartilaginous airways) and lung parenchyma respectively. In both asthma and COPD, the persistence of distinct inflammatory cells initiated by allergen or cigarette smoke, respectively, is probably responsible for most of the structural change and usually referred to as 'remodelling': interactions with the effects of acute and chronic infection and genetic predisposition are clearly important also.

The chapter focuses on the patterns of infiltrating inflammatory cells in asthma and COPD and the associated remodelling of the airway wall. First, airway wall thickening is considered, particularly in asthma, remodelling is defined and the relationship between inflammation and remodelling discussed briefly. Lumenal secretions obtained as sputum or lavage and asphyxic plugging of the airways with mixtures of mucus and inflammatory exudate are discussed briefly. The chapter then divides into two

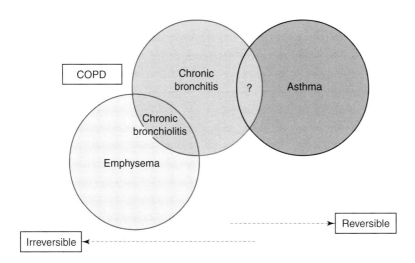

Fig. 1.1 Venn diagram illustrating the overlap between asthma and COPD.

major sections considering first inflammation and then remodelling in asthma and COPD. The results of examination of the conducting airways by flexible fibre-optic bronchoscopy are included as this technique has provided the means by which the early inflammatory and structural alterations of asthma and COPD have been compared, free from the complications of end stage disease[6].

Airway wall thickening

The airway walls in asthma are thickened by the remodelling process by between 50 and 300% of normal and there is lumenal narrowing, which is further compromised by excessive mucus admixed with an inflammatory exudate (Fig. 1.2, see colour plate section). In cases of fatal asthma, the longer the duration of asthma, the thicker becomes the airway wall[7]. However, it has been suggested that airway wall thickness *per se* is not a requirement for asphyxic fatality as a group of relatively young asthmatics (i.e. with a relatively short history of asthma) had an airway wall thickness not significantly different from that of non-asthma controls. Lumenal secretions and plugging are likely the greater contribution to asthmatic death in these young cases of

fatal asthma[7]. All tissue structural components, as well as inflammatory cell infiltration and edema, can contribute to the observed thickening; however, in the last mentioned study it is thickening of the (outer) adventitial layers that was most pronounced in the older group with the longest duration of disease. The airway walls are also thickened in COPD. One systematic study has described changes in large airway dimensions in relation to the lung function of patients with COPD and found wall area internal to the muscle to be significantly thickened over the entire range of cartilaginous airways measured[8]. The relative contributions of the airway wall components contributing to the thickening, however, vary with airway generation.

Inflammation and remodelling

Acute inflammation is the response of vascularized tissue to injury: the inflammatory reaction is designed to protect the host and to restore tissue and its function to normal. One generally accepted proposal is that the accelerated decline in forced expiratory flow over time in COPD, and that which occurs also in an important subset of asthmatics, is the direct result of a switch from acute, episodic, to chronic inflammation and to consequent airway and parenchymal remodelling[1]. The proposal is attractive but, as yet, there is no convincing evidence that the remodelling process is dependent upon the prior development of chronic inflammation. It is equally plausible that the processes responsible for the development of chronic inflammation are distinct to those responsible for remodelling. The last consideration has important implications for the design of disease modifying therapy: thus those agents that are effective antiinflamatory compounds will not necessarily prevent or attenuate the process of remodelling for which new classes of drugs will be required.

Definition

The concept of 'remodelling' implies that a process of 'modelling' must have preceded it. The lung, in utero, undergoes extensive modelling and remodelling yet these processes are entirely appropriate to the normal process of lung development. Many of the cytokines and growth factors thought to be pro-inflammatory in asthma and in COPD are also expressed normally without detriment to the developing lung; these include: members of the fibroblast growth factor family, the transforming growth factor family, epithelial-derived growth factor, granulocyte–macrophage colony stimulating factor, platelet-derived growth factor, vascular endothelial growth factor and hepatocyte growth factor[1,9]. Accordingly the working definition of remodelling proposed herein recognizes that the process of remodelling *per se* is not of necessity abnormal. It is: an alteration in size, mass or number of tissue structural components that occurs during growth or in response to injury and/or inflammation. It may be appropriate, as in normal lung development or that which occurs during acute reaction to injury, or 'inappropriate' when it is chronic and associated with abnormally altered tissue structure and function as, for example, in asthma or COPD.

In wound healing (in the skin) the components of an appropriate response include: clot formation, swelling/edema, rapid restitution of the denuded areas by epithelial dedifferentiation, proliferation and migration from the margins of the wound. This is normally associated with an inflammatory reaction, i.e. early infiltration of the injured tissue by neutrophils and later by lymphocytes and macrophages. Reticulin is deposited within days and this may mature to form interstitial collagen, a scar, within 2–3 weeks. In addition, healing may involve contraction of the surrounding tissue (in the case of an open wound), by myofibroblasts that may proliferate transiently in relatively large numbers[10]. Vasodilatation, congestion and mucosal oedema are also cardinal signs of acute inflammation and the angiogenesis of the granulation tissue is an integral part of the reparative response. Thus, normal tissue architecture and function is restored consequent to an entirely appropriate inflammatory reaction with which there has been an associated remodelling process. Each of these stages in normal wound healing and many of the inflammatory cell types and cytokines involved appear also in asthma and in COPD, but in these last two conditions both the inflammation and remodelling persist and result in exaggerated remodelling inappropriate to the maintenance of normal (airway) function. The reasons for the persistence of the inflammation are unknown but may be the result of repeated inhalation of allergen or exposure to high concentrations of allergen, irritation (e.g. by tobacco smoke) or persistent infection or a genetically influenced abnormal host inflammatory response or a defective repair process.

Lumenal secretions

Sputum and bronchoalveolar lavage

The examination of spontaneously produced or saline-induced sputum has become a much used and relatively non-invasive method for determining the extent of inflammation in the asthmatic airway[11,12] (Fig. 1.3(*a*), 1.2(*b*), see colour plate section). Corkscrew-shaped twists of condensed mucus (Curshmann's spirals), clusters of surface airway epithelial cells (referred to as Creola bodies and named after the first patient in whom they were described)[13], and the presence of Charcot–Leyden crystals, composed of eosinophil cell and granule membrane lysophospholipase (Fig. 1.3(*a*), (*b*), see colour plate section[14]), together with eosinophils and metachromatic cells, are characteristic features of sputa obtained from asthmatic, but not bronchitic patients[15]. Sputum eosinophilia has, however, also been reported in non-asthmatics in the absence of the airways hyper-responsiveness (AHR) characteristic of asthma[16]. In contrast, sputa from bronchitic patients may be mucoid or, during infective exacerbations, purulent when neutrophils may be present in large numbers. BAL in mild (allergic) asthma demonstrates the presence of sloughed epithelial cells, the numbers of which show an association with AHR,[17] and of eosinophils and their highly charged secreted products (such as eosinophil cationic protein (ECP) and major basic protein (MBP))[18]. In contrast, in smoker's bronchitis, macrophages are the most usually reported cell type and neutrophils are numerous as are their secreted products.

Airway plugging

Examination, postmortem, of cases of fatal asthma has shown that the lungs are hyperinflated and remain so on opening the pleural cavities due to the widespread presence of markedly tenacious airway 'plugs' in both large (segmental) and small bronchi (Fig. 1.4(*a*), see colour plate section). Even intra-bronchial inflation with fixative to a 1.5-metre head of pressure hardly moves these sticky lumenal plugs[19]. Histologically the airway plugs in asthma are composed predominantly of inflammatory exudate together with mucus in which lie: eosinophils, lymphocytes and desquamated surface epithelial cells. The arrangement of the eosinophilic elements of the plug is often as concentric, multiple lamellae suggesting that several episodes of inflammation have led to their formation rather than a single terminal event (Fig. 1.4(*b*), see colour section). The non-mucinous, proteinaceous contribution is the result of increased vascular permeability and includes a fibrin. Electrostatic interaction of positively charged (cationic) eosinophil products and serum constitu-

ents and negatively charged (due to carboxyl and sulfate groups) mucin likely contributes to the particular stickiness of the airway plug. There are, however, reports of sudden death in asthmatics in which intraluminal plugs are absent[20] but these are rare. In the absence of a history of smoking, emphysema in fatal asthma and right ventricular hypertrophy is uncommon. However, areas of atelectasis and petechial hemorrhages may be present in asthma due to bronchial obstruction, reabsorption collapse and repeated forced inspiratory efforts. The asthmatic who has smoked will likely have features which overlap between asthma and COPD and, in these cases, there may be focal evidence of centriacinar (i.e.bronchocentric) alveolar destruction (see Fig. 1.4(*a*), colour plate section).

Inflammation

To the physiologist, inflammation is characterized by cardinal signs: redness, heat, swelling, pain and loss of normal function. To the pathologist, inflammation is recognized in tissue sections as congestion of vessels together with the recruitment (i.e. margination within and emigration from vessels) of a variety of morphologically and immuno-phenotypically distinct inflammatory cells. It is now recognized that both asthma[21,22] and COPD are inflammatory conditions albeit the relative magnitude and site of the inflammatory infiltrate and the predominant inflammatory cell phenotype differs.

Asthma

Studies of biopsies obtained by fibreoptic bronchoscopy or at open lung biopsy in asthma demonstrate the presence of an inflammatory cell infiltrate even in patients with newly diagnosed asthma[23]. The infiltrate comprises CD3 immuno-positive (T) lymphocytes of the CD4 (i.e. T-helper) subset and eosinophils[17,24–26]. An increase in leukocytes, including lymphocytes and eosinophils, occurs in relatively mild atopic, occupational and intrinsic asthma and it is associated with an increase of 'activation' markers for both lymphocytes (CD25 + cells) and eosinophils (EG2 + cells)[21,24,26–28]. In symptomatic atopic asthmatics, in electron microscopic studies, irregularly shaped lymphomononuclear cells appear and these may represent ultrastructural forms of the CD25 + (activated) lymphocyte. EG2 is a marker for the cleaved ('secreted') form of eosinophil cationic protein that can be found both within eosinophils and diffusely in the wall, often in association with the epithelial reticular basement membrane. Eosinophil-derived products such as major basic protein[29] together with toxic oxygen radicals and proteases probably all contribute to the epithelial fragility described in asthma (see below). Eosinophil cytolysis or disintegration and release of granules[30,31] and of cytokines may also stimulate nearby fibroblasts to produce additional reticulin and so induce thickening of the reticular basement membrane.

In fatal asthma there is a marked infiltrate throughout the airway wall, in sputum and also in the occluding plug. Compare Fig. 1.5(a) and (b), see colour plate section, see Figs. 1.3(a) and 1.4(b), see colour plate section: lymphocytes are abundant[22,32,33] and (EG2 +)eosinophils are characteristic (Fig. 1.6, see colour plate section)[22,34,35]. Neutrophils are sparse in mild asthma[21] albeit they are present in relatively large numbers in sputa during infective exacerbations[36], in biopsies of severe asthmatics refractory to high dose treatment with corticosteroids[37] and in status asthmaticus when death is sudden (i.e. within 24 hours of the attack)[38]. It has been suggested based on examination of biopsy tissue that two forms of asthma may be usefully distinguished: those with a relatively high eosinophil count and those with predominant neutrophilia[39]. The inflammation of the airway wall may involve the adjacent pulmonary artery[33] and, in small (distal) airways, may spread to surrounding alveolar septae[40]. Alveolar walls may thus show evidence of eosinophilic infiltration[40] and alveolar spaces may contain a fibrillar-rich component, most likely fibrin (author's unpublished observations). However, destruction of the parenchyma (i.e. emphysema) is not a feature of asthma. Thus, both small and large airways may be inflamed in asthma:

transbronchial biopsy studies of relatively severe asthma and studies of resection tissue in asthmatics have demonstrated infiltration of bronchioli by eosinophils and lymphocytes[40,41]. There are also recent data in severe asthma that demonstrate the inner wall to be infiltrated by neutrophils in numbers considerably greater than in larger airways[42]. Thus the pattern of inflammation in severe asthma appears to be different from that in mild and, in order to be effective, treatment needs to be tailored accordingly. The association of tissue eosinophilia and asthma is a strong one. However, the extent of tissue eosinophilia varies greatly with each case and with the duration of the terminal episode[22,38,43]. The variation may be due, in part, to eosinophil degranulation, which makes cell identification difficult. In comparison with mild asthma, fatal asthma is reported to be associated with a higher concentration of eosinophils in the large airways and a reduction of lymphocytes in the peripheral (smaller) airways[35].

The role of the activated T-helper (Th) lymphocyte in controlling and perpetuating the chronic inflammatory reaction in asthma has received much attention[24,44]. The T-lymphocyte is thought to control allergic inflammation via the selective release of the proinflammatory cytokines (interleukins) IL-4 and IL-5, which characterize the T-helper (type 2) phenotype[45]. IL-5 gene expression has been shown to be increased in bronchial biopsies from symptomatic atopic asthmatic subjects[46] (Fig. 1.10), and this is supported by studies of cells obtained at bronchoalveolar lavage[47,48] and peripheral blood[49]. IL5 appears to be a key cytokine required to induce terminal differentiation of eosinophils and, together with IL4, enhances their vascular retention and longevity in tissues. It is also a key cytokine in the late phase reaction to allergen challenge[48]. IL4 is also increased in atopic asthma[50,51] and may be important in both the initiation and persistence of allergic inflammation. IL4 encourages the selective recruitment of eosinophils by up-regulating adhesion molecules (V-CAM) on bronchial endothelium whose ligand on the eosinophil cell surface is VLA-4. The last is absent from the surface of neutrophils and helps to explain the eosinophil predominance in mild asthma. There is currently debate as to the involvement of IL4 in asthma of the intrinsic (i.e. non-atopic) form[52]. IL4 and IL5 are not, however, unique to asthma and may occur in other inflammatory conditions such as fibrosing alveolitis[53]. Whilst IL5 may be important in promoting eosinophil terminal differentiation, and the release of eosinophils into the blood from bone marrow, other molecules such as eotaxin and RANTES (regulated on activation normal T-cell expressed and secreted) are involved as selective chemokines inducing eosinophil emigration from blood vessels and their migration through the mucosa to the airway lumen from whence they are cleared[54–56]. The same or distinct molecules may be involved in eosinophil activation, a process about which little is as yet known. Symptomatic asthma is associated with the production of additional cytokines including TNFα, GM–CSF, IL1β, IL2 and IL6[45,57]. GM–CSF has also been reported to increase during the late phase reaction to allergen[58]. In addition to their production of toxins and lipid-derived mediators, eosinophils themselves may also produce proinflammatory cytokines and growth factors as evidenced by their gene expression for TNFα, IL6 and GM-CSFβ[45,59,60]. Macrophages have been reported to increase in number in more severe asthma of the intrinsic form[28].

Mast cells have long been thought to play a key role in the immediate (type I sensitivity) reaction in asthma through their release of a variety of mediators including those which bronchoconstrict i.e. histamine, prostaglandin D$_2$ and leukotriene D4. Mast cells are now thought to act as an important source of IL4 and other proinflammatory cytokines whose secretion may act as a trigger to the induction of subsequent persistent production of IL4 and IL5 by lymphocytes[61,62.] There are reports of decreases, increases and no change of mast cell numbers. Early biopsy studies demonstrated an apparent reduction in bronchial mast cell numbers in asthma due to their degranulation[63]. Studies of bronchoalveolar lavage report increased intralumenal mast cell numbers together with increased numbers of T-helper cells and eosinophils and evidence of histamine release and of eosinophil degranulation[18,64,65].

Although considered to be important in allergic conditions, little is known of the role of basophils in these conditions albeit there is evidence for increased recruitment of basophils and their precursors to sites of allergic reaction in atopic patients[66]. Asthma is also characterized by infiltration of the bronchial surface epithelium by dendritic cells (i.e. Langerhans' cell equivalent)[67]. These non-phagocytic histiocytes are rich in surface receptors and their functions are thought to include the presentation of antigenic information to T lymphocytes; very few Langerhans' cells are found in the normal lung although there is a rich network of their probable precursor dendritic cells[68]. Thus lymphocytes of the T-helper (CD4 +) subset appear to be key to the controller cell and eosinophils the prime effector cell in mild asthma. However, with increasing severity of asthma and in infective exacerbations there is an increasing involvement of neutrophils and perhaps also of macrophages and these changes appear to be more refractory to conventional treatment with inhaled or even oral corticosteroids. Alternative approaches would seem to be required to treat more severe than mild asthma and the reasons for this may in part be explained by the altered pattern of inflammation.

COPD

T-lymphocytes appear also to be key controller cells in COPD but in contrast to asthma it is the CD8 + cells that are the predominant cells in COPD[69]. It is currently presumed that the majority of these CD8 + cells are T-lymphocytes of the cytotoxic/suppressor subset, but this is as yet unproven and these may also include natural killer cells and even a dendritic cell sub-type. The altered CD8:CD4 + cell ratio appears, however, to be a fundamental distinction between the CD4 + T-cell, allergen-driven process of allergic asthma in non-smokers and the CD8 + T-cell, cigarette smoked-induced inflammation of COPD[70].

Smoking tobacco *per se* induces an inflammatory

response. Smoking shortens the transit time of neutrophils through the bone marrow, causes a leukocytosis and alters the immunoregulatory balance of T-cell subsets found in blood, bronchoalveolar lavage (BAL), and tissues of the conducting airways and lung[71–73]. Smoking initiates a peripheral blood leukocytosis and a reversible decrease in the normally high CD4 to CD8 cell ratio in blood of heavy smokers (i.e. > 50 pack–years). There is also a significant reduction of the CD4:CD8 + cell ratio in BAL fluid but not blood of a group of milder smokers (i.e. on average who have smoked 14 pack–years). The increase in the number of BAL and tissue CD8 + T-cells is positively associated with pack–years smoked[72,74,75].

Chronic bronchitis

Histological examination of airway tissues (taken at resection for tumour) from smokers demonstrates that inflammatory cells are present in and around the area of mucus-secreting submucosal glands and that scores of inflammation show a better association with the subjects who have symptoms of mucus hypersecretion than does gland size *per se*[76]. In bronchial biopsies of subjects with mild stable chronic bronchitis and COPD there is infiltration of the mucosa by inflammatory cells[75,77–79] (Fig. 1.7, see colour plate section): this is associated with up-regulation of cell surface adhesion molecules of relevance to the inflammatory process[80]. In the surface epithelium where, in contrast to the subepithelium, CD8 + cells normally predominate, Fournier and colleagues have demonstrated by comparison with non-smokers, an increase in all inflammatory cell types in smokers with chronic bronchitis and mild COPD[81]. In a subepithelial zone (also referred to as the lamina propria), bronchial lymphomononuclear cells appear to form the predominant cell type with scanty neutrophils (in the absence of an exacerbation): the lymphomononuclear component is composed of lymphocytes, plasma cells and macrophages. Significant increases are reported in the numbers of CD45 (total leukocytes), CD3 (T-lymphocytes), CD25 (i.e.activated) and VLA-1 (late activation) positive

cells, presumed to be T-lymphocytes and of macrophages. The endobronchial biopsy studies of O'Shaughnessy and co-workers have demonstrated that by comparison with normal non-smokers, T-lymphocytes and neutrophils increase in the surface epithelium whilst T-lymphocytes and macrophages increase in the subepithelium of smokers with COPD[79,82]. In contrast to asthma, in COPD it is the CD8 + cell and not the CD4 + T-cell subset, which increases in number and proportion to become the predominant T-cell subset. Furthermore, the increase of CD8 + cells shows a negative association with the forced expiratory volume in one second (FEV1 expressed as a percentage of predicted). This novel distinction between the relative proportions in T-cell subsets of smokers with mild stable COPD and non-smoking mild asthmatics has received the support of subsequent studies of both resected tissues and bronchial biopsies[74,83,84]. The increase of the CD8 + phe‴ notype and of the CD8/CD4 ratio seen in the mucosa also occurs deeper in the airway wall in association with submucosal mucus-secreting glands in bronchitic smokers[83]. In addition neutrophils increase in the surface epithelium and glands especially when the disease increases in severity (Fig. 1.8, see colour plate section).

Similarity between COPD and asthma

COPD and asthma would seem to differ at the tissue level in a number of respects; for example the marked tissue eosinophilia and thickening of the reticular basement membrane of asthma (see below) is not usually a feature of COPD[85]. However, compared to normal healthy control tissue, there are a number of studies that report a small but significant increase in the number of tissue eosinophils in subjects with chronic bronchitis or COPD[76,79,86]. Sputum eosinophilia is also reported in cases of 'eosinophilic bronchitis', i.e. patients without a history of asthma and without bronchial hyper-responsiveness[12,87]. Furthermore, in mild COPD, the numbers of tissue eosinophils are markedly and significantly increased when there is an exacerbation of bronchitis (defined as a need by the patient to seek medical attention due to a sudden worsening of dyspnoea or an increase in sputum volume or purulence[88,89]. In such mild cases of COPD the exacerbation is associated with an increase in eosinophil chemoattractants, especially RANTES[90]. The bronchial mucus-secreting glands of smokers may also show gene expression for both IL4 and IL5 and the numbers of these cells are significantly higher in smokers with chronic hypersecretion as compared with their asymptomatic controls[91]. Thus, IL4, IL5 and eosinophil chemoattractant gene expression is not restricted to asthma and, like the recent reports of fibrosing lung disease[92], these regulatory cytokines can be expressed also in chronic bronchitic smokers.

Chronic bronchiolitis

Histologically, the earliest observed effects of cigarette smoke in small airways and surrounding alveoli is a marked increase in the number of macrophages and neutrophils, both in human and experimentally in animal studies. The increase is seen within both the tissue and lumena and can be detected in bronchoalveolar lavage fluid (BAL)[93]. Examination of small airway tissue in lungs resected from smokers also shows that the same profile of CD8-predominant inflammation reported in bronchial biopsies of the larger airways occurs deeper in the lung in both the 'small' airways[74,84] and also the lung parenchyma[94,95]. As with the findings in the large conducting airways there are significant negative associations of the numbers of CD8 + cells and FEV1% of predicted in both the small (peripheral) conducting airways and lung parenchyma. However, at these sites the negative correlations are stronger than in the large airways. Thus the patterns of inflammation are similar at both proximal and distal sites. However, in contrast to the larger airways, the CD8 + T-cell predominance in the small airways and lung parenchyma is more closely associated with decreased lung function in these subjects with COPD.

The infiltration of the airway wall by lymphocytes is associated with loss of alveolar attachments to the outer wall of small airways, a characteristic of centriacinar emphysema. The accompanying loss of radial traction and lung elastic recoil leads to early airway closure during expiration (Fig. 1.9(a), (b), see colour plate section). The loss of alveolar–bronchiolar attachments is thought to be due to the circumferential spread of small airway wall inflammation.

Emphysema

In the normal, the macrophage is the resident phagocyte of the alveolus: neutrophils are rarely present[96]. Neutrophils are recruited to the lung in smokers, albeit the extent of tissue neutrophilia is highly variable. On exposure to cigarette smoke, there is recruitment of macrophages and phagocytosis of cigarette smoke components. A macrophage alveolitis and respiratory bronchiolitis are the early changes in young cigarette smokers[97,98]. As in the large and small conducting airways in COPD, CD8 + cells also become the predominant inflammatory cell phenotype in the parenchyma and their numbers show a strong inverse correlation with FEV1% of predicted[95].

Inflammation and the pathogenesis of COPD

The neutrophil, the macrophage and the CD8 + cell may each be involved in the destruction of the lung parenchyma by distinct mechanisms.

The neutrophil

The alveolar microcirculation is composed of a network of short interconnecting tubules of average diameter 5 μm. The average diameter of circulating neutrophils is 7.0 μm, which necessitates their deformation as they squeeze through capillary segments. Neutrophil traffic through the capillaries of the lung is normally slower (i.e. there is a higher transit time) than that of red blood cells as they are 700 times less deformable than RBCs[99]. Studies with radioactively labelled neutrophils have demonstrated that the normal delay in neutrophil transit is further exaggerated, transiently, even in healthy subjects during smoking. Exposure of neutrophils to cigarette smoke in vitro and in vivo results in decreased deformability associated with polymerization of actin microfilaments[99,100]. This is the likely mechanism of the observed cigarette smoke-induced increase in transit time. Factors chemotactic for neutrophils, and which will induce their emigration from the microcirculation are released by the alveolar macrophages of smokers and the alveolar neutrophil population may increase from 1% to 5% of inflammatory cells. Cigarette smoke itself may contain substances chemoattractant for neutrophils, a possibility that is supported by the associated peripheral blood leukocytosis widely reported[101]. Cigarette smoke or factors released from cigarette smoke-exposed macrophages encourage the release of neutrophil elastase which may degrade lung elastin even in the presence of antiprotease[102–104]. Such neutrophil-derived serine proteases have been implicated in the pathogenesis of COPD since the appreciation of the emphysematous change that results from alpha-1 antitrypsin (AAT) deficiency in man. AAT protects against the proteolytic effects of neutrophil elastase, cathepsin G and proteinase 3, each of which has been shown to induce emphysematous change in experimental animal models of emphysema. These and earlier results led to the protease/antiprotease hypothesis in which emphysema develops if there is an imbalance favouring proteolytic digestion of the elastic framework of the lung (Fig. 1.10). Recent studies have shown that, when released from the cell, the concentrations of neutrophil elastase far outweigh the antiprotease in the immediate vicinity of the neutrophil cell surface. In the absence or reduction of the antiprotease this pericellular zone of proteolysis is greatly increased[105].

The macrophage

The role of the macrophage in the pathogenesis of COPD has been controversial. However, the data of recent studies support the hypothesis that the

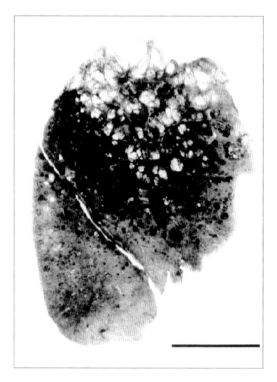

Fig. 1.10 Gross appearance of the cut surface of a lung in which the distribution of centracinar emphysema caused by proteolytic digestion is characteristically restricted to the upper aspects of each lobe. Scale = 10 cm. (By courtesy of Professor B. Heard.)

macrophage may play a critical role in regulating the inflammatory response and also directly in the tissue destruction associated with COPD[106,107]. Macrophages are able to synthesize significant amounts of matrix metalloproteinases (MMPs) including macrophage elastase (MMP12), collagenase 1 (MMP1), gelatinase B (MMP9) and others[106,108]. The hypothesis is that dysregulated expression of macrophage MMPs, induced either directly or indirectly by cigarette smoke, leads to the lung destruction characteristic of human emphysema. There is support for the hypothesis from experimental animal work using gene manipulated strains in conjunction with exposure to passive cigarette smoke[106]. MMP1 over expression in mice is associated with enlargement of airspaces suggesting that collagen degradation may also be important in the generation of emphysema. Moreover, when macrophage MMP12-deficient (-/-)mice are exposed chronically to cigarette smoke, they fail to develop emphysema and fail to recruit macrophages to the lung: in contrast the smoke-exposed MMP12 intact (+/+) mice developed it[109]. Also in humans there are data from cultured macrophages of patients with COPD that show that there is increased expression of MMP1, MMP9 and MMP12[110]. MMP12 can be detected by immunohistochemistry and in situ hybridization in the alveolar macrophages of patients with emphysema but not in normal lung[106]. It appears that macrophage elastase is required for both macrophage accumulation and the emphysema that results from inhalation of cigarette smoke. The current working hypothesis is that cigarette smoke induces constitutive macrophages to produce MMPs that cleave lung elastin, generating fragments chemotactic for monocytes. This positive feed-back loop would perpetuate the accumulation of macrophages and lung tissue destruction. Zinc-containing metalloproteases released from the cigarette smoke-stimulated macrophages are not inhibited by the normal antiprotease of the alveolus and may thus also degrade alpha$_1$-antitrypsin *per se*[111].

The CD8 + cell

There are several differences between the CD4 + and CD8 + subsets of T-lymphocytes[112]. CD4 + T-cells have been well studied in the context of asthma and the Th2-type allergic response. However, until recently relatively little has been known about the CD8 + cell and smokers with COPD. CD8 + T-cells are generally associated with Th1-type immunity and play a role in generating protective immunity to *Mycobacterium* sp.[113]. LPS from gram negative bacteria cause selective activation of the CD8 + T-cell subset. Currently there is more speculation than knowledge about the role of this predominant cell in COPD. A recent study has shown they may interact

with virus infected epithelial cells in a way that generates a chemotactic factor (MCP-1) for macrophages, an accumulation of which may then destroy host tissue[107]. CD8 + T-lymphocytes produce interferon gamma a cytokine that when overexpressed has been shown to induce emphysema experimentally in mice[114]. In addition, the CD8 + T-cell can produce perforin and granzymes, which may contribute to the apoptosis and cell destruction reported in emphysema[115]. Consequently the parenchymal damage associated with COPD could also be CD8 + cell driven.

One hypothesis is that individuals with a genetically determined low CD4 + /CD8 + T-cell ratio and those who smoke would be more likely to have an exaggerated CD8 + T-cytotoxic response to viral infection. Increased frequency of virally-associated exacerbations in this group would likely lead to lung tissue destruction and the development of COPD. In this respect the prevailing balance of CD4 + and CD8 + cells in the tissues is likely to be critical[70,116]. Finally, there are recent interesting data on the role of retinoic acid in influencing alveolar number and the repair of established emphysematous lung suggesting that nutrition may also act as an important additive factor in the emphysematous process[117]. Thus the patterns of inflammation in mild COPD in smokers and mild asthma in non-smokers differ but the distinctions become less clear when there is an exacerbation in mild COPD when eosinophilia develops in association with up-regulation of RANTES, an eosinophil chemoattractant usually thought of as characteristic of asthma. These alterations in COPD may explain why exacerbations in COPD may be responsive to corticosteroid treatment whereas the inflammation of ongoing mild to moderate COPD is not[118,119].

Vascular inflammation

There are few studies that examine the inflammatory process in pulmonary arteries of subjects with COPD. There is inflammation of these vessels due

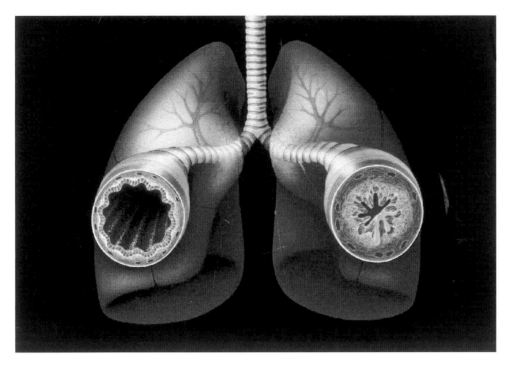

Fig. 1.2 Cartoon representation of the airways in the normal (left) and in asthma (right) demonstrating the thickening of the airway wall in asthma due to chronic inflammation and remodelling of epithelium and subepithelial tissue. The result is encroachment of the airway lumen and a marked increase in resistance to airflow.

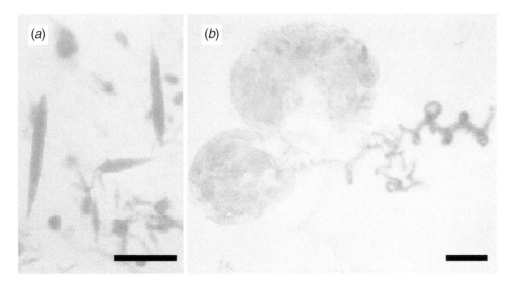

Fig. 1.3 Sputum showing the presence of: (*a*) Charcot–Leyden crystals and eosinophilia. Scale = 20 μm. (*b*) clusters of sloughed epithelial cells (i.e. Creola bodies) and a Curschman spiral characteristic of the asthmatic. Scale = 20 μm.

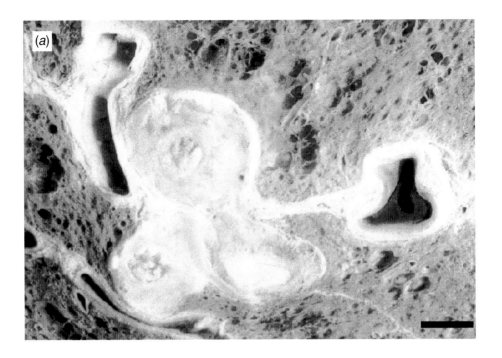

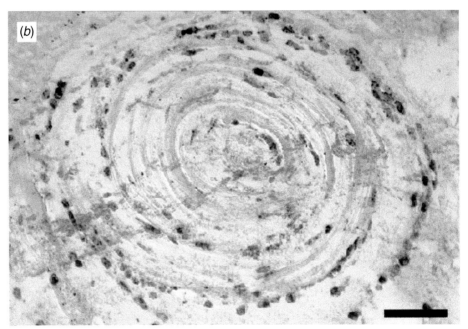

Fig. 1.4 Plugging of the airways in fatal asthma: (*a*) showing the gross appearance of the cut surface of the lung with the airways completely blocked by secretions. Scale = 400 μm. (*b*) an immunostain (i.e. anti-EG2) demonstrating the inclusion within the secretions of concentric lamellae of activated eosinophils. Scale = 50 μm.

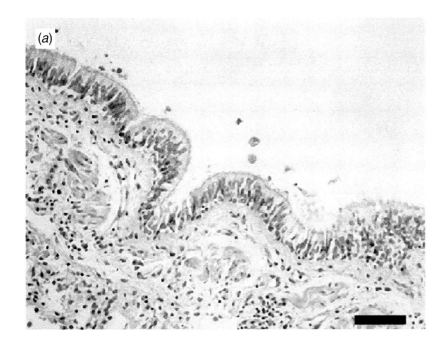

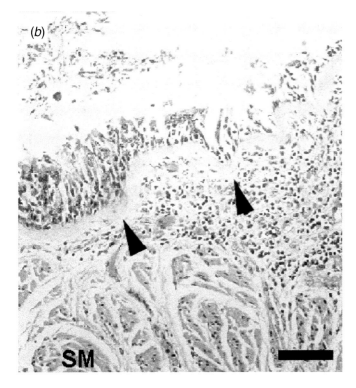

Fig. 1.5 Histological sections of part of the airway wall stained by haematoxylin and eosin (H&E): (*a*) an intrapulmonary airway from a road traffic accident death in a non-asthmatic showing intact pseudostratified ciliated columnar epithelium, isolated inflammatory cells and small blocks of bronchial smooth muscle. Scale = 80 μm. (*b*) by comparison the airway mucosa in a case of fatal asthma has lost much of the surface epithelium, there is a distinct homogeneously thickened reticular basement membrane (arrowheads), an infiltration of the mucosa by lymphocytes and eosinophils and the blocks of smooth muscle (SM) are greatly thickened. Scale = 80 μm.

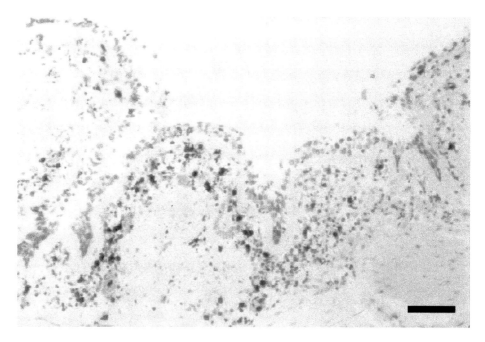

Fig. 1.6 Immunohistochemical staining for activated (i.e EG2 +) eosinophils in the airway wall of a case of fatal asthma. The cells are clustered beneath the RBM and surface epithelium, which is damaged (airway lumen = L). Scale = 80 µm.

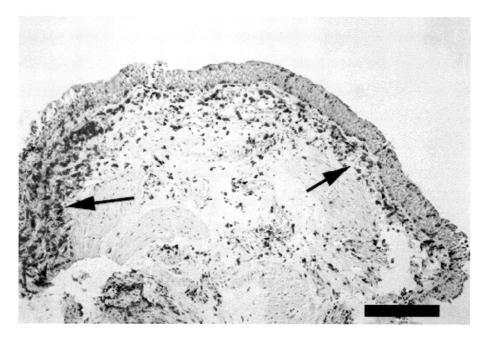

Fig. 1.7 A section through a bronchial biopsy from a smoker with chronic bronchitis and COPD. It has been immunostained (arrows) to demonstrate the CD8 + (cytotoxic / suppressor) cells that predominate in COPD. This contrasts with asthma where CD4 + T-lymphocytes predominate. Scale = 150 µm.

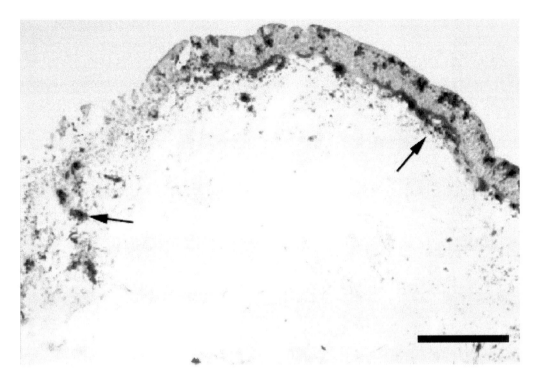

Fig. 1.8 Neutrophil infiltration of a smoker with cough productive of sputum. Compared with an asymptomatic individual there is an increase in the number of neutrophils. Immunostaining with antihuman neutrophil elastase (arrows). Scale = 150 μm.

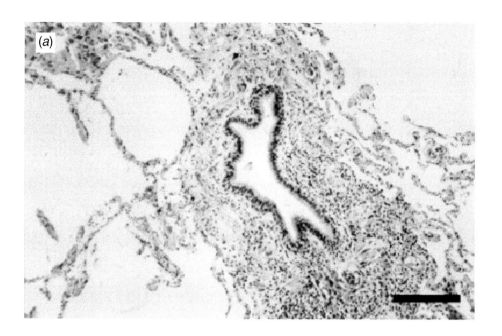

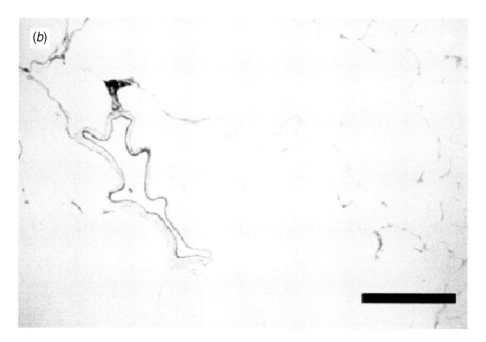

Fig. 1.9 Small airways disease: (*a*) transverse section of a small airway showing peribronchiolitis consisting predominantly of lymphocytes. Scale = 250 μm. (*b*) Loss of alveolar-bronchiolar attachments due to centriacinar emphysema and consequent collapse of the conducting airway. H&E. Scale = 1.0 mm.

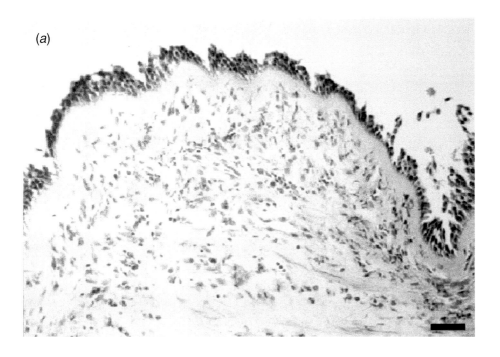

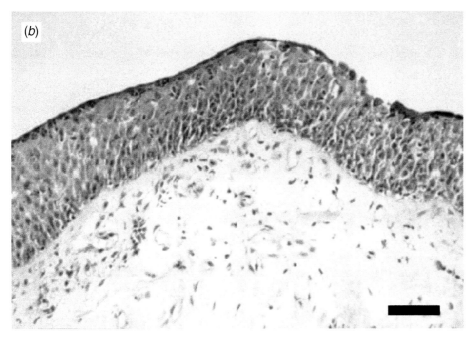

Fig. 1.11 The airway mucosa: as it appears by light microscopy (LM) in sections of bronchial biopsies in: (*a*) an atopic asthmatic showing loss of surface epithelium and early thickening of the reticular basement membrane. Scale = 60 μm. (*b*) A heavy smoker with COPD (FEV1 = 40% of predicted) demonstrating epithelial squamous metaplasia. Stained with hematoxylin–eosin (H&E). Scale = 60 μm.

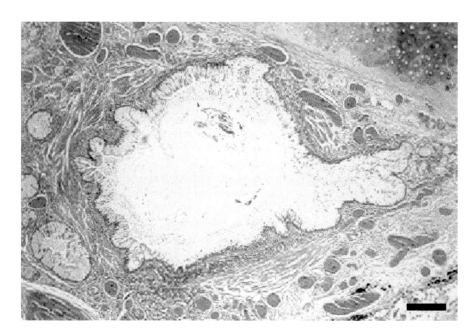

Fig. 1.15 Histological transverse section of a segmental bronchus of a case of fatal asthma stained with H&E to show a lumen plugged with secretions, epithelial goblet cell hyperplasia, inflammation of the airway wall and dilatation and congestion of bronchial vessels. Scale = 180 μm.

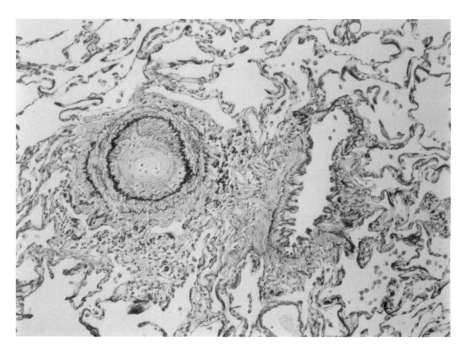

Fig. 19.3 Histological section demonstrating the obliteration of the lumen of a small precapillary pulmonary artery. Tissue section is taken from the lung of a patient with primary pulmonary hypertension. The pentachrome stain shows collagen (yellow) and elastin (black).

probably to the close approximation of airways and pulmonary arteries and the spread of the inflammatory process from the bronchiolar wall to the adjacent pulmonary artery. An inflammatory process similar to that present in the conducting airways and in the lung parenchyma, consisting predominantly of CD8 + T-lymphocytes, has been reported in the adventitia of pulmonary arteries in smokers with COPD[95,120]. The vascular infiltration of CD8 + T-lymphocytes correlates with the degree of airflow limitation in these subjects[95], supporting a role for vascular inflammation in the progression of the disease. The vascular inflammatory process is also associated with impairment of endothelium-dependent vascular relaxation. The endothelium plays a crucial role in the regulation of vascular cell growth and tone through the release of endothelium-derived relaxing factors. Endothelial dysfunction, which results in an impaired release of these factors, has been shown in patients with end-stage COPD undergoing lung transplantation[121]. In this study, the degree of endothelial dysfunction was correlated with both the severity of pulmonary vascular remodelling and the arterial oxygen tension, suggesting that in end-stage obstructive lung disease, hypoxemia is the principal factor determining the endothelial dysfunction that leads to vasoconstriction. However, endothelial dysfunction and intimal thickening may be present also in smokers with mild COPD[122] who are not hypoxemic, indicating that factors other than hypoxemia might be capable of producing the vascular changes in smokers. It is possible that endothelial damage by cigarette smoking is the first vascular alteration occurring in COPD. This early alteration may predispose smokers to develop further vascular damage due to additional factors such as hypoxemia and inflammation, ultimately leading to the development of pulmonary hypertension[120].

Further studies of the distinctive patterns inflammation, cytokine gene expression and protein secretion in the airways and vessel walls of asthma and COPD should prove to be of scientific, clinical and therapeutic interest.

Remodelling

Surface epithelium

Histologically, damage and shedding of the airway surface epithelium are reported in asthma postmortem (compare Fig. 1.5(a), (b)) (Fig. 1.11(*a*), (*b*), see colour plate section) but this change is highly variable with some airways having completely intact surface epithelium in the presence of marked inflammation and other structural changes[123]. Subepithelial edema has been suggested to be one mechanism responsible for lifting of the overlying surface epithelium where this occurs[32]. Repeated loss of the epithelium induces a healing process as evidenced by squamous cell metaplasia and/or goblet cell hyperplasia. Histologically, damage and shedding of airway surface epithelium appears to be an early feature of asthma, particularly of the allergic form[124]: it has been reported in biopsy specimens of patients with stable mild disease and is not a usual feature of smokers with bronchitis or COPD (see Fig. 1.11(*a*), (*b*))[17,24,25,125]. Loss of superficial epithelium is accompanied by mitotic activity in the remaining epithelial cells in normal healthy individuals[126]. There is repeated epithelial regeneration in the form of simple and then stratified cells prior to restoration of the normal ciliated and goblet cell phenotypes, the entire process taking approximately 2 weeks. However, there are reports that such mitotic activity is deficient in asthma and this has led to the suggestion that there may be defective repair of epithelium in asthma with the consequent release of a range of factors that would promote a remodelling response[126,127]. These factors include epithelial-derived growth factor and granulocyte–macrophage colony stimulating factor and would induce alterations to the epithelial reticular basement membrane, via activation of adjacent fibroblasts/myofibroblasts, and deeper structures including bronchial smooth muscle, mucus-secreting glands and wall vessels. The release of these and other molecules including IL8, eotaxin and RANTES would also provide a chemoattractant gradient to both inflammatory and phenotypically altered structural cells. Aggregations of platelets together with fibrillary material, thought to be fibrin have been observed in association with the damaged surface[24]. Such fibrin deposits are also seen during the late phase response following allergen challenge (author's unpublished results). The greater the loss of surface epithelium in biopsy specimens the greater appears to be the degree of airways hyper-responsiveness[24].

It is recognized that there is inevitably artefactual loss of surface epithelium during the taking and preparation of such small biopsy pieces, even normally, which makes interpretation of the epithelial loss seen in bronchial biopsies controversial. In the author's opinion, the observed loss reflects the fragility of the epithelium in vivo that facilitates sloughing during the bronchoscopy procedure. The fragility of the epithelium in vivo in asthma is supported by the frequent appearance of clusters of sloughed epithelial cells in sputa (see Fig. 1.3(b), see colour plate[124]) and the increased presence of bronchial epithelial cells in bronchoalveolar lavage of asthmatics with mild disease[17]. Other researchers have found no significant loss of epithelium in biopsies of mild asthmatics[128,129]: this may be due to differing methods of measurement of such loss or to differences in the severity of the patients sampled.

The fragility of the surface may be associated with disruption of epithelial cell tight junctions[130,131] and this may be facilitated by allergens per se, several of which have been shown to have proteolytic activity[132]. Tight junctions normally act as a selective barrier to the passage of ions, molecules and water between cells: their disruption may lower the threshold for stimulation of intraepithelial nerves leading to axonal reflexes, stimulation of mucus-secreting submucosal glands, vasodilatation and oedema through the release of sensory neuropeptides (i.e. referred to as neurogenic inflammation)[133,134]. Experimentally there is also evidence that the sensitivity of bronchial smooth muscle to substances placed in the airway lumen correlates strongly with the integrity of the surface epithelium[135]. Loss or damage of surface epithelium in asthma would thus lead to a reduction in the concentration of factors normally relaxant to bronchial smooth muscle with resultant increased sensitivity and 'reactivity' of bronchial smooth muscle.

Apart from their role as stem cells, the basal cells of normal pseudostratified surface epithelium have been suggested to act as a bridge, enhancing the adhesion of 'superficial' cells to epithelial basement membrane[136]. When superficial cells are lost in asthma the preferential plane of cleavage appears to be between superficial and basal cells[137], leaving basal cells still attached to their basement membrane. Epithelial cells also act as effector cells by their synthesis and release of cytokines such as IL-6, IL-8, GM-CSF and chemokines such as RANTES[138] and eotaxin. Disruption of the epithelium and attempts at repair may increase production of these proinflammatory cytokines by those cells that remain.

In contrast, epithelial loss is a less often reported feature of bronchial biopsies taken from smokers with bronchitis or COPD when goblet cell hyperplasia and/or squamous metaplasia are often seen (Fig. 1.11(b), see colour plate section)[139,140].

Reticular basement membrane

Thickening of the reticular basement membrane (i.e. the lamina reticularis) which lies external to (or below) the epithelium has long been recognized as a consistent change in allergic, non-allergic and occupational forms of asthma[24,32,141–143]: this may occur in response to repeated loss and healing of the surface epithelium (see Fig. 1.12(a)(b) and 1.5 (a)(b), see colour plate). Whilst there may be focal and variable thickening of the reticular layer in COPD and other inflammatory chronic diseases of the lung such as bronchiectasis and tuberculosis[143], the lesion, when homogenous and hyaline in appearance, is highly characteristic of asthma and is not usually found in COPD. The reticular layer appears to be absent in the fetus (at least up to 18 weeks of gestation)[144] but develops in normal, healthy individuals, presumably during early childhood: its thickening in asthma begins early[145], even before asthma is diag-

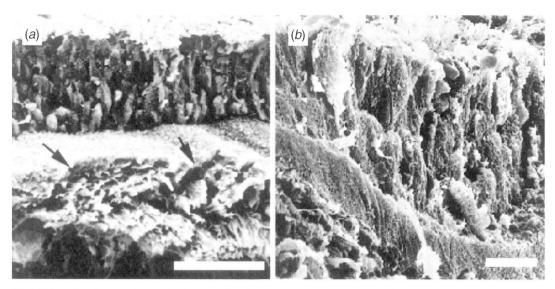

Fig. 1.12 Scanning electron micrographs demonstrating the airway mucosa in (*a*) the non-asthmatic with epithelium attached to a reticular basement membrane (RBM) of normal thickness (arrows) beneath which there is interstitial collagen. Scale = 50 μm. (*b*) A subject with a 25-year history of asthma, but who died of non-respiratory cause demonstrating the thickened RBM and damaged epithelium. Scale = 10 μm.

nosed[146]. The thickening remains even when asthma is mild and well controlled by antiasthma treatment[147] and is present in patients with a long history of asthma but who have not died of their asthma[142]. The extent of thickening is maximal early on in the development of asthma and does not appear to increase significantly with age, duration or severity of disease[7,145].

It should be noted that the basal lamina (i.e. the so-called 'true' epithelial basement membrane), which consists mainly of type IV collagen, glycosaminoglycans and laminin, is not thickened in either asthma or COPD. The thickening of the lamina reticularis (i.e. reticular basement membrane) (Fig. 1.13(*a*)(*b*)) which is immuno-positive for collagen types III and V together with tenascin[148] and fibronectin but not laminin has been referred to as 'subepithelial fibrosis'[141]. In the author's opinion this is an unfortunate use of the term as the thickened layer of reticulin is ultrastructurally different from the banded collagen that lies deeper in the airway wall or that which is characteristic of scarring. The reticular layer is composed of thinner fibres of reticulin linked to a

tenascin-rich matrix in which there are sugars together with entrapped molecules such as heparin sulphate and serum-derived components such as fibronectin: these molecules may modulate the state of differentiation and function of overlying epithelium. In the author's opinion, swelling of this subepithelial reticular layer may also contribute to its thickening in asthma. Interestingly the thickened layer does not behave as a barrier to the transmigration of inflammatory cells, which by the release of enzymes (such as matrix metalloproteinases) or by the presence of pre-existing pores[149] can pass through it with apparent ease (see Fig. 1.13(*b*)). An association between the numbers of 'myofibroblasts' underlying the reticular layer and the thickness of the reticular layer has been demonstrated in asthma indicating these cells may secrete additional material contributing to its thickening[150].

In contrast to asthma, a study of bronchial biopsies, in carefully characterized patients with COPD, reports that the reticular layer is not thickened[140]. A recent report confirms this and demonstrates that the reticular layer in smokers with irreversible

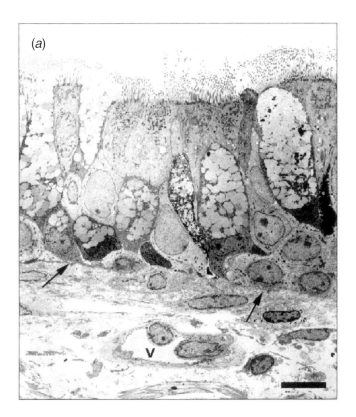

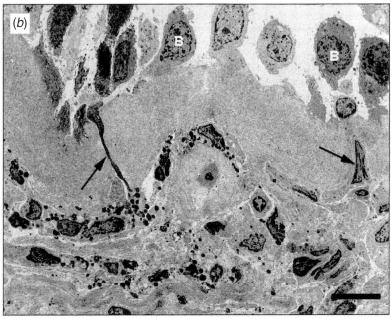

Fig. 1.13 Transmission electron micrographs of the epithelium and basement membrane: (*a*) normal epithelium of ciliated and goblet cells resting on the basal lamina (arrows) with relatively thin RBM and bronchial blood vessel (V) beneath. Scale = 10 μm. (*b*) Mild atopic asthmatic showing sloughing of basal epithelial cells (B) and thickened RBM and eosinophils with electron-dense granules beneath. Two mononuclear inflammatory cells (probably lymphocytes) are traversing the RBM (arrows). Scale = 10 μm.

disease is similar to that in normal healthy non-smokers and is significantly thinner than that of asthmatics who had been treated with inhaled corticosteroids[147]. There are, however, subpopulations of non-asthmatic smokers with COPD, defined by their smoking history and irreversibility to inhaled beta-2 agonist, who show significant airways reversibility (within the asthma range) to a 14-day course of oral prednisolone. These 'responders' have a thicker reticular basement membrane than normal and evidence of BAL eosinophilia: neither are present in the 'non-responder' group[151]. This interesting COPD group with a significant degree of reversibility demonstrates further the potential overlap that may exist between asthma and COPD at the tissue level.

Connective tissue

There is no consensus as to whether there is increased interstitial collagen in asthma or whether it increases with disease severity or duration. A recent study of bronchial biopsies obtained from asthmatics of varying severity reports increasing scores for collagen[152], whereas another reports no difference in collagen content[153]. Electron microscopic quantitative assessment of interstitial collagen in biopsies of mild asthmatics found no difference in the area of the mucosa occupied by collagen fibres[26]. There is similar controversy over loss of elastic tissue in asthma, one study demonstrating there is not[26] and others indicating that there is either elastolysis or altered ultrastructure of elastic tissue[154,155]. In contrast, airway wall fibrosis is generally, but not always, considered a feature of the airways in smokers who develop COPD, albeit these studies have focused on small rather than large airways[156–158].

Bronchial smooth muscle

The percentage of bronchial wall occupied by bronchial smooth muscle often increased substantially in fatal asthma[19] (Fig. 1.14(*a*), (*b*)). The absolute increase in muscle mass is reported to be particularly striking in large intrapulmonary bronchi of lungs obtained following a fatal attack as compared with that in asthmatic subjects dying of other causes[123]: it is an important contributor to the thickening of the airway wall and hence to the marked increase in resistance to airflow which may become life threatening[159–162]. Using a morphometric technique Dunnill showed that approximately 12% of the wall in segmental bronchi obtained from cases of fatal asthma was composed of muscle compared with about 5% in normals. Other studies have confirmed this trend in airways larger than 2 mm diameter and demonstrated a three- to fourfold increase over normal in the area of the wall occupied by bronchial smooth muscle[7,163,164]. The increase in muscle mass in small airways is not as great in absolute terms as in the large airways although as a percentage of the airway wall airway smooth muscle occupies a relatively larger percentage in the smaller than in the larger airway. Thus small increases of muscle in small airways may have a more significant effect functionally than similar increases in more proximal bronchi. In the absence of wheeze, values for muscle mass in segmental bronchi in chronic bronchitis and emphysema fall largely within the normal range but intermediate levels are present in so-called wheezy bronchitis[165,166].

Few studies in COPD have focused attention on the larger (cartilaginous) airways. One systematic study has described changes in large airway dimensions in relation to the lung function of patients with COPD[8]. These authors found that the wall area internal to the muscle was significantly thickened over the entire range of cartilaginous airways measured and that this was associated with a reduction in FEV/FVC. However, alterations in large airway smooth muscle mass were not observed and there was no correlation between muscle mass and airflow limitation. There was a positive association between peripheral airway inflammation and large airway inner wall area and the authors argued that their findings and those of others favour inflammation as the cause of the increasing inner airway wall thickness that occurs in both large and small airways in COPD. Airway smooth muscle increases significantly in the small airways in COPD[84,98,158,167]. In a

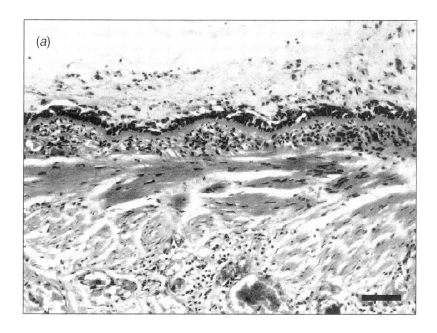

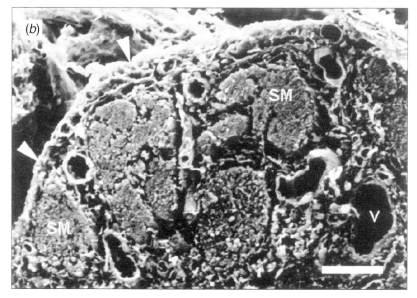

Fig. 1.14 Increased bronchial smooth muscle: (*a*) a histological section of the airway wall of a case of fatal asthma stained with H&E to show enlarged smooth muscle blocks lying relatively close to the surface epithelium. Scale = 80 μm. (*b*) Scanning electron microscopy of part of the mucosa in fatal asthma demonstrating the three-dimensional appearance of the enlarged blocks of bronchial smooth muscle (SM) and dilatation of bronchial vessels (V) which both contribute to thickening of the airway wall. The arrowheads show the position of the RBM from which the epithelium has been lost. Scale = 70 μm.

study of small (membranous) airways of 15 patients with COPD compared to the lungs of non-obstructed subjects and a group of asthmatic patients, it was only the airway smooth muscle area that was significantly increased in COPD[168]. In asthma, the increase in the wall area occupied by muscle, in absolute terms, is not as striking in small airways as in the large[123]. It is considered that the increased muscle mass that occurs at all generations of airway is likely to be the most important abnormality responsible for the increased airflow resistance observed in response to bronchoconstricting stimuli in both asthma and COPD[169]. Further studies and a greater understanding of the changes occurring in small airways is required as is a means of effective delivery of anti-inflammatory and antiremodelling therapy to this distal anatomic site. Whether the increase in muscle mass in asthma is due to muscle fibre proliferation (i.e. hyperplasia)[170] or hypertrophy is at present unclear. Two patterns of distribution of increased muscle mass have been described in asthma: one in which the increase is restricted to the largest airways and another in which the increase occurs throughout the airways: it is suggested that in the former hyperplasia of muscle fibres predominates whereas hypertrophy predominates when there is increased muscle occurring throughout the bronchial tree[171].

A newly proposed mechanism involves dedifferentiation of existing smooth muscle bundles. Cells that have ultrastructural features of both a contractile and secretory phenotype have been found in substantial numbers in the late phase response to allergen challenge. It has been suggested that, with repeated exposure to allergen, these may contribute to the increased mass of bronchial smooth muscle by a process of differentiation of existing smooth muscle and its migration to a subepithelial site where new muscle is formed[172]. The mechanisms involved in this response are likely to be similar to those occurring in atherosclerosis where there is vascular smooth muscle dedifferentiation and migration to form a neo-intima of increased vascular smooth muscle[173].

Mucus-secreting elements

The sources of the lumenal mucus that contributes to the airway mucus in both asthma and COPD are the submucosal glands and epithelial goblet cells. There is submucosal gland enlargement in both fatal asthma and COPD[19] and excessive production of mucus. The eosinophilic inflammatory exudate of asthma is probably responsible for the particularly sticky tenacious plugs that plug the airways and are associated with asphyxic death[174]. In asthma, there is dilatation of submucosal gland ducts, referred to as bronchial gland ectasia[175]. Whilst the characteristic condensed twists of mucus in asthma referred to as Curshman spirals (see Fig. 1.3(b) see colour plate section) are often said to represent the casts of small airways, their size is more in keeping with that of gland ducts which is their more likely origin. The normal proportion of serous and mucous secretory acini is retained in asthma whereas in COPD there is a shift towards a greater than normal predominance of mucous acini[176]. Goblet cell hyperplasia is a feature of both asthma[177] and bronchitis[178]. The mucous metaplasia that results in newly differentiated goblet cells in small bronchi and bronchioli of less than 2 mm diameter, where they are normally absent or sparse, is a feature of small airways disease in COPD[167]: whether mucous metaplasia also occurs in asthma is debated. It is considered by some that the mucus present at this distal site in asthma may have been aspirated from larger airways. In cases of fatal asthma where mucous metaplasia has occurred, the lumenal mucus secreted from surface goblet cells appears to remain adherent maintaining continuity between the cell's secretions and the plug, suggesting the secretory process or the mucin itself is altered in fatal asthma[177,179].

Airway vessels

Dilatation of bronchial mucosal blood vessels, congestion and wall edema are consistently reported features of fatal asthma and these can account for considerable swelling and stiffening of the airway wall

(Fig. 1.14(*b*), 1.15, see colour plate section[168,169,180]). There are indications that the increased proportion of the wall occupied by vessel may be due in part to a proliferation of bronchial vessels (angiogenesis)[181]. Whilst angiogenesis has been reported in mild asthma[182] it is particularly marked in severe corticosteroid-dependent asthma[183]. Whether these changes are the consequence of chronic allergic inflammation or due to the response to chronic (or latent) viral, mycoplasm or bacterial infection is not known.

Whilst proliferation of the bronchial vasculature is a feature of bronchiectasis and occurs in response to infection, changes to the bronchial vasculature have not been reported as a particular feature of COPD[168]. However, patients with moderate to severe COPD do have elevated pulmonary vascular pressures during exercise and there are structural changes in the pulmonary arteries consistent with endothelial dysfunction and pulmonary hypertension when compared with patients with minimal or no disease. Small (<500 μm) pulmonary vessels in airway obstructed smokers show intimal thickening as compared with those of non-obstructed non-smokers: in severely obstructed smokers, there is medial hypertrophy also[122,184,185]. Such structural changes likely contribute to the narrower lumens and vascular obstruction of these vessels. There is infiltration of the pulmonary arterial wall by T-lymphocytes. The CD8(+) T-cell phenotype is increased in both non-obstructed smokers and smokers with COPD compared with non-smokers and the intensity of the inflammatory infiltrate has been shown to correlate with both endothelium-dependent relaxation and intimal thickness[120].

Emphysema

Destruction of the lung parenchyma can be detected microscopically in the alveolar walls of smokers even when there is no evidence of airspace enlargement on gross examination (see Fig. 1.16). The microscopic measurement of such parenchymal destruction can, therefore, allow early identification of the disease, at a time when emphysema is not detectable macroscopically. The functional signifi-

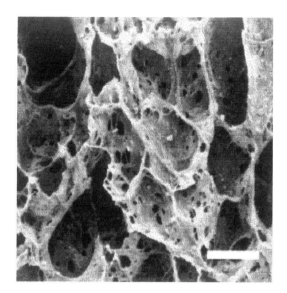

Fig. 1.16 SEM of human lung parenchyma illustrating microscopic emphysema in a smoker. Alveolar walls are peppered by fenestrae too small to be seen by the naked eye. Such early lesions probably result in loss of lung elastic recoil. Scale = 150 μm.

cance of such early destruction is demonstrated by its correlation with indices of airflow limitation and loss of elastic recoil of the lung[186].

The two major forms of emphysema, centriacinar and panacinar, have distinct mechanical properties and distinct peripheral airway involvement[187]. In particular, lung compliance is greater in panacinar than in centriacinar emphysema, whereas the extent of peripheral airway inflammation is greater in the centriacinar than in the panacinar form. It is possible that, in centriacinar emphysema, airflow limitation is primarily a function of peripheral airway inflammation, as supported by the correlation between reduced expiratory flow and increased airway inflammation observed in this form of emphysema. By contrast, in panacinar emphysema, airflow limitation seems to be primarily a function of loss of elastic recoil, as supported by the correlation between reduced expiratory flow and increased compliance observed in this form of emphysema[187].

The current emphasis in smoking-related disease is on emphysema associated with loss of alveolar-bronchiolar attachments. Bronchioles are supported within the lung by attachment of the adjacent alveolar walls. Loss of these attached alveolar walls and an increase in the interalveolar attachment distance (IAAD) appear to be associated with functional abnormalities, including a decrease in forced expiratory volume in 1 second (FEV_1) and abnormalities of tests of small airway function[188–191]. There is likely to be a role for airway wall inflammation in the selective loss of alveolar–bronchiolar attachments. It is possible that inflammatory cell activity may weaken the alveolar tissue and facilitate its rupture, particularly at the point where alveolar walls and airway adventitia meet and where the mechanical stress is likely to be greatest. This mechanism might provide an explanation for the relationship of airway inflammation and abnormalities of pulmonary function reported in smokers. Surprisingly, the majority of studies examining the pathology of COPD have been performed in subjects with mild to moderate disease, while pathological studies on subjects with severe COPD are few. The largest study, performed by Nagai and colleagues[192], showed that in subjects who had had severe disease both emphysema and peripheral airway abnormalities were present. Although the relative role of each of these pathologic lesions in the development of airflow limitation was difficult to establish, the authors concluded that emphysema was the more important. However, the findings of Nagai and colleagues should be interpreted with caution[156]. Their data indicate that, when emphysema is severe, loss of elastic recoil assumes overwhelming importance as the mechanism of airflow limitation, thus masking the effects of peripheral airway abnormalities. By contrast, when emphysema is mild, peripheral airways abnormalities do appear to play a role in causing airflow limitation.

While earlier suggestions that distinct clinical patterns of disease, referred to as 'pink puffers' and 'blue bloaters', represented morphologically different patterns of pathology detected postmortem, more recent studies have shown no correlation between the amount of macroscopic emphysema and chronic hypoxemia.

Studies of the relationships of macroscopically assessed emphysema and gas transfer or radiological changes have shown only moderate correlations. With microscopically assessed emphysema, however, carbon monoxide transfer coefficient (KCO) shows a strong linear correlation ($r = 0.86$) in a group of patients, of whom only half showed macroscopic emphysema. When the microscopic assessment of emphysema is expressed in terms of an estimate of the density of alveolar tissue per unit volume of lung (AWUV), there is good correlation with assessment of emphysema using computed tomography (CT)[189,193]. Such studies, based on microscopic assessment of emphysema, represent a significant advance in the ability to identify early emphysema in life, and to follow its progression[194]. By application of combinations of quantitative histology and CT-determined lung volume data, Coxson and colleagues have been able to provide quantitative estimates of the extent of lung destruction in patients that may be followed longitudinally in the future: this will allow pathogenesis to be better understood and the effects of treatment to be determined[195,196]. Recent application of these methods has allowed the number of inflammatory cells present per unit surface area of lung parenchyma to be investigated in COPD. The data from these investigations indicate that emphysematous lung destruction is associated with a marked amplification of the inflammatory response in patients with emphysema compared to the lungs of smokers without emphysema but with equivalent smoking histories[195].

Emphysema in COPD, is also the likely consequence of a chronic CD8 + cell inflammatory process. The current definition of emphysema excludes the presence of obvious fibrosis, yet it is now known that fibrosis may also occur even in the presence of alveolar wall loss[197,198]. The enlargement of alveolar spaces, distal to the terminal bronchiolus, in COPD may thus represent the consequence of lung injury and a failure to repair rather than of destruction *per se*. The focal fibrosis that may be identified in some cases of emphysema may represent the remainder of a repair component. Further studies of the mechanisms that balance the production and degradation of collagen that occurs during the reparative and remodelling response to lung injury may yield important findings applicable to the treatment or prevention of the parenchymal lesions so important to COPD.

Airway wall nerves

The topic of airway wall innervation and its relation to asthma is a large one[133,134]. There are data suggesting that in fatal asthma there is an absence of (relaxant) vasoactive intestinal polypeptide (VIP)-containing nerve fibres and an increase in the numbers of substance P-containing fibres (stimulatory to bronchial smooth muscle) contrasting markedly with the innervation of the control lungs taken at resection from chronic smokers[199,200]. The reduction has not, however, been confirmed in examination of bronchial biopsies in mild asthma[201]. Whilst Sharma and colleagues have described a reduction of airway VIP and β-adrenoreceptors in cystic fibrosis, the densities of both VIP receptors and β-adrenoreceptors are reported to be similar in asthma to those of grossly normal tissue of the lungs of smokers resected for carcinoma[202,203].

Conclusions

The key points of comparison between asthma and COPD are summarized in Tables 1.1 and 1.2. There is evidence of airways inflammation in both asthma and COPD but there are marked differences in terms of the predominant anatomic site involved, the predominant pattern of inflammatory cells and the structural consequences of such inflammation. It will be of interest to learn whether further studies confirm or refute the hypothesis that chronic asthma and COPD are two distinct conditions that require equally distinct approaches to their management. This notion has received support from the recent findings of long-term trials of mild to moderate disease in which inhaled corticosteroids have been shown to be effective in the treatment of

Table 1.1. Asthma summary

The airway walls in asthma are thickened by inflammation and 'remodelling' and there is lumenal narrowing.

The association of tissue eosinophilia and asthma is a strong one and activated T-helper (CD4 +) lymphocytes perpetuate the chronic eosinophilia.

Neutrophils are sparse in mild asthma but they are present in relatively large numbers in severe asthma

Mast cells play a role in the immediate (type I sensitivity) reaction in asthma: little is known of the role of basophils albeit they are considered important.

Epithelial fragility and loss are often but not always reported in asthma: healing or abnormal repair may be driving subsequent remodelling.

Thickening of the reticular basement membrane (i.e. the lamina reticularis but not the lamina densa) is a consistent change in allergic, non-allergic and occupational forms of asthma.

There is no consensus as to increased interstitial collagen in asthma.

The percentage of bronchial wall occupied by bronchial smooth muscle increases substantially in fatal asthma: there are several mechanisms that could explain the increase and there may be parallels with the changes in vessel walls in atheroma.

There is submucosal gland enlargement in fatal asthma and excessive production of mucus that, together with the inflammatory exudate, forms the sticky tenacious plugs that block airway lumena.

Dilatation of bronchial mucosal blood vessels, congestion and wall oedema are consistently reported features of fatal asthma: these can account for considerable swelling of the airway wall.

While corticosteroids are effective in treating the eosinophilic inflammation of mild asthma new treatments need to be found to treat the altered inflammation and the remodelling of severe asthma.

Inflammation and remodelling may respond to distinct classes of drug.

mild/moderate asthma but not so in COPD. However, the author predicts that the responses to any one treatment will vary from patient to patient depending not only on the diagnosis of 'asthma' of 'COPD' *per se* but rather on the particular prevailing patterns of inflammatory cells, cytokines and

Table 1.2. COPD summary

The relationship between cigarette smoking and COPD is a strong one statistically: smoking tobacco *per se* induces an inflammatory response

COPD is a CD8 + cell and monocyte/macrophage predominant inflammatory condition of large and small airways and of the alveolar walls.

The increase of CD8 + cells shows a negative association with FEV1

A macrophage alveolitis and respiratory bronchiolitis are early changes in young cigarette smokers

The neutrophil, the macrophage and the CD8 + cell may each be involved in the destruction of the lung parenchyma by distinct mechanisms

The infiltration of the airway wall by lymphocytes is associated with loss of alveolar attachments to the outer wall of small airways, a characteristic of centriacinar emphysema.

When there is an exacerbation of bronchitis, there is a change in the pattern of inflammation (i.e. an eosinophilia develops), which more closely resembles that of asthma.

Airflow limitation usually occurs late in the course of cigarette smoke-related events, whereas inflammation in small airways occurs relatively early.

Loss of surface epithelium is not a feature of COPD but there is often squamous or mucous metaplasia

Thickening of the reticular basement membrane does not occur unless there is evidence of airway reversibility (in response to corticosteroid treatment)

Collagen is reported to be increased and smooth muscle mass increased in small airways

Submucosal glands are increased in amount to the same extent as in asthma

Corticosteroids do not alter the rate of decline of lung function in COPD but they may be effective in the treatment of exacerbations. New treatments need to be found for COPD.

remodelling. The emerging data indicate that inflammation will differ markedly in relation to exacerbation and severity and perhaps also in response to chronic but less than effective treatment. It is also likely that the remodelling process will require new classes of drug that target it more specifically: it is likely more than a consequence of chronic inflammation alone. The development, results and consideration of a range of such agents is now considered in the chapters that follow.

Acknowledgements

The author warmly thanks Mr Andrew Rogers for his expert assistance with the illustrations and the numerous clinical and research colleagues with whom I work.

REFERENCES

1 Bousquet J, Jeffery PK, Busse WW, Johnson M, Vignola AM. Asthma. From bronchoconstriction to airways inflammation and remodeling. *Am J Resp Crit Care Med* 2000; 161:1720–1745.

2 Jeffery PK. Comparison of the structural and inflammatory features of COPD and asthma (Giles F. Filley Lecture). *Chest* 2000; 117:251s–260s.

3 Global Initiative for Asthma. Global strategy for asthma management and prevention. NHLBI/WHO workshop report (based on a March 1993 meeting). NHBLI 1995; 1.

4 Pauwels R, Anthonisen N, Barnes PJ et al. In Lenfant C and Khaltaev N, eds. *Global Initiative for Chronic Obstructive Lung Disease*. National Institues of Health; National Heart, Lung, and Blood Institute; 2001. 1p.

5 Orie NGM, Sluiter HJ, De Vries K et al. The host factor in bronchitis. In Orie NGM, Sluiter HJ, eds. *Bronchitis, An International Symposium*. Assen, The Netherlands: Royal Van Gorcum; 1961; 43–59.

6 Jeffery PK. Bronchial biopsies and airway inflammation. *Eur Respir J* 1996; 9:1583–1587.

7 Bai TR. Abnormalities in airway smooth muscle in fatal asthma. *Am Rev Respir Dis* 1990; 141:552–557.

8 Tiddens HAWM, Pare PD, Hogg JC, Hop WCJ, Lambert R, De Jongste JC. Cartilagenous airway dimensions and airflow obstruction in human lungs. *Am J Resp Crit Care Med* 1995; 152:260–266.

9 Cardoso WV. Molecular regulation of lung development. *Annu Rev Physiol* 1901; 63:471–494.

10 Serini G, Gabbiani G. Mechanisms of myofibroblast activity and phenotypic modulation. *Exp Cell Res* 1999; 250:273–283.

11 Pizzichini MNN, Pizzichini E, Morris M, Efthimiadis A, Berman L, Dolovich J, Hargreaves FE. Indicies of airway inflammation in sputum of smokers with non-obstructive and obstructive bronchitis. *Eur Respir J* 1996; 9:126S.

12 Gibson PG, Hargreaves FE, Girgis-Gabardo A, Morris M, Denburg JA, Dolovich J. Chronic cough with eosinophilic bronchitis and examination for variable airflow

obstruction and reponse to corticosteroid. *Allergy* 1995; 25:127–132.

13 Naylor B. The shedding of the mucosa of the bronchial tree in asthma. *Thorax* 1962; 17:69–72.

14 Weller PF, Bach DS, Austen KF. Biochemical characterization of human eosinophil Charcot–Leyden crystal protein (lysophospholipase). *J Biol Chem* 1984; 259:15100–15105.

15 Gibson PG, Girgis-Gabardo A, Morris MM et al. Cellular characteristics of sputum from patients with asthma and chronic bronchitis. *Thorax* 1989; 44:693–699.

16 Gibson PG, Dolivich J, Denburg J, Ramsdale EH, Hargreave FE. Chronic cough: eosinophilic bronchitis without asthma. *Lancet* 1989; 1:1346–1348.

17 Beasley R, Roche W, Roberts JA, Holgate ST. Cellular events in the bronchi in mild asthma and after bronchial provocation. *Am Rev Respir Dis* 1989; 139:806–817.

18 Wardlaw AJ, Dunnett S, Gleich GJ, Collins JV, Kay AB. Eosinophils and mast cells in bronchoalveolar lavage in mild asthma: relationship to bronchial hyperreactivity. *Am Rev Respir Dis* 1988; 137:62–69.

19 Dunnill MS, Massarella GR, Anderson JA. A comparison of the quantitative anatomy of the bronchi in normal subjects, in status asthmaticus, in chronic bronchitis, and in emphysema. *Thorax* 1969; 24:176–179.

20 Reid LM. The presence or absence of bronchial mucus in fatal asthma. *J Allergy Clin Immunol* 1987; 80:415–416.

21 Azzawi M, Bradley B, Jeffery PK et al. Identification of activated T lymphocytes and eosinophils in bronchial biopsies in stable atopic asthma. *Am Rev Respir Dis* 1990; 142:1407–1413.

22 Azzawi M, Johnston PW, Majumdar S, Kay AB, Jeffery PK. T lymphocytes and activated eosinophils in asthma and cystic fibrosis. *Am Rev Respir Dis* 1992; 145:1477–1482.

23 Laitinen LA, Laitinen A, Haahtela T. Airway mucosal inflammation even in patients with newly diagnosed asthma. *Am Rev Respir Dis* 1993; 147:697–704.

24 Jeffery PK, Wardlaw A, Nelson FC, Collins JV, Kay AB. Bronchial biopsies in asthma: an ultrastructural quantification study and correlation with hyperreactivity. *Am Rev Respir Dis* 1989; 140:1745–1753.

25 Laitinen LA, Heino M, Laitinen A, Kava T, Haahtela T. Damage of the airway epithelium and bronchial reactivity in patients with asthma. *Am Rev Respir Dis* 1985; 131:599–606.

26 Jeffery PK, Godfrey RWA, Adelroth E, Nelson F, Rogers A, Johansson S-A. Effects of treatment on airway inflammation and thickening of reticular collagen in asthma: a quantitative light and electron microscopic study. *Am Rev Respir Dis* 1992; 145:890–899.

27 Bentley AM, Maestrelli P, Saetta M et al. Activated T lymphocytes and eosinophils in the bronchial mucosa in isocyanate-induced asthma. *J Allergy Clin Immunol* 1992; 89:821–829.

28 Bentley AM, Menz G, Storz C. et al. Identification of T-lymphocytes, macrophages and activated eosinophils in the bronchial mucosa in intrinsic asthma: relationship to symptoms and bronchial responsiveness. *Am Rev Respir Dis* 1992; 146:500–506.

29 Filley WV, Holley KE, Kephart GM, Gleich GJ. Identification by immunofluorescence of eosinophil granule major basic protein in lung tissue of patients with bronchial asthma. *Lancet* 1982; 1:11–16.

30 Persson CGA, Erjefalt JS. Eosinophil lysis and free granules: an in vivo paradigm for cell activation and drug development. *Trends Pharmacol Sci* 1997; 18: 117–123.

31 Erjefalt JS, Andersson M, Greiff L et al. Cytolysis and piecemeal degranulation as distinct modes of activation of airway mucosal eosinophils. *J Allergy Clin Immunol* 1998; 102:286–294.

32 Dunnill MS. The pathology of asthma, with special reference to changes in the bronchial mucosa. *J Clin Pathol* 1960; 13:27–33.

33 Saetta M, Di Stefano A, Rosina C, Thiene G, Fabbri LM. Quantitative structural analysis of peripheral airways and arteries in sudden fatal asthma. *Am Rev Respir Dis* 1991; 143:138–143.

34 Carroll N, Carello S, Cooke C, James A. Airway structure and inflammatory cells in fatal attacks of asthma. *Eur Respir J* 1996; 9:709–715.

35 Synek M, Beasley R, Frew AJ et al. Cellular infiltration of the airways in asthma of varying severity. *Am J Resp Crit Care Med* 1996; 154:224–230.

36 Fahy JV, Kim KW, Liu J, Boushey HA. Prominent neutrophilic inflammation in sputum from subjects with asthma exacerbation. *J Allergy Clin Immunol* 1995; 95:843–852.

37 Wenzel SE, Szefler SJ, Leung DYM, Sloan SI, Rex MD, Martin RJ. Bronchoscopic evaluation of severe asthma. Persistent inflammation associated with high dose glucocorticoids. *Am J Resp Crit Care Med* 1997; 156:737–743.

38 Sur S, Crotty TB, Kephart GM et al. Sudden onset fatal asthma: a distinct entity with few eosinophils and relatively more neutrophils in the airway submucosa? *Am Rev Respir Dis* 1993; 148:713–719.

39 Wenzel SE, Schwartz LB, Langmack EL et al. Evidence that severe asthma can be divided pathologically into two inflammatory subtypes with distinct physiologic and clinical characteristics. *Am J Respir Crit Care Med* 1999; 160:1001–1008.

40 Kraft M, Djukanovic R, Wilson S, Holgate ST, Martin RJ. Alveolar tissue inflammation in asthma. *Am J Respir Crit Care Med* 1996; 154:1505–1510.

41 Hamid Q, Song Y, Kotsimbos TC et al. Inflammation of small airways in asthma. *J Allergy Clin Immunol* 1997; 100:44–51.

42 Wenzel S, Balzar S, Gibbs R, Chu HW. Small airway inflammation in refractory asthmatics and the relationship to physiologic abnormalities. *Am J Respir Crit Care Med* 2001; 163:A19

43 Gleich GJ, Motojima S, Frigas E, Kephart GM, Fujisawa T, Kravis LP. The eosinophilic leucocyte and the pathology of fatal bronchial asthma: evidence for pathologic heterogeneity. *J Allergy Clin Immunol* 1980; 80:412–415.

44 Kay AB. Asthma and inflammation. *J Allergy Clin Immunol* 1991; 87:893–910.

45 Robinson DS, Durham SR, Kay AB. Cytokines: 3-cytokines in asthma. *Thorax* 1993; 48:845–853.

46 Hamid Q, Azzawi M, Ying S et al. IL-5 mRNA in bronchial biopsies from asthmatic subjects. *J Clin Invest* 1991; 87:1541–1546.

47 Robinson DS, Hamid Q, Ying S et al. Predominant TH2-like bronchoalveolar T-lymphocyte population in atopic asthma. *N Engl J Med* 1992; 326:298–304.

48 Ohnishi T, Kita H, Weiler D et al. IL-5 is the predominant eosinophil-active cytokine in the antigen-induced pulmonary late-phase reaction. *Am Rev Respir Dis* 1993; 147:901–907.

49 Corrigan CJ, Haczku A, Gemou-Engesaeth V et al. CD4 T-lymphocyte activation in asthma is accompanied by increased serum concentrations of interleukin-5. *Am Rev Respir Dis* 1993; 147:540–547.

50 Walker C, Bode E, Boer L, Hansel TT, Blaser K, Virchow J-C, Jr. Allergic and nonallergic asthmatics have distinct patterns of T-cell activation and cytokine production in peripheral blood and bronchoalveolar lavage. *Am Rev Respir Dis* 1992; 146:109–115.

51 Ackerman V, Marini M, Vittori E, Bellini A, Vassali G, Mattoli S. Detection of cytokines and their cell sources in bronchial biopsy specimens from asthmatic patients: relationship to atopic status, symptoms and level of airway hyperresponsiveness. *Chest* 1994; 105:687–696.

52 Humbert M, Durham SR, Ying S et al. IL-4 and IL-5 mRNA and protein in bronchial biopsies from atopic and non-atopic asthma. Evidence against 'intrinsic' asthma being a distinct immunopathological entity. *Am J Resp Crit Care* Med. 1996; 154:1497–1504.

53 Jeffery PK, Hamid Q, Majumdar S et al. Antigen-primed T cells and expression of cytokine mRNA for IL4, IL5 and INF-gamma in fibrosing alveolitis associated with systemic sclerosis. [Abstract] *J Pathol* 1993; 170:380A.

54 Jose PJ, Griffiths-Johnson DA, Collins PD et al. Eotaxin: a potent eosinophil chemoattractant cytokine detected in a guinea pig model of allergic airways inflammation. *J Exp Med* 1994; 179:881–887.

55 Collins PD, Marleau S, Griffiths-Johnson DA, Jose PJ, Williams TJ. Cooperation between interleukin-5 and the chemokine eotaxin to induce eosinophil accumulation in vivo. *J Exp Med* 1995; 182:1169–1174.

56 Li D, Wang D, Griffiths-Johnson DA et al. Eotaxin protein gene expression in guinea-pigs: constitutive expression and upregulation after allergen challenge. *Eur Respir J* 1997; 10:1946–1954.

57 Broide DH, Lotz M, Cuomo AJ, Coburn DA, Federman EC, Wasserman SI. Cytokines in symptomatic asthma airways. *J Allergy Clin Immunol* 1992; 89:958–967.

58 Woolley KL, Adelroth E, Woolley MJ, Ellis R, Jordana M, O'Byrne PM. Granulocyte-macrophage colony-stimulating factor, eosinophils and eosinophil cationic protein in subjects with and without mild, stable atopic asthma. *Eur Resp J* 1994; 9: 1576–1584.

59 Holgate ST, Howarth PH, Church MK et al. Austen KF, In Lichtenstein L, Kay AB, Holgate ST, editors. *Asthma*, Vol. IV, *Physiology, immunopharmacology and treatment.* Oxford: Blackwell Scientific Publications; 1993; Mechanisms of acute and chronic mucosal inflammation in asthma. p. 287–298.

60 Hamid Q, Barkans J, Meng Q et al. Human eosinophils synthesize and secrete interleukin-6, in vitro. *Blood* 1992; 80:1496–1501.

61 Bradding P, Feather IH, Howarth PH et al. Interleukin 4 is localized to and released by human mast cells. *J Exp Med* 1992; 176:1381–1386.

62 Bradding P, Feather IH, Wilson S et al. Immunolocalization of cytokines in the nasal mucosa of normal and perennial rhinitic subjects. *J Immunol* 1993; 151:3853–3865.

63 Salvato G. Some histological changes in chronic bronchitis and asthma. *Thorax* 1968; 23:168–172.

64 Gerblich AA, Campbell AE, Schuyler MR. Changes in T-lymphocyte subpopulations after antigenic bronchial provocation in asthmatics. *N Engl J Med* 1984; 310:1349–1352.

65 Adelroth E, Rosenhall L, Johansson S-A, Linden M, Venge P. Inflammatory cells and eosinophilic activity in asthmatics investigated by bronchoalveolar lavage: the effects of anti-asthmatic treatment with budesonide or terbutaline. *Am Rev Respir Dis* 1990; 142:91–99.

66 Denburg JA, Telizyn S, Belda A, Dolovich J, Bienenstock J.

Increased numbers of circulating basophil progenitors in atopic patients. *J Allergy Clin Immunol* 1985; 76:466–472.

67 Bellini A, Vittori E, Marini M, Ackerman V, Mattoli S. Intraepithelial dendritic cells and selective activation of Th2-like lymphocytes in patients with atopic asthma. *Chest* 1993; 103:997–1005.

68 Holt PG. Regulation of antigen-presenting cell function(s) in lung and airway tissues. *Eur Respir J* 1993; 6:120–129.

69 O'Shaughnessy TC, Ansari TW, Barnes NC, Jeffery PK. Inflammation in bronchial biopsies of subjects with chronic bronchitis. inverse relationship of CD8 + T lymphocytes with FEV1. *Am J Respir Crit Care Med* 1997; 155:852–857.

70 Jeffery PK. Lymphocytes, chronic bronchitis and chronic obstructive pulmonary disease. In Chadwick D, Goode JA, eds.*Chronic obstructive pulmonary disease: pathogenesis to treatment*. Chichester: John Wiley; 2001; 149–168.

71 Miller LG, Goldstein G, Murphy M, Ginns LC. Reversible alterations in immunoregulatory T cells in smoking. Analysis by monoclonal antibodies and flow cytometry. *Chest* 1982; 82:526–529.

72 Costabel U, Bross KJ, Reuter C, Ruhle K-H, Matthys H. Alterations in immunoregulatory T-cell subsets in cigarette smokers. A phenotypic analysis of bronchoalveolar and blood lymphocytes. *Chest* 1986; 90:39–44.

73 van Eeden SF, Hogg JC. The response of human bone marrow to chronic cigarette smoking. *Eur Respir J* 2000; 15:915–921.

74 Lams BEA, Sousa AR, Rees PJ, Lee TH. Immunopathology of the small-airway submucosa in smokers with and without chronic obstructive pulmonary disease. *Am J Respir Crit Care Med* 1998; 158:1518–1523.

75 Lams BE, Sousa AR, Rees PJ, Lee TH. Subepthelial immunopathology of large airways in smokers with and without chronic obstructive pulmonary disease. *Eur Respir J* 2000; 15:512–516.

76 Mullen JBM, Wright JL, Wiggs BR, Pare PD, Hogg JC. Reassessment of inflammation of airways in chronic bronchitis. *Br Med J* 1985; 291:1235–1239.

77 Saetta M, Di Stefano A, Maestrelli et al. Activated T-lymphocytes and macrophages in bronchial mucosa of subjects with chronic bronchitis. *Am Rev Respir Dis* 1993; 147:301–306.

78 Di Stefano A, Turato G, Maestrelli P et al. Airflow limitation in chronic bronchitis is associated with T-lymphocyte and macrophage infiltration of the bronchial mucosa. *Am J Respir Crit Care Med* 1996; 153:629–632.

79 O'Shaughnessy T, Ansari TW, Barnes NC, Jeffery PK. Inflammation in bronchial biopsies of subjects with chronic bronchitis: inverse relationship of CD8 + T lymphocytes with FEV$_1$. *Am J Resp Crit Care Med* 1997; 155:852–857.

80 Di Stefano A, Maestrelli P, Roggeri A et al. Upregulation of adhesion molecules in the bronchial mucosa of subjects with chronic obstructive bronchitis. *Am J Respir Crit Care Med* 1994; 149:803–810.

81 Fournier M, Lebargy F, Le Roy Ladurie F, Lenormand E, Pariente R. Intraepithelial T-lymphocyte subsets in the airways of normal subjects and of patients with chronic bronchitis. *Am Rev Respir Dis* 1989; 140:737–742.

82 O'Shaughnessy TC, Ansari TW, Barnes NC, Jeffery PK. Inflammatory cells in the airway surface epithelium of smokers with and without bronchitic airflow obstruction. *Eur Respir J* 1996; 9 (suppl 23):14s.

83 Saetta M, Turato G, Facchini FM et al. Inflammatory cells in the bronchial glands of smokers with chronic bronchitis. *Am J Respir Crit Care Med* 1997; 156:1633–1639.

84 Saetta M. CD8 + T-lymphocytes in peripheral airways of smokers with chronic obstructive pulmonary disease. *Am J Respir Crit Care Med* 1998; 157:822–826.

85 Jeffery PK. Differences and similarities between chronic obstructive pulmonary disease and asthma. *Clin Exp Allergy* 1999; 29(S2):14–26.

86 Lacoste J-Y, Bousquet J, Chanez P et al. Eosinophilic and neutrophilic inflammation in asthma, chronic bronchitis, and chronic obstructive pulmonary disease. *J Allergy Clin Immunol* 1993; 92:537–548.

87 Pizzichini E, Pizzichini MMM, Gibson P et al. Sputum eosinophilia predicts benefit from prednisone in smokers with chronic obstructive bronchitis. *Am J Respir Crit Care Med* 1998; 158:1511–1517.

88 Saetta M, Di Stefano A, Maetrelli P et al. Airway eosinophilia in chronic bronchitis during exacerbations. *Am J Respir Crit Care Med* 1994; 150:1646–1652.

89 Saetta M, Di Stefano A, Maestrelli P et al. Airway eosinophilia and expression of interleukin-5 protein in asthma and in exacerbations of chronic bronchitis. *Clin Exp Allergy* 1996; 26:766–774.

90 Zhu J, Qui YS, Majumdar S, et al. Bronchial eosinophilia in gene expression for IL-4, Il-5 and eosinophilia chemoattractants in bronchitis. *Am J Respir Crit Care Med* 2001; 164:109–116.

91 Zhu J, Majumdar S, Ansari T et al. IL-4 and IL-5 mRNA in the bronchial wall of smokers. *Am J Resp Crit Care Med* 1999; 159:A450.

92 Majumdar S, Li D, Ansari T et al. Different cytokine profiles in cryptogenic fibrosing alveolitis and fibrosing alveolitis associated with systemic sclerosis. *Eur Respir J* 1999; 14:251–257.

93 Reynolds HY. Bronchoalveolar lavage. *Am Rev Respir Dis* 1987; 135:250–263.

94 Finkelstein R, Fraser RS, Ghezzo H, Cosio MG. Alveolar inflammation and its relation to emphysema in smokers. *Am J Respir Crit Care Med* 1995; 152:1666–1672.

95 Saetta M, Baraldo S, Corbino L et al. CD8 + cells in the lungs of smokers with chronic obstructive pulmonary disease. *Am J Respir Crit Care Med* 1999; 160:711–717.

96 Saltini C, Hance AJ, Ferrans VJ, Basset F, Bitterman PB, Crystal RG. Accurate quantification of cells recovered by bronchoalveolar lavage. *Am Rev Respir Dis* 1984; 130:650–658.

97 Niewoehner DE, Klienerman J, Rice D. Pathologic changes in the peripheral airways of young cigarette smokers. *N Engl J Med* 1974; 291:755–758.

98 Cosio MG, Hale KA, Niewoehner DE. Morphologic and morphometric effects of prolonged cigarette smoking on the small airways. *Am Rev Respir Dis* 1980; 122:265–271.

99 MacNee W, Selby C. New perspectives on basic mechanisms in lung disease: 2.Neutrophil traffic in the lungs: role of haemodynamics, cell adhesion and deformability. *Thorax* 1993; 48:79–88.

100 Drost EM, Selby C, Lannan S, Lowe GDO, MacNee W. Changes in neutrophil deformability following in vitro smoke exposure : mechanisms and protection. *Am J Respir Cell Mol Biol* 1992; 6:287–295.

101 Ludwig WP, Hoidal JR. Alterations in leucocyte oxidative metabolism in cigarette smokers. *Am Rev Respir Dis* 1982; 126:977–980.

102 Eliraz A, Kimbell P, Weinbaum G. Canine alveolar macrophage and neutrophil exposure to cigarette smoke: regulation of elastase secretion. *Chest* 1977; 72:239.

103 Cohen AB, James HL. Reduction of the elastase inhibitory capacity of alpha 1-antitrypsin by peroxides in cigarette smoke: an analysis of brands and filters. *Am Rev Respir Dis* 1982; 126:25–30.

104 Sandhaus RA. Migration-induced elastolysis: directed migration of human neutrophils causes connective tissue proteolysis in the absence of alpha 1-protease inhibitor. *Am Rev Respir Dis* 1983; 127:2815.

105 Stockley RA. Proteases and antiproteases. In Chadwick D, Goode JA, eds.*Chronic Obstructive Pulmonary Disease: Pathogenesis to Treatment.* Chichester: John Wiley; 2001; 189–204.

106 Shapiro SD. The pathogenesis of emphysema: the elastase:antielastase hypothesis 30 years later. *Proc Assoc Am Physicians* 1995; 107:346–352.

107 Zhao MQ, Stoler MH, Liu AN et al. Alveolar epithelial cell chemokine expression triggered by antigen-specific cyto-

lytic CD8 + T cell recognition. [Abstract] *J Clin Invest* 2000; 106:R49-R58

108 Cawston T, Carrere S, Catterall J et al. Matrix metalloproteinases and TIMPs properties and implications for treatment of chronic obstructive pulmonary disease. In: Chadwick D, Goode A, eds.*Chronic Obstructive Pulmonary Disease: Pathogenesis to Treatment.* Novartis Foundation Symposium 234 Chichester: John Wiley; 2001; 205–228.

109 Hautamaki RD, Kobayashi DK, Senior RM, Shapiro SD. Requirement for macrophage elastase for cigarette smoke-induced emphysema in mice. *Science* 1997; 277:2002–2004.

110 Finlay GA, O'Driscoll LR, Russell KJ et al. Matrix metalloproteinase expression and production by alveolar macrophages in emphysema. *Am J Respir Crit Care Med* 1997; 156:240–7.

111 Niederman MS, Fritts LL, Merrill WM et al. Demonstration of a free elastolytic metallo-enzyme in human lung lavage fluid and its relationship to alplha 1-antiprotease. *Am Rev Respir Dis* 1984; 129:943–947.

112 Vukmanovic-Stejic M, Vyas B, Gorak-Stolinska P, Noble A, Kemeny DM. Human Tc1 and Tc2/Tc0 CD8 T-cell clones display distinct cell surface and functional phenotypes. *Blood* 2000; 95:231–240.

113 Kemeny DM, Noble A, Holmes BJ, Diaz-Sanchez D. Immune regulation: a new role for the CD8 + T cell. *Immunol Today* 1994; 15:107–110.

114 Wang Z, Zheng T, Zhu Z et al. Interferon gamma induction of pulmonary emphysema in the adult murine lung. *J Exp Med* 2000; 192:1587–1600.

115 Tuder RM, Wood K, Taraseviciene L, Flores SC, Voekel NF. Cigarette smoke extract decreases the expression of vascular endothelial growth factor by cultured cells and triggers apoptosis of pulmonary endothelial cells. *Chest* 2000; 117:241S-242S.

116 Amadori A, Zamarchi R, De Silvestro G. Genetic control of the CD4/CD8 T-cell ratio in humans. *Nat Med* 1995; 1:1279–1283.

117 Massaro D, Massaro GD. Pulmonary alveolus formation: critical period, retinoid regulation and plasticity. In: Chadwick D, Goode A, eds. *Chronic Obstructive Pulmonary Disease: Pathogenesis to Treatment.* Novartis Foundation Symposium 234 ed. Chichester: John Wiley; 2001; 229–249.

118 Hattotuwa K, Ansari T, Gizycki M, Barnes N, Jeffery PK. A double blind placebo-controlled trial of the effect of inhaled corticosteroids on the immunopathology of COPD. *Am J Respir Crit Care Med* 1999; 159:A523.

119 Burge PS, Calverley PM, Jones PW, Spencer S, Anderson JA, Maslen TK. Randomised, double blind, placebo controlled

study of fluticasone propionate in patients with moderate to severe chronic obstructive pulmonary disease: the ISOLDE trial. *Br Med J* 2000; 320:1297–303.

120 Peinado VI, Barbera JA, Abate P et al. Inflammatory reaction in pulmonary muscular arteries of patients with mild chronic obstructive pulmonary disease. *Am J Respir Crit Care Med* 1999; 159:1605–1611.

121 Dinh-Xuan AT, Higenbottam TW, Clelland CA et al. Impairment of endothelium-dependent pulmonary-artery relaxation in chronic obstructive lung disease. *N Engl J Med* 1991; 324:1539–1547.

122 Peinado VI, Barbera JA, Ramirez J et al. Endothelial dysfunction in pulmonary arteries of patients with mild COPD. *Am J Physiol* 1998; 274:L908-L913.

123 Carroll N, Elliot A, Morton A, James A. The structure of large and small airways in nonfatal and fatal asthma. *Am Rev Respir Dis* 1993; 147:405–410.

124 Amin K, Ludviksdottir D, Janson C et al. Inflammation and structural changes in the airways of patients with atopic and nonatopic asthma. *Am J Respir Crit Care Med* 2000; 162:2295–2301.

125 Naylor B. The shedding of the mucosa of the bronchial tree in asthma. *Thorax* 1962; 17:69–72.

126 Holgate ST. Epithelial damage and response. *Clin Exp Allergy* 2000; 30 Suppl 1:37–41.

127 Holgate ST, Lackie PM, Davies DE, Roche WR, Walls AF. The bronchial epithelium as a key regulator of airway inflammation and remodelling in asthma. *Clin Exp Allergy* 1999; 29 Suppl 2:90–95.

128 Lozewicz S, Wells C, Gomez E et al. Morphological integrity of the bronchial epithelium in mild asthma. *Thorax* 1990; 45:12–15.

129 Ordonez C, Ferrando R, Hyde DM, Wong HH, Fahy JV. Epithelial desquamation in asthma. Artifact or pathology? *Am J Respir Crit Care Med* 2000; 162:2324–2329.

130 Elia C, Bucca C, Rolla G, Scappaticci E, Cantino D. A freeze–fracture study of tight junctions in human bronchial epithelium in normal, bronchitic and asthmatic subjects. *J Submic Cytol Pathol* 1988; 20:509–517.

131 Godfrey RWA, Severs NJ, Jeffery PK. Freeze-fracture morphology and quantification of human bronchial epithelial tight junctions. *Am J Respir Cell Molec Biol* 1992; 6:453–458.

132 Wan H, Winton HL, Soeller C et al. The transmembrane protein occludin of epithelial tight junctions is a functional target for serine peptidases from faecal pellets of *Dermatophagoides pteronyssinus*. *Clin Exp Allergy* 2001; 31:279–294.

133 Barnes PJ. State of art: neural control of human airways

in health and disease. *Am Rev Respir Dis* 1986; 134:1289–1314.

134 Jeffery PK. Goldie R, eds.Innervation of the airway mucosa: Structure, function and changes in airway disease. In *Immunopharmacology of Epithelial Barriers*. Vol 8 *Handbook of Immunopharmacology* (series ed. C. Page). London: Academic Press; 1994; 4:85–118.

135 Sparrow MP, Mitchell HW. The epithelium acts as a barrier modulating the extent of bronchial narrowing produced by substances perfused through the lumen. *Br J Pharmacol* 1991; 103:1160–1164.

136 Evans MJ, Plopper CG. The role of basal cells in adhesion of columnar epithelium to airway basement membrane. *Am Rev Respir Dis* 1988; 138:481–482.

137 Montefort S, Roberts JA, Beasley R, Holgate ST, Roche WR. The site of disruption of the bronchial epithelium in asthmatic and non-asthmatic subjects. *Thorax* 1992; 47:499–503.

138 Bellini A, Yoshimura H, Vittori E, Marini M, Mattoli S. Bronchial epithelial cells of patients with asthma release chemoattractant factors for T-lymphocytes. *J Allerg.Clin Immunol* 1993; 92:412–424.

139 Jeffery PK. Structural and inflammatory changes in COPD: a comparison with asthma. *Thorax* 1998; 53:129–136.

140 Ollerenshaw SL, Woolcock AJ. Characteristics of the inflammation in biopsies from large airways of subjects with asthma and subjects with chronic airflow limitation. *Am Rev Respir Dis* 1992; 145:922–927.

141 Roche WR, Beasley R, Williams JH, Holgate ST. Subepithelial fibrosis in the bronchi of asthmatics. *Lancet* 1989; 1:520–523.

142 Sobonya RE. Quantitative structural alterations in long-standing allergic asthma. *Am Rev Respir Dis* 1984; 130:289–292.

143 Crepea SB, Harman JW. The pathology of bronchial asthma. I. The significance of membrane changes in asthmatic and non-allergic pulmonary disease. *J Allergy* 1955; 26:453–460.

144 Jeffery PK. The development of large and small airways. *Am J Respir Crit Care Med* 1998; 157:S174–S180.

145 Payne D, Rogers A, Adelroth E et al. Reticular basement membrane thickness in children with difficult asthma. [Abstract] *Am J Respir Crit Care Med* 2001; 163:A19.

146 Pohunek P, Roche WR, Turzikova J et al. Eosinophilic inflammation in the bronchial mucosa of children with bronchial asthma. [Abstract] *Eur Resp J* 1997; 11:160s.

147 O'Shaughnessy TC, Ansari TW, Barnes NC et al. Reticular basement membrane thickness in moderately severe asthma and smokers' chronic bronchitis with and without

airflow obstruction. [Abstract] *Am J Resp Crit Care Med* 1996; 153:A879.

148 Laitinen A, Altraja A, Kampe M, Linden M, Virtanen I, Laitinen L. Tenascin is increased in airway basement membrane of asthmatics and decreased by an inhaled steroid. *Am J Respir Crit Care Med* 1997; 156(3 Pt 1):951–958.

149 Howat WJ, Holmes JA, Holgate ST, Lackie PM. Basement membrane pores in human bronchial epithelium: a conduit for infiltrating cells? *Am J Pathol* 2001; 158:673–680.

150 Brewster CEP, Howarth PH, Djukanovic R, Wilson J, Holgate ST, Roche WR. Myofibroblasts and subepithelial fibrosis in bronchial asthma. *Am J Respir Cell Mol Biol* 1990; 3:507–511.

151 Chanez P, Vignola AM, O'Shaughnessy T et al. Corticosteroid reversibility in COPD is related to features of asthma. *Am J Respir Crit Care Med* 1997; 155:1529–1534.

152 Minshall EM, Leung DYM, Martin RJ et al. Eosinophil-associated TGF-beta1 mRNA expression and airways fibrosis in bronchial asthma. *Am J Respir Cell Mol Biol* 1997; 17:326–333.

153 Chu HW, Halliday JL, Martin RJ, Leung DYM, Szefler SJ, Wenzel SE. Collagen deposition in large airways may not differentiate severe asthma from milder forms of the disease. *Am J Respir Crit Care Med* 1998; 158:1936–1944.

154 Bousquet J, Lacoste J-Y, Chanez P, Vic P, Godard P, Michel F-B. Bronchial elastic fibers in normal subjects and asthmatic patients. *Am J Respir Crit Care Med* 1996; 153:1648–1654.

155 Mauad T, Xavier AC, Saldiva PH, Dolhnikoff M. Elastosis and fragmentation of fibers of the elastic system in fatal asthma. *Am J Respir Crit Care Med* 1999; 160:968–915.

156 Snider GL. Chronic obstructive pulmonary disease – a continuing challenge. *Am Rev Respir Dis* 1986; 133:942–944.

157 Cosio M, Ghezzo H, Hogg JC et al. The relations between structural changes in small airways and pulmonary-function tests. *N Engl J Med* 1977; 298:1277–1281.

158 Bosken CH, Wiggs BR, Pare PD, Hogg JC. Small airway dimensions in smokers with obstruction to airflow. *Am Rev Respir Dis* 1990; 142:563–570.

159 James AL, Pare PD, Hogg JC. The mechanics of airway narrowing in asthma. *Am Rev Respir Dis* 1989; 139:242–246.

160 Moreno RH, Hogg JC, Pare PD. Mechanisms of airway narrowing. *Am Rev Respir Dis* 1986; 133:1171–1180.

161 Wiggs BR, Moreno R, Hogg JC, Hilliam C, Pare PD. A model of the mechanics of airway narrowing. *J Appl Physiol* 1990; 69:849–860.

162 Wiggs BR, Bosken C, Pare PD, James A, Hogg JC. A model of airway narrowing in asthma and in chronic obstructive pulmonary disease. *Am Rev Respir Dis* 1992; 145:1215–1218.

163 Hogg J. Austen KF, Lichtenstein L, Kay AB, Holgate ST, editors. *Asthma,* Vol. IV, *Physiology, Immunopharmacology and Treatment.* Oxford: Blackwell Scientific Publications; 1993; *The pathology of asthma.* p. 17–25.

164 Pare PD, Wiggs BR, James A, Hogg JC, Bosken C. The comparative mechanics and morphology of airways in asthma and chronic obstructive pulmonary disease. *Am J Resp Crit Care Med* 1991; 143:1189–1193.

165 Thurlbeck WM, Petty TL, eds. *Chronic Obstructive Pulmonary Disease.* 2nd edn Dekker; 1985; 6, *Chronic Airflow Obstruction. Correlation of Structure and Function.* pp. 129–203.

166 Takizawa T, Thurlbeck WM. Muscle and mucous gland size in the major bronchi of patients with chronic bronchitis, asthma and asthmatic bronchitis. *Am Rev Respir Dis* 1971; 104:331–336.

167 Saetta M, Turato G, Baraldo S et al. Goblet cell hyperplasia and epithelial inflammation in peripheral airways of smokers with both symptoms of chronic bronchitis and chronic airflow limitation. *Am J Respir Crit Care Med* 2000; 161:1016–1021.

168 Kuwano K, Bosken CH, Pare PD, Bai TR, Wiggs BR, Hogg JC. Small airways dimensions in asthma and in chronic obstructive pulmonary disease. *Am J Resp Crit Care Med* 1993; 148:1220–1223.

169 Lambert RK, Wiggs BR, Kuwano K, Hogg JC, Pare PD. Functional significance of increased airway smooth muscle in asthma and COPD. *J Appl Physiol* 1991; 74:2771–2781.

170 Heard BE, Hossain S. Hyperplasia of bronchial muscle in asthma. *J Pathol* 1983; 110:319–331.

171 Ebina M, Takahashi T, Chiba T, Motomiya M. Cellular hypertrophy and hyperplasia of airway smooth muscles underlying bronchial asthma – A 3-D morphometric study. *Am Rev Respir Dis* 1993; 148:720–726.

172 Gizycki MJ, Adelroth E, Rogers AV, O'Byrne PM, Jeffery PK. Myofibroblast involvement in the allergen-induced late response in mild atopic asthma. *Am J Respir Cell Mol Biol* 1997; 16:664–673.

173 Jeffery PK. Page C, Black J, eds. *Airways and Vascular Remodelling in Asthma and Cardiovascular Disease.* London: Academic Press; 1994; *Structural changes in asthma.* p. 3–19.

174 Wanner A. Middleton E, Reed CE, Ellis EF, Adkinson NF, Uunginer JW, eds. Airway mucus and the mucociliary system. In *Allergy: Principles and Practice.* St. Loius, Washington DC, Toronto: C.V.Mosby; 1988; 541–8.

175 Cluroe A, Holloway L, Thomson K, Purdie G, Beasley R. Bronchial gland duct ectasia in fatal bronchial asthma:

association with interstitial emphysema. *J Clin Pathol* 1989; 42:1026–1031.

176 Glynn AA, Michaels L. Bronchial biopsy in chronic bronchitis and asthma. *Thorax* 1960; 15:142–153.

177 Aikawa T, Shimura S, Sasaki H, Ebina M, Takishima T. Marked goblet cell hyperplasia with mucus accumulation in the airways of patients who died of severe acute asthma attack. *Chest* 1992; 101:916–921.

178 Reid L. Pathology of chronic bronchitis. *Lancet* 1954; i:275–279.

179 Shimura S, Andoh Y, Haraguchi M, Shirato K. Continuity of airway goblet cells and intraluminal mucus in the airways of patients with bronchial asthma. *Eur Respir J* 1996; 9:1395–401.

180 Carroll NG, Cooke C, James AL. Bronchial blood vessel dimensions in asthma. *Am J Respir Crit Care Med* 1997; 155:689–695.

181 Charan NB, Baile EM, Pare PD. Bronchial vascular congestion and angiogenesis. *Eur Respir J* 1997; 10.

182 Orsida BE, Li X, Hickey B, Thien F, Wilson JW, Walters EH. Vascularity in the asthmatic airways: relation to inhaled steroids. *Thorax* 1999; 54:289–295.

183 Vrugt B, Wilson S, Bron A, Holgate ST, Djukanovic R, Aalbers R. Bronchial angiogenesis in severe glucocorticoid-dependent asthma [In Process Citation]. *Eur Respir J* 2000; 15(6):1014–1021.

184 Magee F, Wright JL, Wiggs BR, Pare PD, Hogg JC. Pulmonary vascular structure and function in chronic obstructive pulmonary disease. *Thorax* 1988; 43:183–189.

185 Barbera JA, Riverola A, Roca J et al. Pulmonary vascular abnormalities and ventilation–perfusion relationship in mild chronic obstructive pulmonary disease. *Am J Resp Crit Care Med* 1994; 149:423–429.

186 Saetta M, Shiner RJ, Angus GE et al. Destructive index: a measurement of lung parenchymal destruction in smokers. *Am Rev Respir Dis* 1985; 131:764–769.

187 Kim WD, Eidelman DH, Izquierdo JL, Ghezzo H, Saetta MP, Cosio MG. Centrilobular and panlobular emphysema in smokers. Two distinct morphologic and functional entities. *Am Rev Respir Dis* 1991; 144:1385–1390.

188 Petty TL, Silvers GW, Stanford RE. Functional correlations with mild and moderate emphysema in excised human lungs. *Am Rev Respir Dis* 1981; 124:700–704.

189 Gould GA, MacNee W, McLean A et al. CT measurements of lung density in life can quantitate distal airspace enlargement—an essential defining feature of human emphysema. *Am Rev Respir Dis* 1988; 137:380–392.

190 Petty TL, Silvers GW, Stanford RE. Radial traction and small

airways disease in excised human lungs. *Am Rev Respir Dis* 1986; 133:132–135.

191 Nagai A, Yamawaki I, Takizawa T, Thurlbeck WM. Alveolar attachments in emphysema of human lungs. *Am Rev Respir Dis* 1991; 144:888–891.

192 Nagai A, West WW, Thurlbeck WM. The National Institutes of Health intermittent positive-pressure breathing trial: pathology studies. II.Correlation between morphologic findings, clinical findings, and evidence of expiratory airflow obstruction. [Abstract] *Am Rev Respir Dis* 1985; 132:946–953.

193 MacNee W, Gould G, Lamb D. Quantifying emphysema by CT scanning. Clinicopathologic correlates. *Ann N Y Acad Sci* 1991; 624:179–194.

194 Hayhurst MD, MacNee W, Flenley DC et al. Diagnosis of pulmonary emphysema by computerised tomography. *Lancet* 1984; 2:320–322.

195 Hogg JC. Chadwick D, Goode A, eds. Chronic obstructive pulmonary disease: pathogenesis to treatment. Novartis Foundation Symposium 234 ed. Chichester: John Wiley & Sons Ltd; 2001; Chronic obstructive pulmonary disease: an overview of pathology and pathogenesis. p. 4–26.

196 Coxson HO, Rogers RM, Whittall KP et al. A quantification of the lung surface area in emphysema using computed tomography. *Am J Respir Crit Care Med* 1999; 159:851–856.

197 Lang MR, Fiaux GW, Gilooly M, Stewart JA, Hulmes DJS, Lamb D. Collagen content of alveolar wall tissue in emphysematous and non-emphysematous lungs. *Thorax* 1994; 49:319–326.

198 Vlahovic G, Russell ML, Mercer RR, Crapo JD. Cellular and connective tissue changes in alveolar septal walls in emphysema. *Am J Respir Crit Care Med* 1999; 160:2086–2092.

199 Ollerenshaw SL, Woolcock AJ. Quantification and location of vasoactive intestinal peptide immunoreactive nerves in bronchial biopsies from subjects with mild asthma. *Am Rev Respir Dis* 1993; 147:A285.

200 Ollerenshaw SL, Jarvis D, Sullivan CE, Woolcock AJ. Substance P immunoreactive nerves in airways from asthmatics and non-asthmatics. *Eur Respir J* 1991; 4:673–682.

201 Howarth PS, Springall DR, Redington AE, Djukanovic R, Holgate ST, Polak JM. Neuropeptide-containing nerves in endobronchial biopsies from asthmatic and non-asthmatic subjects. *Am J Respir Cell Molec Biol* 1995; 13:288–296.

202 Sharma R, Jeffery PK. Airway β-adrenoceptor number in cystic fibrosis and asthma. *Clin Sci* 1990; 78:409–417.

203 Sharma RK, Jeffery PK. Airway V.I.P. receptor number is reduced in cystic fibrosis but not asthma. *Am Rev Respir Dis* 1990; 141:A726.

204 MacNee W, Wiggs B, Belzberg AS, Hogg JC. The effect of cigarette smoking on neutrophil kinetics in human lungs. *N Engl J Med* 1989; 321:924–928.

Glucocorticosteroids

Peter J. Barnes

Department of Thoracic Medicine, National Heart and Lung Institute, Imperial College School of Medicine, London, UK

Introduction

Corticosteroids are the most effective therapy currently available for asthma and improvement with corticosteroids is one of the hallmarks of asthma. By contrast, corticosteroids have little or no place in the management of COPD[1]. Inhaled corticosteroids have revolutionized asthma treatment and have become the mainstay of therapy for patients with chronic disease[2,3]. There is now a much better understanding of the molecular mechanisms whereby corticosteroids suppress inflammation in asthma and this has led to changes in the way corticosteroids are used and may point the way to the development of more specific therapies in the future[4]. This chapter discusses current understanding of the mechanism of action of corticosteroids and how corticosteroids are used in the management of asthma. The lack of benefit of corticosteroids in COPD is also discussed.

Molecular mechanisms

Corticosteroids are highly effective anti-inflammatory therapy in asthma and the molecular mechanisms involved in suppression of airway inflammation in asthma are now better understood[4]. Corticosteroids are effective in asthma because they block many of the inflammatory pathways that are abnormally activated in asthma and they have a wide spectrum of anti-inflammatory actions.

Glucocorticoid receptors

Corticosteroids bind to a single class of glucocorticoid receptors (GR) which are localized to the cytoplasm of target cells. Corticosteroids bind at the C-terminal end of the receptor, whereas the N-terminal end of the receptor is involved in regulating gene transcription. Between these domains is the DNA-binding domain which has two finger-like projections formed by a zinc molecule bound to four cysteine residues that bind to the DNA double helix. The inactive GR is bound to a protein complex that includes two molecules of 90 kDa heat shock protein (hsp90) and various other proteins that act as a 'molecular chaperone' preventing the unoccupied GR moving into the nuclear compartment. Once corticosteroids bind to GR, conformational changes in the receptor structure result in dissociation of these molecules, thereby exposing nuclear localization signals on GR which then results in rapid nuclear localization of the activated GR–corticosteroid complex and its binding to DNA. Two GR molecules bind to DNA as a dimer, resulting in changed transcription. There is a splice variant of GR, termed GR-β, that has been identified that does not bind corticosteroids, but binds to DNA and may theoretically interfere with the action of corticosteroids[5].

Effects on gene transcription

Corticosteroids produce their effect on responsive cells by activating GR to directly or indirectly regulate the transcription of certain target genes[6]. The number of genes per cell directly regulated by corticosteroids is estimated to be between 10 and 100, but many genes are regulated indirectly through an interaction with other transcription factors. GR dimers bind to DNA at consensus sites termed glucocorticoid response elements (GREs) in the 5'-upstream promoter region of steroid-responsive genes. This interaction changes the rate of transcription, resulting in either induction or occasionally repression of the gene. Interaction of the activated GR homodimer with GRE usually increases transcription, resulting in increased protein synthesis. GR may increase transcription by interacting with a large coactivator molecule, CREB binding protein (CBP), which is bound at the start site of transcription and switches on RNA polymerase, resulting in formation of messenger RNA (mRNA) and then synthesis of protein.

However, in controlling inflammation, the major effect of corticosteroids is to inhibit the synthesis of inflammatory proteins, such as cytokines. This was originally believed to be through interaction of GR with negative GRE sites, resulting in repression of transcription. However, such negative GREs have rarely been demonstrated. GR may also affect protein synthesis by altering the stability of messenger RNA, through effects on ribonucleases that break down mRNA.

Interaction with transcription factors

Activated GRs may bind directly with several other activated transcription factors as a protein–protein interaction. This could be an important determinant of corticosteroid responsiveness and is a key mechanism whereby corticosteroids switch off inflammatory genes. Most of the inflammatory genes that are activated in asthma do not appear to have GREs in their promoter regions yet are repressed by corticosteroids. There is increasing evidence that this may be due to interaction between the activated GR and transcription factors that regulate the expression of genes, that code for inflammatory proteins, such as cytokines, inflammatory enzymes, adhesion mole-

cules and inflammatory receptors. These 'inflammatory' transcription factors include activator protein-1 (AP-1) and nuclear factor-κB (NF-κB) which may regulate many of the inflammatory genes that are switched on in asthmatic airways[7,8].

Effects on chromatin structure

There is increasing evidence that corticosteroids may have effects on the chromatin structure. DNA in chromosomes is wound around histone molecules in the form of nucleosomes. Several transcription factors interact with large coactivator molecules, such as CBP, and the related molecule p300, which bind to the basal transcription factor apparatus. Several transcription factors have now been shown to bind directly to CBP, including AP-1, NF-κB and GR[9]. Since binding sites on this molecule may be limited, this may result in competition between transcription factors for the limited binding sites available, so that there is an indirect rather than a direct protein–protein interaction (Fig. 2.1). At a microscopic level that chromatin may become dense or opaque due to the winding or unwinding of DNA around the histone core. CBP and p300 have histone acetylation activity, which is activated by the binding of transcription factors, such as AP-1 and NF-κB. Acetylation of histone residues results in unwinding of DNA coiled around the histone core, thus opening up the chromatin structure, which allows transcription factors to bind more readily, thereby increasing transcription. Repression of genes reverses this process by histone deacetylation[10]. Deacetylation of histone increases the winding of DNA round histone residues, resulting in dense chromatin structure and reduced access of transcription factors to their binding sites, thereby leading to repressed transcription of inflammatory genes. Activated GR may bind to several transcription co-repressor molecules that associate with proteins that have histone deacetylase activity, resulting in deacetylation of histone, increased winding of DNA round histone residues and thus reduced access of transcription factors to their binding sites and therefore repression of inflammatory genes[11].

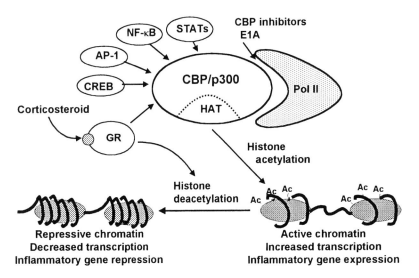

Fig. 2.1 Effect of corticosteroids on chromatin structure. Transcription factors, such as STATs, AP-1 and NF-κB, bind to coactivator molecules, such as CREB binding protein (CBP) or p300, which have intrinsic histone acetyltransferase (HAT) activity, resulting in acetylation (-Ac) of histone residues. This leads to unwinding of DNA and allows increased binding of transcription factors resulting in increased gene transcription. Glucocorticoid receptors (GR) after activation by corticosteroids bind to a glucocorticoid receptor co-activator which is bound to CBP. This results in deacetylation of histone, with increased coiling of DNA around histone, thus preventing transcription factor binding leading to gene repression.

Target genes in inflammation control

Corticosteroids may control inflammation by inhibiting many aspects of the inflammatory process through increasing the transcription of anti-inflammatory genes and decreasing the transcription of inflammatory genes (Table 2.1).

Anti-inflammatory proteins

Corticosteroids may suppress inflammation by increasing the synthesis of anti-inflammatory proteins. For example, corticosteroids increase the synthesis of lipocortin-1, a 37 kDa protein that has an inhibitory effect on phospholipase A_2 (PLA_2), and therefore may inhibit the production of lipid mediators. Corticosteroids induce the formation of lipocortin-1 in several cells and recombinant lipocortin-1 has acute anti-inflammatory properties. However, lipocortin-1 does not appear to be increased by inhaled corticosteroid treatment in asthma[12]. Corticosteroids increase the expression of other potentially anti-inflammatory proteins, such as interleukin (IL)-1 receptor antagonist (which inhibits the binding of IL-1 to its receptor), secretory leukoprotease inhibitor (which inhibits proteases, such as tryptase), neutral endopeptidase (which degrades bronchoactive peptides such as kinins) CC-10 (an immunomodulatory protein), an inhibitor of NF-κB (IκB-α) and IL-10 (an anti-inflammatory cytokine).

β_2-adrenoceptors

Corticosteroids increase the expression of β_2-adrenoceptors by increasing the rate of transcription and the human β_2-receptor gene has three potential GREs. Corticosteroids double the rate of β_2-receptor gene transcription in human lung in vitro, resulting in increased expression of β_2-receptors [13]. This may be relevant in asthma as corticosteroids may prevent down-regulation of β-receptors in response to prolonged treatment with β_2-agonists. In rats corticosteroids prevent down-regulation and

Table 2.1. Effect of corticosteroids on gene transcription[115]

Increased transcription

Lipocortin-1 (phospholipase A$_2$ inhibitor)

β_2-Adrenoceptor

Secretory leukoprotease inhibitor

Clara cell protein (CC10; phospholipase A$_2$ inhibitor)

IL-1 receptor antagonist

IL-1R2 (decoy receptor)

IκB-α (inhibitor of NF-κB)

Decreased transcription

Cytokines

  IL-1, IL-2, IL-3, IL-4, IL-5,IL-6, IL-11, IL-12, IL-13, TNFα, GM-CSF, SCF

Chemokines

  IL-8, RANTES, MIP-1α, MCP-1, MCP-3, MCP-4, eotaxin

Inducible nitric oxide synthase (iNOS)

Inducible cyclooxygenase (COX-2)

Cytoplasmic phospholipase A$_2$ (cPLA$_2$)

Endothelin-1

NK$_1$-receptors, NK$_2$-receptors

Adhesion molecules (ICAM-1, E-selectin)

---

reduced transcription of β_2-receptors in response to chronic β-agonist exposure[14].

Cytokines

The inhibitory effect of corticosteroids on cytokine synthesis is likely to be of particular importance in the control of inflammation in asthma. Corticosteroids inhibit the transcription of many cytokines and chemokines that are relevant in asthma (Table 2.1). These inhibitory effects are due, at least in part, to an inhibitory effect on the transcription factors that regulate induction of these cytokine genes, including AP-1 and NF-κB. For example, eotaxin which is important in selective attraction of eosinophils from the circulation into the airways is regulated in part by NF-κB and its expression in airway epithelial cells is inhibited by corticosteroids[15]. Many transcription factors are likely to be involved in the regulation of inflammatory genes in asthma in addition to AP-1 and NF-κB. IL-4 and IL-5 expression in T-lymphocytes plays a

critical role in allergic inflammation, but NF-κB does not play a role, whereas the transcription factor nuclear factor of activated T-cells (NF-AT) is important[16]. AP-1 is a component of the NF–AT transcription complex, so that corticosteroids inhibit IL-5, at least in part, by inhibiting the AP-1 component of NF-AT.

There may be marked differences in the response of different cells and of different cytokines to the inhibitory action of corticosteroids and this may be dependent on the relative abundance of transcription factors within different cell types. Thus in alveolar macrophages and peripheral blood monocytes GM–CSF secretion is more potently inhibited by corticosteroids than IL-1β or IL-6 secretion.

Inflammatory enzymes

Nitric oxide (NO) synthase may be induced by proinflammatory cytokines, resulting in NO production. NO may amplify asthmatic inflammation and contribute to epithelial shedding and airway hyperresponsiveness through the formation of peroxynitrite. The induction of the inducible form of NOS (iNOS) is inhibited by corticosteroids. In cultured human pulmonary epithelial cells proinflammatory cytokines result in increased expression of iNOS and increased NO formation, due to increased transcription of the iNOS gene, and this is inhibited by corticosteroids acting through inhibition of NF-κB. Corticosteroids inhibit the synthesis of several other inflammatory mediators implicated in asthma through an inhibitory effect on the induction of enzymes such as cyclo-oxygenase-2 (COX-2) and cytosolic PLA$_2$[17,18].

Corticosteroids also inhibit the synthesis of endothelin-1 in lung and airway epithelial cells and this effect may also be via inhibition of transcription factors that regulate its expression.

Inflammatory receptors

Corticosteroids also decrease the transcription of genes coding for certain receptors. Thus the gene for the NK$_1$-receptor, which mediates the inflammatory effects of tachykinins in the airways, has an increased expression in asthma and is inhibited by

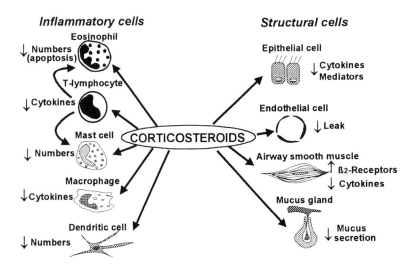

Fig. 2.2 Cellular effect of corticosteroids.

corticosteroids, probably via an inhibitory effect on AP-1[19]. Corticosteroids also inhibit the transcription of the NK_2-receptor which mediates the broncho-constrictor effects of tachykinins[20].

Adhesion molecules

Adhesion molecules play a key role in the trafficking of inflammatory cells to sites of inflammation. The expression of many adhesion molecules on endo-thelial cells is induced by cytokines and corticoster-oids may lead indirectly to a reduced expression via their inhibitory effects on cytokines, such as IL-1β and TNFα. Corticosteroids may also have a direct inhibitory effect on the expression of adhesion molecules, such as ICAM-1 and E-selectin at the level of gene transcription. ICAM-1 and VCAM-1 expression in bronchial epithelial cell lines and monocytes is inhibited by corticosteroids[21].

Apoptosis

Corticosteroids markedly reduce the survival of certain inflammatory cells, such as eosinophils. Eosinophil survival is dependent on the presence of certain cytokines, such as IL-5 and GM–CSF. Exposure to corticosteroids blocks the effects of these cytokines and leads to programmed cell death

or apoptosis, although the corticosteroid-sensitive molecular pathways have not yet been defined[22].

Effects on cell function

Corticosteroids may have direct inhibitory actions on several inflammatory cells and structural cells that are implicated in asthma (Fig. 2.2).

Macrophages

Corticosteroids inhibit the release of inflammatory mediators and cytokines from alveolar macro-phages in vitro. Inhaled corticosteroids reduce the secretion of chemokines and proinflammatory cyto-kines from alveolar macrophages from asthmatic patients, whereas the secretion of IL-10 is increased[23].

Eosinophils

Corticosteroids have a direct inhibitory effect on mediator release from eosinophils, although they are only weakly effective in inhibiting secretion of reactive oxygen species and eosinophil basic pro-teins. More importantly corticosteroids induce apoptosis by inhibiting the prolonged survival due to IL-3, IL-5 and GM–CSF[22], resulting in an increased number of apoptotic eosinophils in induced sputum of asthmatic patients[24]. One of the best described actions of corticosteroids in asthma is a reduction in circulating eosinophils, which may reflect an action on eosinophil production in the bone marrow.

T-lymphocytes

T-helper 2 lymphocytes (Th2) play an important orchestrating role in asthma through the release of cytokines such as IL-4 and IL-5 and may be an important target for corticosteroids in asthma therapy.

Mast cells

While corticosteroids do not appear to have a direct inhibitory effect on mediator release from lung mast cells, chronic corticosteroid treatment is associated with a marked reduction in mucosal mast cell number. This may be linked to a reduction in IL-3 and stem cell factor (SCF) production, which are necessary for mast cell expression at mucosal surfaces. Mast cells also secrete various cytokines (TNF-α, IL-4, IL-5, IL-6, IL-8), and this may also be inhibited by corticosteroids.

Dendritic cells

Dendritic cells in the epithelium of the respiratory tract appear to play a critical role in antigen presentation in the lung as they have the capacity to take up allergen, process it into peptides and present it via MHC molecules on the cell surface for presentation to uncommitted T-lymphocytes. In experimental animals the number of dendritic cells is markedly reduced by systemic and inhaled corticosteroids, thus dampening the immune response in the airways[25].

Neutrophils

Neutrophils, which are not prominent in the biopsies of asthmatic patients, are not sensitive to the effects of corticosteroids. Systemic corticosteroids increase peripheral neutrophil counts, which may reflect an increased survival time due to an inhibitory action of neutrophil apoptosis (in complete contrast to the increased apoptosis seen in eosinophils)[26].

Endothelial cells

GR gene expression in the airways is most prominent in endothelial cells of the bronchial circulation and airway epithelial cells. Corticosteroids do not appear to directly inhibit the expression of adhesion molecules, although they may inhibit cell adhesion indirectly by suppression of cytokines involved in the regulation of adhesion molecule expression. Corticosteroids may have an inhibitory action on airway microvascular leak induced by inflammatory mediators. This appears to be a direct effect on post-capillary venular epithelial cells. The mechanism for this antipermeability effect has not been fully elucidated, but there is evidence that synthesis of a 100 kDa protein distinct from lipocortin-1 termed vasocortin may be involved. Although there have been no direct measurements of the effects of corticosteroids on airway microvascular leakage in asthmatic airways, regular treatment with inhaled corticosteroids decreases the elevated plasma proteins found in bronchoalveolar lavage fluid of patients with stable asthma.

Epithelial cells

Epithelial cells may be an important source of many inflammatory mediators in asthmatic airways and may drive and amplify the inflammatory response in the airways through the secretion of proinflammatory cytokines, chemokines and inflammatory peptides. Airway epithelium may be one of the most important targets for inhaled corticosteroids in asthma[27,28] (Fig. 2.3). Inhaled corticosteroids inhibit the increased expression of many inflammatory proteins in airway epithelial cells[27]. An example is iNOS, which has an increase expressed in airway epithelial and inflammatory cells in asthma and is reduced by inhaled corticosteroids [29]. This is reflected by a reduction in the elevated levels of exhaled NO in asthma after inhaled corticosteroids[30].

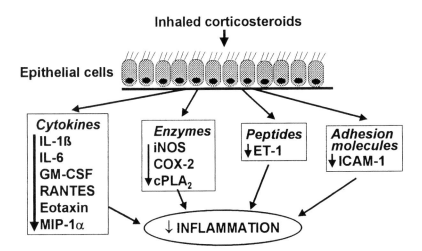

Fig. 2.3 Inhaled corticosteroids may inhibit the transcription of several 'inflammatory' genes in airway epithelial cells and thus reduce inflammation in the airway wall.

Mucus secretion

Corticosteroids inhibit mucus secretion in airways and this may be a direct action of corticosteroids on submucosal gland cells. Corticosteroids may also inhibit the expression of mucin genes, such as MUC2 and MUC5AC[31]. In addition, there are indirect inhibitory effects due to the reduction in inflammatory mediators that stimulate increased mucus secretion.

Effects on asthmatic inflammation

Corticosteroids are remarkably effective in controlling the inflammation in asthmatic airways and it is likely that they have multiple cellular effects. Biopsy studies in patients with asthma have now confirmed that inhaled corticosteroids reduce the number and activation of inflammatory cells in the airway mucosa and in bronchoalveolar lavage[27]. These effects may be due to inhibition of cytokine synthesis in inflammatory and structural cells and suppression of adhesion molecules. The disrupted epithelium is restored and the ciliated to goblet cell ratio is normalized after 3 months of therapy with inhaled corticosteroids. There is also some evidence for a reduction in the thickness of the basement membrane, although in asthmatic patients taking inhaled corticosteroids for over 10 years the characteristic thickening of the basement membrane was still present.

Effects on airway hyper-responsiveness

By reducing airway inflammation inhaled corticosteroids consistently reduce airway hyper-responsiveness (AHR) in asthmatic adults and children[32]. Chronic treatment with inhaled corticosteroids reduces responsiveness to histamine, cholinergic agonists, allergen (early and late responses), exercise, fog, cold air, bradykinin, adenosine and irritants (such as sulfur dioxide and metabisulfite). The reduction in AHR takes place over several weeks and may not be maximal until several months of therapy. The magnitude of reduction is variable between patients and is in the order of one to two doubling dilutions for most challenges and often fails to return to the normal range. This may reflect suppression of the inflammation but persistence of structural changes which cannot be reversed by corticosteroids. Inhaled corticosteroids not only make the airways less sensitive to spasmogens, but they also limit the maximal airway narrowing in response to spasmogens.

Clinical efficacy of inhaled corticosteroids

Inhaled corticosteroids are very effective in control-ling asthma symptoms in asthmatic patients of all ages and severity [7,33,34] (Table 2.2). Inhaled cortico-steroids improve the quality of life of patients with asthma and allow many patients to lead normal lives, improve lung function, reduce the frequency of exacerbations and may prevent irreversible airway changes. They were first introduced to reduce the requirement for oral corticosteroids in patients with severe asthma and many studies have confirmed that the majority of patients can be weaned off oral corticosteroids[35].

Studies in adults

As experience has been gained with inhaled corti-costeroids they have been introduced in patients with milder asthma, with the recognition that inflammation is present even in patients with mild asthma. Inhaled anti-inflammatory drugs have now become first-line therapy in any patient who needs to use a β_2-agonist inhaler more than once a day, and this is reflected in national and international guide-lines for the management of chronic asthma. In patients with newly diagnosed asthma inhaled cor-ticosteroids (budesonide 600 µg twice daily) reduced symptoms and β_2-agonist inhaler usage and improved peak expiratory flows. These effects persisted over the 2 years of the study, whereas in a parallel group treated with inhaled β_2-agonists alone there was no significant change in symptoms or lung function[36]. In another study patients with mild asthma treated with a low dose of inhaled cortico-steroid (budesonide 400 µg daily) showed fewer symptoms and a progressive improvement in lung function over several months and many patients became completely asymptomatic[37]. There was also a significant reduction in the number of exacerba-tions. Although the effects of inhaled corticosteroids on AHR may take several months to reach a plateau, the reduction in asthma symptoms occurs more rapidly[38].

High dose inhaled corticosteroids have now been

Table 2.2. Effects of inhaled corticosteroids in asthma

Control symptoms
Improve quality of life
Improve lung function
Prevent exacerbations
Reduce mortality (probably)
Prevent irreversible airway changes
Alter natural history of asthma?

introduced for the control of more severe asthma. This markedly reduces the need for maintenance oral corticosteroids and has revolutionized the manage-ment of more severe and unstable asthma. Inhaled corticosteroids are the treatment of choice in noctur-nal asthma, which is a manifestation of inflamed airways, reducing night-time awakening and reduc-ing the diurnal variation in airway function.

High doses of inhaled corticosteroids may also substitute for a course of oral steroids in controlling acute exacerbations of asthma. High dose flutica-sone propionate (FP; 2000 µg daily) was as effective as a course of oral prednisolone in controlling acute exacerbations of asthma in general practice[39].

Inhaled corticosteroids effectively control asth-matic inflammation but must be taken regularly. When inhaled corticosteroids are discontinued there is usually a gradual increase in symptoms and airway responsiveness back to pretreatment values[38], although in patients with mild asthma who have been treated with inhaled corticosteroids for a long time symptoms may not recur in some patients[40].

Studies in children

Inhaled corticosteroids are equally effective in chil-dren. In an extensive study of children aged 7–17 years there was a significant improvement in symp-toms, peak flow variability and lung function com-pared to a regular inhaled β_2-agonist which was maintained over the 22 months of the study[41], but asthma deteriorated when the inhaled corticoster-oids were withdrawn[42]. There was a high proportion of dropouts (45%) in the group treated with inhaled β_2-agonist alone. Inhaled corticosteroids are more effective than a long-acting β_2-agonist in controlling asthma in children[43]. Inhaled corticosteroids are also effective in younger children. Nebulized budesonide reduces the need for oral corticosteroids and also improved lung function in children under the age of three[44]. Inhaled corticosteroids given via a large volume spacer improve asthma symptoms and reduce the number of exacerbations in preschool children and in infants.

Dose–response studies

Surprisingly, the dose–response curve for the clinical efficacy of inhaled corticosteroids is relatively flat and, while all studies have demonstrated a clinical benefit of inhaled corticosteroids, it has been difficult to demonstrate differences between doses, with most benefit obtained at the lowest doses used[33,35,45]. This is in contrast to the steeper dose–response for systemic effects, implying that while there is little clinical benefit from increasing doses of inhaled corticosteroids the risk of adverse effects is increased. However, the dose response effect of inhaled corticosteroids may depend on the parameters measured and, while it is difficult to discern a dose–response when traditional lung function parameters are measured, there may be a dose–response effect in prevention of asthma exacerbations. Thus, in a recent study there was a significantly greater effect of budesonide 800 μg daily compared to 200 μg daily in preventing severe and mild asthma exacerbations[46]. Normally, a fourfold or greater difference in dose has been required to detect a statistically significant (but often small) difference in effect on commonly measured outcomes such as symptoms, PEF, use of rescue β_2-agonist and lung function and even such large differences in dose are not always associated with significant differences in response. These findings suggest that pulmonary function tests or symptoms may have a rather low sensitivity in the assessment of the effects of inhaled corticosteroids. This is obviously important for the interpretation of clinical comparisons between different inhaled corticosteroids or inhalers. It is also important to consider the type of patient included in clinical studies. Patients with relatively mild asthma may have relatively little room for improvement with inhaled corticosteroids, so that maximal improvement is obtained with relatively low doses. Patients with more severe asthma or with unstable asthma may have more room for improvement and may therefore show a greater response to increasing doses, but it is often difficult to include such patients in controlled clinical trials.

More studies are needed to assess whether other outcome measures such as AHR or more direct measurements of inflammation, such as sputum eosinophils or exhaled NO, may be more sensitive than traditional outcome measures such as symptoms or lung function tests[47–49]. A recent study showed that higher doses of inhaled corticosteroids are needed to control AHR than to improve symptoms and lung function, but that this may have a better long-term outcome in terms of reduction in structural changes of the airways[50].

Prevention of irreversible airway changes

Some patients with asthma develop an element of irreversible airflow obstruction, but the pathophysiological basis of these changes is not yet understood. It is likely that they are the result of chronic airway inflammation and that they may be prevented by treatment with inhaled corticosteroids. There is some evidence that the annual decline in lung function may be slowed by the introduction of inhaled corticosteroids[51]. Increasing evidence also suggests that delay in starting inhaled corticosteroids may result in less overall improvement in lung function in both adults and children[52–54]. These studies suggest that introduction of inhaled corticosteroids at the time of diagnosis is likely to have the greatest impact[53,54]. Several large studies are now under way to assess the benefit of very early introduction of inhaled corticosteroids in children and adults. So far there is no evidence that early use of inhaled corticosteroids is curative and even when inhaled corticosteroids are introduced at the time of diagnosis, symptoms and lung function revert to pretreatment levels when corticosteroids are withdrawn[52].

Reduction in mortality

Inhaled corticosteroids may reduce the mortality from asthma but prospective studies are almost impossible to conduct. In a retrospective review of the risk of mortality and prescribed antiasthma medication, there was a significant apparent protection provided by regular inhaled beclomethasone dipropionate (BDP) therapy (adjusted odds ratio of 0.1), although numbers were small[55].

Comparison between inhaled corticosteroids

Several inhaled corticosteroids are currently prescribable in asthma, although their availability varies between countries. There have been relatively few studies comparing efficacy of the different inhaled corticosteroids, and it is important to take into account the delivery system and the type of patient under investigation when such comparisons are made. Because of the relatively flat dose–response curve for the clinical parameters normally used in comparing doses of inhaled corticosteroids, it may be difficult to see differences in efficacy of inhaled corticosteroids and most comparisons have concentrated in differences in systemic effects at equally efficacious doses, although it has often proved difficult to establish true clinical efficacy. In the UK BDP, budesonide and FP are available, whereas in the USA BDP, flunisolide, triamcinolone, FP and budesonide are available. There are few studies comparing different doses of inhaled corticosteroids in asthmatic patients. Budesonide has been compared with BDP and in adults and children appears to have comparable antiasthma effects at equal doses, whereas FP appears to be approximately twice as potent as BDP and budesonide. There do appear to be some differences between inhaled corticosteroids in terms of their systemic effects at comparable antiasthma doses, however.

Clinical use of inhaled corticosteroids in asthma

Inhaled corticosteroids are now recommended as first-line therapy for all patients with persistent symptoms. Inhaled corticosteroids should be started in any patient who needs to use a β_2-agonist inhaler for symptom control more than once daily (or possibly three times weekly). It is conventional to start with a low dose of inhaled corticosteroid and to increase the dose until asthma control is achieved. However, this may take time and a preferable approach is to start with a dose of corticosteroids in the middle of the dose range (400 µg twice daily) to establish control of asthma more rapidly[56]. Once control is achieved (defined as normal or best possible lung function and infrequent need to use an inhaled β_2-agonist) the dose of inhaled corticosteroid should be reduced in a stepwise manner to the lowest dose needed for optimal control. It may take as long as three months to reach a plateau in response and any changes in dose should be made at intervals of three months or more. This strategy ('start high – go low') is emphasized in the most recent US and UK guidelines[57,58]. When daily doses of ≥800 µg daily are needed, a large volume spacer device should be used with an MDI and mouth washing with a dry powder inhaler in order to reduce local and systemic side effects. Inhaled corticosteroids are usually given as a twice daily dose in order to increase compliance. When asthma is more unstable four times daily dosage is preferable[59]. For patients who require ≤400 µg daily once daily dosing appears to be as effective as twice daily dosing, at least for budesonide[60].

The dose of inhaled corticosteroid should be increased to 2000 µg daily if necessary, but higher doses may result in systemic effects and it may be preferable to add a low dose of oral corticosteroid, since higher doses of inhaled corticosteroids are expensive and have a high incidence of local side effects. Nebulized budesonide has been advocated in order to give an increased dose of inhaled corticosteroid and to reduce the requirement for oral corticosteroids[61], but this treatment is expensive and may achieve its effects largely via systemic absorption.

Additional bronchodilators

Conventional advice was to increase the dose of inhaled corticosteroids if asthma was not controlled, on the assumption that there was residual inflammation of the airways. However, it is now apparent that the dose response effect of inhaled corticosteroids is relatively flat, so that there is little improvement in lung function after doubling the dose of inhaled corticosteroids. An alternative strategy is to add some other call of controller drug. In patients in general practice who were not controlled on BDP 200 μg twice daily, addition of salmeterol 50 μg twice daily was more effective than increasing the dose of inhaled corticosteroid to 500 μg twice daily, in terms of lung function improvement, use of rescue β_2-agonist use and symptom control[62]. This surprising result was confirmed in a more severe group of patients who were not controlled on 800–1000 μg BDP daily[63]. Similar results have been found with another long-acting inhaled β_2-agonist formoterol, which in addition reduced the frequency of mild and severe asthma exacerbations[46]. This has led to the development of fixed combinations of corticosteroids and long-acting β_2-agonists, such as FP and salmeterol (Seretide), which may be more convenient for patients[64]. Recent studies have also shown that addition of low doses of theophylline (giving plasma concentrations of < 10 mg/l) were more effective than doubling the dose of inhaled budesonide, either in mild or severe asthma[65,66]. Similar data are now emerging with antileukotrienes[67]. The reason why these alternative treatments are more effective than higher doses of inhaled corticosteroids remains to be elucidated, but does suggest that there is a reversible component of asthma that may not be steroid-sensitive inflammation. It is possible that this may be an abnormality in airway smooth muscle itself (as a result of remodelling), edematous swelling of the airway or production of cysteinyl–leukotrienes that is not sensitive to inhibition by inhaled corticosteroids[68].

Cost effectiveness

Although inhaled corticosteroids may be more expensive than short-acting inhaled β_2-agonists, they are the most cost-effective way of controlling asthma, since reducing the frequency of asthma attacks will save on total costs[69]. Inhaled corticosteroids also improve the quality of life of patients with asthma and allow many patients a normal lifestyle, thus saving costs indirectly[70].

Corticosteroid-sparing therapy

In patients who have serious side effects with maintenance corticosteroid therapy there are several treatments which have been shown to reduce the requirement for oral corticosteroids[71]. These treatments are commonly termed corticosteroid-sparing, although this is a misleading description that could be applied to any additional asthma therapy (including bronchodilators). The amount of corticosteroid sparing with these therapies is not impressive.

Several immunosuppressive agents have been shown to have corticosteroid effects, including methotrexate, oral gold and cyclosporin A. These therapies all have side effects that may be more troublesome than those of oral corticosteroids and are therefore only indicated as an additional therapy to reduce the requirement of oral corticosteroids. None of these treatments is very effective, but there are occasional patients who appear to show a good response. Because of side effects these treatments cannot be considered as a way to reduce the requirement for inhaled corticosteroids. Several other therapies, including azathioprine, dapsone and hydroxychloroquine have not been found to be beneficial. The macrolide antibiotic troleandomycin is

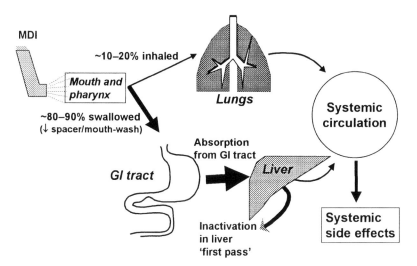

Fig. 2.4 Pharmacokinetics of inhaled corticosteroids.

also reported to have corticosteroid-sparing effects, but this is only seen with methylprednisolone and is due to reduced metabolism of this corticosteroid, so that there is little therapeutic gain[72].

Pharmacokinetics

The pharmacokinetics of inhaled corticosteroids is important in determining the concentration of drug reaching target cells in the airways and in the fraction of drug reaching the systemic circulation and therefore causing side effects[35]. Beneficial properties in an inhaled corticosteroid are a high topical potency, a low systemic bioavailability of the swallowed portion of the dose and rapid metabolic clearance of any corticosteroid reaching the systemic circulation. After inhalation a large proportion of the inhaled dose (80–90%) is deposited on the oropharynx and is then swallowed and therefore available for absorption via the liver into the systemic circulation (Fig. 2.4). This fraction is markedly reduced by using a large volume spacer device with a metered dose inhaler (MDI) or by mouth washing and discarding the washing with dry powder inhalers. Between 10% and 20% of inhaled drug enters the

respiratory tract, where it is deposited in the airways and this fraction is available for absorption into the systemic circulation. Most of the early studies on the distribution of inhaled corticosteroids were conducted in healthy volunteers, and it is not certain what effect inflammatory disease, airway obstruction, age of the patient or concomitant medication may have on the disposition of the inhaled dose. There may be important differences in the metabolism of different inhaled corticosteroids. BDP is metabolized to its more active metabolite beclomethasone monopropionate in many tissues including lung, but there is no information about its absorption or metabolism of this metabolite in humans. Flunisolide and budesonide are subject to extensive first-pass metabolism in the liver so that less reaches the systemic circulation. Little is known about the distribution of triamcinolone. FP is almost completely metabolized by first-pass metabolism, which reduces systemic effects.

When inhaled corticosteroids were first introduced, it was recommended that they should be given four times daily, but several studies have now demonstrated that twice daily administration gives comparable control, although four times daily administration may be preferable in patients with

Table 2.3. Side effects of inhaled corticosteroids

Local side effects
Dysphonia
Oropharyngeal candidiasis
Cough

Systemic side effects
Adrenal suppression
Growth suppression
Bruising
Osteoporosis
Cataracts
Glaucoma
Metabolic abnormalities (glucose, insulin, triglycerides)
Psychiatric disturbances

more severe asthma. However, patients may find it difficult to comply with such frequent administration unless they have troublesome symptoms. For patients with mild asthma who require ≤400 μg daily, once daily therapy may be sufficient.

Side effects of inhaled corticosteroids

The efficacy of inhaled corticosteroids is now established in short- and long-term studies in adults and children, but there are still concerns about side effects, particularly in children and when high inhaled doses are needed. Several side effects have been recognized (Table 2.3).

Local side effects

Side effects due to the local deposition of the inhaled corticosteroid in the oropharynx may occur with inhaled corticosteroids, but the frequency of complaints depends on the dose and frequency of administration and on the delivery system used.

Dysphonia

The commonest complaint is of hoarseness of the voice (dysphonia) and may occur in over 50% of patients using MDI. Dysphonia is not appreciably reduced by using spacers, but may be less with dry powder devices. Dysphonia may be due to myopathy of laryngeal muscles and is reversible when treatment is withdrawn[73]. For most patients it is not troublesome, but may be disabling in singers and lecturers.

Oropharyngeal candidiasis

Oropharyngeal candidiasis (thrush) may be a problem in some patients, particularly in the elderly, with concomitant oral corticosteroids and more than twice daily administration[74]. Large volume spacer devices protect against this local side effect by reducing the dose of inhaled corticosteroid that deposits in the oropharynx.

Other local complications

There is no evidence that inhaled corticosteroid, even in high doses, increases the frequency of infections, including tuberculosis, in the lower respiratory tract. There is no evidence for atrophy of the airway epithelium and even after 10 years of treatment with inhaled corticosteroids there is no evidence for any structural changes in the epithelium. Cough and throat irritation, sometimes accompanied by reflex bronchoconstriction, may occur when inhaled corticosteroids are given via a metered dose inhaler. These symptoms are likely to be due to surfactants in pressurized aerosols as they disappear after switching to a dry powder corticosteroid inhaler device.

Systemic side effects

The efficacy of inhaled corticosteroids in the control of asthma is undisputed, but there are concerns about systemic effects of inhaled corticosteroids, particularly as they are likely to be used over long periods and in children of all ages[33]. The safety of inhaled corticosteroids has been extensively investigated since their introduction 30 years ago[35]. One of the major problems is to decide whether a measurable systemic effect has any significant clinical consequence and this necessitates careful long-term follow-up studies. As biochemical markers of systemic corticosteroid effects become more sensitive, then systemic effects may be seen more often, but this does not mean that these effects are clinically relevant. There are several case reports of adverse systemic effects of inhaled corticosteroids, and these may be idiosyncratic reactions, which may be due to abnormal pharmacokinetic handling of the inhaled corticosteroid. The systemic effect of an inhaled corticosteroid will depend on several factors, including the dose delivered to the patient, the site of delivery (gastrointestinal tract and lung), the delivery system used and individual differences in the patient's response to the corticosteroid.

Effect of delivery systems

The systemic effect of an inhaled corticosteroid is dependent on the amount of drug absorbed into the systemic circulation. Approximately 90% of the inhaled dose from an MDI deposits in the oropharynx and is swallowed and subsequently absorbed from the gastrointestinal tract. Use of a large volume spacer device markedly reduces the oropharyngeal deposition, and therefore the systemic effects of inhaled corticosteroids, although this is less important when oral bioavailability is minimal, as with FP. For dry powder inhalers similar reductions in systemic effects may be achieved with mouth-washing and discarding the fluid. All patients using a daily dose of $\geq$800 µg of an inhaled corticosteroid should therefore use either a spacer or mouth-washing to reduce systemic absorption. Approximately 10% of an MDI enters the lung and this fraction (which presumably exerts the therapeutic effect) may be absorbed into the systemic circulation. As the fraction of inhaled corticosteroid deposited in the oropharynx is reduced, the proportion of the inhaled dose entering the lungs is increased. More efficient delivery to the lungs is therefore accompanied by increased systemic absorption, but this is offset by a reduction in the dose needed for optimal control of airway inflammation. For example, a multiple dry powder delivery system, the Turbuhaler, delivers approximately twice as much corticosteroid to the lungs as other devices, and therefore has increased systemic effects. However,

this is compensated for by the fact that only half the dose is required.

Hypothalamic–pituitary–adrenal axis

Corticosteroids may cause hypothalamic–pituitary–adrenal (HPA) axis suppression by reducing corticotrophin (ACTH) production, which reduces cortisol secretion by the adrenal gland. The degree of HPA suppression is dependent on dose, duration, frequency and timing of corticosteroid administration. There is no evidence that cortisol responses to the stress of an asthma exacerbation or insulin-induced hypoglycemia are impaired, even with high doses of inhaled corticosteroids. However, measurement of HPA axis function provides evidence for systemic effects of an inhaled corticosteroid. Basal adrenal cortisol secretion may be measured by a morning plasma cortisol, 24 h urinary cortisol or by plasma cortisol profile over 24 h. Other tests measure the HPA response following stimulation with tetracosactrin (which measures adrenal reserve) or stimulation with metyrapone and insulin (which measure the response to stress).

There are many studies of HPA axis function in asthmatic patients with inhaled corticosteroids, but the results are inconsistent as they have often been uncontrolled and patients have also been taking courses of oral corticosteroids (which may affect the HPA axis for weeks)[35]. BDP, budesonide and FP at high doses by conventional MDI ($>$1600 µg daily) give a dose-related decrease in morning serum cortisol levels and 24 h urinary cortisol, although values still lie well within the normal range. However, when a large volume spacer is used doses of 2000 µg daily of BDP or budesonide have little effect on 24 h urinary cortisol excretion. Stimulation tests of HPA axis function similarly show no consistent effects of doses of 1500 µg or less of inhaled corticosteroid. At high doses ($>$1500 µg daily) budesonide and FP have less effect than BDP on HPA axis function. In children no suppression of urinary cortisol is seen with doses of BDP of 800 µg or less. In studies where plasma cortisol has been measured at frequent intervals there was a significant reduction in cortisol peaks with doses of inhaled BDP as low as 400 µg daily, although this does not appear to be dose related in the range 400–1000 µg. The clinical significance of these effects is not certain, however.

Overall, the studies which are not confounded by concomitant treatment with oral corticosteroids, have consistently shown that there are no significant suppressive effects on HPA axis function at doses of ≤1500 µg in adults and ≤400 µg in children.

Effects on bone metabolism

Corticosteroids lead to a reduction in bone mass by direct effects on bone formation and resorption and indirectly by suppression of the pituitary–gonadal and HPA axes, effects on intestinal calcium absorption, renal tubular calcium reabsorption and secondary hyperparathyroidism[75]. The effects of oral corticosteroids on osteoporosis and increased risk of vertebral and rib fractures are well known, but there are no reports suggesting that long-term treatment with inhaled corticosteroids is associated with an increased risk of fractures. Bone densitometry has been used to assess the effect of inhaled corticosteroids on bone mass. Although there is evidence that bone density is less in patients taking high dose inhaled corticosteroids, interpretation is confounded by the fact that these patients are also taking intermittent courses of oral corticosteroids.

Changes in bone mass occur very slowly and several biochemical indices have been used to assess the short-term effects of inhaled corticosteroids on bone metabolism. Bone formation has been measured by plasma concentrations of bone-specific alkaline phosphatase, serum osteocalcin or procollagen peptides. Bone resorption may be assessed by urinary hydroxyproline after a 12-hour fast, urinary calcium excretion and pyridinium cross-link excretion. It is important to consider the age, diet, time of day and physical activity of the patient in interpreting any abnormalities. It is also necessary to choose appropriate control groups as asthma itself may have an effect on some of the measurements, such as osteocalcin. Inhaled corticosteroids, even at doses up to 2000 µg daily, have no significant effect on calcium excretion, but acute and reversible dose-related suppression of serum osteocalcin has been reported with BDP and budesonide when given by conventional MDI in several studies. Budesonide consistently has less effect than BDP at equivalent doses and only BDP increases urinary hydroxyproline at high doses. With a large volume spacer even doses of 2000 µg daily of either BDP or budesonide are without effect on plasma osteocalcin concentrations, however. Urinary pyridinium and deoxypyridinoline cross-links, which are a more accurate and stable measurement of bone and collagen degradation, are not increased with inhaled corticosteroids (BDP > 1000 µg daily), even with intermittent courses of oral corticosteroids. It is important to monitor changes in markers of bone formation as well as bone degradation, as the net effect on bone turnover is important.

There has been particular concern about the effect of inhaled corticosteroids on bone metabolism in growing children. A very low dose of oral corticosteroids (prednisolone 2.5 mg) causes significant changes in serum osteocalcin and urinary hydroxyproline excretion, whereas daily BDP and budesonide at doses up to 800 µg daily have no effect. It is important to recognize that the changes in biochemical indices of bone metabolism are less than those seen with even low doses of oral corticosteroids. This suggests that even high doses of inhaled corticosteroids, particularly when used with a spacer device, are unlikely to have any long-term effect on bone structure. Careful long-term follow-up studies in patients with asthma are needed.

There is no evidence that inhaled corticosteroids increase the frequency of fractures. Long-term treatment with high dose inhaled corticosteroids has not been associated with any consistent change in bone density. In elderly patients there may be an increase in bone density due to increased mobility.

Effects on connective tissue

Oral and topical corticosteroids cause thinning of the skin, telangiectasiae and easy bruising, probably as a result of loss of extracellular ground substance within the dermis, due to an inhibitory effect on dermal fibroblasts. There are reports of increased skin bruising and purpura in patients using high doses of inhaled BDP, but the amount of intermittent oral corticosteroids in these patients is not known. Easy bruising in association with inhaled cortico-steroids is more frequent in elderly patients[76] and there are no reports of this problem in children. Long-term prospective studies with objective meas-urements of skin thickness are needed with different inhaled corticosteroids.

Ocular effects

Long-term treatment with oral corticosteroids increase the risk of posterior subcapsular cataracts and there are several case reports describing cata-racts in individual patients taking inhaled cortico-steroids[35]. In a recent cross-sectional study in patients aged 5–25 years taking either inhaled BDP or budesonide no cataracts were found on slit-lamp examination, even in patients taking 2000 μg daily for over 10 years[77]. However, epidemiological studies have identified an increased risk of cataracts in patients taking high dose inhaled steroids over pro-longed periods[78]. A slight increase in the risk of glau-coma in patients taking very high does of inhaled corticosteroids has also been identified[79].

Growth

There has been particular concern that inhaled cor-ticosteroids may cause stunting of growth and several studies have addressed this issue. Asthma itself (as with other chronic diseases) may have an effect on the growth pattern and has been asso-ciated with delayed onset of puberty and decelera-tion of growth velocity that is more pronounced with more severe disease. However, asthmatic children appear to grow for longer, so that their final height is normal. The effect of asthma on growth makes it difficult to assess the effects of inhaled corticoster-oids on growth in cross-sectional studies, particu-larly as courses of oral corticosteroids is a confounding factor. Longitudinal studies have dem-onstrated that there is no significant effect of inhaled corticosteroids on statural growth in doses of up to 800 μg daily and for up to 5 years of treat-ment[35]. A meta-analysis of 21 studies, including over 800 children, showed no effect of inhaled BDP on statural height, even with higher doses and long duration of therapy[80] and in a large study of asth-matics treated with inhaled corticosteroids during childhood there was no difference in statural height compared to normal children[81].

Short-term growth measurements (knemometry) have demonstrated that even a low dose of an oral corticosteroid (prednisolone 2.5 mg) is sufficient to give complete suppression of lower leg growth. However, inhaled budesonide up to 400 μg is without effect, although some suppression is seen with 800 μg and with 400 μg BDP. The relationship between knemometry measurements and final height are uncertain since low doses of oral corticos-teroid that have no effect on final height cause pro-found suppression.

Metabolic effects

Several metabolic effects have been reported after inhaled corticosteroids, but there is no evidence that these are clinically relevant at therapeutic doses. In adults fasting glucose and insulin are unchanged after doses of BDP up to 2000 μg daily and in chil-dren with inhaled budesonide up to 800 μg daily. In normal individuals high dose inhaled BDP may slightly increase resistance to insulin. However, in patients with poorly controlled asthma high doses of BDP and budesonide paradoxically decrease insulin resistance and improve glucose tolerance, suggest-ing that the disease itself may lead to abnormalities in carbohydrate metabolism. Neither BDP 2000 μg daily in adults nor budesonide 800 μg daily in chil-dren have any effect on plasma cholesterol or trigly-cerides.

Hematological effects

Inhaled corticosteroids may reduce the numbers of circulating eosinophils in asthmatic patients, pos-sibly due to an effect on local cytokine generation in the airways. Inhaled corticosteroids may cause a small increase in circulating neutrophil counts.

Central nervous system effects

There are various reports of psychiatric disturbance, including emotional lability, euphoria, depression, aggressiveness and insomnia, after inhaled cortico-steroids. Only eight such patients have so far been reported, suggesting that this is very infrequent and a causal link with inhaled corticosteroids has usually not been established.

Safety in pregnancy

Based on extensive clinical experience inhaled corticosteroids appear to be safe in pregnancy, although no controlled studies have been performed. There is no evidence for any adverse effects of inhaled corticosteroids on the pregnancy, the delivery or on the fetus[35,82]. It is important to recognize that poorly controlled asthma may increase the incidence of perinatal mortality and retard intra-uterine growth, so that more effective control of asthma with inhaled corticosteroids may reduce these problems.

Systemic corticosteroids

Oral or intravenous corticosteroids may be indicated in several situations. Prednisolone, rather than prednisone, is the preferred oral corticosteroid as prednisone has to be converted in the liver to the active prednisolone. In pregnant patients prednisone may be preferable as it is not converted to prednisolone in the fetal liver, thus diminishing the exposure of the foetus to corticosteroids. Enteric-coated preparations of prednisolone are used to reduce side effects (particularly gastric side effects) and give delayed and reduced peak plasma concentrations, although the bioavailability and therapeutic efficacy of these preparations is similar to uncoated tablets. Prednisolone and prednisone are preferable to dexamethasone, betamethasone or triamcinolone, which have longer plasma half-lives and therefore an increased frequency of adverse effects.

Short courses of oral corticosteroids (30–40 mg prednisolone daily for 1–2 weeks or until the peak flow values return to best attainable) are indicated for exacerbations of asthma, and the dose may be tailed off over 1 week once the exacerbation is resolved. The tail-off period is not strictly necessary, but some patients find it reassuring.

Maintenance oral corticosteroids are only needed in a small proportion of asthmatic patients with the most severe asthma that cannot be controlled with maximal doses of inhaled corticosteroids (2000 μg daily) and additional bronchodilators. The minimal dose of oral corticosteroid needed for control should be used and reductions in the dose should be made slowly in patients who have been on oral corticosteroids for long periods (e.g. by 2.5 mg per month for doses down to 10 mg daily and thereafter by 1 mg per month). Oral corticosteroids are usually given as a single morning dose as this reduces the risk of adverse effects since it coincides with the peak diurnal concentrations. There is some evidence that administration in the afternoon may be optimal for some patients who have severe nocturnal asthma[83]. Alternate day administration may also reduce adverse effects, but control of asthma may not be as good on the day when the oral dose is omitted in some patients.

Intramuscular triamcinolone acetonide (80 mg monthly) has been advocated in patients with severe asthma as an alternative to oral corticosteroids[84,85]. This may be considered in patients in whom compliance is a particular problem, but the major concern is the high frequency of proximal myopathy associated with this fluorinated corticosteroid. Some patients who do not respond well to prednisolone are reported to respond to oral betamethasone, presumably because of pharmacokinetic handling problems with prednisolone.

Acute severe asthma

Intravenous hydrocortisone is given in acute severe asthma. The recommended dose is 200 mg i.v.[86]. While the value of corticosteroids in acute severe asthma has been questioned, others have found that they speed the resolution of attacks[87]. There is no apparent advantage in giving very high doses of intravenous corticosteroids (such as methylprednisolone 1 g). Intravenous corticosteroids have occasionally been associated with an acute severe myopathy[88]. In a recent study no difference in recovery from acute severe asthma was seen whether i.v. hydrocortisone in doses of 50, 200 or 500 mg 6 hourly were used[89] and another placebo controlled study showed no beneficial effect of i.v. corticosteroids[90]. Intravenous corticosteroids are indicated in acute asthma if lung function is < 30% predicted and in whom there is no significant improvement with nebulized β_2-agonist. Intravenous therapy is usually given until a satisfactory response is obtained and then oral prednisolone may be substituted. Oral prednisolone (40–60 mg) has a similar effect to intravenous hydrocortisone and is easier to administer[87,91]. Oral prednisolone is the preferred treatment for acute severe asthma, providing there are no contraindications to oral therapy[57].

Corticosteroid-resistant asthma

Although glucocorticoids are highly effective in the control of asthma and other chronic inflammatory or immune diseases, a small proportion of patients with asthma fail to respond even to high doses of oral glucocorticoids[92,93]. Resistance to the therapeutic effects of glucocorticoids is also recognized in other inflammatory and immune diseases, including rheumatoid arthritis and inflammatory bowel disease. Corticosteroid-resistant patients, although uncommon, present considerable management problems. Recently, new insights into the mechanisms whereby corticosteroids suppress chronic inflammation has shed new light on the molecular basis of corticosteroid-resistant asthma.

Corticosteroid-resistant asthma is defined as a failure to improve FEV_1 or PEF by > 15% after treatment with oral prednisolone 30–40 mg daily for 2 weeks, providing the oral steroid is taken (verified by plasma prednisolone level or a reduction in early morning cortisol level). These patients are not Addisonian and they do not suffer from the abnormalities in sex hormones described in the very rare familial glucocorticoid resistance. Plasma cortisol and adrenal suppression in response to exogenous cortisol is normal in these patients, so they suffer from side effects of corticosteroids.

Complete corticosteroid resistance in asthma is very rare, with a prevalence of < 1:1000 asthmatic patients. Much more common is a reduced responsiveness to corticosteroids, so that large inhaled or oral doses are needed to control asthma adequately (corticosteroid-dependent asthma). It is likely that there is a range of responsiveness to corticosteroids and that corticosteroid resistance is at one extreme of this range.

It is important to establish that the patient has asthma, rather than chronic obstructive pulmonary disease (COPD), 'pseudoasthma' (a hysterical conversion syndrome involving vocal cord dysfunction)[94], left ventricular failure or cystic fibrosis that do not respond to corticosteroids. Asthmatic patients are characterized by a variability in PEF and, in particular, a diurnal variability of > 15% and episodic symptoms. It is also important to identify provoking factors (allergens, drugs, psychological problems) that may increase the severity of asthma and its resistance to therapy. Biopsy studies have demonstrated the typical eosinophilic inflammation of asthma in these patients[93].

Mechanisms of corticosteroid resistance

There may be several mechanisms for resistance to the effects of glucocorticoids. Certain cytokines (particularly IL-2, IL-4 and IL-13) may induce a reduction in affinity of glucocorticoid receptors in inflammatory cells such as T-lymphocytes, resulting in local resistance to the anti-inflammatory actions of corticosteroids[93]. Another mechanism is an increased activation of the transcription factor AP-1 by inflammatory cytokines, so that AP-1 may consume activated glucocorticoid receptors and thus reduce their availability for suppression of inflammation at inflamed sites[95]. There is an increased expression of c-Fos, one of the components of AP-1[96]. The reasons for this excessive activation of AP-1 by activating enzymes is currently unknown, but may be genetically determined.

Corticosteroids in COPD

Inhaled corticosteroids are now widely used in the treatment of COPD. In my opinion this is incorrect and indeed patients may suffer from systemic side effects.

COPD as an inflammatory disease

There is increasing evidence that COPD is associated with chronic inflammation in the airways and parenchyma. This has been used as a rationale for the use of inhaled corticosteroids in COPD by analogy with the striking suppressive effects of inhaled corticosteroids on airway inflammation and symptoms in asthma. But the inflammatory pattern in COPD differs markedly from that seen in asthma, with a preponderance of macrophages and $CD8^+$ T-lymphocytes in the airways and lung parenchyma, and an increase in macrophages and neutrophils in sputum and bronchoalveolar lavage, in contrast to the increase in eosinophils and activation of mast cells and $CD4^+$ T-cells that are characteristic of asthma[97,98]. In both chronic diseases there is an increased production of cytokines, but the pattern differs with IL-8 and TNF-α predominating in COPD, compared to IL-4, IL-5 and IL-13 in asthma.

Corticosteroids do not suppress inflammation in COPD

Corticosteroids are very effective at suppressing airway inflammation in asthma and have potent inhibitory effects on eosinophilic inflammation, with reduced production, recruitment, activation and particularly survival of eosinophils[35]. By contrast, double-blind placebo-controlled studies in carefully characterized patients with COPD have shown that even high doses of inhaled corticosteroids do not reduce inflammatory cell numbers, concentrations of cytokines or proteases[99,100]. Even high doses of oral corticosteroids, given because there was concern that the inhaled steroid may not reach inflammatory sites in patients with severe COPD, were without any effect[99]. Another study found a small inhibitory effect of inhaled corticosteroids on neutrophil counts in induced sputum of patients with COPD, but this study was not controlled and there was a high eosinophil count, suggesting that asthmatic patients had been included[101]. The lack of effect of corticosteroids on inflammatory markers in induced sputum has been confirmed in a preliminary study showing no effect in bronchial biopsies[102]. It appears that COPD is a steroid-resistant disease.

Clinical studies with inhaled corticosteroids in COPD

Since inhaled corticosteroids are so clearly effective in asthma, it is important that patients with asthma are rigorously excluded from any trial of inhaled corticosteroids. Approximately 10% of patients are likely to have both asthma and COPD and share features of the two diseases; these patients may show a beneficial response to steroids and should be labelled as asthmatic. A 2-week course of oral steroids and perhaps a 3-month trial of inhaled corticosteroids are indicated in order to exclude any asthmatic component. Several studies that purport to show a benefit of inhaled steroids in COPD include a large proportion of patients with asthma[51,103]. The remaining patients, with 'pure' COPD, do not appear to respond to corticosteroids. Several studies have failed to show any beneficial effect of inhaled corticosteroids in patients with COPD where asthma has been rigorously excluded. Inhaled steroids do not improve airway responsiveness to bronchoconstriction and have little or no effect on spirometry in COPD[104,105]. Three recent studies examined the effects of inhaled corticosteroids in controlled trials of large numbers of patients over 2–3 years and showed no significant reduction in the accelerated decline in lung function, indicating that there is no effect of inhaled steroids on the progressive inflammatory disease process[106–108]. A high dose of inhaled steroids does not reduce the total number of acute exacerbations in patients with severe COPD, although they were less severe[109].

Why are inhaled corticosteroids ineffective in COPD?

There are several possible reasons why corticosteroids may not be effective in suppressing the inflammatory disease process in COPD, while they are highly effective in asthma. Neutrophilic inflammation is generally resistant to corticosteroids, whereas eosinophilic inflammation is suppressed. Corticosteroids decrease the survival of eosinophils in vitro, whereas they prolong the survival of neutrophils by inhibiting apoptosis[26,110]. In normal subjects ozone inhalation induces a neutrophilic inflammatory response (with an increase in neutrophils of a similar magnitude to that seen in patients with COPD) and this is unaffected by high doses of inhaled corticosteroids[111]. There may even be an active resistance to the effects of inhaled corticosteroids in COPD, since corticosteroid therapy fails to suppress cytokines, such as TNF-α and IL-8, that are inhibited by steroids in vitro. The molecular mechanisms underlying this resistance are currently under investigation.

Adverse effects of inhaled corticosteroids

As patients with COPD respond so poorly to inhaled corticosteroids, they are commonly prescribed high doses that may be associated with systemic side effects. Patients with COPD may be particularly vulnerable to these systemic effects as they are often elderly, immobile and have poor nutrition, thus increasing the risks of osteoporosis. Elderly patients may also have an increased risk of developing cataracts, glaucoma and diabetes. In a recent large study of inhaled corticosteroids in patients with mild COPD 10% of patients developed skin bruising compared to 4% in the control group[107]. Any discussion of the use of inhaled corticosteroids in patients with COPD must weigh the real risk of systemic side effects against the minimal clinical value provided

by this treatment. High doses of inhaled corticosteroids are expensive and, as they provide little or no benefit, cannot be justified in terms of cost-effectiveness.

Systemic corticosteroids in COPD

In contrast to the lack of effects of inhaled corticosteroids, oral corticosteroids have a well-established place in the treatment of acute exacerbation. There is evidence that systemic steroids (intravenous methylprednisolone for 3 days followed by oral prednisolone) improve the time of recovery from an acute exacerbation, although the risk of systemic side effects, such as hyperglycemia, is high[112]. Oral steroids speed the recovery from acute exacerbations, so that patients may be discharged home earlier, although the effect is rather small[113]. The reasons why steroids are effective in acute exacerbations but not chronic disease may be related to differences in the inflammatory process in acute exacerbations, where there is evidence for an eosinophil component[114].

REFERENCES

1 Barnes PJ. Inhaled corticosteroids in COPD. *Am J Respir Crit Care Med* 2000; 161:(in press).

2 Barnes PJ. Inhaled glucocorticoids for asthma. *N Engl J Med* 1995; 332:868–875.

3 Barnes PJ. Efficacy of inhaled corticosteroids in asthma. *J Allergy Clin Immunol* 1998; 102:531–538.

4 Barnes PJ. Antiinflammatory actions of glucocorticoids: molecular mechanisms. *Clin Sci* 1998; 94:557–572.

5 Bamberger CM, Bamberger AM, de Castr M, Chrousos GP. Glucocorticoid receptor b, a potential endogenous inhibitor of glucocorticoid action in humans. *J Clin Invest* 1995; 95:2435–2441.

6 Reichardt HM, Kaestner KH, Tuckermann J et al. DNA binding of the glucocorticoid receptor is not essential for survival. *Cell* 1998; 93:531–541.

7 Barnes PJ, Karin M. Nuclear factor-κB: a pivotal transcription factor in chronic inflammatory diseases. *N Engl J. Med* 1997; 336:1066–1071.

8 Barnes PJ, Adcock IM. Transcription factors and asthma. *Eur Respir J* 1998; 12:221–34.

9 Kamei Y, Xu L, Heinzel T et al. A CBP integrator complex mediates transcriptional activation and AP-1 inhibition by nuclear receptors. *Cell* 1996; 85:403–414.

10 Karin M. New twists in gene regulation by glucocorticoid receptor: is DNA binding dispensable?. *Cell* 1998; 93:487–490.

11 Ito K, Adcock IM, Barnes PJ. Different histone acetylation induced by glucocorticoids and IL-1β in human epithelial cells (A549). *Am J Respir Crit Care Med* 1999; 159:A442.

12 Hall SE, Lim S, Witherden IR, Tetley TD, Barnes PJ, Kamal AM, Smith SF. Lung type II cell and macrophage annexin I release: differential effects of two glucocorticoids. *Am J Physiol* 1999; 276:L114–21.

13 Mak JCW, Nishikawa M, Barnes PJ. Glucocorticosteroids increase β_2-adrenergic receptor transcription in human lung. *Am J Physiol* 1995; 12:L41–L46.

14 Mak JCW, Nishikawa M, Shirasaki H, Miyayasu K, Barnes PJ. Protective effects of a glucocorticoid on down-regulation of pulmonary β_2-adrenergic receptors *in vivo*. *J Clin Invest* 1995; 96:99–106.

15 Lilly CM, Nakamura H, Kesselman H et al. Expression of eotaxin by human lung epithelial cells: induction by cytokines and inhibition by glucocorticoids. *J Clin Invest* 1997; 99:1767–1773.

16 Rao A, Luo C, Hogan PG. Transcription factors of the NFAT family: regulation and function. *Annu Rev Immunol* 1997; 15:707–47:707–747.

17 Mitchell JA, Belvisi MG, Akarasereemom P et al. Induction of cyclo-oxygenase-2 by cytokines in human pulmonary epithelial cells: regulation by dexamethasone. *Br J Pharmacol* 1994; 113:1008–1014.

18 Newton R, Kuitert LM, Slater DM, Adcock IM, Barnes PJ. Cytokine induction of cytosolic phosholipase A$_2$ and cyclooxygenase-2 mRNA by proinflammatory cytokines is suppressed by dexamethasone in human epithelial cells. *Life Sci* 1997; 60:67–78.

19 Adcock IM, Peters M, Gelder C, Shirasaki H, Brown CR, Barnes PJ. Increased tachykinin receptor gene expression in asthmatic lung and its modulation by steroids. *J Mol Endocrinol* 1993; 11:1–7.

20 Katsunuma T, Mak JCW, Barnes PJ. Glucocorticoids reduce tachykinin NK$_2$-receptor expression in bovine tracheal smooth muscle. *Eur J Pharmacol* 1998; 344:99–107.

21 Atsuta J, Plitt J, Bochner BS, Schleimer RP. Inhibition of VCAM-1 expression in human bronchial epithelial cells by glucocorticoids. *Am J Respir Cell Mol Biol* 1999; 20:643–650.

22 Walsh GM. Mechanisms of human eosinophil survival and apoptosis. *Clin Exp Allergy* 1997; 27:482–487.

23 John M, Lim S, Seybold J et al. Inhaled corticosteroids increase IL-10 but reduce MIP-1α, GM-CSF and IFN-γ release from alveolar macrophages in asthma. *Am J Respir Crit Care Med* 1998; 157:256–262.

24 Woolley KL, Gibson PG, Carty K, Wilson AJ, Twaddell SH, Woolley MJ. Eosinophil apoptosis and the resolution of airway inflammation in asthma. *Am J Respir Crit Care Med* 1996; 154:237–243.

25 Nelson DJ, McWilliam AS, Haining S, Holt PG. Modulation of airway intraepithelial dendritic cells following exposure to steroids. *Am J Respir Crit Care Med* 1995; 151:475–481.

26 Cox G. Glucocorticoid treatment inhibits apoptosis in human neutrophils. *J Immunol* 1995; 193:4719–4725.

27 Barnes PJ. Mechanism of action of glucocorticoids in asthma. *Am J Respir Crit Care Med* 1996; 154:S21–S27.

28 Schweibert LM, Stellato C, Schleimer RP. The epithelium as a target for glucocorticoid action in the treatment of asthma. *Am J Respir Crit Care Med* 1996; 154:S16–S20.

29 Saleh D, Ernst P, Lim S, Barnes PJ, Giaid A. Increased formation of the potent oxidant peroxynitrite in the airways of asthmatic patients is associated with induction of nitric oxide synthase: effect of inhaled glucocorticoid. *FASEB J* 1998; 12:929–937.

30 Kharitonov SA, Yates DH, Barnes PJ. Regular inhaled budesonide decreases nitric oxide concentration in the exhaled air of asthmatic patients. *Am J Respir Crit Care Med* 1996; 153:454–457.

31 Kai H, Yoshitake K, Hisatsune A et al. Dexamethasone suppresses mucus production and MUC-2 and MUC-5AC gene expression by NCI-H292 cells. *Am J Physiol* 1996; 271:L484–L484.

32 Barnes PJ. Effect of corticosteroids on airway hyperresponsiveness. *Am Rev Respir Dis* 1990; 141:S70–6.

33 Kamada AK, Szefler SJ, Martin RJ et al. Issues in the use of inhaled steroids. *Am J Respir Crit Care Med* 1996; 153:1739–1748.

34 Barnes PJ. Therapeutic strategies for allergic diseases. *Nature* 1999; 402:31–38.

35 Barnes PJ, Pedersen S, Busse WW. Efficacy and safety of inhaled corticosteroids: an update. *Am J Respir Crit Care Med* 1998; 157:S1–S53.

36 Haahtela T, Jarvinen M, Kava T et al. Comparison of a β_2-agonist terbutaline with an inhaled steroid in newly detected asthma. *N Engl J Med* 1991; 325:388–392.

37 Juniper EF, Kline PA, Vanzieleghem MA, Ramsdale EH, O'Byrne PM, Hargreave FE. Effect of long-term treatment with an inhaled corticosteroid (budesonide) on airway hyperresponsiveness and clinical asthma in nonsteroid-dependent asthmatics. *Am Rev Respir Dis* 1990; 142:832–836.

38 Vathenen AS, Knox AJ, Wisniewski A, Tattersfield AE. Time course of change in bronchial reactivity with an inhaled corticosteroid in asthma. *Am Rev Respir Dis* 1991; 143:1317–1321.

39 Levy ML, Stevenson C, Maslen T. Comparison of short courses of oral prednisolone and fluticasone propionate in the treatment of adults with acute exacerbations of asthma in primary care. *Thorax* 1996; 51:1987–1092.

40 Juniper EF, Kline PA, Vanzielegmem MA, Hargreave FE. Reduction of budesonide after a year of increased use: a randomized controlled trial to evaluate whether improvements in airway responsiveness and clinical asthma are maintained. *J Allergy Clin Immunol* 1991; 87:483–489.

41 van Essen-Zandvliet EE, Hughes MD, Waalkens HJ, Duiverman EJ, Pocock SJ, Kerrebijn KF. Effects of 22 months of treatment with inhaled corticosteroids and/or β_2-agonists on lung function, airway responsiveness and symptoms in children with asthma. *Am Rev Respir Dis* 1992; 146:547–554.

42 Waalkens HJ, van Essen-Zandvliet EE, Hughes MD et al. Cessation of long-term treatment with inhaled corticosteroids (budesonide) in children with asthma results in deterioration. *Am Rev Respir Dis* 1993; 148:1252–1257.

43 Simons FE. A comparison of beclomethasone, salmeterol, and placebo in children with asthma. Canadian Beclomethasone Dipropionate-Salmeterol Xinafoate Study Group [see comments]. *N Engl J Med* 1997; 337:1659–1665.

44 Ilangovan, P, Pedersen S, Godfrey S, Nikander K, Novisky N, Warner JO. Nebulised budesonide suspension in severe steroid-dependent preschool asthma. *Arch Dis Child* 1993; 68:356–359.

45 Busse WW, Chervinsky P, Condemi J et al. Budesonide delivered by Turbuhaler is effective in a dose-dependent fashion when used in the treatment of adult patients with chronic asthma. *J Allergy Clin Immunol* 1998; 101:457–463.

46 Pauwels RA, Lofdahl C-G, Postma DS et al. Effect of inhaled formoterol and budesonide on exacerbations of asthma. *N Engl J Med* 1997; 337:1412–1418.

47 Lim, S, Jatakanon A, John M, Gilbey T, O'Connor BJ, Chung KF, Barnes PJ. Effect of inhaled budesonide on lung function and airway inflammation. Assessment by various inflammatory markers in mild asthma. *Am J Respir Crit Care Med* 1999; 159:22–30.

48 Jatakanon A, Lim S, Chung KF, Barnes PJ. An inhaled steroid improves markers of inflammation in asymptomatic steroid-naive asthmatic patients. *Eur Respir J* 1998; 12:1084–1088.

49 Jatakanon A, Kharitonov S, Lim S, Barnes PJ. Effect of differing doses of inhaled budesonide on markers of airway inflammation in patients with mild asthma. *Thorax* 1999; 54:108–114.

50 Sont JK, Willems LN, Bel EH, van Krieken JH, Vandenbroucke JP, Sterk PJ. Clinical control and histopathologic outcome of asthma when using airway hyperresponsiveness as an additional guide to long-term treatment. The AMPUL Study Group. *Am J Respir Crit Care Med* 1999; 159:1043–1051.

51 Dompeling E, Van Schayck CP, Molema J, Folgering H, van Grusven PM, van Weel C. Inhaled beclomethasone improves the course of asthma and COPD. *Eur Resp J* 1992; 5:945–952.

52 Haahtela T, Järvinsen M, Kava T et al. Effects of reducing or discontinuing inhaled budesonide in patients with mild asthma. *N Engl J Med* 1994; 331:700–705.

53 Agertoft L, Pedersen S. Effects of long-term treatment with an inhaled corticosteroid on growth and pulmonary function in asthmatic children. *Resp Med* 1994; 5:369–372.

54 Selroos O, Pietinalcho A, Lofroos A-B, Riska A. Effect of early and late intervention with inhaled corticosteroids in asthma. *Chest* 1995; 108:1228–1234.

55 Ernst P, Spitzer WD, Suissa S et al. Risk of fatal and near fatal asthma in relation to inhaled corticosteroid use. *J Am Med Assoc* 1992; 268:3462–3464.

56 Barnes PJ. Inhaled glucocorticoids: new developments relevant to updating the Asthma Management Guidelines. *Resp Med* 1996; 90:379–384.

57 British Thoracic Society. The British guidelines on asthma management. *Thorax* 1997; 52(Suppl 1):S1-S21.

58 Expert Panel Report 2. Guidelines for the diagnosis and management of asthma. Washington D.C. National Institutes of Health, 1997.

59 Malo J, Cartier A, Merland N et al. Four-times-a-day dosing frequency is better than twice-a-day regimen in subjects requiring a high-dose inhaled steroid, budesonide, to control moderate to severe asthma. *Am Rev Respir Dis* 1989; 140:624–628.

60 Jones AH, Langdon CG, Lee PS, Lingham SA, Nankani JP, Follows RMA, Tollemar U, Richardson PDI. Pulmicort Turbohaler once daily as initial prophylactic therapy for asthma. *Resp Med* 1994; 88:293–299.

61 Otulana BA, Varma N, Bullock A, Higenbottam T. High dose nebulized steroid in the treatment of chronic steroid-dependent asthma. *Resp Med* 1992; 86:105–108.

62 Greening AP, Ind PW, Northfield M, Shaw G. Added salmeterol versus higher-dose corticosteroid in asthma patients with symptoms on existing inhaled corticosteroid. *Lancet* 1994; 344:219–224.

63 Woolcock A, Lundback B, Ringdal N, Jacques L. Comparison of addition of salmeterol to inhaled steroids with doubling the dose of inhaled steroids. *Am J Respir Crit Care Med* 1996; 153:1481–1488.

64 Chapman KR, Ringdal N, Backer V, Palmqvist M, Saarelainen S, Briggs M. Salmeterol and fluticasone propionate (50/250 mg) administered via combination diskus inhaler: As effective as when given via separate diskus inhalers. *Can Respir J* 1999; 6:45–51.

65 Evans DJ, Taylor DA, Zetterstrom O, Chung KF, O'Connor BJ, Barnes PJ. A comparison of low-dose inhaled budesonide plus theophylline and high-dose inhaled budesonide for moderate asthma. *N Engl J Med* 1997; 337:1412–1418.

66 Ukena D, Harnest U, Sakalauskas R et al. Comparison of addition of theophylline to inhaled steroid with doubling of the dose of inhaled steroid in asthma. *Eur Respir J* 1997; 10:2754–2760.

67 Virchow J, Hassall SM, Summerton L, Klim J, Harris A. Reduction of asthma exacerbations with zafirlukast in patients on inhaled corticosteroids. *Eir Respir J* 1997; 10(supl 25):420S.

68 O'Shaughnessy KM, Wellings R, Gillies B, Fuller RW. Differential effects of fluticasone proprionate on allergen-induced bronchoconstriction and increased urinary leukotriene E_4 excretion. *Am Rev Respir Dis* 1993; 147:1472–1476.

69 Barnes PJ, Jonsson B, Klim J. The costs of asthma. *Eur Respir J* 1996; 9:636–642.

70 van Schayk CP, Dompeling E, Rutten MP, Folgering H, van den Boom G, van Weel C. The influence of an inhaled steroid on quality of life in patients with asthma or COPD. *Chest* 1995; 107:1199–1205.

71 Hill SJ, Tattersfield AE. Corticosteroid sparing agents in asthma. *Thorax* 1995; 50:577–582.

72 Nelson HS, Hamilos DL, Corsello PR, Levesque NV, Buchameier AD, Bucher BL. A double-blind study of troleandamycin and methylprednisolone in asthmatic patients who require daily corticosteroids. *Am Rev Respir Dis* 1993; 147:398–404.

73 Williamson IJ, Matusiewicz SP, Brown PH, Greening AP, Crompton GK. Frequency of voice problems and cough in patients using pressurised aerosol inhaled steroid preparations. *Eur Resp J* 1995; 8:590–592.

74 Toogood JA, Jennings B, Greenway RW, Chung L. Candidiasis and dysphonia complicating beclomethasone treatment of asthma. *J Allergy Clin Immunol* 1980; 65:145–153.

75 Efthimou J, Barnes PJ. Effect of inhaled corticosteroids on bone and growth. *Eur Respir J* 1998; 11:1167–1177.

76 Roy A, Leblanc C, Paquette L et al. Skin bruising in asthmatic subjects treated with high doses of inhaled steroids: frequency and association with adrenal function. *Eur Respir J* 1996; 9:226–231.

77 Simons FER, Persaud MP, Gillespie CA, Cheang M, Shuckett EP. Absence of posterior subcapsular cataracts in young patients treated with inhaled glucocorticoids. *Lancet* 1993; 342:736–738.

78 Cumming RG, Mitchell P, Leeder SR. Use of inhaled corticosteroids and the risk of cataracts. *N Engl J Med* 1997; 337:8–14.

79 Garbe E, LeLovier J, Boivin J, Suissa S. Inhaled and nasal glucocorticoids and the risks of ocular hypertension or open-angle glaucoma. *J Am Med Assoc* 1997; 227:722–722.

80 Allen DB, Mullen M, Mullen B. A meta-analysis of the effects of oral and inhaled corticosteroids on growth. *J Allergy Clin Immunol* 1994; 93:967–976.

81 Silverstein MD, Yunginger JW, Reed CE et al. Attained adult height after childhood asthma: effect of glucocorticoid therapy. *J Allergy Clin Immunol* 1997; 99:466–474.

82 Schatz M, Zeiger RS, Harden K, Hoffman CC, Chilingar L, Petitti D. The safety of asthma and allergy medications during pregnancy. *J Allergy Clin Immunol* 1997; 100:301–306.

83 Beam WR, Ballard RD, Martin RJ. Spectrum of corticosteroid sensitivity in nocturnal asthma. *Am Rev Respir Dis* 1992; 145:1082–1086.

84 McLeod DT, Capewell SJ, Law J, MacLaren W, Seaton A. Intramuscular triamcinolone acetamide in chronic severe asthma. *Thorax* 1985; 40:840–845.

85 Ogirala RG, Aldrich TK, Prezant DJ, Sinnett MJ, Enden JB, Williams MH. High dose intramuscular triamcinolone in severe life-threatening asthma. *N Engl J Med* 1991; 329:585–589.

86 British Thoracic Society. Guidelines on the management of asthma. *Thorax* 1993; 48S (Supl):S1–S24.

87 Engel T, Heinig JH. Glucocorticoid therapy in acute severe asthma – a critical review. *Eur Respir J* 1991; 4:881–889.

88 Decramer M, Lacquet LM, Fagard R, Rogiers P. Corticosteroids contribute to muscle weakness in chronic airflow obstruction. *Am J Respir Crit Care Med* 1995; 150:11–16.

89 Bowler SD, Mitchell CA, Armstrong JG. Corticosteroids in acute severe asthma: effectiveness of low doses. *Thorax* 1992; 47:584–587.

90 Morell F, Orkiols R, de Gracia J, Curul V, Pujol A. Controlled trial of intravenous corticosteroids in severe acute asthma. *Thorax* 1992; 47:588–591.

91 Harrison BDN, Stokes TC, Hart GJ, Vaughan DA, Ali NJ,

Robinson AA. Need for intravenous hydrocortisone in addition to oral prednisolone in patients admitted to hospital with severe asthma without ventilatory failure. *Lancet* 1986; i:181–184.

92 Barnes PJ. Pathophysiology of asthma. *Br J Clin Pharmacol* 1996; 42:3–10.

93 Szefler SJ, Leung DY. Glucocorticoid-resistant asthma: pathogenesis and clinical implications for management. *Eur Respir J* 1997; 10:1640–1647.

94 Thomas PS, Geddes DM, Barnes PJ. Pseudo-steroid resistant asthma. *Thorax* 1999; 54:352–356.

95 Adcock IM, Brown CR, Shirasaki H, Barnes PJ. Effects of dexamethasone on cytokine and phorbol ester stimulated c-Fos and c-Jun DNA binding and gene expression in human lung. *Eur Resp J* 1994; 7:2117–2123.

96 Lane SJ, Adcock IM, Richards D, Hawrylowicz C, Barnes PJ, Lee TH. Corticosteroid-resistant bronchial asthma is associated with increased *c-Fos* expression in monocytes and T-lymphocytes. *J Clin Invest* 1998; 102:2156–2164.

97 Jeffery PK. Structural and inflammatory changes in COPD: a comparison with asthma. *Thorax* 1998; 53:129–136.

98 Keatings VM, Collins PD, Scott DM, Barnes PJ. Differences in interleukin-8 and tumor necrosis factor-a in induced sputum from patients with chronic obstructive pulmonary disease or asthma. *Am J Respir Crit Care Med* 1996; 153:530–534.

99 Keatings VM, Jatakanon A, Worsdell YM, Barnes PJ. Effects of inhaled and oral glucocorticoids on inflammatory indices in asthma and COPD. *Am J Respir Crit Care Med* 1997; 155:542–548.

100 Culpitt SV, Nightingale JA, Barnes PJ. Effect of high dose inhaled steroid on cells, cytokines and proteases in induced sputum in chronic obstructive pulmonary disease. *Am J Respir Crit Care Med* 1999; 160:1635–1639.

101 Confalonieri M, Mainardi E, Della Porta R et al. Inhaled corticosteroids reduce neutrophilic bronchial inflammation in patients with chronic obstructive pulmonary disease. *Thorax* 1998; 53:583–585.

102 Hattotuwa K, Ansari T, Gizycki M, Barnes N, Jeffery PK. A double-blind placebo-controlled trial of the effect of inhaled corticosteroids on the immunopathology of COPD. *Am J Respir Crit Care Med* 1999; 159:A523.

103 Kertjens HAM, Brand PLP, Hughes MD et al. A comparison of bronchodilator therapy with or without inhaled corticosteroid therapy for obstructive airways disease. *N Engl J Med* 1992; 327:1413–1419.

104 Watson A, Lim TK, Joyce H, Pride NB. Failure of inhaled corticosteroids to modify bronchoconstrictor or bronchodilator responses in middle-aged smokers with mild airflow obstruction. *Chest* 1992; 101:350–355.

105 Weir DC, Burge PS. Effects of high dose inhaled beclomethasone dipropionate 750mg and 1500mg twice daily and 40 mg oral prednisolone on lung function, symptoms and bronchial hyperresponsiveness in patients with non-asthmatic airflow obstruction. *Thorax* 1993; 48:309–316.

106 Vestbo J, Sorensen T, Lange P, Brix A, Torre P, Viskum K. Long-term effect of inhaled budesonide in mild and moderate chronic obstructive pulmonary disease: a randomised controlled trial. *Lancet* 1999; 353:1819–1823.

107 Pauwels RA, Lofdahl CG, Laitinen LA et al. Long-term treatment with inhaled budesonide in persons with mild chronic obstructive pulmonary disease who continue smoking. European Respiratory Society Study on Chronic Obstructive Pulmonary Disease. *N Engl J Med* 1999; 340:1948–1953.

108 Burge PS. EUROSCOP, ISOLDE and the Copenhagen City Lung Study. *Thorax* 1999; 54:287–288.

109 Paggiaro PL, Dahle R, Bakran I, Frith L, Hollingworth K, Efthimou J. Multicentre randomised placebo-controlled trial of inhaled fluticasone propionate in patients with chronic obstructive pulmonary disease. *Lancet* 1998; 351:773–80.

110 Meagher LC, Cousin JM, Seckl JR, Haslett C. Opposing effects of glucocorticoids on the rate of apoptosis in neutrophilic and eosinophilic granulocytes. *J Immunol* 1996; 156:4422–4428.

111 Nightingale JA, Rogers DF, Chung KF, Barnes PJ. Effect of inhaled budesonide on the response to inhaled ozone in normal subjects. *Am J Respir Crit Care Med* 1999; 160:

112 Niewoehner DE, Erbland ML, Deupree RH et al. Effect of systemic glucocorticoids on exacerbations of chronic obstructive pulmonary disease. Department of Veterans Affairs Cooperative Study Group. *N Engl J Med* 1999; 340:1941–1947.

113 Davies L, Angus RM, Calverley PM. Oral corticosteroids in patients admitted to hospital with exacerbations of chronic obstructive pulmonary disease: a prospective randomised controlled trial. *Lancet* 1999; 354:456–460.

114 Saetta M, Di Stefano A, Maestrelli P et al. Airway eosinophilia and expression of interleukin-5 protein in asthma and in exacerbations of chronic bronchitis. *Clin Exp Allergy* 1996; 26:766–774.

β_2-adrenoceptor agonists

Domenico Spina, Clive P. Page[1] & Brian J. O'Connor

The Sackler Institute of Pulmonary Pharmacology, Department of Respiratory Medicine and Allergy, GKT School of Medicine, King's College London, UK. [1]Division of Pharmacology and Therapeutics, GKT School of Biomedical Sciences, Guy's Campus, London, UK

Introduction

β_2-adrenoceptor agonists afford symptomatic bronchodilator relief against a wide range of stimuli including antigen, exercise, pharmacological agonists, physiological stimuli and chemical irritants and are therefore the agents of first choice in the treatment of the symptoms of asthma. The major action attributed to these agonists is functional antagonism of airway smooth muscle contraction. However, it is also recognized that these agonists inhibit the activity of various cell types within the lung including mast cells, which may also contribute toward their beneficial action. The relatively short duration of action of bronchodilator agonists including salbutamol, terbutaline and fenoterol has led to the development of longer acting agonists including salmeterol and formoterol. These agents have a considerably longer duration of action that is advantageous in the treatment of nocturnal asthma and in the day-to-day management of asthma and chronic obstructive pulmonary disease (COPD). There is no doubting the effectiveness of this drug class in acute exacerbation of asthma. However, a number of studies have raised concerns that regular chronic treatment with β_2-adrenoceptor agonists may also have a detrimental impact in asthma, a controversy which has intensified following the introduction of salmeterol and formoterol. This chapter will summarize our current understanding of the pharmacology of this drug class and their use in the chronic treatment of asthma and COPD.

Structure and metabolism

The majority of the β_2-adrenoceptor agonists currently used in asthma are derived from the known structure of adrenaline and share a phenylethylamine structure, with a catechol, resorcinol or related moiety that confers potency and an ethanolamine side chain, which confers selectivity to the molecule. The chemical structure of a number of these agonists is illustrated in Fig. 3.1.

Adrenaline

Adrenaline possesses a benzene ring structure that is hydroxylated in the 3 and 4 position (catechol). It also contains a methyl ethanolamine side chain. Hence, adrenaline possesses activity at both α- and β-adrenoceptors, the latter of greater importance in the clinical efficacy of this drug in asthma. The pharmacological action of adrenaline is predominantly terminated by tissue uptake (extraneuronal uptake) in airway smooth muscle, gut and liver. However, adrenaline is also sequestered into storage vesicles of nerve endings (neuronal uptake), although this is the smaller of the two uptake compartments[1]. Following uptake into sympathetic nerve terminals, adrenaline is metabolized by deamination and oxidation by monoamine oxidase (MAO) to 3,4 dihydroxymandelic acid[1]. Adrenaline is predominantly metabolized by catechol-O-methyl transferase (COMT) following uptake into extraneuronal sites, resulting in the formation of 3-O-methyl adrenaline (metanephrine). Thus, the combined effects of the two metabolic pathways result in the secretion of

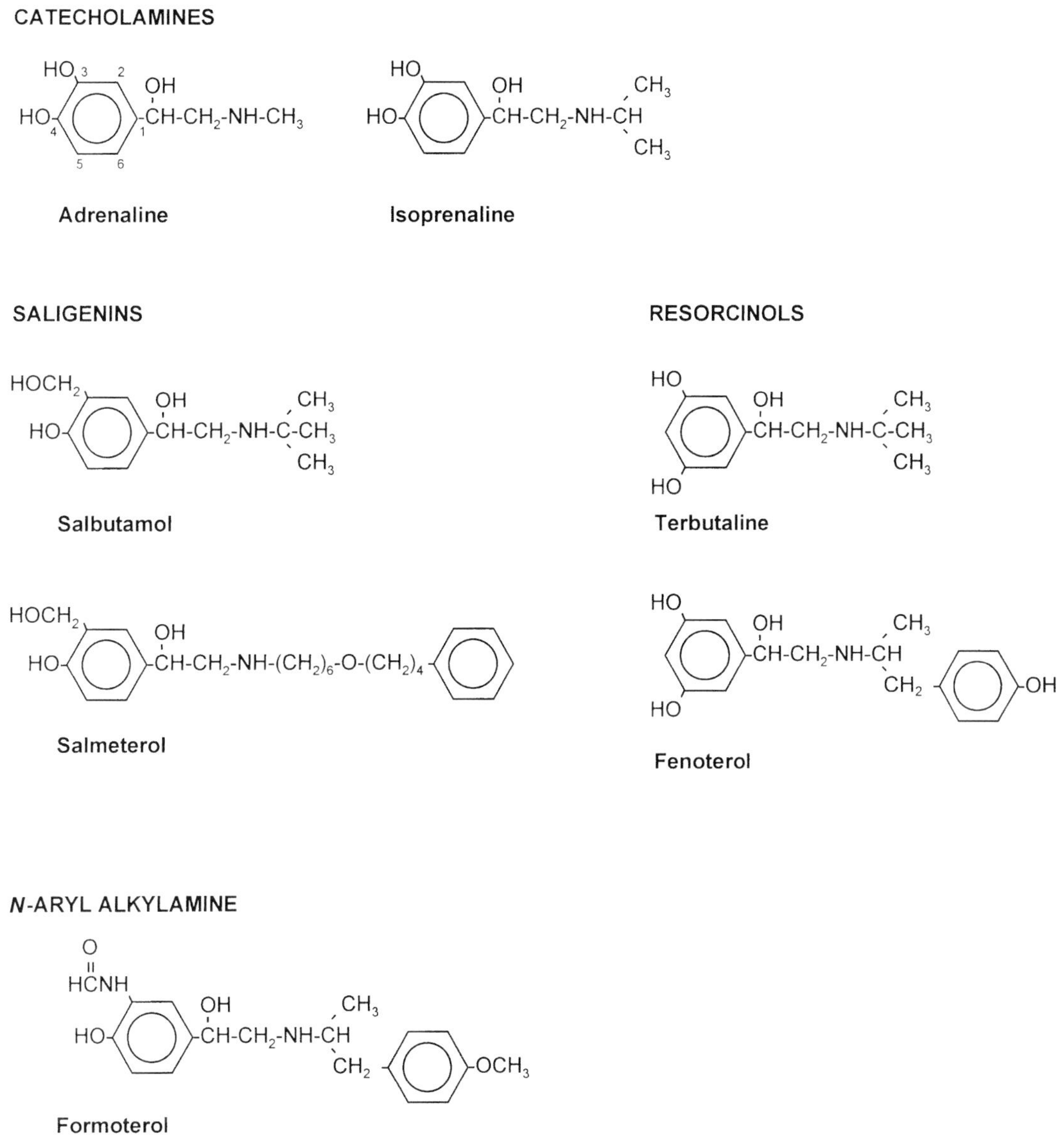

CATECHOLAMINES

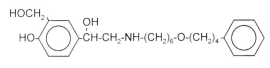

Adrenaline   Isoprenaline

SALIGENINS

Salbutamol

Salmeterol

RESORCINOLS

Terbutaline

Fenoterol

N-ARYL ALKYLAMINE

Formoterol

Fig. 3.1 Chemical structures of catecholamines and currently used β_2-adrenoceptor agonists.

3-methoxy-4-hydroxy mandelic acid (vanillyl mandelic acid)[1]. Adrenaline is a short-acting but potent bronchodilator that is active following inhaled and parenteral but not oral administration.

Isoprenaline

Isoprenaline, like adrenaline, is a catecholamine and was developed in an attempt to increase agonist selectivity for β-adrenoceptors. Significantly greater β-adrenergic selectivity was achieved with isoprenaline by the incorporation of an isopropyl ethanolamine side chain. Following oral administration, large doses are required to produce pharmacological effects since isoprenaline undergoes sulphate conjugation in the gut and liver[2,3] while mainly unchanged drug is excreted in the urine following intravenous administration[3]. However, the powerful cardiovascular stimulatory effect of isoprenaline can preclude its intravenous use. Isoprenaline also undergoes significant 3-O-methylation when administered intrabronchially or by inhalation in man[3,4]. Only approximately 10% of a conventionally delivered metered inhaled dose (MDI) of isoprenaline is deposited into the lungs, while the remainder is swallowed and largely inactivated by sulphate conjugation[3]. Hence, a greater selectivity for pulmonary β-adrenoceptors is achieved when the agonist is given by the inhaled route.

Salbutamol

In an attempt to minimize enzymatic degradation, a number of modifications were made to the basic structure of the catecholamines. Resistance to COMT degradation was achieved by the addition of a methyl group to the 3-hydroxyl group, forming a saligen derivative (e.g. salbutamol). Furthermore, greater selectivity for β_2 over β_1-adrenoceptors was achieved following the addition of a tertiary butyl group to the ethanolamine side chain[5].

Salbutamol is orally active, although it remains susceptible to 4-O'-sulphate conjugation in the intestinal wall and liver in man[6,7]. Following intrabronchial administration of salbutamol there is rapid clearance with no metabolism across the airway wall[8]. Both the free drug and sulfate metabolite appear in the urine following aerosol administration, indicating that much of the aerosol dose is swallowed[6,7]. Salbutamol is also active following intravenous administration of this drug, with lesser amounts of the sulfate conjugate appearing in the urine compared with the inhaled and oral route[6,7].

Salbutamol exists as a racemic mixture of the R (eutomer) and S isomer (distomer) and, while the pharmacological activity of this drug resides with the eutomer, there is increasing evidence that the distomer may exert pharmacological activity unrelated to β_2-adrenoceptor occupancy. This may contribute to the possible adverse effects observed following regular therapy with short-acting agonists[9]. Oral dosing of R,S salbutamol is characterized by significantly greater plasma levels and reduced excretion of the distomer over the eutomer which would be consistent with a greater first pass metabolism and elimination of the eutomer over the distomer[10,11]. In vitro studies have shown that the rate of sulfate conjugation of the eutomer is an order of magnitude greater than for the distomer in liver, gastrointestinal tract[12] and human airway epithelial cells.[13] This would account for the preferential accumulation of the distomer over the eutomer via the oral route of administration.

The administration of R,S-salbutamol by the inhaled route is also associated with greater plasma levels of the distomer over the eutomer. However, a majority of any inhaled dose is swallowed and this difference is most likely attributed to preferential sulphate conjugation of the eutomer across the gastrointestinal tract and in the liver[11]. Moreover, a recent study has demonstrated the preferential retention of the distomer by the lung following inhalation with a metered dose inhaler and a holding chamber to minimize gastrointestinal deposition[14], suggest that the S isomer may accumulate in the lung following regular treatment.

Terbutaline

Another method employed to confer resistance to metabolism by COMT led to the synthesis of terbutaline, a β_2-adrenoceptor agonist that possesses a resorcinol ring structure[15]. Its β_2-selectivity is defined by the tertiary butyl group on the N terminus as for salbutamol. Terbutaline is also susceptible to sulphate conjugation when given by the oral route in man[16,17]. Predominantly unchanged drug is detected in plasma following intratracheal administration of terbutaline in rats, indicating the absence of metabolism across the airway wall[18,19]. Thus, terbutaline is effective when given by the inhaled, oral or intravenous route[20]. In contrast to salbutamol, S-terbutaline shows preferential sulphate conjugation in the liver[21], although it is not known whether the distomer is preferentially retained in the lung.

Fenoterol

Fenoterol has a resorcinol ring structure and thus, like salbutamol and terbutaline, is also resistant to metabolism via COMT. Fenoterol has increased selectivity for β_2- over β_1-adrenoceptors by virtue of a large cyclic structure attached to the N terminal. However, fenoterol appears to be less selective for β_2-adrenoceptors than salbutamol and terbutaline[5]. Fenoterol is effective orally although it is susceptible to 5-O'-sulfation[22,23]. Fenoterol is also effective by intravenous injection and by inhalation and is excreted in the urine relatively slowly, with 12% of a inhaled dose excreted after 24 h[22,23].

Salmeterol

Salmeterol is derived from salbutamol and consists of a phenylethanolamine head and a long non-polar N-substituent (Fig. 3.1) that confers a substantial increase in duration of activity of this molecule[24]. There is a paucity of published papers concerning the pharmacokinetics of salmeterol. Salmeterol is significantly bound to plasma protein in vitro, extensively metabolized by aliphatic oxidation and slowly eliminated in urine and feces[25,26]. Following inhalation of salmeterol (400 μg), oral bioavailability accounted for 28–36% of the systemic response to this drug[27] and indicates that systemic side effects of this drug are predominantly attributed to the inhaled route. The enantiomeric disposition of salmeterol following inhalation remains to be established.

Formoterol

Formoterol contains a formamide group in the 3 position on the benzene ring and an N-aralkyl side chain (Fig. 3.1). Only 10% and 24% of an oral and inhaled dose, respectively, of formoterol was recovered in the urine after 24 h[28,29]. Following oral administration of formoterol (80 mg), 6% and 8% of

the dose was recovered over a 10 h period, as the unchanged and glucuronide conjugate, respectively[29]. The appearance of formoterol in the systemic circulation following inhalation of 120 μg dose in healthy subjects is described by a two-compartment model. A consequence of rapid absorption from the airways and mucosal surfaces, accounting for approximately 70% of the concentration of formoterol detected systemically and a delayed appearance with slower time course, from the gastrointestinal tract[30]. A similar model (see below, abstracted papers) was required to describe the systemic appearance of formoterol following oral administration. It is unclear whether differences in enantiomeric metabolism of formoterol occur but may be inferred since pharmacodynamic modelling shows that formoterol is significantly less potent in reducing plasma potassium levels via the inhaled compared with oral route[30]. Moreover, if like salbutamol preferential sulfate conjugation of the eutomer and retention of the distomer within the lung is known to occur[11,14], this might account for the lower levels of *RR* formoterol detected in the urine[31]. However, further studies are required to quantify the levels of *RR* and *SS* formoterol in the plasma to confirm whether the distomer is preferentially retained within the lung.

Mechanism of action

β_2-adrenoceptor agonists mediate their effects by binding to cell surface glycoproteins which belong to the family of guanosine nucleotide binding protein (G protein) coupled receptors characterized by 7 transmembrane spanning regions (Fig. 3.2). The agonist/receptor complex stabilizes the receptor in its active conformation resulting in the stimulation of heterotrimeric guanine nucleotide regulatory (G) proteins. The G proteins dissociate into α and $\beta\gamma$ subunits which modulate the activity of a variety of effectors including adenylyl cyclase. The activation of adenylyl cyclase results in the production of the second messenger, cyclic-3',5'-adenosine monophosphate (cAMP) and subsequent action of protein

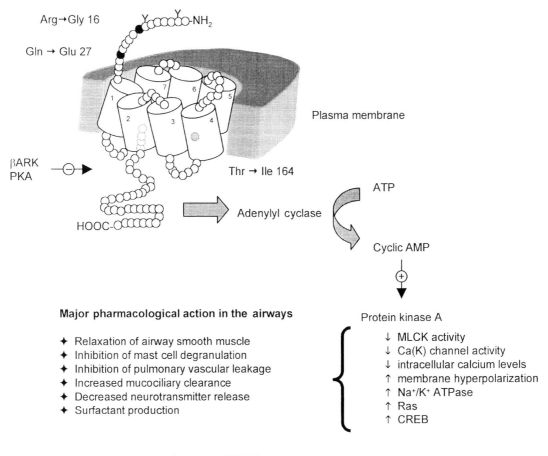

Major pharmacological action in the airways

+ Relaxation of airway smooth muscle
+ Inhibition of mast cell degranulation
+ Inhibition of pulmonary vascular leakage
+ Increased mucociliary clearance
+ Decreased neurotransmitter release
+ Surfactant production

Protein kinase A

↓ MLCK activity
↓ Ca(K) channel activity
↓ intracellular calcium levels
↑ membrane hyperpolarization
↑ Na+/K+ ATPase
↑ Ras
↑ CREB

Major clinical action in asthma/COPD

+ Bronchodilation
+ Bronchoprotection

Fig. 3.2 Diagrammatic representation of the β_2-adrenoceptor highlighting the characteristic seven transmembrane (TSM) spanning regions of the protein together with the localization of three polymorphisms at amino acid positions 16, 27 and 164. For the sake of clarity, the intracellular loops linking TSM5/6 and TSM6/7 are not shown. The amino acids critical for the binding of isoprenaline to the β_2-adrenoceptor are located within the core of the receptor protein.[451] Asp113 (TSM3) and Ser204, 207 (TSM5) are anchoring points for the amine group and hydroxyl groups on the catechol ring, respectively; while interaction between Asn293 (TSM6) binds and the β-hydroxyl group confers stereoselectivity of catecholamine binding. Specific amino acid sequences within TSM4, 6 and 7 are thought to play an important role in anchoring the aliphatic chain of salmeterol (see text). As a consequence of ligand binding, conformational change by the receptor leads to signalling via G protein (not shown), activation of adenylyl cyclase and formation of the intracellular messenger, cyclic AMP. Phosphorylation of the receptor by G-protein coupled receptor kinases (e.g. βARK) leads to homologous desensitization and termination of G-protein signalling. Cyclic AMP in turn, activates protein kinase A which can activate multiple pathways that account for the pharmacological action of β_2-adrenoceptor agonists in the airways. Abbreviations: Arg, arginine; Gly, glycine; Gln, glutamine; Glu, glutamate; Thr, threonine; Ile, isoleucine; PKA, protein kinase A; MLCK, myosin light chain kinase; Ca(K) channel, calcium-activated potassium channel; CREB, cyclic AMP response element binding protein.

kinase (PK)A. PKA phosphorylates a number of proteins including Na^+/K^+ ATPase, myosin light chain kinase (MLCK), large conductance Ca(K) channels, calcium channels and transcription factors (cyclic AMP response element binding protein; CREB)[32,33]. Activation of the β-adrenoceptor has recently been shown to stimulate tyrosine phosphorylation of adaptor proteins and signalling via the Ras pathway, implicated in cell growth and differentiation[34], although the consequence of this novel signalling pathway in the clinical efficacy of these drugs remains to be established.

Specific regions within the receptor core are essential for agonist binding and the subsequent conformational change induced by this interaction leads to activation of the receptor and intracellular signalling. Alterations to the structure of the adrenaline molecule has led to the development of agonists with significantly greater selectivity and potency for the $β_2$-adrenoceptor and improved duration of action, which is considerable for formoterol and salmeterol. In vitro studies demonstrate that formoterol is more potent than salmeterol in relaxing human airway smooth muscle[35,36] reflected by the greater efficacy of formoterol than salmeterol[37] since both drugs have similar affinity for $β_2$-adrenoceptors[38]. Despite this, salmeterol has considerably longer duration of action compared with formoterol in vitro[35,39] but both drugs have long duration of action in vivo[40,41]. The long duration of action of salmeterol is attributed to an interaction between the non-polar N-substituent of salmeterol and the hydrophobic core of the $β_2$-adrenoceptor[24]. This was confirmed in studies using site-directed mutagenesis showing that removal of amino acids 149–173 within transmembrane spanning domain (TSM)4, significantly reduced the ability of salmeterol to persist at the $β_2$-adrenoreceptor[42]. However, binding of salmeterol to this chimeric receptor was not abolished and led investigators to further probe other sites within the receptor protein that might account for the 'tethering' of this molecule to the receptor. Recent studies have suggested that specific amino acid sequences within TSM6 and/or 7 may also be important loci for 'exosite' binding by salmeterol[43,44]. The hypothesis of tethering to the receptor is not universally accepted and another view is that the lipophilic nature of salmeterol is a major determinant of its long duration of action[45,46]. The tethering of salmeterol to the receptor does not apply to formoterol since it lacks the non-polar N-substituent and its duration of actions is thought to be a consequence of retention within the plasma membrane[47].

Prolonged incubation of $β_2$-adrenoceptors with their agonist results in a dose- and time-dependent loss in agonist activity due to receptor phosphorylation, uncoupling from G proteins, receptor internalization and down-regulation of receptor protein. Agonist binding to receptor leads to the activation by G protein coupled receptor kinases (GRKs) and phosphorylation of serine and threonine residues on the C terminus of the protein. This facilitates binding of a cytoplasmic inhibitory protein, β-arrestin which uncouples the receptor from G protein and subsequent internalization, a process known as homologous desensitization (Fig. 3.2). Phosphorylation of the $β_2$-adrenoceptor can also occur via a PKA dependent pathway that can also mediate desensitization of other G protein-coupled receptors, and is termed heterologous desensitization[48]. High efficacy agonists including adrenaline, isoprenaline, fenoterol and formoterol are more efficient than low efficacy agonists like salmeterol in causing $β_2$-adrenoceptor desensitization, internalization and phosphorylation[49–51], as these events are determined by the ability of an agonist to stabilize the receptor in the activated state. Thus, one might predict tolerance to low efficacy agonists would require a longer period of time to develop in vivo.

Receptor desensitization also appears to be tissue dependent. Thus, airway smooth muscle is resistant to desensitization compared with inflammatory cells including mast cells and lymphocytes. The level of β-adrenoceptor receptor kinase (βARK) mRNA in airway smooth muscle was 11% of the level found in mast cells and little βARK protein was found in airway smooth muscle compared with mast cells. GRK activity was tenfold greater in mast cells despite similar levels of PKA activity. These differences in enzyme activity may explain why β_2-adrenoceptors on mast cells are more susceptible to desensitization than airway smooth muscle[52]. It has been suggested that the ability of agonists to induce desensitization is not dependent upon receptor number[50]. However, it is clear that tissues with a greater receptor reserve exhibit a greater degree of resistance to desensitization[53]. Thus, in the clinical setting, β_2-adrenoceptor desensitization will have a greater impact on the function of cell types with low receptor reserve, while airway smooth muscle function would be more resistant to the development of tolerance.

At least nine different variants (polymorphisms) of the β_2-adrenoceptor exist and the three most common polymorphisms are changes in amino acid 16, from arginine to glycine (Gly16); amino acid 27 from glutamine to glutamic acid (Glu27); and amino acid 164, from threonine to isoleucine (Ile164) (Fig. 3.2). The allelic frequencies of these polymorphisms are 54%, 24% and 1% respectively, in asthmatic subjects with moderate to severe asthma, which is similar to that observed in healthy subjects[54]. The functional consequences of these polymorphisms has been investigated and it has been shown that the downregulation of the β_2-adrenoceptor is influenced by two common polymorphisms in the β_2-adrenoceptor gene, which alter the N-terminal domain of the receptor. The Gly16 polymorphism undergoes enhanced receptor down-regulation while Glu27 polymorphism confers resistance to down-regulation. Receptors expressing both Gly16 and Glu27 are also susceptible to desensitization in vitro[55,56]. The Ile164 polymorphism results in a receptor with a fourfold loss in binding affinity for adrenaline, reduced coupling to G protein and desensitization[57]. The clinical significance of the Gly16 allele include a greater frequency in the occurrence of nocturnal symptoms[58]; asthmatic subjects are more likely to be glucocorticosteroid dependent[54]; and asthmatic children are less likely to bronchodilate in response to salbutamol[59]. However, this allele is not a major determinant of the prevalence of asthma in children or adults[54,59–62] and therefore is not a major factor in

the pathophysiology of asthma but may be an important pharmacogenetic factor in the treatment of asthmatic subjects. In contrast, asthmatic subjects with the Glu27 polymorphism are less likely to demonstrate bronchial hyperresponsiveness[62,63] and there is an association between Gln27 polymorphism and childhood asthma[61], total IgE[64] and bronchial hyperresponsiveness[63]. While these studies have investigated the associations between single polymorphisms and the asthma phenotype, population based studies have begun to examine haplotypes of the β_2-adrenoceptor gene and their association with bronchial hyperresponsiveness. It appears that the β_2-adrenoceptor haplotype with Gly16/Gln27 polymorphism is associated with bronchial hyperresponsiveness[65], although in another study, the Gly16/Glu27/Thr164 haplotype appeared to be protective for bronchial hyperresponsiveness[66]. The need to repeat these studies in populations solely consisting of asthmatic subjects with bronchial hyperresponsiveness will be critical in furthering our understanding of the role of β_2-adrenoceptor polymorphism in asthma.

Route of administration

Maximal bronchodilator activity can be achieved by the oral, intravenous or inhaled route resulting in a dose-dependent increase in forced expiratory volume in 1 second (FEV_1) for a number of agonists including isoprenaline and salbutamol[67], terbutaline[68], fenoterol[23] and formoterol[69]. The increase in heart rate observed with maximal bronchodilator doses of the non-catecholamine agonists are considerably lower than those achieved for isoprenaline. However, to achieve maximal bronchodilation by the systemic route, cardiac stimulation is unavoidable as a consequence of a reduction in total peripheral resistance resulting in reflex activation of cardiac β_1-adrenoceptors[70]. Furthermore, because a significant population of β_2-adrenoceptors exists in the human heart some cardiac activation is to be expected for even very selective β_2-adrenoceptor agonists[71–73].

The inhaled route offers a number of advantages over the systemic route including direct access to the lung and rapid onset of action with considerably lower systemic activity. Comparison of the dose–effect curves for terbutaline[68], salbutamol[74] and formoterol[75] given systemically or by inhalation, demonstrate that at maximal levels of bronchodilation, the systemic side effects are considerably less significant by the inhaled than by the systemic route.

In mild asthmatic subjects, inhaled salbutamol was shown to provide better bronchodilator relief than intravenous salbutamol[74]. In contrast, patients with acute severe asthma who responded poorly to inhaled salbutamol, responded favourably to intravenous salbutamol[76,77]. The diminished bronchodilator efficacy observed in severe asthma is possibly a consequence of reduced penetration of the bronchodilator due to mucus plugging and edema[78]. In contrast, a number of studies have shown the inhaled route to be as effective as the intravenous route in acute severe or moderately severe asthma[79–81]. The difference in the results may be related to the severity of the disease and the size of the population studied. Recently a large multicentre study demonstrated that in severe acute asthma, salbutamol was more efficacious by the inhaled route than by the intravenous route. Consequently, it has been recommended that nebulized bronchodilator should be used in the treatment of severe acute asthma[82].

Duration of action by inhaled route

Baseline FEV$_1$

Catecholamines including isoprenaline and isoetharine exert their maximal bronchodilator effect within 5 min. In contrast, the non-catecholamines including salbutamol, terbutaline and fenoterol produce 80% maximal bronchodilation within 5 min, with maximal bronchodilation between 15 and 60 min.[1] The duration of bronchodilation for equieffective doses of the non-catecholamine β_2-adrenoceptor agonists is sustained for approxi-mately 2–6 h[23,83–91]. In contrast, both formoterol[40,41,75,92] and salmeterol[40,41,93] are potent bronchodilator agonists compared with salbutamol, although the onset of the bronchodilator response to salmeterol is much slower than for salbutamol and formoterol[40,41]. These clinical findings are consistent with in vitro functional studies documenting that formoterol and salmeterol are considerably more potent than salbutamol in relaxing human airway smooth muscle in vitro[35,36,94] and the onset time for salmeterol is slower than for formoterol and salbutamol[35].

The duration of bronchodilation is also considerably longer for salmeterol and formoterol compared with short acting β_2-adrenoceptor agonists. Both formoterol[75,92,95–97] and salmeterol[91,93,98] provide sustained bronchodilation for 6–12 h in adult asthmatic subjects. Formoterol also provides sustained bronchodilation in asthmatic children for a similar length of time[99,100]. Since the duration of drug activity is dependent on the dose,[101] it is possible that the long duration of action of these drugs in vivo, might be attributed to the use of maximal doses of bronchodilator. However, formoterol[40,99] and salmeterol[40] produce sustained bronchodilation for 6–12 h compared with 2–6 h for an equieffective dose of salbutamol. In vitro studies in human airways demonstrate that salmeterol has a considerably longer duration of action compared with formoterol[35,36]. However, equieffective doses of formoterol and salmeterol cause sustained bronchodilation for at least 12 h[40,41]. Interestingly, the duration of bronchodilation for equieffective doses of orally administered salbutamol and formoterol are similar[69], although the reason for this is unclear.

Bronchospasm

The duration of action of β_2-adrenoceptor agonists following spasmogen-induced bronchoconstriction has also been investigated and is of particular interest as an exacerbation of asthma can be triggered by many provoking stimuli and it is desirable to obtain prolonged and effective bronchoprotection, thereby reducing the severity of asthma symptoms.

The duration of action of a number of non-catecholamine β_2-adrenoceptor agonists at clinically relevant doses against histamine-[90,91,102], exercise-[103] and eucapnic and isocapnic hyperventilation-induced[104,105] bronchospasm peaks between 1 and 2 h and resolve by 4 h. Hence, these agonists provide less protection against bronchoconstriction to provoking stimuli compared with their prolonged effect on baseline FEV_1. This presumably reflects the inability of these drugs to functionally antagonize bronchospastic agonists at a time when the concentration at effector sites is reduced, although high enough to induce maximal reduction of baseline FEV_1[90].

In contrast to the short acting β_2-adrenoceptor agonists, both salmeterol[91,98,106] and formoterol[99,106–108] provide significant bronchoprotection against direct acting stimuli including histamine and methacholine for up to 24 h. Furthermore, significant protection against exercise-induced bronchospasm was afforded for up to 12 h by salmeterol[103,109–114] and formoterol[115–118] which is considerably greater than the protection (less than 4 h) provided by an equieffective dose of salbutamol. Similarly, formoterol afforded protection against cold air hyperventilation-induced bronchospasm for 8 h, while the beneficial effect of salbutamol had resolved after 4 h[119]. Salmeterol provided significant protection against bronchoconstriction induced by sulfur dioxide[120] and distilled water[121] for up to 20 h. This substantially longer duration of action by salmeterol and formoterol compared with shorter duration β_2-adrenoceptor agonists is obviously of clinical importance in providing symptomatic relief over a prolonged period of time to stimuli which asthmatic subjects are likely to encounter in their environment.

In the clinical setting β_2-adrenoceptor agonists are generally taken during an exacerbation of asthma and the onset of action is of considerable importance. In this regard, it has been shown that salmeterol is significantly slower than both salbutamol and formoterol in reversing bronchoconstriction induced by methacholine[122,123] and therefore salmeterol should not be used as rescue medication.

β-adrenoceptor agonist selectivity and efficacy

Selectivity

Isoprenaline provides fast bronchodilator relief, although it possesses powerful cardiac stimulatory activity. It was subsequently shown that the rise in asthma deaths during the 1960s was correlated with the consumption of isoprenaline and while providing short-term bronchodilator relief, contributed to the delay in the introduction of corticosteroid therapy in patients whose asthma was deteriorating because of worsening inflammation or tolerance[124,125]. It was also thought that the powerful cardiac stimulatory effects may have been a contributing factor[126]. The demonstration of β-adrenoceptor subtypes[127] prompted the development of more β_2-selective and potent bronchodilators such as salbutamol, fenoterol and terbutaline.

Fenoterol is a full agonist compared with salbutamol and terbutaline in relaxing airway smooth muscle obtained from asthmatic[128] and non-diseased lung[36,37,128]. Functional studies in the guinea-pig trachea and atria reveal that while fenoterol is significantly more potent than salbutamol and terbutaline on guinea-pig trachea, both salbutamol and terbutaline are approximately twofold more β_2-selective than fenoterol[5,129,130]. Similarly, a recent radioligand binding study has confirmed that salbutamol is 2.9-fold more selective for β_2 than β_1-adrenoceptors compared with fenoterol.[38] This increase in β_2-adrenoceptor selectivity might be expected to confer airway vs. systemic selectivity and thereby reduce systemic side effects. However, this receptor subtype is present on human cardiac muscle that also is responsible for mediating both chronotrophic and inotrophic effects[131]. Thus, β_2-adrenoceptor agonists can have both direct cardiac stimulation and reflex action due to stimulation of presynaptic β_2-adrenoceptors.

A number of studies have shown that fenoterol has greater inotrophic, chronotrophic, electrocardiographic and hypokalaemic effects than salbutamol and terbutaline in both healthy individuals[132–135] and asthmatic subjects[136–138]. Fenoterol is approximately twofold more potent than salbutamol with regard to increasing heart rate and reducing plasma levels of potassium[132,134,138]. The cardiostimulatory and hypokalemic effect of β_2-selective agonists observed in the studies cited above occurs at doses that are not recommended by the manufacturers. However, under conditions of severe exacerbation of asthma large doses of these agonists may be consumed, which might result in cardiostimulatory and hypo-kalaemic side effects. This is particularly relevant for fenoterol since it is marketed at a higher equivalent dose than salbutamol and, as a consequence, side effects are more likely to be manifested in asthmatic subjects who undergo acute exacerbation of asthma[138]. However, it is important to recognize that tolerance to these extrapulmonary effects occurs following chronic β_2-adrenoceptor agonist therapy[131,139].

Formoterol and salmeterol are considerably more potent than salbutamol. A number of studies have shown that formoterol and salmeterol are 116–323 and 2–62 fold more potent, respectively, than salbu-tamol in relaxing human airway smooth muscle.[35–37] In rat atria, salmeterol is three orders of magnitude less potent than isoprenaline as a cardiac stimulant and behaves as a partial agonist[94]. In contrast, for-moterol is 12-fold more β_2-selective than salbutamol and is a full agonist in guinea-pig atria[130], and radio-ligand binding studies have confirmed that formot-erol and salmeterol are 60 and 190 times, respectively, more selective for β_2- than β_1-adreno-ceptors[38].

While it is clear that formoterol and salmeterol are more potent than salbutamol on airway smooth muscle, they are not devoid of systemic side effects. In healthy volunteers, both formoterol (24 µg) and salbutamol (200 µg) increased cardiovascular parameters including heart rate and QTc interval to a similar degree, although less than for fenoterol (400 µg)[140]. In contrast, fenoterol and formoterol were more effective than salbutamol in reducing serum potassium levels. Similarly, salmeterol is at least eight times more potent than salbutamol at producing systemic side effects in healthy volun-teers[141]. In asthmatic subjects, significant falls in

serum potassium and increased tremor was observed following inhalation of high doses of for-moterol (60–120 µg) and salmeterol (500 µg)[142]. Together, these studies show that formoterol and salmeterol also demonstrate airway vs. systemic selectivity, but are not devoid of systemic side effects, particularly at doses not recommended by the guidelines.

Efficacy

Efficacy is a dimensionless proportionality factor that describes the ability of an agonist to induce a response in a particular tissue. Hence, an agonist with high efficacy can elicit a maximal response by occupying relatively fewer receptors (greater pro-portion of spare receptors) than an agonist with low efficacy[143].

A number of in vitro studies using airway smooth muscle have demonstrated an inverse relationship between the level of contraction induced by a spas-mogen and the potency and maximum degree of relaxation induced by β_2-adrenoceptor ago-nists[144–147]. Thus, under normal contractile condi-tions, β_2-adrenoceptor agonists may induce maximal relaxation, but the capacity of these ago-nists to induce relaxation of highly contracted muscle may differ[146]. The ability of these agonists to induce maximal relaxation was significantly reduced in maximally contracted preparations of human bronchus[148], guinea pig trachea[146,149], bovine trachea[145] and canine trachea[147]. Other studies have examined whether application of these drugs prior to the addition of a bronchoconstrictor agonist pre-empted contraction of airway smooth muscle. Contraction induced by methacholine was func-tionally antagonized by isoprenaline in bovine trachea[145] and by salbutamol and fenoterol[149] but not terbutaline[150] in guinea pig tracheal tissue. The reasons for the failure of Gustafsson and Persson[150] to observe similar phenomena with terbutaline are puzzling, but may be due to the use of low concen-trations of these agonists. These studies indicate that β_2-adrenoceptor agonists are effective at inhibiting the development of contraction, and the ability to functionally antagonize spasmogen-induced contractile responses is also dependent on the contractile agonist used as demonstrated in vitro[144,145,151] and in vivo[152]. Very few studies have compared the efficacy of the different β_2-adrenoceptor agonists. The efficacy of fenoterol is twice that of salbutamol in guinea-pig trachea[149]; and while equieffective doses of salbutamol, fenoterol and terbutaline are indistinguishable with respect to their ability to increase baseline FEV_1[88,153,154], salbutamol and fenoterol were more potent than terbutaline in antagonizing histamine-induced bronchospasm in asthmatic subjects[138].

Salmeterol is less effective than formoterol and salbutamol in reversing baseline tone in human airways,[35–37] which suggests that salmeterol has lower efficacy than formoterol and this difference in efficacy is highlighted further if bronchial tone is increased[36,37,155,156]. The clinical implications of the differences in efficacy between formoterol and salmeterol remain to be established. However, while equieffective doses of these agonists produces a similar degree of bronchodilation in asthmatic subjects, formoterol produced a greater degree of bronchoprotection than salmeterol[142], and the implications of this study is that, during a severe exacerbation of asthma, formoterol will afford better bronchoprotection than salmeterol. The potential disadvantage of a high efficacy β_2-adrenoceptor agonist is that, during exacerbations of asthma when consumption may be high, drugs like fenoterol[138] and formoterol[142] have the potential to produce greater cardiovascular side effects than drugs with lower efficacy including salbutamol and salmeterol.

Sites of action

Airway smooth muscle

A variety of functional, biochemical, radioligand binding and autoradiographic techniques have confirmed the presence of β_2-adrenoceptors on human airway smooth muscle[157]. Activation of these receptors leads to relaxation, which is a consequence of inhibition of myosin light chain kinase, membrane hyperpolarization, reduction in intracellular calcium, inhibition of phosphoinositide hydrolysis and stimulation of $Na^+/K^+ATPase$[32,33]. Both salmeterol and formoterol are potent inhibitors of airway smooth muscle function, characterized by long duration of action. The inhibition of contractile responses elicited by cholinergic nerve stimulation is abolished for at least 12 h following termination of exposure with salmeterol[94]. The duration of action of formoterol is longer than salbutamol but considerably shorter than salmeterol, as assessed against reversal of basal tone in human isolated bronchus[35,36]. The difference in duration of action between formoterol and salmeterol in vitro is probably a consequence of the tethering of salmeterol to the receptor, a feature not exhibited by formoterol. The greater potency of formoterol and retention within the plasma membrane may help explain its long duration of action in vivo. The proliferation of human airway smooth muscle is also a function of considerable importance in the context of airway remodelling that occurs in asthma. β_2-Adrenoceptor agonists have been demonstrated to attenuate the proliferation of human airway smooth muscle cells in culture in response to various mitogens[158,159], although it remains to be established whether this class of drug has significant antiproliferative action in asthma.

Mast cells

In 1968, it was shown that isoprenaline inhibited histamine release from leukocytes isolated from allergic individuals.[160] It was subsequently demonstrated that β_2-adrenoceptor agonists inhibit histamine release from passively sensitized chopped human lung[161–164], human dispersed mast cells[165,166] and human mast cells in culture.[167] The activation of β_2-adrenoceptors present on mast cells inhibits not only the release of histamine, but also prostaglandin (PG)D_2, cysteinyl leukotriene (LT)C_4 and LTD_4[162,164,166–168]. Similarly, both salmeterol[169] and formoterol[39] are potent inhibitors of mediator release from human lung mast cells following stimulation of IgE-dependent pathways. β_2-Adrenoceptor agonists are potent mast cell stabilizers, approximately 2000 – 30 000 times more potent than the putative mast cell stabilizer disodium cromoglycate, with respect to inhibiting mediator release from human lung mast cells in vitro[162,163,166]. Similarly, formoterol was shown to be approximately 12 000 times more potent than disodium cromoglycate with respect to inhibiting IgE-dependent release of slow releasing substance of anaphylaxis from rat peritoneal mast cells[170].

Mast cells are also repositories for various cytokines (e.g. tumour necrosis factor (TNF)α, interleukin (IL)-4 and IL-5) and chemokines (e.g. monocyte inflammatory protein (MIP)1α), which are thought to play an important role in airway inflammation. The release of TNFα from human skin mast cells by antigen is inhibited by salbutamol[171] and salmeterol, an effect that is blocked by β-adrenoceptor antagonists[172]. Similarly, granulocyte monocyte colony stimulating factor (GMCSF), IL-5 and MIP1α release from human mast cells in culture, is also inhibited by salbutamol[173]. Together, these studies demonstrate that, as a class, β_2-adrenoceptor agonists are potent inhibitors of mast cell function and therefore have the potential to inhibit mast cell-dependent pathways in vivo.

Following acute allergen provocation in asthmatic subjects, a rise in circulating plasma levels of histamine and neutrophil chemotactic factor[174,175] and a rise in the level of histamine, PGD_2, and cysteinyl leukotrienes in bronchoalveolar lavage (BAL) fluid have been documented[176–179]. In asthmatic subjects, salbutamol inhibits the allergen-induced rise in plasma histamine and neutrophil chemotactic factor[174,176] and is two orders of magnitude more effective than disodium cromoglycate (a drug considered to be a mast cell stabilizing agent) at inhibiting allergen-induced mediator release in vivo[176]. In contrast, both salbutamol and salmeterol failed to attenuate the allergen-induced rise in urinary excreted LTE_4, which may suggest that β_2-adrenoceptor agonists have little effect on mast cell mediator release in vivo, although it is far from clear whether urinary LTE_4

levels reflect only mast cell-derived LTE_4[180]. A number of cells including airway epithelial cells, macrophages and eosinophils secrete sulfidopeptide leukotrienes[181] and activation of the β_2-adrenoceptor residing on these cells may impart a lesser inhibitory response than for mast cells.

Despite a significant improvement in morning peak expiratory flow (PEF) and reduced nocturnal symptom scores following 6-week treatment with salmeterol (50 µg b.i.d.), there was no reduction in mast cell number in bronchial biopsies or levels of mast cell-derived mediators in BAL fluid[182]. Similarly, regular treatment with formoterol had no effect on mast cell number in bronchial biopsies, and failed to reduce the level of tryptase in BAL fluid[183]. However, despite a reduction in mast cell number following regular budesonide treatment, this was not accompanied by a fall in tryptase levels in BAL fluid. Thus, the effect of long-acting β_2-adrenoceptor agonists on mast cell function in vivo, remains to be established. While there are several challenges in determining whether these agonists inhibit mast cell function in vivo, it seems likely that β_2-adrenoceptor agonists do have an action upon mast cells. These cells are accessible to antigens within the inspired air, and therefore would also be accessible to inhaled β_2-adrenoceptor agonist. Furthermore, their location close to airway epithelium, would make them a potential target for these drugs.

Other evidence also supports the notion that mast cells are targets for inhaled β_2-adrenoceptor agonists. Adenosine or the water soluble precursor, adenosine monophosphate (AMP), mediates indirect bronchoconstriction via degranulation of mast cells and/or activation of afferent nerves. It is of interest that terbutaline[184,185], salbutamol[152,186] and formoterol[187] functionally antagonized the bronchoconstriction to adenosine to a significantly greater extent than direct acting stimulants like histamine and methacholine. This has been interpreted as an indication that these drugs have actions additional to inhibition of airway smooth muscle function, including an inhibitory action of these drugs on mast cell degranulation induced by adenosine. In contrast, salmeterol did not demonstrate preferential bronchoprotection to AMP compared with histamine[186,188] and might be a reflection of the low efficacy demonstrated by salmeterol compared with agonists of greater efficacy (e.g. formoterol[189]). In cells with low β-adrenoceptor density, activation of adenylyl cyclase by salmeterol is considerably less efficient compared with adrenaline which has greater efficacy[50]. This situation is likely to occur in mast cells, which are known to have low receptor reserve[53] and under these circumstances, salmeterol will be a poor inhibitor of mast cell function in vivo.

Endothelial cells

Local instillation of allergen onto the bronchial mucosa of asthmatic subjects causes acute swelling and narrowing of the airways as visualized through a bronchoscope[178,190,191]. It appears that this response is mediated by smooth muscle constriction and bronchial wall edema. A number of pharmacological agonists, including histamine, bradykinin, cysteinyl leukotrienes and capsaicin or activation of IgE bearing cells, are capable of increasing plasma protein extravasation and edema within the bronchial wall, as documented in studies in experimental animals[192,193]. Vascular leakage is a consequence of endothelial cell contraction, thereby promoting gap formation between endothelial cells in pulmonary venules. It is presumed that the 'anti-edema' property of β_2-adrenoceptor agonists is a consequence of functional antagonism of endothelial cell contraction[194]. Systemic administration of terbutaline attenuated topically applied histamine-, bradykinin- and capsaicin-induced plasma protein extravasation and/or edema in bronchial wall or lumen[192,193,195].

Several studies have failed to demonstrate this 'anti-edema' property. Intravenously administered salbutamol failed to attenuate airway edema in guinea-pigs induced by intravenously administered PAF[196] or topically applied LTD_4[197]. However, the bronchospasm mediated by intravenously administered LTD_4 was inhibited. A number of factors including hemodynamic changes mediated by the intravenous administration of these agonists and the failure to take into account residual blood volume remaining within the pulmonary vasculature, may confound analysis[193]. Such methodological problems can be minimized by measuring plasma protein extravasation and edema within the bronchial lumen and/or introducing β_2-adrenoceptor agonist directly to the lung[193,198]. It has subsequently been demonstrated that formoterol inhibits plasma protein extravasation and lumenal edema in response to allergen, bradykinin[193] and histamine[199]. The 'anti-edema' effect of formoterol was greater than that of salbutamol in terms of potency and duration of activity[193]. Similarly, salmeterol was also effective against histamine-induced plasma protein extravasation in guinea-pigs[200].

The expression of adhesion molecules on vascular endothelium plays a critical step for the transmigration of cells into sites of inflammation and the effect of β_2-adrenoceptor agonists on the expression of adhesion molecules has received scant attention. The expression of E-selectin following stimulation of human microvascular endothelium with TNFα was not inhibited by salbutamol, although the combination of salbutamol with a phosphodiesterase (PDE)4 inhibitor, rolipram, did attenuate the expression of the adhesion molecule E-selectin but not ICAM-1 or VCAM-1[201].

In healthy individuals, the wheal response to intradermal injection of bradykinin[202], histamine[202], and both the wheal and flare response to intradermal injection of anti-IgE[203–205] are attenuated by prior injection of β_2-adrenoceptor agonists. A similar finding has also been reported for the allergen-induced early cutaneous response in atopic subjects[204,206]. Furthermore, formoterol[204] and salmeterol[207] produce a longer lasting protection against anti-IgE-induced wheal and flare response and late cutaneous reaction than terbutaline in healthy individuals[205]. It is possible that the effect of formoterol on the edema response is secondary to inhibition of mediator release from mast cells. However, if formoterol is administered 30 min after the induction of mast cell degranulation, the anti-edema properties of formoterol were still evident[208].

Moreover, salmeterol inhibited the extravasation of a plasma-derived protein, alpha$_2$-macroglobulin, into skin chambers induced by blisters on the forearm of allergic rhinitis subjects[209].

The inhibitory effect of β_2-adrenoceptor agonists on edema in the respiratory system has only recently been investigated in the human. Analogous to studies in the skin, edema can be assessed by measuring the level of plasma derived proteins, including albumin and alpha$_2$-macroglobulin that is extravasated into the airways by an inflammatory stimulus. High doses of terbutaline[210] and salmeterol[211,212] administered to the nasal mucosa prior to antigen challenge, significantly attenuated plasma protein extravasation in response to intranasal antigen challenge. This effect was attributed to a direct action on endothelial cells as there was no reduction in the release of mast cell-derived mediators following antigen challenge[212]. Similarly, inhalation of a single dose of formoterol (18 µg) significantly attenuated the increase in sputum levels of alpha$_2$-macroglobulin induced by histamine in healthy volunteers[213].

Inflammatory cells

A number of inflammatory cells are thought to contribute toward the pathogenesis of asthma, including eosinophils[214], lymphocytes[215], platelets[216], and macrophages[217]. Since increasing the intracellular level of cyclic AMP inhibits the function of many inflammatory cells[218], the role of β_2-adrenoceptors in modulating the function of inflammatory cells has been investigated.

Platelets

Human platelets contain β_2-adrenoceptors, although they appear to be poorly coupled to adenylyl cyclase.[219] It is therefore of interest that salbutamol has been demonstrated to inhibit exercise-induced platelet activation in subjects with asthma[220].

Eosinophils

The effect of β_2-adrenoceptor agonists on eosinophil function remains the subject of considerable debate.

Eosinophils obtained from individuals with blood eosinophilia contain β_2-adrenoceptors which are coupled to adenylyl cyclase, although activation of these receptors by salbutamol failed to inhibit superoxide generation and the release of eosinophil peroxidase (EPO) using a number of stimuli, including C5a and IL-5[221,222]. However, EPO release induced by FMLP was attenuated by salbutamol[222–224]. Similarly, respiratory burst[225,226] and LTC$_4$ synthesis[227] from human eosinophils was inhibited by salbutamol and isoprenaline. Salmeterol has been documented to inhibit a variety of eosinophil functions in human including respiratory burst[222], adhesion[222], EPO release[223], chemotaxis[228] but not PAF and LTC$_4$ synthesis[228]. Eosinophil apoptosis appears to be delayed by salbutamol, fenoterol and salmeterol, but inhibited by theophylline and dibutyryl cyclic AMP[229], suggesting a non-β_2-adrenoceptor-dependent mechanism in the ability of these agonists to delay apoptosis.

The anti-eosinophilic activity of salmeterol may be unrelated to β_2-adrenoceptor occupancy, since the action of salmeterol was not reversed by beta-adrenoceptor blockade[222]. Furthermore, salmeterol failed to inhibit chemotaxis of rat eosinophils in vitro in response to LTB$_4$ and PAF, despite raising intracellular levels of cyclic AMP[230], nor inhibit respiratory burst in guinea-pig eosinophils[231]. In contrast, other studies have shown that salmeterol did inhibit aggregation of guinea-pig eosinophils in response to C5a and PAF via stimulation of β_2-adrenoceptors[232]. Since salmeterol is a partial agonist, it can be shown, in some circumstances, to act as an antagonist in the presence of drugs with higher efficacy and the ability of salbutamol[223] and formoterol[231] to attenuate eosinophil activity was antagonized following pretreatment with salmeterol.

A number of clinical studies have assessed the effect of β_2-adrenoceptor agonist therapy on pulmonary eosinophil number and activation in asthma. Regular 4-week treatment with inhaled terbutaline (500 µg, *q.i.d.*) failed to alter the number of circulating eosinophils[233] or to significantly reduce the level of eosinophil cationic protein (ECP) recovered in BAL fluid in mild asymptomatic asthmatic subjects[234].

Quantitative light and electron microscopic analysis of bronchial biopsies from these patients also revealed that regular treatment with terbutaline failed to alter the number of eosinophils or foci of eosinophil-derived granules[235,236]. Similarly, 16 weeks of regular treatment with salbutamol failed to significantly reduce the number of activated eosinophils (positive for EG2) in bronchial biopsies[237]. In contrast, anti-inflammatory agents, including budesonide and disodium cromoglycate reduced the levels of ECP[234] and the number of eosinophils[238] in BAL fluid from asthmatic subjects. Furthermore, inhaled glucocorticosteroids are also effective in reducing the number of eosinophils and foci of eosinophil-derived granules in bronchial biopsies obtained from asthmatic subjects and are associated with clinical improvements in their asthma[235,236,239]. Acute antigen challenge results in a significant increase in eosinophils and EG2 + cells recovered in sputum that is reduced in asthmatic subjects treated with inhaled glucocorticosteroid[240]. In contrast, the number of eosinophils and EG2 + eosinophils in sputum observed 7 h after antigen challenge was significantly increased following 7-day treatment with salbutamol (200 μg, *q.i.d.*)[241]. Together, these studies demonstrate that regular treatment with short-acting β_2-adrenoceptor agonists fails to exert any significant anti-eosinophilic action, which is in direct contrast to inhaled glucocorticosteroids.

Similarly, acute administration of salmeterol (50 μg or 100 μg), while inhibiting the early and late asthmatic response, had no effect on blood eosinophil number and serum ECP levels[242,243], while the number of eosinophils and ECP levels in sputum was attenuated 24 h following treatment[244]. However, the variability between the different treatment groups was considerable in this study. Seven-day treatment with salmeterol (50 μg *b.i.d.*) also had no effect on blood eosinophil number but did result in a twofold fall in serum ECP levels[245]. In contrast, despite significant improvements in a variety of clinical indices including diurnal variation in PEF and improved morning PEF following 3-week treatment with salmeterol (100 μg/day), there was no significant reduction in sputum eosinophil number and

ECP levels. In contrast, treatment with beclomethasone was effective against both clinical parameters and markers of inflammation[246]. Similarly, 8-week treatment with salmeterol (50 μg *b.i.d.*) failed to significantly reduce the number of eosinophils in BAL fluid in asthmatic subjects regularly taking glucocorticosteroids[247]. Conversely, salmeterol failed to prevent the rise in sputum eosinophils following stepwise reduction of inhaled glucocorticosteroid in asthmatic subjects who required high dose glucocorticosteroid for control of their symptoms.[248] The administration of salmeterol during this period led to stable asthma symptoms and significant improvements in FEV$_1$ and PEF; however, this was at the expense of worsening airway inflammation as reflected by an increase in sputum eosinophil number. Similarly, while a significant reduction in nocturnal awakening was observed after 6-week treatment with salmeterol (100 μg *b.i.d.*), this was not accompanied by a significant reduction in the number of eosinophils in BAL fluid nor in levels of eosinophil derived cationic proteins[249]. A recent study has revealed that 8-week treatment with formoterol (24 μg, *t.i.d.*) failed to significantly reduce the number of activated eosinophils in bronchial biopsies, although in those subjects with a high degree of activated eosinophils, formoterol had a significant anti-inflammatory activity.[183] However, the interpretation of the data is difficult given that budesonide treatment was without significant effect on the number of activated eosinophils. Moreover, it has also been shown that 6-week[182] and 12-week[250] treatment with salmeterol (50 μg *b.i.d.*) failed to reduce the number of eosinophils or levels of EG2 + eosinophils, despite significant improvements in morning and evening PEF and reduced asthma symptoms compared with placebo control.

Thus, while there is some evidence that β_2-adrenoceptor agonists can influence eosinophil function in vitro, these anti-eosinophilic properties are poorly translated in the clinical setting and, compared with glucocorticosteroids, which have proven anti-inflammatory activity, are considerably less effective. This assessment is also valid for long-acting β_2-adrenoceptor agonists, which have little if any demonstrable anti-eosinophilic properties in asthma.

Macrophages

Human alveolar macrophages may play a role in asthma as they contain low affinity IgE receptors[251] and are a potential source of inflammatory mediators[217]. The role of β_2-adrenoceptors on human alveolar macrophages is controversial. Radioligand binding studies indicate that a small population of β_2-adrenoceptors reside on human alveolar macrophages and activation of these receptors results in a two to sixfold increase in cyclic AMP[252,253]. Isoprenaline and salbutamol failed to inhibit zymosan- or IgE-induced release of mediators or superoxide anions by human alveolar macrophages[253–255]. Similarly, salbutamol, terbutaline, formoterol and salmeterol were without effect upon LTB_4 release from human alveolar macrophages stimulated by LPS or zymosan[256]. While salmeterol was shown to inhibit the release of thromboxane from human alveolar macrophages, this appeared to be independent of the activation of β_2-adrenoceptors and attributed to the stabilizing action of the aliphatic tail[254].

A number of in vitro studies have investigated the role of β_2-adrenoceptors upon the release of cytokines and chemokines from macrophages. The release of $TNF\alpha$ and IL6 was decreased, while IL10 was increased in differentiated U937 cells by clenbuterol via a β_2-adrenoceptor dependent mechanism[257]. Similarly, $MIP1\alpha$ release from RAW264.7 macrophages stimulated by LPS was inhibited by isoprenaline[258]. In contrast, salbutamol, terbutaline, formoterol and salmeterol were without effect upon $IL1\beta$ release from human alveolar macrophages stimulated by LPS or zymosan[256]. Further studies are required to determine whether β_2-adrenoceptor agonists inhibit the release of other cytokines and chemokines from human alveolar macrophages.

Lymphocytes

There is increasing evidence that lymphocytes play an important role in asthma[215] and COPD[259]. Human lymphocytes contain β_2-adrenoceptors, which are coupled to adenylyl cyclase and are susceptible to desensitization[260–262]. Stimulation of these receptors leads to an alteration in lymphocyte function including inhibition of lymphocyte proliferation, cytokine generation, expression of cytokine receptors and antibody production in vitro[263,264]. In asthma, lymphocyte β-adrenoceptor density and function are reduced as a consequence of disease[265–267] and following regular treatment with β_2-adrenoceptor agonists[260–262]. The consequences of these changes in asthma are not known.

Lymphocytes are a heterogeneous population of cells including B- and T-cells. The latter group may be further subdivided into T-helper (Th, CD4+), T-suppressor/cytotoxic (CD8+) and natural killer (NK) cells. Radioligand binding studies demonstrate that B-cells contain a large number of β-adrenoceptors that are poorly coupled to adenylyl cyclase. In contrast, T-cell subsets possess β-adrenoceptors that are functionally linked to adenylyl cyclase[268]. Following 7 days' treatment with terbutaline (500 µg, *t.i.d.*) in healthy individuals, there was a greater reduction in cell number, β-adrenoceptor density and adenylyl cyclase activity in circulating CD8+ than CD4+ cells, resulting in an increase in the CD4+/CD8+ ratio[268,269]. These data suggest that there is differential regulation of T-cell subsets following β-adrenoceptor stimulation with a greater antiproliferative action on CD8+ than CD4+ T-cells[270]. The ramification of these changes in the context of asthma has yet to be established. An increase in CD4+ cells with a concomitant reduction in CD8+ cells is thought to participate in the exacerbation of asthma[271].

However, different functional subsets of CD4+ T lymphocytes have been classified on the panel of cytokines they release and skewing of cytokine production to a Th2 phenotype is implicated in the pathogenesis of allergic disease[215]. Therefore, it is of interest that β-adrenoceptor agonists inhibit the production of IL-12 from human monocytes, a cytokine implicated in the development of a Th1 response[272] and consistent with the findings that murine Th1 but not Th2 cells contain functional β_2-adrenoceptors, the density of which increases following activation[273,274]. During priming of neonatal T-lymphocytes, the presence of β-adrenoceptor agonist promoted the development of Th2 cells[272] and augments the ability of PDE4 inhibitors to attenuate the release of Th1 cytokines, IFNγ and IL-2 from human peripheral blood mononuclear cells[275]. Furthermore, it has recently been documented that β_2-adrenoceptor agonists facilitate the release of Th2 cytokines from human mononuclear cells, presumably by inhibiting IFNγ production from Th1 cells[276].

A number of studies have shown that high concentrations of salmeterol, salbutamol and isoprenaline inhibited the proliferation of human peripheral blood mononuclear cells and appeared to inhibit IL4 production[277]. However, the effect of salmeterol upon human T-cell proliferation was not inhibited by a β_2-receptor antagonist[278]. In another study, salbutamol and fenoterol potentiated the effect of IL4 on IgE production[279], presumably a consequence of the ability of β-adrenoceptor agonists to inhibit IFNγ production, a known inhibitor of B cell function[275,277,279]. Isoprenaline downregulated the expression of mRNA for IFNγ and upregulated mRNA for IL5 in peripheral blood T-cells[280].

T lymphocytes have been implicated as playing a significant role in the pathogenesis of asthma[281] and it is clear that anti-inflammatory agents including glucocorticosteroids[239,282] and theophylline[283] reduce the number of activated T-lymphocytes in bronchial biopsies from asthmatic subjects. Few studies have investigated the effect of regular treatment with β_2-adrenoceptor agonists on T-lymphocyte activation in asthma. Regular treatment with terbutaline for a 3-month period significantly reduced the number of T-lymphocytes in bronchial epithelium,[236] although this was not a consistent finding[235]. Regular treatment with salmeterol[182,250] or formoterol[183] also failed to reduce the number of CD4 or CD8 positive lymphocytes or the proportion of activated (CD25 +) T-lymphocytes in bronchial biopsies from mild asthmatic subjects. Thus, unlike glucocorticosteroids and theophylline, β_2-adrenoceptor agonists do not appear to exert any significant anti-lymphocytic activity in asthma.

Neutrophils

A role for neutrophils in the pathophysiology of asthma is less clearly defined, as some studies have shown no difference in the number of neutrophils in bronchial biopsies in atopic asthmatic subjects and healthy individuals[284–286]. However, increased numbers of neutrophils are observed in severe asthma[287], during nocturnal asthma[288] and in COPD[289]. Human neutrophils possess β_2-adrenoceptors, which are linked to adenylyl cyclase[290–292], and the release of lysosomal β-glucuronidase, generation of superoxide anions and inflammatory mediators from human neutrophils activated by zymosan-treated serum and by calcium ionophore A23187 are inhibited by β_2-adrenoceptor agonists[293,294]. Similarly, fenoterol inhibited C5a-induced neutrophil migration in vitro, although it did not modify the expression of various adhesion molecules and did not affect intracellular killing of bacteria or phagocytosis[295]. The ability of salmeterol to inhibit respiratory burst in human neutrophils stimulated with FMLP was not reversed by a β-adrenoceptor antagonist[296–298]. Formoterol produced a modest inhibition of respiratory burst in human neutrophils but unlike salmeterol possessed only weak membrane stabilizing activity[297].

The adhesion of human neutrophils to bronchial epithelium was attenuated by salmeterol and isoprenaline in the presence of the non-selective PDE inhibitor, IBMX[299], and salbutamol (200 µg) inhibited the pulmonary sequestration of radiolabelled neutrophils induced by PAF in healthy volunteers[300].

Beneficial clinical effects of β-adrenoceptor agonists

Acute bronchospasm

Acute administration of β_2-adrenoceptor agonists in subjects with asthma results in a significant loss in airway sensitivity to spasmogens. For example, salbutamol reduced airway sensitivity to various spasmogens including histamine in both a dose-[90,102,301,302] and time-dependent[90,91,102] manner, without an alteration in slope of the spasmogen dose–response curve[90,102,152,303]. In contrast, some studies have shown an increase in the slope of the histamine dose–response curve following inhalation of these agonists.[302,304] The short-acting β_2-adrenoceptor agonists also afford protection against bronchospasm induced by a wide range of provocative stimuli, including allergen[174,176,260,305,306], eucapnic and isocapnic hyperventilation[104,105,307], exercise[308–310], and hypo-osmolar[311] and hyperosmolar stimuli[312]. Similarly, salmeterol and formoterol also reduce airways responsiveness to inhaled spasmogens including histamine and methacholine[91,97–99] and are potent inhibitors of the bronchoconstriction induced by allergen[97,98,243], cold air hyperventilation[119,313,314], and exercise[103,113–115,118,315]. This functional antagonism persists well after the effects of shorter-acting β_2-adrenoceptor agonists have resolved and is a reflection of prolonged retention of salmeterol and formoterol in the lung compared with salbutamol.

A number of studies have shown that there is apparently no direct relationship between the ability of β_2-adrenoceptor agonists to induce an increase in baseline FEV_1 and their ability to reduce the potency of bronchoconstrictor agents[102,152,302,316–318]. This inability to obtain a direct relationship might be attributed to the use of maximal bronchodilator doses of β_2-adrenoceptor agonist in these studies[102,302]. A direct relationship between reduction in baseline FEV_1 and the decrease in spasmogen potency was found with submaximal doses of these agonists[301]. However, the muscarinic receptor antagonist, ipratropium bromide, failed to alter airway sensitivity to histamine despite causing an increase in baseline FEV_1[301]. These studies, together with the demonstration of a difference in the effectiveness of β_2-adrenoceptor agonists against changes in FEV_1 and spasmogen potency in time course studies[90,102], illustrate that bronchodilation *per se* is not necessary for the bronchoprotection against a variety of bronchoconstrictor stimuli. It is therefore the ability of these agonists to functionally antagonize the response to spasmogens that is important.

Late asthmatic response

A characteristic feature of some asthmatic subjects is the development of a late phase airway obstruction 4–10 h following exposure to allergen that is associated with pulmonary recruitment of eosinophils[319] and increased bronchial responsiveness to spasmogens[305]. Clinically relevant doses of short-acting β_2-adrenoceptor agonists, including salbutamol, do not inhibit the development of the allergen-induced late asthmatic response[305,320]. In contrast, glucocorticosteroids, disodium cromoglycate[305], theophylline[321,322] and cysteinyl leukotriene (cysLT)$_1$ receptor antagonists[323] inhibit the development of the late asthmatic response via mechanisms unrelated to bronchodilation. Due to the relatively short duration of action of the short-acting β_2-adrenoceptor agonists, it is perhaps not surprising that they are ineffective during the late asthmatic response particularly when administered just prior to antigen challenge. However, these agonists can attenuate the late asthmatic response if administered at the appropriate time. Both fenoterol and salbutamol were shown to reverse the fall in baseline FEV_1 when administered during the late asthmatic response to house dust mite or occupational sensitizing agents[119,324].

The failure of salbutamol to attenuate the late asthmatic response[305], could be attributed to the use of doses of salbutamol which are too low, since duration of action is dose dependent[86]. Inhalation of high dose nebulized terbutaline (5 mg)[325] and salbutamol (2.5 mg)[326], or high dose salbutamol by MDI (500 µg)[327] prior to allergen challenge, appeared to attenuate the development of the late asthmatic response. More recently it has been shown that, at clinically relevant doses, both salmeterol[98,243,328] and formoterol[97,327] inhibit the late asthmatic response when given prior to allergen inhalation. It has been suggested that the attenuation of the late response by high dose salbutamol and salmeterol is due to a putative anti-inflammatory effect based on the diminished bronchodilator activity of β_2-adrenoceptor agonists at the time of the late response[98,326]. However, these data only provide circumstantial evidence of anti-inflammatory activity, since the recruitment of inflammatory cells, notably lymphocytes and eosinophils, was not assessed during the late response. An alternative explanation of the data is that these drugs mask the expression of the late response due to functional antagonism of the allergen-induced changes in FEV_1[97,243]. Despite significant attenuation of the late asthmatic response, salmeterol failed to inhibit the rise in sputum eosinophils observed 7–48 h following antigen challenge[328]. These observations are consistent with the overwhelming evidence that this class of drug has weak anti-eosinophilic properties in asthma.

Bronchial hyperresponsiveness

The allergen-induced increase in airway responsiveness that commonly accompanies the late response is not modified by inhaled salbutamol. In contrast, both glucocorticosteroids and disodium cromoglycate attenuate this increase in airway responsiveness[305]. These data suggest that β_2-adrenoceptor agonists fail to modify the underlying inflammatory process presumably responsible for the exacerbation of bronchial hyperresponsiveness. However, inhalation of nebulized salbutamol (2.5 mg), significantly attenuated the allergen-induced increase in airways responsiveness to histamine over a 3.5–7.5 h period[326]. Similarly, salmeterol and formoterol have both been demonstrated to attenuate the allergen-induced exacerbation of bronchial hyperresponsiveness observed during, and 24–32 h following, inhalation of allergen[97,98]. However, contradictory conclusions have been drawn from these studies. The inhibitory effect of high dose salbutamol[326] and salmeterol[98] on exacerbation of bronchial hyperresponsiveness was attributed to the possible anti-inflammatory properties of these drugs. This conclusion was based on the fact that the bronchodilator effect of high dose salbutamol during the late asthmatic response and of salmeterol 32 h after allergen inhalation, was minimal[98]. In contrast, the beneficial effect provided by formoterol at 24 h

could be explained in terms of functional antagonism of changes in airway tone[97].

Asthmatic subjects are extremely responsive to spasmogens, and this is reflected by dose-response curves that are positioned to the left and described by an increase in maximum bronchoconstrictor response, compared with healthy individuals[329,330]. This excessive airway narrowing observed in asthma, which is reflected by an increase in the maximum response to spasmogens, is thought to be a consequence of the inflammatory process[330]. It is therefore of interest that 4 weeks' regular treatment with budesonide in mild asthmatic subjects resulted in a small decrease in airways sensitivity to methacholine, but more importantly, was associated with a significant reduction in the level of maximal airway narrowing[302]. In contrast, 8 weeks regular treatment with salmeterol caused a substantial decrease in airways sensitivity to methacholine, but without affecting the level of maximal airway narrowing[331]. These data also suggest that β_2-adrenoceptor agonists lack anti-inflammatory activity and illustrate the effectiveness of glucocorticosteroids in this regard.

Nocturnal asthma

In normal individuals lung function varies in a circadian rhythm with modest bronchoconstriction occurring during the night. This is significantly exaggerated in most asthmatic subjects who are woken at least occasionally by nocturnal wheeze and cough with the frequency increasing in moderate to severe asthma. It has been demonstrated that clinically stable patients with nocturnal asthma become hypoxemic during the night and have poorer daytime cognitive performance and poorer subjective and objective sleep quality than normal subjects. A decrement in sleep quality leads to muscle fatigue and hypoxaemia, events which can be fatal in patients with severe acute exacerbations[332,333].

Nocturnal exacerbations of asthma are associated with increased vagal activity[334], platelet activation[335], reduced inhibitory non-adrenergic non-cholinergic activity[336] and with increased recruitment and activation of inflammatory cells notably neutrophils, eosinophils and T-lymphocytes[249,337,338]. The exaggerated bronchoconstriction observed in nocturnal asthma can be attenuated by β_2-adrenoceptor agonists, ipratropium bromide, theophylline and glucocorticosteroids[332,333]. However, the choice of drug is determined by the patient's ability to tolerate side effects and, in the case of β_2-adrenoceptor agonists, duration of action is an important consideration. Slow release[339] and maintenance salbutamol[340] were not entirely effective against nocturnal asthma, presumably due to a decline in clinically effective levels of salbutamol in the airways. In contrast, oral terbutaline significantly protected asthmatic subjects against nocturnal asthma, which was associated with a marginal reduction in the use of inhaler during the night[341–243]. Comparisons between different bronchodilators is futile unless equieffective doses are used. However, the protective effect of terbutaline was associated with no improvement in the quality of sleep, as assessed by electroencephalography[342]. These studies demonstrate that protection against nocturnal asthma can be afforded by short-acting agonists if used in high concentrations, although this in itself may be a limiting factor. Moreover, it may not be possible to provide effective bronchoprotection during the night if bedtime is early as is the case for children, and the duration of effect wanes in the early hours of the morning. It then becomes obvious that drugs with considerable duration of action, like formoterol and salmeterol would be far superior to conventional β_2-adrenoceptor agonists in the treatment of nocturnal asthma.

Formoterol provided significant protection against nocturnal bronchoconstriction following a single inhalation[96], and significantly reduced the frequency of sleep disturbances during 1-month[344] and 3-month[345] treatment periods. Similarly, 2-week treatment with salmeterol provided better subjective sleep quality than salbutamol in asthmatic subjects without nocturnal asthma[346], while 1-week treatment provided significant protection against the fall in lung function during the night and improved objective sleep quality[347], although the latter effect has been disputed[348]. Longer treatment with salmeterol over a 6-week period provided significant protection against nocturnal airway obstruction, reduced the circadian variation in PEF, reduced bronchial hyper-responsiveness to methacholine[349], reduced nocturnal awakenings[249] and improved daytime cognitive performance[350]. These improvements attributed to salmeterol were also observed with fluticasone with no difference between treatment groups[349,350]. Objective measurements of improvements in the quality of sleep, length of sleep or number of interruptions of sleep were not made and it is difficult to ascribe the improvements in daytime cognitive performance to suppression of airways responsiveness and improvements in baseline FEV_1. A recent study has shown that regular treatment with salmeterol is associated with improvements in sleep quality global scores[351].

COPD

Bronchodilator drugs are currently used in the treatment of COPD, a disease characterized by chronic airflow obstruction, which leads to a gradual decline in maximum expiratory flow and slow forced emptying of the lung. The obstruction is often non-reversible, although there can be a small degree of airway reversibility[352]. Short-acting β_2-adrenoceptor agonists produce modest improvements in airflow obstruction and exercise performance in COPD and most likely reflects their short-effect duration[352]. In contrast, a number of studies have reported sustained bronchodilation for 12 h following inhalation of a single dose of salmeterol and formoterol in COPD subjects[353–355]. Similarly, regular treatment with salmeterol for periods of up to 16 weeks is often associated with a clear improvement in quality of life and walking distance in COPD subjects, which appears to be accompanied by modest increases in pulmonary function[356–360]. This suggests that mechanisms additional to functional antagonism of

airway smooth muscle, including increased mucociliary clearance, pulmonary vasodilation and
decrease in neurotransmission, may account for the
beneficial action of these drugs in COPD. It remains
to be established whether treatment with long-
acting β_2-adrenoceptor agonists reduces the decline
in lung function in this airway disease.

Chronic β-adrenoceptor agonist therapy

While there is no doubt concerning the clinical efficacy of β_2-adrenoceptor agonists in the symptomatic relief of asthma and COPD, there is some
evidence that chronic treatment may produce a
number of untoward effects including loss of bronchodilator and bronchoprotective effectiveness and
increased bronchial hyper-responsiveness in
asthma. The clinical significance of these findings
has not been resolved.

Bronchodilator tolerance

The clinical response to inhaled β_2-adrenoceptor
agonists has been shown to diminish as the severity
of the disease increases[361]. A number of factors
accounting for this phenomenon include reduced
penetration of drug to the airways as lung function
deteriorates[78]; the increasing influence of inflammation and mucus plugging in determining airway
calibre which is not modified by this class of agonist
or loss of bronchodilator function due to increased
severity of bronchospasm[361]; and/or a consequence
of receptor desensitization[362].

Healthy individuals continually exposed to β_2-
adrenoceptor agonists become refractory to
β_2-adrenoceptor stimulation[363,364]. However, asthmatic subjects chronically treated with salbutamol[139,260,364,365], or terbutaline[74,346] do not develop
tolerance to the bronchodilator activity of these agonists as assessed by measurements of changes in
FEV_1 and airways conductance. In the studies cited
above, bronchodilator dose–response curves were
performed to determine whether regular agonist
treatment exerted any bronchodilator tolerance.

However, in one study, the duration of the bronchodilator effect to salbutamol was monitored in
subjects who received salbutamol (180 μg, *q.i.d.*) for
13 weeks[366]. Of particular interest was the finding
that, while the peak bronchodilator response to
inhaled salbutamol was not altered, there was a significant decrease in the duration of the bronchodilation. Thus, under appropriate conditions,
bronchodilator tolerance can be observed in asthmatic subjects following regular treatment with salbutamol. However, it is clear that airway smooth
muscle β_2-adrenoceptors are relatively resistant to
development of bronchodilator tolerance and this
may be a consequence of the presence of a large
receptor reserve, which can mask any loss in β_2-
adrenoceptor function due to desensitization[367]. In
contrast, desensitization is observed in leukocytes
from asthmatic subjects following regular β_2-
adrenoceptor agonist therapy [260] and extrapulmonary responses including tremor and increased
heart rate are subject to tachyphylaxis[74,139,260]. This
would be consistent with the hypothesis that receptor reserve is less in cells other than airway smooth
muscle. With the introduction of long-acting β-
adrenoceptor agonists into the clinic, a number of
studies have evaluated whether there is any loss in
bronchodilator activity of these drugs. Regular treatment with formoterol[344,368] and salmeterol[331] did not
reduce the ability of these drugs to induce bronchodilation *per se* although this is not a consistent
observation[369].

Under the current asthma guidelines, rescue medication with short-acting β_2-adrenoceptor agonists
is used in asthmatic subjects regularly treated with
salmeterol and formoterol and a number of studies
have addressed the issue of whether bronchodilator
potency to rescue medication is altered in these
patients. Asthmatic subjects who received salmeterol (50 μg *b.i.d.*) for a 4-week period became tolerant
to the bronchodilator effects of salbutamol[370],
although this was not confirmed in a recent study[371].
Similarly, no loss in bronchodilator potency to salbutamol is observed in subjects who have regularly
taken formoterol[368], although loss in bronchodilator
efficacy to formoterol was observed following 2-

week regular treatment with this drug[369]. This discrepancy in the literature may be due to confounding by an increase in baseline FEV_1 following treatment with long-acting β_2-adrenoceptor agonist, which would leave little room for improvement in baseline FEV_1 by inhalation of salbutamol, and therefore could be interpreted as a loss in bronchodilator function. Alternatively, patients selected in these studies may have differential susceptibility to desensitization because of differences in β_2-adrenoceptor polymorphisms. Individuals with Gly16 genotype undergo a greater loss in bronchodilation to formoterol[372] but not to salbutamol[373] following regular treatment with formoterol. Asthmatic children with Gly16 allele were also less likely to bronchodilate in response to single inhaled dose of salbutamol[59], although it was not clear whether these subjects responded by increasing the dose of salbutamol. Therefore, loss in bronchodilator function may be influenced by these polymorphisms in selected patient groups.

The clinical significance of some of the reported changes in bronchodilator sensitivity to rescue medication following regular treatment with β_2-adrenoceptor agonist appears to be small and may only be of clinical relevance in subjects with the Gly16 allele. However, increasing the dose of rescue medication would be predicted to overcome this problem. Even if there were impaired beta-adrenoceptor function, as only a small percentage of the total receptor pool is required for maximal bronchodilation, there would have to be a considerable reduction in receptor number to have any significant impact on bronchodilator potency. For asthmatic subjects undergoing a severe exacerbation of asthma, the impact of mucus plugging and edema would pose a far greater problem in impeding access of bronchodilator to airway smooth muscle than any putative loss in bronchodilator efficacy secondary to desensitization.

Loss in bronchoprotection

The effect of regular β_2-adrenoceptor agonist therapy on bronchoprotection to offending stimuli is of more concern, since a loss in the ability of these drugs to act as a functional antagonist to the effects of spasmogens could leave individuals less protected during an exacerbation of asthma. This loss in bronchoprotection can be studied in a variety of ways, either the PC_{20} to spasmogen is determined at various times during regular treatment with these agonists[374]; or the ability to protect against bronchoconstriction is measured at various times during the regular treatment protocol[331].

A number of studies have failed to demonstrate any significant loss in bronchoprotection against histamine following 3–5 week regular treatment with salbutamol and terbutaline[260,364,365]. Conversely, other studies have demonstrated this phenomenon against histamine[375] and methacholine[184,374,376–378]. The discrepancies in the literature may reflect differences in methodology, patient selection, duration of treatment and whether sufficient time is allowed for bronchodilator to be eliminated from the airways prior to the measurement of airways responsiveness, which may confound attempts to establish loss in bronchoprotection. Similarly, various studies have investigated the effect of antiasthma drugs on the shape of the dose–response curve to inhaled spasmogens. Salbutamol and salmeterol steepen the dose–response curve to methacholine[302,379] and this may be of significance since the slope of the dose–response curve is thought to reflect the degree of airway narrowing and may represent an index of thickened airway wall secondary to inflammation[330]. These findings suggest that β_2-adrenoceptor agonists, while providing effective bronchoprotection acutely, may mask the potential for rapid bronchoconstriction following exacerbation of airway narrowing particularly following regular therapy. In contrast, glucocorticosteroids like budesonide[302] and fluticasone[380] reduce the slope and restore the plateau of the dose–response curve to methacholine, observations which have been taken as evidence that, unlike β_2-adrenoceptor agonists, glucocorticosteroids can reduce airway wall thickening by virtue of their anti-inflammatory properties. A reduction in protection afforded by salmeterol was found following an 8-week treatment period. The loss in protection from 3.3 doubling doses (DD) after a single dose to 1.1 DD was observed after 4 and 8 weeks of treatment[331], a finding that has been confirmed in a number of studies[379,381–384]. Similarly, bronchoprotection by formoterol was significantly reduced 12 h after the first dose from 3.4 DD to 0.5 DD after 2 weeks' treatment with formoterol (24 μg *b.i.d.*)[374].

While methacholine and histamine are often used to assess loss in bronchoprotection, a number of studies have investigated whether loss in bronchoprotection occurs to more clinically relevant stimuli like exercise or antigen or to stimuli that activate cellular components of the asthma response like mast cells. Regular treatment with salbutamol or terbutaline resulted in a significant loss in bronchoprotection to AMP[184,185]; exercise[385,386]; acute bronchoconstriction to antigen challenge[261,376,378]; and increased the magnitude of the late asthmatic response induced by allergen[377]. Loss in protection against bronchoconstriction to adenosine[189] and antigen[387,388] is also observed following 1 week's treatment with formoterol and salmeterol, respectively. Similarly, 1–4 weeks' regular treatment with salmeterol (50 μg *b.i.d.*) also lead to a loss in protection against bronchospasm induced by exercise[110,113,114]. In general, the use of indirect acting stimuli including allergen, AMP and exercise are more sensitive indicators of loss in bronchoprotection to regularly administered β_2-adrenoceptor agonists. The mechanism of this effect remains to be established; however, the loss in bronchoprotection to exercise observed following regular administration of salbutamol [386] or salmeterol[110,113,114] was reversed by acute administration of bronchodilator. These studies suggest that airway smooth muscle β_2-adrenoceptor function is not unduly compromised during regular treatment, and loss, if any, of receptor function on airway smooth muscle can be overcome by increasing concentrations of β_2-adrenoceptor agonist at effector sites.

The loss in bronchoprotection afforded by regular treatment with β_2-adrenoceptor agonists might also have implications during an exacerbation of asthma when rescue medication with salbutamol is often employed. Regular treatment with terbutaline (1 mg *b.i.d.*) for 6 weeks led to a twofold loss in the ability of salbutamol to reverse an established increase in baseline FEV_1 with inhaled methacholine, in order to mimic an exacerbation of asthma[389]. This suggests that subjects may have to resort to using higher doses of their rescue medication following regular treatment with short-acting bronchodilator drugs. Similarly, following a single dose or regular treatment with salmeterol or formoterol, there was a significant loss in bronchoprotection to rescue medication with salbutamol when administered up to 1.6 mg[390–392]. Whether these findings of loss in efficacy to rescue medication following regular treatment with β_2-adrenoceptor agonists have an impact in the clinical setting remains to be established. A recent study has shown that subjects who were taking regular salmeterol as part of their medication responded to high dose salbutamol as rescue medication in the emergency room[393].

It is clear that an overwhelming number of studies provide evidence that a loss in bronchoprotection can occur following regular β_2-adrenoceptor agonist treatment; however, it is recognized that not all subjects are susceptible to this loss in bronchoprotection[383,388,394] and this may reflect differences in β_2-adrenoceptor polymorphisms. In one study, the loss in bronchoprotection to AMP following regular treatment with formoterol did not appear to be linked to Gly16 allele[189], although the small sample size precludes any definitive assessment of these polymorphisms and loss in bronchoprotection to AMP. In a more recent study, the bronchoprotection efficacy of salbutamol was attenuated after a single administration of formoterol or salmeterol, which appeared to correlate with those individuals with Gly16 allele[391]. More studies with a greater number of subjects are required to investigate the relationship between loss in bronchoprotection following regular treatment and β_2-adrenoceptor polymorphism. Thus, while a number of these studies seem artificial, it may closely model the situation in the general population where asthmatic subjects will be less compliant with their medication. Under these conditions, the loss of protection afforded by β_2-

adrenoceptor agonists will be manifested under conditions of elevated basal tone, as would be expected during an exacerbation of asthma. The exact mechanism contributing to this loss in protection against bronchospastic stimuli following regular bronchodilator therapy might be a consequence of the inability of these agonists to control the inflammatory process and/or desensitization.

If exacerbation of the inflammatory response and/or desensitization are explanations for the loss in bronchoprotection afforded by β_2-adrenoceptor agonists, then presumably concurrent treatment with glucocorticosteroids may ameliorate this phenomenon. Glucocorticosteroids control the synthesis of β_2-adrenoceptors by increasing gene transcription and protein density in a variety of cells within the lung and have the potential to reverse desensitization and augment bronchodilator efficacy in asthmatic subjects[395]. However, despite these mechanisms of action, glucocorticosteroids failed to reverse isoprenaline-induced desensitization in human airway smooth muscle in vitro[396] or desensitization in alveolar macrophages during oral treatment with terbutaline in healthy volunteers[367]. It is unclear whether regular high doses of β_2-adrenoceptor agonist promote the sequestration of the glucocorticosteroid–glucocorticosteroid receptor complex from promoter regions within the β_2-adrenoceptor gene, and thereby reduce the ability of glucocorticosteroids to normalize receptor function[395].

It is therefore of considerable interest that the loss in bronchoprotection to exercise[113], acute allergen challenge[397], AMP[185], and methacholine[389] following regular treatment with short- and long-acting β_2-adrenoceptor agonists was not abolished following treatment with inhaled glucocorticosteroids in steroid-naïve asthmatic subjects. Similarly, in asthmatic subjects regularly taking glucocorticosteroids as part of their therapy, loss in bronchoprotection to AMP[398] and methacholine[374,382,383] was still evident following regular treatment with salmeterol and formoterol. In contrast, the loss in bronchoprotection against antigen challenge following regular treatment with salmeterol is only partially restored when subjects are treated with inhaled glucocorticosteroid[388]. However, loss in bronchoprotection to AMP following regular treatment with formoterol is reversed by an acute bolus dose of inhaled budesonide (1.6 mg)[398]. Similarly, loss in bronchodilator potency to formoterol following regular treatment with this drug is reversed following acute (1 h) administration of systemic glucocorticosteroid[399]. The differences in the reported efficacy of glucocorticosteroids between these studies does not appear to be dependent upon the Gly16 polymorphism, since the ability of glucocorticosteroid to reverse the loss in bronchoprotection to AMP was independent of this polymorphism[398]. While this loss in bronchoprotection seen with regular β_2-adrenoceptor treatment is relatively resistant to glucocorticosteroid treatment, it is reassuring that high dose or systemic administration of glucocorticosteroid can overcome any deleterious action of β_2-adrenoceptor agonists on bronchoprotection[398,399].

Bronchial hyperresponsiveness

The apparent lack of protection afforded by regular β_2-adrenoceptor agonist therapy against bronchospastic stimuli was investigated further in studies assessing the effect of long-term treatment with these agonists on bronchial hyperresponsiveness. Initial studies found no significant change in bronchial responsiveness following regular 4-week treatment with salbutamol (100–500 µg, q.i.d.)[364,365] or terbutaline (300 µg, t.i.d.)[260] and following regular 2-year treatment with terbutaline (375 µg, b.i.d.)[400]. In contrast, regular administration of terbutaline (750 µg t.i.d.) for 2 weeks followed by cessation of administration for 23 h, resulted in a rebound increase in bronchial responsiveness to histamine[375]. This effect was attributed to desensitization that was not sufficient to reduce the response to inhaled β_2-adrenoceptor agonists. However, it was sufficient to reduce the protective effect of endogenous catecholamines in the lung and thus cause rebound bronchial hyperresponsiveness[375].

In other chronic studies, a small increase in bronchial responsiveness was observed following regular

2-week (500 μg, *q.i.d.*)[233] and 6-month treatment with terbutaline (500 μg, *q.i.d.*)[401]; and regular 2-month treatment with fenoterol (200 μg, *t.i.d.*)[402]. Similarly, a small increase in airway responsiveness to histamine was observed following regular 1-year treatment with salbutamol (400 μg, *q.i.d.*)[403]. Note that the small increase in bronchial hyper-responsiveness to histamine was not attributable to desensitization (as reflected by changes in baseline lung function to salbutamol) and was not observed following regular treatment with ipratropium bromide[403]; indicating that bronchodilation was not responsible for the observed effect. The effect of regular treatment with β_2-adrenoceptor agonists on bronchial hyper-responsiveness is conflicting, possibly due to patient selection, number and/or the dose of agonist. One criticism of some of these studies is the absence of a control group and the clinical significance of these small changes. The increase in bronchial hyperresponsiveness might simply reflect a deterioration of the disease over time. Bronchial hyperresponsiveness to histamine was significantly reduced when the same patients[234,404] or a parallel group of patients[233,401] were treated with glucocorticosteroid. Furthermore, the change in bronchial hyperresponsiveness in response to glucocorticosteroids was of a similar magnitude to that observed with β_2-adrenoceptor agonist but in the opposite direction[233,401,404]. These changes produced by glucocorticosteroids have often been used to argue the beneficial anti-inflammatory nature of this class of drug.

The magnitude of the changes in bronchial hyper-responsiveness produced by regular treatment with β_2-adrenoceptor agonists is small, ranging from 0.6–1.5 DD of spasmogen[233,375,400–402]. The clinical significance of these small changes in airway responsiveness is not known. During the pollen season, airway responsiveness is increased by a similar order of magnitude and is associated with exacerbation of symptoms that is reversible by glucocorticosteroid treatment[405,406]. Furthermore, a small change in bronchial hyperresponsiveness in the population may significantly increase the proportion of patients with severe asthma (Fig. 3.3)[407].

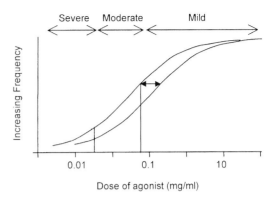

Fig. 3.3 Frequency distribution of asthma severity based on the dose of agonist which causes a 20% fall in FEV_1. On theoretical grounds, small changes in bronchial hyper-responsiveness (double-headed arrow) in a population leads to a small increase in the number of patients with mild to moderate asthma, but a substantial increase in the proportion of subjects with severe asthma. The question of whether regular treatment with β_2-adrenoceptor agonists increases asthma morbidity is a hotly debated issue. (Modified from Mitchell et al., 1989.[407])

In some studies, bronchial hyperresponsiveness was not altered following regular agonist therapy, although a deterioration in lung function[408] and an increase in asthma symptoms[400] were observed. In contrast, regular treatment with glucocorticosteroids not only significantly improves bronchial hyper-responsiveness, but also improves lung function and reduces symptoms[400,404]. Together, these studies indicate that, unlike glucocorticosteroids, regular treatment with β_2-adrenoceptor agonists fail to control the disease.

Very few studies have investigated the effect of regular treatment with salmeterol and formoterol on airway responsiveness to bronchoconstrictor stimuli. Rebound bronchial hyperresponsiveness has not been documented after cessation of regular treatment with salmeterol[331,409] or formoterol[410].

Regular vs. symptomatic therapy

Short-acting β-adrenoceptor agonists
Since the 1980s there has been a considerable debate as to whether β_2-adrenoceptor agonists

should be used on a regular basis or only when circumstances are such that symptomatic treatment is necessary. The general consensus is that short-acting β_2-adrenoceptor agonists should only be used when required, since regular use provides no clinical advantage, and in some circumstances can lead to deterioration in disease.

Regular 2-week treatment with inhaled salbutamol was shown to provide better control of asthma symptoms than salbutamol *p.r.n*[411]. However, closer examination of the results demonstrate that, for a similar degree of control of asthma symptoms, the total aerosol consumption per day was 10.8 compared with 5.7 puffs/day in the regular and *p.r.n.* group, respectively. These findings indicate that there was no advantage in taking regular salbutamol over *p.r.n.* use. Conversely, better control of symptoms and lung function was apparently observed in asthmatic subjects taking salbutamol regularly compared with the 'as needed' use of salbutamol for 1 year, although none of the data was analysed statistically[412]. However, the apparent beneficial effect afforded with regular treatment with salbutamol was at the expense of more bronchodilator; 5.0 compared with 1.7 doses of salbutamol in the prophylactic compared with the symptomatic group, respectively. Furthermore, the FEV_1 values in the intermittent group tended to fall, together with an increase in the consumption of rescue β_2-adrenoceptor agonist medication when this group of patients was crossed over to regular bronchodilator use. Conversely, the regularly treated group demonstrated improved FEV_1 with less consumption of these drugs when crossed over to the intermittent arm of the experiment[412].

A number of studies have demonstrated that regular treatment with β_2-adrenoceptor agonists is no better or worse than symptomatic treatment. No significant difference in symptoms was observed in asthmatic subjects taking regular or *p.r.n.* salbutamol for 1 month[413]. However, to achieve comparable control of symptoms and lung function, less bronchodilator was consumed when asthmatic subjects were taking salbutamol 'as needed'[413]. The effect of 6-month dry-powder inhaled fenoterol taken either

regularly (200 μg, *q.i.d.*) or *p.r.n.* in a double-blind, placebo-controlled, randomized crossover study was investigated. It was shown that asthmatic subjects on regular compared with *p.r.n.* treatment had improved daytime measurements of lung function. However, this was at the expense of poorer control of their asthma as assessed by a number of variables and a 3.4-fold increase in total daily bronchodilator use[414]. More importantly, these findings were also observed in asthmatic subjects who were taking glucocorticosteroid or disodium cromoglycate, and bronchial hyperresponsiveness was higher in 34% of the patients taking regular compared with symptomatic fenoterol[414]. A criticism of this study is the absence of quantitative data. All comparisons are in terms of the percentage of patients showing better control during each of the two treatment arms. No indication of the magnitude of the differences or their possible clinical significance is made. Furthermore, it has been suggested that, since the patients in the study did not require frequent β_2-adrenoceptor agonist medication at the start of the trial, these patients would be susceptible to desensitization, which might account for the observed results[415]. However, this seems unlikely given that a deterioration in asthma was observed following regular treatment with terbutaline for 2 years, in the absence of desensitization[400].

In a further study comparing regular and *p.r.n.* use of bronchodilators, a 3–4 times greater annual decline in FEV_1 was observed in asthmatic subjects treated regularly with salbutamol (400 μg *q.i.d.*) for 2 years[408]. The perception of quality of life and the number and duration of exacerbations was similar in the two groups of patients, despite the fall in FEV_1. This suggests that patients taking regular β_2-adrenoceptor agonist treatment may be unaware of a true deterioration of disease[408]. A similar finding was observed with ipratropium bromide, suggesting that the decline in FEV_1 is a feature common to bronchodilators. Patients preferred salbutamol treatment, indicating that these drugs are better at masking deterioration in asthma.

Despite an average consumption of 9.3 puffs/day compared with 1.6 puffs/day in mild asthmatic subjects for a period of 16 weeks, there was no difference in morning or evening peak flow, FEV_1, no difference in symptom score or quality-of-life score[416]. Those individuals taking regular salbutamol were associated with significantly greater peak-flow variability and increased airways responsiveness to methacholine. These changes did not lead to a worsening of their asthma and is not surprising given that these subjects had mild asthma. More importantly, these data clearly show that there is no advantage in regular salbutamol treatment in mild asthmatic subjects. The loss in symptom control and lung function cannot be simply a consequence of desensitization as these findings were more readily observed in asthmatic subjects with the Arg16 and not Gly16 phenotype, the latter linked to susceptibility to desensitization[417,418].

Similar studies have also been undertaken in subjects with increased asthma severity. Mild to moderate asthmatics who received salbutamol (400 μg *q.i.d.*) for 24 weeks had significantly greater evening PEF, improvements in daytime symptom score and reduction in rescue medication, but the overall control of asthma was no different to placebo[409]. However, it is clear that there was a general decline in the control of asthma during the course of treatment as reflected by a significant increase in the days spent during a major exacerbation of asthma during the last 4 weeks of the study and the percentage of subjects with one or more exacerbations was significantly greater than placebo. There was also a trend for a greater consumption of rescue prednisone and number of major exacerbations. There was no evidence of an increase in bronchial hyperresponsiveness to methacholine, nor rebound changes in methacholine PC20. Since many of these subjects were taking glucocorticosteroid medication it is possible that this may have negated any untoward change in airways responsiveness observed in previous studies. Consistent with this view is the finding that there was no difference in asthma exacerbation rates in subjects receiving glucocorticosteroid treatment and regularly treated with salbutamol (400 μg *q.i.d.*) vs. p.r.n., despite a PEF recording 3% higher in the regular treated

group[419] and suggests no advantage in regular consumption of short-acting β_2-agonist in overall symptom control in subjects taking glucocorticosteroids prophylactically.

Together, these studies suggest that regular treatment with short-acting β_2-adrenoceptor agonists offers no advantage over 'as needed' medication. In many cases this can lead to deterioration in disease control that may be of concern in subjects with more severe asthma (Fig. 3.3) and therefore β_2-agonists should only be used in the symptomatic relief of asthma.

Long-acting β-adrenoceptor agonists
Regular treatment with salmeterol (4 weeks; 12.5, 50, 100 μg, *b.i.d.*) was associated with significant improvements in various physiological and clinical indices[420] and more effective than regular salbutamol[421–424]. In a study of mild asthmatic children, there were significant improvements in various lung function parameters during 12 months' treatment with salmeterol (50 μg *b.i.d.*) compared with placebo, despite the fact that there was no difference in the overall control of symptoms[425]. There was no change in bronchial hyperresponsiveness to methacholine during this period and no evidence of rebound bronchial hyperresponsiveness. Of particular interest, however, was the finding that regular treatment with beclomethasone was similar to salmeterol with respect to improvements in various spirometric indices, but far superior regarding overall symptom scores and improving baseline responsiveness to methacholine[425].

A recent study comparing the effect of regular treatment with salmeterol and salbutamol vs. placebo demonstrated fewer minor and major exacerbations, improved day-time and night-time symptom score and better control of asthma than either salbutamol or placebo[409]. Moreover, there was no evidence of increased bronchial hyper-responsiveness to methacholine nor rebound hyperresponsiveness following termination of the study and no evidence of loss in rescue bronchodilator potency to salbutamol[409]. This particular study does not support the view that loss in bronchodilator activity to rescue medication is an important consequence of long-term salmeterol treatment. Similarly, no evidence of loss in bronchoprotection to methacholine was observed during 1–6 months treatment with salmeterol compared with salbutamol p.r.n. in mild asthmatic subjects, as reflected by day-time asthma symptoms of wheezing, shortness of breath and chest tightness[426]. Thus, while there were significant but small improvements in morning and evening PEF, subject-related symptoms, greater number of symptom free days and reduced night-time awakenings compared with salbutamol p.r.n., those individuals taking salbutamol p.r.n. had similar exacerbation rates as the salmeterol group and more importantly, did not become progressively worse during the course of their treatment[426].

Regular treatment with formoterol (3 months, 12 μg b.i.d.[345] or 12 months, 12 μg, b.i.d.[368]) resulted in greater increases in spirometry and/or peak flow than placebo or salbutamol, and the number of asthma episodes and sleep disruption were less with formoterol than salbutamol[345]. In a 24-week study in moderate asthmatics who were maintained on inhaled glucocorticosteroid therapy (approx. 740 μg/day), regular treatment with formoterol (12 μg b.i.d.) significantly reduced night-time and day-time symptom scores, improved PEF compared with on demand salbutamol treatment and was not associated with loss in bronchoprotection to methacholine over the treatment period. In addition, no evidence of rebound bronchial hyper-responsiveness following termination of the study was observed[427]. Similarly, 52-week treatment with salmeterol (50 μg b.i.d.) in mild to moderate asthmatics taking inhaled glucocorticosteroids were shown to have greater changes in baseline lung function than salbutamol p.r.n., despite the fact that daily symptom scores were not significantly different[428]. A small rebound increase in airway responsiveness to methacholine was observed following termination of the study, but this was not associated with a deterioration in symptom scores. Together, these studies suggest that regular treatment with long-acting β_2-adrenoceptor agonists does not lead to a worsening of asthma symptoms, loss in bronchoprotection or increased bronchial hyper-responsiveness when used in conjunction with glucocorticosteroids.

The inability to observe any loss in bronchoprotection or increase in baseline hyperresponsiveness following regular treatment with long-acting β_2-adrenoceptor agonists may be due to a number of confounding factors. Following the termination of bronchodilator treatment, there is a quick re-establishment of baseline airways responsiveness to prestudy levels[409,423,425–427]. This suggests that, during chronic dosing with long-acting β_2-adrenoceptor agonists, the presence of drug within the lung, despite attempts to minimize this by withholding drug treatment prior to challenge test, may confound any attempts to detect a loss in bronchoprotection and/or exacerbation of baseline hyper-responsiveness. Secondly, while no evidence of worsening of asthma was evident during regular treatment, the continual presence of glucocorticosteroid would tend to mask this phenomenon. The termination of beclomethasone (2 weeks) after regular treatment resulted in a small loss in bronchoprotection to methacholine, whereas a greater loss in bronchoprotection to methacholine was observed in subjects who received salmeterol only[425] and asthma control failed to improve or, indeed, worsened following discontinuation of their inhaled glucocorticosteroids and replaced with regular administered salmeterol[429] indicative of the disease modifying characteristics of glucocorticosteroids compared with β_2-adrenoceptor agonists.

A number of studies have investigated the impact of supplementing regular glucocorticosteroid treatment with salmeterol[429–431] and formoterol[432] and, in general, have shown that addition of bronchodilator to glucocorticosteroid significantly improves control of asthma symptoms compared with either treatment or increasing the dose of glucocorticosteroid. The molecular mechanism of the β_2-adrenoceptor agonist/glucocorticosteroid interaction on asthma control remains to be established, although one study has reported that β_2-adrenoceptor agonists facilitate glucocorticosteroid receptor translocation to the nucleus in vitro, following activation of the receptor and signalling via PKA[433]. Since there is overwhelming evidence that salmeterol and formoterol have no significant anti-eosinophilic or lymphocytic activity in asthma[182,183,249,250], it suggests that this novel signalling pathway still requires the presence of exogenously administered glucocorticosteroid for the functional effect of this interaction to be revealed in a clinical setting. Alternatively, the extra beneficial action of these drugs in reducing symptom scores is solely due to the added benefit of the ability of β_2-adrenoceptor agonists to induced functional antagonism of airway smooth muscle function and/or mast cell degranulation against the background of the disease-modifying effect of glucocorticosteroids.

Asthma deaths

Case control studies

During the 1960s an increase in asthma mortality was correlated with the consumption of isoprenaline. An over-reliance on the use of isoprenaline contributing to a delay in the use of glucocorticosteroids has been suggested as a possible cause[124,125]. A similar rise in asthma deaths was also observed during the 1970s in New Zealand, which was correlated with the sale of fenoterol[134,434]. A number of explanations were forwarded to account for the deaths including the combined use of β-adrenoceptor agonists and theophylline replacing inhaled glucocorticosteroid and disodium chromoglycate[435]; over-reliance on domiciliary nebulizers[436,437]; under-estimation of the severity of the disease, poor compliance; and the number not the choice of drugs[437–440].

A large case-control study was performed to determine the contribution of drug therapy in asthma deaths in New Zealand. It was subsequently demonstrated that, in 117 fatal cases of asthma, there was a 1.55-fold increased risk of death in patients taking fenoterol by MDI[134]. Patients were not at risk of death in any of the groups of patients taking salbutamol by MDI, corticosteroids or theophylline. Further analysis of subgroups defining markers of asthma severity, revealed that the risk of death in patients prescribed fenoterol was twofold higher in patients taking drugs in three or more categories of asthma therapy or with a previous hospital admission. Furthermore, the association between risk of death and the use of fenoterol was six- and 13-fold higher in patients prescribed oral corticosteroid alone or together with a recent hospital admission, respectively[134]. The authors suggested that the use of fenoterol by MDI in severe asthma increased the risk of death. However, the nature of the experimental design raises a number of criticisms. These include the inappropriate use of controls from a less severe patient category, the inability to determine which bronchodilator drug was used near or at death and the misleading use of subgroups which define asthma severity. An alternative conclusion from this study is that fenoterol is prescribed for patients with severe asthma and thus is a marker of disease severity. In order to answer these criticisms, another case-control study was performed in which information relating to drug prescription was obtained from prior hospital admission for both cases and controls and the severity of controls and cases were more closely matched. As with the previous study, there was a twofold increase in the risk of death in patients prescribed fenoterol. In patients taking fenoterol and who were also prescribed oral corticosteroid, or together with a recent hospital admission, the risk factor was increased by six- and tenfold, respectively[441]. In contrast to their previous study[134], oral corticosteroids and theophylline (prescribed at discharge) were associated with an increased risk of death in some subgroups defined by markers of asthma severity. However, when the influence of fenoterol was removed from the analysis, the increased risk of death in patients prescribed these drugs was also removed in these subgroups. A further case-control study assessing different methods of matching cases and controls also showed that severe asthmatic subjects taking fenoterol were at a greater risk of death[442].

Similar findings were reported in a large case-control study in Canada. The use of fenoterol, salbutamol, oral but not inhaled corticosteroids and theophylline was associated with an increased risk of death and near-death from asthma[443]. In this study it was demonstrated that case patients tended to have more severe asthma than the controls. On this basis alone, the data would suggest that *β*$_2$-adrenoceptor agonists are not a risk factor and that the extent of their use is more likely to be a marker of severity. However, when the data was adjusted for exposure to other antiasthma drugs and the number of hospitalizations, the use of fenoterol and salbutamol was associated with increased risk in morbidity and mortality. In contrast, following adjustment, oral corticosteroids were confined to a small increased risk in morbidity[443]. An interesting finding from this study was that, on a microgram equivalent basis, the risk factor for asthma death was similar for both fenoterol and salbutamol. In contrast to these studies, attempts made to remove confounding by various severity markers appear to remove the association between *β*$_2$-adrenoceptor consumption and mortality[444].

Because of the design of these studies it is difficult to determine whether there is a causal relationship between *β*$_2$-adrenoceptor agonist consumption and increased asthma mortality/morbidity. However, it does seem reasonable to suggest that the sole reliance on *β*$_2$-adrenoceptor agonist therapy may delay the introduction of anti-inflammatory drugs, which might place patients at risk. A concern reflected in the current asthma guidelines whereby increased reliance upon *β*$_2$-adrenoceptor agonists is indicative of poor disease control and addition of glucocorticosteroid is recommended. The suggestion that *β*$_2$-adrenoceptor agonists *per se* are responsible for placing patients at risk is highly controversial, and without the proper experimental design this issue will be difficult to resolve.

Mechanisms

A number of mechanism(s) by which *β*$_2$-adrenoceptor agonists could lead to a worsening of asthma have been proposed. It has been hypothesized that these drugs may increase the access of allergen into the airways by virtue of their ability to dilate the airways[414,445]. However, bronchodilation induced by ipratropium bromide was not associated with an increase in airways hyperresponsiveness in asthmatic subjects[403]. Thus, it is more likely that individuals taking *β*-adrenoceptor agonists are able to tolerate greater antigen loads and/or remain exposed to low levels of allergen for greater periods, which may lead to an exacerbation of asthma[174,306,414,445]. Whether this accounted for the increase in magnitude of the late asthmatic response to antigen challenge in asthmatic subjects following 1-week regular treatment with salbutamol remains to be established[241]. The effect of regular treatment with *β*$_2$-adrenoceptor agonists on the ability of asthmatic subjects to tolerate environments which contain sensitizing agents and moreover, whether this leads to increased penetration and/or concentration of sensitizing agents within the lung have yet to be established.

It has also been suggested that mast cell degranulation is a normal defence mechanism. The release of bronchospastic mediators following antigen challenge may limit the further penetration of allergen down the bronchial tree. Furthermore, mast cells release heparin a molecule that possesses anti-inflammatory properties[446]. Inhibition of this normal defence mechanism by these agonists may contribute to the detrimental effects associated with *β*$_2$-adrenoceptor agonist therapy, as this interferes with the normal defence and repair mechanisms of the lung[447]. This would be consistent with the recent findings of increased serum levels of tryptase after allergen challenge in asthmatic subjects who were treated with salbutamol (200 μg *q.i.d.*) over a 10-day period[448].

In animal studies, it has been demonstrated that the intravenous administration of (±) isoprenaline can induce nerve-mediated bronchial hyperresponsiveness to histamine in guinea-pigs. Furthermore, this effect is observed with the distomer and is propranolol insensitive, and it has been suggested that the distomers present in the current formulation of *β*-adrenoceptor agonists may be harmful in asthma. This is supported by data showing that intratracheal administration of distomers of *β*$_2$-adrenoceptor agonists is associated with increased bronchial responsiveness to histamine in guinea-pigs[9]. This hypothesis could explain why the loss in bronchoprotection to various stimuli following regular treatment with β_2-adrenoceptor agonist is resistant to glucocorticosteroid treatment and demands investigation.

Adverse side effects with therapeutic doses

Skeletal muscle tremor

Activation of β_2-adrenoceptors in skeletal muscle results in tremor[124] a common adverse reaction to these agents, although tolerance usually develops following chronic therapy[74,139].

Cardiovascular

When given by inhalation at therapeutic doses, the incidence of tachycardia is minimized. In contrast, when given by the systemic route, significant changes in heart rate and blood pressure can be observed[67]. Furthermore, high inhaled doses of β_2-adrenoceptor agonists can also lead to a dose-dependent increase in heart rate and a fall in diastolic blood pressure[134,138,139]. Tolerance develops to the changes in heart rate following chronic therapy[139]. Untoward cardiovascular effects are more likely to be manifested in patients with serious cardiac problems.

Metabolic changes

Hypokalemia is observed following inhaled and systemic administration of β_2-adrenoceptor agonists. The change in plasma concentration of potassium ions is minimal under normal therapeutic doses, although a dose-dependent decrease in the plasma level of potassium ions is observed with increasing doses of these agonists[138]. Hypokalemia is mediated by uptake of potassium ions in skeletal muscle and tolerance to this effect is observed following chronic therapy[139]. The effect of lowering plasma potassium ions and cardiac stimulation may become significant in patients with heart disease.

β_2-Adrenoceptor activation also can result in glycogenolysis,[449] and ketoacidosis may occur in diabetic patients prescribed these agonists, which depends on the degree of tolerance that has developed to the metabolic effects of β_2-adrenoceptor agonists.

Arterial oxygen tension

β_2-Adrenoceptor agonists may reduce arterial oxygen tension as a consequence of ventilation/perfusion mismatching[450]. Such effects may present problems in individuals who are severely hypoxemic to begin with and may therefore require oxygen supplementation.

Conclusions

β_2-Adrenoceptor agonists provide effective bronchodilator relief in asthmatic subjects undergoing acute bronchospasm. As such, they are the drugs of choice in the symptomatic relief of asthma. Their major influence is the functional antagonism of spasmogen-induced contraction of airway smooth muscle. However, because β_2-adrenoceptors are widely distributed throughout the lung, the beneficial effect of these agonists may also be mediated at sites other than airway smooth muscle, including mast cells and endothelial cells. The effects of β_2-adrenoceptor agonists on mast cells and endothelial cells have been cited by many authors as evidence of an acute anti-inflammatory property of these drugs. However, evidence for anti-inflammatory activity in chronic inflammation is lacking.

More recently, salmeterol and formoterol have been developed which provide significantly longer protection against bronchospasm than currently available shorter-acting β_2-adrenoceptor agonists. In particular, these drugs offer significant protection in nocturnal asthma and COPD. Some studies have suggested that these drugs possess acute anti-inflammatory properties; however, there is little evidence to support this view in light of their poor anti-eosinophilic or anti-lymphocytic activity in asthma. It is intriguing to speculate that the potential anti-neutrophilic action of this class of drug may explain some of the beneficial effects of this treatment in COPD.

Considerable controversy has been raised concerning the regular use of β_2-adrenoceptor agonists in asthma and the possibility that the regular consumption of these drugs may place patients at risk. Although a causal relationship has not been established, a number of studies have observed an association between regular consumption of these drugs and increased asthma mortality/morbidity. More controlled studies are required to clearly establish such a relationship. However, it is obvious that relying solely on β_2-adrenoceptor agonist therapy alone, which provides excellent symptomatic relief, can result in patients perceiving that their asthma is improving, when in reality their delay in receiving anti-inflammatory medication may place them at risk. Current guidelines reflect this view whereby these drugs should only be prescribed as needed and only used regularly with glucocorticosteroid therapy.

It would seem prudent to suggest that β_2-adrenoceptor agonists should only be used for symptomatic relief in patients with mild to moderate asthma,. The role of these drugs in chronic severe asthma is more controversial. Given that no randomized placebo controlled study has been performed which investigates the effect of regular β-adrenoceptor agonist treatment with this group of patients, the suggestion from case-controlled studies of the possible risk factors posed by these drugs should be tempered. However, what these studies do suggest is that, in this group of patients, it is imperative that therapeutic strategies directed to the more frequent and early use of anti-inflammatory drugs which can be accompanied by β_2-adrenoceptor agonists taken as needed.

REFERENCES

1 Reed CE. Adrenergic bronchodilators: Pharmacology and toxicology. *J Allergy Clin Immunol* 1985; 76:335–41.

2 George CF, Blackwell EW, Davies DS. Metabolism of isoprenaline in the intestine. *J Pharm Pharmacol* 1974; 26:265–76.

3 Davies DS. Pharmacokinetics of inhaled substances. *Postgrad Med J* 1975; 51(suppl 7):69–71.

4 Blackwell EW, Briant RH, Conolly ME, Davies DS, Dollery CT. Metabolism of isoprenaline after aerosol and direct intrabronchial administration in man and dog. *Br J Pharmacol* 1974; 50:587–591.

5 Brittain RT, Dean CM, Jack D. Sympathomimetic bronchodilator drugs. *Pharmacol Ther* 1976; 2:423–462.

6 Evans ME, Walker SR, Brittain RT, Paterson JW. The metabolism of salbutamol in man. *Xenobiotica* 1973; 3:113–20.

7 Morgan DJ, Paull JD, Richmond BH, Wison-Evered E, Ziccone SP. Pharmacokinetics of intravenous and oral salbutamol and its sulphate conjugate. *Br J Clin Pharmacol* 1986; 22:587–593.

8 Shenfield GM, Evans ME, Paterson JW. Absorption of drugs by the lung. *Br J Clin Pharmacol* 1976; 3:583–589.

9 Handley DA, McCullough JR, Crowther SD, Morley J. Sympathomimetic enantiomers and asthma. *Chirality* 1998; 10:262–72.

10 Boulton DW, Fawcett JP. Enantioselective disposition of salbutamol in man following oral and intravenous administration. *Br J Clin Pharmacol* 1996; 41:35–40.

11 Schemekel B, Rydberg I, Norlander B, Sjosward KN, Ahlner J, Andersson RGG. Stereoselective pharmacokinetic of S-salbutamol after administration of the racemate in healthy volunteers. *Eur Respir J* 1999; 13:1230–1235.

12 Walle UK, Pesulo GR, Walle T. Stereoselective sulphate conjugation of salbutamol in humans: comparison of hepatic, intestinal and platelet activity. *Br J Clin Pharmacol* 1993; 35:413–418.

13 Eaton EA, Walle UK, Wilson HM, Aberg G, Walle T. Stereoselective sulphate conjugation of salbutamol by human lung and bronchial epithelial cells. *Br J Clin Pharmacol* 1996; 41:201–206.

14 Dhand R, Goode M, Reid R, Fink JB, Fahey PJ, Tobin MJ. Preferential pulmonary retention of (S)-albuterol after inhalation of racemic albuterol. *Am J Respir Crit Care Med* 1999; 160:1136–1141.

15 Bergman J, Persson H, Wetterlin K. Two new groups of selective stimulants of adrenergic β-receptors. *Experientia* 1969; 25:899–901.

16 Nilsson HT, Persson K, Tegner K. The metabolism of terbutaline by man. *Xenobiotica* 1972; 2:363–75.

17 Davies DS, George CF, Blackwell E, Conolly ME, Dollery CT. Metabolism of terbutaline in man and dog. *Br J Clin Pharmacol* 1974; 1:129–136.

18 Ryrfeldt A, Nilsson E. Physiological disposition of albuterol and terbutaline in the isolated perfused rat lung. *Acta Pharmacol Toxicol* 1976; 39:39–45.

19 Ryrfeldt A, Nilsson E. Uptake and biotransformation of albuterol and terbutaline in isolated perfused rat and guinea pig lungs. *Biochem.Pharmacol.* 1978; 27:301–305.

20 Leifer KN, Wittig HJ. The beta-2 sympathomimetic aerosols in the treatment of asthma. *Ann Allergy* 1975; 35:69–80.

21 Walle T, Walle UK. Stereoselective sulphate conjugation of racemic terbutaline by human liver cytosol. *Br J Clin Pharmacol* 1990; 30:127–133.

22 Heel RC, Brogden RN, Speight TM, Avery GS. Fenoterol: a review of its pharmacological properties and therapeutic efficacy in asthma. *Drugs* 1978; 15:3–32.

23 Svedmyr N. Fenoterol: A beta2-adrenergic agonist for use in asthma. Pharmacology, pharmacokinetics, clinical efficacy and adverse effects. *Pharmacotherapy* 1985; 5:109–126.

24 Jack D. A way of looking at agonism and antagonism: Lessons from salbutamol, salmeterol and other beta-adrenoceptor agonists. *Br J Clin Pharmacol* 1991; 31:501–514.

25 Brogden RN, Faulds D. Salmeterol xinafoate: A review of its pharmacological properties and therapeutic potential in reversible obstructive airways disease. Drugs 1991; 42:895–912.

26 Manchee GR, Barrow A, Kulkarni S et al. Disposition of salmeterol xinafoate in laboratory animals and humans. *Drug Metab Dispos* 1993; 21:1022–1028.

27 Bennett JA, Harrison TW, Tattersfield AE. The contribution of the swallowed fraction of an inhaled dose of salmeterol to it systemic effects. *Eur Respir J* 1999; 13:445–448.

28 Yokoi K, Murase K, Shiobara Y. The development of a radioimmunoassay for formoterol. *Life Sci* 1983; 33:1665–1672.

29 Faulds D, Hollingshead LM, Goa KL. Formoterol. A review of its pharmacological properties and therapeutic potential in reversible obstructive airways disease. *Drugs* 1991; 42:115–137.

30 Derks MGM, Van den Berg BTJ, Van der Zee JS, Braat MCP, Van Boxtel CJ. Biphasic effect-time courses in man after formoterol inhalation: Eosinopenic and hypokalemic effects and inhibition of allergic skin reactions. *J Pharmacol Exp Ther* 1997; 283:824–832.

31 Butter JJ, Van den Berg BTJ, Portier EJG, Kaiser G, Van Boxtel CJ. Determination by HPLC with electrochemical detection of formoterol RR and SS enantiomers in urine. *J Liquid Chromatog Rel Tech* 1996; 19:993–1005.

32 Torphy TJ. Beta-adrenoceptors, cAMP and airway smooth muscle relaxation: challenges to the dogma. *Trends Pharmacol Sci* 1994; 15:370–374.

33 Johnson M. The beta-adrenoceptor. *Am J Respir Crit Care Med* 1998; 158:S146-S153.

34 Luttrell LM, Daaka Y, Lefkowitz RJ. Regulation of tyrosine kinase cascades by G-protein-coupled receptors. *Curr Opin Cell Biol* 1999; 11:177–183.

35 Nials AT, Coleman RA, Johnson M, Magnussen H, Rabe KF, Vardey CJ. Effects of beta-adrenoceptor agonists in human bronchial smooth muscle. *Br J Pharmacol* 1993; 110:1112–1116.

36 Naline E, Zhang Y, Qian Y et al. Relaxant effects and durations of action of formoterol and salmeterol on the isolated human bronchus. *Eur Respir J* 1994; 7:914–920.

37 Molimard M, Naline E, Zhang Y, Le G, V, Begaud B, Advenier C. Long- and short-acting beta2 adrenoceptor agonists: Interactions in human contracted bronchi. *Eur Respir J* 1998; 11:583–588.

38 Roux FJ, Grandordy B, Douglas JS. Functional and binding characteristics of long-acting beta2-agonists in lung and heart. *Am J Respir Crit Care Med* 1996; 153:1489–1495.

39 Nials AT, Ball DI, Butchers PR et al. Formoterol on airway smooth muscle and human lung mast cells: A comparison with salbutamol and salmeterol. *Eur J Pharmacol* 1994; 251:127–135.

40 Van Noord JA, Smeets JJ, Raaijmakers JAM, Bommer AM, Maesen FPV. Salmeterol versus formoterol in patients with moderately severe asthma: Onset and duration of action. *Eur Respir J* 1996; 9:1684–1688.

41 Palmqvist M, Persson G, Lazer L, Rosenborg J, Larsson P, Lotvall J. Inhaled dry-powder formoterol and salmeterol in asthmatic patients: Onset of action, duration of effect and potency. *Eur Respir J* 1997; 10:2484–2489.

42 Green SA, Spasoff AP, Coleman RA, Johnson M, Liggett SB. Sustained activation of a G protein-coupled receptor via 'anchored' agonist binding. Molecular localization of the salmeterol exosite within the beta2-adrenergic receptor. *J Biol Chem* 1996; 271:24029–24035.

43 Isogaya M, Yamagiwa Y, Fujita S, Sugimoto Y, Nagao T, Kurose H. Identification of a key amino acid of the beta2-adrenergic receptor for high affinity binding of salmeterol. *Mol Pharmacol* 1998; 54:616–622.

44 Rong Y, Arbabian M, Thiriot DS, Seibold A, Clark RB, Ruoho AE. Probing the salmeterol binding site on β_2-adrenergic receptor using a novel photoaffinity ligand, [^{125}I]iodoazidosalmeterol. *Biochemistry* 1999; 38:11278–11286.

45 Bergendal A, Linden A, Skoogh B-E, Gerspacher M, Anderson GP, Lofdahl C-G. Extent of salmeterol-mediated

reassertion of relaxation in guinea-pig trachea pretreated with aliphatic side chain structural analogues. *Br J Pharmacol* 1996; 117:1009–1015.

46 Teschemacher A, Lemoine H. Kinetic analysis of drug-receptor interactions of long-acting beta2 sympathomimetics in isolated receptor membranes: evidence against prolonged effects of salmeterol and formoterol on receptor-coupled adenylyl cyclase. *J Pharmacol Exp Ther* 1999; 288:1084–1092.

47 Anderson GP, Linden A, Rabe KF. Why are long-acting beta-adrenoceptor agonists long-acting? *Eur Respir J* 1994; 7:569–578.

48 Pitcher JA, Freedman NJ, Lefkowitz RJ. G protein-coupled receptor kinases. *Ann Rev Biochemistry* 1998; 67:-692

49 January B, Seibold A, Whaley B et al. beta2-Adrenergic receptor desensitization, internalization, and phosphorylation in response to full and partial agonists. *J Biol Chem* 1997; 272:23871–23879.

50 January B, Seibold A, Allal C et al. Salmeterol-induced desensitization, internalization and phosphorylation of the human β_2-adrenoceptor. *Br J Pharmacol* 1998; 123:701–711.

51 Kallal L, Gagnon AW, Penn RB, Benovic JL. Visualization of agonist-induced sequestration and down-regulation of a green fluorescent protein-tagged beta2-adrenergic receptor. *J Biol Chem* 1998; 273:322–328.

52 McGraw DW, Liggett SB. Heterogeneity in beta-adrenergic receptor kinase expression in the lung accounts for cell-specific desensitization of the beta2-adrenergic receptor. *J Biol Chem* 1997; 272:7338–7344.

53 Drury DEJ, Chong LK, Ghahramani P, Peachell PT. Influence of receptor reserve on beta-adrenoceptor-mediated responses in human lung mast. *Br J Pharmacol* 1998; 124:711–718.

54 Reihsaus E, Innis M, MacIntyre N, Liggett SB. Mutations in the gene encoding for the β_2-adrenergic receptor in normal and asthmatic subjects. *Am J Respir Cell Mol Biol* 1993; 8:334–339.

55 Green SA, Turki J, Innis M, Liggett SB. Amino-terminal polymorphisms of the human beta2-adrenergic receptor impart distinct agonist-promoted regulatory properties. *Biochemistry* 1994; 33:9414–9419.

56 Green SA, Turki J, Hall IP, Liggett SB. Implications of genetic variability of human beta2-adrenergic receptor structure. *Pulmon Pharmacol* 1995; 8:1–10.

57 Green SA, Cole G, Jacinto M, Innis M, Liggett SB. A polymorphism of the human beta2-adrenergic receptor within the fourth transmembrane domain alters ligand binding

and functional properties of the receptor. *J Biol Chem* 1993; 268:23116–23121.

58 Turki J, Pak J, Green SA, Martin RJ, Liggett SB. Genetic polymorphisms of the beta2-adrenergic receptor in nocturnal and nonnocturnal asthma. Evidence that Gly16 correlates with the nocturnal phenotype. *J Clin Immunol* 1995; 95:1635–1641.

59 Martinez FD, Graves PE, Baldini M, Solomon S, Erickson R. Association between genetic polymorphisms of the b2-adrenoceptor and response to albuterol in children with and without a history of wheezing. *J Clin Invest* 1997; 100:3184–3188.

60 Hancox RJ, Sears MR, Taylor DR. Polymorphism of the β_2-adrenoceptor and the response to long-term β_2-agonist therapy in asthma. *Eur Respir J* 1998; 11:589–593.

61 Hopes E, McDougall C, Christie G et al. Association of glutamine 27 polymorphism of β_2 adrenoceptor with reported childhood asthma: population based study. *Br Med J* 1998; 316:664

62 Ramsay CE, Hayden CM, Tiller KJ, Burton PR, Goldblatt J, Lesouef PN. Polymorphisms in the β_2-adrenoceptor gene are associated with decreased airway responsiveness. *Clin Exp Allergy* 1999; 29:1195–1203.

63 Hall IP, Wheatley A, Wilding P, Liggett SB. Association of Glu 27 beta2-adrenoceptor polymorphism with lower airway reactivity in asthmatic subjects. *Lancet* 1995; 345:1213–1214.

64 Dewar JC, Wilkinson J, Wheatley A et al. The glutamine 27 β_2-adrenoceptor polymorphism is associated with elevated IgE levels in asthmatic families. *J Allergy Clin Immunol* 1997; 100:261–265.

65 D'Amato M, Vitiani LR, Petrelli G, Ferrigno L, di Pietro A, Trezza R, et al. Association of persistent bronchial hyperresponsiveness with β_2-adrenoceptor (ADRB2) haplotypes. *Am J Respir Crit Care Med* 1998; 158:1968–1973.

66 Ulbrecht M, Hergeth MT, Wjst M et al. Association of β_2-adrenoceptor variants with bronchial hyperresponsiveness. *Am J Respir Crit Care Med* 2000; 161:469–474.

67 Svedmyr N, Thiringer G. The effects of salbutamol and isoprenaline on beta-receptors in patients with chronic obstructive lung disease. *Br Med J* 1971; 47(suppl):44–46.

68 Thiringer G, Svedmyr N. Comparison of infused and inhaled terbutaline in patients with asthma. *Scand J Respir* 1976; 57:17–22.

69 Lofdahl C-G, Svedmyr N. Formoterol fumarate, a new beta2-adrenoceptor agonist. Acute studies of selectivity and duration of effect after inhaled and oral administration. *Allergy* 1989; 44:264–271.

70 Gibson D, Coltart DJ. Haemodynamic effects of intravenous salbutamol in patients with mitral valve disease: comparison with isoprenaline and atropine. *Postgrad Med J* 1971; 47(Suppl):40–44.

71 Heitz A, Schwartz J, Velly J. β-Adrenoceptors of the human myocardium: Determination of beta1 and beta2 subtypes by radioligand binding. *Br J Pharmacol* 1983; 80:

72 Robberecht P, Delhaye M, Taton G. The human heart beta-adrenergic receptors. I. Heterogeneity of the binding sites: Presence of 50% beta1- and 50% beta2-adrenergic receptors. *Mol Pharmacol* 1983; 24.

73 Corea L, Bentivoglio M, Verdecchia P. Noninvasive assessment of chronotropic and inotropic response of preferential beta-1 and beta-2 adrenoceptor stimulation. *Clin Pharmacol Therap* 1984; 35.

74 Larsson S, Svedmyr N. Bronchodilating effect and side-effects of beta2-adrenoceptor stimulants by different modes of administration (tablets, metered aerosol and combinations thereof). A study with salbutamol in asthmatics. *Am Rev Respir Dis* 1977; 116:861–869.

75 Lofdahl CG, Chung KF. Long-acting beta2-adrenoceptor agonists: A new perspective in the treatment of asthma. *Eur Respir J* 1991; 4:218–226.

76 Hertzel MR, Clark TJH. Comparison of intravenous and aerosol salbutamol. *Br Med J* 1976; ii:919.

77 Cheong B, Reynolds SR, Rajan G, Ward MJ. Intravenous beta agonist in severe acute asthma. *Br Med J* 1988; 297:448–450.

78 Barnes PJ, Pride NB. Dose-response curves to inhaled beta-adrenoceptor agonists in normal and asthmatic subjects. *Br J Clin Pharmacol* 1983; 15:677–682.

79 Bloomfield P, Carmichael J, Petrie GR, Jewell NP, Crompton GK. Comparison of salbutamol given intravenously and by intermittent positive-pressure breathing in life-threatening asthma. *Br Med J* 1979; 1:848–850.

80 Pierce RJ, Payne CR, Williams SJ, Denison DM, Clark TJH. Comparison of intravenous and inhaled terbutaline in the treatment of asthma. *Chest* 1981; 79:506–511.

81 Williams SJ, Winner SJ, Clark TJH. Comparison of inhaled and intravenous terbutaline in acute severe asthma. *Thorax* 1981; 36:629–631.

82 Swedish Society of Chest Medicine. High-inhaled versus intravenous salbutamol combined with theophylline in severe acute asthma. *Eur Respir J* 1990; 3:163–170.

83 Freedman BJ. Trial of a terbutaline aerosol in the treatment of asthma and a comparison of its effects with those of a salbutamol aerosol. *Br J Dis Chest* 1972; 66:222-229.

84 Choo-Kang YFJ, MacDonald HL, Horne NW. A comparison of salbutamol and terbutaline aerosols in bronchial asthma. *Practitioner* 1973; 211:801–813.

85 Hartnett BJS, Marlin GE. Comparison of terbutaline and salbutamol aerosols. *Aust NZ J Med* 1977; 7:13–15.

86 Ruffin RE, Montgomery JM, Newhouse MT. Site of beta-adrenergic receptors in the respiratory tract. *Chest* 1978; 74:256–260.

87 Fairshter RD, Novey HS, Wilson AF. Site and duration of bronchodilation in asthmatic patients after oral administration of terbutaline. *Chest* 1981; 79:50–57.

88 Gray BJ, Frame MH, Costello JF. A comparative double-blind study of the bronchodilator effects and side effects of inhaled fenoterol and terbutaline administered in equipotent doses. *Br J Dis Chest* 1982; 76:341–250.

89 Webb J, Rees J, Clark TJH. A comparison of the effects of different methods of administration of beta-2 sympathomimetics in patients with asthma. *Br J Dis Chest* 1982; 76:351–257.

90 Ahrens RC, Harris JB, Milavetz G. Use of bronchial provocation with histamine to compare the pharmacodynamics of inhaled albuterol and metaproterenol in patients with asthma. *J Allergy Clin Immunol* 1987; 79:876–882.

91 Gongora HC, Wisniewski AFZ, Tattersfield AE. A single-dose comparison of inhaled albuterol and two formulations of salmeterol on airway reactivity in asthmatic subjects. *Am Rev Respir Dis* 1991; 144:626–629.

92 Derom EY, Pauwels RA, Van der Straeten MEF. The effect of inhaled salmeterol on methacholine responsiveness in subjects with asthma up to 12 hours. *J Allergy Clin Immunol* 1992; 89:811–815.

93 Ullman A, Svedmyr N. Salmeterol, a new long acting inhaled beta2 adrenoceptor agonist: Comparison with salbutamol in adult asthmatic patients. *Thorax* 1988; 43:674–678.

94 Ball DI, Brittain RT, Coleman RA et al. Salmeterol, a novel, long-acting beta2-adrenoceptor agonist: Characterization of pharmacological activity in vitro and in vivo. *Br J Pharmacol* 1991; 104:665–671.

95 Sykes AP, Ayres JG. A study of the duration of the bronchodilator effect of 12 mug and 24 mug of inhaled formoterol and 200 mug inhaled salbutamol in asthma. *Respir Med* 1990; 84:135–138.

96 Maesen FPV, Smeets JJ, Gubbelmans HLL, Zweers PGMA. Bronchodilator effect of inhaled formoterol vs salbutamol over 12 hours. *Chest* 1990; 97:590–594.

97 Wong BJ, Dolovich J, Ramsdale EH et al. Formoterol compared with beclomethasone and placebo on allergen-induced asthmatic responses. *Am Rev Respir Dis* 1992; 146:1156–1160.

98 Twentyman OP, Finnerty JP, Harris A, Palmer J, Holgate ST. Protection against allergen-induced asthma by salmeterol. *Lancet* 1990; 336:1338–1342.

99 Becker AB, Simons FER. Formoterol, a new long-acting selective beta2-adrenergic receptor agonist: Double-blind comparison with salbutamol and placebo in children with asthma. *J Allergy Clin Immunol* 1989; 84:891–895.

100 Graff-Lonnevig V, Browaldh L. Twelve hours' bronchodilating effect of inhaled formoterol in children with asthma: A double-blind cross-over study versus salbutamol. *Clin Exp Allergy* 1990; 20:429–432.

101 Ruffin RE, Obminski G, Newhouse MT. Aerosol salbutamol administration by IPPB: lowest effective dose. *Thorax* 1978; 33:689–693.

102 Salome CM, Schoeffel RE, Yan K, Woolcock AJ. Effect of aerosol fenoterol on the severity of bronchial hyperreactivity in patients with asthma. *Thorax* 1983; 38:854–858.

103 Anderson SD, Rodwell LT, Du TJ, Young IH. Duration of protection by inhaled salmeterol in exercise-induced asthma. *Chest* 1991; 100:1254–1260.

104 Smith CM, Anderson SD, Seale JP. The duration of action of the combination of fenoterol hydrobromide and ipratropium bromide in protecting against asthma provoked by hyperpnea. *Chest* 1988; 94:709–717.

105 Malo J-L, Ghezzo H, Trudeau C, Cartier A, Morris J. Duration of action of inhaled terbutaline at two different doses and of albuterol in protecting against bronchoconstriction induced by hyperventilation of dry cold air in asthmatic subjects. *Am Rev Respir Dis* 1989; 140:817–821.

106 Rabe KF, Jorres R, Nowak D, Behr N, Magnussen H. Comparison of the effects of salmeterol and formoterol on airway tone and responsiveness over 24 hours in bronchial asthma. *Am Rev Respir Dis* 1993; 147:1436–1441.

107 Nix A, Nichol GM, Robson A, Barnes PJ, Chung KF. Effect of formoterol, a long-lasting beta2-adrenoceptor agonist, against methacholine-induced bronchoconstriction. *Br J Clin Pharmacol* 1990; 29:321–224.

108 Ramsdale EH, Otis J, Kline PA, Gontovnick LS, Hargreave FE, O'Byrne PM. Prolonged protection against methacholine-induced bronchoconstriction by the inhaled beta2-agonist formoterol. *Am Rev Respir Dis* 1991; 143:998–1001.

109 Kemp JP, Dockhorn RJ, Busse WW, Bleecker ER, Van As A. Prolonged effect of inhaled salmeterol against exercise-induced bronchospasm. *Am J Respir Crit Care Med* 1994; 150:1612–1615.

110 Ramage L, Lipworth BJ, Ingram CG, Cree IA, Dhillon DP. Reduced protection against exercise induced bronchoconstriction after chronic dosing with salmeterol. *Respir Med* 1994; 88:363–368.

111 De Benedictis FM, Tuteri G, Pazzelli P, Niccoli A, Mezzetti D, Vaccaro R. Salmeterol in exercise-induced bronchoconstriction in asthmatic children: Comparison of two doses. *Eur Respir J* 1996; 9:2099–2103.

112 Schaanning J, Vilsvik J, Henriksen AH, Bratten G. Efficacy and duration of salmeterol powder inhalation in protecting against exercise-induced bronchoconstriction. *Ann Allergy* 1996; 76:57–60.

113 Simons FER, Gerstner TV, Cheang MS. Tolerance to the bronchoprotective effect of salmeterol in adolescents with exercise-induced asthma using concurrent inhaled glucocorticoid treatment. *Pediatrics* 1997; 99:655–659.

114 Nelson JA, Strauss L, Skowronski M, Ciofo R, Novak R, McFadden ER, Jr. Effect of long-term salmeterol treatment on exercise-induced asthma. *N Engl J Med* 1998; 339:141–146.

115 McAlpine LG, Thomson NC. Prophylaxis of exercise-induced asthma with inhaled formoterol, a long-acting beta2-adrenergic agonist. *Respir Med* 1990; 84:293–295.

116 Boner AL, Spezia E, Piovesan P, Chiocca E, Maiocchi G. Inhaled formoterol in the prevention of exercise-induced bronchoconstriction in asthmatic children. *Am J Respir Crit Care Med* 1994; 149:935–939.

117 Daugbjerg P, Nielsen KG, Skov M, Bisgaard H. Duration of action of formoterol and salbutamol dry-powder inhalation in prevention of exercise-induced asthma in children. *Acta Paediatr* 1996; 85:684–687.

118 Patessio A, Podda A, Carone M, Trombetta N, Donner CF. Protective effect and duration of action of formoterol aerosol on exercise-induced asthma. *Eur Respir J* 1991; 4:296–300.

119 Malo J-L, Cartier A, Trudeau C, Ghezzo H, Gontovnick L. Formoterol, a new inhaled beta-2 adrenergic agonist, has a longer blocking effect than albuterol on hyperventilation-induced bronchoconstriction. *Am Rev Respir Dis* 1990; 142:1147–1152.

120 Cong HJ, Linn WS, Shamoo DA et al. Effect of inhaled salmeterol on sulfur dioxide-induced bronchoconstriction in asthmatic subjects. *Chest* 1996; 110:1229–1235.

121 Bootsma GP, Dekhuijen PNR, Festen J, Lammers J-W, Mulder PGH, Van Herwaarden CLA. Sustained protection against distilled water provocation by a single dose of salmeterol in patients with asthma. *Eur Respir J* 1997; 10:2230–2236.

122 Beach JR, Young CL, Stenton SC, Avery AJ, Walters EH, Hendrick DJ. A comparison of the speeds of action of

salmeterol and salbutamol in reversing methacholine-induced bronchoconstriction. *Pulmon Pharmacol* 1992; 5:133–135.

123 Beach JR, Bromly CL, Avery AJ, Reid RWEC, Walters EH, Hendrick DJ. Speeds of action of single doses of formoterol and salbutamol compared with placebo in reversing methacholine-induced bronchoconstriction. *Pulmon Pharmacol* 1996; 9:245–249.

124 Sly RM. Mortality from asthma, 1979–1984. *J Allergy Clin Immunol* 1988; 82:705–717.

125 Sly RM, Anderson JA, Bierman CW. Adverse effects and complications of treatment with beta-adrenergic agonist drugs. *J Allergy Clin Immunol* 1985; 75:443–449.

126 Paterson JW, Lulich KM, Goldie RG. A comment on b2-agonists and their use in asthma. *Trends Pharmacol Sci* 1983; 4:67–69.

127 Lands AM, Arnold A, McAullif JP, Luduena FS, Brown TG. Differentiation of receptor systems activated by sympathomimetic amines. *Nature* 1967; 214:597–598.

128 Goldie RG, Spina D, Henry PJ, Lulich KM, Paterson JW. In vitro responsiveness of human asthmatic bronchus to carbachol, histamine, beta-adrenoceptor agonists and theophylline. *Br J Clin Pharmacol* 1986; 22:669–676.

129 O'Donnell SR. An examination of some β-adrenoceptor stimulants for selectivity using the isolated trachea and atria of the guinea-pig. *Eur J Pharmacol* 1972; 19:371–279.

130 Decker N, Quennedey MC, Rouot B. Effects of N-aralkyl substitution of beta-agonists on alpha- and beta-adrenoceptor subtypes: Pharmacological studies and binding assays. *J Pharmacy Pharmacol* 1982; 34:107–112.

131 Lipworth BJ, McDevitt DG. Inhaled beta2-adrenoceptor agonists in asthma: Help or hindrance? *Br J Clin Pharmacol* 1992; 33:129–138.

132 Scheinin M, Koulu M, Laurikainen E, Allonen H. Hypokalaemia and other non-bronchial effects of inhaled fenoterol and salbutamol: A placebo-controlled dose-response study in healthy volunteers. *Br J Clin Pharmacol* 1987; 24:645–653.

133 Deenstra M, Haalboom JRE, Struyvenberg A. Decrease of plasma potassium due to inhalation of beta-2-agonists: Absence of an additional effect of intravenous theophylline. *Europ J Clin Investig* 1988; 18:162–165.

134 Crane J, Burgess C, Beasley R. Cardiovascular and hypokalaemic effects of inhaled salbutamol, fenoterol, and isoprenaline. *Thorax* 1989; 44:136–140.

135 Flatt A, Crane J, Purdie G, Kwong T, Beasley R, Burgess C. The cardiovascular effects of beta adrenergic agonist drugs administered by nebulisation. *Postgrad Med J* 1990; 66:98–101.

136 Tandon MK. Cardiopulmonary effects of fenoterol and salbutamol aerosols. *Chest* 1980; 77:429–431.

137 Bellamy D, Penketh A. A cumulative dose comparison between salbutamol and fenoterol metered dose aerosols in asthmatic patients. *Postgrad Med J* 1987; 63:459–461.

138 Wong CS, Pavord ID, Williams J, Britton JR, Tattersfield AE. Bronchodilator, cardiovascular, and hypokalaemic effects of fenoterol, salbutamol, and terbutaline in asthma. *Lancet* 1990; 336:1396–1399.

139 Lipworth BJ, Struthers AD, McDevitt DG. Tachyphylaxis to systemic but not to airway responses during prolonged therapy with high dose inhaled salbutamol in asthmatics. *Am Rev Respir Dis* 1989; 140:586–592.

140 Bremner P, Woodman K, Burgess C et al. A comparison of the cardiovascular and metabolic effects of formoterol, salbutamol and fenoterol. *Eur Respir J* 1993; 6:204–210.

141 Bennett J, Tattersfield AE. Several studies have shown salmeterol to be more potent than salbutamol for systemic effects [4]. *Br Med J* 1997; 315:121

142 Palmqvist M, Ibsen T, Mellen A, Lotvall J. Comparison of the relative efficacy of formoterol and salmeterol in asthmatic patients. *Am J Respir Crit Care Med* 1999; 160:244–249.

143 Kenakin T. Efficacy in drug receptor theory: outdated concept or under-valued tool? *Trends Pharmacol Sci* 1999; 20:400–405.

144 Van den Brink FG. The model of functional interaction. I. Development and first check of a new model of functional synergism and antagonism. *Eur J Pharmacol* 1973; 22:278

145 Van den Brink FG. The model of functional interaction. II. Experimental verification of a new model: the antagonism of β-adrenoceptor stimulants and other agonists. *Eur J Pharmacol* 1973; 22:279–286.

146 Buckner CK, Saini RK. On the use of functional antagonism to estimate dissociation constants for β-adrenoceptor agonists in isolated guinea-pig trachea. *J Pharmacol Exp Ther* 1975; 194:565–574.

147 Torphy TJ, Rinard GA, Rietow MG, Mayer SE. Functional antagonism in canine tracheal smooth muscle: Inhibition by methacholine of the mechanical and biochemical responses to isoproterenol. *J Pharmacol Exp Ther* 1983; 227:694–699.

148 Advenier C, Naline E, Matran R, Toty L, Bakdach H. Interaction between fenoterol, ipratropium, and acetylcholine on human isolated bronchus. *J Allergy Clin Immunol* 1988; 82:40–46.

149 O'Donnell SR, Wanstall JC. Evidence that the efficacy (intrinsic activity) of fenoterol is higher than that of salbu-

tamol on β-adrenoceptors in guinea-pig trachea. *Eur J Pharmacol* 1978; 47:333–340.

150 Gustafsson B, Persson CGA. Effect of different bronchodilaters on airway smooth muscle responsiveness to contractile agents. *Thorax* 1991; 46:360–365.

151 Mitchell HW, Denborough MA. Drug interactions in cat isolated tracheal smooth muscle. *Clin Exp Pharmacol Physiol* 1979; 6:249–257.

152 Phillips GD, Finnerty JP, Holgate ST. Comparative protective effect of the inhaled beta2-agonist salbutamol (albuterol) on bronchoconstriction provoked by histamine, methacholine, and adenosine 5'-monophosphate in asthma. *J Allergy Clin Immunol* 1990; 85:755–762.

153 Madsen BW, Tandon MK, Paterson JW. Crossover study of the efficacy of four beta-2 sympathomimetic bronchodilator aerosols. *Br J Clin Pharmacol* 1979; 8:75–82.

154 Hockley B, Johnson NM. Fenoterol versus salbutamol nebulisation in asthma. *Postgrad Med J* 1983; 59:504–505.

155 Linden A, Bergendal A, Ullman A, Skoogh B-E, Lofdahl C-G. Salmeterol, formoterol, and salbutamol in the isolated guinea pig trachea: Differences in maximum relaxant effect and potency but not in functional antagonism. *Thorax* 1993; 48:547–553.

156 Kallstrom B-L, Sjoberg J, Waldeck B. The interaction between salmeterol and beta2-adrenoceptor agonists with higher efficacy on guinea-pig trachea and human bronchus in vitro. *Br J Pharmacol* 1994; 113:687–692.

157 Goldie RG, Paterson JW, Lulich KM. Adrenoceptors in airway smooth muscle. *Pharmacol Therap* 1990; 48:295–322.

158 Tomlinson PR, Wilson JWSAG. Inhibition by salbutamol of the proliferation of human airway smooth muscle cells grown in culture. *Br J Pharmacol* 1994; 111:641–647.

159 Young PG, Skinner SJM, Black PN. Effects of glucocorticoids and beta-adrenoceptor agonists on the proliferation of airway smooth muscle. *Eur J Pharmacol* 1995; 273:137–143.

160 Lichtenstein LM, Margolis S. Histamine release in vitro: inhibition by catecholamines and methylxanthines. *Science* 1968; 161:902–903.

161 Assem ESK, Schild HO. Inhibition by sympathomimetic amines of histamine release induced by antigen in passively sensitized human lung. *Nature* 1969; 224:1028–1029.

162 Butchers PR, Skidmore IF, Vardey CJ, Wheeldon A. Characterization of the receptor mediating the antianaphylactic effects of beta-adrenoceptor agonists in human lung tissue in vitro. *Br J Pharmacol* 1980; 71:663–667.

163 Church MK, Young KD. The characteristics of inhibition of

histamine release from human lung fragments by sodium cromoglycate, salbutamol and chlorpromazine. *Br J Pharmacol* 1983; 78:671–679.

164 Undem BJ, Peachell PT, Lichtenstein LM. Isoproterenol-induced inhibition of immunoglobulin E-mediated release of histamine and arachidonic acid metabolites from the human lung mast cell. *J Pharmacol Exp Ther* 1988; 247:209–217.

165 Peters SP, Schulman ES, Schleimer RP. Dispersed human lung mast cells. Pharmacologic aspects and comparison with human lung tissue fragments. *Am Rev Respir Dis* 1982; 126:1034–1039.

166 Church MK, Hiroi J. Inhibition of IgE-dependent histamine release from human dispersed lung mast cells by anti-allergic drugs and salbutamol. *Br J Pharmacol* 1987; 90:421–429.

167 Shichijo M, Inagaki N, Nakai N, Kimata M, Nakahata T, Serizawa I, et al. The effects of anti-asthma drugs on mediator release from cultured human mast cells. *Clin Exp Allergy* 1998; 28:1228–1236.

168 Butchers PR, Fullerton JR, Skidmore IF, Thompson LE, Vardey CE, Wheeldon A. A comparison of the anti-anaphylactic actions of salbutamol and disodium cromoglycate in the rat, the rat mast cell and human lung tissue. *Br J Pharmacol* 1979; 67:23–32.

169 Butchers PR, Vardey CJ, Johnson M. Salmeterol: A potent and long-acting inhibitor of inflammatory mediator release from human lung. *Br J Pharmacol* 1991; 104:672–676.

170 Tomioka K, Yamada T, Tachikawa S. Effects of formoterol (BD 40A), a beta-adrenoceptor stimulant, on isolated guinea-pig lung parenchymal strips and antigen-induced STS-A release in rats. *Arch Internat Pharmacodyn Therap* 1984; 267:91–102.

171 Plaut M, Pierce JH, Watson CJ, Hanley-Hyde J, Nordan R, Paul WE. Mast cell lines produce lymphokines in response to cross-linkage of FcepsilonRI or to calcium ionophores. *Nature* 1989; 339:64–67.

172 Bissonnette EY, Befus AD. Anti-inflammatory effect of beta2-agonists: Inhibition of TNF-alpha release from human mast cells. *J Allergy Clin Immunol* 1997; 100:825–831.

173 Shichijo M, Inagaki N, Kimata M, Serizawa I, Saito H, Nagai H. Role of cyclic 3',5'-adenosine monophosphate in the regulation of chemical mediator release and cytokine production from cultured human mast cells. *J Allergy Clin Immunol* 1999; 103:S421-S428.

174 Martin GL, Atkins PC, Dunsky EH, Zweiman B. Effects of theophylline, terbutaline, and prednisone on antigen-

induced bronchospasm and mediator release. *J Allergy Clin Immunol* 1980; 66:204–212.

175 Nagy L, Lee TH, Kay AB. Neutrophil chemotactic activity in antigen-induced late asthmatic reactions. *N Engl J Med* 1982; 306:497–501.

176 Howarth PH, Durham SR, Lee TH. Influence of albuterol, cromolyn sodium and ipratropium bromide on the airway and circulating mediator reponses to allergen bronchial provocation in asthma. *Am Rev Respir Dis* 1985; 132:986–992.

177 Murray JJ, Tonnel AB, Brash AR. Release of prostaglandin D2 into human airways during acute antigen challenge. *N Engl J Med* 1986; 315:800–804.

178 Miadonna A, Tedeschi A, Brasca C, Folco G, Sala A, Murphy RC. Mediator release after endobronchial antigen challenge in patients with respiratory allergy. *J Allergy Clin Immunol* 1990; 85:906–913.

179 Wenzel SE, Westcott JY, Larsen GL. Bronchoalveolar lavage fluid mediator levels 5 minutes after allergen challenge in atopic subjects with asthma: Relationship to the development of late asthmatic responses. *J Allergy Clin Immunol* 1991; 87:540–548.

180 Taylor IK, O'Shaughnessy KM, Choudry NB, Adachi M, Palmer JBD, Fuller RW. A comparative study in atopic subjects with asthma of the effects of salmeterol and salbutamol on allergen-induced bronchoconstriction, increase in airway reactivity, and increase in urinary leukotriene E4 excretion. *J Allergy Clin Immunol* 1992; 89:575–583.

181 Holtzman MJ. Arachidonic acid metabolism: Implications of biological chemistry for lung function and disease. *Am Rev Respir Dis* 1991; 143:188–203.

182 Roberts JA, Bradding P, Britten KM et al. The long-acting β_2-agonist salmeterol xinafoate: effects on airway inflammation in asthma. *Eur Respir J* 1999; 14:275–282.

183 Wallin A, Sandstrom T, Soderberg M et al. The effects of regular inhaled formoterol, budesonide, and placebo on mucosal inflammation and clinical indices in mild asthma. *Am J Respir Crit Care Med* 1999; 159:79–86.

184 O'Connor BJ, Aikman SL, Barnes PJ. Tolerance to the non-bronchodilator effects of inhaled beta2-agonists in asthma. *N Engl J Med* 1992; 327:1204–1208.

185 Yates DH, Worsdell M, Barnes PJ. Effect of inhaled glucocorticosteroid on mast cell and smooth muscle β_2 adrenergic tolerance in mild asthma. *Thorax* 1998; 53:110–113.

186 Taylor DA, Jensen MW, Aikman SL, Harris JG, Barnes PJ, O'Connor BJ. Comparison of salmeterol and albuterol-induced bronchoprotection against adenosine monophosphate and histamine in mild asthma. *Am J Respir Crit Care Med* 1997; 156:1731–1737.

187 Nightingale JA, Rogers DF, Barnes PJ. Differential effect of formoterol on adenosine monophosphate and histamine reactivity in asthma. *Am J Respir Crit Care Med* 1999; 159:1786–1790.

188 Soler M, Joos L, Bolliger CT, Elsasser S, Perruchoud AP. Bronchoprotection by salmeterol: Cell stabilization or functional antagonism? Comparative effects on histamine- and AMP-induced bronchoconstriction. *Eur Respir J* 1994; 7:1973–1977.

189 Aziz I, Tan KS, Hall IP, Devlin MM, Lipworth BJ. Subsensitivity to bronchoprotection against adenosine monophosphate challenge following regular once-daily formoterol. *Eur Respir J* 1998; 12:580–584.

190 Fick RBJ, Richerson HB, Zavala DC, Hunninghake GW. Bronchoalveolar lavage in allergic asthmatics. *Am Rev Respir Dis* 1987; 135:1204–1209.

191 Metzger WJ, Zavala D, Richerson HB. Local allergen challenge and bronchoalveolar lavage of allergic asthmatic lungs. Description of the model and local airway inflammation. *Am Rev Respir Dis* 1987; 135:433–440.

192 Persson CGA. Role of plasma exudation in asthmatic airways. *Lancet* 1986; ii:1126–1128.

193 Erjefalt I, Persson CGA. Long duration and high potency of antiexudative effects of formoterol in guinea-pig tracheobronchial airways. *Am Rev Respir Dis* 1991; 144:788–791.

194 Grega GJ, Adamski SW, Dobbins DE. Physiological and pharmacological evidence for the regulation of permeability. *Fed Proc* 1986; 45:96–100.

195 Persson CGA, Erjefalt I. Terbutaline and adrenaline inhibit leakage of fluid and protein in guinea-pig lung. *Eur J Pharmacol* 1979; 55:199–201.

196 Boschetto P, Roberts NM, Rogers DF, Barnes PJ. Effect of antiasthma drugs on microvascular leakage in guinea pig airways. *Am Rev Respir Dis* 1989; 139:416–421.

197 Woodward DF, Weichman BM, Wasserman MA. Differential inhibition of LTD4-mediated bronchopulmonary effects by salbutamol. *Eur J Pharmacol* 1984; 100:219–222.

198 Erjefalt I, Persson CGA. Inflammatory passage of plasma macromolecules into airway wall and lumen. *Pulmon Pharmacol* 1989; 2:93–102.

199 Tokuyama K, Lotvall JO, Lofdahl C-G, Barnes PJ, Chung KF. Inhaled formoterol inhibits histamine-induced airflow obstruction and airway microvascular leakage. *Eur J Pharmacol* 1991; 193:35–39.

200 Whelan CJ, Johnson M. Inhibition by salmeterol of increased vascular permeability and granulocyte accumulation in guinea-pig lung and skin. *Br J Pharmacol* 1992; 105:831–838.

201 Blease K, Burke-Gaffney A, Hellewell PG. Modulation of

cell adhesion molecule expression and function on human lung microvascular endothelial cells by inhibition of phosphodiesterases 3 and 4. *Br J Pharmacol* 1998; 124:229–237.

202 Basran GS, Paul W, Morley J, Turner-Warwick M. Adrenoceptor-agonist inhibition of the histamine-induced cutaneous response in man. *Br J Dermat* 1982; 107:140–142.

203 Gronneberg R, Strandberg K, Stalenheim G, Zetterstrom O. Effect in man of anti-allergic drugs on the immediate and late phase cutaneous allergic reactions induced by anti-IgE. *Allergy* 1981; 36:201–208.

204 Gronneberg R, Zetterstrom O. Inhibition of anti-IgE induced skin response in normals by formoterol, a new beta2-adrenoceptor agonist, and terbutaline. 2. Effect on the late phase reaction. *Allergy* 1990; 45:340–346.

205 Gronneberg R, Strandberg K, Hagermark O. Effect of terbutaline, a b-adrenergic receptor stimulating compound, on cutaneous responses to histamine, allergen, compound 48/80 and trypsin. *Allergy* 1979; 34:303–309.

206 Ting S, Zweiman B, Lavker R. Terbutaline modulation of human allergic skin reactions. *J Allergy Clin Immunol* 1983; 71:437–441.

207 Gronneberg R, Raud J. Effects of local treatment with salmeterol and terbutaline on anti-IgE-induced wheal, flare, and late induration in human skin. *Allergy* 1996; 51:685–692.

208 Gronneberg R, Zetterstrom O. Inhibitory effects of formoterol and terbutaline on the development of late phase skin reactions. *Clin Exp Allergy* 1992; 22:257–263.

209 Gronneberg R, Van Hage-Hamsten M, Hallden G, Hed J, Raud J. Effects of salmeterol and terbutaline on IgE-mediated dermal reactions and inflammatory events in skin chambers in atopic patients. *Allergy* 1996; 51:640–646.

210 Svensson C, Greiff L, Andersson M, Alkner U, Gronneberg R, Persson CGA. Antiallergic actions of high topical doses of terbutaline in human nasal airways. *Allergy* 1995; 50:884–890.

211 Birchall MA, O'Connell F, Henderson J et al. Topical salmeterol reduces protein content of nasal lavage fluid in response to allergen and histamine challenge: Double-blind cross-over placebo-controlled studies in adults. *Am J Rhinol* 1996; 10:251–256.

212 Proud D, Reynolds CJ, Lichtenstein LM, Kagey-Sobotka A, Togias A. Intranasal salmeterol inhibits allergen-induced vascular permeability but not mast cell activation or cellular infiltration. *Clin Exp Allergy* 1998; 28:868–875.

213 Greiff L, Wollmer P, Andersson M, Svensson C, Persson CGA. Effects of formoterol on histamine induced plasma exudation in induced sputum from normal subjects. *Thorax* 1998; 53:1010–1013.

214 Martin LB, Kita H, Leiferman KM, Gleich GJ. Eosinophils in allergy: Role in disease, degranulation, and cytokines. *Int Arch Allergy Immunol* 1996; 109:207–215.

215 Kay AB. Allergy and allergic diseases. *N Engl J Med* 2001; 344:30–37.

216 Herd CM, Page CP. Pulmonary immune cells in health and disease: Platelets. *Eur Respir J* 1994; 7:1145–1160.

217 Fuller RW. Pharmacological regulation of airway macrophage function. *Clin Exp Allergy* 1991; 21:651–654.

218 Torphy TJ. Phosphodiesterase isozymes molecular targets for novel antiasthma agents. *Am J Respir Crit Care Med* 1998; 157:351–270.

219 Cook N, Nahorski SR, Jagger C, Barnett DB. Is the human platelet beta2 adrenoceptor coupled to adenylate cyclase? *Naunyn-Schmied Arch Pharmacol* 1988; 238–240.

220 Johnson CE, Belfield PW, Davis S, Cooke NJ, Spencer A, Davies JA. Platelet activation during exercise induced asthma: Effect of prophylaxis with cromoglycate and salbutamol. *Thorax* 1986; 41:290–294.

221 Yukawa T, Ukena D, Kroegel C et al. Beta2-adrenergic receptors on eosinophils. Binding and functional studies. *Am Rev Respir Dis* 1990; 141:1446–1452.

222 Ezeamuzie CI, Al-Hage M. Differential effects of salbutamol and salmeterol on human eosinophil responses. *J Pharmacol Exp Ther* 1998; 284:25–31.

223 Munoz NM, Rabe KF, Vita AJ et al. Paradoxical blockade of beta adrenergically mediated inhibition of stimulated eosinophil secretion by salmeterol. *J Pharmacol Exp Ther* 1995; 273:850–854.

224 Leff AR, Herrnreiter A, Naclerio RM, Baroody FM, Handley DA, Munoz NM. Effect of enantiomeric forms of albuterol on stimulated secretion of granular protein from human eosinophils. *Pulmon Pharmacol Ther* 1997; 10:97–104.

225 Dent G, Giembycz MA, Evans PM, Rabe KF, Barnes PJ. Suppression of human eosinophil respiratory burst and cyclic AMP hydrolysis by inhibitors of type IV phosphodiesterase: Interaction with the beta adrenoceptor agonist albuterol. *J Pharmacol Exp Ther* 1994; 271:1167–1174.

226 Hadjokas NE, Crowley JJ, Bayer CR, Nielson CP. beta-Adrenergic regulation of the eosinophil respiratory burst as detected by lucigenin-dependent luminescenc. *J Allergy Clin Immunol* 1995; 95:735–741.

227 Tenor H, Hatzelmann A, Church MK, Schudt C, Shute JK. Effects of theophylline and rolipram on leukotriene C4 (LTC4) synthesis and chemotaxis of human eosinophils from normal and atopic subjects. *Br J Pharmacol* 1996; 118:1727–1735.

228 Tool ATJ, Mul FPJ, Knol EF, Verhoeven AJ, Roos D. The effect of salmeterol and nimesulide on chemotaxis and synthesis of PAF and LTC4 by human eosinophils. *Eur Respir J* – Suppl 1996; 9:141S-145S.

229 Kankaanranta H, Lindsay MA, Giembycz MA, Zhang X, Moilanen E, Barnes PJ. Delayed eosinophil apoptosis in asthma. *J Allergy Clin Immunol* 2000; 106:77–83.

230 Alves AC, Pires ALA, Cruz HN et al. Selective inhibition of phosphodiesterase type IV suppresses the chemotactic responsiveness of rat eosinophils in vitro. *Eur J Pharmacol* 1996; 312:89–96.

231 Rabe KF, Giembycz MA, Dent G, Perkins RS, Evans P, Barnes PJ. Salmeterol is a competitive antagonist at beta-adreno-ceptors mediating inhibition of respiratory burst in guinea-pig eosinophil. *Eur J Pharmacol* 1993; 231:305–308.

232 Teixeira MM, Rossi AG, Giembycz MA, Hellewell PG. Effects of agents which elevate cyclic AMP on guinea-pig eosino-phil homotypic aggregation. *Br J Pharmacol* 1996; 118:2099–2106.

233 Kraan J, Koeter GH, Van Der Mark T, Sluiter HJ, De Vries K. Changes in bronchial hyperreactivity induced by 4 weeks of treatment with antiasthmatic drugs in patients with allergic asthma: A comparison between budesonide and terbutaline. *J Allergy Clin Immunol* 1985; 76:628–636.

234 Adelroth E, Rosenhall L, Johansson S-A, Linden M, Venge P. Inflammatory cells and eosinophilic activity in asthmatics investigated by bronchoalveolar lavage. The effects of anti-asthmatic treatment with budesonide or terbutaline. *Am Rev Respir Dis* 1990; 142:91–99.

235 Jeffery PK, Godfrey RW, Adelroth E, Nelson A, Rogers A, Johansson S-A. Effects of treatment on airway inflamma-tion and thickening of basement membrane reticular col-lagen in asthma. *Am Rev Respir Dis* 1992; 145:890–899.

236 Laitinen LA, Laitinen A, Haahtela T. A comparative study of the effects of an inhaled corticosteroid, budesonide and a β_2 agonist, terbutaline, on airway inflammation in newly diagnosed asthma: a randomised double-blind, parallel-group controlled study. *J Allergy Clin Immunol* 1992; 90:32–42.

237 Manolitsas ND, Wang J, Devalia JL, Trigg CJ, McAulay AE, Davies RJ. Regular albuterol, nedocromil sodium, and bronchial inflammation in asthma. *Am J Respir Crit Care Med* 1995; 151:1925–1930.

238 Diaz P, Galleguillos FR, Gonzalez MC, Pantin CFA, Kay AB. Bronchoalveolar lavage in asthma: The effect of disodium cromoglycate (cromolyn) on leukocyte counts, immuno-globulins, and complement. *J Allergy Clin Immunol* 1984; 74:41–48.

239 Djukanovic R, Wilson JW, Britten KM et al. Effect of an inhaled corticosteroid on airway inflammation and symp-toms in asthma. *Am Rev Respir Dis* 1992; 145:669–674.

240 Gauvreau GM, Doctor J, Watson RM, Jordana M, O'Byrne PM. Effects of inhaled budesonide on allergen-induced airway responses and airway inflammation. *Am J Respir Crit Care Med* 1996; 154:1267–1271.

241 Gauvreau GM, Jordana M, Watson RM, Cockcroft DW, O'Byrne PM. Effect of regular inhaled albuterol on aller-gen-induced late responses and sputum eosinophils in asthmatic subjects. *Am J Respir Crit Care Med* 1997; 156:1738–1745.

242 Pedersen B, Dahl R, Larsen BB, Venge P. The effect of sal-meterol on the early- and late-phase reaction to bronchial allergen and postchallenge variation in bronchial reactiv-ity, blood eosinophils, serum eosinophil cationic protein, and serum eosinophil protein X. *Allergy* 1993; 48:377–382.

243 Weersink EJM, Aalbers R, Koeter GH, Kauffman HF, De Monchy JGR, Postma DS. Partial inhibition of the early and late asthmatic response by a single dose of salmeterol. *Am J Respir Crit Care Med* 1994; 150:1262–1267.

244 Dente FL, Bancalari L, Bacci E et al. Effect of a single dose of salmeterol on the increase in airway eosinophils induced by allergen challenge in asthmatic subjects. *Thorax* 1999; 54:622–624.

245 Di Lorenzo G, Morici G, Norrito F et al. Comparison of the effects of salmeterol and salbutamol on clinical activity and eosinophil cationic protein serum levels during the pollen season in atopic asthmatics. *Clin Exp Allergy* 1995; 25:951–956.

246 Turner MO, Johnston PR, Pizzichini E, Pizzichini MMM, Hussack PA, Hargreave FE. Anti-inflammatory effects of salmeterol compared with beclomethasone in eosino-philic mild exacerbations of asthma: A randomized, placebo controlled trial. *Can Respir J* 1998; 5:261–268.

247 Gardiner PV, Ward C, Booth H, Allison A, Hendrick DJ, Walters EH. Effect of eight weeks of treatment with salmet-erol on bronchoalveolar lavage inflammatory indices in asthmatics. *Am J Respir Crit Care Med* 1994; 150:1006–1011.

248 McIvor RA, Pizzichini E, Turner MO, Hussack P, Hargreave FE, Sears MR. Potential masking effects of salmeterol on airway inflammation in asthma. *Am J Respir Crit Care Med* 1998; 158:924–930.

249 Kraft M, Wenzel SE, Bettinger CM, Martin RJ. The effect of salmeterol on nocturnal symptoms, airway function, and inflammation in asthma. *Chest* 1997; 111:1249–1254.

250 Li X, Ward C, Thien F et al. An antiinflammatory effect of salmeterol, a long-acting β_2 agonist, assessed in airway

biopsies and bronchoalveolar lavage in asthma. *Am J Respir Crit Care Med* 1999; 160:1493–1499.

251 Capron M, Jouault T, Prin L. Functional study of a monoclonal antibody to IgE Fc receptor (FcepsilonR2) of eosinophils, platelets, and macrophages. *J Exp Med* 1986; 164:72–89.

252 Liggett SB. Identification and characterization of a homogeneous population of beta2-adrenergic receptors on human alveolar macrophages. *Am Rev Respir Dis* 1989; 139:552–555.

253 Fuller RW, O'Malley G, Baker AJ, MacDermot J. Human alveolar macrophage activation: inhibition by forskolin but not b-adrenoceptor stimulation or phosphodiesterase inhibition. *Pulmon Pharmacol* 1988; 1:101–106.

254 Baker AJ, Palmer J, Johnson M, Fuller RW. Inhibitory actions of salmeterol on human airway macrophages and blood monocytes. *Eur J Pharmacol* 1994; 264:301–206.

255 Calhoun WJ, Stevens CA, Lambert SB. Modulation of superoxide production of alveolar macrophages and peripheral blood mononuclear cells by beta-agonists and theophyllin. *J Laborat Clin Med* 1991; 117:514–522.

256 Zetterlund A, Linden M, Larsson K. Effects of beta2-agonists and budesonide on interleukin-1beta and leukotriene B4 secretion: Studies of human monocytes and alveolar macrophages. *J Asthma* 1998; 35:565–573.

257 Izeboud CA, Mocking JAJ, Monshouwer M, Van Miert ASJ, Witkamp RF. Participation of beta-adrenergic receptors on macrophages in modulation of LPS-induced cytokine release. *J Receptor Signal Transduction Res* 1999; 19:191–202.

258 Hasko G, Shanley TP, Egnaczyk G et al. Exogenous and endogenous catecholamines inhibit the production of macrophage inflammatory protein (MIP) 1alpha via a beta adrenoceptor mediated mechanism. *Br J Pharmacol* 1998; 125:1297–1303.

259 Kemeny DM, Vyas B, Vukmanovi-Stejic M et al. CD8 + T cell subsets and chronic obstructive pulmonary disease. *Am J Respir Crit Care Med* 1999; 160:S33-S37.

260 Tashkin DP, Conolly ME, Deutsch RI. Subsensitization of beta-adrenoceptors in airways and lymphocytes of healthy and asthmatic subjects. *Am Rev Respir Dis* 1982; 125:185–193.

261 Sano Y, Watt G, Townley RG. Decreased mononuclear cell beta-adrenergic receptors in bronchial asthma: Parallel studies of lymphocyte and granulocyte desensitization. *J Allergy Clin Immunol* 1983; 72:495–503.

262 Motojima S, Fukuda T, Makino S. Measurement of beta-adrenergic receptors on lymphocytes in normal subjects and asthmatics in relation to beta-adrenergic hyperglycaemic response and bronchial responsiveness. *Allergy* 1983; 38:331–237.

263 Bourne HR, Lichtenstein LM, Melmon KL, Henney CS, Weinstein Y, Shearer GM. Modulation of inflammation and immunity by cyclic AMP. *Science* 1974; 184:19–28.

264 Kammer GM. The adenylate cyclase-cAMP-protein kinase A pathway and regulation of the immune response. *Immunol Today* 1988; 9:222-229.

265 Brooks SM, McGowan K, Bernstein IL, Altenau P, Peagler J. Relationship between numbers of beta-adrenergic receptors in lymphocytes and disease severity in asthma. *J Allergy Clin Immunol* 1979; 63:401–406.

266 Koeter GH, Meurs H, Kauffman HF, De Vries K. The role of the adrenergic system in allergy and bronchial hyperreactivity. *Eur J Respir Dis* 1982; 63:72–78.

267 Meurs H, Koeter GH, De Vries K, Kauffman HF. The beta-adrenergic system and allergic bronchial asthma: Changes in lymphocyte beta-adrenergic receptor number and adenylate cyclase activity after an allergen-induced asthmatic attack. *J Allergy Clin Immunol* 1982; 70:272-280.

268 Maisel AS, Fowler P, Rearden A, Motulsky HJ, Michel MC. A new method for isolation of human lymphocyte subsets reveals differential regulation of beta-adrenergic receptors by terbutaline treatment. *Clin Pharmacol Therap* 1989; 46:429–439.

269 Maisel AS, Knowlton KU, Fowler P, Rearden A, Ziegler MG, Motulsky HJ, et al. Adrenergic control of circulating lymphocyte subpopulations. Effects of congestive heart failure, dynamic exercise, and terbutaline treatment. *J Clin Immunol* 1990; 85:462–467.

270 Maisel AS, Michel MC. β-adrenoceptor control of immune function in congestive heart failure. *Br J Clin Pharmacol* 1990; 30:49S-53S.

271 Gonzalez MC, Diaz P, Galleguillos FR, Ancic P, Cromwell O, Kay AB. Allergen-induced recruitment of bronchoalveolar helper (OKT4) and suppressor (OKT8) T-cells in asthma. Relative increases in OKT8 cells in single early responders compared with those in late-phase responders. *Am Rev Respir Dis* 1987; 136:600–604.

272 Panina-Bordignon P, Mazzeo D, Di Lucia P et al. Beta2-agonists prevent Th1 development by selective inhibition of interleukin 12. *J Clin Immunol* 1997; 100:1513–1519.

273 Sanders VM, Baker RA, RamerQuinn DS, Kasprowicz DJ, Fuchs BA, Street NE. Differential expression of the beta(2)-adrenergic receptor by Th1 and Th2 clones – implications for cytokine production and B cell help. *J Immunol* 1997; 158:4200–4210.

274 Ramer-Quinn DS, Baker RA, Sanders VM. Activated T helper 1 and T helper 2 cells differentially express the beta-2-adrenergic receptor – a mechanism for selective modulation of T helper 1 cell cytokine production. *J Immunol* 1997; 159:4857–4867.

275 Yoshimura T, Nagao T, Nakao T et al. Modulation of Th1- and Th2-like cytokine production from mitogen-stimulated human peripheral blood mononuclear cells by phosphodiesterase inhibitors. *Gen Pharmacol* 1998; 30:175–180.

276 Agarwal SK, Marshall GD. beta-adrenergic modulation of human type-1/type-2 cytokine balance. *J Allergy Clin Immunol* 2000; 105:91–98.

277 Mohede ICM, Van A, I, Brons FM, Van Oosterhout AJM, Nijkamp FP. Salmeterol inhibits interferon-gamma and interleukin-4 production by human peripheral blood mononuclear cells. *Int J Immunopharmacol* 1996; 18:193–201.

278 Sekut L, Champion BR, Page K, Menius JJ, Connolly KM. Anti-inflammatory activity of salmeterol: Down-regulation of cytokine production. *Clin Exp Immunol* 1995; 99:461–466.

279 Coqueret O, Dugas B, Mencia-Huerta JM, Braquet P. Regulation of IgE production from human mononuclear cells by beta2-adrenoceptor agonist. *Clin Exp Allergy* 1995; 25:304–311.

280 Borger P, Jonker G-J, Vellenga E, Postma DS, De Monchy JGR, Kauffman HF. Allergen challenge primes for IL-5 mRNA production and abrogates beta-adrenergic function in peripheral blood T lymphocytes from asthmatics. *Clin Exp Allergy* 1999; 29:933–940.

281 Kay AB. Role of T cells in asthma. *Chem Immunol* 1998; 71:191

282 Wilson JW, Djukanovic R, Howarth PH, Holgate ST. Inhaled beclomethasone dipropionate downregulates airway lymphocyte activation in atopic asthma. *Am J Respir Crit Care Med* 1994; 149:86–90.

283 Jaffar ZH, Sullivan P, Page C, Costello J. Low-dose theophylline modulates T-lymphocyte activation in allergen-challenged asthmatics. *Eur Respir J* 1996; 9:456–462.

284 Beasley R, Roche WR, Roberts JA, Holgate ST. Cellular events in the bronchi in mild asthma and after bronchial provocation. *Am Rev Respir Dis* 1989; 139:806–817.

285 Azzawi M, Bradley B, Jeffery PK et al. Identification of activated T lymphocytes and eosinophils in bronchial biopsies in stable atopic asthma. *Am Rev Respir Dis* 1990; 142:1407–1413.

286 Bradley BL, Azzawi M, Jacobson M et al. Eosinophils, T-lymphocytes, mast cells, neutrophils, and macrophages in bronchial biopsy specimens from atopic subjects with asthma: Comparison with biopsy specimens from atopic subjects without asthma and normal control subjects and relationship to bronchial hyperresponsiveness. *J Allergy Clin Immunol* 1991; 88:661–674.

287 Jatakanon A, Uasuf C, Maziak M, Lim S, Chung KF, Barnes PJ. Neutrophilic inflammation in severe persistent asthma. *Am J Respir Crit Care Med* 1999; 160:1532–1539.

288 Martin RJ, Cicutto LC, Smith HR, Ballard RD, Szefler SJ. Airways inflammation in nocturnal asthma. *Am Rev Respir Dis* 1991; 143:351–257.

289 Saetta M. Airway inflammation in chronic obstructive pulmonary disease. *Am J Respir Crit Care Med* 1999; 160:S17-S20

290 Galant SP, Duriset L, Underwood S, Allfred S, Insel PA. Beta-adrenergic receptors of polymorphonuclear particulates in bronchial asthma. *J Clin Invest* 1980; 65:577–585.

291 Davis PB, Simpson DM, Paget GL, Turi V. Beta-adrenergic responses in drug-free subjects with asthma. *J Allergy Clin Immunol* 1986; 77:871–879.

292 Nielson CP, Vestal RE, Sturm RJ, Heaslip R. Effects of selective phosphodiesterase inhibitors on the polymorphonuclear leukocyte respiratory burst. *J Allergy Clin Immunol* 1990; 86:801–808.

293 Busse WW, Sosman JM. Isoproterenol inhibition of isolated human neutrophil function. *J Allergy Clin Immunol* 1984; 73:404–410.

294 Mack JA, Nielson CP, Stevens DL, Vestal RE. beta-Adrenoceptor-mediated modulation of calcium ionophore activated polymorphonuclear leucocytes. *Br J Pharmacol* 1986; 88:417–423.

295 Silvestri M, Oddera S, Lantero S, Rossi GA. Beta2-agonist-induced inhibition of neutrophil chemotaxis is not associated with modification of LFA-1 and Mac-1 expression or with impairment of polymorphonuclear leukocyte antibacterial activity. *Respir Med* 1999; 93:416–423.

296 Ottonello L, Morone P, Dapino P, Dallegri F. Inhibitory effect of salmeterol on the respiratory burst of adherent human neutrophils. *Clin Exp Immunol* 1996; 106:97–102.

297 Anderson R, Feldman C, Theron AJ, Ramafi G, Cole PJ, Wilson R. Anti-inflammatory, membrane-stabilizing interactions of salmeterol with human neutrophils in vitro. *Br J Pharmacol* 1996; 117:1387–1394.

298 Nials AT, Coleman RA, Johnson M, Vardey CJ. The duration of action of non-beta2-adrenoceptor mediated responses to salmeterol. *Br J Pharmacol* 1997; 120:961–967.

299 Bloemen PGM, Van den Tweel MC, Henricks PAJ et al.

Increased cAMP levels in stimulated neutrophils inhibit their adhesion to human bronchial epithelial cells. *Am J Physiol Lung Cell Mol Physiol* 1997; 272:L580-L587.

300 Masclans JR, Barbera JA, MacNee W et al. Salbutamol reduces pulmonary neutrophil sequestration of platelet-activating factor in humans. *Am J Respir Crit Care Med* 1996; 154:529–532.

301 Britton J, Hanley SP, Garrett HV, Hadfield JW, Tattersfield AE. Dose related effects of salbutamol and ipratropium bromide on airway calibre and reactivity in subjects with asthma. *Thorax* 1988; 43:300–305.

302 Bel EH, Zwinderman AH, Timmers MC, Dijkman JH, Sterk PJ. The protective effect of beta2 agonist against excessive airway narrowing in response to bronchoconstrictor stimuli in asthma and chronic obstructive lung disease. *Thorax* 1991; 46:9–14.

303 Salome CM, Schoeffel RE, Woolcock AJ. Effect of aerosol and oral fenoterol on histamine and methacholine challenge in asthmatic subjects. *Thorax* 1981; 36:580–584.

304 Chung KF, Morgan B, Keyes SJ, Snashall PD. Histamine dose-response relationships in normal and asthmatic subjects. The importance of starting airway caliber. *Am Rev Respir Dis* 1982; 126:849–854.

305 Cockcroft DW, Murdock KY. Comparative effects of inhaled salbutamol, sodium cromoglycate, and beclomethasone dipropionate on allergen-induced early asthmatic responses, late asthmatic responses, and increased bronchial responsiveness to histamine. *J Allergy Clin Immunol* 1987; 79:734–740.

306 Lai CKW, Twentyman OP, Holgate ST. The effect of an increase in inhaled allergen dose after rimiterol hydrobromide on the occurrence and magnitude of the late asthmatic response and the associated change in nonspecific bronchial responsiveness. *Am Rev Respir Dis* 1989; 140:917–923.

307 Latimer KM, O'Byrne PM, Morris MM. Bronchoconstriction stimulated by airway cooling. Better protection with combined inhalation of terbutaline sulphate and cromolyn sodium than with either alone. *Am Rev Respir Dis* 1983; 128:440–443.

308 Anderson SD, Bye PTP, Schoeffel RE. Arterial plasma histamine levels at rest, and during and after exercise in patients with asthma: Effects of terbutaline aerosol. *Thorax* 1981; 36:259–267.

309 Neijens HJ, Kerrebijn KF. Variation with time in bronchial responsiveness to histamine and to specific allergen provocation. *Eur J Respir Dis* 1983; 64:591–597.

310 Morton AR, Scott CA, Fitch KD. Rimiterol and the prevention of exercise-induced asthma. *J Allergy Clin Immunol* 1989; 83:61–65.

311 Moscato G, Rampulla C, Dellabianca A, Zanotti E, Candura S. Effect of salbutamol and inhaled sodium cromoglycate on the airway and neutrophil chemotactic activity in 'fog'-induced bronchospasm. *J Allergy Clin Immunol* 1988; 82:382–388.

312 Boulet L-P, Turcotte H, Tennina S. Comparative efficacy of salbutamol, ipratropium, and cromoglycate in the prevention of bronchospasm induced by exercise and hyperosmolar challenges. *J Allergy Clin Immunol* 1989; 83:882–887.

313 Malo J-L, Ghezzo H, Trudeau C, L'Archeveque J, Cartier A. Salmeterol, a new inhaled beta2-adrenergic agonist, has a longer blocking effect than albuterol on hyperventilation-induced bronchoconstriction. *J Allergy Clin Immunol* 1992; 89:567–574.

314 Cartier A, Ghezzo H, L'Archeveque J, Trudeau C, Malo J-L. Duration and magnitude of action of 50 and 100 mug of inhaled salmeterol in protecting against bronchoconstriction induced by hyperventilation of dry cold air in subjects with asthma. *J Allergy Clin Immunol* 1993; 92:488–492.

315 Blake K, Pearlman DS, Scott C, Wang Y, Stahl E, Arledge T. Prevention of exercise-induced bronchospasm in pediatric asthma patients: a comparison of salmeterol powder with albuterol. *Ann Allergy* 1999; 82:205–211.

316 Casterline CL, Evans R, Ward GW. The effect of atropine and albuterol aerosols on the human bronchial response to histamine. *J Allergy Clin Immunol* 1976; 58:607–613.

317 Cockcroft DW, Killian DN, Mellon JJA, Hargreave FE. Protective effect of drugs on histamine induced asthma. *Thorax* 1977; 32:429–437.

318 Bandouvakis J, Cartier A, Roberts R. The effect of ipratropium and fenoterol on methacholine- and histamine-induced bronchoconstriction. *Br J Dis Chest* 1981; 75:295–305.

319 De Monchey JGR, Kauffman HF, Venge P et al. Bronchoalveolar eosinophilia during allergen-induced late asthmatic reactions. *Am Rev Respir Dis* 1985; 131:373–376.

320 Booij-Noord H, De Vries K, Sluiter HJ, Van Der Straeten M, Johannesson N, Persson CGA. Late bronchial obstructive reaction to experimental late asthmatic reactions. *Clin Allergy* 1972; 2:43–61.

321 Pauwels R, Van Renterghem D, Van Der Straeten M. The effect of theophylline and enprofylline on allergen-induced bronchoconstriction. *J Allergy Clin Immunol* 1985; 76:583–590.

322 Ward AJM, McKenniff M, Evans JM, Page CP, Costello JF.

Theophylline – an immunomodulatory role in asthma? *Am Rev Respir Dis* 1993; 147:518–523.

323 Diamant Z, Grootendorst DC, Veselic-Charvat M et al. The effect of montelukast (MK-0476), a cysteinyl leukotriene receptor antagonist, on allergen-induced airway responses and sputum cell counts in asthma. *Clin Exp Allergy* 1999; 29:42–51.

324 Van Bever HP, Desager KN, Stevens WJ. The effect of inhaled fenoterol, administered during the late asthmatic reaction to house dust mite (*Dermatophagoides pteronyssinus*). *J Allergy Clin Immunol* 1990; 85:700–703.

325 Hegardt B, Pauwels R, Van Der Straeten M. Inhibitory effect of KWD 2131, terbutaline, and DSCG on the immediate and late allergen-induced bronchoconstriction. *Allergy* 1981; 36:115–122.

326 Twentyman OP, Finnerty JP, Holgate ST. The inhibitory effect of nebulized albuterol on the early and late asthmatic reactions and increase in airway responsiveness provoked by inhaled allergen in asthma. *Am Rev Respir Dis* 1991; 144:782–787.

327 Palmqvist M, Balder B, Lowhagen O, Melander B, Svedmyr N, Wahlander L. Late asthmatic reaction decreased after pretreatment with salbutamol and formoterol, a new long-acting beta2-agonist. *J Allergy Clin Immunol* 1992; 89:844–849.

328 Pizzichini MMM, Kidney JC, Wong BJO et al. Effect of salmeterol compared with beclomethasone on allergen-induced asthmatic and inflammatory responses. *Eur Respir J* 1996; 9:449–455.

329 Woolcock AJ, Salome CM, Yan K. The shape of the dose-response curve to histamine in asthmatic and normal subjects. *Am Rev Respir Dis* 1984; 130:71–75.

330 Sterk PJ, Bel EH. The shape of the dose-response curve to inhaled bronchoconstrictor agents in asthma and in chronic obstructive pulmonary disease. *Am Rev Respir Dis* 1991; 143:1433–1437.

331 Cheung D, Timmers MC, Zwinderman AH, Bel EH, Dijkman JH, Sterk PJ. Long-term effects of a long-acting beta2-adrenoceptor agonist, salmeterol, on airway hyper-responsiveness in patients with mild asthma. *N Engl J Med* 1992; 327:1198–1203.

332 Fitzpatrick MF, Jokic R. Nocturnal asthma. *Eur Respir Monog* 1998; 3:285–302.

333 Silkoff PE, Martin RJ. Pathophysiology of nocturnal asthma. *Ann Allergy* 1998; 81:378–387.

334 Morrison JFJ, Pearson SB. The effect of the circadian rhythm of vagal activity on bronchomotor tone in asthma. *Br J Clin Pharmacol* 1989; 28:545–549.

335 Morrison JFJ, Pearson SB. The parasympathetic nervous system and the diurnal variation of lung mechanics in asthma. *Respir Med* 1991; 85:285–289.

336 Mackay TW, Fitzpatrick MF, Douglas NJ. Nonadrenergic, noncholinergic nervous-system and overnight airway caliber in asthmatic and normal subjects. *Lancet* 1991; 338:1289–1292.

337 Kraft M, Torvik JA, Trudeau JB, Wenzel SE, Martin RJ. Theophylline: Potential antiinflammatory effects in nocturnal asthma. *J Allergy Clin Immunol* 1996; 97:1242–1246.

338 Kraft M, Martin RJ, Wilson S, Djukanovic R, Holgate ST. Lymphocyte and eosinophil influx into alveolar tissue in nocturnal asthma. *Am J Respir Crit Care Med* 1999; 159:228–234.

339 Fairfax AJ, McNabb WR, Davies HJ, Spiro SG. Slow-release oral salbutamol and aminophylline in nocturnal asthma: Relation of overnight changes in lung function and plasma drug levels. *Thorax* 1980; 35:526–530.

340 Joad JP, Ahrens RC, Lindgren SD, Weinberger MM. Relative efficacy of maintenance therapy with theophylline, inhaled albuterol, and the combination for chronic asthma. *J Allergy Clin Immunol* 1987; 79:78–85.

341 Westermann CJJ, Van Weelden BM, Laros CD. Sustained release terbutaline in nocturnal asthma. *Allergy* 1986; 41:308–310.

342 Stewart IC, Rhind GB, Power JT, Flenley DC, Douglas NJ. Effect of sustained-release terbutline on symptoms and sleep quality in patients with nocturnal asthma. *Thorax* 1987; 42:797–800.

343 Postma DS, Koeter GH, Keyzer JJ, Meurs H. Influence of slow-release terbutaline on the circadian variation of catecholamines, histamine, and lung function in nonallergic patients with partly reversible airflow obstruction. *J Allergy Clin Immunol* 1986; 77:471–477.

344 Wallin A, Melander B, Rosenhall L, Sandstrom T, Wahlander L. Formoterol, a new long acting beta2 agonist for inhalation twice daily, compared with salbutamol in the treatment of asthma. *Thorax* 1990; 45:259–261.

345 Kesten S, Chapman KR, Broder I et al. A three-month comparison of twice daily inhaled formoterol versus four times daily inhaled albuterol in the management of stable asthma. *Am Rev Respir Dis* 1991; 144:622–625.

346 Ullman A, Hedner J, Svedmyr N. Inhaled salmeterol and salbutamol in asthmatic patients. An evaluation of asthma symptoms and the possible development of tachyphylaxis. *Am Rev Respir Dis* 1990; 142:571–575.

347 Fitzpatrick MF, Mackay T, Driver H, Douglas NJ. Salmeterol in nocturnal asthma: A double blind, placebo controlled trial of a long acting inhaled beta2 agonist. *Br Med J* 1990; 301:1365–1368.

348 Sarin S, Shami S, Cheatle T. Salmeterol in nocturnal asthma. *Br Med J* 1991; 302:347

349 Weersink EJM, Douma RR, Postma DS, Koeter GH. Fluticasone propionate, salmeterol xinafoate, and their combination in the treatment of nocturnal asthma. *Am J Respir Crit Care Med* 1997; 155:1241–1246.

350 Weersink EJM, Van Zomeren EH, Koeter GH, Postma DS. Treatment of nocturnal airway obstruction improves cognitive performance in asthmatics. *Am J Respir Crit Care Med* 1997; 156:1144–1150.

351 Wiegand L, Mende CN, Zaidel G et al. Salmeterol vs theophylline: Sleep and efficacy outcomes in patients with nocturnal asthma. *Chest* 1999; 115:1525–1532.

352 Cazzola M, Spina D, Matera MG. The use of bronchodilators in stable chronic obstructive pulmonary disease. *Pulmon Pharmacol Ther* 1997; 10:129–144.

353 Cazzola M, Santagelo G, Piccolo A et al. Effect of salmeterol and formoterol in patients with chronic obstructive pulmonary disease. *Pulmon Pharmacol Ther* 1994; 7:103–107.

354 Cazzola M, Matera MG, Santangelo G, Vinciguerra A, Rossi F, D'Amato G. Salmeterol and formoterol in partially reversible severe chronic obstructive pulmonary disease: a dose–response study. *Respir Med* 1995; 89:357–362.

355 Maesen BLP, Westermann CJJ, Duurkens VAM, Van den Bosch JMM. Effects of formoterol in apparently poorly reversible chronic obstructive pulmonary disease. *Eur Respir J* 1999; 13:1103–1108.

356 Ulrik CS. Efficacy of inhaled salmeterol in the management of smokers with chronic obstructive pulmonary disease. A single center randomized, double-blind, placebo-controlled, crossover study. *Thorax* 1995; 50:750–754.

357 Grove A, Lipworth BJ, Reid P et al. Effects of regular salmeterol on lung function and exercise capacity in patients with chronic obstructive airways disease. *Thorax* 1996; 51:689–693.

358 Boyd G, Morice AH, Pounsford JC, Siebert M, Peslis N, Crawford C. An evaluation of salmeterol in the treatment of chronic obstructive pulmonary disease (COPD). *Eur Respir J* 1997; 10:815–821.

359 Jones PW, Bosh TK. Quality of life changes in COPD patients treated with salmeterol. *Am J Respir Crit Care Med* 1997; 155:1283–1289.

360 Mahler DA, Donohue JF, Barbee RA et al. Efficacy of salmeterol xinafoate in the treatment of COPD. *Chest* 1999; 115:957–965.

361 Paterson JW, Lulich KM, Goldie RG. Drug effects on beta-adrenoceptor function in asthma. In: Morley J, ed. *Perspectives in Asthma: Beta-adrenoceptors in Asthma.* Vol 2. New York: Academic Press, 1984:245–268.

362 Conolly ME, Davies DS, Dollery CT, George CF. Resistance to β-adrenoceptor stimulants, a possible explanation for the rise in asthma deaths. *Br J Pharmacol* 1971; 43:389–402.

363 Holgate ST, Baldwin CJ, Tattersfield AE. β-adrenergic agonist resistance in normal human airways. *Lancet* 1977; 2:375–377.

364 Harvey JE, Tattersfield AE. Airway response to salbutamol: effect of regular salbutamol inhalations in normal, atopic, and asthmatic subjects. *Thorax* 1982; 37:280–287.

365 Peel ET, Gibson GJ. Effects of long-term inhaled salbutamol therapy on the provocation of asthma by histamine. *Am Rev Respir Dis* 1980; 121:973–978.

366 Repsher LH, Anderson JA, Bush RK. Assessment of tachyphylaxis following prolonged therapy of asthma with inhaled albuterol aerosol. *Chest* 1984; 85:34–38.

367 Hjemdahl P, Zetterlund A, Larsson K. β_2-agonist treatment reduces b2-sensitivity in alveolar macrophages despite corticosteroid treatment. *Am J Respir Crit Care Med* 1996; 153:576–581.

368 Arvidsson P, Larsson S, Lofdahl C-G, Melander B, Svedmyr N, Wahlander L. Inhaled formoterol during one year in asthma: A comparison with salbutamol. *Eur Respir J* 1991; 4:1168–1173.

369 Newnham DM, McDevitt DG, Lipworth BJ. Bronchodilator subsensitivity after chronic dosing with eformoterol in patients with asthma. *Am J Med* 1994; 97:29–37.

370 Grove A, Lipworth BJ. Bronchodilator subsensitivity to salbutamol after twice daily salmeterol in asthmatic patients. *Lancet* 1995; 346:201–206.

371 Nelson HS, Berkowitz RB, Tinkelman DA, Emmett AH, Rickard KA, Yancey SW. Lack of subsensitivity to albuterol after treatment with salmeterol in patients with asthma. *Am J Respir Crit Care Med* 1999; 159:1556–1561.

372 Tan KS, Hall IP, Dewar J, Dow E, Lipworth B. Association between beta2-adrenoceptor polymorphism and susceptibility to bronchodilator desensitisation in moderately severe stable asthmatics. *Lancet* 1997; 350:995–999.

373 Aziz I, Hall IP, McFarlane LC, Lipworth BJ. beta2-Adrenoceptor regulation and bronchodilator sensitivity after regular treatment with formoterol in subjects with stable asthma. *J Allergy Clin Immunol* 1998; 101:337–341.

374 Lipworth B, Tan S, Devlin M, Aiken T, Baker R, Hendrick D. Effects of treatment with formoterol on bronchoprotection against methacholine. *Am J Med* 1998; 104:431–438.

375 Vathenen AS, Higgins BG, Knox AJ, Britton JR, Tattersfield AE. Rebound increase in bronchial responsiveness after treatment with inhaled terbutaline. *Lancet* 1988; 1:554–557.

376 Cockcroft DW, McParland CP, Britto SA, Swystun VA,

Rutherford BC. Regular inhaled salbutamol and airway responsiveness to allergen. *Lancet* 1993; 342:833–837.

377 Cockcroft DW, Bhagat R, Kalra S, Swystun VA. Inhaled beta2-agonists and allergen-induced airway responses [1]. *J Allergy Clin Immunol* 1995; 96:1013–1014.

378 Bhagat R, Swystun VA, Cockcroft DW. Salbutamol-induced increased airway responsiveness to allergen and reduced protection versus methacholine: Dose response. *J Allergy Clin Immunol* 1996; 97:47–52.

379 Wong AG, O'Shaughnessy AD, Walker CM, Sears MR. Effects of long-acting and short-acting beta-agonists on methacholine dose-response curves in asthmatics. *Eur Respir J* 1997; 10:330–336.

380 Overbeek SE, Rijnbeek PR, Vons C, Mulder PGH, Hoogsteden HC, Bogaard JM. Effects of fluticasone propionate on methacholine dose-response curves in non-smoking atopic asthmatics. *Eur Respir J* 1996; 9:2256–2262.

381 Bhagat R, Kalra S, Swystun VA, Cockcroft DW. Rapid onset of tolerance to the bronchoprotective effect of salmeterol. *Chest* 1995; 108:1235–1239.

382 Kalra S, Swystun VA, Bhagat R, Cockcroft DW. Inhaled corticosteroids do not prevent the development of tolerance to the bronchoprotective effect of salmeterol. *Chest* 1996; 109:953–956.

383 Booth H, Bish R, Walters J, Whitehead F, Walters EH. Salmeterol tachyphylaxis in steroid treated asthmatic subjects. *Thorax* 1996; 51:1100–1104.

384 Verberne AAPH, Hop WCJ, Creyghton FBM et al. Airway responsiveness after a single dose of salmeterol and during four months of treatment in children with asthma. *J Allergy Clin Immunol* 1996; 97:938–946.

385 Gibson GJ, Greenacre JK, Konig P, Conolly ME, Pride NB. Use of exercise challenge to investigate possible tolerance to beta-adrenoceptor stimulation in asthma. *Br J Dis Chest* 1978; 72:199–206.

386 Inman MD, O'Byrne PM. The effect of regular inhaled albuterol on exercise-induced bronchoconstriction. *Am J Respir Crit Care Med* 1996; 153:65–69.

387 Giannini D, Carletti A, Dente FL, Bacci E, Di Franco A, Vagaggini B, et al. Tolerance to the protective effect of salmeterol on allergen challenge. *Chest* 1996; 110:1452–1457.

388 Giannini D, Bacci E, Dente FL et al. Inhaled beclomethasone dipropionate reverts tolerance to the protective effect of salmeterol on allergen challenge. *Chest* 1999; 115:629–634.

389 Hancox RJ, Aldridge RE, Cowan JO, Flannery EM, Herbison GP, McLachlan CR, et al. Tolerance to beta-agonists during acute bronchoconstrichmatic subjects receiving regular salmeterol or formoterol. *J Allergy Clin Immunol* 1999; 103:88–92.

390 Yates DH, Worsdell M, Barnes PJ. Effect of regular salmeterol treatment on albuterol-induced bronchoprotection in mild asthma. *Am J Respir Crit Care Med* 1997; 156:988–991.

391 Aziz I, Lipworth BJ. In vivo effect of albuterol on methacholine-contracted bronchi in conjunction with salmeterol and formoterol. *J Allergy Clin Immunol* 1999; 103:816–822.

392 Lipworth BJ, Aziz I. A high dose of albuterol does not overcome bronchoprotective subsensitivity in asthmatic subjects receiving regular salmeterol or formoterol. *J Allergy Clin Immunol* 1999; 103:88–92.

393 Korosec M, Novak RD, Myers E, Skowronski M, McFadden ER. Salmeterol does not compromise the bronchodilator response to albuterol during acute episodes of asthma. *Am J Med* 1999; 107:209–213.

394 Booth H, Fishwick K, Harkawat R, Devereux G, Hendrick DJ, Walters EH. Changes in methacholine induced bronchoconstriction with the long acting beta2 agonist salmeterol in mild to moderate asthmatic patients. *Thorax* 1993; 48:1121–1124.

395 Barnes PJ. Beta-adrenergic receptors and their regulation. *Am J Respir Crit Care Med* 1995; 152:838–860.

396 Hall IP, Daykin K, Widdop S. β_2-adrenoceptor desensitization in cultured human airway smooth muscle. *Clin Sci* 1993; 84:151–157.

397 Cockcroft DW, Swystun VA, Bhagat R. Interaction of inhaled beta2 agonist and inhaled corticosteroid on airway responsiveness to allergen and methacholine. *Am J Respir Crit Care Med* 1995; 152:1485–1489.

398 Aziz I, Lipworth BJ. A bolus of inhaled budesonide rapidly reverses airway subsensitivity and beta2-adrenoceptor down-regulation after regular inhaled formoterol. *Chest* 1999; 115:623–628.

399 Tan KS, Grove A, McLean A, Gnosspelius Y, Hall IP, Lipworth BJ. Systemic corticosteroid rapidly reverses bronchodilator subsensitivity induced by formoterol in asthmatic subjects. *Am J Respir Crit Care Med* 1997; 156:28–35.

400 Haahtela T, Jarvinen M, Kava T et al. Comparison of a beta2-agonist, terbutaline, with an inhaled corticosteroid, budesonide, in newly detected asthma. *N Engl J Med* 1991; 325:388–392.

401 Kerrebijn KF, Van Essen-Zandvliet EEM, Neijens HJ. Effect of long-term treatment with inhaled corticosteroids and beta-agonists on the bronchial responsiveness in children with asthma. *J Allergy Clin Immunol* 1987; 79:653–659.

402 Raes M, Mulder P, Kerrebijn KF. Long-term effect of ipratropium bromide and fenoterol on the bronchial hyperres-

ponsiveness to histamine in children with asthma. *J Allergy Clin Immunol* 1989; 84:874–879.

403 Van Schayck CP, Graafsma SJ, Visch MB, Dompeling E, Van Weel C, Van Herwaarden CLA. Increased bronchial hyper-responsiveness after inhaling salbutamol during 1 year is not caused by subsensitization to salbutamol. *J Allergy Clin Immunol* 1990; 86:793–800.

404 Waalkens HJ, Gerritsen J, Koeter GH, Krouwels FH, Van Aalderen WMC, Knol K. Budesonide and terbutaline or ter-butaline alone in children with mild asthma: Effects on bronchial hyperresponsiveness and diurnal variation in peak flow. *Thorax* 1991; 46:499–503.

405 Boulet LP, Cartier A, Thomson NC, Roberts RS, Dolovich J, Hargreave FE. Asthma and increases in nonallergic bron-chial responsiveness from seasonal pollen exposure. *J Allergy Clin Immunol* 1983; 71:399–406.

406 Sotomayor H, Badier M, Vervloet D, Orehek J. Seasonal increase of carbachol airway responsiveness in patients allergic to grass pollen: Reversal by corticosteroids. *Am Rev Respir Dis* 1984; 130:56–58.

407 Mitchell EA. Is current treatment increasing asthma mor-tality and morbidity? *Thorax* 1989; 44:81–84.

408 Van Schayck CP, Dompeling E, Van Herwaarden CLA et al. Bronchodilator treatment in moderate asthma or chronic bronchitis: Continuous or on demand? A randomised con-trolled study. *Br Med J* 1991; 303:1426–1431.

409 Taylor DR, Town GI, Herbison GP et al. Asthma control during long term treatment with regular inhaled salbuta-mol and salmeterol. *Thorax* 1998; 53:744–752.

410 Yates DH, Sussman HS, Shaw MJ, Barnes PJ, Chung KF. Regular formoterol treatment in mild asthma: Effect on bronchial responsiveness during and after treatment. *Am J Respir Crit Care Med* 1995; 152:1170–1174.

411 Shepherd GL, Hetzel MR, Clark TJH. Regular versus symp-tomatic aerosol bronchodilator treatment of asthma. *Br J Dis Chest* 1981; 75:215–217.

412 Beswick KBJ, Pover GM, Sampson S. Long-term regularly inhaled salbutamol. *Curr Med Res Opin* 1986; 10:228–234.

413 Patakas D, Maniki E, Tsara V, Daskalopoulou E. Intermittent and continuous salbutamol rotacaps inhala-tion in asthmatic patients. *Respiration* 1988; 54:174–178.

414 Sears MR, Taylor DR, Print CG et al. Regular inhaled beta-agonist treatment in bronchial asthma. *Lancet* 1990; 336:1391–1396.

415 Nelson HS, Szefler SJ, Martin RJ. Regular inhaled beta-adrenergic agonists in the treatment of bronchial asthma: Beneficial or detrimental? *Am Rev Respir Dis* 1991; 144:249–250.

416 Drazen JM, Israel E, Boushey HA et al. Comparison of reg-ularly scheduled with as-needed use of albuterol in mild asthma. *N Engl J Med* 1996; 335:841–847.

417 Israel E, Drazen JM, Liggett SB et al. The effect of polymor-phisms of the beta(2)-adrenergic receptor on the response to regular use of albuterol in asthma. *Am J Respir Crit Care Med* 2000; 162:75–80.

418 Taylor DR, Drazen JM, Herbison GP, Yandava CN, Hancox RJ, Town GI. Asthma exacerbations during long term beta agonist use: influence of beta(2) adrenoceptor polymor-phism. *Thorax* 2000; 55:762–767.

419 Dennis SM, Sharp SJ, Vickers MR et al. Regular inhaled sal-butamol and asthma control: the TRUST randomised trial. *Lancet* 2000; 355:1675–1679.

420 Dahl R, Earnshaw JS, Palmer JBD. Salmeterol: A four week study of a long-acting beta-adrenoceptor agonist for the treatment of reversible airways disease. *Eur Respir J* 1991; 4:1178–1184.

421 Pearlman DS, Chervinsky P, LaForce C et al. A comparison of salmeterol with albuterol in the treatment of mild-to-moderate asthma. *N Engl J Med* 1992; 327:1420–1425.

422 D'Alonzo GE, Nathan RA, Henochowicz S, Morris RJ, Ratner P, Rennard SI. Salmeterol xinafoate as maintenance therapy compared with albuterol in patients with asthma. *J Am Med Asssoc* 1994; 271:1412–1416.

423 Verberne AAPH, De Jongste JC. The role of inhaled long-acting bronchodilator therapy. *Eur Respir Rev* 1996; 6:199–203.

424 Boulet L-P, Laviolette M, Boucher S, Knight A, Hebert J, Chapman KR. A twelve-week comparison of salmeterol and salbutamol in the treatment of mild-to-moderate asthma: A Canadian multicenter study. *J Allergy Clin Immunol* 1997; 99:13–21.

425 Simons FER. A comparison of beclomethasone, salmete-rol, and placebo in children with asthma. *N Engl J Med* 1997; 337:1659–1665.

426 Rosenthal RR, Busse WW, Kemp JP et al. Effect of long-term salmeterol therapy compared with as-needed albuterol use on airway hyperresponsiveness. *Chest* 1999; 116:595–602.

427 FitzGerald JM, Chapman KR, Della CG et al. Sustained bronchoprotection, bronchodilatation, and symptom control during regular formoterol use in asthma of moder-ate or greater severity. *J Allergy Clin Immunol* 1999; 103:427–435.

428 Kemp JP, DeGraff AC, Pearlman DS et al. A 1-year study of salmeterol powder on pulmonary function and hyperres-ponsiveness to methacholine. *J Allergy Clin Immunol* 1999; 104:1189–1197.

429 Shapiro G, Lumry W, Wolfe J et al. Combined salmeterol 50

μg and fluticasone proprionate 250 μg in the Diskus device for the treatment of asthma. *Am J Respir Crit Care Med* 2000; 161:527–534.

430 Greening AP, Wind P, Northfield M, Shaw G. Added salmeterol versus higher-dose corticosteroid in asthma patients with symptoms on existing inhaled corticosteroid. *Lancet* 1994; 344:219–224.

431 Woolcock A, Lundback B, Ringdal N, Jacques LA. Comparison of addition of salmeterol to inhaled steroids with doubling of the dose of inhaled steroids. *Am J Respir Crit Care Med* 1996; 153:1481–1488.

432 Pauwels RA, Lofdahl C-G, Postma DS et al. Effect of inhaled formoterol and budesonide on exacerbations of asthma. *N Engl J Med* 1997; 337:1405–1411.

433 Eickelberg O, Roth M, Lorx R et al. Ligand-independent activation of the glucocorticoid receptor by β_2-adrenergic receptor agonists in primary human lung fibroblasts and vascular smooth muscle cells. *J Biol Chem* 1999; 274:1005–1010.

434 Jackson RT, Beaglehole R, Rea HH, Sutherland DC. Mortality from asthma: a new epidemic in New Zealand. *Br Med J* 1982; 285:771–774.

435 Wilson JD, Sutherland DC, Thomas AC. Has the change to beta-agonists combined with oral theophylline increased cases of fatal asthma? *Lancet* 1981; 1:1235–1237.

436 Grant IWB. Asthma in New Zealand. *NZ Med J*, 1983; 167–170.

437 Sears MR, Rea HH, Fenwick J. 75 Deaths in asthmatics prescribed home nebulisers. *Br Med J* 1987; 294:477–480.

438 Sears MR, Rea HH, Beaglehole R. Asthma mortality in New Zealand: a two year national study. *NZ Med J* 1985; 98:271–275.

439 Sears MR, Rea HH, Rothwell RPG. Asthma mortality: comparison between New Zealand and England. *Br Med J* 1986; 293:1342–1345.

440 Rea HH, Scragg R, Jackson R. A case-control study of deaths from asthma. *Thorax* 1986; 41:833–839.

441 Pearce N, Grainger J, Atkinson M et al. Case-control study of prescribed fenoterol and death from asthma in New Zealand, 1977–81. *Thorax* 1990; 45:170–175.

442 Grainger J, Woodman K, Pearce N et al. Prescribed fenoterol and death from asthma in New Zealand, 1981–7: A further case-control study. *Thorax* 1991; 46:105–111.

443 Spitzer WO, Suissa S, Ernst P et al. The use of beta-agonists and the risk of death and near death from asthma. *N Engl J Med* 1992; 326:501–506.

444 Rea HH, Garrett JE, Lanes SF, Birmann BM, Kolbe J. The association between asthma drugs and severe-life threatening attacks. *Chest* 1996; 110:1446–1451.

445 Morley J, Sanjar S, Newth C. Viewpoint- Untoward effects of beta-adrenoceptor agonists in asthma. *Eur Respir J* 1990; 3:228–233.

446 Tyrrell DJ, Horne AP, Holme KR, Preuss JMH, Page CP. Heparin in Inflammation: potential therapeutic applications beyond coagulation. *Adv.Pharmacol.* 1999; 46:151–208.

447 Page CP. Inhibition of natural anti-inflammatory mechanism by beta2-agonists [4]. *Lancet* 1991; 337:1285–1286.

448 Swystun VA, Gordon JR, Davis EB, Zhang X, Cockcroft DW. Mast cell tryptase release and asthmatic responses to allergen increase with regular use of salbutamol. *J Allergy Clin Immunol* 2000; 106:57–64.

449 Smith SR, Kendall MJ. Metabolic responses to beta2-stimulants. *J.R.Coll.Phys Lond.* 1984; 18:190–194.

450 Paterson JW, Woolcock AJ, Shenfield GM. Bronchodilator drugs. *Am Rev Respir Dis* 1979; 120:1149–1188.

451 Zuurmond HM, Hessling J, Bluml K, Lohse M, Ijzerman AP. Study of interaction between agonists and Asn293 in Helix VI of human β_2-adrenergic receptor. *J Pharmacol Exp Ther* 1999; 56:909–916.

4

Anticholinergic bronchodilators

Jeremy M. Segal[1] and Nicholas J. Gross[2]

[1] Departments of Medicine and Molecular Biochemistry, Stritch School of Medicine, Loyola University of Chicago, IL, USA
and [2] Hines Veterans Affairs Hospital, Hines, IL, USA

Introduction

Anticholinergic alkaloid agents, such as atropine and scopolamine, exist in the roots, seeds and leaves of a variety of plants. *Atropa belladonna* (deadly nightshade) and *Datura stromonium* (jimsonweed, stinkweed, devil's apple or thorn apple) contain atropine, whereas the alkaloid scopolamine (hyoscine) is found in the shrub *Hyoscyamus niger* and *Scopolia carnolica*[1]. These plants have been used in herbal remedies for many centuries. The earliest written record of their medical use is from seventeenth-century Aryuvedic literature discussing the use of *Datura* specifically for asthma. They were introduced into Europe in 1802 by General Gent who, while stationed in Madras, had found that smoking stramonium alleviated his asthma as well as in others[2]. In 1859, it was reported that a severe asthma attack was successfully treated by injection of atropine into the vagus nerve[3 quoted in 4]. By the end of the nineteenth century, anticholinergic alkaloids enjoyed enormous use as bronchodilators. Their use declined after the discovery of adrenaline in the 1920s, followed soon by ephedrine, other adrenergic agents and then methylxanthines. Natural anticholinergic agents such as atropine produced many side effects that resulted in poor acceptability by patients. More recently, advances in the understanding of the role of the parasympathetic system in controlling airway tone, and the improved side effect profile of synthetic topically active derivatives of atropine have renewed interest in anticholinergic agents, particularly in the therapy of COPD[5].

Rationale for use of anticholinergic bronchodilators

Autonomic control of airway calibre

Most of the efferent autonomic nerves supplying human airways are cholinergic[6]. Branches of the vagus nerve travel along the airways. At the peribronchial ganglia they synapse with the short postganglionic nerves which innervate smooth muscle cells and mucus glands, predominantly in the central airways. Muscarinic receptors are activated by the release of acetylcholine from varicosities and terminals of the postganglionic nerves. This signal stimulates smooth muscle contraction, and release of mucus from mucus glands and may cause ciliary beat frequency to accelerate. In experimental animals at rest there is a low level of cholinergic, vagal (bronchomotor) tone. A variety of stimuli can cause considerable augmentation of this vagal output[5]. Anticholinergic agents competitively inhibit acetylcholine at muscarinic receptors. The consequent withdrawal of tonic and phasic cholinergic activity permits airways to dilate. These drugs neither affect smooth muscle contraction caused by other mediators, nor do they modulate most of the mediators of airway obstruction in abnormal states such as asthma.

Cholinergic bronchomotor activity can be augmented by a variety of stimuli by means of the neural pathways shown in Fig. 4.1. Mechanical irritation, many irritant gases, aerosols, particles, cold dry air and specific mediators such as histamine and bronchoconstricting eicosanoids[7,8] can induce

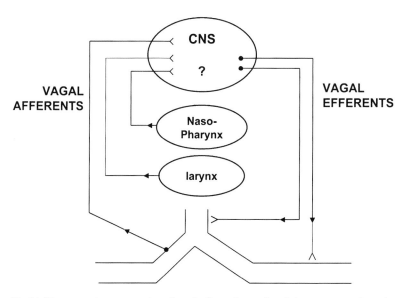

Fig. 4.1 Diagrammatic representation of vagal reflex pathways from irritant receptors through vagal afferents, central nervous system (CNS), and vagal efferents to effector cells in the airways. Reproduced from *Am Rev Respir Dis* 1984; 129:856–870 , ref 5, with permission.

afferent activity from irritant receptors and C fibres. These are found throughout the upper and lower airways, and also in the carotid bodies and esophagus. The impulses are transmitted via vagal afferents, through the vagal nuclei to vagal efferents which supply the larger airways. Vagally mediated bronchoconstriction has been shown in animals, and also to some extent in humans. There is evidence that cholinergic bronchomotor tone is increased in both asthma[9] and COPD[10], but it is not clear how much such mechanisms actually contribute to airflow limitation in these patients. Abolition of cholinergic activity by anticholinergic agents usually produces a degree of bronchodilatation, but airflow limitation is seldom completely reversed. The response also varies widely among patients. In patients with asthma or chronic obstructive pulmonary disease (COPD) vagal activity probably accounts for only a part of the airflow obstruction.

Muscarinic receptor subtypes in airways

Cholinergic nerves are the dominant neural bronchoconstrictor pathways in human and animal airways[11]. There are at least three muscarinic receptor subtypes, known as M_1, M_2 and M_3, expressed in the human lung, each of which appears to play a role in the control of airway calibre (Fig. 4.2). Briefly, M_1 receptors, located in peribronchial ganglia, and M_3 receptors, located on submucosal glands and smooth muscle cells, mediate smooth muscle contraction[12]. M_2 receptors, on the postganglionic nerves, are autoreceptors whose stimulation provides feedback inhibition of further acetylcholine release from cholinergic nerves, and thus tend to limit the bronchoconstriction. Adrenergic terminals on these structures are absent, or at most, sparse, except in the upper trachea; however, sympathetic nerves do terminate on parasympathetic ganglion cells in the peribronchial plexa, and thus could affect the function of postganglionic parasympathetic fibres[5]. Expression of M_2 receptors is reduced by certain viruses, and cytokines, including gamma interferon[13.] Also, inflammatory cell products such as eosinophil major basic protein, act as functional antagonists to M_2 receptor function[14]. These observations may account, at least partly, for the bronchospasm associated with viral infections and

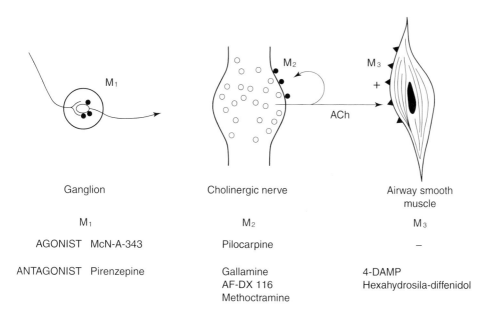

Ganglion   Cholinergic nerve   Airway smooth
                                                                muscle

	M_1	M_2	M_3
AGONIST	McN-A-343	Pilocarpine	–
ANTAGONIST	Pirenzepine	Gallamine	4-DAMP
		AF-DX 116	Hexahydrosila-diffenidol
		Methoctramine	

Fig. 4.2 Muscarinic receptor subtypes in airways M_1 receptors are localized to parasympathetic ganglia, M_2 receptors to postganglionic cholinergic nerves (autoreceptors), and M_3 receptors to airway smooth muscle. Reproduced from *Chest* 1999; 115(5):1338–1345 , ref 95, with permission.

asthma. Another possible implication of this data is that currently available anticholinergic bronchodilators, none of which is selective for muscarinic receptor subtypes, may be suboptimal. Attempts to develop other synthetic anticholinergic agents have resulted in one, tiotropium bromide, that, dissociates more rapidly from M_2 receptors, rendering it functionally selective for both M_1 and M_3 receptors[15–17]. For this reason, tiotropium may prove relatively more potent as a bronchodilator than currently available agents.

Pharmacology

Anticholinergic agents are classed as tertiary or quaternary ammonium compounds depending on the valency of the nitrogen atom on the tropane ring (Fig. 4.3). The three-valent tertiary ammonium compounds, such as atropine and scopolamine, occur naturally and are freely soluble in water and lipids. This facilitates their absorption from the skin and mucosal surfaces and they are thus widely distributed in the body and cross the blood–brain barrier. They counteract parasympathetic in multiple sites throughout the body and can cause severe systemic effects. Atropine, for example, in the dose that results in bronchodilatation (1.0–2.5 mg in adults) frequently produces skin flushing, mouth dryness and possibly tachycardia. In slightly higher doses it produces blurred vision, urinary retention and mental effects such as irritability, confusion and hallucinations. Because their therapeutic range is so narrow, atropine and its natural congeners are difficult to use.

Ipratropium, oxitropium bromide (Oxivent), atropine methonitrate, glycopyrrolate bromide (Robinul) and tiotropium bromide are quaternary congeners, and are all synthetic. These molecules are poorly absorbed from mucosal surfaces because of the charge associated with the five-valent tropane nitrogen atom. These agents are fully anticholinergic at the site of deposition and are able, for example, to dilate the pupil if delivered to the eye or dilate the bronchi when inhaled. Their limited absorption

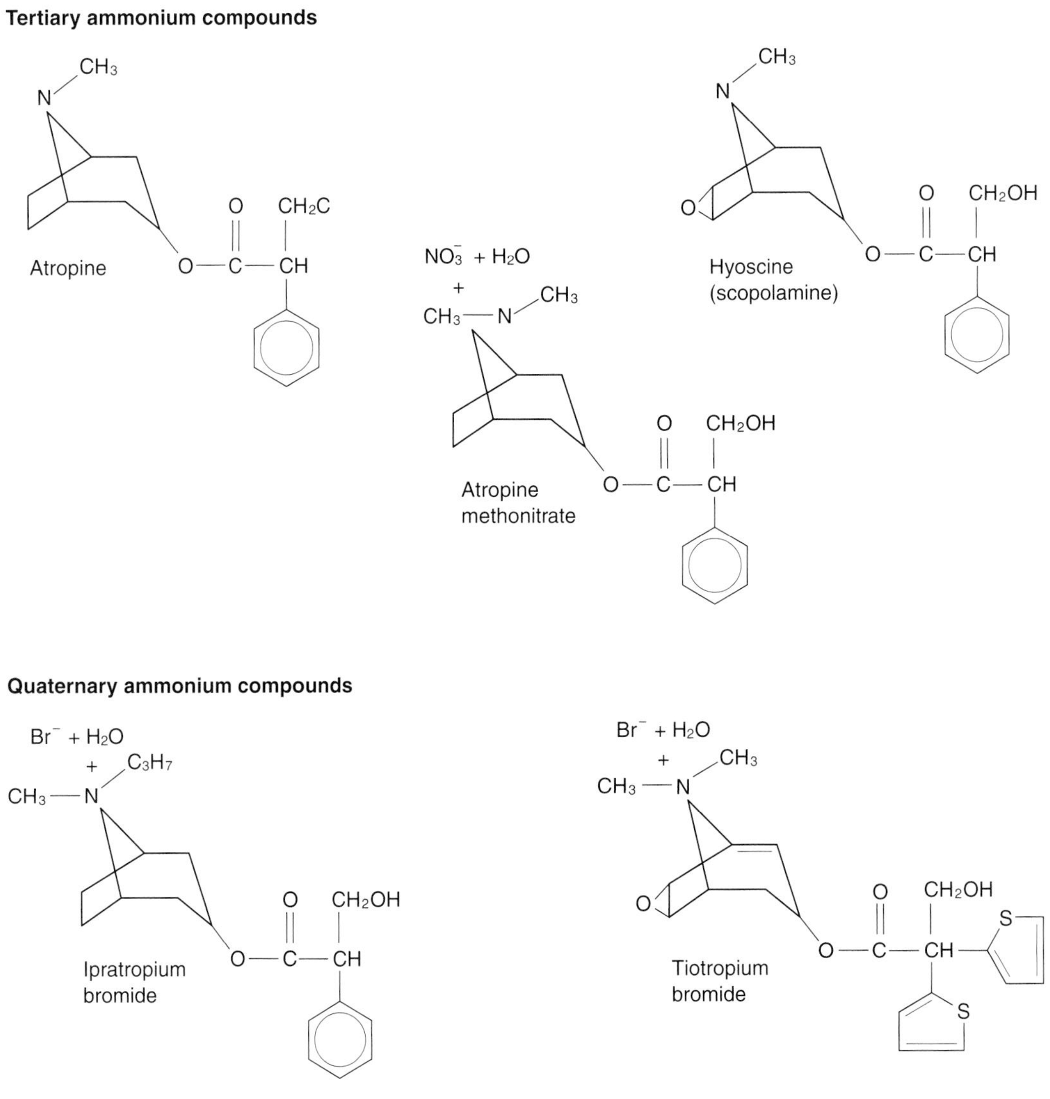

Tertiary ammonium compounds

Quaternary ammonium compounds

Fig. 4.3 Structures of some anticholinergic agents.

from these sites does not produce either detectable blood levels or systemic effects, even when delivered in supramaximal doses[18]. For practical purposes, these drugs can be regarded as topical forms of atropine. Tiotropium is of particular interest in that it is a functionally selective antagonist of the muscarinic receptor subtypes that mediate bronchoconstriction (see above) and is also extremely long acting. It has been shown to be active at least 32 hours after

administration in patients with COPD[15,16], and protects against inhaled methacholine for up to 48 hours after a single dose[17].

Pharmacokinetics

Atropine and its natural congeners exist in two optical isomeric forms, only one of which is physiologically active, whereas the quaternary agents are generally synthesized in the active isomeric form, resulting in apparently greater activity of the latter. Atropine is quantitatively absorbed from the airways, reaching peak blood levels in 1 hour. The half-life in the circulation is about 3 hours in adults, but longer in children and the elderly[5.] Small concentrations can be measured in the feces and in breast milk. Radiolabelling studies of ipratropium pharmacokinetics in humans show that, following oral or inhaled doses, the serum levels are very low, with a peak at about 1–2 hours and a half-life of about 4 hours. Most of the drug is excreted unchanged in the urine. Its bronchodilator action is somewhat longer, probably because it is not removed from the airways by absorption. Most of an oral dose is recovered in the feces, a small amount as inactive metabolites in the urine. Very little reaches the central nervous system.

Clinical efficacy

Dose–response

The dose–response of anticholinergic agents given by various inhalational methods is provided in a previous review[19]. The optimal dose of ipratropium in adults is 500 μg when administered by nebulizer and in younger adults with asthma it is 40–80 μg by MDI. The optimal MDI dose in older adults with severe airflow limitation is two to four times higher, probably 160 μg. Newer inhalers will employ a dry powder form without propellants, rather than the suspension that is currently more widely used. The optimal dose of the dry powder form may be a little lower than that for the suspension. For instance, 10 μg of ipratropium delivered by turbuhaler, was equipotent to 20 μg delivered by MDI[20]. The optimal dose of oxitropium MDI, is approximately 200 μg. For less commonly used agents, the optimal doses are as follows: atropine, 0.25–0.4 mg/kg; atropine methonitrate, 0.015–0.02 mg/kg; glycopyrrolate, 0.02 mg/kg. Tiotropium has been studied at doses ranging from 10 to 80 μg as a lactose powder, with demonstrable dose related improvements in airflow limitation[16].

Against specific stimuli

When given in advance of bronchospastic stimuli, anticholinergic agents provide variable degrees of protection.[5] They protect more or less completely against cholinergic agonists such as methacholine. In asthmatics they can prevent bronchospasm induced by β-blocking agents and by psychogenic factors. They provide only partial protection against bronchospasm due to most other stimuli, e.g. histamine[21,22], prostaglandins, non-specific dusts and irritant aerosols, exercise and hyperventilation with cold, dry air, most of which are better prevented by adrenergic agents. Ipratropium has no prophylactic effect on leukotriene induced asthma[23].

Stable asthma

A very large number of studies have compared the bronchodilator potential of the anticholinergic agents with that of adrenergic agents. While many of these studies are flawed by the fact that they used recommended doses rather than optimal doses, they provide the clinician with useful information about the comparative actions of these bronchodilators[24]. Figure 4.4, which is typical of most such studies, illustrates many of these points. Anticholinergic agents are slower to reach peak effect, typically 1–2 hours, compared with about 15 minutes for many adrenergic agents. At their peak effect they almost invariably result in less bronchodilation in patients with asthma. The quaternary forms may be slightly longer acting than agents such as salbutamol. Among asthmatic patients there is, however, substantial variation in responsiveness, some patients responding very little to anticholinergic agents, others responding almost as well to them as to adrenergic agents.

It has been difficult to identify subgroups of asthmatic patients who are most likely to respond to anticholinergic therapy. The bronchodilating effect of ipratropium may increase with age, in contrast to the decline in response to salbutamol[25]. However, children aged 10–18 years do respond favourably[26] (see below). Individuals with intrinsic asthma and

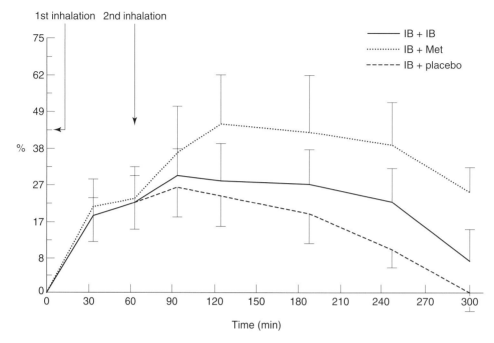

Fig. 4.4 Mean values of FEV$_1$ in ten patients with allergic asthma treated with ipratropium 40 μg followed by a second inhalation of either ipratropium 40 μg, metaproterenol 1 250 μg or placebo. Reproduced from *Chest* 1983; 83(2):208–210 , ref 97, with permission.

those with longer duration of asthma may also respond better than individuals with extrinsic asthma[27], although these appear to be poor predictors of response. An individual trial remains the best way to identify responsiveness[28].

Recently, attention has been focused on the role of nasal symptoms in exacerbation of asthma. Ipratropium nasal spray is commercially available and effective at reducing rhinorrhea[29].

Acute severe asthma

Most studies suggest that β-agonists are more effective bronchodilators in the setting of acute severe asthma. There has been a lot of interest in determining whether anticholinergic agents can add to the bronchodilatation achieved by adrenergic agonists. In a large study ($n = 199$), Rebuck et al[30]. found that the combination of 500 μg nebulized ipratropium with 1.25 mg nebulized fenoterol resulted in significantly more bronchodilatation over the first 90 min of treatment than either agent alone. The combina-

tion was most efficacious in patients with more severe airway obstruction. A recent meta-analysis of ten similar studies, involving 1377 patients concluded that the addition of ipratropium reduced hospital admissions (relative risk = 0.73), and increased FEV1 by 7.5% (on average 100cm^3, 95%CI 50 to 149 ml) when compared with groups receiving β2 stimulants alone. These benefits, albeit modest, were statistically significant[31]. The optimal duration of combination therapy in this setting is somewhere between 12 and 36 hours[32].

It seems appropriate to recommend that both classes of bronchodilators be given in acute severe asthma, especially in the early hours of treatment and particularly in patients with more severe airflow obstruction.

Pediatric airways disease

Studies of acute severe asthma in children have compared salbutamol alone with the combination of ipratropium and salbutamol. In the 1980s two well-designed studies showed that the addition of ipratropium accelerated the rate of improvement in airflow[33,34]. Others have, however, failed to show much benefit from the addition of ipratropium[35–37]. A large study of the same question[38] showed a clear dose-related decrease in hospital admission for children with more severe bronchospasm at presentation. Another large trial demonstrated that the addition of ipratropium was associated with a faster discharge from the emergency room, and a decreased need for albuterol nebulizations. The admission rate (18% in the ipratropium group, vs. control, 22%) was not significant[39]. A similar trial found that combination therapy decreased admission rates overall (27.4% vs. 36.5%), and was most beneficial in severe attacks (37.5% vs. 52.6%)[40]. As in adult status asthmaticus, therefore, the combination of ipratropium with an adrenergic agent is probably more effective than salbutamol monotherapy, particularly in severe exacerbations.

There is less clear evidence to support the addition of ipratropium to salbutamol in stable childhood asthma. Two consensus reports concluded that although ipratropium was safe for this purpose in the pediatric population, its benefit compared with an adrenergic agent alone was slight at best[41,42]. In cystic fibrosis ipratropium decreases methacholine-induced airway hyperreactivity[43]. There are scattered reports of ipratropium use in other paediatric conditions such as viral bronchiolitis, exercise-induced bronchospasm and bronchopulmonary dysplasia, but these do not provide strong and consistent evidence for the benefit of ipratropium over alternative bronchodilators.

Stable COPD

A large number of studies have compared anticholinergic agents with other bronchodilators in patients with COPD[44,45]. Although patients with COPD usually do not exhibit as much improvement in airflow limitation to any agent or combination of agents as do patients with asthma, most studies show that the anticholinergic agent provides at least as great and prolonged an increase in airflow as other agents[46], including the long acting β_2 agonist salmeterol[47]. Most studies show that the anticholinergic agent is a more potent bronchodilator[28,48–50]. Even when large cumulative doses, of each agent, rather than recommended doses are given, the anticholinergic agent alone achieves all the available bronchodilatation in these patients[51]. As this is clearly not the case in asthmatic patients, there is thus likely to be a systematic difference between asthmatic and COPD patients with respect to their responsiveness to bronchodilators. Lefcoe and associates performed one of a few studies in which bronchodilator responsiveness was compared in patients with asthma and COPD who had similar baseline airflows. As illustrated in Fig. 4.5 patients with bronchitis had a better response to ipratropium than to the combination of fenoterol and theophylline (change in FEV_1 0.29L vs. 0.18 l), whereas in asthmatics ipratropium was a less effective bronchodilator than the combination[52]. The difference between the two groups of patients is probably due to the fact that airflow obstruction in asthma results from airway inflammation that is, at least partially, modified by adrenergic agents but not by anticholinergics. In patients with COPD the major reversible component is bronchomotor tone, which is best reversed by anticholinergic agents[51]. Whatever the reason, COPD represents the group of patients in whom anticholinergic agents are the most potent bronchodilators. It is not possible to predict which patients with COPD will respond to therapy with ipratropium, although a retrospective study involving 296 patients suggested that older patients with an isolated volume response were more likely to benefit[53]. Other authors described a greater response in patients with more severe airflow limitation, and in those who continued to smoke[49].

Using bronchodilators, patients often report improvement in symptoms and functional capacity[54] in the absence of spirometric changes. Consequently, rather than relying on FEV_1 as their primary end-point, several studies have focused on the effect of inhaled anticholinergic medications on exercise tolerance. One such study, involving 18 patients given 144 µg of ipratropium by MDI showed

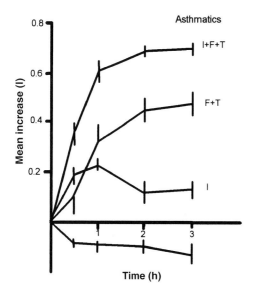

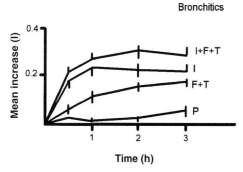

Fig. 4.5 Comparison of responses to bronchodilator combinations in asthmatics and bronchitics. Mean increases in FEV_1 for four treatment groups + / - standard error of the mean. Reproduced from *Chest* 1982; 82(3):300–305, ref 52, with permission. I, ipratropium bromide; F, fenoterol; T. theophylline; P, Placebo.

no increase in effort tolerance as measured by treadmill testing, despite a 25% increase in FEV_1[55]. A study using salbutamol found a similar lack of correlation between increases in FEV_1 and exercise tolerance [56] and another study showed that inhaled metaproterenol increased exercise tolerance in the absence of measurable bronchodilation[57]. A recent study involving 29 patients with advanced COPD showed

that improvements in exercise endurance and breathlessness following inhalation of ipratropium correlated better with measurements of inspiratory capacity than with FEV_1[58].

Ipratropium is currently recommended as first-line treatment for stable COPD in the most recent official statements of the European Respiratory Society[59] and the American Thoracic Society[60]. Bronchodilation produced by inhaled ipratropium bromide is accompanied by decreased dyspnea and increased exercise capacity[61–63], although this finding was not confirmed in another study[64]. The Lung Health Study, a large multicentre trial was unable to show that these improvements in pulmonary symptoms modify the age-related decline in lung function in healthy smokers[65].

Acute exacerbations of COPD

Three studies comparing the efficacy of bronchodilators in acute exacerbations of COPD found no significant differences between adrenergic and anticholinergic agents or their combination[30,66,67].

Effects on sleep quality

Sleep disturbance is surprisingly common in patients with chronic bronchitis and asthma. In the Tucson Epidemiological Study, 41% of patients with obstructive airways disease reported at least one symptom of disturbed sleep[68]. Patients with stable COPD frequently experience nocturnal oxygen desaturation, particularly during REM sleep, even in the absence of concomitant obstructive sleep apnea[69]. This contributes to the development of pulmonary hypertension, polycythemia and predisposes patients to cardiac arrhythmias[70]. Sleep disturbance in children with asthma is associated with psychological problems and impairment of memory[71]. A randomized double blind study involving 36 patients with moderate to severe COPD showed that ipratropium increased total sleep time, decreased the severity of nocturnal desaturation (Fig. 4.6) and improved the patient's perceptions of sleep quality.

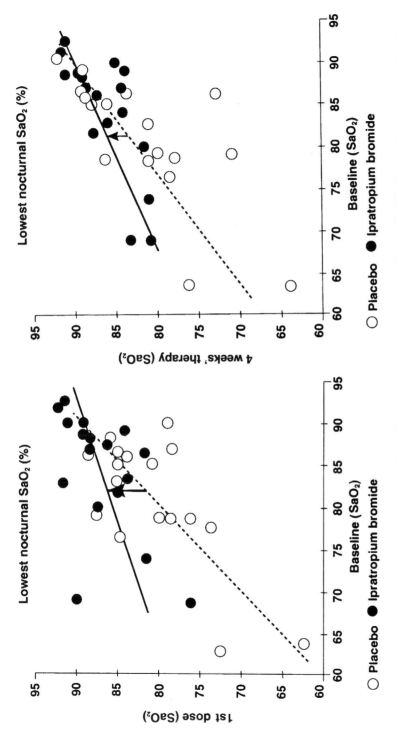

Fig. 4.6 The relationship between SaO$_2$ before treatment and after the first dose of ipratropium, and after 4 weeks of double-blind therapy (right). Reproduced from *Chest* 1999; 115(5):1338–1345, ref 96, with permission.

Combinations with other bronchodilators

Combinations of different classes of bronchodilators often provide more bronchodilatation than single agents, and this effect is seen in many of the studies cited. This may be due to the fact that most clinical studies are performed with recommended rather than optimal doses of the agents. Consequently, when two or more classes of agents are given together the effects may simply be additive rather than potentiating. However, since anticholinergic, adrenergic and methylxanthine agents work by different mechanisms, affect different-sized airways and have different pharmacodynamic and pharmacokinetic properties, their combination is rational and is likely to result in improved bronchodilatation. No unfavourable interactions between these three classes of agents have been reported, so the greater bronchodilation achieved by their combination is achieved without increasing the risk of side effects. In practice, it is common to use two or even all of these agents simultaneously to manage severe airways obstruction.

Single MDIs combining different classes of inhaled bronchodilator have been in use for over 40 years. Ipratropium and the β_2 agonist fenoterol have been widely available as a single inhaler (Berodual and DuoVent) and have been in wide use since the l970s. Because of the concerns about the safety of fenoterol, a new combination MDI containing ipratropium and salbutamol, both in recommended dosage, has been developed (Combivent). In 863 patients with moderately severe COPD, nebulization of a combination of ipratropium bromide and albuterol sulfate (Dey combination, Dey LP, Napa, California, USA) resulted in 30% more improvement in bronchodilation than was seen by albuterol alone, and 32% more than with ipratropium alone. However, the 6-minute walking distance was unchanged[72]. For patients who need two agents, a single MDI containing two agents is likely to be less expensive than two MDIs, easier and more convenient for the patient to use, and therefore more likely to improve patient compliance. Clinical trials with this combination in patients with COPD[73–75] suggest it possesses all the advantages mentioned above. A

post hoc review of two trials, involving 1067 patients over an 85-day period, concluded that this approach appears to be cost-effective[76]. Bronchodilatation is greater during the first 4–5 h after administration, but not much prolonged over that achieved by single agents, and no increase in side effects is incurred.

Side effects

Atropine produces numerous systemic side effects related to the inhibition of physiological functions of the parasympathetic system, as mentioned above. These effects occur in doses at or only slightly above the bronchodilator dose. Atropine is contraindicated in patients with glaucoma or prostatism. The principal advantage of quaternary anticholinergic agents is that they are so poorly absorbed from mucosae that the risk of such effects is insignificant. Even massive, inadvertent overdosage of one such agent resulted in trivial effects[18]. Ipratropium, the most widely studied quaternary anticholinergic, has been exonerated after extensive exploration for atropine-like side effects[77]. It can, for example, be given to patients with glaucoma without affecting intraocular tension[78] (provided it is not sprayed directly into the eye). It has been found not to affect urinary flow characteristics in older men. Nor has it been found to alter the viscosity and elasticity of respiratory mucus, or mucociliary clearance, as does atropine[79]. It has negligible effects on hemodynamics, minute ventilation[62] and the pulmonary circulation.[80] Consequently, quaternary anticholinergics do not carry the risk of potentially increasing hypoxemia, as do adrenergic agents[81–83], an important consideration in exacerbations of asthma and COPD. In normal clinical use the only side effects that the patient might experience with ipratropium are dryness of the mouth and a brief coughing spell, which has been reported to occur in 5% of patients[50]. Rarely, it can result in paradoxical bronchoconstriction. This has been variously attributed to hypotonicity of the nebulized solution, idiosyncracy to the bromine radical, the benzalkonium preservative[84,85], the soya lecithin (in a patient allergic to soy and peanuts)[86] and a selective effect on the M2 receptor. Paradoxical bronchoconstriction may also occur with other anticholinergic agents. Although rare, occurring in possibly 0.3% of patients[87] the possibility of paradoxical bronchoconstriction in a patient warrants withdrawal of the drug from that patient. Rarely, ipratropium contributes to urinary retention, usually in elderly men with prostatic hypertrophy[88]. Other case reports describe cases of bowel dysmotility[89], anisocoria[90] and supraventricular tachycardia[91]. Other than these effects, very extensive investigation and the worldwide use of ipratropium for over two decades demonstrate a remarkably low incidence of untoward reactions. There is no reason at present to believe that the safety profile of the newer quaternary anticholinergic agents will be different from that of ipratropium.

Clinical recommendations

The use of anticholinergic bronchodilators is best limited to the poorly absorbed quaternary forms, e.g. ipratropium, oxitropium, atropine methonitrate, glycopyrrolate, and tiotropium, administered by inhalation. They are sometimes useful in stable asthma as adjuncts to other bronchodilator therapy, and have a demonstrated role in combination with adrenergic agents in the treatment of acute severe asthma. Their principal indication is for the long-term management of stable COPD, where they are probably the most efficacious bronchodilators. Because of their slow onset of action they are best used on a regular, maintenance basis, rather than p.r.n. The usual dose, of ipratropium, two puffs of 20 μg each, is probably suboptimal[92] for many patients with COPD and can safely be doubled or quadrupled[93].

REFERENCES

1 Brown JHTP. Muscarinic receptor agonists and antagonists. In: Hardman JG, editor. *Goodman and Gillman's The pharmacological basis of therapeutics*. New York: McGraw-Hill, 1996; 141.

2 Gandevia B. Historical review of the use of parasympatholytic agents in the treatment of respiratory disorders. *Postgrad Med J* 1975; 517 (Suppl):13–20.

3 Courty MA. Treatment of asthma. *Edin Med J* 1859; 5:665.

4 Dweik RA. Anticholinergic therapy in COPD. *UpToDate* 1999; 7(2).

5 Gross NJ, Skorodin SM. Anticholinergic, antimuscarinic bronchodilators. *Am Rev Respir Dis* 1984; 129:856–870.

6 Richardson JB. The innervation of the lung. *Eur J Respir Dis suppl.* 1982; 117:13–31.

7 Widdicombe JG. The parasympathetic nervous system in airways disease. *Scand J Respir Dis Suppl.* 1979; 103:38–43.

8 Nadel JA. Autonomic regulation of airway smooth muscle. In: Nadel JA, editor. *Physiology and pharmacology of the airways.* New York: Marcel Dekker, 1980; 217–257.

9 Shah PK, Lakhotia M, Mehta S, Jain SK, Gupta GL. Clinical dysautonomia in patients with bronchial asthma. Study with seven autonomic function tests. *Chest* 1990; 98(6):1408–1413.

10 Gross NJ, Co E, Skorodin MS. Cholinergic bronchomotor tone in COPD. Estimates of its amount in comparison with that in normal subjects. *Chest* 1989; 96(5):984–987.

11 Barnes PJ. Neural control of human airways in health and disease. *Am Rev Respir Dis* 1986; 134(6):1289–1314.

12 Gross NJ, Barnes PJ. A short tour around the muscarinic receptor. *Am Rev Respir Dis* 1988; 138(4):765–767.

13 Fryer AD, Jacoby DB. Parainfluenza virus infection damages inhibitory M2 muscarinic receptors on pulmonary parasympathetic nerves in the guinea-pig. *Br J Pharmacol* 1991; 102(1):267–271.

14 Fryer AD, Jacoby DB. Effect of inflammatory cell mediators on M2 muscarinic receptors in the lungs. *Life Sci* 1993; 52(5–6):529–536.

15 O'Connor BJ, Towse LJ, Barnes PJ. Prolonged effect of tiotropium bromide on methacholine-induced bronchoconstriction in asthma. *Am J Respir Crit Care Med* 1996; 154(4 Pt 1):876–880.

16 Maesen FP, Smeets JJ, Sledsens TJ, Wald FD, Cornelissen PJ. Tiotropium bromide, a new long-acting antimuscarinic bronchodilator: a pharmacodynamic study in patients with chronic obstructive pulmonary disease (COPD). Dutch Study Group. *Eur Respir J* 1995; 8(9):1506–1513.

17 Barnes PJ, Belvisi MG, Mak JC, Haddad EB, O'Connor B. Tiotropium bromide (Ba 679 BR), a novel long-acting muscarinic antagonist for the treatment of obstructive airways disease. *Life Sci* 1995; 56(11–12):853–859.

18 Gross NJ, Skorodin MS. Massive overdose of atropine methonitrate with only slight untoward effects [letter]. *Lancet* 1985; 2(8451):386.

19 Gross NJ SM. Anticholinergic agents. In: Jenne JWMS, editor.

Drug therapy. New York: Marcel Dekker, 1987: 615–668.

20 Bollert FG, Matusiewicz SP, Dewar MH, Brown GM, McLean A, Greening AP et al. Comparative efficacy and potency of ipratropium via Turbuhaler and pressurized metered-dose inhaler in reversible airflow obstruction. *Eur Respir J* 1997; 10(8):1824–1828.

21 Ayala LE, Ahmed T. Is there loss of protective muscarinic receptor mechanism in asthma?. *Chest* 1989; 96(6):1285–1291.

22 Azevedo M, da Costa JT, Fontes P, da Silva JP, Araujo O. Effect of terfenadine and ipratropium bromide on ultrasonically nebulized distilled water-induced asthma. *J Int Med Res* 1990; 18(1):37–49.

23 Ayala LE, Choudry NB, Fuller RW. LTD4-induced broncho-constriction in patients with asthma: lack of a vagal reflex. *Br J Clin Pharmacol* 1988; 26(1):110–112.

24 Ruffin RE, Fitzgerald JD, Rebuck AS. A comparison of the bronchodilator activity of Sch 1000 and salbutamol. *J Allergy Clin Immunol* 1977; 59(2):136–141.

25 Ullah MI, Newman GB, Saunders KB. Influence of age on response to ipratropium and salbutamol in asthma. *Thorax* 1981; 36(7):523–529.

26 Vichyanond P, Sladek WA, Sur S, Hill MR, Szefler SJ, Nelson HS. Efficacy of atropine methylnitrate alone and in combination with albuterol in children with asthma. *Chest* 1990; 98(3):637–642.

27 Jolobe OM. Asthma vs. non-specific reversible airflow obstruction: clinical features and responsiveness to anti-cholinergic drugs. *Respiration* 1984; 45(3):237–242.

28 Brown IG, Chan CS, Kelly CA, Dent AG, Zimmerman PV. Assessment of the clinical usefulness of nebulised ipratro-pium bromide in patients with chronic airflow limitation. *Thorax* 1984; 39(4):272-276.

29 Baroody FM, Majchel AM, Roecker MM et al. Ipratropium bromide (Atrovent nasal spray) reduces the nasal response to methacholine. *J Allergy Clin Immunol* 1992; 89(6):1065–1075.

30 Rebuck AS, Chapman KR, Abboud R et al. Nebulized anti-cholinergic and sympathomimetic treatment of asthma and chronic obstructive airways disease in the emergency room. *Am J Med* 1987; 82(1):59–64.

31 Stoodley RG, Aaron SD, Dales RE. The role of ipratropium bromide in the emergency management of acute asthma exacerbation: a metaanalysis of randomized clinical trials [see comments]. *Ann Emerg Med* 1999; 34(1):8–18.

32 Brophy C, Ahmed B, Bayston S, Arnold A, McGivern D, Greenstone M. How long should Atrovent be given in acute asthma? *Thorax* 1998; 53(5):363–367.

33 Beck R, Robertson C, Galdes-Sebaldt M, Levison H. Combined salbutamol and ipratropium bromide by inhala-tion in the treatment of severe acute asthma. *J Pediatr* 1985; 107(4):605–608.

34 Reisman J, Galdes-Sebalt M, Kazim F, Canny G, Levison H. Frequent administration by inhalation of salbutamol and ipratropium bromide in the initial management of severe acute asthma in children. *J Allergy Clin Immunol* 1988; 81(1):16–20.

35 Storr J, Lenney W. Nebulised ipratropium and salbutamol in asthma. *Arch Dis Child* 1986; 61(6):602–603.

36 Boner AL, De Stefano G, Niero E, Vallone G, Gaburro D. Salbutamol and ipratropium bromide solution in the treat-ment of bronchospasm in asthmatic children. *Ann Allergy* 1987; 58(1):54–58.

37 Ducharme FM, Davis GM. Randomized controlled trial of ipratropium bromide and frequent low doses of salbutamol in the management of mild and moderate acute pediatric asthma. *J Pediatr* 1998; 133(4):479–485.

38 Schuh S, Johnson DW, Callahan S, Canny G, Levison H. Efficacy of frequent nebulized ipratropium bromide added to frequent high-dose albuterol therapy in severe childhood asthma. *J Pediatr* 1995; 126(4):639–645.

39 Zorc JJ, Pusic MV, Ogborn CJ, Lebet R, Duggan AK. Ipratropium bromide added to asthma treatment in the pediatric emergency department. *Pediatrics* 1999; 103(4 Pt 1):748–752.

40 Qureshi F, Pestian J, Davis P, Zaritsky A. Effect of nebulized ipratropium on the hospitalization rates of children with asthma. *N Engl J Med* 1998; 339(15):1030–1035.

41 Warner JO, Gotz M, Landau LI, Levison H, Milner AD, Pedersen S et al. Management of asthma: a consensus state-ment. *Arch Dis Child* 1989; 64(7):1065–1079.

42 Hargreave FE, Dolovich J, Newhouse MT. The assessment and treatment of asthma: a conference report. *J Allergy Clin Immunol* 1990; 85(6):1098–1111.

43 Avital A, Sanchez I, Chernick V. Efficacy of salbutamol and ipratropium bromide in decreasing bronchial hyperreactiv-ity in children with cystic fibrosis. *Pediatr Pulmonol* 1992; 13(1):34–37.

44 Thiessen B, Pedersen OF. Maximal expiratory flows and forced vital capacity in normal, asthmatic and bronchitic subjects after salbutamol and ipratropium bromide. *Respiration* 1982; 43(4):304–316.

45 Passamonte PM, Martinez AJ. Effect of inhaled atropine or metaproterenol in patients with chronic airway obstruction and therapeutic serum theophylline levels. *Chest* 1984; 85(5):610–615.

46 Ashutosh K, Dev G, Steele D. Nonbronchodilator effects of pirbuterol and ipratropium in chronic obstructive pulmo-nary disease. *Chest* 1995; 107(1):173–178.

47 Cazzola M, Matera MG, Di Perna F, Calderaro F, Califano C, Vinciguerra A. A comparison of bronchodilating effects of salmeterol and oxitropium bromide in stable chronic obstructive pulmonary disease. *Respir Med* 1998; 92(2):354–357.

48 Bleecker ER, Britt EJ. Acute bronchodilating effects of ipratropium bromide and theophylline in chronic obstructive pulmonary disease. *Am J Med* 1991; 91(4A):24S-27S.

49 Braun SR, McKenzie WN, Copeland C, Knight L, Ellersieck M. A comparison of the effect of ipratropium and albuterol in the treatment of chronic obstructive airway disease [published erratum appears in *Arch Intern Med* 1990 Jun;150(6):1242]. *Arch Intern Med* 1989; 149(3):544–547.

50 Tashkin DP, Ashutosh K, Bleecker ER et al. Comparison of the anticholinergic bronchodilator ipratropium bromide with metaproterenol in chronic obstructive pulmonary disease. A 90-day multi-center study. *Am J Med* 1986; 81(5A):81–90.

51 Gross NJ, Skorodin MS. Role of the parasympathetic system in airway obstruction due to emphysema. *N Engl J Med* 1984; 311(7):421–425.

52 Lefcoe NM, Toogood JH, Blennerhassett G, Baskerville J, Paterson NA. The addition of an aerosol anticholinergic to an oral beta agonist plus theophylline in asthma and bronchitis. A double-blind single dose study. *Chest* 1982; 82(3):300–305.

53 Barros MJ, Rees PJ. Bronchodilator responses to salbutamol followed by ipratropium bromide in partially reversible airflow obstruction. *Respir Med* 1990; 84(5):371–275.

54 Hay JG, Stone P, Carter J et al. Bronchodilator reversibility, exercise performance and breathlessness in stable chronic obstructive pulmonary disease. *Eur Respir J* 1992; 5(6):659–664.

55 Shivaram U, Cash ME, Mateo F, Shim C. Effects of high-dose ipratropium bromide and oral aminophylline on spirometry and exercise tolerance in COPD. *Respir Med* 1997; 91(6):327–334.

56 Papiris S, Galavotti V, Sturani C. Effects of beta-agonists on breathlessness and exercise tolerance in patients with chronic obstructive pulmonary disease. *Respiration* 1986; 49(2):101–108.

57 Berger R, Smith D. Effect of inhaled metaproterenol on exercise performance in patients with stable 'fixed' airway obstruction. *Am Rev Respir Dis* 1988; 138(3):624–629.

58 O'Donnell DE, Lam M, Webb KA. Spirometric correlates of improvement in exercise performance after anticholinergic therapy in chronic obstructive pulmonary disease. *Am J Respir Crit Care Med* 1999; 160(2):542–549.

59 Siafakas NM, Vermeire P, Pride NB et al. Optimal assessment and management of chronic obstructive pulmonary disease (COPD). The European Respiratory Society Task Force. *Eur Respir J* 1995; 8(8):1398–1420.

60 Standards for the diagnosis and care of patients with chronic obstructive pulmonary disease. American Thoracic Society. *Am J Respir Crit Care Med* 1995; 152(5 Pt 2):S77–121.

61 Patakas D, Andreadis D, Mavrofridis E, Argyropoulou P. Comparison of the effects of salmeterol and ipratropium bromide on exercise performance and breathlessness in patients with stable chronic obstructive pulmonary disease. *Respir Med* 1998; 92(9):1116–1121.

62 Tobin MJ, Hughes JA, Hutchison DC. Effects of ipratropium bromide and fenoterol aerosols on exercise tolerance. *Eur J Respir Dis* 1984; 65(6):441–446.

63 Teramoto S, Fukuchi Y, Orimo H. Effects of inhaled anticholinergic drug on dyspnea and gas exchange during exercise in patients with chronic obstructive pulmonary disease. *Chest* 1993; 103(6):1774–1782.

64 Leitch AG, Hopkin JM, Ellis DA, Merchant S, McHardy GJ. The effect of aerosol ipratropium bromide and salbutamol on exercise tolerance in chronic bronchitis. *Thorax* 1978; 33(6):711–713.

65 Anthonisen NR, Connett JE, Kiley JP et al. Effects of smoking intervention and the use of an inhaled anticholinergic bronchodilator on the rate of decline of FEV1. The Lung Health Study. *J Am Med Assoc* 1994; 272(19):1497–1505.

66 Karpel JP, Pesin J, Greenberg D, Gentry E. A comparison of the effects of ipratropium bromide and metaproterenol sulfate in acute exacerbations of COPD. *Chest* 1990; 98(4):835–839.

67 Patrick DM, Dales RE, Stark RM, Laliberte G, Dickinson G. Severe exacerbations of COPD and asthma. Incremental benefit of adding ipratropium to usual therapy. *Chest* 1990; 98(2):295–297.

68 Klink M, Quan SF. Prevalence of reported sleep disturbances in a general adult population and their relationship to obstructive airways diseases. *Chest* 1987; 91(4):540–546.

69 Douglas NJ, Calverley PM, Leggett RJ, Brash HM, Flenley DC, Brezinova V. Transient hypoxaemia during sleep in chronic bronchitis and emphysema. *Lancet* 1979; 1(8106):1–4.

70 Douglas NJ. Sleep in patients with chronic obstructive pulmonary disease. *Clin Chest Med* 1998; 19(1):115–125.

71 Stores G, Ellis AJ, Wiggs L, Crawford C, Thomson A. Sleep and psychological disturbance in nocturnal asthma. *Arch Dis Child* 1998; 78(5):413–419.

72 Gross N, Tashkin D, Miller R, Oren J, Coleman W, Linberg S. Inhalation by nebulization of albuterol–ipratropium combination (Dey combination) is superior to either agent alone in the treatment of chronic obstructive pulmonary disease.

Dey Combination Solution Study Group. *Respiration* 1998; 65(5):354–362.

73 Petty TL. In chronic obstructive pulmonary disease, a combination of ipratropium and albuterol is more effective than either agent alone. An 85-day multicenter trial. COMBIVENT Inhalation Aerosol Study Group. *Chest* 1994; 105(5):1411–1419.

74 Ikeda A, Nishimura K, Koyama H, Izumi T. Bronchodilating effects of combined therapy with clinical dosages of ipratropium bromide and salbutamol for stable COPD: comparison with ipratropium bromide alone [see comments]. *Chest* 1995; 107(2):401–405.

75 Routine nebulized ipratropium and albuterol together are better than either alone in COPD. The COMBIVENT Inhalation Solution Study Group. *Chest* 1997; 112(6):1514–1521.

76 Friedman M, Serby CW, Menjoge SS, Wilson JD, Hilleman DE, Witek TJ, Jr. Pharmacoeconomic evaluation of a combination of ipratropium plus albuterol compared with ipratropium alone and albuterol alone in COPD. *Chest* 1999; 115(3):635–641.

77 Gross NJ. Ipratropium bromide. *N Engl J Med* 1988; 319(8):486–494.

78 Watson WT, Shuckett EP, Becker AB, Simons FE. Effect of nebulized ipratropium bromide on intraocular pressures in children. *Chest* 1994; 105(5):1439–1441.

79 Pavia D, Bateman JR, Sheahan NF, Clarke SW. Effect of ipratropium bromide on mucociliary clearance and pulmonary function in reversible airways obstruction. *Thorax* 1979; 34(4):501–507.

80 Chapman KR, Smith DL, Rebuck AS, Leenen FH. Haemodynamic effects of inhaled ipratropium bromide, alone and combined with an inhaled beta 2-agonist. *Am Rev Respir Dis* 1985; 132(4):845–847.

81 Ashutosh K, Dev G, Steele D. Nonbronchodilator effects of pirbuterol and ipratropium in chronic obstructive pulmonary disease. *Chest* 1995; 107(1):173–178.

82 Gross NJ, Bankwala Z. Effects of an anticholinergic bronchodilator on arterial blood gases of hypoxaemic patients with chronic obstructive pulmonary disease. Comparison with a beta-adrenergic agent. *Am Rev Respir Dis* 1987; 136(5):1091–1094.

83 Khoukhaz G, Gross NJ. Effects of salmeterol on arterial blood gases in patients with stable chronic obstructive pulmonary disease. Comparison with albuterol and ipratropium. *Am J Respir Crit Care Med* 1999; 160(3):1028–1030.

84 Beasley R, Fishwick D, Miles JF, Hendeles L. Preservatives in nebulizer solutions: risks without benefit. *Pharmacotherapy* 1998; 18(1):130–139.

85 Boucher M, Roy MT, Henderson J. Possible association of benzalkonium chloride in nebulizer solutions with respiratory arrest. *Ann Pharmacother* 1992; 26(6):772–774.

86 Bone WD, Amundson DE. An unusual case of severe anaphylaxis due to ipratropium bromide inhalation [letter]. *Chest* 1993; 103(3):981–982.

87 Bryant DH, Rogers P. Effects of ipratropium bromide nebulizer solution with and without preservatives in the treatment of acute and stable asthma. *Chest* 1992; 102(3):742–747.

88 Pras E, Stienlauf S, Pinkhas J, Sidi Y. Urinary retention associated with ipratropium bromide. *DICP* 1991; 25(9):939–940.

89 Markus HS. Paralytic ileus associated with ipratropium [letter]. *Lancet* 1990; 335(8699):1224.

90 Helprin GA, Clarke GM. Unilateral fixed dilated pupil associated with nebulised ipratropium bromide [letter]. *Lancet* 1986; 2(8521–22):1469.

91 O'Driscoll BR. Supraventricular tachycardia caused by nebulised ipratropium bromide. *Thorax* 1989; 44(4):312.

92 Gross NJ, Petty TL, Friedman M, Skorodin MS, Silvers GW, Donohue JF. Dose response to ipratropium as a nebulized solution in patients with chronic obstructive pulmonary disease. A three-center study. *Am Rev Respir Dis* 1989; 139(5):1188–1191.

93 Leak A, O'Connor T. High dose ipratropium bromide: is it safe? *Practitioner* 1988; 232(1441):9–10.

94 Barnes PJ, Minette P, Maclagan J. Muscarinic receptor subtypes in airways. *Trends Pharmacol Sci* 1988; 9(11):412–416.

95 Martin RJ, Bartelson BL, Smith P et al. Effect of ipratropium bromide treatment on oxygen saturation and sleep quality in COPD. *Chest* 1999; 115(5):1338–1345.

96 Bruderman I, Cohen-Aranovski R, Smorzik J. A comparative study of various combinations of ipratropium bromide and metaproteranol in allergic asthmatic patients. *Chest* 1983; 83 (2): 208–210.

5

Antiallergic drugs

Masakazu Ichinose

Department of Respiratory and Infectious Diseases, Tohoku University School of Medicine, Sendai, Japan

Introduction

Bronchial asthma is a disease of the airways that is characterized by increased responsiveness of the tracheobronchial tree to a multiplicity of stimuli[1]. A number of causes have been postulated for the increased airway responsiveness; however, the basic mechanism remains unknown. The most popular hypothesis at present is that of airway inflammation, in which allergic mechanisms seem to play a key role. Therefore, the modulation of allergic mechanisms should be a fruitful approach to treating asthma.

Allergic reaction are dependent on an IgE response controlled by T- and B-lymphocytes and are activated by the interaction of antigen with mast cell-bound IgE molecules. After that, eosinophil recruitment into the airways occurs via cytokine- and adhesion molecule-dependent mechanisms. Thus, for the modulation of allergic responses there are many possible approaches, including interfering with IgE production, modulation of inflammatory cell activation, and antagonism to mediators.

In this book, IgE modifiers and mediator antagonists, namely receptor antagonists for lipid mediators, tachykinins, and bradykinin, are described elsewhere. Therefore, in this chapter I will discuss cromones and some other agents which are used for the clinical treatment of asthma as antiallergic drugs.

Chromones

The drugs cromolyn sodium and nedocromil sodium, traditionally referred to as mast cell stabilizing agents, comprise an important group of anti-inflammatory drugs useful in the treatment of bronchial asthma[2–4]. Although cromolyn sodium is a chromone, whereas nedocromil sodium belongs to the structural class of pyranoquinolines, they share many clinical characteristics.

Cromolyn sodium

Cromolyn sodium is a bischromone antiallergic drug first discovered in 1965 as a result of a series of pharmacological experiments on the antispasmodic agent khelin[2,5], and the drug has become accepted as a first-line anti-inflammatory agent in national and international asthma treatment guidelines[3,4].

Mechanisms of action

Cromolyn sodium functions through several pathways[2]. The most widely recognized mechanism of action for cromolyn sodium is its mast cell stabilizing effect because it was found to inhibit the influx of extracellular calcium[6]. Cromolyn sodium inhibits the release of various mediators from human mast cells and other inflammatory cells involved in airway inflammation in vitro, particularly when the release is triggered by IgE[5,7–10]. Therefore, this agent has potent effects in preventing both early and late asthmatic responses to inhaled allergens such as pollen, and it reduces airway reactivity resulting from exposure to a range of inhaled irritants such as sulfur dioxide and cold air.

Cromolyn sodium inhibits both the early and late airway reactions after allergen challenge by its effect on inflammatory cells other than mast cells[2]. Cromolyn sodium attenuates the in vitro activation of human neutrophils, eosinophils, and monocytes and the end organ effects of platelet activating factor, all of which are important in the late-phase allergic reaction[2].

Cromolyn sodium also is effective in treating asthmatic attacks induced by metabisulfites, diisocyanates, western red cedar, and colophany fumes, which may occur as the result of reflex bronchoconstriction through the stimulation of irritant or sensory C-fibres in the airways[2], possibly by attenuating sensory and cholinergic nerve activation. In guinea pig, cromolyn sodium partially inhibits the leukotriene D4-induced bronchoconstrictor response, via the attenuation of the cholinergic reflex pathway[11]. The inhibitory effect of cromolyn sodium on SO_4^- or distilled water-induced bronchoconstriction also seems to be mediated via the cholinergic pathway[2]. Further, cromolyn sodium inhibits sensory C-fibre activation resulting in the attenuation of tachykinin release from the nerves.

Clinical utility in asthma therapy

Based on the unique bimodal pharmacology outlined above, cromolyn sodium has an established place in asthma management in two distinct clinical situations[3,4]. Early investigations of the use of inhaled cromolyn sodium for asthma therapy focused on its ability to decrease airway hyperresponsiveness[2]. Cromolyn sodium inhibits both the early and late phase airway allergic reactions via its direct mast cell stabilizing effect that prevents inflammatory cell migration into the airways[12]. Cromolyn sodium also prevents exercise-induced asthma. This agent controls asthmatic airway inflammation, reduces bronchial hyperresponsiveness, reduces symptomatology, and gradually improves pulmonary function.

In one analysis of 175 children using cromolyn sodium for mild to moderately severe asthma, the long-term prognosis was improved and the deterioration in spirometry over time was prevented when compared with bronchodilators used alone on an as-needed basis[13]. Both cromolyn sodium and, to a greater extent, inhaled corticosteroids conferred sig-

nificant protection against exacerbations of asthma leading to hospitalization in an analysis of 16,941 eligible persons in a managed health-care setting[14]. This supports the widespread clinical impression that inhaled corticosteroids are more efficacious than chromones, but that chromones can also play a major role in the management of asthma. Cromolyn sodium may be used as long-term therapy early in the course of asthma[4,15]. It reduces symptoms and the frequency of exacerbations. Although there is insufficient knowledge about the mechanisms of action to predict which patients will achieve a beneficial response to cromolyn sodium, this agent seems to be effective in mild to moderate allergic asthma[4,16]. To determine the efficacy of this agent, 4 to 8 weeks of administration may be required[4]. The side effects of cromolyn sodium are only minimal. This drug causes coughing occasionally upon inhalation of the powder formulation[4].

Nedocromil sodium

Nedocromil sodium generally has displayed greater potency in protecting patients against non-immunological stimuli and was thus introduced as an anti-inflammatory agent with a broader spectrum than cromolyn sodium. Nedocromil sodium is a disodium salt of pyranoquinoline dicarboxylic acid.

Mechanisms of action

Nedocromil sodium has been found to work through several pathways similar to those of cromolyn sodium, but many of its actions are still incompletely understood[2]. Nedocromil sodium has been demonstrated to inhibit histamine release from human dispersed lung tissue and mast cells obtained by bronchoalveolar lavage in a dose-dependent manner[17]. It was less effective in inhibiting histamine release from human colonic mucosal and submucosal mast cells and it had no effect on inhibiting mast cell release from cutaneous mast cells or basophils[18,19]. Nedocromil sodium also inhibits both leukotriene C4 and prostaglandin D2 release from human mast cells[20].

Both nedocromil sodium and cromolyn sodium have been demonstrated to inhibit intermediate conductance chloride channels in cultured RBL-2H3 mucosal mast cells[21]. Chloride ion influx results in cell membrane hyperpolarization, which is necessary for calcium ion influx and subsequent mast cell activation[21].

Nedocromil sodium reduces the chemotaxis of neutrophils in the presence of chemotactic agents such as platelet activating factor and leukotriene B4[22]. For eosinophils, nedocromil sodium shows an effect against the chemotactic actions induced by platelet activating factor and leukotriene B4 but has no effect on those induced by interleukin-3 (IL-3), IL-5, or granulocyte macrophage-colony stimulating factor[22].

Nedocromil sodium has been shown to inhibit airway sensory nerve activation[23] as does in cromolyn sodium. Therefore, this agent may be useful to manage coughing observed in airway inflammatory diseases.

Clinical utility in asthma therapy
The prevention by nedocromil sodium of bronchoconstriction that would otherwise result from acute airway challenges such as antigen inhalation and exercise has been reported. Treatment with nedocromil from a metered dose inhaler several minutes before an anticipated challenge is usually sufficient to provide protection.

In the long-term maintenance therapy for asthma, most clinical trials evaluating the efficacy of nedocromil sodium have demonstrated an improvement in symptoms as well as pulmonary function such as peak expiratory flow rate[24]. Both national and international asthma treatment guidelines have shifted their recommendations towards the use of cromones for less severe asthma, particularly episodic asthma and mild persistent asthma[3,4]. However, in patients already receiving inhaled corticosteroid, nedocromil sodium has been reported to have a more potent steroid-sparing effect than cromolyn sodium[25,26].

Histamine H1-receptor antagonists

Histamine has been thought to be an important inflammatory mediator of asthma because of its variety of airway actions, namely airway smooth muscle contraction, mucus secretion, vasodilation, and vagal nerve activation, which are involved in the pathogenesis of asthma[27]. Therefore, oral antihistamines (histamine H1-receptor antagonists) are frequently used in asthma therapy. However, at present, the effect of this class of drugs on asthma therapy has been disappointing. A recent meta-analysis study has shown that antihistamines do not cause a significant bronchodilatory effect as assessed by peak expiratory flow rate, but do result in a slight reduction in the need for inhaled bronchodilator use[28].

In the international asthma treatment guidelines, several drugs that have a histamine H1-receptor antagonistic activity and other effects are listed[4]. These drugs will be described in the next section.

Oral antiallergic compounds

Ketotifen

Mechanisms of action
Ketotifen antagonizes histamine H1-receptors. Ketotifen also inhibits mast cell activation and mast cell mediator release. In addition, other pharmacological activities of this agent have mainly been shown in animal models[29]; however, the efficacy of ketotifen has not yet been sufficiently documented[4].

Clinical utility in asthma therapy
Controlled clinical studies comparing the therapeutic efficacy of ketotifen in asthma to a placebo or cromolyn sodium have shown variable results[4]. Most studies suggest that ketotifen results in a slow but significant improvement of asthma symptomatology and a reduction in the need for concomitant antiasthma medication[30]. It has been reported that the clinical efficacy of ketotifen can be observed after 2 months of drug administration[31]. This delay

in the onset of the therapeutic activity has also been observed in other studies. The most frequent side effect of ketotifen is sedation.

Other antiallergic drugs

Other oral antiallergic drugs, such as tranilast, repirinast, tazanolast, pemirolast, ozagrel, azelastine, amlexanox, and ibudilast, are used for asthma therapy, especially in Japan. These compounds have been reported to inhibit mast cell activation, interfere with the synthesis of allergic inflammatory mediators, or act as antagonists of mediators, such as histamine, leukotriene, and thromboxane. However, further studies on the relative efficacy of these compounds are needed before recommendations can be made about the inclusion of these oral antiallergic compounds in the long-term treatment of asthma[4].

Down-regulation of TH2 cell-mediated responses

The recently developed suplatast tosilate[32] has been reported to inhibit Th2 cytokine, IL4 and IL5, synthesis in vitro and the allergen-induced increase in peritoneal eosinophils in mice[33]. In an uncontrolled trial, 6 weeks' treatment of patients with suplatast tosilate was reported to reduce airway hyper-responsiveness and eosinophil infiltration into the airways[34]. A steroid sparing effect by suplatast tosilate also has been recently shown[35] in a limited trial. To assess the long-term efficacy of suplatast tosilate, a well-controlled, multi-centre trial seems to be needed.

Conclusion

In this chapter I have discussed cromones and other agents which are used for the clinical treatment of asthma as antiallergic drugs, IgE modifiers or antagonists for lipid mediators, tachykinins, and bradykinin, are described elsewhere in this book. The recent worldwide use of inhaled corticosteroids for asth-

matic patients has largely improved disease management. Actually, the combination of inhaled steroids and long acting β2-adrenoreceptor agonists seem to be effective for the majority of asthmatic patients. In contrast, the efficacy of antiallergic drugs are weak compared with inhaled low dose steroids. However, from the point of view of tolerability, oral drugs, if possible once per day, are more desirable for asthma therapy, especially in children and older persons. The development of antiallergic drugs that cause strong anti-inflammatory effects on asthmatic airways comparable to those of inhaled steroids is needed.

REFERENCES

1 McFadden Jr, ER. Asthma. In: Fauci AS, Braunwald E et al eds, *Principles of internal medicine*, McGraw-Hill, New York, 1998; pp. 1419–1426.
2 Bernstein JA, Bernstein IL. Cromones. In: Barnes PJ, Grunstein MM et al. eds, *Asthma*, Lippincott-Raven Publishers, Philadelphia, 1997; pp. 1647–1665.
3 Expert Panel Report 2. Guidelines for the diagnosis and management of asthma. US Department of Health and Human Services, NIH Publication No 97–4051, April 1997.
4 Global Strategy for Asthma Management and Prevention (GINA). NHLBI/WHO Workshop Report. National Institutes of Health Publication No. 96–3659A, December 1995
5 Murphy S. Cromolyn sodium: Basic mechanisms and clinical usage. *Pediatr Asthma Allergy Immunol* 1988; 2:237–254.
6 Foreman JC, Hallett MB, Mongar, JL. Site of action of the anti-allergic drugs cromoglycate and doxantrazole. *Br J Pharmacol* 1977; 59:473p-474p.
7 Leung KB, Flint KC, Brostoff J et al. Effects of sodium cromoglycate and nedocromil sodium on histamine secretion from human lung mast cells. *Thorax* 1988; 43:756–761.
8 Church MK. Is inhibition of mast cell mediator release relevant to the clinical activity of anti-allergic drugs? *Agents Action* 1986; 18:288–293.
9 Edwards AM. Sodium cromoglycate (Intal) as an anti-inflammatory agent for the treatment of chronic asthma. *Clin Exp Allergy* 1994; 24:612–623.
10 Loh RKS, Jabara HH, Geha RS. Disodium cromoglycate inhibits S mu→S epsilon deletional switch recombination and IgE synthesis in human B cells. *J Exp Med* 1994; 180:663–671.

11 Advenier C, Rizk NW, Boushey HA, Bethel RA. Sodium cromoglycate, verapamil and nicardipine antagonism to leukotriene D4 bronchoconstriction. *Br J Pharmacol* 1983; 78:301–206.

12 Cockcroft DW, Murdock KY. Comparative effects of inhaled salbutamol, sodium cromoglycate and beclomethasone dipropionate on allergen-induced early asthmatic responses, late asthmatic responses, and increased bronchial responsiveness. *J Allergy Clin Immunol* 1987; 79:734–740.

13 König P, Shaffer J. The effect of drug therapy on long-term outcome of childhood asthma: a possible preview of the international guidelines. *J Allergy Clin Immunol* 1996; 98:1103–1111.

14 Foreman JC, Pearce FL. Cromolyn and nedocromil. In: Middleton E, Reed CE, Ellis EF et al (eds), *Allergy: Principles and Practice*, Mosby, St. Louis, 1993; pp. 926–940

15 Altounyan ER. Review of clinical activity and mode of action of sodium cromoglycate. *Clin Allergy* 1980; 10:s481–s489.

16 Eigen H, Reid JJ, Dahl R et al. Evaluation of the addition of cromolyn sodium to bronchodilator maintenance therapy in the long-term management of asthma. *J Allergy Clin Immunol* 1987; 80:612–621.

17 Leung KB, Flint KC, Brostoff J, Hudspith BN, Johnson NM, Pearce FL. A comparison of nedocromil sodium and sodium cromoglycate on human lung mast cells obtained by bronchoalveolar lavage and by dispersion of lung fragments. *Eur J Respir Dis* 1986; 69:223–226.

18 Liu WL, Bosman L, Boulos PB, Lau HY, Pearce FL. Mast cells from human colonic mucosa and submucosa/muscle: a comparison with the human lung mast cells. *Agents Actions* 1990; 30:70–73.

19 Tainsh KR, Lau HY, Liu WL, Pearce FL. The human skin mast cell: a comparison with the human lung cell and novel mast cell type, the uterine mast cell. *Agents Actions* 1991; 33:16–19

20 Pearce FL. Effect of nedocromil sodium on mediator release from mast cells. *J Allergy Clin Immunol* 1993; 92:155–158.

21 Barnes PJ, Holgate ST, Laitinen LA, Payels R. Asthma mechanisms, determinants of severity and treatment: the role of nedocromil sodium. *Clin Exp Allergy* 1995; 25:771–787.

22 Bruijnzeel PL, Warringa RA, Kok PT, Hamelink ML, Kreukniet H, Koenderman L. Effects of nedocromil sodium on in vitro induced migration, activation, and mediator release from human granulocytes. *J Allergy Clin Immunol* 1993; 92:159–154.

23 Barnes PJ. Effect of nedocromil sodium on airway sensory nerves. *J Allergy Clin Immunol* 1993; 92:182–186.

24 Ruggieri F, Patalano F. Nedocromil sodium: a review of clinical studies. *Eur Respir J* 1989; 2:568s-571s.

25 Marin JM, Carrizo SJ, Garcia R, Ejea MV. Effects of nedocromil sodium in steroid-resistant asthma: a randomized controlled trial. *J Allergy Clin Immunol* 1996; 97:602–610.

26 Svendsen UG, Jorgensen H. Inhaled nedocromil sodium as additional treatment to high dose inhaled corticosteroids in the management of bronchial asthma. *Eur Respir J* 1991; 4:992–999.

27 Barnes PJ, Chung KF, Page CP. Inflammatory mediators of asthma: an update. *Pharmacol Rev* 1998; 50:515–596.

28 Van Ganse E, Kaufman L, Derde MP, Yernault JC, Vincken W. Effects of antihistamines in adult asthma: a meta-analysis of clinical trials. *Eur Respir J* 1997; 10:2216–2224.

29 Grant SM, Goa KL, Fitton A, Sorkin EM. Ketotifen. A review of its pharmacodynamic and pharmacokinetic properties, and therapeutic use in asthma and allergic disorders. *Drugs* 1990; 40:412–48.

30 Medici TC, Radielovic P, Morley J. Ketotifen in the prophylaxis of extrinsic bronchial asthma. A multicenter controlled double-blind study with a modified-release formulation. *Chest* 1989; 96:252–257.

31 Tinkelman DG, Moss BA, Bukantz SC et al. A multicenter trial of the prophylactic effect of ketotifen, theophylline, and placebo in atopic asthma. *J Allergy Clin Immunol* 1985; 76:487–497.

32 Koda A, Yanagihara Y, Matsuura N. IPD-1151T: a prototype drug of IgE antibody synthesis modulation. *Agents Actions* 1991; 34:369–378.

33 Yamaya H, Basaki Y, Togawa M, Kojima M, Kiniwa M, Matsuura N. Down-regulation of Th2 cell-mediated murine peritoneal eosinophilia by antiallergic agents. *Life Sci* 1995; 19:1647–1654.

34 Sano Y, Miyamoto T, Makino S. Anti-inflammatory effect of suplatast tosilate on mild asthma. *Chest* 1997; 112:862–863.

35 Tamaoki J, Kondo M, Sakai N et al. Effect of suplatast tosilate, a Th2 cytokine inhibitor, on steroid-dependent asthma: a double-blind randomised study. *Lancet* 2000; 356:273–278.

6

Drugs affecting the synthesis and action of leukotrienes

Paul M. O'Byrne

Firestone Institute for Respiratory Health, St Joseph's Heathcare, Hamilton, Ontario, Canada

Introduction

In 1938, Feldberg and Kellaway[1] reported an activity in the perfusate of guinea pigs' lungs stimulated with cobra venom, which caused slow onset, but very sustained, contraction of smooth muscle. The time course of the contraction was subsequently demonstrated to be distinct from histamine and Kellaway and Trethewie named the mediator Slow Reacting Substance of Anaphylaxis (SRS-A)[2]. In 1960, Brocklehurst[3] reported that SRS-A was released from lung fragments from an asthmatic subject, when these fragments were exposed to allergen. This raised the possibility that SRS-A was important in causing symptoms in allergic asthmatics after allergen inhalation, because of its ability to contract airway smooth muscle with a much longer duration of action than other smooth muscle constrictors. Subsequent studies demonstrated the potency of SRS-A as a bronchoconstrictor agonist in animals[4]. In the late 1970s, the identity of the component molecules of SRS-A was reported to consist of the cysteinyl leukotrienes C_4, D_4 and E_4[5].

Synthetic pathways of the leukotrienes

The leukotrienes are derived from the ubiquitous membrane constituent arachidonic acid and are members of a larger group of biomolecules known as eicosanoids[5,6]. Arachidonic acid-(5,8,11,14-*cis*-eicosatetraenoic acid), is found esterified, in the *sn*-2 position, to cell-membrane phospholipids in a wide variety of mammalian cells[7,8]. The synthesis of leukotrienes is initiated by the action of phospholipase A_2, which selectively cleaves arachidonic acid from cell membranes. Arachidonic acid is converted sequentially to 5-hydroperoxyeicosatetraenoic acid (5-HPETE) and then to leukotriene A_4 (5,6-oxido-7,9-*trans*-11,14-*cis*-eicosatetraenoic acid) by a catalytic complex consisting of 5-lipoxygenase (5-LO)[9,10] and the 5-lipoxygenase activating protein (FLAP)[11]. In the intracellular microenvironment, and in the presence of leukotriene C_4 synthase[12], glutathione is adducted at the C6 position of leukotriene A_4 to yield the molecule known as leukotriene C_4 (5(S)-hydroxy-6(R)-glutathionyl-7,9-*trans*-11,14-*cis*-eicosatetraenoic acid)[13]. Leukotriene C_4 is exported from the cytosol to the extracellular microenvironment[14] where the glutamic acid moiety is cleaved by -glutamyltranspeptidase to form leukotriene D_4 (5(S)-hydroxy-6(R)-cysteinyl-glycyl-7,9 *trans*-11,14-*cis*-eicosatetraenoic acid)[14]. Cleavage of the glycine moiety from leukotriene D_4 by a variety of dipeptidases results in the formation of leukotriene E_4 (5(S)-hydroxy-6(R)-cysteinyl-7,9-*trans*-11,14-*cis*-eicosatetraenoic acid)[15]. Because they each contain cysteine, leukotriene C_4, leukotriene D_4, and leukotriene E_4, are known as the cysteinyl leukotrienes; together these molecules constitute the material formerly known as SRS-A. All three cysteinyl leukotrienes have the same range of biological effects; however, leukotriene E_4 is much less potent than its precursor molecules. Among the cells in the

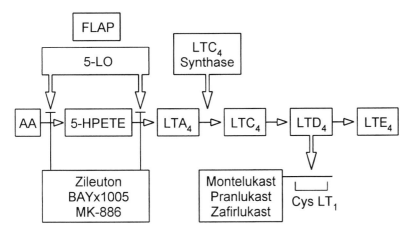

Fig. 6.1 The 5-lipoxygenase pathway of arachidonic acid metabolism, indicating the other enzymes, 5-lipoxygenase activating protein and LTC$_4$ synthetase, necessary for the production of the cysteinyl leukotrienes. Also 5-lipoxygenase activating protein antagonists such as BAYx1005 and MK-886, 5-lipoxygenase inhibitors such as Zileuton and *Cys LT$_1$* antagonists, such as Zafirulast inhibit the production or action of the cysteinyl leukotrienes. (Reproduced with permission.)[99]

lung that possess the enzymatic activities to produce the cysteinyl leukotrienes are mast cells[16], eosinophils[17] and alveolar macrophages[18].

Inhibition of leukotriene production or action

The only enzyme in the biosynthetic pathway of the cysteinyl leukotrienes (Fig. 6.1) that has been selectively inhibited is 5-lipoxygenase[19], thereby preventing their production. It has also been possible to interrupt leukotriene production by preventing the binding of arachidonic acid to FLAP[20].

The cysteinyl leukotrienes cause airway obstruction in humans through stimulation of specific receptors now termed the cysteinyl leukotriene receptor Type 1(CysLT$_1$)[21]. The CysLT$_1$ receptor is a seven transmembrane spanning, G-protein coupled receptor, whose gene has been mapped to the X chromosome[22]. Stimulation of the CysLT$_1$ receptor results in smooth muscle constriction, with signal transduction occurring by stimulation of phosphoinositide turnover[23,24]. A number of chemically distinct, specific, selective antagonists have been identified[25–29] and used in studies in human asthma. A distinct cysteinyl leukotriene receptor Type

2(CysLT$_2$) has also recently been characterized[30], which has 38% amino acid identity to the CysLT$_1$ receptor, whose gene has been mapped to chromosome 13q14. The biological role of this receptor has not yet been identified.

Several antileukotrienes are now available by prescription to treat asthma. Only one of these is a synthesis inhibitor. This is the 5-lipoxygenase inhibitor, zileuton[31], which is available for prescription in the United States. The CysLT$_1$ receptor antagonists are much more widely available; zafirlukast[32] and montelukast[33] in most countries, while pranlukast[34] is available currently in Japan and Korea.

Importance of leukotrienes in asthma

Asthmatic airway obstruction

Spontaneous bronchoconstriction has been used as a model for examination of the role of leukotrienes in airway narrowing in asthma. The capacity of a CysLT1 receptor antagonist to reverse asthmatic bronchoconstriction was first demonstrated by Hui and Barnes[35], in a group of patients with moderately severe asthma, most of whom were using inhaled steroids. They demonstrated that the administration of zafirlukast resulted in a 5–10% improvement in the FEV_1. In these same subjects, inhalation of a β_2-agonist increased in the FEV_1 by 20–30%. However, the effects of the β_2-agonist were additive with the effects of the $CysLT_1$ receptor antagonist; this observation suggested that distinct contractile mechanisms are involved in each response. In a trial of similar design in which MK-571, a chemically distinct $CysLT_1$ receptor antagonist, was given intravenously, similar results were obtained[36]. Also, the 5-lipoxygenase inhibitor zileuton, has been demonstrated to increase the FEV_1 by 10–15% in asthmatic subjects[37]. These data indicate that a significant component of asthmatic bronchoconstriction is directly due to the action of leukotrienes at their receptors, and that the stimuli resulting in leukotriene synthesis are continuously activated.

Airway hyperresponsiveness

The capacity of leukotrienes to cause airway hyperresponsiveness in stable asthmatics is not fully resolved. Exogenously administered inhaled leukotriene D_4 has been shown in one[38], but not another study[39] to increase airway responsiveness. However, a study from Fischer et al.[40] has demonstrated that regular treatment with the 5-lipoxygenase inhibitor, zileuton for 13 weeks, improved airway responsiveness to cold air for up to 10 days after completion of treatment, which is much longer than the expected duration of zileuton's pharmacological action. This study suggests that inhibition of leukotriene generation can improve airway hyperresponsiveness, possibly by improving airway inflammation.

Airway inflammation

Airway inflammation is central to the pathogenesis of asthma symptoms, bronchoconstriction, and airway hyperresponsiveness. Many studies have demonstrated the presence of activated eosinophils and of mast cells in the airway lumen and airway wall of patients with asthma, even those with mild disease[41,42]. Activated eosinophils and mast cells

have the capacity to release the cysteinyl leukotrienes, and measurements of urinary leukotrienes in asthmatic children suggest that persistent generation of leukotrienes are a consequence of persisting airway inflammation[43]. In addition, inhaled leukotriene E_4 markedly increased numbers of eosinophils in induced sputum[44] and in airway biopsies from asthmatic subjects. These studies confirm in vitro studies that the cysteinyl leukotrienes can cause eosinophil chemotaxis[45], and suggest that the cysteinyl leukotrienes may be involved in causing the airway eosinophilia of asthma. This concept is supported by studies which have demonstrated a reduction in airway eosinophils and leukotriene E_4 levels associated with an improvement in lung function, in patients with nocturnal asthma during treatment with zileuton, when measurements were made during the night[46], as well as in less severe asthmatic patients[33], and a reduction in eosinophils in induced sputum in asthmatics during treatment with montelukast[47]. These interesting results, taken together with the study which indicates an improvement in airway hyperresponsiveness after zileuton treatment[40], suggest that inhibition of leukotriene biosynthesis not only improves airway inflammation, but also its consequent physiological effect on airway hyperresponsiveness. However, further studies are needed to demonstrate that the improvements in airway inflammation and airway hyperresponsiveness are occurring in the same patients.

Exercise and cold air hyperventilation

Exercise-induced bronchoconstriction occurs in 70–80% of patients with symptomatic asthma[48]. The cysteinyl leukotrienes play an important role in causing exercise- and cold air-induced bronchoconstriction, as is demonstrated by the effects of a variety of different $CysLT_1$-receptor antagonists and leukotriene synthesis inhibitors in attenuating these bronchoconstrictor responses. The receptor antagonists, such as MK-571[49], montelukast[50], or zafirlukast, given either orally[51] or by inhalation[52], inhibit the maximal bronchoconstrictor response after exercise by between 50 and 70%, greatly shorten the

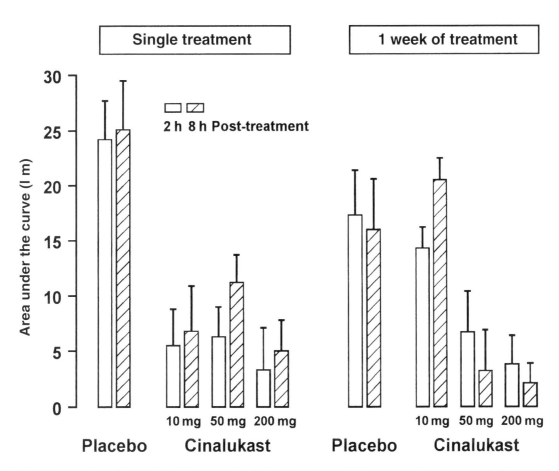

Fig. 6.2 The protection afforded by Cinalukast on exercise-induced bronchoconstriction as measured by the area under the FEV_1-time curve. On the first day of treatment, the protective effect at each dose is maintained for at least 8 h. After 1 week of treatment the protective effect is lost for the lowest (10 mg) dose, but preserved for the two higher doses. (Reproduced with permission.)[53]

time to recovery of normal lung function, and thereby markedly reduce the time response curve; in 30–50% of asthmatic subjects studied, these agents completely inhibit the response. Administration of the potent and long-lasting receptor antagonist, cinalukast, resulted in a reduction in exercise-induced bronchoconstriction measured as the area under the time response curve after exercise by >80% in asthmatic subjects, and this effect lasted more than 8 hours after dosing[53](Fig. 6.2).

Similar effects have been demonstrated when cold air hyperventilation has been used as the stim-ulus to provoke bronchoconstriction. Israel et al.[54] have shown that treatment with zileuton attenuates this bronchoconstrictor response. Taken together, these studies indicate that cooling and drying the airways results in the generation of leukotrienes, presumably from resident airway cells, such as mast cells, which results in bronchoconstriction. The observation by multiple investigative groups of het-erogeneity among subjects, that is that in some sub-jects interruption of the leukotriene cascade results in a complete inhibition of the bronchospastic response to exercise while in others this intervention has no effect, indicates that the pathways leading to bronchoconstriction after exercise vary in different asthmatics, and that in some, mediators other than the leukotrienes may be more important bronchoconstrictor agonists.

The currently available treatment for exercise-induced bronchoconstriction is not optimal for all patients. The most usual approach to treatment for such patients is to take two puffs of a rapid-acting inhaled β_2-agonist, 5–10 min before exercise, or inhaled cromoglycate 15–20 min before exercise[55]. These interventions have, however, a limited duration of effect. Long acting inhaled β_2-agonist (such as salmeterol) have been demonstrated to provide more prolonged protection against exercise-induced bronchoconstriction. However, the regular use of both short acting inhaled β_2-agonists[56], as well as long-acting inhaled β_2-agonists[57], rather than their use as prophylaxis, results in reduced protection against exercise-induced bronchoconstriction. This loss of efficacy against exercise-induced bronchoconstriction does not occur when anti-leukotrienes are used as regular treatment[50].

Other types of antiasthma treatments are not very effective in protecting against exercise-induced bronchoconstriction. For example oral β_2-agonists and methylxanthines are marginally effective or ineffective in almost all patients[58,59]. Thus, for the patients in whom leukotriene inhibition has a salutary effect, having an orally available treatment, which provides prolonged protection against exercise-induced bronchoconstriction will be a therapeutic advance. In the only comparisons published, the leukotriene antagonist SK&F 104353 was as effective as cromoglycate in preventing exercise-induced bronchconstriction[60], and montelukast provided prolonged protection[61] without the development of tolerance, which did develop with the long-acting inhaled β_2-agonist, salmeterol, with regular use[62].

Aspirin-induced asthma

The cysteinyl leukotrienes are the main cause of the bronchoconstriction that develops in aspirin-sensitive asthmatics following exposure to aspirin. In clinical trials in which aspirin-sensitive asthmatics were pretreated with the inhaled leukotriene receptor antagonist SKF104353[63], or the receptor antagonist MK-679[64], many tolerated, without developing significant bronchoconstriction, the doses of inhaled lysine aspirin that had previously caused bronchoconstriction. When aspirin is given systemically to patients with aspirin-sensitive asthma, naso-ocular, dermal, gastrointestinal and bronchospastic responses occur. However, pretreatment of these individuals with zileuton[65] completely ablated all physiological responses observed after aspirin challenge. These data clearly implicate products of the 5-lipoxygenase pathway as the primary effector molecules in aspirin-induced asthma. Dahlen and coworkers[66] obtained additional evidence for this hypothesis by demonstrating that the systemic administration of a $CysLT_1$ receptor antagonist is associated with improvement in lung function in individuals with ASA-induced asthma in the absence of specific ASA provocation. Finally, anti-leukotrienes have been demonstrated to improve overall asthma control in patients with ASA-induced asthma[67].

Allergen-induced asthma

Inhalation of specific allergens by sensitized patients results in acute bronchoconstriction which usually resolves within 2 hours; this is known as the early asthmatic response. In up to 50% of adult subjects the early asthmatic response is followed by a second period of bronchoconstriction, beginning 3–4 hours after inhalation and lasting up to 24 hours; this is known as the late asthmatic response[68]. The late asthmatic response is associated with increases in airway hyperresponsiveness, which can last several days to weeks[69].

Cysteinyl leukotrienes are generated during the early asthmatic response[70] and the magnitude of leukotriene generation, as indicated by increases in urinary excretion of the metabolite leukotriene E_4, directly correlates with the magnitude of the early asthmatic response[71]. Many studies using antileuko-

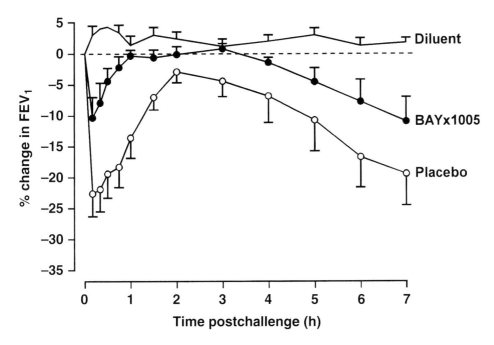

Fig. 6.3 The protection afforded by BAYx1005 on allergen-induced early and late asthmatic responses. The results are expressed as mean ($\pm$ SEM) % change in FEV_1 from baseline during the early and late asthmatic response to allergen inhalation after BAYx1005 (closed circles) and placebo (open circles) pretreatment and after inhaled diluent (open squares).* $P<0.05$; ** $P<0.001$. (Reproduced with permission.)[77]

triene drugs have shown that most of the broncho-constriction during the early asthmatic response is attenuated and the late asthmatic response is partially attenuated by such treatments. These studies have included a variety of antileukotriene agents including receptor antagonists, such as zafirlukast[72], MK-571[73] or pranlukast[74], and biosynthesis inhibitors, such as MK-886[75], MK-591[76] and BAYx 1005[77](Fig. 6.3). The magnitude of the protection afforded by these drugs during the early asthmatic response has varied from 58%[76] to 84%[77]; taken together, these results demonstrate that the cysteinyl leukotrienes are the mediators responsible for the majority of the bronchoconstriction during the early asthmatic response. Similarly, treatment with antileukotriene agents has demonstrated varied effectiveness in the magnitude of the protection afforded during the late asthmatic response from 49%[78] to 60%[77], suggesting that, as inhaled leuko-

triene D_4 does not itself cause the development of late responses[39], newly generated cysteinyl leukotrienes, possibly from inflammatory cells, such as eosinophils[79], mast cells or basophils[80] recruited into the airways during the late asthmatic response, are partially responsible for the bronchoconstriction during this response. Finally, the leukotriene receptor antagonist. pranlukast, has been demonstrated to attenuate allergen-induced airway hyperresponsiveness[74].

Efficacy of antileukotriene drugs in asthma

Several different antileukotrienes have been used in clinical trials where the primary goal was to assess the capacity of these agents to control of chronic stable asthma. In the first of these, LY171883, a relatively non-potent receptor antagonist that shifted the LTD_4 dose-response curve about 5-fold in nonasthmatic subjects, was given to patients with mild asthma in a 6-week parallel group placebo-controlled trial[81]. Patients receiving the leukotriene D_4 receptor antagonist had a small, but statistically significant, increase in FEV_1 of approximately 300 ml during the trial. Moreover, in those patients using inhaled β_2-agonists more frequently before randomized treatment was begun, this use decreased while their FEV_1 increased. In two other trials of 4–6 weeks' duration, the effectiveness of treatment with zileuton[37] or zafirlukast[32] was compared with placebo treatment. Each study used a randomized, double-blind, parallel group design with a run-in period, in which patients were treated with placebo (single blind) followed by 4 or 6 weeks of double-blind randomized treatment. Patients receiving higher doses of either antileukotriene had a significantly greater increase in FEV_1 than did patients taking placebo, while patients receiving the lower doses of treatment had an increase of intermediate magnitude. Chronic treatment with either antileukotriene was also associated with significant decrements in asthma medication use, in asthma symptoms, and an increase in morning peak flow. The final shorter-term study compared the *Cys LT₁*-antagonist, montelukast compared to placebo in a crossover design for 1.5 weeks of treatment demonstrated a mean 16% improvement in FEV_1[82]. These data, taken together, indicate that, in patients with mild chronic stable asthma, the leukotrienes mediate a clinically significant component of airway obstruction.

These findings have been confirmed and extended in longer studies in patients with mild -to-moderate chronic stable asthma in which the efficacy of treatment with zileuton (400 mg *q.i.d.* or 600 mg *q.i.d.*) was compared to placebo[31,83]. All patients were receiving treatment only with inhaled β_2-agonists and had prebronchodilator FEV_1 values that were approximately 60% of predicted normal. Zileuton treatment was associated with approximately a 15% improvement in the FEV_1, decreased asthma symptoms and decreased β_2-agonist use. More importantly in both trials over 2.5-fold more patients receiving placebo treatment required steroid 'rescue' treatment than did patients receiv-

ing high-dose zileuton treatment. There was no significant deterioration in the improvement in the FEV_1 during the course of either study, thus extending the previous findings that patients do not become 'tolerant' to the effects of 5-lipoxygenase inhibition. Other longer term studies have been reported with the receptor antagonists zafirlukast[84], montelukast[85] and pranlukast[34] and demonstrating clinical benefit.

Safety of antileukotriene drugs

Since this entire class of drugs is new, the total patient exposure to these agents is limited. Nevertheless a number of issues have emerged. In a safety study in over 3000 patients, about 4.5% of patients receiving zileuton, compared to 1.1% of patients receiving placebo, had reversible elevations in hepatic transaminases to over three times the upper limit of the reference range. These elevations occur in the first 2–3 months after initiation of treatment; after this time, the incidence of increased hepatic transaminases falls to the levels observed in the placebo treatment group[31]. In addition, several cases of Churg–Strauss syndrome have been reported after initiation of treatment with both zafirlukast and montelukast[86,87], mostly, but not exclusively[88], in patients with severe asthma on oral corticosteroid therapy, in whom the oral corticosteroids were being reduced. This raises the possibility that the treatment with the antileukotrienes allowed a reduction in oral corticosteroid dosage, which unmasked previously unrecognized Churg–Strauss syndrome[89].

Role of antileukotriene drugs in asthma treatment

The studies described above were designed to evaluate the efficacy of antileukotrienes in asthma treatment, and used study designs required to obtain registration of the drugs to allow them to be available for prescription. These studies have demonstrated that antileukotrienes improve asthma control, but they were not designed to show how they fit in asthma management schemes.

There is no evidence to support the use of anti-leukotrienes in patients with very mild, intermittent asthma, in whom infrequent inhaled β_2-agonist use is adequate to control symptoms. In patients with mild persistent asthma, in whom another treatment is needed, the currently available consensus guidelines on asthma management suggest that regular treatment with inhaled corticosteroids or anti-leukotrienes or cromoglycate be considered[90–92]. If an antileukotriene is chosen as the next line of treatment, a therapeutic trial of 6–8 weeks will allow a decision to be made about the efficacy of the treatment. If the treatment is not effective, there is no currently available evidence that it should be continued beyond this time.

There is some preliminary evidence that the anti-leukotrienes may be even more effective in patients with more severe asthma. Their additive effect to the bronchodilation achieved even with high doses of inhaled β_2-agonists[35,36] suggest that they may have a place in the treatment of the severe bronchoconstriction associated with acute severe asthma. Also, clinical benefit has been demonstrated with their addition to the treatment of patients with poor asthma control, already taking high doses of inhaled corticosteroids[93]. In addition, there is evidence that antileukotrienes can reduce the doses of inhaled corticosteroids required for asthma control[94]. Finally, antileukotrienes have been demonstrated, in several different studies, to reduce the risks of acute severe asthma exacerbations[31,95,96].

More recent studies using antileukotrienes have focused on comparisons with inhaled corticosteroids, or their additive effects to inhaled corticosteroids. Several studies have directly compared leukotriene-receptor antagonists and a recent meta-analysis has evaluated these[97]. Ten studies met the inclusion criteria to be included in the meta-analysis, of which only a few are currently published as full papers. Most of the studies focused on subjects with mild-to-moderate persistent asthma and two studies included children. The duration of the blinded studies ranged from 6 to 12 weeks. The doses

of inhaled corticosteroids ranged from 250 to 400 µg of beclomethasone-equivalent per day and various antileukotrienes were tested. The conclusions of the meta-analysis were that the inhaled corticosteroid provided better lung function and quality of life, as well as reduced symptoms, night awakenings and need for rescue β_2-agonist. The rate of asthma exacerbations were similar when the antileukotrienes were compared to the inhaled corticosteroids.

The possible added benefit of adding leukotriene-receptor antagonists to inhaled corticosteroids has also been evaluated in two studies. The first compared the effects of adding pranlukast or placebo to half the usual dose of inhaled corticosteroids in patients with moderate-to-severe persistent asthma[98]. The study demonstrated loss of asthma control over 6 weeks in the placebo group, but maintained control in the group receiving the receptor antagonist. Another study[96] compared, after removal of inhaled corticosteroids, montelukast or placebo plus continuing inhaled corticosteroids, to montelukast or placebo tablet, plus inhaled placebo. The removal of the inhaled corticosteroid caused worsening of asthma control. The treatment with montelukast resulted in improved asthma control, while the combination of the two treatments provided the best control. Taken together, the studies suggest that leukotriene-receptor antagonists can provide additional benefits when added to inhaled corticosteroids. However, the effectiveness of this approach when compared to the addition of a long-acting inhaled β_2-agonist to an inhaled corticosteroid has not yet been studied.

The published studies also support two other indications for the use of anti-leukotrienes. One of these is in patients with aspirin-sensitive asthma, where these drugs are effective in blocking aspirin-induced asthmatic responses[64,65], which can be life threatening and are not prevented by any other currently available antiasthma treatment. Thus, antileukotrienes should be used in all patients with aspirin-induced asthma, together with other antiasthma treatment needed to control other manifestations of their asthma. The second indication is in patients taking regular inhaled β_2-agonists and who have exercise-induced bronchoconstriction. In these patients, the regular use of inhaled β_2-agonists will reduce the ability of inhaled β_2-agonists to protect against exercise-induced bronchoconstriction[56,57], and anti-leukotrienes have been shown to be effective, without loss of protection, in this setting[61].

These studies have helped to support the positioning of the leukotriene-receptor antagonists in the management of asthma in the most recent iteration of the Asthma Consensus Guidelines as drugs that are useful as additional therapy to inhaled corticosteroids or that should be considered to be the first-line therapy in patients who cannot or will not use the most effective therapy, which is inhaled corticosteroids.

Conclusions

Antileukotrienes are an important novel therapy for asthma. Currently available data indicated that inhibition of leukotriene synthesis or action has a salutary effect in the treatment of both induced and spontaneously occurring asthma. These results provide strong biological proof of the concept that leukotrienes are important mediators of the asthmatic response. The clinical trials of the anti-leukotrienes have demonstrated efficacy in patient populations with asthma severity ranging from mild persistent to severe persistent, and more recent studies have helped to provide guidelines for the optimal clinical use of antileukotrienes in asthma treatment.

REFERENCES

1 Feldberg W, Kellaway CH. Liberation of histamine and formation of lysocithin-like substances by cobra venom. *J Physiol* 1938; 94:13–20.

2 Kellaway CH, Trethewie ER. The liberation of a slow-reacting smooth muscle-stimulating substance in anaphylaxis. *Q J Exp Physiol* 1940; 30:121–145.

3 Brocklehurst WE. The release of histamine and formation of a slow reacting substance (SRS-A) during anaphylactic shock. *J Physiol* 1960; 151:416–435.

4 Drazen JM, Austen KF. Effects of intravenous administration of slow reacting substance of anaphylaxis, histamine, bradykinin, and prostaglandin F2 alpha on pulmonary mechanics in the guinea pig. *J Clin Invest* 1974; 53:1679–1685.

5 Samuelsson B. Leukotrienes: mediators of immediate hypersensitivity reactions and inflammation. *Science* 1983; 220:568–575.

6 Samuelsson B, Dahlen B, Lindgren JA, Rouzer CA, Serhan CN. Leukotrienes and lipoxins: structures, biosynthesis, and biological side effects. *Science* 1987; 237:1171–1176.

7 Dennis EA. Modification of the arachidonic acid cascade through phospholipase A2 dependent mechanisms. *Adv Prost Thromb Leuko Res* 1990; 20:217–223.

8 Ferguson JE, Hanley MR. The role of phospholipases and phospholipid-derived signals in cell activation. *Curr Opin Cell Biol* 1991; 3:206–212.

9 Matsumoto T, Funk CD, Radmark O, Hoog JO, Jornvall H, Samuelsson B. Molecular cloning and amino acid sequence of human 5-lipoxygenase. *Proc Natl Acad Sci USA* 1988; 85:26–30.

10 Rouzer CA, Rands E, Kargman S, Jones RE, Register RB, Dixon RA. Characterization of cloned human leukocyte 5-lipogenase expressed in mammalian cells. *J Biol Chem* 1988; 263:10135–10140.

11 Dixon RA, Diehl RE, Opas E et al. Requirement of a 5-lipoxygenase-activating protein for leukotriene synthesis. *Nature* 1990; 343:282-284.

12 Lam BK, Penrose JF, Freeman GJ, Austen KF. Expression cloning of a cDNA for human luekotriene C4 synthase, an integral membrane protein conjugating reduced glutathione to leukotriene A4. *Proc Natl Acad Sci USA* 1994; 91:7663–7667.

13 Lewis RA, Drazen JM, Austen KF, Clark DA, Corey EJ. Identification of the C^6- S-conjugate of leukotriene A with cysteine as a naturally occurring slow reacting substance of anaphylaxis (SRS-A). Importance of the 11-*cis*-geometry for biological activity. *Biochem Biophys Res Commun* 1980; 96:271–277.

14 Lam BK, Owen WFJr, Austen KF, Soberman RJ. The identification of a distinct export step following the biosynthesis of leukotriene C4 by human eosinophils. *J Biol Chem* 1989; 264:12885–12889.

15 Parker CW, Koch D, Huber MM, Falkenhein SF. Formation of the cysteinyl form of slow reacting substance (leukotriene E4) in human plasma. *Biochem Biophys Res Commun* 1980; 97:1038–1046.

16 Schleimer RP, MacGlashan DWJr, Peters SP, Pinckard RN, Adkinson NFJr, Lichtenstein LM. Characterization of inflammatory mediator release from purified human lung mast cells. *Am Rev Respir Dis* 1986; 133:614–617.

17 Weller PF, Lee CW, Foster DW, Corey EJ, Austen KF, Lewis RA. Generation and metabolism of 5-lipoxygenase pathway leukotrienes by human eosinophils: predominant production of leukotriene C4. *Proc Natl Acad Sci USA* 1983; 80:7626–7630.

18 Rankin JA, Hitchcock M, Merrill W, Bach MK, Brashler JR, Askenase PW. IgE- dependent release of leukotriene C4 from alveolar macrophages. *Nature* 1982; 297:329–331.

19 Carter GW, Young PR, Albert DH et al. 5-lipoxygenase inhibitory activity of zileuton. *J Pharmacol Exp Ther* 1991; 256:929–937.

20 Ford-Hutchinson AW. FLAP: a novel drug target for inhibiting the synthesis of leukotrienes. *TiPS* 1991; 12:68–70.

21 Coleman RA, Eglen RM, Jones RL et al. Prostanoid and leukotriene receptors: a progress report from the IUPHAR working parties on classification and nomenclature. *Prostaglandins related Compounds* 1996; 23:280–285.

22 Lynch KR, O'Neill GP, Liu Q et al. Characterization of the human cysteinyl leukotriene CysLT1 receptor. *Nature* 1999; 399:789–793.

23 Crooke ST, Mattern M, Sarau HM et al. The signal transduction system of the leukotriene D$_4$ receptor. *TiPS* 1989; 10:103- 107.

24 Mong S, Hoffman K, Wu HL, Crooke ST. Leukotriene-induced hydrolysis of inositol lipids in guinea pig lung: mechanism of signal transduction for leukotriene-D4 receptors. *Mol Pharmacol* 1987; 31:35–41.

25 Fleisch JH, Rinkema LE, Haisch KD et al. LY171883, 1,2-hydroxy-3-propyl-4-<4-(¹H-tetrazol-5-yl) butoxy>phenyl >ethanone, an orally active leukotriene D4 antagonist. *J Pharmacol Exp Ther* 1985; 233:148–157.

26 Hay DW, Muccitelli RM, Tucker SS et al. Pharmacologic profile of SK&F 104353: a novel, potent and selective pertidoleukotriene receptor antagonist in guinea pig and human airways. *J Pharmacol Exp Ther* 1987; 243:474–481.

27 Jones TR, Zamboni R, Belley M et al. Pharmacology of L-660,711 (MK-571): a novel potent and selective leukotriene D4 receptor antagonist. *Can J Physiol Pharmacol* 1989; 67:17–28.

28 O'Donnell M, Crowley HJ, Yaremko B, Oneil N, Welton AF. Pharmacologic actions of RO 24–59113, a novel antagonist of leukotriene-D(4). *J Pharmacol Exp Ther* 1991; 259:751–759.

29 Snyder DW, Giles RE, Keith RA, Yee YK, Krell RD. In vitro pharmacology of ICI 198,615; a novel, potent and selective peptide leukotriene antagonist. *J Pharmacol Exp Ther* 1987; 243:548–556.

30 Heise CE, O'Dowd BF, Figueroa DJ et al. Characterization of the human cysteinyl leukotriene 2 receptor. *J Biol Chem* 2000; 275:30531–20536.

31 Israel E, Cohn J, Dube L, Drazen JM. Effects of treatment with zileuton, a 5-lipoxygenase inhibitor, in patients with asthma. *J Am Med* 1996; 275:931–936.

32 Spector SL, Glass M, Birmingham BK et al. Effects of 6 weeks of therapy with oral doses of ICI 204,219 a leukotriene D4 receptor antagonist, in subjects with bronchial asthma. *Am J Respir Crit Care Med* 1994; 150:618–623.

33 Malmstrom K, Rodriguez Gomez G, Guerra J et al. Oral montelukast, inhaled beclomethasone, and placebo for chronic asthma. A randomized, controlled trial. *Ann Intern Med* 1999; 130:487–495.

34 Barnes NC, Pujet JC. Pranlukast, a novel leukotriene receptor antagonist: results of the first European, placebo controlled, multicentre clinical study in asthma. *Thorax* 1997; 52:523–527.

35 Hui KP, Barnes NC. Lung function improvement in asthma with a cysteinyl-leukotriene receptor antagonist. *Lancet* 1991; 337:1062–1063.

36 Gaddy JN, Margolskee DJ, Bush RK, Williams VC, Busse WW. Bronchodilation with a potent and selective leukotriene D4 (LTD4) antagonist (MK-571) in patients with asthma. *Am Rev Respir Dis* 1992; 146:358–363.

37 Israel E, Rubin P, Kemp JP et al. The effect of inhibition of 5-lipoxygenase by zileuton in mild- to-moderate asthma. *Ann Intern Med* 1993; 119:1059–1066.

38 Smith LJ, Greenberger PA, Patterson R, Krell RD, Bernstein PR. The effect of inhaled leukotriene D4 in humans. *Am Rev Respir Dis* 1985; 131:368–372.

39 Manning PJ, O'Byrne PM. The effects of inhaled leukotriene D4 on histamine airway responsiveness in asthmatic subjects. *Am Rev Respir Dis* 145, 287. 1992.

40 Fischer AR, McFadden CA, Frantz R et al. Effect of chronic 5-lipoxygenase inhibition on airway hyperresponsiveness in asthmatic subjects. *J Appl Physiol* 1995; 152:1203–1207.

41 Kirby JG, Hargreave FE, Gleich GJ, O'Byrne PM. Bronchoalveolar cell profiles of asthmatic and nonasthmatic subjects. *Am Rev Respir Dis* 1987; 136:379–383.

42 Beasley R, Roche WR, Roberts JA, Holgate ST. Cellular events in the bronchi in mild asthma and after bronchial provocation. *Am Rev Respir Dis* 1989; 139:806–817.

43 Sampson AP, Castling DP, Green CP, Price JF. Persistent increase in plasma and urinary leukotrienes after acute asthma. *Arch Dis Child* 1995; 73:221–225.

44 Laitinen LA, Laitinen A, Haahtela T, Vikka V, Spur BW, Lee

TH. Leukotriene E4 and granulocytic infiltration into asthmatics' airways. *Lancet* 1993; 341:989–990.

45 Spada CS, Nieves AL, Krauss AH, Woodward DF. Comparison of leukotriene B4 and D4 effects on human eosinophil and neutrophil motility in vitro. *J Leukoc Biol* 1994; 55:183–191.

46 Wenzel SE, Trudeau JB, Kaminsky DA, Cohn J, Martin RJ, Westcott JY. Effect of 5-lipoxygenase inhibition on bronchoconstriction and airway inflammation in nocturnal asthma. *Am J Respir Crit Care Med* 1995; 152:897–905.

47 Pizzichini E, Leff JA, Reiss T et al. Montelukast reduces airway eosinophilic inflammation in asthma: a randomized, controlled trial. *Eur Resp J* 1999; 14:12–18.

48 Anderson SD. Exercise-induced asthma. The State of the Art. *Am Rev Respir Dis* 1985; 87S:191–195.

49 Manning PJ, Watson RM, Margolskee DJ, Williams VC, Schwartz JI, O'Byrne PM. Inhibition of exercise-induced bronchoconstriction by MK-571, a potent leukotriene D4-receptor antagonist. *N Engl J Med* 1990; 323:1736–1739.

50 Leff JA, Busse WW, Pearlman DS et al. Montelukast, a leukotriene-receptor antagonist, for the treatment of mild asthma and exercise-induced bronchoconstriction. *N Engl J Med* 1998; 339:147–152.

51 Finnerty JP, Wood-Baker R, Thomson H, Holgate ST. Role of leukotrienes in exercise-induced asthma. Inhibitory effect of ICI 204219, a potent leukotriene D4 receptor antagonist. *Am Rev Respir Dis* 1992; 145:746–749.

52 Makker HK, Lau LC, Thomson HW, Binks SM, Holgate ST. The protective effect of inhaled leukotriene D4 receptor antagonist ICI 204,219 against exercise-induced asthma. *Am Rev Respir Dis* 1993; 147:1413–1418.

53 Adelroth E, Inman MD, Summers E, Pace D, Modi M, O'Byrne PM. Prolonged protection against exercise-induced bronchoconstriction by the leukotriene D4-receptor antagonist Cinalukast. *J Allergy Clin Immunol* 1997; 99:210–215.

54 Israel E, Dermarkarian R, Rosenberg M et al. The effects of a 5-lipoxygenase inhibitor on asthma induced by cold, dry air. *N Engl J Med* 1990; 323:1740–1744.

55 McFadden ER, Jr., Gilbert IA. Exercise-induced asthma. *N Engl J Med* 1994; 330:1362–1367.

56 Inman MD, O'Byrne PM. The effect of regular inhaled albuterol on exercise-induced bronchoconstriction. *Am J Respir Crit Care Med* 1996; 153:65–69.

57 Ramage L, Lipworth BJ, Ingram CG, Cree IA, Dhillon DP. Reduced protection against exercise induced bronchoconstriction after chronic dosing with salmeterol. *Respir Med* 1994; 88:363–368.

58 Ellis EF. Inhibition of exercise-induced asthma by theophylline. *J Allergy Clin Immunol* 1984; 73:690–692.

59 Fuglsang G, Hertz B, Holm EB. No protection by oral terbutaline against exercise-induced asthma in children: a dose–response study. *Eur Respir J* 1993; 6:527–530.

60 Robuschi M, Riva E, Fuccella LM et al. Prevention of exercise-induced bronchoconstriction by a new leukotriene antagonist (SK&F 104353). A double-blind study versus disodium cromoglycate and placebo. *Am Rev Respir Dis* 1992; 145:1285–1288.

61 Coreno A, Skowronski M, Kotaru C, McFadden ER, Jr. Comparative effects of long-acting beta2-agonists, leukotriene receptor antagonists, and a 5-lipoxygenase inhibitor on exercise-induced asthma. *J Allergy Clin Immunol* 2000; 106(3):500–506.

62 Villaran C, O'Neill SJ, Helbling A et al. Montelukast versus salmeterol in patients with asthma and exercise-induced bronchoconstriction. Montelukast/Salmeterol Exercise Study Group. *J Allergy Clin Immunol* 1999; 104(3 Pt 1):547–553.

63 Christie L, Lee TH. The effects of SKF104353 on aspirin induced asthma. *Am Rev Respir Dis* 1991; 144:957–958.

64 Dahlen B, Kumlin M, Margolskee DJ et al. The leukotriene-receptor antagonist MK-0679 blocks airway obstruction induced by inhaled lysine-aspirin in aspirin-sensitive asthmatics. *Eur Respir J* 1993; 48:1018–1026.

65 Israel E, Fischer AR, Rosenburg MA et al. The pivotal role of 5-lipoxygenase products in the reaction of aspirin-sensitive asthmatics to aspirin. *Am Rev Respir Dis* 1993; 148:1447–1451.

66 Dahlen B, Margolskee DJ, Zetterstrom O, Dahlen SE. Effect of the leukotriene receptor antagonist MK-0679 on baseline pulmonary function in aspirin-sensitive asthmatic subjects. *Thorax* 1993; 48:1205–1210.

67 Yamamoto H, Nagata M, Kuramitsu K et al. Inhibition of analgesic-induced asthma by leukotriene receptor antagonist ONO-1078. *Am J Respir Crit Care Med* 1994; 150(1):254–257.

68 O'Byrne PM, Dolovich J, Hargreave FE. Late asthmatic responses. *Am Rev Respir Dis* 1987; 136:740–751.

69 Cartier A, Thomson NC, Frith PA, Roberts R, Hargreave FE. Allergen-induced increase in bronchial responsiveness to histamine: relationship to the late asthmatic response and change in airway caliber. *J Allergy Clin Immunol* 1982; 70:170–177.

70 Taylor GW, Black P, Turner N et al. Urinary leukotriene E4 after antigen challenge and in acute asthma and allergic rhinitis. *Lancet* 1989; i:585–587.

71 Manning PJ, Rokach J, Malo JL et al. Urinary leukotriene E4 levels during early and late asthmatic responses. *J Allergy Clin Immunol* 1990; 86:211–220.

72 Taylor IK, O'Shaughnessy KM, Fuller RW, Dollery CT. Effect of a cysteinylleukotriene receptor antagonist, ICI 204–219

on allergen-induced bronchoconstriction and airway hyperactivity in atopic subjects. *Lancet* 1991; 337:690–694.

73 Rasmussen JB, Erikson L-O, Margolskee DJ, Tagari P, Williams VC, Andersson K-E. Leukotriene D4 receptor blockade inhibits the immediate and late bronchoconstrictor responses to inhaled antigen in patients with asthma. *J Allergy Clin Immunol* 1992; 90:193–201.

74 Hamilton AL, Faiferman I, Stober P, Watson RM, O'Byrne PM. Pranlukast, a leukotriene receptor antagonist, attenuates allergen-induced early and late phase bronchoconstriction and airway hyperresponsiveness in asthmatic subjects. *J Allergy Clin Immunol* 1998; 102:177–183.

75 Friedman BS, Bel EH, Buntinx A et al. Oral leukotriene inhibitor (MK-886) blocks allergen-induced airway responses. *Am Rev Respir Dis* 1993; 147:839–844.

76 Diamant Z, Timmers MC, van der Veen H et al. The effect of MK-0591, a novel 5-lipoxygenase activating protein inhibitor, on leukotriene biosynthesis and allergen-induced airway responses in asthmatic subjects in vivo. *J Allergy Clin Immunol* 1995; 95:42–51.

77 Hamilton AL, Watson RM, Wyile G, O'Byrne PM. A 5-lipoxygenase activating protein antagonist, Bay x 1005, attenuates both early and late phase allergen-induced bronchoconstriction in asthmatic subjects. *Thorax* 1997; 52:348–354.

78 Chung KF, Aizawa H, Leikauf GD, Ueki IF, Evans TW, Nadel JA. Airway hyperresponsiveness induced by platelet-activating factor: role of thromboxane generation. *J Pharmacol Exp Therap* 1986; 236:580–584.

79 Gauvreau GM, Watson RM, O'Byrne PM. Kinetics of allergen-induced airway eosinophilic cytokine production and airway inflammation. *Am J Respir Crit Care Med* 1999; 160:640–647.

80 Gauvreau GM, Lee LM, Watson RM, Irani AM, Schwartz LB, O'Byrne PM. Increased numbers of both airway basophils and mast cells in sputum after allergen inhalation challenge in atopic asthmatics. *Am J Respir Crit Care Med* 2000; 161:1473–1478.

81 Cloud ML, Enas GC, Kemp J et al. A specific LTD4/LTE4-receptor antagonist improves pulmonary function in patients with mild, chronic asthma. *Am Rev Respir Dis* 1989; 140:1336–1339.

82 Reiss TF, Altman LC, Chervinsky P et al. Effect of montelukast (MK- 0476), a new potent cysteinyl leukotriene (LTD4) receptor antagonist, in patients with chronic asthma. *J Allergy Clin Immunol* 1996; 98:528–534.

83 Liu MC, Dube L, Lancaster J, and the Zileuton Study Group. Acute and chronic effects of a 5-lipoxygenase inhibitor in asthma: a 6 month randomized multicentre trial. *J Allergy Clin Immunol* 1996; 98:859–871.

84 Calhoun WJ. Summary of clinical trials with zafirlukast. *Am J Respir Crit Care Med* 1998; 157(6 Pt 2):S238-S245.

85 Blake KV. Montelukast: data from clinical trials in the management of asthma. *Ann Pharmacother* 1999; 33(12):1299–1314.

86 Wechsler ME, Garpestad E, Flier SR et al. Pulmonary infiltrates, eosinophils, and cardiomyopathy following corticosteroid withdrawal in patients with asthma receiving zafirlukast. *J Am Med Assoc* 1998; 276:455–457.

87 Wechsler ME, Finn D, Gunawardena D et al. Churg–Strauss syndrome in patients receiving montelukast as treatment for asthma. *Chest* 2000; 117(3):708–713.

88 Green RL, Vayonis AG. Churg-Strauss syndrome after zafirlukast in two patients not receiving systemic steroid treatment. *Med J Aust* 1999; 353(9154):725–726.

89 Wechsler ME, Pauwels R, Drazen JM. Leukotriene modifiers and Churg-Strauss syndrome: adverse effect or response to corticosteroid withdrawal? *Drug Saf* 1999; 21(4):241–251.

90 Sheffer AL, Bartal M, Bousquet J et.al. Global strategy for asthma management and prevention. *Nat Inst Health* 1995; 95–3659:70–114.

91 Von Mutius E. Presentation of new GINA guidelines for paediatrics. The Global Initiative on Asthma. *Clin Exp Allergy* 2000; 30 Suppl 1:6–10.

92 Bousquet J. Global initiative for asthma (GINA) and its objectives. *Clin Exp Allergy* 2000; 30 Suppl 1:2–5.

93 Janssen LJ, Sims SM. Ca^{2+}-dependent Cl^- current in canine tracheal smooth muscle cells. *Am J Physiol* 1995; 269:C163-C169.

94 Lofdahl C-G, Reiss T, Leff JA et al. Randomized, placebo controlled trial of effect of a leukotriene receptor antagonist, montelukast, on tapering inhaled corticosteroids in asthmatic patients. *Br Med J* 1999; 319:87–90.

95 Barnes NC, Miller CJ. Effect of leukotriene receptor antagonist therapy on the risk of asthma exacerbations in patients with mild to moderate asthma: an integrated analysis of zafirlukast trials. *Thorax* 2000; 55(6):478–483.

96 Laviolette M, Malmstrom K, Lu S et al. Montelukast added to inhaled beclomethasone in treatment of asthma. *Am J Respir Crit Care Med* 1999; 160:1862–1866.

97 Ducharme FM, Hicks GC. Anti-leukotriene agents compared to inhaled corticosteroids in the management of recurrent and/or chronic asthma. *Cochrane Database Syst Rev* 3[CD 002314]. 2000.

98 Tamaoki J, Kondo M, Sakai N et al. Leukotriene antagonist prevents exacerbations of asthma during reduction of high-dose inhaled corticosteroid. *Am J Respir Crit Care Med* 1997; 155:1235–1240.

99 O'Byrne PM, Israel E, Drazen JM. Anti-leukotrienes in the treatment of asthma. *Ann Inter Med* 1997; 127:427–480.

7

Theophylline and selective phosphodiesterase inhibitors in the treatment of respiratory disease

Neil A. Jones, Domenico Spina[1] and Clive P. Page

The Sackler Institute of Pulmonary Pharmacology, Pharmacology and Therapeutics Division, GKT School of Biomedical Sciences, Hodgkin Building, Guy's Campus, London, UK

[1] Department of Respiratory Medicine and Allergy, GKT School of Medicine, King's College London, UK

Introduction

At least 11 families of PDE including PDE1–7[1] and PDE8–11[2] are known to exist based upon a variety of criteria including substrate specificity, inhibitor potency, enzyme kinetics and amino acid sequence. These enzymes are distributed widely throughout the body, differentially expressed in cells and localized to different compartments within cells. The functional significance of the subcellular localization of PDEs is not completely understood, although there is a considerable body of evidence to suggest that the expression of PDE in cellular domains can tightly regulate the levels of cyclic nucleotides in the vicinity of effector proteins and is therefore implicated in the regulation of cell function[3].

Classification of phosphodiesterase enzymes

PDE enzymes function by hydrolysing the phosphodiester bond of the second messenger molecules cyclic 3′,5′-adenosine monophosphate (cAMP) and cyclic 3′,5′-guanosine monophosphate (cGMP). This converts cAMP and cGMP to their inactive 5′-mononucleotides; adenosine monophosphate (AMP) and guanosine monophosphate (GMP). These products are incapable of activating specific cyclic nucleotide-dependent protein kinase cascades.

The PDE enzyme family consists of a growing number of genetically heterologous isoenzymes (Table 7.1).

Regarding substrate affinities, PDE4 and PDE7 are highly selective for cAMP. Although PDE3 hydrolyses cAMP and cGMP with equal affinity (K_m:0.1–0.5 μM), its V_{max} ('Velocity' of action) for cAMP is five-fold greater than for cGMP. Functionally, then, PDE3 favours cAMP. Conversely, cGMP is the preferred substrate for PDE5 and PDE6, whereas PDE1 and PDE2 hydrolyse either cyclic nucleotide. Adding further complexity to the functional role taken by various PDEs in intact tissues is the fact that several are subject to short-term allosteric regulation by endogenous activators or inhibitors. For example, PDE1 is allosterically activated by Ca^{2+}/calmodulin[4].

Each of the families of PDE isoenzymes is populated by at least one, and as many as four, distinct gene products, thus isoenzymes are further subdivided into subtypes, which have a high percentage genetic homology (70–90%). Subtypes may also undergo further post-translational modification and this can result in a large number of splice variants. The result of this is an array of enzymes with distinct kinetic characteristics, regulatory properties and subcellular distributions, allowing specific drug design and targeting of specific isoenzymes or subtypes in affected cells or tissues. Isoenzyme-selective inhibitors are available for most PDE families. Generally, these compounds are at least 30-fold selective for the PDE against which they are directed. Most are substrate site directed competitive inhibitors, but a few act at allosteric sites[5].

Table 7.1. Characteristics and properties of PDE isoenzymes

Family	Specific property	$K_m(\mu M)$cAMP	$K_m(\mu M)$cGMP
1	Ca2$^+$/calmodulin-stimulated	1–30	3
2	cGMP-stimulated	50	50
3	cGMP-inhibited	0.2	0.3
4	cAMP-specific	4	>100.0
5	cGMP-specific	150	1
6	Photoreceptor	60	>100
7	High affinity cAMP-specific	0.2	>100
8	High affinity cAMP-specific	0.055	124
9	High affinity cGMP-specific	230	0.17
10	Unknown	0.05	3
11	Unknown	1.04	0.52

Theophylline in the treatment of respiratory disease

The archetypal non-selective PDE inhibitor theophylline has now been in clinical use for more than a century, although it is only during the last 50 years that this drug has been in regular use for the treatment of respiratory diseases. In 1886, Henry Hyde Salter described the efficacious use of strong coffee taken on an empty stomach as a treatment for asthma[6]. The principal agent in coffee producing the bronchodilatory effect observed was the methylxanthine caffeine. Theophylline has a similar chemical structure to caffeine and was first used in the treatment of asthma as early as 1922, when it was found to be effective in the treatment of three asthmatic subjects[7]. In 1937, theophylline was administered i.v. for the treatment of acute asthma and in 1940 theophylline was first used orally in combination with ephedrine. There are now many studies in the literature describing the effects of theophylline in the treatment of both asthma[8] and COPD[9]. Theophylline is presently used in various slow-release formulations to overcome rapid metabolism and maintain constant plasma levels. However, over the last decade, the number of prescriptions being written for theophylline has declined as newer medications have been introduced for the treatment of respiratory disease. This decline has mainly come about due to concerns raised over the narrow therapeutic window of theophylline, which has typically been classified as being 10–20 μg/ml in plasma[8].

Whilst theophylline has traditionally been classified as a bronchodilator drug, it is becoming increasingly apparent that this drug has a range of other pharmacological effects of potential therapeutic value in the treatment of respiratory diseases[10], that occur independently of the bronchodilator actions, including anti-inflammatory and immunomodulatory actions[11,12], and increased respiratory drive[9]. These effects often occur at plasma levels below 10 μg/ml suggesting that lower levels of theophylline than have previously been used to obtain bronchodilation may be of benefit in the treatment of lung diseases, thus reducing the side effect profile and improving the safety margin of this drug. These actions have caused the therapeutic window to be reduced to 5–15 μg/ml in plasma in many countries.

A number of studies have reported that intravenous administration of theophylline or the related xanthine enprophylline prior to allergen challenge can inhibit the development of the late asthmatic response without any significant effect on the acute bronchoconstrictor response[11,13–15] and associated bronchial hyperresponsiveness to methacholine[16]. Thus, neither functional antagonism of airway smooth muscle shortening nor inhibition of mast cell degranulation accounted for the attenuated late asthmatic response by theophylline and enprofylline, although, in allergic rhinitis, 1 week's treatment with theophylline reduced histamine release during pollen exposure[17], which indicated that theophylline inhibited mast cell and basophil degranulation in this disorder or reduced the number of mast cells as has been shown with glucocorticosteroids.

Individuals exposed for long periods of time to certain industrial chemicals develop asthma-like symptoms that can be duplicated in the clinical laboratory following aerosol challenge with the inciting agent. Thus, susceptible individuals demonstrate acute bronchospasm, late asthmatic responses and bronchial hyperresponsiveness following inhalation of toluene di-isocyanate (TDI)[18]. The inflammatory nature of this response has been confirmed by its sensitivity to inhibition by the glucocorticosteroid, beclomethasone. Theophylline partially modified the acute response and attenuated the late asthmatic response induced by TDI but was ineffective against bronchial hyperresponsiveness[14,18]. This latter finding is consistent with the inability of theophylline to modulate allergen-induced bronchial hyperresponsiveness in asthmatics[11,16].

The late asthmatic response to allergen is known to be accompanied by an influx of inflammatory cells into the airways[19] and this allergen-induced infiltration of activated eosinophils into the airways (assessed as the total number of eosinophils and as an increase in the number of $EG_2 +$ eosinophils in biopsies) was also reduced significantly by 6 weeks of treatment with theophylline[20], an effect that occurred at plasma levels well below the 10–20 μg/ml plasma levels required for bronchodilation (mean plasma levels of 6.7 μg/ml). More recent clinical studies have confirmed these anti-inflammatory properties of theophylline in patients with asthma. In two randomized, placebo controlled studies[11,15], the effect of theophylline or placebo was investigated on various inflammatory indices following once and twice daily treatment for 1 and 5 weeks, respectively. The late asthmatic response was reduced in those subjects treated with theophylline after 5 weeks[11] despite a mean plasma concentration of only 7.8 μg/ml. The lack of effect of theophylline

on the acute response is presumably due to the low plasma levels in these subjects. Inhibition of the late asthmatic response therefore, was unlikely to be due to functional antagonism of airway smooth muscle shortening or inhibition of mast cell degranulation[11]. Similarly, various surrogate markers of nasal inflammation in response to allergen challenge including the late phase response and the accumulation/activation of eosinophils in the nose were significantly attenuated in allergic rhinitis subjects following chronic treatment with theophylline[21], again consistent with an anti-inflammatory property of this drug.

The mechanism whereby theophylline inhibits the recruitment of activated eosinophils into the airways is not known, but several mechanisms have been put forward to explain this observation. The first mechanism relates to an immunomodulatory action of theophylline whereby it is thought that the inhibitory effect of theophylline may be a consequence of a restoration of T-suppressor cell function since it has long been recognized that theophylline can increase T-suppressor cell function[22–24,25,26] and impair graft rejection in vitro[27] and in vivo[28]. Individuals who do not develop a late asthmatic response have been shown to recruit a greater proportion of CD8 + (suppressor) than CD4 + (helper) T-lymphocytes in BAL fluid[29]. It is recognized that T-lymphocytes play a central role in the pathogenesis of allergic asthma, in particular the orchestration of eosinophil migration into the airways, via the release of cytokines such as IL-5[30]. Regular treatment with theophylline has also been reported to inhibit allergen-induced recruitment of T-lymphocytes into the airway[31] and to increase the number of suppressor CD8 cells in peripheral blood[11,23,27]. Furthermore, withdrawal of theophylline from asthmatics has been shown to cause a significant increase in asthma symptoms[12,32], which was associated with an increase in T-lymphocytes in the airways[12], an immunomodulatory effect that again occurred at plasma levels below 10 μg/ml. Regular treatment with theophylline has also been reported to reduce the number of inflammatory cells expressing IL-4 in the airway[33] and to induce the production of IL-10 from peripheral blood mononuclear cells obtained from asthmatics[34], an observation of considerable interest as IL-10 can shorten eosinophil survival[35] and induce tolerance in T-cells[36].

Another suggested mechanism of action of theophylline that occurs at clinically relevant concentrations is the ability of theophylline to alter eosinophil survival. A number of cytokines, including IL-5 have been shown to prolong eosinophil survival[37]. Theophylline has been shown to inhibit IL-5-mediated survival of human eosinophils and to accelerate apoptosis, again at concentrations below 10 μg/ml[38]. Analysis of bronchial biopsies taken from mild asthmatics treated with low dose theophylline over 6 weeks revealed a significant reduction in EG2$^+$ staining cells (activated eosinophils) and total number of eosinophils[20], which may be a consequence of the ability of theophylline to induce apoptosis of human eosinophils in this way[38,39]. Similarly, a reduction in CD3$^+$T lymphocytes and expression of various activation markers on CD4$^+$T lymphocytes including HLA-DR and VLA-1 was observed in BAL fluid[31]. Furthermore, a reduction in CD4$^+$, CD8$^+$T-lymphocytes and IL-4 and IL-5 containing cells was observed in bronchial biopsies from asthmatics who were taking theophylline over a 6-week period[33], while a fall in circulating levels of Th2 cytokines, IL-4 and IL-5, was observed after a single low dose of theophylline[40].

Many of the biological effects of theophylline have been suggested to be via an inhibitory effect on the phosphodiesterase (PDE) family of enzymes[41,42]. However, the effect of theophylline on apoptosis of eosinophils was not shared by the selective PDE4 inhibitor rolipram suggesting that this anti-inflammatory effect of theophylline may not be via inhibition of PDE4[38]. This observation supports other recent work carried out in mononuclear cells obtained from asthmatics where theophylline was able to inhibit mononuclear cell proliferation via mechanisms distinct from selective PDE4 inhibitors[43] and recent data with the related xanthine pentoxyphylline, showing that this drug can inhibit proliferation of fibroblasts via a mechanism unrelated to cAMP generation[44].

Another prominent action of theophylline is the ability of this drug to antagonize adenosine receptors[45]. However, for more than a decade this suggestion was questioned as the related drug enprophylline had similar effects to theophylline clinically[13], yet was claimed to lack adenosine receptor antagonism[45]. However, studies have now reported that enprophylline can act as a selective A$_{2B}$ receptor antagonist on human mast cells[46], a property shared by theophylline, which has been suggested to be of potential importance for the clinical activities of theophylline[47]. However, other studies have shown that whilst asthmatics are very sensitive to inhaled adenosine[48], an effect that is blocked by theophylline[49,50], there is no evidence to date that this effect is mediated via activation of A$_{2B}$ receptors; rather there is evidence from experimental animals that it is the A$_1$ receptor that is upregulated as a result of allergic sensitization[51,52], an observation supported by the study of Nyce and Metzger[53] that an antisense oligonucleutide to A$_1$ receptors blocks allergen-reduced eosinophilia and allergen-induced bronchial hyperresponsiveness in allergic rabbits. In more recent studies, it has been suggested that theophylline has an immunomodulatory effect on neutrophil apoptosis through A$_{2A}$ receptor antagonism at relevant therapeutic concentrations[54]. In contrast to this, inhibition by theophylline of complement C5a-induced degranulation of human eosinophils was significantly reversed by the selective A$_3$ antagonist MRS 1220, but not A$_1$ or A$_2$ antagonists, suggesting that therapeutic concentrations of theophylline inhibit human eosinophil degranulation by acting as an A$_3$ agonist[55]. Conversely, a study investigating the antiproliferative effects of theophylline on human peripheral blood mixed mononuclear cells (HPBMC) in vitro showed that theophylline was only capable of reducing proliferation at higher concentrations than are required to significantly antagonize A$_{2B}$ receptors[56]. This study also demonstrated that exogenous or endogenous adenosine has little impact on HPBMC proliferation, as neither adenosine receptor agonists, antagonists nor adenosine deaminase had a significant effect on the proliferation of HPBMC from either healthy or asthmatic subjects[56]. While it remains plausible that adenosine may be involved in a number of anti-inflammatory functions, which can also be modulated by theophylline, results such as these suggest the anti-inflammatory effects of theophylline to be mediated through mechanisms other than adenosine antagonism.

Recently regular theophylline treatment has been demonstrated to produce anti-inflammatory activity in patients having natural exacerbations of their asthma, in the form of nocturnal asthma. Theophylline treatment significantly improved the overnight deterioration in lung function associated with nocturnal asthma compared with placebo treatment[57], a finding consistent with previous studies using theophylline for the treatment of asthma[58]. Theophylline also inhibited the ability of neutrophils to migrate into the airways of patients undergoing nocturnal attacks of asthma[57], associated with a reduction in the ability of PMNs to release LTB4. This work not only extends the anti-inflammatory actions of theophylline, but also supports earlier work that regular treatment with theophylline can reduce PMN activation[59,60] in addition to the actions of theophylline on eosinophils and lymphocytes discussed above. Theophylline treatment has also been reported to reduce the steepness of methacholine dose-response curves in asthmatics vs. placebo treatment[61,62], a change also seen with glucocorticosteroids[63], but not with β_2 agonists[64], which actually steepen the curve.

The clinical relevance of these anti-inflammatory actions of theophylline is now being evaluated and a number of recent clinical studies lend weight to the suggestion that such activities may offer clinical benefit. Two separate studies have demonstrated that, in asthmatics who were poorly controlled on existing glucocorticosteroid therapy, a significant improvement in a number of clinical outcomes, including peak expiratory flow, FEV1, symptom scores and reduced rescue medication, was observed when patients were taking theophylline together with low dose glucocorticosteroid compared with high dose glucocorticosteroid treatment[65,66]. In both studies, the plasma levels of theophylline measured were unlikely to be sufficient to induce bronchodilation (median 7.8 μg/ml[65] and mean 10.1 μg/ml[66]. In other studies, withdrawing theophylline from asthmatics who were taking glucocorticosteroids resulted in a significant deterioration of their disease[12,32] together with a concomitant rise in the number of CD4[+] and CD8[+] T-lymphocytes in bronchial biopsies[12]. These results suggest that theophylline may offer additional benefit to glucocorticosteroids, as has been previously suggested from other clinical studies by the use of different types of protocol[12,66,67].

Other studies in pediatric asthma have shown that there is a clear effect of theophylline in the treatment of asthma that is comparable to low doses of glucocorticosteroids[68]. This observation is of particular interest given that theophylline is an orally active drug and has been shown to have a better compliance rate than inhaled medications[69], which is particularly relevant to the treatment of asthmatic children. Given the low cost of theophylline, relative to other antiasthma medications[70], the fact that it is still one of the few drugs available for use orally in the treatment of this common disease and the growing body of evidence suggesting that theophylline has anti-inflammatory and immunomodulatory at lower than conventional plasma levels, it may be timely to reconsider the wider use of theophylline in the overall management of asthma[71].

Characteristic features of asthma and COPD

The incidence of respiratory diseases like asthma and COPD continue to increase despite the availability of current treatment modalities and there is therefore a need to improve our understanding of the pathophysiology of these diseases for the development of novel therapeutic agents. While the exact causes of asthma and COPD are not completely understood it is clear that both diseases are characterized by inflammation of the airways and a decline in respiratory function. In asthma, a number of inflammatory cells are thought to contribute toward the pathogenesis of this disease, including eosinophils[72] and CD4+T-lymphocytes[73], while it is thought that CD8 + lymphocytes[74] and neutrophils[75] play an important role in COPD. Another important feature of these diseases is the presence of airway wall remodelling and there is evidence of hyperplasia/hypertrophy of airway smooth muscle, increased collagen deposition beneath the basement membrane, increased mucus production, angiogenesis and alterations in extracellular matrix in asthma[76]. In COPD, there is evidence of mucus gland hyperplasia, increased bronchiolar smooth muscle hypertrophy, fibrosis of the small airways and, in the case of emphysema, destruction of alveolar tissue[77]. The mainstay of treatment for asthma includes bronchodilators like β_2-adrenoceptor agonists and glucocorticosteroids while for COPD, ipratropium bromide and β_2-adrenoceptor agonists are used. Reducing the inflammatory response in the airways is thought to be critical in reversing many of the changes seen in these airway diseases.

PDE expression in allergic disease

Allergy

It had long been recognized that the ability of lymphocytes to raise levels of intracellular cyclic AMP is impaired in mild, severe atopic eczema[78,79] and atopic dermatitis[80,81]. This finding was all the more significant since, unlike asthma, none of the subjects were taking beta-adrenoceptor agonist medication. Therefore, tachyphylaxis of beta-adrenoceptors is not an issue and not a confounding factor in this disease. The increased level of cAMP in mononuclear cells from patients with atopic dermatitis was a consequence of increased cAMP PDE activity as assessed biochemically[81]. The exact splice variant responsible for this activity remains to be established, although, evidence was provided of a putative monocyte derived PDE in atopic dermatitis that had increased cAMP PDE catalytic activity and was Ca^{+2}/calmodulin and Ro201724 sensitive[82].

However, such changes in cAMP PDE activity have not been observed in all studies in cells from patients with atopic dermatitis[83] and it is unclear whether differences in methodology and/or patient selection account for this discrepancy. It has been proposed that this alteration in PDE activity is responsible for the pathogenesis of this disease since functional consequences of increased cAMP PDE activity in atopic dermatitis include increased IgE production by B-lymphocytes, increased histamine and LTC_4 release from basophils, increased IL-4 and reduced IFNγ and IL-10 release by mononuclear cells; physiological responses that can be inhibited by PDE4 inhibitors[84].

An interesting feature of the altered cAMP PDE activity in atopic dermatitis is increased susceptibility of the isoenzyme to inhibition by PDE4 inhibitors. This is reflected by increased inhibitor potency against cAMP catalytic activity[82,85,86] and increased inhibitor potency against the proliferation of mononuclear cells[87]. Interestingly, the anti-proliferative effect of theophylline was not altered in atopic dermatitis. The molecular mechanism(s) responsible for the increased PDE catalytic activity and increased sensitivity to PDE4 inhibitors in atopic dermatitis remain to be established, but conformational changes in PDE4 protein[88], phosphorylation of PDE4[89] and/or expression of a splice variant/novel PDE4[82] could explain such a phenomenon.

Few studies have investigated the effect of methylxanthines in atopic dermatitis. Mononuclear cells from atopic dermatitis patients have increased cAMP PDE activity that is more susceptible to PDE4 inhibitors and is reflected by increased PDE4 inhibitor potency[85]. However, cAMP PDE activity in mononuclear cells was restored to normal values in atopic dermatitis subjects who were taking theophylline to control their asthma[85]. An interpretation of this finding is that prolonged treatment with theophylline altered the activity of cAMP PDE activity to control values. This could be attributed to the anti-inflammatory effect of theophylline resulting in a reduction in the release of inflammatory mediators and cytokines known to increase the activity and expression of PDE4. In a double blind study, the PDE4 inhibitor Ro201724 was shown to improve psoriatic lesions[90] and daily topical treatment with CP80633 on one arm improved clinical scores (erythrema, induration and excoriation) compared with the untreated arm[86] and indicated the potential use of PDE4 inhibitors in the treatment of atopic dermatitis.

Asthma

Despite our understanding of the mechanisms that can alter PDE4 activity, there is a paucity of data concerning whether there is any alteration in the function or expression of PDEs in airway diseases like asthma. The ability of lymphocytes to raise intracellular cAMP and/or increase adenylyl cyclase activity in response to various stimuli, including isoprenaline, sodium fluoride and guanyl-5-yl-imidobiphosphate (GppNHp), was compromised following antigen challenge in atopic asthmatics[91,92]. Similarly, the capacity of alveolar macrophages to raise intracellular cAMP in response to histamine, salbutamol, PGE_2 and 1-methyl-3-isobutylxanthine (IBMX) was reduced in asthmatics[93,94]. These studies suggest that PDE activity may be increased in inflammatory cells in asthma. However, there is no difference in PDE4 activity in alveolar macrophages[95] and eosinophils[96,97] noted between atopic and non-atopic subjects. We documented a 50% increase in total cAMP PDE activity in monocytes isolated from asthmatic subjects compared to healthy individuals[98], a finding that is supported by a previous study in atopic dermatitis subjects with a history of airway disease[99].

While there is a considerable body of evidence of increased PDE4 inhibitor sensitivity observed in inflammatory cell populations obtained from some[82,87] but not all[83,96] subjects with atopic dermatitis, we have failed to document a similar finding in monocytes from mild asthmatic subjects[98]. This is consistent with a study examining the potency of Ro-201724 against zymosan-induced release of glucuronidase from neutrophils obtained from asth-

matic subjects[100]. Similarly, atopic subjects with upper and/or lower airway disease, and who did not suffer from atopic dermatitis, failed to document an increase in PDE4 inhibitor sensitivity against mononuclear cell proliferation[101,102]. In contrast, PDE4 inhibitors attenuated $TNF\alpha$ and IL-10 release from mononuclear cells stimulated by mitogen to a greater extent in atopic rhinitis compared with healthy subjects[103].

Together, these studies highlight an important observation that alterations in PDE4 catalytic activity or inhibitor sensitivity is dependent upon the type of allergic disease under study and extrapolating from atopic disease other than asthma should be made with caution. The increase in total PDE activity observed in our study was unrelated to an increase in PDE4 activity and is consistent with a lack of evidence of an alteration in the expression of mRNA for PDE4A, B and D in monocytes from mild asthmatic subjects[104]. Thus, despite the lack of evidence of an alteration in PDE4 activity in mild asthma, the rational basis for drug targeting PDE4 in the treatment of respiratory disease stems from the finding that inhibitors of PDE4 can down-regulate inflammatory cell function.

Properties and classification of PDE4

The selective targeting of individual PDE isoenzymes has profound implications for the treatment of disease as recently highlighted with the introduction of the PDE5 selective inhibitor, sildenafil, for erectile dysfunction[105]. In the context of lung disease, PDE4 has been selectively targeted using chemical inhibitors on the basis of the clinical efficacy of the archetypal non-selective PDE inhibitor, theophylline which has long been used in the treatment of asthma and COPD. A number of highly potent PDE4 inhibitors have been tested in clinical trials and shown to have some therapeutic potential. However, one of the major stumbling blocks to the development of these inhibitors is the potential side effect profile including emesis that is a characteris-

Table 7.2. Summary of the expression of mRNA for PDE4 genes in human cells

Cell type	PDE4A	PDE4B	PDE4C	PDE4D	Reference
CD4 T cell	+	+ + (B2)		Weak	(83)
Th1 cells	+ +	+ +	−	−	(234)
Th2 cells	+ +	+ +	−	+ +	(234)
CD8 T cell	+ +	+ + (B2)		+ +	(83)
B cell	+	+ + (B2)		+ +	(257)
Monocyte	+	+ + (B2)	−	Weak	(83,125,184,287)
Eosinophil	+ +	+ +	−	+ +	(371,83)
Neutrophil	±	+ + (B2)	−	±	(184,372)
Macrophage	+ +				(116)
Brain	+ +	+ +	±	+ +	(106,372)[a]
Area postrema				+ +	(144)[a](143)[b]
Epithelium	+ (A5)		+ (C1)	+ (D2)	(373)
				+ (D3)	(307)

Notes:

[a] Analysis performed in rat brain.

[b] Immunohistochemical detection using mouse brain.

Text in parenthesis denotes splice variant. + and − denote presence and absence of expression, respectively.

tic feature of many of these drugs, although attempts are being made to reduce these unwarranted side effects.

PDE4 is a cyclic AMP specific isoenzyme (K_m 0.2 – 4 μM), showing very low affinity for cyclic GMP (K_m >1000 μM), the latter without effect on PDE4 catalytic activity. Four PDE4 subtypes (PDE4A–D) have been cloned and expressed, with additional complexity arising as a consequence of mRNA splicing resulting in isoforms with alterations in amino acid sequences within the N-terminal region[3]. In order to gain insights into the functional significance of PDE4, various studies have investigated the distribution of PDE4. It is clear that PDE4C is predominantly localized to the testis, skeletal muscle and human fetal lung[106], while PDE4A, B and D are known to be distributed in many inflammatory cells in man (Table 7.2).

Analysis of the amino acid sequence of PDE4 revealed a catalytic domain and two upstream conserved regions (UCRs) that is unique to this family of PDE. Using deletion analysis, studies have shown that the catalytic domain in PDE4A4B for example, lies between amino acid sequence 332/365 to 680/772[3,107]. Similarly, PDE4B2B has a catalytic domain between amino acid sequence 152–528[108,109]. The atomic structure of the catalytic domain of 4B2B has recently been published, showing important structural features within the binding pocket for cyclic AMP including the presence of two metal ions, most likely zinc and magnesium that is important for binding the cyclic phosphate group and various other amino acids critical for cyclic AMP binding[110].

The cDNAs for PDE4 encode for enzymes that can exist as either the long form, containing both UCR regions and a short form, characterized by either a lack in UCR1 and intact or partially truncated UCR2 region. It is thought that the short and long forms differ with respect to enzyme activity, subcellular localization and activation by different intracellular signalling pathways. Thus, PDE4D3 catalytic activity is increased[111,112] by a protein kinase A dependent mechanism a consequence of phosphorylation of Ser[54]. Additionally, specific sites in the UCR region are also subject to phosphorylation by MAP kinase dependent mechanisms which could have important implications for PDE4 activity[3]. Furthermore, the N-terminal region is implicated in targeting PDE4 to specific domains within the cell by virtue of protein–protein interactions with SH3 domain containing proteins[89]. Regions near the carboxyl terminus are also implicated in the regulation of PDE4 function. Thus, substitution of Ser[487] for Ala resulted in a significant attenuation of MAP kinase dependent phosphorylation of PDE4B2B[108]. Similarly, phosphorylation by ERK2 kinase of PDE4D3 at Ser[579] in the carboxyl terminal region, led to a significant reduction in catalytic activity[113]. Further complexity arises with the findings that alteration in the activity of PDE4 by ERK2 kinase is also influenced by the presence of UCR regions. Thus, while phosphorylation of PDE4D3 at Ser[579] resulted in a reduction in cyclic AMP PDE activity, an increase in catalytic activity was observed following phosphorylation of Ser[491] in PDE4D1, a PDE4 enzyme that lacks a UCR1 domain[114]. These findings suggest that different splice variants of PDE4 may be differentially regulated by intracellular signalling pathways that may have important implications in the regulation of cell function under normal physiological and pathophysiological conditions. Alterations to the N-terminal regions of these proteins has important functional consequences as this may alter their subcellular localization[89], activation[108,111,115] and inhibition by PDE4 inhibitors[111]. Moreover, the observation of alterations in PDE4 expression during cell differentiation[116] or following activation by cytokines, growth factors and lipid mediators[108,117–119] could have important functional consequences during an inflammatory episode.

It has long been recognized that the archetypal PDE4 inhibitor, rolipram, binds with high affinity to brain tissue compared with peripheral organs[120], yet is at least two to three orders of magnitude less potent at inhibiting PDE4 catalytic activity in this tissue[121]. The significance of this discrepancy was later clarified in studies expressing human recombinant PDE4 in yeast and showing that the high affinity rolipram binding site and the PDE4 catalytic domain reside on the same gene product[122,123]. There was little correlation between the ability of a range of compounds to displace rolipram binding from PDE4 and their ability to inhibit PDE4 catalytic activity, raising the possibility of synthesizing compounds that could selectively target these sites. The functional significance of the two domains recognized by PDE4 inhibitors was clarified further in studies examining rolipram binding and PDE4 catalytic activity in N-terminally truncated enzymes expressed in yeast, COS and Sf9 cells[107,109,124]. Specific regions within the N-terminal domain of PDE4A are important for determining high affinity binding by rolipram and the removal of this site from the protein did not abolish catalytic activity nor the ability of rolipram to inhibit PDE4 catalytic activity suggesting that binding to the high affinity site is not a prerequisite for inhibition of catalytic activity[107,124]. Similarly, expression of an N-terminal truncated PDE4B2B[152–564] resulted in a protein which lacked a high affinity binding site for rolipram compared with PDE4B2B[81–564,109], suggesting that specific sequences within the N-terminal domain are necessary for the expression of high affinity binding. However, the binding of another PDE4 inhibitor, RP 73401 to PDE4A was unaffected by the loss of this specific amino acid sequence within the N-terminal domain, but the ability of rolipram to displace RP 73401 binding was characterized by a two-site binding model[107]. The implication of these findings is that specific amino acid sequences outside the catalytic domain of PDE4 can alter the conformation of the protein, such that it binds rolipram with high affinity and therefore the 'high affinity' binding site represents a different conformation of the same protein[107,109,122,124]. There is biochemical evidence supporting the view that PDE4 can exist in different conformational states, as different methods employed to isolate PDE4 from cells can lead to differences in catalytic activity and inhibitor sensitivity[125,126]. A number of intracellular processes including phosphorylation[108,111–114] or the presence of cofactors (e.g. magnesium ions[127]) are known to alter PDE4 catalytic activity.

Pharmacological studies have been used in order to determine structure activity relationships between different PDE4 inhibitors and a number of functional studies have shown correlation between PDE4 inhibitor potency and the ability of PDE4 inhibitors to inhibit various aspects of cell function or rolipram binding. The ability of PDE4 inhibitors to inhibit gastric acid secretion[128]; emesis[129]; fMLP-induced myeloperoxidase release from human neutrophils[130]; inhibition of purified solubilized PDE4 from guinea pig eosinophils and potentiation of isoprenaline-induced cyclic AMP accumulation from guinea pig eosinophils[88], correlated with the ability of these inhibitors to displace high affinity rolipram binding. In contrast, the ability of compounds to inhibit PDE4 catalytic activity correlated with the potency of these agents against LPS-induced TNFα release by human monocytes[125,130], fMLP-induced superoxide production by guinea pig eosinophils[128] and interleukin (IL)-2 release by murine splenocytes[131]. The possibility that PDE4 may exist as different conformers has been used in an attempt to discover novel inhibitors that are selective for the 'low' affinity conformer as this subtype is suggested to be responsible for regulating cell function, while the 'high' affinity conformer is linked to the side effect profile seen with PDE4 inhibitors.

The ability of PDE4 inhibitors to activate emetic centres within the CNS may be a consequence of a peripheral action of these drugs secondary to raising intracellular levels of cyclic AMP in gastric acid secreting cells and/or afferent neurones in the gut. Alternatively, stimulation of the area postrema, a region within the CNS with a poorly developed blood–brain barrier and therefore accessible to substances within the circulation, can lead to activation of the emetic centre within the CNS[129,132]. Since emesis and gastric acid secretion correlate with the potency of PDE4 inhibitors to displace rolipram binding (high affinity PDE) it led to the suggestion that drugs with low affinity for this site may be useful in improving the side effect profile of these drugs[128,130]. However, some aspects of cell function may also correlate with inhibitors that target the 'high' affinity conformer and suggest that this method may be of limited value for the future development of PDE4 inhibitors with low emetic potential[130]. It is therefore of interest that CDP840[133] and SB 207499 (Cilomilast)[134] demonstrate a 'high' to 'low' ratio of 5 and 1.3, respectively. In contrast, rolipram is one to two orders of magnitude more selective for the high affinity binding site compared with inhibition of PDE4 catalytic activity[107,122,133,134]. Accordingly, both compounds have low emetic potential and a low side effect profile in asthma[134–136]. Cilomilast has been shown to inhibit myeloperoxidase release from human neutrophils with an equal potency to rolipram, even though this particular cell function is modulated by the 'high' PDE4 conformer[130]. This[137] suggests that a number of additional factors may govern why these drugs demonstrate a better side effect profile compared with other PDE inhibitors. Cilomilast is negatively charged at normal pH, which may retard its ability to gain access to the area postrema, although clearly not enough to retard access across inflammatory cells[136,137]. It is unclear whether the expression of splice variants of PDE4 in different cells also contribute to the observed correlations between cell function and PDE4 inhibitor potency or high affinity rolipram binding because of the similarities in the expression of PDE4 subtypes in these cells (Table 7.2) and the lack of subtype selectivity of the PDE4 inhibitors tested in these studies.

Another approach that is being investigated is whether compounds can be synthesized which exhibit selectivity for different PDE4 subtypes in an attempt to diminish the side effect profile and selectively target inflammatory cells. While CDP840 does not demonstrate subtype selectivity for PDE4A, B and D[133], Cilomilast shows a fivefold selectivity toward PDE4D compared with the other two subtypes[138,139]. Cilomilast is considerably less emetic than rolipram and is well tolerated by subjects, although it is not free from emesis. Therefore, there is clearly a need to discover highly potent PDE4 inhibitors with an even better side effect profile. Consequently a number of compounds have been synthesized that demonstrate selectivity for either PDE4A/B or PDE4D with a difference of up to 55-fold[138,139] and structure activity relationships have been documented. Thus, a significant correlation was found between PDE4A/B inhibitory potency and inhibition of TNFα release from monocytes, proliferation of T-lymphocytes and oxidative burst from human eosinophils. In contrast, no significant correlation between PDE4D inhibitory potency and inhibition of lymphocyte proliferation and TNFα release from monocytes was observed, consistent with the finding of weak PDE4D expression in these cells[138] (Table 7.2). However, a correlation was observed against human eosinophil function and selectivity for PDE4D, consistent with the presence of PDE4D in these cells[139]. Therefore, it may be possible to synthesize compounds that document greater subtype and cell selectivity. An important question that needs to be addressed is whether selective targeting of PDE4 subtypes will be sufficient to modulate inflammatory cell function, particularly if cells contain multiple PDE4 subtypes.

Pharmacokinetic considerations notwithstanding, there is some evidence that selective targeting of PDE4D significantly improved the ability of compounds to attenuate pulmonary eosinophil recruitment following antigen provocation in allergic rats[139]. In contrast, mice lacking the ability to express PDE4D have impaired growth and fertility, underlying the importance of cyclic AMP signalling in these processes[140]. However, of particular interest was the lack of effect of this gene disruption on lymphocyte proliferation, IgE production, IL-4 production and eosinophil recruitment to the airways in a model of murine inflammation[141], features which are characteristic of an allergic phenotype. This contrasts with the findings that the PDE4 inhibitor, rolipram, inhibited allergen-induced eosinophilia in a murine model of airway inflammation[142]. The lack of effect of this gene disruption upon eosinophil recruitment suggests redundancy concerning PDE4 regulation of cyclic AMP signalling in inflammatory cells or alter-

natively, other PDE4 subtypes play a greater role in regulating allergic inflammation[138].

It remains to be established whether drug targeting of PDE4A/B offers the advantage of suppressing inflammatory cell function in vivo while exhibiting a low emetic profile, considering that PDE4D is expressed in the area postrema in rat and mouse[143,144].

Effect of PDE inhibition on inflammatory cell function

It is readily apparent that PDEs are widely distributed throughout the body and regulate the function of many cells. Particular interest has focused on the role of PDE4 and to a lesser extent PDE3 in disease as these enzymes are found in many inflammatory cells. The following section will highlight the role of PDE isoenzymes in regulating the function of cells thought to participate in the inflammatory process.

Mast cells and basophils

It has been recognized for over 25 years that cyclic AMP elevating drugs inhibit mast cell degranulation[145,146]. The suppression of mast cell and basophil degranulation in response to different stimuli by a range of non-selective PDE inhibitors has been well documented in rodents and man[71,147–150]. IBMX decreases basophil histamine release induced by PAF[151] and theophylline, enprophylline and IBMX have been shown to inhibit anti-IgE-induced histamine release by both human lung mast cells and basophils[71,152,153] and cytokine release in human basophils[154].

The presence of PDE enzymes was confirmed in rat mast cells (PDE1 and PDE3-5)[155] and basophils from healthy human subjects[71] using a variety of pharmacological, biochemical and molecular biochemical techniques. In human basophils, cGMP PDE activity was minimal, appearing to be that of PDE 5, while cAMP PDE activity was considerably greater, comprising of both PDE3 and PDE4[71]. These observations are consistent with functional studies demonstrating inhibition of leukotriene (LT)C_4 and anti-IgE-induced histamine or interleukin (IL)-4 and IL-13 release from human basophils by rolipram[71,137,151,153,154,156], denbufylline, Ro20-1724, RP73401, nitroquazone[153] and Cilomilast[137]. Some of these compounds were found to be ineffective against IgE-induced histamine release by human lung mast cells[153], thus the nature of the PDE regulating human lung mast cell responses remains uncertain. Although agents that induce and sustain elevations in intracellular cAMP appear to attenuate the stimulated release of mediators from both basophils and human lung mast cells, the responsiveness of human lung mast cells and basophils to selected cAMP-active agents differs markedly[157]. In other studies, the PDE4 inhibitor rolipram attenuated LTC_4 and histamine release from murine mast cells[158] and in combination with forskolin, inhibited anti-IgE-induced increase of intracellular calcium levels in human skin mast cells[159].

The inhibitory effect of rolipram in basophils is potentiated by addition of the PDE3 inhibitors siguazodan (SKF95654) or cilostazol[71,154], although the mixed PDE3 and 4 inhibitor zardaverine had little effect over and above the PDE4 inhibitors alone[156]. Similarly, the PDE3/4 inhibitor, benzafentrine (AH21–1321) was observed to inhibit antigen-induced histamine release from human lung fragments[160]. In contrast, neither the PDE3 inhibitors siguazodan, SKF95654 or cilostazol alone[71,151,153,154], nor the PDE5 inhibitor zaprinast (M and B22948)[147,153] affected histamine or cytokine release from human basophils. These compounds also failed to inhibit histamine release by human lung mast cells[153].

Neutrophil

The non-selective PDE inhibitors pentoxifylline, theophylline and IBMX inhibited phagocytosis of latex particles[161], superoxide anion production[60,161–163], chemotaxis[163–167], aggregation[168], adhesion[169], PAF induced CD11b up-regulation and L-selectin shedding[170], degranulation[168,171,172], apoptosis[38] and platelet activating factor (PAF) biosynthesis in neutrophils[173]. The effects of these inhibitors on neutrophil function were associated with an increase in the level of intracellular cAMP, as similar effects are observed with respect to neutrophil adhesion[174,175], chemotaxis[165], apoptosis[38,176–178], superoxide anion production, and degranulation[179] when cAMP analogues or cAMP elevating agents are applied.

A predominant PDE isoenzyme with high affinity for cAMP but insensitive to cGMP and inhibited by rolipram was documented using diethylaminoethyl-sepharose chromatography, suggesting PDE4 activity[180–182]. In addition to this, PDE4B mRNA has been described in human neutrophils[183], with PDE4B2 thought to be the predominant PDE isoform present[184]. A cGMP-specific enzyme, identified as PDE5, has also been purified in human neutrophils[181,185]. These findings support a number of functional studies demonstrating the ability of various PDE4 inhibitors to attenuate respiratory burst[166,180,181,186,187], degranulation[100,130,137,172,186], apoptosis[38,177,178], chemotaxis[166], leukotriene biosynthesis[181,188], chemokine release (IL-8)[189] and surface expression of the beta 2 integrins, CD11a/CD18 and CD11b/CD18[175] in neutrophils. In contrast, the PDE3 inhibitors amrinone, milrinone, imazodan and Cilostamide had no significant effect on neutrophil superoxide anion production[180,186] while both milrinone and bemoradan were ineffective in attenuating the expression of adhesion molecules in human neutrophils[175]; milrinone has also been observed to have no inhibitory effect on human neutrophil degranulation[172]. However, in a more recent study both amrinone and milrinone were observed to reduce superoxide, hydrogen peroxide, and hydroxyl radical levels in neutrophils, while neither was found to impair neutrophil chemotaxis or phagocytosis[190].

Eosinophil

A number of cAMP elevating drugs including the non-selective PDE inhibitors have been shown to affect a wide range of eosinophil functions. Both theophylline[158] and IBMX[191] inhibit zymosan-induced superoxide anion generation by guinea pig eosinophils. Both compounds have also been shown to inhibit the C5a-stimulated formation of reactive oxygen species in intact human eosinophils[163,192]. Low doses of theophylline augmented superoxide anion generation secondary to adenosine A_2-receptor antagonism[158]. Theophylline has been observed to decrease the viability of eosinophils in culture[193], attenuate immunoglobulin (Ig)-[194] and C5a-induced secretion of cationic proteins[192], inhibit PAF and C5a-induced release of LTC_4[96], reduce GM-CSF and IL-8 release in response to sIgA-coated beads[195] and suppress PAF-induced up-regulation of Mac-1[196]. Theophylline has also been shown to inhibit PAF and C5a induced chemotaxis of eosinophils[96], an effect which was substantially reversed by addition of Rp-cAMPs, which in turn suggests PKA-dependence and thus a true PDE inhibitory mechanism. Suppression of eosinophil chemotaxis in vitro by PDE inhibitors may be due to inhibition of adhesion molecule expression as theophylline has been seen to inhibit PAF-induced CD11b upregulation on the eosinophil cell surface[197].

The presence of mRNA for PDE4D was first documented in guinea pig eosinophils using reverse transcription polymerase chain reaction (RT-PCR) with primers designed against specific sequences in rat PDE4 subtype DNA clones[198]. Studies to elucidate the PDE profiles of human eosinophils have shown the presence of high levels of PDE4 activity[83,96,192]; the majority of this activity was observed in the cytosolic fraction of cells with some activity also observed in the particulate fraction[192]. RT-PCR analysis of levels of PDE subtype messenger RNA expression in human eosinophils has revealed total PDE4 activity is a result of PDE4A, PDE4B and PDE4D subtype activity[83]. Selective PDE4 inhibition in eosinophils has been shown to increase the level of intracellular cAMP[88,198,199] and attenuate superoxide anion generation[191,192,198–203], LTB_4-induced thromboxane release[201,204], and Ig- or C5a-induced secretion of cationic proteins[197,198] in both human and guinea pig eosinophils. Moreover, PDE4 inhibitors attenuated PAF, LTB_4 and C5a-induced release of LTC_4 from eosinophils[96], eosinophil chemotaxis in vitro[96,202,205–208] and PAF-induced cell surface CD11b upregulation[197,208]. In some studies, the efficacy of PDE4 inhibitors was significantly increased in the presence of cAMP elevating drugs[96,192,200,203] and although only low levels of PDE3 activity have been observed in eosinophil cytosolic and particulate fractions[192] cotreatment with both a PDE3 and a PDE4 inhibitor has shown increased inhibitory effects on eosinophil function[209]. In one study, cAMP elevating drugs but not rolipram inhibited eosinophil viability in culture[210] while in separate studies, PDE4 selective inhibition has been shown not to inhibit C5a-induced eosinophil degranulation[192,203]. The differing results of these studies suggest that PDE4 inhibitors alone may not be sufficient to elevate cAMP in this cell type and therefore may not inhibit all aspects of eosinophil function.

T-lymphocyte

Methylxanthines

Cyclic AMP elevating agents can modulate development, proliferation, cytokine generation, expression of cytokine receptors, chemotaxis and antibody production in T-lymphocytes[211–214]. Theophylline has been shown to inhibit lymphocyte proliferation in response to a variety of stimuli, including phytohemagglutinin (PHA) and anti-CD3[26,56,102,215,216], which may be secondary to inhibition of IL-2 synthesis[26,217] and downregulation of IL-2 receptor expression[218]. Theophylline has also been observed to inhibit PAF- or IL8 induced human T-lymphocyte chemotaxis in vitro[214], lymphocyte migration through human endothelium, an effect thought to be mediated via inhibition of lymphocyte motility[219] and the release of both IL-4 and IL-5 by PMA- and anti-CD3 stimulated Th2 cells[102]. Furthermore, it has been suggested that theophylline may stimulate a subpopulation of T-lymphocytes with suppressor cell activity[25,220]. Pentoxifylline can attenuate T-lymphocyte responsiveness in an experimental model of autoimmune encephalomyelitis in Lewis rats[221] and in patients with autoimmune disease such as multiple sclerosis[222]. Pentoxifylline has also been observed to inhibit release of cytokines including TNFα, IFNγ and GM-CSF from HIV-specific CD8 + cytotoxic T-cells[223]. Both pentoxifylline and IBMX have been shown to inhibit T-lymphocyte adhesion to HMEC-1 (a human dermal endothelial cell line), an effect mediated by inhibition of LFA-1 and ICAM-1[224]. Moreover, theophylline and enprophylline increased IL-5, yet had no effect on IL-4 production in a Th2 cell line[225]. These studies are consistent with the view that methylxanthines preferentially inhibit Th1 lymphocyte-mediated responses.

Selective inhibitors

Cyclic AMP PDE activity in the soluble and particulate fraction of enriched T-lymphocytes was inhibited by Ro-201724 and the PDE3 inhibitor, Cl-930[79] and both PDE3 and PDE4 have been confirmed in membrane and cytosolic compartments of human CD4 + and CD8 + T lymphocytes[95,226]. On closer inspection, PDE4A, PDE4B, PDE4D were described in CD4$^+$ and CD8$^+$ human T lymphocytes[104,226]. Semiquantitative RT-PCR analyses of mRNA from healthy and mild atopic subjects revealed that PDE4A and PDE4B2 were present in both CD4$^+$ and CD8$^+$ cells and that PDE4D was expressed only in CD8$^+$ cells[83]. Increased PDE4A and PDE4B2 expression was observed in CD4$^+$ cells from atopic subjects, although this did not appear to result in significantly higher cAMP PDE activity[83]. PDE3B has been shown to account for the PDE3 activity in lymphocytes from healthy subjects[227] and a fragment corresponding to PDE7 has also been described[226,228,229].

Functional studies have shown that PDE4, and to a lesser extent PDE3 inhibitors, attenuated mitogen-, antiCD3- and allergen-induced human T-lymphocyte proliferation[83,87,101,102,137,215,216,230–234]. However, inhibition of lymphocyte proliferation was more pronounced if dual inhibitors or a combination of PDE3 and PDE4 inhibitors were used[83,87,231,233,235]. Similarly, rolipram and Ro-201724 inhibited lymphocyte proliferation and contact hypersensitivity in oxazolone treated mice[236]. The PHA- or anti-CD3-induced proliferation of CD4$^+$ and CD8$^+$ T-lymphocytes was inhibited in a concentration-dependent manner by rolipram but not SKF95654, consistent with the ability of rolipram to elevate intracellular cyclic AMP in these cells[226]. SKF95654 increased the inhibitory potency of rolipram against CD4$^+$ and CD8$^+$ T-lymphocyte proliferation, although complete inhibition was not achieved. Similarly, it has been demonstrated that PDE7 activity is increased upon activation of lymphocytes, and that this in turn, correlates with decreased cAMP and increased proliferation[237]. Furthermore, when PDE7 expression is reduced by a PDE7 antisense oligonucleotide, proliferation is reduced[237]. Thus, it appears that PDE4 and to a lesser degree, both PDE3 and PDE7 may all play a role in regulating T-lymphocyte proliferation.

Various studies have shown that elevating the level of intracellular cyclic AMP may preferentially inhibit the synthesis and release of Th1 cytokines. Thus, drugs which elevate intracellular levels of cAMP including forskolin and prostaglandin (PG)E$_2$[238–242] inhibited the production of Th1 but not Th2 cytokines, most likely via inhibition of IL-2 synthesis, reduction in $t_{1/2}$ of IL-2 mRNA and IL-2 receptor (IL2R) expression by a protein kinase A dependent mechanism[230,243–245].

The production of T-lymphocyte derived cytokines is also influenced by antigen presenting cells like monocytes. PGE2 inhibited the release of monocyte derived IL-12, yet augmented the release of IL-10. These cytokines are important for the proliferation of Th1 and Th2 lymphocytes respectively[213,246]. In other studies addition of exogenous PGE$_2$ to purified lymphocytes caused a marked reduction in IFNβ release[247]. Similarly, rolipram attenuated the PHA- or PMA and ionomycin-induced release of IL-2, and IFNγ from CD4$^+$ and CD8$^+$ human T-lymphocytes[248] and IFNγ production by PHA-stimulated human peripheral blood mononuclear cells[244]. On the other hand, rolipram only inhibited T lymphocyte proliferation when the former stimulus was used and suggested the possible involvement of other cytokines in the proliferative response[226]. In LPS stimulated human peripheral blood mononuclear cells, rolipram was observed to inhibit IL-1β and TNF-α production[249]. In each of these studies PDE3 selective inhibitors showed little or no independent efficacy; however, they were observed to augment the efficacy of PDE4 inhibitors. Other studies have shown that rolipram significantly reduced TNFα, and, to a lesser extent, IFNγ production in human and rat autoreactive T-lymphocytes[250] and was only partially effective against TNFα release from encephalitogenic T-cells[251]. In general, these studies support the view that elevation of cAMP inhibits the generation of Th1-like cytokines but that PDE mediated effects are selective.

It has now become increasingly apparent that intracellular cAMP can also regulate the expression and release of cytokines from Th2 cells. It was established in a murine Th2 cell clone that rolipram had minimal effects on anti-CD3 induced IL-4 production but enhanced IL-5 production via a protein kinase A-dependent pathway[225] which is consistent with the ability of dibutyryl cyclic AMP, in combination with PMA, to increase IL-5 mRNA expression and protein levels in a mouse thymoma line EL-4[252]. The effect of cAMP on the expression of IL-5 mRNA is indirect since there does not appear to be a CRE consensus sequence in the IL-5 promoter. Furthermore, dibutyryl cAMP inhibited the production of IL-2, IL-4 and IL-10 in these cells and confirms the ability of cAMP to regulate the expression of Th2 cytokines[252]. Similarly, IBMX inhibited the synthesis of IL-2 and IL-4, yet moderately affected IFNγ production in human T lymphocytes[242] and both Ro-201724 and theophylline inhibited IL-4 and IL-5 secretion in human Th2 cell lines[102]. Rolipram has also been observed to reduce IL-2, IL-4 and IL-5 production in PHA-stimulated human peripheral blood mononuclear cells[244]. The ability of cAMP to regulate Th2 cytokine production is not specific for T cell clones and cell lines. Rolipram inhibited ragweed (Th2)- but not tetanus toxoid (Th1)-driven proliferation of peripheral blood mononuclear cells[101]. This antiproliferative effect of rolipram against ragweed challenge was associated with a reduction in gene expression for IL-5 and IFN-γ but not IL-4[232]. It was initially suggested that the relative resistance to inhibition by rolipram of peripheral blood mononuclear cell proliferation to a Th1 driven stimulus, may be due to the lack of PDE4B in Jurkat cells[232] and that this may account for the inability of rolipram to effect IL-2 mRNA synthesis in these cells[253]. The differential effect of PDE inhibitors on T-lymphocyte cytokine generation was also suggested to be a function of the ability of different populations of T-lymphocytes to elevate cyclic AMP[242,254]. It has since been reported that the enhanced sensitivity of Th2 cells and the relative insensitivity of Th1 to PDE inhibition is more likely to be due to differential expression of PDE4 isoforms in these cell types. Investigation by RT-PCR revealed reduced gene expression for the PDE4C isoform and a lack of gene expression for the PDE4D isoform in Th1 cells when compared to Th2[234].

It is clear, that Th2 cell derived cytokines can be inhibited by cAMP elevating drugs particularly when a physiological stimulus such as antigen is used as opposed to mitogens or anti-CD3. Another factor which may influence whether cAMP up or down-regulates the expression of Th2 cytokines is the availability of IL-2[255]. Finally, cAMP elevating agents including prostaglandin E$_2$ inhibited the expression of monocyte-derived IL-12 yet augmented the expression of IL-10 from monocytes, which would also be a determinant of the expression of Th1 and Th2 cytokines particularly if antigen presenting cells and/or antigen presenting cell-dependent stimuli are used[213].

B-lymphocyte

Initially, studies of RNA from a human lymphocytic B-cell line (43D-C12) revealed a cDNA that encoded a protein with 93% homology to rat PDE4B[256]. It has since been demonstrated that cytosolic PDE4 is the predominant isoenzyme, followed by cytosolic PDE7-like activity, some PDE3 activity was also noted in the particulate fraction[257]. Molecular biology techniques were used in this study allowing further investigation of the PDE profile of human B-lymphocytes. RT-PCR revealed PDE4A, PDE4B and PDE4D to be present; in addition small amounts of PDE3A were also detected[257]. A rise in the level of intracellular cAMP has been shown to inhibit proliferation[211], differentiation[258], apoptosis[259,260] and promote isotype switching by IL-4 in murine and human B lymphocytes[261,262].

PGE2 inhibits IgE production induced by IL-4 in purified human B-cells enriched with T lymphocytes[263]. In contrast, the β_2-adrenoceptor agonist, salbutamol, was reported to potentiate IL-4-induced IgE production in human peripheral blood mononuclear cells[264,265]. The reason for this discrepancy remains to be established. However, the expression of IgE in B cells is regulated by low affinity IgE receptors (CD23) which is expressed on and released (soluble CD23) by B cells, a process that is cAMP-dependent[266]. It is known that PGE2[263] but not salbutamol[265] inhibits the expression of CD23 on B-cells. The role of cAMP in regulating human B-lymphocyte function can only be resolved with purified populations of CD40 + lymphocytes.

Very few studies have investigated the effect of PDE inhibitors on B-lymphocyte function. Peripheral blood mononuclear cells from individuals with atopic dermatitis have a propensity to generate IgE, which is inhibited by Ro-201724 and appeared to be mediated by a direct inhibition of the cAMP PDE activity of B-lymphocytes[267]. This result was reflected in a separate study that showed cAMP PDE activity to be more susceptible to inhibition by both selective PDE4 and non-selective PDE inhibitors in B-lymphocyte homogenates from atopic subjects when compared to healthy subjects[268]. Rolipram and RP73401 (PDE4 inhibitor) increased intracellular cAMP levels and augmented proliferation of LPS- and IL-4 stimulated human B lymphocytes[257]. This effect was reduced by PKA inhibition with PDDE4 activity being reduced by up to 50% in stimulated cells, thus showing stimulation of B-cell proliferation to be dependent on a PDE4-mediated increase in cAMP. PDE3 inhibition was shown to have little effect in this model[257]. In another study,

rolipram and Ro-301724 were shown to be ineffective in inhibiting IL-4 induced IgE production by human B-lymphocytes[269].

Monocyte

In human monocytes, theophylline, IBMX and pentoxifylline inhibited the release of arachidonic acid[270-272], superoxide anion generation[273], TNFα production at the level of gene transcription[98,125,274-276], complement component C2[277], phagocytosis[161], IL-2R expression[218], production of IL-12[213], generation of LTB$_4$[278], prevented adherence dependent expression of platelet derived growth factor (PDGF)β mRNA[279] and facilitated the production of IL-10[213,280]. Some studies have demonstrated that non-selective phosphodiesterase inhibitors and cAMP elevating drugs, have either no effect[274], inhibited[281] or enhanced[282-284] IL-1 production in monocytes. These discrepancies may be accounted by a number of observations. First, cAMP inhibited the release but had no effect on the intracellular concentration of IL-1β in monocytes[276,285]. Secondly, the inhibition of IL-1 production by methylxanthines is not due to a reduction in the level of IL-1 mRNA but to a reduction in IL-1 activity[281].

Many groups using various assay techniques to detect cAMP activity in cell homogenates have studied the isoenzyme profile of human monocytes. Purified human monocytes were found to contain PDE4 almost exclusively in the cytosol[286], consistent with the description of PDE4A, PDE4B (specifically PDE4B2) and PDE4D in these cells[116,125,287]. Small amounts of membrane-bound PDE3 have also been observed, and although investigated, no PDE2, PDE5 or PDE4C expression could be described[116,125,287]. Functional studies demonstrated that rolipram attenuated leukotriene production[158], cytokine secretion[103] and arachidonic acid release[272,288] from human monocytes. Furthermore, PDE4 and, to a lesser extent, PDE3 inhibitors, attenuated endotoxin or lipopolysaccharide (LPS)-induced TNFα production in monocytes[98,116,130,233,251,276,289-295]. Similarly, the PDE4 inhibitor CP80633 inhibited the release of TNFα induced by LPS in human monocytes[202]. The effect of PDE4 inhibitors on TNFα production was a consequence of a reduction in TNFα mRNA expression and protein activity[276,289,292,295]. PDE4 inhibitors either have no effect[289] or inhibited IL-1β release[251,276], but did not inhibit IL-1β mRNA expression[276]. As with non-selective PDE inhibition, rolipram was also observed to enhance IL-10 production, an effect that was reversed by addition of a selective PKA inhibitor[294,295].

Macrophage

The PDE profile of monocyte-derived macrophages from healthy subjects has been determined; PDE4 activity was observed to be lower and PDE1 and PDE3 activities increased in comparison to monocytes[116]. In human alveolar macrophages large amounts of PDE1 and also PDE5 account for cGMP PDE activity, while an equivalent expression of both PDE3 and PDE4 are responsible for the cAMP PDE activities observed[286]. PDE3 is located in both cytosolic and membrane compartments while PDE1, PDE4 and PDE5 are predominantly located in the cytosol[233,286]. Exposure of macrophages to inflammatory stimuli leads to a decrease in intracellular cAMP[93]; in this way LPS-induced secretion of TNFα by monocyte-derived macrophages was inhibited by the cAMP elevators dibutyl cAMP, PGE$_2$ and forskolin[116]. Similarly, 8-bromo cAMP, PGE$_2$ and cholera toxin reduced IL-1α expression and caused a downregulation of TNFα gene expression in LPS-stimulated human macrophages[296], while both dibutyl cAMP and 8-bromo cAMP were observed to cause an inhibition of thromboxane B$_2$ release in alveolar macrophages[297,298].

Functional studies have shown that elevation of intracellular cAMP via inhibition of PDE can also affect the inflammatory response of this cell type. Theophylline and enprophylline inhibited lipoprotein lipase activity, a consequence of reduced synthesis and increased lysosomal acid hydrolase activity in human monocyte-derived macrophages[299]. Furthermore, these drugs inhibited TNFα

release from alveolar macrophages[275], superoxide anion production from guinea pig[300] and rat[301] peritoneal and human alveolar macrophages, respectively[298], and to a lesser extent, attenuated thromboxane (TXB)$_2$ release from human alveolar macrophages[298]. Theophylline was also observed to suppress human alveolar macrophage respiratory burst, an effect reversed by PKA inhibition, suggesting that the functional effect observed here was mediated through elavation of cAMP as a result of PDE inhibition[302]. IBMX in combination with salbutamol, increased LTB$_4$ release from human non-diseased alveolar macrophages but not from macrophages obtained from patients with COPD, although PGE$_2$ release was inhibited[303]. In a separate study, a similar effect was observed in alveolar macrophages from asthmatic subjects, which exhibited reduced responsiveness to PGE$_2$, IBMX and salbutamol[93].

Ro-201724 alone, or in combination with isoprenaline, attenuated zymosan or IgE/anti-IgE complex-induced release of TXB$_2$, LTB$_4$ and superoxide anion[304]. Similarly, rolipram, RP73401 and the dual PDE3/PDE4 inhibitor, zardaverine, inhibited LPS-induced TNFα release from human alveolar macrophages[116,233,305]. In this model, motapizone (PDE3 inhibitor) alone acted as a weak inhibitor, and combination of this compound with either rolipram or RP73401 caused total inhibition of TNFα release[116]. Rolipram has also been shown to reduce LPS-induced TNFα release from macrophages obtained from Lewis rats with experimental autoimmune encephalomyelitis[251], while higher concentrations of both rolipram and zardaverine have been shown to attenuate the release of LTC$_4$ by LPS in murine resident peritoneal macrophages[305]. However, FMLP-induced superoxide anion production in guinea pig peritoneal macrophages remained unaffected by PDE4 inhibition[300].

Bronchial epithelium

The PDE profile of bronchial epithelial cells has been identified. In an early study, PDE1–5 were isolated from airway epithelium with PDE3 predominantly localized to the membrane fraction[306]. In more recent studies, analysis of PCR products from primary airway epithelial cell cultures revealed the presence of several PDE4 splice variants, PDE4A5, PDE4C1, PDE4D2 and PDE4D3, and also provided evidence of PDE7 expression through demonstration of PDE7 mRNA[307]. Alterations in the levels of intracellular cAMP have long been recognized to regulate chloride channel activity in the epithelium. It is of interest, therefore, that airway epithelium chloride channel activity was increased in the presence of the PDE3 inhibitor, milrinone, but neither rolipram, Ro-201724 nor IBMX were active[308]. This effect was mediated by a protein kinase dependent pathway but was found to be unrelated to changes in total cAMP content and once again underlines the possibility that compartmentalization of cAMP in cells is important in regulating protein function[308]. Similarly, in functional studies, PDE inhibitors have been shown to have limited effects on bronchial epithelium. Rolipram was observed to inhibit bacteria-induced epithelial damage of bronchial mucosa[309]. However, in other studies, IBMX had no effect on basal or TNFα-induced IL-8 release[310] and neither IBMX nor rolipram had any effect on bradykinin-induced PGE$_2$ release in human bronchial epithelial cells grown in primary culture[310].

Vascular endothelium

Characterization of cAMP PDE revealed the presence of PDE3 and PDE4 in bovine and pig aortic endothelial cells in culture[311,312] and PDE2–4 in porcine pulmonary artery endothelial cells in culture[313]. Functional studies have revealed the PDE profile of human vascular endothelial cells, which have been shown to express large amounts of PDE2, 3 and 4[314]. An increase in the intracellular level of cAMP within the endothelium attenuated transendothelial cell permeability[315,316]. Both IBMX and pentoxifylline inhibited thrombin-[315] and endotoxin-induced[317] increase in permeability of human umbilical vein and bovine pulmonary artery endothelial cell monolayers in culture, respectively.

Interestingly, the effect of pentoxifylline on endothelial cell permeability was not associated with an increase in intracellular cAMP[317] and might reflect compartmentalization of cAMP within cells. Motapizone, rolipram and zardaverine significantly reduced hydrogen peroxide induced permeability of porcine pulmonary artery endothelial cells[313] implicating a role for PDE3 and PDE4 in this response. Similarly, in human endothelial cell layers, adenylyl cyclase activation by either forskolin, cholera toxin or prostaglandin E1 or treatment with the PDE3 and/or PDE4 inhibitors motapizone, rolipram and zardaverine, was seen to abrogate thrombin or HlyA (*Escherichia coli* hemolysin, a membrane-perturbing bacterial endotoxin) induced hyperpermeability[314].

The endothelium also provides an interface for the adhesion and transmigration of inflammatory cells from the blood into sites of inflammation. The transendothelial migration of lymphocytes but not monocytes through human endothelial cells in culture was attenuated by theophylline and Ro-201724[219]. It remains to be established whether the surface expression of adhesion proteins is inhibited, although an effect on lymphocyte mobility was observed. Similarly, R-rolipram inhibited PMA and TNFα-stimulated guinea-pig eosinophil adhesion to human umbilical cord vein endothelial cells (HUVECs) in culture[318].

IBMX attenuated TNFα-induced expression of endothelial leukocyte adhesion molecule 1 (ELAM-1 or E-selectin), vascular cell adhesion molecule 1 (VCAM-1) but not intercellular adhesion molecule 1 (ICAM-1) in forskolin-treated human umbilical cord vein endothelial cells in culture[319]. Similarly, treatment of HUVECs with selective PDE4 inhibitors has also been shown to inhibit E-selectin but not V-CAM1 expression[320]. In contrast, pentoxifylline in combination with dibutyryl cyclic AMP failed to attenuate the TNFα-induced expression of any of these adhesion molecules[321]. Rolipram in combination with salbutamol has been shown to inhibit TNFα induced E-selectin expression, whilst ICAM-1 and VCAM-1 expression were not affected. In the same study, the PDE 3 inhibitor ORG 9935 had no effect on CAM expression alone, but in combination with rolipram, a synergistic inhibition of VCAM-1 and E-selectin, but not ICAM-1, expression was observed[209]. In this way, a combination of both PDE3 and PDE4 inhibition appears to be more effective in reducing CAM expression than inhibition of either isoenzyme alone. Further studies are required to determine the exact role played by cyclic AMP in expression of adhesion molecules on vascular endothelial cells.

Vascular smooth muscle

Cyclic nucleotide PDE activity in human, bovine and rat aorta was resolved into three peaks characterized by PDE1, PDE3 and PDE5, respectively[322]. In later studies, PDE4 was observed in rat aorta[323] and mesenteric artery[324] and in pig aorta, PDE1 (soluble), PDE3 (soluble and particulate) and PDE4 (predominantly soluble) activity was found[325]. PDE1–5 were detected in the cytosolic fraction of human aorta[326], and in more recent studies, advanced molecular biology techniques on a range of vascular smooth muscle tissues have revealed more specific expression of isoenzyme subtypes. These include PDE5A1 and PDE5A2 in human aortic smooth muscle cells[327], PDE3A and PDE3B in human blood vessel vascular smooth muscle cells[328] and more specifically, PDE3A1 in human aortic myocytes[329]. These biochemical studies are consistent with functional studies showing vasodilation of human mesenteric vessels, coronary, lung and renal arteries[330,331] and rat aorta[323] by PDE3 inhibitors, including milrinone, and vasodilation of rabbit aorta by the mixed PDE3/4 inhibitor ORG20421[201]. Interestingly, the ability of PDE4 and PDE5 inhibitors to induce relaxation of rat aorta is dependent on the presence of endothelium-derived nitric oxide[323,332]. The endothelium-dependence of the relaxant response to PDE4 inhibitors was subsequently shown to be due to nitric oxide-induced elevation of cGMP which inhibited PDE3, thereby increasing the level of intracellular cAMP in vascular smooth muscle[79]. A similar finding was noted for pentoxifylline and theophylline, although relaxa-

tion mediated by theophylline was endothelium-independent and has been attributed to the different affinities these drugs have for PDE3 and PDE4[333]. These studies highlight the cross-talk in vascular tissue between the nitric oxide/cGMP pathway and the cAMP pathway.

There is an abundance of PDE in human pulmonary artery according to the profile: PDE5 = PDE3 > > PDE4, while PDE1 was relatively scarce[334]. Both PDE3 and PDE5 were predominantly located in the cytosolic fraction. The biochemical data is supported by functional studies, which showed that vasodilation of human pulmonary artery by zardaverine and motapizone was greater than rolipram[335]. Recent studies have also revealed expression of PDE2 in human pulmonary artery, more specifically PDE 2A[336].

The role of PDE in regulating vascular smooth muscle proliferation has also been investigated. The PDE3 inhibitor, cilostazol, attenuated growth factor-induced [^{3}H]-thymidine incorporation into DNA and cell growth of rat aortic arterial smooth muscle cells in culture[337]. Similarly, in a cell line derived from embryonic rat aorta that contained both PDE3 and PDE4 activity (~ 30% and 70% respectively), the combined use of PDE3 and PDE4 inhibitors attenuated cell proliferation to a greater extent than either inhibitor alone[338] and IBMX inhibited surgery-induced intimal thickening in organ cultures of human saphenous vein[339].

Airway smooth muscle

Biochemical investigations have documented PDE1–5 in dog[340], bovine[341], guinea pig[342–344] and human airway smooth muscle[345–347] with most of the PDE activity located in the cytosol. Airway smooth muscle relaxation is observed following inhibition of PDE3 and PDE4 in canine[348–350], guinea pig tracheal[342,344,351,352]; and human airway preparations[345–347,353–355]. In contrast, inhibition of PDE4 and not PDE3 correlated with smooth muscle relaxation in bovine trachea[341].

The contribution of PDE3 and PDE4 to human airway smooth muscle relaxation has been investigated. The non-selective PDE inhibitors theophylline, pentoxifylline and IBMX, the PDE4 selective inhibitors rolipram, denbufylline and D22888, and the PDE3 inhibitor ORG9935, have all been observed to relax inherent bronchial smooth muscle tone, while the PDE5 selective inhibitor Zaprinast remained ineffective[310,345,346,353,354]. Similarly, the combination of PDE3 and PDE4 inhibitors, or the use of a dual PDE3/4 inhibitor resulted in significant relaxation of smooth muscle tone[345,346]. In spontaneously contracted human bronchial preparations, relaxation by rolipram was greater than siguazodan[354] and SKF94120 was more potent than rolipram[346]. Thus, the relaxation potency of the PDE3 inhibitor ORG9935 was less when methacholine and not histamine was used as the spasmogen, which was not seen for rolipram[345]. In contrast, siguazodan was more efficacious than rolipram in spasmogen-contracted tissue[347,354]. Histamine, acetylcholine and methacholine-induced contraction of human bronchi were significantly attenuated by aminophylline, T440 (PDE4 inhibitor) and ORG20241 (PDE3/4 inhibitor)[201,355], but although it has been demonstrated that theophylline, IBMX and zardaverine inhibit the contractile response to allergen, RP73401 (PDE4 inhibitor) and motapizone were without effect[356]. Differences in the degree of basal tone, age and source of the tissue, variability in tissue response to relaxant agonists and methodology may account for the conflicting reports. Clearly, the greater efficacy demonstrated by mixed PDE3/4 inhibitors as relaxant agonists compared with subtype selective enzyme inhibitors imply a role for both PDE3 and PDE4 in mediating relaxation of human airway smooth muscle[345,346].

The role of PDE in the regulation of airway smooth muscle proliferation has only received scant attention; nonetheless, IBMX was observed to attenuate thrombin-induced mitogenesis of human cultured airway smooth muscle cells[357]. In another study, the PDE3 inhibitor siguazodan and the non-selective PDE inhibitor IBMX were observed to inhibit both [^{3}H]thymidine incorporation and the increase in cell number induced by platelet-derived growth factor-BB in human cultured airway smooth

muscle cells, while the PDE 4 inhibitor rolipram had no effect[358].

Clinical studies of PDE inhibitors in asthma and COPD

PDE inhibitors are currently being developed for the treatment of asthma and COPD, although side effects including emesis have halted the development of some examples of this class of drug into the clinic. To date, there are a limited number of clinical studies investigating the efficacy of PDE inhibitors in the treatment of asthma. Inhalation of zardaverine was shown to produce a modest bronchodilator effect in patients with asthma, although unacceptable side effects of nausea and emesis were reported in a significant number of patients[359], while oral administration of cilostazol (PDE3 inhibitor) caused bronchodilation and bronchoprotection against methacholine challenge in healthy subjects at the expense of mild to severe headache[360]. AH-2132 (benzafentrine; a mixed PDE3/4 inhibitor) has also been reported to have significant bronchodilator activity in normal volunteers[361]; the PDE4 inhibitor, ibudilast significantly improved baseline airways responsiveness to spasmogens by twofold after 6 months' treatment[362] and MKS492 (PDE3 inhibitor) has been reported to attenuate the early and late asthmatic response in atopic asthmatics[363].

Recently, the orally active PDE4 selective inhibitors, CDP840[135] and Roflumilast[364] have been demonstrated to modestly attenuate the development of the late asthmatic response in mild asthmatics whilst having no effect on the acute response, with no significant side effects being reported in comparison with placebo. The ability of these novel selective PDE4 inhibitors to inhibit the late asthmatic response was not associated with bronchodilation, suggesting actions of this drug other than smooth muscle relaxation. Furthermore, the PDE4 inhibitor RP 73401, has also been shown to have no significant effect on allergen-induced bronchoconstriction in allergic asthmatic subjects[365]. These data are consistent with the suggestion that PDE3 rather than PDE4 may be the important isoenzyme regulating airway smooth muscle tone in asthmatic subjects. However, recent clinical studies with another orally active PDE4 inhibitor, cilomilast have shown that this drug can attenuate bronchoconstriction following exercise in asthmatic subjects[366], an effect mimicked by four weeks of treatment with the selective PDE4 inhibitor, Roflumilast[367], although the effect of the latter drug was accompanied by a reduction in TNFα levels. This would suggest that PDE4 inhibition can influence inflammatory cell function in vivo. The oral administration of V11294 has also been shown to reduce TNFα levels in healthy volunteers[368].

More recently, cilomilast administered to asthmatic subjects taking inhaled glucocorticosteroids[136] or individuals with COPD[369] demonstrated improvements in baseline lung function and was well tolerated with doses up to 15 mg *b.i.d.* The mechanism of the beneficial action observed with cilomilast is unlikely to be due to bronchodilation *per se*, since this drug has modest effects on airway smooth muscle function[370]. An explanation for the beneficial effect of cilomilast might include suppression of bronchial hyper-responsiveness secondary to a reduction of airway inflammation that would lead to improvements in lung function and/or reduction in afferent nerve activity and thereby reducing reflex bronchoconstriction.

Conclusion

Our increasing knowledge of the molecular biology of the expanding PDE family of enzymes provides exciting opportunities for the development of highly selective, even disease specific drugs. It is already apparent that encouraging signs beginning to emerge concerning the development of novel PDE4 inhibitors, will not only assist in our understanding of the role of PDE4 subtypes in the regulation of cell function, but also offer the potential to find novel treatments for respiratory diseases[371].

REFERENCES

1 Torphy TJ. Phosphodiesterase isozymes: molecular targets for novel antiasthma agents. *Am J Respir Crit Care Med* 1998; 157(2):351–370.

2 Soderling SH, Beavo JA. Regulation of cAMP and cGMP signaling: new phosphodiesterases and new functions. *Curr Opin Cell Biol* 2000; 12:174–179.

3 Houslay MD, Sullivan M, Bolger GB. The multienzyme PDE4 cyclic adenosine monophosphate-specific phosphodiesterase family: intracellular targeting, regulation, and selective inhibition by compounds exerting anti-inflammatory and antidepressant actions. In: August JT, Anders MW, Murad F, Coyle JT, eds. *Advances in pharmacology.* London: Academic Press;1998; 225–342.

4 Sharma RK, Wang JH. Purification and characterization of bovine lung calmodulin-dependent cyclic nucleotide phosphodiesterase. An enzyme containing calmodulin as a subunit. *J Biol Chem* 1986; 261(30):14160–14166.

5 Beavo JA. Cyclic nucleotide phosphodiesterases: functional implications of multiple isoforms. *Physiol Rev* 1995; 75(4):725–748.

6 Persson CGA, Pauwels R. Pharmacology of anti-asthma xanthines. In: Page CP, Barnes PJ, eds. *Pharmacology of asthma.* Berlin: Springer-Verlag, 1991; 207–225.

7 Becker AB, Simons KJ, Gillespie CA, Simons FE. The bronchodilator effects and pharmacokinetics of caffeine in asthma. *N Engl J Med* 1984; 310:743–746.

8 Weinberger M, Hendeles L. Theophylline in asthma. *N Engl J Med* 1996; 334(21):1380–1388.

9 Ashutosh K, Sedat M, Fragale-Jackson J. Effects of theophylline on respiratory drive in patients with chronic obstructive pulmonary disease. *J Clin Pharmacol* 1997; 37(12):1100–1107.

10 Spina D, Ferlenga P, Biasini I et al. The effect duration of selective phosphodiesterase inhibitors in the guinea-pig. *Life Sci* 1998; 11:953–965.

11 Ward AJ, McKenniff M, Evans JM, Page CP, Costello JF. Theophylline – an immunomodulatory role in asthma? *Am Rev Respir Dis* 1993; 147(3):518–523.

12 Kidney J, Dominguez M, Taylor PM, Rose M, Chung KF, Barnes PJ. Immunomodulation by theophylline in asthma. Demonstration by withdrawal of therapy. *Am J Respir Crit Care Med* 1995; 151(6):1907–1914.

13 Pauwels R, van Renterghem D, van der Straeten M, Johannesson N, Persson CG. The effect of theophylline and enprofylline on allergen-induced bronchoconstriction. *J Allergy Clin Immunol* 1985; 76(4):583–590.

14 Crescioli S, Spinazzi A, Plebani M et al. Theophylline inhib-

its early and late asthmatic reactions induced by allergens in asthmatic subjects. *Ann Allergy* 1991; 66(3):245–251.

15 Hendeles L, Harman E, Huang D, O'Brien R, Blake K, Delafuente J. Theophylline attenuation of airway responses to allergen: comparison with cromolyn metered-dose inhaler. *J Allergy Clin Immunol* 1995; 95(2):505–514.

16 Cockcroft DW, Murdock KY, Gore BP, O'Byrne PM, Manning P. Theophylline does not inhibit allergen-induced increase in airway responsiveness to methacholine. *J Allergy Clin Immunol* 1989; 83(5):913–920.

17 Naclerio RM, Bartenfelder D, Proud D et al. Theophylline reduces histamine release during pollen-induced rhinitis. *J Allergy Clin Immunol* 1986; 78(5 Pt 1):874–876.

18 Mapp C, Boschetto P, dal Vecchio L et al. Protective effect of antiasthma drugs on late asthmatic reactions and increased airway responsiveness induced by toluene di-isocyanate in sensitized subjects. *Am Rev Respir Dis* 1987; 136(6):1403–1407.

19 De Monchy JG, Kauffman HF, Venge P et al. Bronchoalveolar eosinophilia during allergen-induced late asthmatic reactions. *Am Rev Respir Dis* 1985; 131(3):373–376.

20 Sullivan P, Bekir S, Jaffar Z, Page C, Jeffery P, Costello J. Anti-inflammatory effects of low-dose oral theophylline in atopic asthma [published erratum appears in *Lancet* 1994 Jun 11; 343(8911):1512]. *Lancet* 1994; 343(8904):1006–1008.

21 Aubier M, Neukirch C, Maachi M et al. Effect of slow-release theophylline on nasal antigen challenge in subjects with allergic rhinitis. *Euro Respir J* 1998; 11(5):1105–1110.

22 Limatibul S, Shore A, Dosch HM, Gelfand EW. Theophylline modulation of E-rosette formation: an indicator of T-cell maturation. *Clin Exp Immunol* 1978; 33(3):503–513.

23 Shohat B, Volovitz B, Varsano I. Induction of suppressor T cells in asthmatic children by theophylline treatment. *Clin Allergy* 1983; 13(5):487–493.

24 Pardi R, Zocchi MR, Ferrero E, Ciboddo GF, Inverardi L, Rugarli C. In vivo effects of a single infusion of theophylline on human peripheral blood lymphocytes. *Clin Exp Immunol* 1984; 57(3):722–728.

25 Zocchi MR, Pardi R, Gromo G et al. Theophylline induced non specific suppressor activity in human peripheral blood lymphocytes. *J Immunopharmacol* 1985; 7(2):217–234.

26 Scordamaglia A, Ciprandi G, Ruffoni S et al. Theophylline and the immune response: in vitro and in vivo effects. *Clin Immunol Immunopathol* 1988; 48(2):238–246.

27 Fink G, Mittelman M, Shohat B, Spitzer SA. Theophylline-induced alterations in cellular immunity in asthmatic patients. *Clin Allergy* 1987; 17(4):313–316.

28 Guillou PJ, Ramsden C, Kerr M, Davison AM, Giles GR. A prospective controlled clinical trial of aminophylline as an adjunctive immunosuppressive agent. *Transpl Proc* 1984; 16(5):1218–1220.

29 Gonzalez MC, Diaz P, Galleguillos FR, Ancic P, Cromwell O, Kay AB. Allergen-induced recruitment of bronchoalveolar helper (OKT4) and suppressor (OKT8) T-cells in asthma. Relative increases in OKT8 cells in single early responders compared with those in late-phase responders. *Am Rev Respir Dis* 1987; 136(3):600–604.

30 Hamid Q, Azzawi M, Ying S et al. Expression of mRNA for interleukin-5 in mucosal bronchial biopsies from asthma. *J Clin Invest* 1991; 87(5):1541–1546.

31 Jaffar ZH, Sullivan P, Page CP, Costello J. Low-dose theophylline modulates T-lymphocyte activation in allergen-challenged asthmatics. *Eur Respir J* 1996; 9:456–462.

32 Brenner M, Berkowitz R, Marshall N, Strunk RC. Need for theophylline in severe steroid-requiring asthmatics. *Clin Allergy* 1988; 18(2):143–150.

33 Finnerty JP, Lee C, Wilson S, Madden J, Djukanovic R, Holgate ST. Effects of theophylline on inflammatory cells and cytokines in asthmatic subjects: a placebo-controlled parallel group study. *Eur Respir J* 1996; 9:1672–1677.

34 Mascali JJ, Cvietusa P, Negri J, Borish L. Anti-inflammatory effects of theophylline: modulation of cytokine production. *Ann Allergy Asthma Immunol* 1996; 77(1):34–38.

35 Punnonen J, Punnonen K, Jansen CT, Kalimo K. Interferon (IFN)-alpha, IFN-gamma, interleukin (IL)-2, and arachidonic acid metabolites modulate IL-4-induced IgE synthesis similarly in healthy persons and in atopic dermatitis patients. *Allergy* 1993; 48(3):189–195.

36 Enk AH, Angeloni VL, Udey MC, Katz SI. Inhibition of Langerhans cell antigen-presenting function by IL-10. A role for IL-10 in induction of tolerance. *J Immunol* 1993; 151(5):2390–2398.

37 Yamaguchi Y, Hayashi Y, Sugama Y et al. Highly purified murine interleukin 5 (IL-5) stimulates eosinophil function and prolongs in vitro survival. IL-5 as an eosinophil chemotactic factor. *J Exp Med* 1988; 167(5):1737–1742.

38 Yasui K, Hu B, Nakazawa T, Agematsu K, Komiyama A. Theophylline accelerates human granulocyte apoptosis not via phosphodiesterase inhibition. *J Clin Invest* 1997; 100(7):1677–1684.

39 Ohta K, Yamashita N. Apoptosis of eosinophils and lymphocytes in allergic inflammation. *J Allergy Clin Immunol* 1999; 104(1):14–21.

40 Kosmas EN, Michaelides SA, Polychronaki A et al.

Theophylline induces a reduction in circulating inter-
leukin-4 and interleukin-5 in atopic asthmatics [In Process
Citation]. *Eur Respir J* 1999; 13(1):53–58.

41 Spina D, Landells LJ, Page CP. The role of phosphodieste-
rase isoenzymes in health and in atopic disease. In: August
T, ed. *Advances in Pharmacology*. San Diego: Academic
Press Inc; 1998: 33–89.

42 Barnes PJ, Pauwels RA. Theophylline in the management of
asthma: time for reappraisal? *Eur Respir J* 1994;
7(3):579–591.

43 Banner KH, Page C. Prostaglandins contribute to the anti-
proliferative effect of isoenzyme selective phosphodiesterase 4 inhibitors but not theophylline in human
mononuclear cells. *Br J Pharmacol* 1997; 120.

44 Peterson TC, Slysz G, Isbrucker R. The inhibitory effect of
ursodeoxycholic acid and pentoxifylline on platelet
derived growth factor-stimulated proliferation is distinct
from an effect by cyclic AMP. *Immunopharmacology* 1998;
39(3):181–191.

45 Persson CG, Pauwels R. Pharmacology of anti-asthma xanthines. In Page C, Barnes, PJ, eds London: Academic Press.
Pharmacology of Asthma 1989; 7, 207–225.

46 Feoktistov I, Biaggioni I. Adenosine A_{2B} receptors evoke
interleukin-8 secretion in human mast cells. An enpro-
fylline-sensitive mechanism with implications for asthma.
J Clin Invest 1995; 96(4):1979–1986.

47 Feoktistov I, Polosa R, Holgate ST, Biaggioni I. Adenosine
A2B receptors: a novel therapeutic target in asthma? *Trends
Pharmacol Sci* 1998; 19(4):148–153.

48 Cushley MJ, Tattersfield AE, Holgate ST. Inhaled adenosine
and guanosine on airway resistance in normal and asthmatic subjects. *Br J Clin Pharmacol* 1983; 15(2):161–165.

49 Cushley MJ, Tattersfield AE, Holgate ST. Adenosine-
induced bronchoconstriction in asthma. Antagonism by
inhaled theophylline. *Am Rev Respir Dis* 1984;
129(3):380–384.

50 Mann JS, Holgate ST. Specific antagonism of adenosine-
induced bronchoconstriction in asthma by oral theophylline. *Br J Clin Pharmacol* 1985; 19(5):685–692.

51 el Hashim A, D'Agostino B, Matera MG, Page C.
Characterization of adenosine receptors involved in
adenosine-induced bronchoconstriction in allergic
rabbits. *Br J Pharmacol* 1996; 119(6):1262–1268.

52 Ali S, Mustafa SJ, Metzger WJ. Adenosine receptor-mediated bronchoconstriction and bronchial hyperresponsiveness in allergic rabbit model. *Am J Physiol* 1994; 266(3 Pt
1):L271–L277.

53 Nyce JW, Metzger WJ. DNA antisense therapy for asthma in
an animal model. *Nature* 1997; 385(6618):721–725.

54 Yasui K, Agematsu K, Shinozaki K, Hokibara S, Nagumo H,
Nakazawa T et al. Theophylline induces neutrophil apop-
tosis through adenosine A2A receptor antagonism. *J
Leukoc Biol* 2000; 67(4):529–535.

55 Ezeamuzie CI. Involvement of A(3) receptors in the potentiation by adenosine of the inhibitory effect of theophylline
on human eosinophil degranulation: possible novel mechanism of the anti-inflammatory action of theophylline.
Biochem Pharmacol 2001; 61(12):1551–1559.

56 Landells LJ, Jensen MW, Orr LM, Spina D, O'Connor BJ,
Page CP. The role of adenosine receptors in the action of
theophylline on human peripheral blood mononuclear
cells from healthy and asthmatic subjects. *Br J Pharmacol*
2000; 129(6):1140–1144.

57 Kraft M, Torvik JA, Trudeau JB, Wenzel SE, Martin RJ.
Theophylline: potential antiinflammatory effects in nocturnal asthma. *J Allergy Clin Immunol* 1996; 97(6):1242–1246.

58 D'Alonzo GE, Smolensky MH, Feldman S, Gianotti LA,
Emerson MB, Staudinger H et al. Twenty-four hour lung
function in adult patients with asthma. Chronoptimized
theophylline therapy once-daily dosing in the evening
versus conventional twice-daily dosing. *Am Rev Respir Dis*
1990; 142(1):84–90.

59 Nielson CP, Crowley JJ, Morgan ME, Vestal RE.
Polymorphonuclear leukocyte inhibition by therapeutic
concentrations of theophylline is mediated by cyclic-3′,5′-
adenosine monophosphate. *Am Rev Respir Dis* 1988;
137(1):25–30.

60 Nielson CP, Crowley JJ, Cusack BJ, Vestal RE. Therapeutic
concentrations of theophylline and enprofylline potentiate catecholamine effects and inhibit leukocyte activation. *J Allergy Clin Immunol* 1986; 78(4 Pt 1):660–667.

61 Magnussen H, Reuss G, Jorres R. Theophylline has a dose-
related effect on the airway response to inhaled histamine
and methacholine in asthmatics. *Am Rev Respir Dis* 1987;
136(5):1163–1167.

62 Page CP, Cotter T, Kilfeather S, Sullivan P, Spina D, Costello
JF. Effect of chronic theophylline treatment on the
methacholine dose-response curve in allergic asthmatic
subjects. *Euro Respir J* 1998; 12(1):24–29.

63 Bel EH, Timmers MC, Zwinderman AH, Dijkman JH, Sterk
PJ. The effect of inhaled corticosteroids on the maximal
degree of airway narrowing to methacholine in asthmatic
subjects. *Am Rev Respir Dis* 1991; 143(1):109–113.

64 Bel EH, Zwinderman AH, Timmers MC, Dijkman JH, Sterk
PJ. The protective effect of a beta 2 agonist against excessive airway narrowing in response to bronchoconstrictor
stimuli in asthma and chronic obstructive lung disease.
Thorax 1991; 46(1):9–14.

65 Evans DJ, Taylor DA, Zetterstrom O, Chung KF, O'Connor BJ, Barnes PJ. A comparison of low-dose inhaled budesonide plus theophylline and high-dose inhaled budesonide for moderate asthma. *N Engl J Med* 1997; 337:1412–1418.

66 Ukena D, Harnest U, Sakalauskas R et al. Comparison of addition of theophylline to inhaled steroid with doubling of the dose of inhaled steroid in asthma. *Eur Respir J* 1997; 10:2754–2760.

67 Rivington RN, Boulet LP, Cote J, Kreisman H, Small DI, Alexander M et al. Efficacy of Uniphyl, salbutamol, and their combination in asthmatic patients on high-dose inhaled steroids. *Am J Respir Crit Care Med* 1995; 151(2 Pt 1):325–332.

68 Tinkelman DG, Reed CE, Nelson HS, Offord KP. Aerosol beclomethasone dipropionate compared with theophylline as primary treatment of chronic, mild to moderately severe asthma in children. *Pediatrics* 1993; 92(1):64–77.

69 Kelloway JS, Wyatt RA, Adlis SA. Comparison of patients' compliance with prescribed oral and inhaled asthma medications. *Arch Intern Med* 1994; 154(12):1349–1352.

70 Barnes PJ, Jonsson B, Klim JB. The costs of asthma. *Eur Respir J* 1996; 9(4):636–642.

71 Peachell PT, Undem BJ, Schleimer RP et al. Preliminary identification and role of phosphodiesterase isozymes in human basophils. *J Immunol* 1992; 148(8):2503–2510.

72 Gleich GJ. Mechanisms of eosinophil-associated inflammation. *J Allergy Clin Immunol* 2000; 105:651–663.

73 Romagnani S. The role of lymphocytes in allergic disease. *J Allergy Clin Immunol* 2000; 105:399–408.

74 Kemeny DM, Vyas B, Vukmanovic-Stejic M et al. CD8 + T cell subsets and chronic obstructive pulmonary disease. *Am J Respir Crit Care Med* 1999; 160:S33–S37.

75 Saetta M. Airway inflammation in chronic obstructive pulmonary disease. *Am J Respir Crit Care Med* 1999; 160:S17–S20.

76 Bousquet J, Jeffery PK, Busse WW, Johnson M, Vignola AM. Asthma – from bronchoconstriction to airways inflammation and remodeling. *Am J Respir Crit Care Med* 2000; 161(5):1720–1745.

77 Jeffery PK. Structural and inflammatory changes in COPD: a comparison with asthma. *Thorax* 1998; 53:129–136.

78 Parker CW, Kennedy S, Eisen AZ. Leukocyte and lymphocyte cyclic AMP responses in atopic eczema. *J Invest Dermatol* 1977; 68(5):302–306.

79 Archer CB, Morley J, MacDonald DM. Impaired lymphocyte cyclic adenosine monophosphate responses in atopic eczema. *Br J Dermatol* 1983; 109(5):559–564.

80 Safko MJ, Chan SC, Cooper KD, Hanifin JM. Heterologous desensitization of leukocytes: a possible mechanism of beta adrenergic blockade in atopic dermatitis. *J Allergy Clin Immunol* 1981; 68(3):218–225.

81 Grewe SR, Chan SC, Hanifin JM. Elevated leukocyte cyclic AMP-phosphodiesterase in atopic disease: a possible mechanism for cyclic AMP-agonist hyporesponsiveness. *J Allergy Clin Immunol* 1982; 70(6):452–457.

82 Chan SC, Reifsnyder D, Beavo JA, Hanifin JM. Immunochemical characterization of the distinct monocyte cyclic AMP-phosphodiesterase from patients with atopic dermatitis. *J Allergy Clin Immunol* 1993; 91(6):1179–1188.

83 Gantner F, Tenor H, Gekeler V, Schudt C, Wendel A, Hatzelmann A. Phosphodiesterase profiles of highly purified human peripheral blood leukocyte populations from normal and atopic individuals: a comparative study. *J Allergy Clin Immunol* 1997; 100(4):527–535.

84 Hanifin JM, Chan SC. Monocyte phosphodiesterase abnormalities and dysregulation of lymphocyte function in atopic dermatitis. *J Invest Dermatol* 1995; 105:84S-88S.

85 Giustina TA, Chan SC, Thiel ML, Baker JW, Hanifin JM. Increased leukocyte sensitivity to phosphodiesterase inhibitors in atopic dermatitis: tachyphylaxis after theophylline therapy. *J Allergy Clin Immunol* 1984; 74(3 Pt 1):252–257.

86 Hanifin JM, Chan SC, Cheng JB et al. Type 4 phosphodiesterase inhibitors have clinical and in vitro anti-inflammatory effects in atopic dermatitis. *J Invest Dermatol* 1996; 107:51–56.

87 Banner KH, Roberts NM, Page CP. Differential effect of phosphodiesterase 4 inhibitors on the proliferation of human peripheral blood mononuclear cells from normals and subjects with atopic dermatitis. *Br J Pharmacol* 1995; 116:3169–3174.

88 Souness JE, Scott LC. Stereospecificity of rolipram actions on eosinophil cyclic AMP-specific phosphodiesterase. *Biochem J* 1993; 291(Pt 2):389–395.

89 O'Connell JC, McCallum JF, McPhee I et al. The SH3 domain of Src tyrosyl protein kinase interacts with the N-terminal splice region of the PDE4A cAMP-specific phosphodiesterase RPDE-6 (RNPDE4A5). *Biochem J* 1996; 318:255–262.

90 Stawiski MA, Rusin LJ, Burns TL, Weinstein GD, Voorhees JJ. Ro 20–1724: an agent that significantly improves psoriatic lesions in double-blind clinical trials. *J Invest Dermatol* 1979; 73(4):261–263.

91 Koeter GH, Meurs H, Kauffman HF, de Vries K. The role of the adrenergic system in allergy and bronchial hyperreactivity. *Eur J Respir Dis* Suppl 1982; 121:72–78.

92 Meurs H, Koeter GH, de Vries K, Kauffman HF. The beta-adrenergic system and allergic bronchial asthma: changes in lymphocyte beta-adrenergic receptor number and adenylate cyclase activity after an allergen-induced asthmatic attack. *J Allergy Clin Immunol* 1982; 70(4):272–280.

93 Bachelet M, Vincent D, Havet N et al. Reduced responsiveness of adenylate cyclase in alveolar macrophages from patients with asthma. *J Allergy Clin Immunol* 1991; 88(3 Pt 1):322–328.

94 Beusenberg FD, Van Amsterdam JGC, Hoogsteden HC et al. Stimulation of cyclic AMP production in human alveolar macrophages induced by inflammatory mediators and beta-sympathomimetic. *Eur J Pharmacol-Environ Toxicol Pharmacol* Section 1992; 228(1):57–62.

95 Tenor H, Staniciu L, Schudt C, Hatzelmann A, Wendel A, Djukanovic R et al. Cyclic nucleotide phosphodiesterases from purified human CD4+ and CD8+ T lymphocytes. *Clin Exp Allergy* 1995; 25(7):616–624.

96 Tenor H, Hatzelmann A, Church MK, Schudt C, Shute JK. Effects of theophylline and rolipram on leukotriene C4 (LTC4) synthesis and chemotaxis of human eosinophils from normal and atopic subjects. *Br J Pharmacol* 1996; 118:1727–1735.

97 Aloui R, Gormand F, Prigent AF, PerrinFayolle M, Pacheco Y. Increased respiratory burst and phosphodiesterase activity in alveolar eosinophils in chronic eosinophilic pneumonia. *Eur Respir J* 1996; 9:377–379.

98 Landells LJ, Spina D, Souness JE, O'Connor BJ, Page CP. A biochemical and functional assessment of monocyte phosphodiesterase activity in healthy and asthmatic subjects. *Pulm Pharmacol Ther* 2000; 13(5):231–239.

99 Sawai T, Ikai K, Uehara M. Cyclic adenosine monophosphate phosphodiesterase activity in peripheral blood mononuclear leukocytes from patients with atopic dermatitis: correlation with respiratory atopy. *Br J Dermatol* 1998; 138:846–848.

100 Busse WW, Anderson CL. The granulocyte response to the phosphodiesterase inhibitor RO 20–1724 in asthma. *J Allergy Clin Immunol* 1981; 67(1):70–74.

101 Essayan DM, Huang SK, Undem BJ, Kagey S, Lichtenstein LM. Modulation of antigen- and mitogen-induced proliferative responses of peripheral blood mononuclear cells by nonselective and isozyme selective cyclic nucleotide phosphodiesterase inhibitors. *J Immunol* 1994; 153(8):3408–3416.

102 Crocker IC, Townley RG, Khan MM. Phosphodiesterase inhibitors suppress proliferation of peripheral blood mononuclear cells and interleukin-4 and -5 secretion by human T-helper type 2 cells. *Immunopharmacology* 1996; 31:223–235.

103 Crocker IC, Ohia SE, Church MK, Townley RG. Phosphodiesterase type 4 inhibitors, but not glucocorticoids, are more potent in suppression of cytokine secretion by mononuclear cells from atopic than nonatopic donors. *J Allergy Clin Immunol* 1998; 102:797–804.

104 Landells LJ, Szilagy CM, Jones NA et al. Identification and quantification of phosphodiesterase 4 subtypes in CD4 and CD8 lymphocytes from healthy and asthmatic subjects. *Br J Pharmacol* 2001; 133(5):722–729.

105 Stief CG. Phosphodiesterase inhibitors in the treatment of erectile dysfunction. *Drugs Today* 2000; 36(2–3):93–99.

106 Obernolte R, Ratzliff J, Baecker PA et al. Multiple splice variants of phosphodiesterase PDE4C cloned from human lung and testis. *Biochem Biophys Acta* 1997; 1353:287–297.

107 Jacobitz S, McLaughlin MM, Livi GP, Burman M, Torphy TJ. Mapping the functional domains of human recombinant phosphodiesterase 4A: structural requirements for catalytic activity and rolipram binding. *Mol Pharmacol* 1996; 50:891–899.

108 Lenhard JM, Kassel DB, Rocque WJ et al. Phosphorylation of a cAMP-specific phosphodiesterase (HSPDE4B2B) by mitogen-activated protein kinase. *Biochem J* 1996; 319:751–758.

109 Rocque WJ, Tian G, Wiseman JS et al. Human recombinant phosphodiesterase 4B2B binds (R)-rolipram at a single site with two affinities. *Biochemistry* 1997; 36:14250–14261.

110 Xu RX, Hassell AM, Vanderwall D et al. Atomic structure of PDE4: insights into phosphodiesterase mechanism a specificity. *Science* 2000; 288:1822–1825.

111 Alvarez R, Sette C, Yang D et al. Activation and selective inhibition of a cyclic AMP-specific phosphodiesterase, PDE-4D3. *Mol Pharmacol* 1995; 48(4):616–622.

112 Sette C, Conti M. Phosphorylation and activation of cAMP-specific phosphodiesterase by the cAMP-dependent protein kinase. *J Biol Chem* 1996; 271:16526–16534.

113 Hoffman R, Baillie GS, MacKenzie SJ, Yarwood SJ, Houslay MD. The MAP kinase ERK2 inhibits the cyclic AMP-specific phosphodiesterase HSPDE3D3 by phosphorylating it at Ser579. *EMBO J* 1999; 18:893–903.

114 MacKenzie SJ, Baillie GS, McPhee I, Bolger GB, Houslay MD. ERK2 mitogen-activated protein kinase binding, phosphorylation, and regulation of the PDE4D cAMP-specific phosphodiesterases. *J Biol Chem* 2000; 275:16609–16617.

115 Sette C, Vicini E, Conti M. The rat PDE3/IVd phosphodiesterase gene codes for muliple proteins differentially activated by cAMP-dependent protein kinase. *J Biol Chem* 1994; 269:18271–18274.

116 Gantner F, Kupferschmidt R, Schudt C, Wendel A, Hatzelmann A. In vitro differentiation of human monocy-

tes to macrophages: Change of PDE profile and its relationship to suppression of tumour necrosis factor-alpha release by PDE inhibitors. *Br J Pharmacol* 1997; 121(2):221–231.

117 Li SH, Chan SC, Toshitani A, Leung DY, Hanifin JM. Synergistic effects of interleukin 4 and interferon-gamma on monocyte phosphodiesterase activity. *J Invest Dermatol* 1992; 99(1):65–70.

118 Li SH, Chan SC, Kramer SM, Hanifin JM. Modulation of leukocyte cyclic AMP phosphodiesterase activity by recombinant interferon-gamma: evidence for a differential effect on atopic monocytes. *J Interferon Res* 1993; 13(3):197–202.

119 DiSanto ME, Glaser KB, Heaslip RJ. Phospholipid regulation of a cyclic AMP-specific phosphodiesterase (PDE4) from U937 cells. *Cell Signal* 1995; 7(8):827–835.

120 Schneider HH, Schmiechen R, Brezinski M, Seidler J. Stereospecific binding of the antidepressant rolipram to brain protein structures. *Eur J Pharmacol* 1986; 127(1–2):105–115.

121 Nemoz G, Moueqqit M, Prigent AF, Pacheco H. Isolation of similar rolipram-inhibitable cyclic-AMP-specific phosphodiesterases from rat-brain and heart. *Eur J Biochem* 1989; 184(3):511–520.

122 Torphy TJ, Stadel JM, Burman M et al. Coexpression of human cAMP-specific phosphodiesterase activity and high affinity rolipram binding in yeast. *J Biol Chem* 1992; 267(3):1798–1804.

123 McLaughlin MM, Cieslinski LB, Burman M, Torphy TJ, Livi GP. A low K(M), rolipram-sensitive, cAMP-specific phosphodiesterase from human brain. Cloning and expression of cDNA, biochemical characterization of recombinant protein, and tissue distribution of messenger-RNA. *J Biol Chem* 1993; 268(9):6470–6476.

124 Owens RJ, Caterall C, Batty D et al. Human phosphodiesterase 4A: characterization of full-length and truncated enzymes expressed in COS cells. *Biochem J* 1997; 326:53–60.

125 Souness JE, Griffin M, Maslen C et al. Evidence that cyclic AMP phosphodiesterase inhibitors suppress TNFα generation from human monocytes by interacting with a 'low-affinity' phosphodiesterase 4 conformer. *Br J Pharmacol* 1996; 118:649–658.

126 Kelly JR, Barnes PJ, Giembycz MA. Phosphodiesterase 4 in macrophages: relationship between cAMP accumulation, suppression of cAMP hydrolysis and inhibition of [³H]R-(-)-rolipram binding by selective inhibitors. *Biochem J* 1996; 318:425–436.

127 Laliberte F, Han Y, Govindaragan A et al. Conformational difference between PDE4 apoenzyme and haloenzyme. *Biochemistry* 2000; 39:6449–6458.

128 Barnette MS, Grous M, Cieslinski LB, Burman M, Christensen SB, Torphy TJ. Inhibitors of phosphodiesterase IV (PDE IV) increase acid secretion in rabbit isolated gastric glands: correlation between function and interaction with a high-affinity rolipram binding site. *J Pharmacol Exp Ther* 1995; 273(3):1396–1402.

129 Duplantier AJ, Biggers MS, Chambers RJ et al. Biarylcarboxylic acids and amides: inhibition of phosphodiesterase type IV versus [3H]rolipram binding activity and their relationship to emesis in the ferret. *J Med Chem* 1996; 39:120–125.

130 Barnette MS, Bartus JO, Burman M et al. Association of the anti-inflammatory activity of phosphodiesterase 4 (PDE4) inhibitors with either inhibition of PDE4 catalytic activity or competition for [³H]rolipram binding. *Biochem Pharmacol* 1996; 51(7):949–956.

131 Souness JE, Houghton C, Sardar N, Withnall MT. Evidence that cyclic AMP phosphodiesterase inhibitors suppress interleukin-2 release from murine splenocytes by interacting with a 'low-affinity' phosphodiesterase 4 conformer. *Br J Pharmacol* 1997; 121(4):743–750.

132 Carpenter DO, Briggs DB, Knox AP, Strominger N. Excitation of area postrema neurones by transmitters, peptides and cyclic nucleotides. *J Neurophysiol* 1988; 59:358–369.

133 Hughes B, Howat D, Lisle H et al. The inhibition of antigen-induced eosinophilia and bronchoconstriction by CDP840, a novel stereo-selective inhibitor of phosphodiesterase type 4. *Br J Pharmacol* 1996; 118:1183–1191.

134 Christensen SB, Guider A, Forster CJ et al. 1,4-Cyclohexanecarboxylates: potent and selective inhibitors of phosphodiesterase 4 for the treatment of asthma. *J Med Chem* 1998; 41(6):821–835.

135 Harbinson PL, MacLeod D, Hawksworth R et al. The effect of a novel orally active selective PDE4 isoenzyme inhibitor (CDP840) on allergen-induced responses in asthmatic subjects. *Eur Respir J* 1997; 10(5):1008–1014.

136 Torphy TJ, Barnette MS, Underwood DC et al. Ariflow™ (SB 207499), a second generation phosphodiesterase 4 inhibitor for the treatment of asthma and COPD: from concept to clinic. *Pulm Pharmacol Ther* 1999; 12:131–135.

137 Barnette MS, Christensen SB, Essayan DM et al. SB 207499 (Ariflo), a potent and selective second-generation phosphodiesterase 4 inhibitor: in vitro anti-inflammatory actions. *J Pharmacol Exp Ther* 1998; 284(1):420–426.

138 Manning CD, Burman M, Christensen SB et al. Suppression of human inflammatory cell function by subtype-selective PDE4 inhibitors correlates with inhibition of PDE4A and PDE4B. *Br J Pharmacol* 1999; 128(7):1393–1398.

139 Hersperger R, Bray-French K, Mazzoni L, Muller T.

Palladium-catalyzed cross-coupling reactions for the synthesis of 6, 8-disubstituted 1,7-naphthyridines: a novel class of potent and selective phosphodiesterase type 4D inhibitors. *J Med Chem* 2000; 43(4):675–682.

140 Jin SL, Richard FJ, Kuo WP, D'Ercole AJ, Conti M. Impaired growth and fertility of cAMP-specific phosphodiesterase PDE4D-deficient mice. *Proc Natl Acad Sci USA* 1999; 96(21):11998–12003.

141 Hansen G, Jin S, Umetsu DT, Conti M. Absence of muscarinic cholinergic airway responses in mice deficient in the cyclic nucleotide phosphodiesterase PDE4D. *Proc Natl Acad Sci USA* 2000; 97(12):6751–6756.

142 Kung TT, Crawley Y, Luo B, Young S, Kreutner W, Chapman RW. Inhibition of pulmonary eosinophilia and airway hyperresponsiveness in allergic mice by rolipram: involvement of endogenously released corticosterone and catecholamines. *Br J Pharmacol* 2000; 130:457–463.

143 Cherry JA, Davis RL. Cyclic AMP phosphodiesterases are localized in regions of the mouse brain associated with reinforcement, movement and affect. *J Comp Neurol* 1999; 407:287–301.

144 Takahashi M, Terwilliger R, Lane C, Mezes PS, Conti M, Duman RS. Chronic antidepressant administration increases the expression of cAMP-specific phosphodiesterase 4A and 4B isoforms. *J Neurosci* 1999; 19:610–618.

145 Lichtenstein LM, Margolis S. Histamine release in vitro: inhibition by catecholamines and methylxanthines. *Science* 1968; 161(844):902–903.

146 Orange RP, Kaliner MA, Laraia PJ, Austen KF. Immunological release of histamine and slow reacting substance of anaphylaxis from human lung. II. Influence of cellular levels of cyclic AMP. *Fed Proc* 1971; 30(6):1725–1729.

147 Frossard N, Landry Y, Pauli G, Ruckstuhl M. Effects of cyclic AMP- and cyclic GMP-phosphodiesterase inhibitors on immunological release of histamine and on lung contraction. *Br J Pharmacol* 1981; 73(4):933–938.

148 Pearce FL, Befus AD, Gauldie J, Bienenstock J. Mucosal mast cells. II. Effects of anti-allergic compounds on histamine secretion by isolated intestinal mast cells. *J Immunol* 1982; 128(6):2481–2486.

149 Louis RE, Radermecker MF. Substance P-induced histamine release from human basophils, skin and lung fragments: effect of nedocromil sodium and theophylline. *Int Arch Allergy Appl Immunol* 1990; 92(4):329–333.

150 Louis R, Bury T, Corhay JL, Radermecker M. LY 186655, a phosphodiesterase inhibitor, inhibits histamine release from human basophils, lung and skin fragments. *Int J Immunopharmacol* 1992; 14(2):191–194.

151 Columbo M, Horowitz EM, McKenzie W, Kagey S, Lichtenstein LM. Pharmacologic control of histamine release from human basophils induced by platelet-activating factor. *Int Arch Allergy Immunol* 1993; 102(4):383–390.

152 Peachell PT, MacGlashan DW, Jr., Lichtenstein LM, Schleimer RP. Regulation of human basophil and lung mast cell function by cyclic adenosine monophosphate. *J Immunol* 1988; 140(2):571–579.

153 Weston MC, Anderson N, Peachell PT. Effects of phosphodiesterase inhibitors on human lung mast cell and basophil function. *Br J Pharmacol* 1997; 121(2):287–295.

154 Shichijo M, Shimizu Y, Hiramatsu K, Inagaki N, Tagaki K, Nagai H. Cyclic AMP-elevating agents inhibit mite-antigen-induced IL-4 and IL-13 release from basophil-enriched leukocyte preparation. *Int Arch Allergy Immunol* 1997; 114(4):348–353.

155 Alfonso A, Estevez M, Louzao MC, Vieytes MR, Botana LM. Determination of phosphodiesterase activity in rat mast cells using the fluorescent cAMP analogue anthraniloyl cAMP. *Cell Signal* 1995; 7(5):513–518.

156 Kleine T, Wicht L, Gagne H et al. Inhibition of IgE-mediated histamine release from human peripheral leukocytes by selective phosphodiesterase inhibitors. *Agents Actions* 1992; 36(3–4):200–206.

157 Weston MC, Peachell PT. Regulation of human mast cell and basophil function by cAMP. *Gen Pharmacol* 1998; 31(5):715–719.

158 Griswold DE, Webb EF, Breton J, White JR, Marshall PJ, Torphy TJ. Effect of selective phosphodiesterase type IV inhibitor, rolipram, on fluid and cellular phases of inflammatory response. *Inflammation* 1993; 17(3):333–344.

159 Columbo M, Botana LM, Horowitz EM, Lichtenstein LM, MacGlashan DW, Jr. Studies of the intracellular Ca2 + levels in human adult skin mast cells activated by the ligand for the human c-kit receptor and anti-IgE. *Biochem Pharmacol* 1994; 47(12):2137–2145.

160 Nagai H, Takeda H, Iwama T, Yamaguchi S, Mori H. Studies on anti-allergic action of AH 21–132, a novel isozyme-selective phosphodiesterase inhibitor in airways. *Jap J Pharmacol* 1995; 67:149–156.

161 Bessler H, Gilgal R, Djaldetti M, Zahavi I. Effect of pentoxifylline on the phagocytic activity, cAMP levels, and superoxide anion production by monocytes and polymorphonuclear cells. *J Leukoc Biol* 1986; 40(6):747–754.

162 Carletto A, Biasi D, Bambara LM et al. Studies of skin-window exudate human neutrophils: increased resistance to pentoxifylline of the respiratory burst in primed cells. *Inflammation* 1997; 21(2):191–203.

163 Yasui K, Agematsu K, Shinozaki K et al. Effects of theophylline on human eosinophil functions: comparative study with neutrophil functions. *J Leukoc Biol* 2000; 68(2):194–200.

164 Rivkin I, Neutze JA. Influence of cyclic nucleotides and a phosphodiesterase inhibitor on in vitro human blood neutrophil chemotaxis. *Arch Int Pharmacodyn Ther* 1977; 228(2):196–204.

165 Harvath L, Robbins JD, Russell AA, Seamon KB. cAMP and human neutrophil chemotaxis. Elevation of cAMP differentially affects chemotactic responsiveness. *J Immunol* 1991; 146(1):224–232.

166 Ferretti ME, Spisani S, Pareschi MC et al. Two new formylated peptides able to activate chemotaxis and respiratory burst selectively as tools for studying human neutrophil responses. *Cell Signal* 1994; 6(1):91–101.

167 Elferink JG, Huizinga TW, de-Koster BM. The effect of pentoxifylline on human neutrophil migration: a possible role for cyclic nucleotides. *Biochem Pharmacol* 1997; 54(4):475–480.

168 Schmeichel CJ, Thomas LL. Methylxanthine bronchodilators potentiate multiple human neutrophil functions. *J Immunol* 1987; 138(6):1896–1903.

169 Franzini E, Sellak H, Babin CC, Hakim J, Pasquier C. Effects of pentoxifylline on the adherence of polymorphonuclear neutrophils to oxidant-stimulated human endothelial cells: involvement of cyclic AMP. *J Cardiovasc Pharmacol* 1995; 25 Suppl 2:S92–S95.

170 Spoelstra FM, Berends C, Dijkhuizen B, De Monchy JGR, Kauffman HF. Effect of theophylline on CD11b and L-selectin expression and density of eosinophils and neutrophils in vitro. *Euro Respir J* 1998; 12(3):585–591.

171 Paul E, Pene J, Bousquet J, Dugas B. Role of cyclic nucleotides and nitric oxide in blood mononuclear cell IgE production stimulated by IL-4. *Cytokine* 1995; 7(1):64–69.

172 Jones NA, Page C, Lever R. The effect of selective phosphodiesterase (PDE) isoenzyme inhibition on F-Met-Leu-Phe (fMLP) and tumor necrosis factor-alpha induced human neutrophil elastase release. *Am J Resp Crit Care Med* 163. 2001.

173 Fonteh AN, Winkler JD, Torphy TJ, Heravi J, Undem BJ, Chilton FH. Influence of isoproterenol and phosphodiesterase inhibitors on platelet-activating factor biosynthesis in the human neutrophil. *J Immunol* 1993; 151(1):339–350.

174 Bloemen PG, van-den-Tweel MC, Henricks PA et al. Increased cAMP levels in stimulated neutrophils inhibit their adhesion to human bronchial epithelial cells. *Am J Physiol* 1997; 272(4 Pt 1):L580–L587.

175 Derian CK, Santulli RJ, Rao PE, Solomon HF, Barrett JA. Inhibition of chemotactic peptide-induced neutrophil adhesion to vascular endothelium by cAMP modulators. *J Immunol* 1995; 154(1):308–317.

176 Rossi AG, Cousin JM, Dransfield I, Lawson MF, Chilvers ER, Haslett C. Agents that elevate cAMP inhibit human neutrophil apoptosis. *Biochem Biophys Res Commun* 1995; 217(3):892–899.

177 Ottonello L, Gonella R, Dapino P, Sacchetti C, Dallegri F. Prostaglandin E2 inhibits apoptosis in human neutrophilic polymorphonuclear leukocytes: role of intracellular cyclic AMP levels. *Exp Hematol* 1998; 26(9):895–902.

178 Niwa M, Hara A, Kanamori Y, Matsuno H, Kozawa O, Yoshimi N et al. Inhibition of tumor necrosis factor-alpha induced neutrophil apoptosis by cyclic AMP: involvement of caspase cascade. *Eur J Pharmacol* 1999; 371(1):59–67.

179 Nourshargh S, Hoult JR. Inhibition of human neutrophil degranulation by forskolin in the presence of phosphodiesterase inhibitors. *Eur J Pharmacol* 1986; 122(2):205–212.

180 Nielson CP, Vestal RE, Sturm RJ, Heaslip R. Effects of selective phosphodiesterase inhibitors on the polymorphonuclear leukocyte respiratory burst. *J Allergy Clin Immunol* 1990; 86(5):801–808.

181 Schudt C, Winder S, Forderkunz S, Hatzelmann A, Ullrich V. Influence of selective phosphodiesterase inhibitors on human neutrophil functions and levels of cAMP and Cai. *Naunyn-Schmiedeberg's Arch Pharmacol* 1991; 344(6):682–690.

182 Schudt C, Winder S, Eltze M, Kilian U, Beume R. Zardaverine: a cyclic AMP specific PDE III/IV inhibitor. *Agents Actions* Suppl 1991; 34:379–402.

183 Muller T, Engels P, Fozard JR. Subtypes of the type 4 cAMP phosphodiesterases: structure, regulation and selective inhibition. *Trends Pharmacol Sci* 1996; 17:294–298.

184 Wang P, Wu P, Ohleth KM, Egan R, Billah MM. Phosphodiesterase 4B2 is the predominant phosphodiesterase species and undergoes differential regulation of gene expression in human monocytes and neutrophils. *Mol Pharmacol* 1999; 56:170–174.

185 Prigent AF, Fonlupt P, Dubois M et al. Cyclic nucleotide phosphodiesterases and methyltransferases in purified lymphocytes, monocytes and polymorphonuclear leucocytes from healthy donors and asthmatic patients. *Eur J Clin Invest* 1990; 20(3):323–329.

186 Wright CD, Kuipers PJ, Kobylarz S, Devall LJ, Klinkefus BA, Weishaar RE. Differential inhibition of human neutrophil functions. Role of cyclic AMP-specific, cyclic GMP-insensitive phosphodiesterase. *Biochem Pharmacol* 1990; 40(4):699–707.

187 Ottonello L, Morone P, Dapino P, Dallegri F. Inhibitory effect of salmeterol on the respiratory burst of adherent human neutrophils. *Clin Exp Immunol* 1996; 106(1):97–102.

188 Cortijo J, Villagrasa V, Navarrete C et al. Effects of SCA40 on human isolated bronchus and human polymorphonuclear leukocytes: comparison with rolipram, SKF94120 and levcromakalim. *Br J Pharmacol* 1996; 119(1):99–106.

189 Au BT, Teixeira MM, Collins PD, Williams TJ. Effect of PDE4 inhibitors on zymosan-induced IL-8 release from human neutrophils: synergism with prostanoids and salbutamol. *Br J Pharmacol* 1998; 123(6):1260–1266.

190 Mikawa K, Akamatsu H, Nishina K et al. The effect of phosphodiesterase III inhibitors on human neutrophil function. *Crit Care Med* 2000; 28(4):1001–1005.

191 Dent G, Giembycz MA, Rabe KF, Barnes PJ. Inhibition of eosinophil cyclic nucleotide PDE activity and opsonised zymosan-stimulated respiratory burst by 'type IV'-selective PDE inhibitors. *Br J Pharmacol* 1991; 103(2):1339–1346.

192 Hatzelmann A, Tenor H, Schudt C. Differential effects of non-selective and selective phosphodiesterase inhibitors on human eosinophil functions. *Br J Pharmacol* 1995; 114(4):821–831.

193 Hossain M, Okubo Y, Sekiguchi M. Effects of various drugs (staurosporine, herbimycin A, ketotifen, theophylline, FK506 and cyclosporin A) on eosinophil viability. *Arerugi* 1994; 43(6):711–717.

194 Kita H, Abu G, Gleich GJ, Abraham RT. Regulation of Ig-induced eosinophil degranulation by adenosine 3',5'-cyclic monophosphate. *J Immunol* 1991; 146(8):2712–2718.

195 Shute JK, Tenor H, Church MK, Holgate ST. Theophylline inhibits the release of eosinophil survival cytokines - Is Raf-1 the protein kinase A target? *Clin Exp Allergy*, Suppl 1998; 28(3):47–52.

196 Sagara H, Fuiuda T, Okada T, Ishikawa A, Makino S. Theophylline at therapeutic concentration suppresses PAF-induced upregulation of Mac-1 on human eosinophils. *Clin Exp Allergy* Suppl 1996; 26:16–21.

197 Momose T, Okubo Y, Horie S, Suzuki J, Isobe M, Sekiguchi M. Effects of intracellular cyclic AMP modulators on human eosinophil survival, degranulation and CD11b expression. *Int Arch Allergy Immunol* 1998; 117(2):138–145.

198 Souness JE, Maslen C, Webber S et al. Suppression of eosinophil function by RP 73401, a potent and selective inhibitor of cyclic AMP-specific phosphodiesterase: comparison with rolipram. *Br J Pharmacol* 1995; 115(1):39–46.

199 Dent G, Giembycz MA, Evans PM, Rabe KF, Barnes PJ.

Suppression of human eosinophil respiratory burst and cyclic AMP hydrolysis by inhibitors of type IV phosphodiesterase: interaction with the beta adrenoceptor agonist albuterol. *J Pharmacol Exp Ther* 1994; 271(3):1167–1174.

200 Hadjokas NE, Crowley JJ, Bayer CR, Nielson CP. beta-Adrenergic regulation of the eosinophil respiratory burst as detected by lucigenin-dependent luminescence. *J Allergy Clin Immunol* 1995; 95:735–741.

201 Nicholson CD, Shahid M, Bruin J et al. Characterization of ORG 20241, a combined phosphodiesterase IV/III cyclic nucleotide phosphodiesterase inhibitor for asthma. *J Pharmacol Exp Ther* 1995; 274(2):678–687.

202 Cohan VL, Showell HJ, Fisher DA et al. In vitro pharmacology of the novel phosphodiesterase type 4 inhibitor, CP-80633. *J Pharmacol Exp Ther* 1996; 278:1356–1361.

203 Ezeamuzie CI. Requirement of additional adenylate cyclase activation for the inhibition of human eosinophil degranulation by phosphodiesterase IV inhibitors. *Eur J Pharmacol* 2001; 417(1–2):11–18.

204 Souness JE, Villamil ME, Scott LC, Tomkinson A, Giembycz MA, Raeburn D. Possible role of cyclic AMP phosphodiesterases in the actions of ibudilast on eosinophil thromboxane generation and airways smooth muscle tone. *Br J Pharmacol* 1994; 111(4):1081–1088.

205 Kaneko T, Alvarez R, Ueki IF, Nadel JA. Elevated intracellular cyclic AMP inhibits chemotaxis in human eosinophils. *Cell Signal* 1995; 7(5):527–534.

206 Alves AC, Pires ALA, Cruz HN, Serra MF, Diaz BL, Cordeiro RSB et al. Selective inhibition of phosphodiesterase type IV suppresses the chemotactic responsiveness of rat eosinophils in vitro. *Eur J Pharmacol* 1996; 312:89–96.

207 Alves AC, Pires AL, Lagente V, Cordeiro RS, Martins MA, Silva PM. Effect of selective phosphodiesterase inhibitors on the rat eosinophil chemotactic response in vitro. *Mem Inst Oswaldo* Cruz 1997; 92 Suppl 2:201–204.

208 Santamaria LF, Palacios JM, Beleta J. Inhibition of eotaxin-mediated human eosinophil activation and migration by the selective cyclic nucleotide phosphodiesterase type 4 inhibitor rolipram. *Br J Pharmacol* 1997; 121(6):1150–1154.

209 Blease K, Burke-Gaffney A., Hellewell PG. Modulation of cell adhesion molecule expression and function on human lung microvascular endothelial cells by inhibition of phosphodiesterases 3 and 4. *Br J Pharmacol* 1998; 124(1):229–237.

210 Hallsworth MP, Giembycz MA, Barnes PJ, Lee TH. Cyclic AMP-elevating agents prolong or inhibit eosinophil survival depending on prior exposure to GM-CSF. *Br J Pharmacol* 1996; 117:79–86.

211 Kammer GM. The adenylate cyclase-cAMP-protein kinase

A pathway and regulation of the immune response. *Immunol Today* 1988; 9(7–8):222–229.

212 Scherer LJ, Diamond RA, Rothenberg EV. Developmental regulation of cAMP signaling pathways in thymocyte development. *Thymus* 1994; 23:231–257.

213 van der Pouw K, Boeije LC, Smeenk RJ, Wijdenes J, Aarden LA. Prostaglandin-E2 is a potent inhibitor of human interleukin 12 production. *J Exp Med* 1995; 181(2):775–779.

214 Hidi R, Timmermans S, Liu E et al. Phosphodiesterase and cyclic adenosine monophosphate-dependent inhibition of T-lymphocyte chemotaxis. *Eur Respir J* 2000; 15(2):342–349.

215 Banner KH, Harbinson P, Costello JF, Page CP. Effect of PDE inhibitors on the proliferation of human peripheral blood mononuclear cells (HPBM) from mild asthmatics and normals [Abstract]. *Am J Resp Crit Care Med* 1997; 155: A542.

216 Banner KH, Hoult JR, Taylor MN, Landells LJ, Page CP. Possible contribution of prostaglandin E2 to the antiproliferative effect of phosphodiesterase 4 inhibitors in human mononuclear cells. *Biochem Pharmacol* 1999; 58(9):1487–1495.

217 Mary D, Aussel C, Ferrua B, Fehlmann M. Regulation of interleukin 2 synthesis by cAMP in human T cells. *J Immunol* 1987; 139(4):1179–1184.

218 Hancock WW, Pleau ME, Kobzik L. Recombinant granulocyte-macrophage colony-stimulating factor down-regulates expression of IL-2 receptor on human mononuclear phagocytes by induction of prostaglandin E. *J Immunol* 1988; 140(9):3021–3025.

219 Lidington E, Nohammer C, Dominguez M, Ferry B, Rose ML. Inhibition of the transendothelial migration of human lymphocytes but not monocytes by phosphodiesterase inhibitors. *Clin Exp Immunol* 1996; 104:66–71.

220 Shore A, Dosch H, Gelfand EW. Induction and separation of antigen-dependent T helper and T suppressor cells in man. *Nature* 1978; 274(5671):586–587.

221 Rott O, Cash E, Fleischer B. Phosphodiesterase inhibitor pentoxifylline, a selective suppressor of T helper type 1- but not type 2-associated lymphokine production, prevents induction of experimental autoimmune encephalomyelitis in Lewis rats. *Eur J Immunol* 1993; 23(8):1745–1751.

222 Rieckmann P, Weber F, Gunther A et al. Pentoxifylline, a phosphodiesterase inhibitor, induces immune deviation in patients with multiple sclerosis. *J Neuroimmunol* 1996; 64(2):193–200.

223 Heinkelein M, SchneiderSchaulies J, Walker BD, Jassoy C. Inhibition of cytotoxicity and cytokine release of CD8 + HIV-specific cytotoxic T lymphocytes by pentoxifylline. *J Acq Immune Def Syn Hum Retrovirol* 1995; 10:417–424.

224 Bruynzeel I, Van der Raaij LMH, Willemze R, Stoof TJ. Pentoxifylline inhibits human T-cell adhesion to dermal endothelial cells. *Arch Dermatol Res* 1997; 289(4):189–193.

225 Schmidt J, Hatzelmann A, Fleissner S, Heimann W, Lindstaedt R, Szelenyi I. Effect of phosphodiesterase inhibition on IL-4 and IL-5 production of the murine TH2-type T cell clone D10.G4.1. *Immunopharmacology* 1995; 30(3):191–198.

226 Giembycz MA. Phosphodiesterase 4 and tolerance to β_2-adrenoceptor agonists in asthma. *Trends Pharmacol Sci* 1996; 17:331–336.

227 Sheth SB, Chaganti K, Bastepe M et al. Cyclic AMP phosphodiesterases in human lymphocytes. *Br J Haematol* 1997; 99(4):784–789.

228 Ichimura M, Kase H. A new cyclic nucleotide phosphodiesterase isozyme expressed in the T-lymphocyte cell lines. *Biochem Biophys Res Commun* 1993; 193(3):985–990.

229 Bloom TJ, Beavo JA. Identification and tissue-specific expression of PDE7 phosphodiesterase splice variants. *Proc Natl Acad Sci USA* 1996; 93(24):14188–14192.

230 Averill LE, Stein RL, Kammer GM. Control of human T-lymphocyte interleukin-2 production by a cAMP- dependent pathway. *Cell Immunol* 1988; 115(1):88–99.

231 Robicsek SA, Blanchard DK, Djeu JY, Krzanowski JJ, Szentivanyi A, Polson JB. Multiple high-affinity cAMP-phosphodiesterases in human T- lymphocytes. *Biochem Pharmacol* 1991; 42(4):869–877.

232 Essayan DM, Huang SK, Kagey S, Lichtenstein LM. Effects of nonselective and isozyme selective cyclic nucleotide phosphodiesterase inhibitors on antigen-induced cytokine gene expression in peripheral blood mononuclear cells. *Am J Respir Cell Mol Biol* 1995; 13(6):692–702.

233 Schudt C, Tenor H, Hatzelmann A. PDE isoenzymes as targets for anti-asthma drugs. *Eur Respir J* 1995; 8(7):1179–1183.

234 Essayan DM, Kagey-Sobotka A, Lichtenstein LM, Huang S-K. Differential regulation of human antigen-specific Th1 and Th2 lymphocyte responses by isozyme selective cyclic nucleotide phosphodiesterase inhibitors. *J Pharmacol Exp Therap* 1997; 282(1):505–512.

235 Marcoz P, Prigent AF, Lagarde M, Nemoz G. Modulation of rat thymocyte proliferative response through the inhibition of different cyclic nucleotide phosphodiesterase isoforms by means of selective inhibitors and cGMP-elevating agents. *Mol Pharmacol* 1993; 44(5):1027–1035.

236 Moodley I, Sotsios Y, Bertin B. Modulation of oxazolone-induced hypersensitivity in mice by selective PDE inhibitors. *Mediators Inflammation* 1995; 4:112–116.

237 Li L, Yee C, Beavo JA. CD3- and CD28-dependent induction

of PDE7 required for T cell activation. *Science* 1999; 283(5403):848–849.

238 Munoz E, Zubiaga AM, Merrow M, Sauter NP, Huber BT. Cholera toxin discriminates between T helper 1 and 2 cells in T cell receptor-mediated activation: role of cAMP in T cell proliferation. *J Exp Med* 1990; 172(1):95–103.

239 Novak TJ, Rothenberg EV. cAMP inhibits induction of interleukin 2 but not of interleukin 4 in T cells. *Proc Natl Acad Sci USA* 1990; 87(23):9353–9357.

240 Betz M, Fox BS. Prostaglandin E2 inhibits production of Th1 lymphokines but not of Th2 lymphokines. *J Immunol* 1991; 146(1):108–113.

241 van der Pouw K, van Kooten C, Rensink I, Aarden L. Interleukin (IL)-4 production by human T cells: differential regulation of IL-4 vs. IL-2 production. *Eur J Immunol* 1992; 22(5):1237–1241.

242 Snijdewint FG, Kalinski P, Wierenga EA, Bos JD, Kapsenberg ML. Prostaglandin E2 differentially modulates cytokine secretion profiles of human T helper lymphocytes. *J Immunol* 1993; 150(12):5321–5329.

243 Anastassiou ED, Paliogianni F, Balow JP, Yamada H, Boumpas DT. Prostaglandin E2 and other cyclic AMP-elevating agents modulate IL-2 and IL-2R alpha gene expression at multiple levels. *J Immunol* 1992; 148(9):2845–2852.

244 Yoshimura T, Nagao T, Nakao T et al. Modulation of Th1- and Th2-like cytokine production from mitogen-stimulated human peripheral blood mononuclear cells by phosphodiesterase inhibitors. *Gen Pharmacol* 1998; 30(2):175–180.

245 Kanda N, Watanabe S. Gangliosides GD1b, GT1b, and GQ1b enhance IL-2 and IFN-gamma production and suppress IL-4 and IL-5 production in phytohemagglutinin-stimulated human T cells. *J Immunol* 2001; 166(1):72–80.

246 Van der Pouw Kraan TCTM, Boeije LCM, Snijders A, Smeenk RJT, Wijdenes J, Aarden LA. Regulation of IL-12 production by human monocytes and the influence of prostglandin E2. *Ann NY Acad Sci* 1996; 795: 147–157.

247 Chan SC, Henderson WR, Jr., Shi-Hua L, Hanifin JM. Prostaglandin E2 control of T cell cytokine production is functionally related to the reduced lymphocyte proliferation in atopic dermatitis. *J Allergy Clin Immunol* 1996; 97:85–94.

248 Giembycz MA, Corrigan CJ, Seybold J, Newton R, Barnes PJ. Identification of cyclic AMP phosphodiesterases 3,4 and 7 in human CD4$^+$ and CD8$^+$ T-lymphocytes: role in regulating proliferation and the biosynthesis of interleukin-2. *Br J Pharmacol* 1996; 118:1945–1958.

249 Yoshimura T, Kurita C, Nagao T et al. Effects of cAMP-phosphodiesterase isozyme inhibitor on cytokine production

by lipopolysaccharide-stimulated human peripheral blood mononuclear cells. *Gen Pharmacol* 1997; 29(4):633–638.

250 Sommer N, Loschmann PA, Northoff GH et al. The antidepressant rolipram suppresses cytokine production and prevents autoimmune encephalomyelitis. *Nat Med* 1995; 1(3):244–248.

251 Molnar K, Yonno L, Heaslip R, Weichman B. Modulation of TNF alpha and IL-1 beta from endotoxin-stimulated monocytes by selective PDE isozyme inhibitors. *Agents Actions* 1993; 39 Spec No:C77–C79.

252 Lee HJ, Koyano N, Naito Y et al. cAMP activates the IL-5 promoter synergistically with phorbol ester through the signaling pathway involving protein kinase A in mouse thymoma line EL-4. *J Immunol* 1993; 151(11):6135–6142.

253 Lewis GM, Caccese RG, Heaslip RJ, Bansbach CC. Effects of rolipram and CI-930 on IL-2 mRNA transcription in human Jurkat cells. *Agents Actions* 1993; 39 Spec No:C89–C92.

254 Knudsen JH, Kjaersgaard E, Christensen NJ. Individual lymphocyte subset composition determines cAMP response to isoproterenol in mononuclear cell preparations from peripheral blood. *Scand J Clin Lab Invest* 1995; 55:9–14.

255 Hilkens CM, Vermeulen H, van Neerven RJ, Snijdewint FG, Wierenga EA, Kapsenberg ML. Differential modulation of T helper type 1 (Th1) and T helper type 2 (Th2) cytokine secretion by prostaglandin E2 critically depends on interleukin-2. *Eur J Immunol* 1995; 25(1):59–63.

256 Obernolte R, Bhakta S, Alvarez R et al. The cDNA of a human lymphocyte cyclic-AMP phosphodiesterase (PDE IV) reveals a multigene family. *Gene* 1993; 129(2):239–247.

257 Gantner F, Gotz C, Gekeler V, Schudt C, Wendel A, Hatzelmann A. Phosphodiesterase profile of human B lymphocytes from normal and atopic donors and the effects of PDE inhibition on B cell proliferation. *Br J Pharmacol* 1998; 123:1031–1038.

258 Huang R, Cioffi J, Berg K et al. B cell differentiation factor-induced B cell maturation: regulation via reduction in cAMP. *Cell Immunol* 1995; 162(1):49–55.

259 Mentz F, Merle B, Ouaaz F, Binet JL. Theophylline, a new inducer of apoptosis in B-CLL: role of cyclic nucleotides. *Br J Haematol* 1995; 90(4):957–959.

260 Baixeras E, GarciaLozano E, Martinez AC. Decrease in cAMP levels promoted by CD48–CD2 interaction correlates with inhibition of apoptosis in B cells. *Scand J Immunol* 1996; 43:406–412.

261 Roper RL, Conrad DH, Brown DM, Warner GL, Phipps RP. Prostaglandin E2 promotes IL-4-induced IgE and IgG1 synthesis. *J Immunol* 1990; 145(8):2644–2651.

262 Roper RL, Brown DM, Phipps RP. Prostaglandin E2 promotes B lymphocyte Ig isotype switching to IgE. *J Immunol* 1995; 154(1):162–170.

263 Pene J, Rousset F, Briere F et al. IgE production by normal human lymphocytes is induced by interleukin 4 and suppressed by interferons gamma and alpha and prostaglandin E2. *Proc Natl Acad Sci USA* 1988; 85(18):6880–6884.

264 Paul E, Kolb JP, Calenda A et al. Functional interaction between beta 2-adrenoceptor agonists and interleukin-4 in the regulation of CD23 expression and release and IgE production in human. *Mol Immunol* 1993; 30(2):157–164.

265 Coqueret O, Dugas B, Mencia H, Braquet P. Regulation of IgE production from human mononuclear cells by beta 2-adrenoceptor agonists. *Clin Exp Allergy* 1995; 25(4):304–311.

266 Paul E, Kolb JP, Damais C et al. Beta 2-adrenoceptor agonists regulate the IL-4-induced phenotypical changes and IgE-dependent functions in normal human monocytes. *J Leukoc Biol* 1994; 55(3):313–320.

267 Cooper KD, Kang K, Chan SC, Hanifin JM. Phosphodiesterase inhibition by Ro 20–1724 reduces hyper-IgE synthesis by atopic dermatitis cells in vitro. *J Invest Dermatol* 1985; 84(6):477–482.

268 Chan SC, Hanifin JM. Differential inhibitor effects on cyclic adenosine monophosphate-phosphodiesterase isoforms in atopic and normal leukocytes. *J Lab Clin Med* 1993; 121(1):44–51.

269 Coqueret O, Boichot E, Lagente V. Selective type IV phosphodiesterase inhibitors prevent IL-4-induced IgE production by human peripheral blood mononuclear cells. *Clin Exp Allergy* 1997; 27:816–823.

270 Godfrey RW, Manzi RM, Gennaro DE, Hoffstein ST. Phospholipid and arachidonic acid metabolism in zymosan-stimulated human monocytes: modulation by cAMP. *J Cell Physiol* 1987; 131(3):384–392.

271 Godfrey RW, Manzi RM, Jensen BD, Hoffstein ST. FMLP-induced arachidonic acid release, phospholipid metabolism, and calcium mobilization in human monocytes. Regulation by cyclic AMP. *Inflammation* 1988; 12(3):223–230.

272 Hichami A, Boichot E, Germain N, Legrand A, Moodley I, Lagente V. Involvement of cyclic AMP in the effects of phosphodiesterase IV inhibitors on arachidonate release from mononuclear cells. *Eur J Pharmacol* 1995; 291(2):91–97.

273 Elliott KR, Leonard EJ. Interactions of formylmethionyl-leucyl-phenylalanine, adenosine, and phosphodiesterase inhibitors in human monocytes. Effects on superoxide release, inositol phosphates and cAMP. *FEBS Lett* 1989; 254(1–2):94–98.

274 Endres S, Fulle HJ, Sinha B et al. Cyclic nucleotides differentially regulate the synthesis of tumour necrosis factor-alpha and interleukin-1 beta by human mononuclear cells. *Immunology* 1991; 72(1):56–60.

275 Spatafora M, Chiappara G, Merendino AM, D'Amico D, Bellia V, Bonsignore G. Theophylline suppresses the release of tumour necrosis factor-alpha by blood monocytes and alveolar macrophages. *Eur Respir J* 1994; 7(2):223–228.

276 Verghese MW, McConnell RT, Strickland AB et al. Differential regulation of human monocyte-derived TNF alpha and IL-1 beta by type IV cAMP-phosphodiesterase (cAMP-PDE) inhibitors. *J Pharmacol Exp Ther* 1995; 272(3):1313–1320.

277 Lappin D, Riches DW, Damerau B, Whaley K. Cyclic nucleotides and their relationship to complement-component-C2 synthesis by human monocytes. *Biochem J* 1984; 222(2):477–486.

278 Jeurgens UR, Overlack A, Vetter H. Theophylline inhibits the formation of leukotriene B_4 (LTB_4) by enhancement of cyclic-AMP and prostaglandin E_2 (PGE_2) production in normal human monocytes *in vitro*. *Eur Resp J* 17S, 3685. 1993.

279 Kotecha S, Taylor IK, Shaw RJ. Pharmacological modulation of platelet-derived growth factor (B) mRNA expression in alveolar macrophages and adherent monocytes. *Pulm Pharmacol* 1994; 7(6):383–391.

280 Platzer C, Meisel C, Vogt K, Platzer M, Volk HD. Up-regulation of monocytic IL-10 by tumor necrosis factor-alpha and cAMP elevating drugs. *Int Immunol* 1995; 7(4):517–523.

281 Knudsen PJ, Dinarello CA, Strom TB. Prostaglandins post-transcriptionally inhibit monocyte expression of interleukin 1 activity by increasing intracellular cyclic adenosine monophosphate. *J Immunol* 1986; 137(10):3189–3194.

282 Kassis S, Lee JC, Hanna N. Effects of prostaglandins and cAMP levels on monocyte IL-1 production. *Agents Actions* 1989; 27(3–4):274–276.

283 Sung SS, Walters JA. Increased cyclic AMP levels enhance IL-1 alpha and IL-1 beta mRNA expression and protein production in human myelomonocytic cell lines and monocytes. *J Clin Invest* 1991; 88(6):1915–1923.

284 Lorenz JJ, Furdon PJ, Taylor JD, Verghese MW, Chandra G, Kost TA et al. A cyclic adenosine 3′,5′-monophosphate signal is required for the induction of IL-1 beta by TNF-alpha in human monocytes. *J Immunol* 1995; 155(2):836–844.

285 Viherluoto J, Palkama T, Silvennoinen O, Hurme M. Cyclic adenosine monophosphate decreases the secretion, but not the cell-associated levels, of interleukin-1 beta in

lipopolysaccharide-activated human monocytes. *Scand J Immunol* 1991; 34(1):121–125.

286 Tenor H, Hatzelmann A, Kupferschmidt R et al. Cyclic nucleotide phosphodiesterase isoenzyme activities in human alveolar macrophages. *Clin Exp Allergy* 1995; 25(7):625–633.

287 Manning CD, McLaughlin MM, Livi GP, Cieslinski LB, Torphy TJ, Barnette MS. Prolonged beta adrenoceptor stimulation up-regulates cAMP phosphodiesterase activity in human monocytes by increasing mRNA and protein for phosphodiesterases 4A and 4B. *J Pharmacol Exp Ther* 1996; 276(2):810–818.

288 Hichami A, Boichot E, Germain N, Coqueret O, Lagente V. Interactions between cAMP- and cGMP-dependent protein kinase inhibitors and phosphodiesterase IV inhibitors on arachidonate release from human monocytes. *Life Sci* 1996; 59(16):L255–L261.

289 Prabhakar U, Lipshutz D, Bartus JO et al. Characterization of cAMP-dependent inhibition of LPS-induced TNF alpha production by rolipram, a specific phosphodiesterase IV (PDE IV) inhibitor. *Int J Immunopharmacol* 1994; 16(10):805–816.

290 Seldon PM, Barnes PJ, Meja K, Giembycz MA. Suppression of lipopolysaccharide-induced tumor necrosis factor-alpha generation from human peripheral blood monocytes by inhibitors of phosphodiesterase 4: interaction with stimulants of adenylyl cyclase. *Mol Pharmacol* 1995; 48(4):747–757.

291 Sinha B, Semmler J, Eisenhut T, Eigler A, Endres S. Enhanced tumor necrosis factor suppression and cyclic adenosine monophosphate accumulation by combination of phosphodiesterase inhibitors and prostanoids. *Eur J Immunol* 1995; 25(1):147–153.

292 Greten TF, Sinha B, Haslberger C, Eigler A, Endres S. Cicaprost and the type IV phosphodiesterase inhibitor, rolipram, synergize in suppression of tumor necrosis factor-alpha synthesis. *Eur J Pharmacol* 1996; 299:229–233.

293 Souness JE, Griffin M, Maslen C et al. Evidence that cyclic AMP phosphodiesterase inhibitors suppress TNF-alpha generation from human monocytes by interacting with a 'low affinity' phosphodiesterase 4 conformer. *Br J Pharmacol* 1996; 118:649–658.

294 Eigler A, Siegmund B, Emmerich U, Baumann KH, Hartmann G, Endres S. Anti-inflammatory activities of cAMP-elevating agents: enhancement of IL-10 synthesis and concurrent suppression of TNF production. *J Leukoc Biol* 1998; 63(1):101–107.

295 Siegmund B, Eigler A, Moeller J, Greten TF, Hartmann G,

Endres S. Suppression of tumor necrosis factor-alpha production by interleukin-10 is enhanced by cAMP-elevating agents. *Eur J Pharmacol* 1997; 321(2):231–239.

296 Zhong WW, Burke PA, Drotar ME, Chavali SR, Forse RA. Effects of prostaglandin E2, cholera toxin and 8-bromo-cyclic AMP on lipopolysacchaside-induced gene expression of cytokines in human macrophages. *Immunology* 1995; 84(3):446–452.

297 Fuller RW. Control of mediator release from the human alveolar macrophage: Role of cyclic AMP. *Eur J Pharmacol* 1990; 183(2):621.

298 Baker AJ, Fuller RW. Effect of cyclic adenosine monophosphate, 5′-(N- ethylcarboxyamido)-adenosine and methylxanthines on the release of thromboxane and lysosomal enzymes from human alveolar macrophages and peripheral blood monocytes in vitro. *Eur J Pharmacol* 1992; 211(2):157–161.

299 Gardette J, Margelin D, Maziere JC, Bertrand J, Picard J. Effect of dibutyryl cyclic AMP and theophylline on lipoprotein lipase secretion by human monocyte-derived macrophages. *FEBS Lett* 1987; 225(1–2):178–182.

300 Turner CR, Esser KM, Wheeldon EB. Therapeutic intervention in a rat model of ARDS: IV. Phosphodiesterase IV inhibition. *Circ Shock* 1993; 39(3):237–245.

301 Lim LK, Hunt NH, Weidemann MJ. Reactive oxygen production, arachidonate metabolism and cyclic AMP in macrophages. *Biochem Biophys Res Commun* 1983; 114(2):549–555.

302 Dent G, Giembycz MA, Rabe KF, Wolf B, Barnes PJ, Magnussen H. Theophylline suppresses human alveolar macrophage respiratory burst through phosphodiesterase inhibition. *Am J Respir Cell Mol Biol* 1994; 10(5):565–572.

303 Beusenberg FD, Hoogsteden HC, Bonta IL, van Amsterdam JG. Cyclic AMP enhancing drugs modulate eicosanoid release from human alveolar macrophages. *Life Sci* 1994; 54(17):1269–1274.

304 Fuller RW, O'Malley G, Baker AJ, MacDermot J. Human alveolar macrophage activation: inhibition by forskolin but not beta-adrenoceptor stimulation or phosphodiesterase inhibition. *Pulm Pharmacol* 1988; 1(2):101–106.

305 Schade FU, Schudt C. The specific type III and IV phosphodiesterase inhibitor zardaverine suppresses formation of tumor necrosis factor by macrophages. *Eur J Pharmacol* 1993; 230(1):9–14.

306 Rousseau E, Gagnon J, Lugnier C. Biochemical and pharmacological characterization of cyclic nucleotide phosphodiesterase in airway epithelium. *Mol Cell Biochem* 1994; 140(2):171–175.

307 Fuhrmann M, Jahn H-U, Seybold J, Neurohr C, Barnes PJ, Hippenstiel S et al. Identification and function of cyclic nucleotide phosphodiesterase isoenzymes in airway epithelial cells. *Am J Respir Cell Mol Biol* 1999; 20:292–302.

308 Kelley TJ, al Nakkash L, Drumm ML. CFTR-mediated chloride permeability is regulated by type III phosphodiesterases in airway epithelial cells. *Am J Respir Cell Mol Biol* 1995; 13(6):657–664.

309 Dowling RB, Johnson M, Cole PJ, Wilson R. The effect of rolipram, a type IV phosphodiesterase inhibitor, on Pseudomonas aeruginosa infection of respiratory mucosa. *J Pharmacol Exp Therap* 1997; 282(3):1565–1571.

310 Dent G, White SR, Tenor H et al. Cyclic nucleotide phosphodiesterases in human bronchial epithelial cells: characterization of isoenzymes and functional effects of PDE inhibitors. *Pulm Pharmacol Ther* 1998; 11:47–56.

311 Lugnier C, Schini VB. Characterization of cyclic nucleotide phosphodiesterases from cultured bovine aortic endothelial cells. *Biochem Pharmacol* 1990; 39(1):75–84.

312 Souness JE, Diocee BK, Martin W, Moodie SA. Pig aortic endothelial-cell cyclic nucleotide phosphodiesterases. Use of phosphodiesterase inhibitors to evaluate their roles in regulating cyclic nucleotide levels in intact cells. *Biochem J* 1990; 266(1):127–132.

313 Suttorp N, Weber U, Welsch T, Schudt C. Role of phosphodiesterases in the regulation of endothelial permeability in vitro. *J Clin Invest* 1993; 91(4):1421–1428.

314 Suttorp N, Ehreiser P, Hippenstiel S et al. Hyperpermeability of pulmonary endothelial monolayer: protective role of phosphodiesterase isoenzymes 3 and 4. *Lung* 1996; 174(3):181–194.

315 Casnocha SA, Eskin SG, Hall ER, McIntire IV. Permeability of human endothelial monolayers: effect of vasoactive agonists and cAMP. *J Appl Physiol* 1989; 67(5):1997–2005.

316 Stelzner TJ, Weil JV, O'Brien RF. Role of cyclic adenosine monophosphate in the induction of endothelial barrier properties. *J Cell Physiol* 1989; 139(1):157–166.

317 Sato K, Stelzner TJ, O'Brien RF, Weil JV, Welsh CH. Pentoxifylline lessens the endotoxin-induced increase in albumin clearance across pulmonary artery endothelial monolayers with and without neutrophils. *Am J Respir Cell Mol Biol* 1991; 4(3):219–227.

318 Torphy TJ, Barnette MS, Hay DW, Underwood DC. Phosphodiesterase IV inhibitors as therapy for eosinophil-induced lung injury in asthma. *Environ Health Perspect* 1994; 102 Suppl 10:79–84.

319 Pober JS, Slowik MR, De Luca LG, Ritchie AJ. Elevated cyclic AMP inhibits endothelial cell synthesis and expression of TNF-induced endothelial leukocyte adhesion molecule- 1, and vascular cell adhesion molecule-1, but not intercellular adhesion molecule-1. *J Immunol* 1993; 150(11):5114–5123.

320 Morandini R, Ghanem G, Portier-Lemarie A, Robaye B, Renaud A, Boeynaems JM. Action of cAMP on expression and release of adhesion molecules in human endothelial cells. *Am J Physiol* 1996; 270:H807–H816.

321 Deisher TA, Garcia I, Harlan JM. Cytokine-induced adhesion molecule expression on human umbilical vein endothelial cells is not regulated by cyclic adenosine monophosphate accumulation. *Life Sci* 1993; 53(4):365–370.

322 Lugnier C, Schoeffter P, Le Bec A, Strouthou E, Stoclet JC. Selective inhibition of cyclic nucleotide phosphodiesterases of human, bovine and rat aorta. *Biochem Pharmacol* 1986; 35(10):1743–1751.

323 Yu SM, Cheng ZJ, Kuo SC. Antiproliferative effects of A02011–1, an adenylyl cyclase activator, in cultured vascular smooth muscle cells of rat. *Br J Pharmacol* 1995; 114(6):1227–1235.

324 Komas N, Lugnier C, Andriantsitohaina R, Stoclet JC. Characterisation of cyclic nucleotide phosphodiesterases from rat mesenteric artery. *Eur J Pharmacol* 1991; 208(1):85–87.

325 Xiong Y, Westhead EW, Slakey LL. Role of phosphodiesterase isoenzymes in regulating intracellular cyclic AMP in adenosine-stimulated smooth muscle cells. *Biochem J* 1995; 305(Pt 2):627–633.

326 Miyahara M, Ito M, Itoh H et al. Isoenzymes of cyclic nucleotide phosphodiesterase in the human aorta: characterization and the effects of E4021. *Eur J Pharmacol* 1995; 284(1–2):25–33.

327 Loughney K, Hill TR, Florio VA et al. Isolation and characterization of cDNAs encoding PDE5A, a human cGMP-binding, cGMP-specific 3′,5′-cyclic nucleotide phosphodiesterase. *Gene* 1998; 216(1):139–147.

328 Palmer D, Maurice DH. Dual expression and differential regulation of phosphodiesterase 3A and phosphodiesterase 3B in human vascular smooth muscle: implications for phosphodiesterase 3 inhibition in human cardiovascular tissues. *Mol Pharmacol* 2000; 58(2):247–252.

329 Choi YH, Ekholm D, Krall J et al. Identification of a novel isoform of the cyclic-nucleotide phosphodiesterase PDE3A expressed in vascular smooth-muscle myocytes. *Biochem J* 2001; 353(Pt 1):41–50.

330 Lindgren S, Andersson KE, Belfrage P, Degerman E, Manganiello VC. Relaxant effects of the selective

phosphodiesterase inhibitors milrinone and OPC 3911 on isolated human mesenteric vessels. *Pharmacol Toxicol* 1989; 64(5):440–445.

331 Lindgren S, Andersson KE. Effects of selective phosphodiesterase inhibitors on isolated coronary, lung and renal arteries from man and rat. *Acta Physiol Scand* 1991; 142(1):77–82.

332 Lugnier C, Komas N. Modulation of vascular cyclic nucleotide phosphodiesterases by cyclic GMP: role in vasodilatation. *Eur Heart J* 1993; 14 Suppl I:141–148.

333 Marukawa S, Hatake K, Wakabayashi I, Hishida S. Vasorelaxant effects of oxpentifylline and theophylline on rat isolated aorta. *J Pharm Pharmacol* 1994; 46(5):342–345.

334 Rabe KF, Magnussen H, Dent G. Theophylline and selective PDE inhibitors as bronchodilators and smooth muscle relaxants. *Eur Respir J* 1995; 8(4):637–642.

335 Rabe KF, Tenor H, Dent G, Schudt C, Nakashima M, Magnussen H. Identification of PDE isozymes in human pulmonary artery and effect of selective PDE inhibitors. *Am J Physiol* 1994; 266(5 Pt 1):L536–L543.

336 Sadhu K, Hensley K, Florio VA, Wolda SL. Differential expression of the cyclic GMP-stimulated phosphodiesterase PDE2A in human venous and capillary endothelial cells. *J Histochem Cytochem* 1999; 47(7):895–906.

337 Takahashi S, Oida K, Fujiwara R et al. Effect of cilostazol, a cyclic AMP phosphodiesterase inhibitor, on the proliferation of rat aortic smooth muscle cells in culture. *J Cardiovasc Pharmacol* 1992; 20(6):900–906.

338 Pan X, Arauz E, Krzanowski JJ, Fitzpatrick DF, Polson JB. Synergistic interactions between selective pharmacological inhibitors of phosphodiesterase isozyme families PDE III and PDE IV to attenuate proliferation of rat vascular smooth muscle cells. *Biochem Pharmacol* 1994; 48(4):827–835.

339 Revel L, Colombo S, Ferrari F, Folco G, Rovati LC, Makovec F. CR 2039, a new bis-(1H-tetrazol-5-yl)phenylbenzamide derivative with potential for the topical treatment of asthma. *Eur J Pharmacol* 1992; 229(1):45–53.

340 Torphy TJ, Cieslinski LB. Characterization and selective inhibition of cyclic nucleotide phosphodiesterase isozymes in canine tracheal smooth muscle. *Mol Pharmacol* 1990; 37(2):206–214.

341 Shahid M, van Amsterdam RG, de Boer J, ten Berge RE, Nicholson CD, Zaagsma J. The presence of five cyclic nucleotide phosphodiesterase isoenzyme activities in bovine tracheal smooth muscle and the functional effects of selective inhibitors. *Br J Pharmacol* 1991; 104(2):471–477.

342 Harris AL, Connell MJ, Ferguson EW et al. Role of low Km cyclic AMP phosphodiesterase inhibition in tracheal relaxation and bronchodilation in the guinea pig. *J Pharmacol Exp Ther* 1989; 251(1):199–206.

343 Burns F, Stevens PA, Pyne NJ. The identification of apparently novel cyclic AMP and cyclic GMP phosphodiesterase activities in guinea-pig tracheal smooth muscle. *Br J Pharmacol* 1994; 113(1):3–4.

344 Miyamoto K, Kurita M, Sakai R, Sanae F, Wakusawa S, Takagi K. Cyclic nucleotide phosphodiesterase isoenzymes in guinea-pig tracheal muscle and bronchorelaxation by alkylxanthines. *Biochem Pharmacol* 1994; 48(6):1219–1223.

345 de Boer J, Philpott AJ, van Amsterdam RG, Shahid M, Zaagsma J, Nicholson CD. Human bronchial cyclic nucleotide phosphodiesterase isoenzymes: biochemical and pharmacological analysis using selective inhibitors. *Br J Pharmacol* 1992; 106(4):1028–1034.

346 Rabe KF, Tenor H, Dent G, Schudt C, Liebig S, Magnussen H. Phosphodiesterase isozymes modulating inherent tone in human airways: identification and characterization. *Am J Physiol* 1993; 264(5 Pt 1):L458–L464.

347 Torphy TJ, Undem BJ, Cieslinski LB, Luttmann MA, Reeves ML, Hay DW. Identification, characterization and functional role of phosphodiesterase isozymes in human airway smooth muscle. *J Pharmacol Exp Ther* 1993; 265(3):1213–1223.

348 Silver PJ, Hamel LT, Perrone MH, Bentley RG, Bushover CR, Evans DB. Differential pharmacologic sensitivity of cyclic nucleotide phosphodiesterase isozymes isolated from cardiac muscle, arterial and airway smooth muscle. *Eur J Pharmacol* 1988; 150(1–2):85–94.

349 Torphy TJ, Burman M, Huang LB, Tucker SS. Inhibition of the low km cyclic AMP phosphodiesterase in intact canine trachealis by SK&F 94836: mechanical and biochemical responses. *J Pharmacol Exp Ther* 1988; 246(3):843–850.

350 Torphy TJ, Undem BJ. Phosphodiesterase inhibitors: new opportunities for the treatment of asthma. *Thorax* 1991; 46(7):512–523.

351 Tomkinson A, Karlsson JA, Raeburn D. Comparison of the effects of selective inhibitors of phosphodiesterase types III and IV in airway smooth muscle with differing beta-adrenoceptor subtypes. *Br J Pharmacol* 1993; 108(1):57–61.

352 Spina D, Harrison S, Page CP. Regulation by phosphodiesterase isoenzymes of non-adrenergic non-cholinergic contraction in guinea-pig isolated main bronchus. *Br J Pharmacol* 1995; 116(4):2334–2340.

353 Cortijo J, Bou J, Beleta J et al. Investigation into the role of phosphodiesterase IV in bronchorelaxation, including studies with human bronchus. *Br J Pharmacol* 1993; 108(2):562–568.

354 Qian Y, Naline E, Karlsson JA, Raeburn D, Advenier C. Effects of rolipram and siguazodan on the human isolated bronchus and their interaction with isoprenaline and sodium nitroprusside. *Br J Pharmacol* 1993; 109(3):774–778.

355 Fujii K, Kohrogi H, Iwagoe H et al. Novel phosphodiesterase 4 inhibitor T-440 reverses and prevents human bronchial contraction induced by allergen. *J Pharmacol Exp Therap* 1998; 284(1):162–169.

356 Schmidt D, Watson N, Morton BE, Dent G, Magnussen H, Rabe KF. Effect of selective and non-selective phoshodiesterase inhibitors on allergen-induced contractions in passively sensitized human airways. *Eur Resp J* 1997; 10(Suppl 25):314S.

357 Tomlinson PR, Wilson JW, Stewart AG. Salbutamol inhibits the proliferation of human airway smooth muscle cells grown in culture: Relationship to elevated cAMP levels. *Biochem Pharmacol* 1995; 49:1809–1819.

358 Billington CK, Joseph SK, Swan C, Scott MG, Jobson TM, Hall IP. Modulation of human airway smooth muscle proliferation by type 3 phosphodiesterase inhibition. *Am J Physiol* 1999; 276(3 Pt 1):L412–L419.

359 Brunnee T, Engelstatter R, Steinijans VW, Kunkel G. Bronchodilatory effect of inhaled zardaverine, a phosphodiesterase III and IV inhibitor, in patients with asthma. *Eur Respr J* 1992; 5(8):982–985.

360 Fujimura M, Kamio Y, Saito M, Hashimoto T, Matsuda T. Bronchodilator and bronchoprotective effects of cilostazol in humans in vivo. *Am J Respir Crit Care Med* 1995; 151:222–225.

361 Foster RW, Rakshi K, Carpenter JR, Small RC. Trials of the bronchodilator activity of the isoenzyme-selective phosphodiesterase inhibitor AH 21–132 in healthy volunteers during a methacholine challenge test. *Br J Clin Pharmacol* 1992; 34(6):527–534.

362 Kawasaki A, Hoshino K, Osaki R, Mizushima Y, Yano S. Effect of ibudilast: a novel antiasthmatic agent, on airway hypersensitivity in bronchial asthma. *J Asthma* 1992; 29(4):245–252.

363 Bardin PG, Dorward MA, Lampe FC, Franke B, Holgate ST. Effect of selective phosphodiesterase 3 inhibition on the early and late asthmatic responses to inhaled allergen. *Br J Clin Pharmacol* 1998; 45(4):387–391.

364 Nell H, Louw C, Leichtl S, Rathgeb F, Neuhauser M, Bardin PG. Acute anti-inflammatory effect of the novel phosphodiesterase 4 inhibitor roflumilast on allergen challenge in asthmatics after a single dose. *Am J Respir Crit Care Med* 161, A200. 2000.

365 Jonker GJ, Tijhuis GJ, de Monchey JGR. RP 73401 (a phosphodiesterase IV inhibitor) single does not prevent allergen induced bronchoconstriction during the early phase reaction in asthmatics. *Eur Respir J* 1996; 9:82s.

366 Nieman RB, Fisher BD, Amit O, Dockhorn RJ. SB 207499 (Ariflow™), a second-generation, selective oral phosphodiesterase type 4 (PDE4) inhibitor, attenuates exercise induced bronchoconstriction in patients with asthma. *Am J Respir Crit Care Med* 157, A413. 1998.

367 Timmer W, Leclerc V, Birraux G et al. The new phosphodiesterase 4 inhibitor roflumilast is efficacious in excercise-induced asthma and leads to suppression of LPS-stimulated TNF-alpha ex-vivo. *J Clin Pharmacol* 2002; 42: 297–303.

368 Landells LJ, Jensen MW, Spina D et al. Oral administration of the phosphodiesterase (PDE)4 inhibitor, V11294A inhibits ex-vivo agonist-induced cell activation. *Eur Respir J* 12[Suppl 28]. 2001.

369 Compton CH, Gubbs J, Nieman R. Cilomilast a selective phosphodiesterase-4 inhibitor for treatment of patients with chronic obstructive pulmonary disease, a randomized, dose-ranging study. *Lancet* 2001; 358: 265–270.

370 Underwood DC, Bochnowicz S, Osborn RR et al. Antiasthmatic activity of the second-generation phosphodiesterase 4 (PDE4) inhibitor SB 207499 (Ariflo) in the guinea pig. *J Pharmacol Exp Ther* 1998; 287:988–995.

371 Torphy TJ, Page C. Phosphodiesterases: the journey toward therapeutics. *Trends Pharmacol Sci* 2000; 21:157–159.

372 Engels P, Fichtel K, Lubbert H. Expression and regulation of human and rat phosphodiesterase type IV isogenes. *FEBS Lett* 1994; 350(2–3):291–295.

373 Wright LC, Seybold J, Robichaud A, Adcock IM, Barnes PJ. Phosphodiesterase expression in human epithelial cells. *Am J Physio–lung Cell Molec Physio* 1998; 275(4 19–4):L694–L700.

8

Potential therapeutic effects of potassium channel openers in respiratory diseases

Ahmed Z. El-Hashim

Department of Applied Therapeutics, Faculty of Pharmacy, Kuwait University

Introduction

The pharmaceutical industry is always in hot pursuit of new therapies to combat diseases and other ailments. Generally, the route is difficult and costly involving the identification of novel disease targets and the design of novel compounds for these targets. An alternative option is that new drugs can be designed from modification of currently existing molecules to achieve compounds with an overall superior therapeutic profile. However, sometimes a class of a drug, designed for a specific indication, can be fortuitously shown to have therapeutic effects in a completely different disease state. In most of these cases, it is the mode of action of the drug and not necessarily similarities in the disease mechanisms *per se* that make these compounds useful across a spectrum of diseases. This is the case for potassium channel openers (KCOs), compounds originally developed as anti-hypertensive agents as they are able to relax vascular smooth muscle. They act by opening potassium channels in cell membranes resulting in membrane hyperpolarization and consequently relaxation of the muscle cells[1]. Cromakalim is one of the earliest used KCOs and is a benzopyran prototype. In addition to its ability to relax vascular smooth muscle cromakalim was shown to also relax airway smooth muscle (ASM). Because of this property, this class of drugs has been receiving increasing attention due to their potential use in respiratory diseases and many studies have been undertaken to investigate this.

The success of KCOs in respiratory diseases will probably depend on whether they will offer advantages over currently existing therapy. In the case of asthma, for example, there is no doubt that currently available therapy is not adequately controlling this disease and hence there is an unmet medical need. However, the question is whether KCOs will have a superior therapeutic profile that is not shared by standard therapy such as β_2 agonist or corticosteroids, currently the most widely used drugs in asthma treatment.

Potassium channels

Potassium (K^+) channels form a discrete group of membrane proteins of diverse structures and biophysical characteristics that have at least one functional feature in common: cation permeability with a high degree of selectivity for K^+ ions. They can be found in many tissues such as vascular and ASM, nerves, pancreatic β-cells and immunologically competent cells such as alveolar macrophages. They are known to have important regulatory function in both excitable and non-excitable cells. In mammalian cells, K^+ ions are found at significantly higher levels intracellularly (150 mM) in comparison to extracellular levels (5 mM). Hence the opening of K^+ ion channels in the cell membrane would allow K^+ ions to move, out of cells, down their concentration gradient which is normally maintained by the ion transporter K^+/Na^+ adenosine triphosphatase

(ATPase). Moreover, the K^+ potential gradient is further regulated by the small pore K^+ channels having a greater probability of being closed than open thus limiting their efflux from cells. On non-excitable tissue K^+ channels are believed to play a role in signal transduction and membrane transport, maintaining resting potential as well as regulating cell volume. On excitable tissue, the channels are thought to play a role in stabilization of the membrane potential such that they set the membrane potential, repolarize action potentials and end periods of action potential firing and in the regulation of neurotransmitter release.

The realization that K^+ channels are ubiquitously expressed proteins has increased interest in attempting to elucidate their function. More recently, this interest has extended to elucidating the role of K^+ channels in certain respiratory diseases with a view to revealing a potentially new class of therapeutic agent.

Types of K channels

Molecular and electrophysiological technologies have led to an expansion in the field of K^+ channels. Over ten types of K^+ channels have been identified so far[2]. Currently K^+ channel families[3] are characterized based on their biophysical properties such as their activation and inactivation kinetics, their current–voltage profiles, and their regulation by certain modulators such as intracellular adenosine triphosphate (ATP) and Ca^{2+}. Studies on native channels, and more recently cloned K^+ channels have led to pharmacological characterization of these channels. For example several K^+ channel blockers, many derived from natural sources, such as scorpion and snake toxins, have been discovered[4]. In addition to blockers, openers of several types of K^+ channels have been discovered. These openers can modulate the activity of channels found in several types of tissue. These openers come from natural sources but have also been derived synthetically[5]. Due to the relatively large number of types of

K^+ channels and their ubiquitous expression, this chapter will focus primarily on the two main types of K^+ channels with some relevance to respiratory diseases, Ca^{2+}-activated K^+ channels and K_{ATP} channels.

Ca^{2+} activated K^+ channels

Ca^{2+}-activated K^+ channels are widely distributed and characterized by their selectivity for K^+ and their dependence on intracellular Ca^{2+} for activation. It is this latter property that separates them from other K^+ channels and demonstrates their importance particularly in the context of excitable tissue and neurotransmitter release. There are possibly two distinct families of Ca^{2+}-activated K channels. The small conductance Ca^{2+}-activated K^+ channels (SK_{Ca}) and the large conductance Ca^{2+}-activated K^+ channels (maxi-K or BK_{Ca})[6].

Small Ca^{2+}-activated K^+ channel (SK_{Ca})

SK_{Ca} play a fundamental role in all excitable tissue. They are selective for K^+, have relatively low single-channel conductance values (5–15 pS), are highly sensitive to $[Ca^{2+}]_{in}$ and they are usually voltage insensitive[7-9]. SK_{Ca} are potently inhibited by certain peptidyl toxins, most notably the bee toxin, apamin[10]. Action potentials increase the levels of intracellular Ca^{2+} consequently activating SK_{Ca}. This results in long hyperpolarization termed afterhyperpolarization (AHP) and contributes to spike afterpolarization and burst termination in neurons[11,12]. This spike-frequency adaptation process protects the cell from the deleterious effects of continuous tetanic activity and is crucial for normal neurotransmission[13,14]. Studies of vertebrate neuronal somata have shown that after each spike in motor neurons, the membrane may hyperpolarize twice, an initial fast AHP lasting for 1 to 2 ms, and a later slow AHP, lasting 50 to 1000 ms. Both are due to elevated K^+ conductance. The slow AHP is generated by SK_{Ca} channels activated by Ca^{2+} influxes occurring during each action potential and lasts presumably as long as it takes for any excess Ca^{2+} ions to be removed. It is thought that the slow AHP limits the firing frequency of repetitive action potentials and hence SK_{Ca}, functionally, transduces fluctuations in intracellular calcium concentrations into changes in membrane potential[15].

Large Ca^{2+}-activated K channels (BK_{Ca} or maxi-K channels)

BK_{Ca} are ubiquitous channels found in both excitable and non-excitable tissue. They are so named because of their large conductances which range from 100 to 300 pS yet are able to maintain a high degree of specificity for potassium ions[8]. They comprise a diverse group of voltage-dependent ion channels with a range of single-channel conductive values and sensitivities to $[Ca^{2+}]_{in}$. On excitable tissue, BK_{Ca} channels have been described on nerve cells[16] where they may regulate neurotransmitter release[17]. Opening of BK_{Ca} channels appears to repolarize the terminal, shortening the action potential and restrict Ca^{2+} entry thereby limiting release. On ASM, they are thought to regulate the membrane potential and intrinsic tone[18,19]. Although the effect of BK_{Ca} opening on resting membrane potential is small, they have a considerably greater effect on action potentials which is most pronounced on very active cells. Moreover, in ASM it is believed that BK_{Ca} channels are responsible for the repolarizing phase of the action potential, control of slow wave activity[20,21]. In this tissue, BK_{Ca} channels mediate a slow outward current which is blocked by tetraethylammonium (TEA), charybdotoxin and iberiotoxin. BK_{Ca} channels are also present in striated muscle where it is thought that they contribute to repolarization and stabilization of transverse tubule membrane[22]. There is also evidence that these channels are, at least partly, involved in mediating the relaxant effect of β-adrenergic agonists on ASM[23].

K_{ATP} channels

ATP sensitive potassium channels were first described in the heart[24]. Subsequently, similar K^+ channels, all with unitary conductances in the range of 40–80 pS, were found to exist in insulin-secreting pancreatic β cells and in skeletal muscle[25–27]. They are also found in many other tissues such as neuronal, immunologically competent cells such as alveolar macrophages and vascular and airway smooth muscle. K_{ATP} confer a degree of metabolic sensitivity to the membrane properties on cells in which they are located. K_{ATP} channels are so named because of their inhibition by physiological (μM) concentrations of intracellular ATP $[ATP]_{in}$ and activation as $[ATP]_{in}$ decreases. They are also Ca^{2+} insensitive and generally show little voltage sensitivity. Under normal circumstances $[ATP]_{in}$ levels are well maintained and are only altered under conditions of high metabolic demand. Hence it is possible that the normal levels of ATP maintain a low open probability against which background changes in other regulatory factors serve to control channel activity. Although these channels are sometimes described as ATP dependent, the term ATP sensitive is probably a better description as phosphorylation via ATP can modify the opening of large conductance calcium-dependent K^+ channels. Moreover, although the opening of K_{ATP} channels can be experimentally modulated by $[ATP]_{in}$, the physiological control of these channels in many tissues may be primarily associated with other nucleotides, G-proteins and various ligands[28]. K_{ATP} channels are inhibited by sulfonylureas such as glibenclamide[29,30] and by phentolamine[31].

Potassium channel openers

The term K^+ channel opener was first used in 1985 in the context of the smooth muscle relaxant effects of the benzopyran, cromakalim. Such a vague pharmacological term was used as it reflected the unknown mechanism by which cromakalim opened K^+ channels. The family comprises a large number of molecules that can be classified into three main groups: (i) agents like cromakalim that open the small conductance (10–30 pS) K_{ATP} channels; (ii) hybrid molecules like nicorandil which open K_{ATP} channels and activate the enzyme, soluble guanylyl cyclase; and (iii) molecules like NS1619 which open the large conductance (100–300 pS) BK_{Ca}. For SK_{Ca} channels, selective openers are not known. Nonetheless the opening of any type of K^+ channel will result in cell membrane hyperpolarization. One significant characteristic of the synthetic KCO is that they not only shift the membrane potential towards E_K but they also tend to voltage clamp the membrane potential at E_K. Therefore in the presence of a KCO any depolarizing stimulus results in further K^+ efflux via the open K^+ channels, and the membrane either remains in the region or quickly returns to E_K.

Openers of the ATP-sensitive K⁺ channels

These agents comprise the largest number of KCOs. Members of this family can be distinguished from other types of KCO as their actions are susceptible to inhibition by glibenclamide but not charybdotoxin or apamin. Moreover, based on differences in the chemical structure of KCOs in this family, they have been further divided into several groups.

Benzopyrans

After the description of the pharmacology of the racemate cromakalim[32], analogues of this molecule have been synthesized more than any other KCOs[33]. The group includes levcromakalim, the more active enantiomer of cromakalim, bimakalim, rilmakalim SDZ PCO 400, SDZ 217–744, and BRL 55834. Generally compounds in this group can open K_{ATP} channels in ASM, vascular smooth muscle and cardiac cells (at higher concentration), but have no (or very little) effect in pancreatic cells.

Thioformamides

The prototypes of this group is aprikalim, the more active enantiomer of the racemate RP49356. Many of the molecules in this group contain both a chiral carbon and a chiral sulphur atom, which results in a complex stereochemistry.

Pyrimidines

The prototype member of this group is minoxidil[34]. Early organ bath studies suggested that members of this group may have potassium channel opening properties[35] and this was subsequently confirmed by ion flux and membrane potential measurements[36]. The potassium channel opening ability of another pyrimidine derivative, LP 805 have been reported[37].

Cyanoguanidines

These compounds were initially developed in the early 1970s; however, their mechanism of action was not known until much later[38,39]. The prototype molecule is the racemate pinacidil. Other closely related derivatives are the achiral P1060 and the highly potent P1075.

Benzothiadiazines

Diazoxide is the most characterized molecule in this group. However, derivatives of this molecule have recently been described[40]. The hyperglycemic actions of diazoxide in pancreatic β cells[41] and vascular smooth muscle, and its vasodilator effects are due to its ability to open K^+ channels[42]. Diazoxide demonstrates antagonistic activity in cardiac cells in contrast to pinacidil and cromakalim.

Openers of the large conductance calcium-activated K-channel (BK_{Ca})

This is a relatively new family of KCOs but is a potentially very exciting one and is currently the subject of intense investigation. NS004, a benzimiadazole, has been shown to activate BK_{Ca} on neuronal cells[43], in airways and vascular smooth muscle[44,45] and in hippocampal cells[46]. It has been suggested[47] that the most interesting advance made in this area is the development of the triterpenoid glycoside derivative, dehydrosaponin 1[48]. Interestingly, although this agent is an opener of BK_{Ca}, it only does so when applied to the inner surface of the cells[48].

Potassium channels on ASM

If a depolarizing current is applied to the membrane of an ASM cell, the plasma membrane limits the degree of depolarization demonstrating that the plasma membrane has inherent rectifying ability. This 'rectifying' behaviour tends to limit depolarization and consequently, smooth muscle contraction from taking place. This membrane potential rectification is due to the opening of K^+ channels. As the membrane begins to depolarize, the K^+ channels open and K^+ ions move down their concentration gradient out of the cell thereby repolarizing the membrane and limiting the potential change and development in muscle tension[49].

In addition to channels that are activated by changes in the membrane potential, BK_{Ca} and K_{ATP}, channels also play a major role in limiting ASM contractility. The presence of BK_{Ca} channels on inside-out patches of bovine tracheal smooth muscle cells was confirmed by conductance of about 240 pS, selectivity for K^+, dependence of channel activity on Ca^{2+} levels and sensitivity to the selective BK_{Ca} channel blocker iberiotoxin. Moreover, the BK_{Ca} channel openers increased the open state probability of BK_{Ca} in a dose-dependent manner[50]. Furthermore, in guinea pigs, tracheal spontaneous tone was markedly suppressed by atrial natriuretic peptide (ANP). The relaxant effects of ANP on spontaneous tone was markedly suppressed in the presence of iberiotoxin. Moreover, the inhibitory effects of iberiotoxin on relaxation induced by ANP were diminished in the presence of nifedipine, an antagonist of voltage-operated Ca^{2+} channels[51]. Therefore as intracellular Ca^{2+} begins to rise, either due to membrane depolarization or through an agonist-induced mechanism, BK_{Ca} channels are activated,

resulting in membrane hyperpolarization and consequently limiting further Ca^{2+} influx through the voltage-operated calcium channels hence decreasing ASM contractility.

The K_{ATP} CO bimakalim has been reported to relax spontaneous tone of guinea pig tracheal rings and also inhibit bombesin-induced bronchoconstriction in anesthetized guinea pig[52]. Moreover, HOE 234 and lemakalim were found to produce concentration-dependent relaxation of both spontaneous tone and tone increased by methacholine in human bronchi; effects that could be inhibited by glibenclamide, suggesting a mechanism involving KCOs[53]. Furthermore, other studies using intraluminal pressure recording[54] or recording of tension changes from segments of trachea[55] have shown that cromakalim can directly inhibit ASM contraction.

K$^+$ channels on airway nerves

Studies have shown that K_{ATP} and BK_{Ca} are present in airway nerves and may play a role in regulating neurotransmitter release from both cholinergic and peptidergic neurones. Studies using isolated guinea pig trachea have shown that pressor responses to preganglionic stimulation of extrinsic vagal nerves are reduced by cromakalim[56,57]. It was reported that cromakalim did not inhibit responses to postganglionic stimulation of cholinergic nerves which would suggest that the mechanism of action is through inhibition of transmitter release[56].

Other studies have demonstrated that KCOs decrease the activity of excitatory non-adrenergic non-cholinergic (eNANC) nerves. The intravenous administration of cromakalim (10–400 µg/kg) reduced eNANC-mediated bronchoconstriction to bilateral vagal stimulation in anaesthetized guinea pigs in a dose dependent fashion. Similar doses of cromakalim did not block substance P (SP)-mediated bronchoconstriction which would indicate that cromakalim inhibits release of the peptidergic neurotransmitter at doses that did not affect the direct action of SP[58]. In vitro experiments have confirmed that K_{ATP} COs can inhibit eNANC-mediated effects through a prejunctional site of action. Transmural stimulation of isolated trachea or bronchus pre-treated with atropine and indomethacin results in NANC-mediated contractions which were inhibited by cromakalim, lemakalim, pinacidil and RP 52891 (the active enantiomer of RP49356)[55,59]. Furthermore, studies have also shown that the action of the K_{ATP} COs is suppressed by glibenclamide consistent with an action on K_{ATP} channels in sensory airway nerves.

There is also evidence that BK_{Ca} channels play an important role in the regulation of neurotransmitter release. Thus charybdotoxin significantly inhibited the μ-opioid agonist-induced prejunctional inhibition of cholinergic nerve induced contraction in human airways[60]. Furthermore, NS1619 inhibited electrically induced NANC induced contraction of isolated guinea-pig bronchi but not contraction induced by exogenous neurokinin A (NKA). Moreover, the effects of NS1619 were prevented by iberiotoxin[17]. NS1619 also inhibited electrical field stimulation (EFS)-induced cholinergic contractile responses without affecting responses to exogenous acetylcholine[61].

KCO in the treatment of respiratory diseases

Due to the ability of KCO to induce cell membrane hyperpolarization particularly in ASM and airway nerves, it is anticipated that these molecules will induce bronchodilation, reduce C-fibre driven neurogenic inflammation and mucus hyper-secretion, decrease airway hyperresponsiveness (AHR) and have antitussive effects. These effects are predicted to have some beneficial action in respiratory conditions such as asthma and chronic obstructive pulmonary diseases (COPD).

KCO and bronchodilation

Few clinical investigations have addressed the bronchospasmolytic capacity of KCOs and these have been namely the K_{ATP} COs. A study using healthy vol-unteers has shown that a 2 mg dose of cromakalim significantly increased the PEFR (PC_{40}) to hista-mine[62]. Furthermore, there is evidence suggesting that KCOs may have an impact on nocturnal asthma. In a randomized double-blind cross-over study, asthmatic subjects given cromakalim orally, significantly reduced the fall in early morning lung function[63]. In neither of these studies did cromakalim have any effects on blood pressure or heart rate. Also cromakalim administered orally has been reported to reduce histamine-induced bronchocon-striction in healthy volunteers[62]. However, in a more recent double-blind, placebo-controlled study in patients with mild to moderate asthma, levcromak-alim did not result in significant bronchodilation or changes in airway responsiveness[64]. Moreover, headache was a major side effect reported by most of the patients possibly due to vasodilation of cere-bral vasculature[64]. In another study with bimakalim, it was reported that no bronchodilation was seen at doses below the threshold for headache induction[65]. This lack of bronchodilator effect in this study may have been due to low doses administered by the inhaler device or indeed due to a real lack of bron-chodilator effect of bimakalim[65]. Moreover, the side-effect problem was not solved by local administration[65].

Therefore these studies do not support the notion that K_{ATP} COs are effective bronchodilators in humans, particularly when compared with β_2 agonist but other types of KCO have not yet been tested clinically.

KCO and airway hyperresponsiveness

The effects of K_{ATP} COs on AHR are well documented. Generally, AHR to numerous airway stimuli can be precipitated through administration of several types of chemically unrelated molecules such as allergen, platelet activating factor (PAF), ozone (±) salbuta-mol and immune complexes. In guinea pigs it was shown that AHR to histamine following intravenous injection of immune complexes is suppressed fol-lowing treatment with either cromakalim or the benzopyran KCO SDZ PCO 400 at doses that did not inhibit the broncoconstrictor responses to histamine in normal animals[66]. Moreover, PCO400 was shown to abolish the airway obstruction to intravenously injected immune complex and also the expression of AHR[67]. It was shown that K_{ATP} COs could suppress AHR without producing significant bronchodilation. Infusion of PAF in guinea pigs induces AHR to histamine but the airway responsiveness of these animals to acetylcholine remains unaltered. Following infusion of PAF, SDZ PCO 400 suppressed the exaggerated response to histamine but not to acetylcholine[68].

Also, it was reported that the KCOs levocromakalim, bimakalim, rilmakalim and SDZ PCO 400 all reversed the bombesin-induced bronchoconstriction. Further, these KCOs reversed immune complex-induced AHR with ED_{50} values that were considerably lower than those for the reversal of bombesin-induced bronchoconstriction. Also bimakalim, levcromakalim and SDZ PCO 400 did not inhibit histamine-induced bronchoconstriction in normoreactive guinea pigs at doses that suppressed immune complex-induced AHR to histamine. Airway responsiveness of normal animals was only slightly susceptible to inhibition by K_{ATP} CO[69]. This would suggest that the bronchodilation was not the mechanism for suppression of AHR. Moreover, KCO such as bimakalim and SDZ 217–744 produced an almost complete suppression of ozone-induced AHR, although other openers such as BRL 55834 and YM 934 were inactive[70], indicating that there are significant differences between the potencies of KCOs in their ability to reverse AHR.

The ability of the second generation KCOs like SDZ 217–744 to inhibit salbutamol-induced AHR was addressed in guinea pigs[70]. In animals that were treated for 10 days with salbutamol (0.2 mg/kg/day) and/or SDZ 217–744 administered by subcutaneously implanted minipumps, the dose response curves to histamine and methacholine performed, after the removal of the minipumps, were considerably enhanced in animals treated with salbutamol alone. However, in animals treated with SDZ 217–744 instead of salbutamol, their airway respon-siveness was unaltered. More significantly concurrent treatment with SDZ 217–744 almost completely prevented salbutamol-induced AHR[70].

The mechanisms by which KCOs produce their anti-AHR effect are not fully understood but are thought to be independent of their bronchospasmolytic effects. It was shown that there was a poor correlation between the ED_{50} values of KCOs for inhibition of histamine- or bombesin-induced bronchoconstriction in normoreactive guinea pigs and the reversal of immune complex-induced AHR[69]. There is a good body of evidence to suggest the involvement of altered neural reflexes[71–73]. Studies have shown that pretreatment of sensitized rabbits with capsaicin, in order to chemically inactivate a subpopulation of afferent nerves, the C-fibres, abolished AHR to histamine following allergen challenge[71] and also in naïve rabbits exposed to PAF[72]. Furthermore, in some animal models, it has been demonstrated that bilateral vagotomy before treatment with immune complexes abolished the AHR to histamine[74]. These data point to enhanced excitability of airway neural tissue as a major contributor to AHR and the mechanism of action of KCOs in suppressing AHR could be at the level of excitatory nerves. There is evidence that KCOs can modulate neural function and consequently neural mediated effects. Studies have reported that cromakalim abrogates NANC but not substance P-mediated bronchoconstriction[58] and inhibits the contraction induced by vagal stimulation of guinea pig isolated trachea at lower concentration than are needed to inhibit responses to exogenous acetylcholine-induced airway responses[58]. This would suggest that the main mechanism of action of this class of drug is not through functional antagonism of airway smooth muscle but rather by a prejunctional mechanism of action on afferent and/or cholinergic nerves and thereby impairing reflex bronchoconstriction.

On AHR, preclinical studies would suggest that K_{ATP} COs are much more effective as suppressing AHR agents than in inducing bronchodilation. However, one criticism of such findings is that the studies reported were all conducted on models of acute AHR and clinical studies have shown this type of AHR is easily controlled by low doses of steroids. However, chronic AHR, the more troublesome type, is only partly steroid sensitive and if KCOs should prove to be efficacious in chronic AHR then they would certainly offer an advantage.

KCO and mucus secretion

Mucus hypersecretion is a characteristic feature of asthma and COPD and contributes significantly to the airway obstruction that is evident in both diseases. It is thought that, in these diseases, the mechanisms that regulate mucus secretion are defective. Therefore, agents which suppress mucus hypersecretion would improve airway calibre. In mammalian airways, the major neural control is cholinergic with a minor adrenergic component[75]. Sensory afferent nerves have also been shown to contribute to the neural control of secretions[76]. A study looking at neuroregulation of mucus secretion in ferret trachea has shown that opening of BK_{Ca} and K_{ATP} channels inhibited neurogenic mucus secretion[77]. NS1619 was more active than levcromakalim suggesting perhaps a more important role for BK_{Ca} channels. Furthermore, only opening of BK_{Ca} inhibited acetylcholine-evoked secretion of mucus. Another study has demonstrated that vasoactive intestinal peptide (VIP) induces an inhibitory effect on cholinergic and tachykininergic neurogenic mucus secretion. The effect appears to be mediated through inhibition of neurotransmitter release consequent to opening of BK_{Ca} as the effect was inhibited by iberiotoxin but not apamin or glibenclamide[78]. These studies point to an important role for potassium channels in regulating the amount of mucus released from mammalian airways such that opening of BK_{Ca} or K_{ATP} may be a physiological mechanism involved in limiting excessive airway mucus secretion. Therefore use of either a BK_{ca} or K_{ATP} channel opener in respiratory disease in which mucus hypersecretion is implicated in the pathophysiology would theoretically reduce mucus output and improve airway calibre.

KCO and cough

Perhaps one of the most common symptoms of respiratory tract infections and respiratory diseases is cough. Although antitussive medicaments are readily available over the counter, unfortunately they are not very potent, are non-specific, have many side effects and cannot be administered for long periods of time. Therefore there is a definite need for specific and potent antitussive therapy. In a study examining the antitussive effects of cromakalim on capsaicin-induced cough reflex in rats, it was reported that cromakalim (0.1 to 10 mg/kg/ i.p.) decreased the number of induced cough in a dose-dependent manner[79]. A more recent study, in guinea pigs, looking at both cromakalim and another K_{ATP} opener, pinacidil, showed that both drugs, administered subcutaneously 45 min before citric acid challenge, inhibited the cough response, with cromakalim being the more potent of the two[80]. The antitussive effects of pinacidil and cromakalim were not due to bronchodilation as this was absent at the doses used. Moreover, the combination of cromakalim and pinacidil with codeine produced an additive effect. Further, the BK_{Ca} channel activator NS1619 has also been shown to inhibit citric acid-induced cough in guinea pigs together with inhibition of C-fibre activity and eNANC-mediated bronchoconstriction[17]. This would suggest that both types of potassium channels K_{ATP} and BK_{Ca} may play a role in regulating sensory nerve function and hence openers of both channels could be of benefit in the treatment of cough.

Conclusions

The objective of this chapter was to provide the reader with an understanding of the types of potassium channels that may be of relevance to respiratory diseases, outline the types of KCOs available and to appreciate areas in respiratory disease where KCO could be of therapeutic use.

Although the case for the clinical use of KCO as bronchodilators is not a strong one, their capacity to suppress AHR, suppression of mucus hypersecre-tion and their antitussive effect are more encourag-ing but require further preclinical verification. Moreover, clinical studies comparing their effects with steroids and other established respiratory drugs will be required to establish the efficacy of KCO as antiasthma therapy.

Agents that open K_{ATP} or BK_{Ca} channels offer a novel therapeutic avenue to decrease excitability of cells. The currently available preclinical and limited clinical evidence would suggest that KCO may be useful in respiratory diseases such as asthma and COPD. However, until compounds that are tissue selective are available, it may be some time before these drugs are on the market. As a consequence of the ubiquitous nature of the targets for KCOs, a lack of tissue selectivity has been observed. The current generation of K^+ channels have serious safety con-cerns. Headaches and flushes are common side effects and cardiovascular side effects can be seen when high doses are used indicating a low therapeu-tic window for this class of compounds. This would imply that there is a need to attempt to identify target subtypes of potassium channels so that KCOs are more respiratory selective. Currently available technology will hopefully aid our understanding of these channels. There is evidence that K_{ATP} isoforms may exist and this will offer realistic potential for therapy. This may help to design K^+ channel subtype specific-openers and determine the degree to which the classes of channels (K_{ATP} and BK_{Ca}) represent a realistic therapeutic target.

REFERENCES

1 Southerton JS, Weston AH, Bray KM, Newgreen DT, Taylor SG. The potassium channel opening action of pinacidil; studies using biochemical, ion flux and microelectrode techniques. *Naunyn Schmiedebergs Arch Pharmacol* 1988; 338(3):310–318.

2 Watson S, Abbott A. TiPS receptor nomenclature supple-ment. *Trends Pharmacol Sci* 1990; Suppl:1–20.

3 Kaczorowski GJ, Garcia ML. Pharmacology of voltage-gated and calcium-activated potassium channels. *Curr Opin Chem Biol* 1999; 3(4):448–458.

4 Knaus HG, Eberhart A, Glossmann H, Munujos P, Kaczorowski GJ, Garcia ML. Pharmacology and structure of high conductance calcium-activated potassium channels. *Cell Signal* 1994; 6(8):861–870.

5 Olesen SP, Munch E, Moldt P, Drejer J. Selective activation of Ca^{2+}-dependent $K+$ channels by novel benzimidazolone. *Eur J Pharmacol* 1994; 251(1):53–59.

6 Latorre R, Oberhauser A, Labarca P, Alvarez O. Varieties of calcium-activated potassium channels. *Annu Rev Physiol* 1989; 51:385–399.

7 Blatz AL, Magleby KL. Ion conductance and selectivity of single calcium-activated potassium channels in cultured rat muscle. *J Gen Physiol* 1984; 84(1):1–23.

8 Malik-Hall M, Ganellin CR, Galanakis D, Jenkinson DH. Compounds that block both intermediate-conductance (IK(Ca)) and small-conductance (SK(Ca)) calcium-activated potassium channels. *Br J Pharmacol* 2000; 129(7):1431–1438.

9 Capiod T, Ogden DC. The properties of calcium-activated potassium ion channels in guinea-pig isolated hepatocytes. *J Physiol (Lond)* 1989; 409:285–295.

10 Quast U, Cook NS. Moving together: K^+ channel openers and ATP-sensitive K^+ channels. *Trends Pharmacol Sci* 1989; 10(11):431–435.

11 Lancaster B, Nicoll RA, Perkel DJ. Calcium activates two types of potassium channels in rat hippocampal neurons in culture. *J Neurosci* 1991; 11(1):23–30.

12 Zhang L, McBain CJ. Potassium conductances underlying repolarization and after-hyperpolarization in rat CA1 hippo-campal interneurones. *J Physiol (Lond)* 1995; 1:488 (3):661–672.

13 Bond CT, Maylie J. Adelman JP. Small-conductance calcium-activation potassium channels. *Ann N Y Acad Sci* 1999; 868:370–378.

14 Kohler M, Hirshberg B, Bond CT et al. Small-conductance, calcium-activated potassium channels from mammalian brain. *Science* 1996; 273(5282):1709–1714.

15 Xia XM, Falker B, Rivard A et al. Mechanism of calcium gating in small-conductance calcium-activated potassium channels. *Nature* 1998; 395(6701):503–507.

16 Reinhart PH, Chung S, Levitan IB. A family of calcium-dependent potassium channels from rat brain. *Neuron* 1989; 2(1):1031–1041, 4343.

17 Fox AJ, Barnes PJ, Venkatesan P, Belvisi MG. Activation of large conductance potassium channels inhibits the afferent and efferent function of airway sensory nerves in the guinea pig. *J Clin Invest* 1997; 99(3):513–519.

18 Murray MA, Berry JL, Cook SJ, Foster RW, Green KA, Small RC. Guinea-pig isolated trachealis: the effects of charybdotoxin on mechanical activity, membrane potential changes and the activity of plasmalemmal K$^+$-channels. *Br J Pharmacol* 1991; 103(3):1814–1818.

19 Kotlikoff MI. Potassium channels in airway smooth muscle: a tale of two channels. *Pharmacol Ther* 1993; 58(1):1–12.

20 Singer JJ and Walsh, J V. Characterization of calcium-activated potassium channels in single smooth muscle cells using patch-clamp technique. *Pfluegers Arch* 1987; 408:98–111.

21 Walsh JV, Singer J J. Ca^{2+} activated K channels in vertebrate smooth muscle cells. *Cell calcium* 1983; 4:321–320.

22 Blatz AL, Magleby KL. Single apamin-blocked Ca-activated K$^+$ channels of small conductance in cultured rat skeletal muscle. *Nature* 1986; 323(6090):718–720.

23 Miura M, Belvisi MG, Stretton CD, Yacoub MH, Barnes PJ. Role of potassium channels in bronchodilator responses in human airways. *Am Rev Respir Dis* 1992; 146(1):132–136.

24 Noma A, Shibasaki T. Membrane current through adenosine-triphosphate-regulated potassium channels in guinea-pig ventricular cells. *J Physiol (Lond)* 1985; 363:463–480.

25 Cook DL, Bryan J. ATP-sensitive K$^+$ channels come of age. *Trends Pharmacol Sci* 1998; 19(12):477–478.

26 Spruce AE, Standen NB, Stanfield PR. Studies of the unitary properties of adenosine-5'-triphosphate-regulated potassium channels of frog skeletal muscle. *J Physiol (Lond)* 1987; 382:213–236.

27 Spruce AE, Standen NB, Stanfield PR. Voltage-dependent ATP-sensitive potassium channels of skeletal muscle membrane. *Nature* 1985; 316(6030):736–738.

28 Edwards G, Weston AH. The pharmacology of ATP-sensitive potassium channels. *Annu Rev Pharmacol Toxicol* 1993; 33:597–637.

29 Schmid-Antomarchi H, de Weille J, Fosset M, Lazdunski M. The antidiabetic sulfonylurea glibenclamide is a potent blocker of the ATP-modulated K$^+$ channel in insulin secreting cells. *Biochem Biophys Res Commun* 1987; 146(1):21–25.

30 Sturgess NC, Kozlowski RZ, Carrington CA, Hales CN, Ashford ML. Effects of sulphonylureas and diazoxide on insulin secretion and nucleotide-sensitive channels in an insulin-secreting cell line. *Br J Pharmacol* 1988; 95(1):83–94.

31 Plant TD, Henquin JC. Phentolamine and yohimbine inhibit ATP-sensitive K$^+$ channels in mouse pancreatic beta-cells. *Br J Pharmacol* 1990; 101(1):115–120.

32 Hamilton TC, Weir SW, Weston AH. Comparison of the effects of BRL 34915 and verapamil on electrical and mechanical activity in rat portal vein. *Br J Pharmacol* 1986; 88(1):103–111.

33 Weston AH, Edwards G. Recent progress in potassium channel opener pharmacology. *Biochem Pharmacol* 1992; 43(1):47–54.

34 McCall JM, Aiken JW, Chidester CG, DuCharme DW, Wendling MG. Pyrimidine and triazine 3-oxide sulfates: a new family of vasodilators. *J Med Chem* 1983; 26(12):1791–1793.

35 Melsheri KD, Cipkus LA, Taylor CJ, Mechanism of action of minoxidil sulfate-induced vasodilation: a role for increased K$^+$ permeability. *J Pharmacol Exp Ther* 1988; 245: 751–760.

36 Newgreen DT Bray KM, McHarg AD et al. The action of diazoxide and minoxidil sulphate on rat blood vessels: a comparison with cromakalim. *Br J Pharmacol* 1990; 100(3):605–613.

37 Kamouchi M, Kajioka S, Sakai T, Kitamura K, Kuriyama H. A target K$^+$ channel for the LP-805-induced hyperpolarization in smooth muscle cells of the rabbit portal vein. *Naunyn Schmiedebergs Arch Pharmacol* 1993; 347(3):329–335.

38 Bray KM, Newgreen DT, Small RC et al. Evidence that the mechanism of the inhibitory action of pinacidil in rat and guinea-pig smooth muscle differs from that of glyceryl trinitrate. *Br J Pharmacol* 1987; 91(2):421–429.

39 Weston AH, Southerton JS, Bray KM, Newgreen DT, Taylor SG. The mode of action of pinacidil and its analogs P1060 and P1368: results of studies in rat blood vessels. *J Cardiovasc Pharmacol* 1988; 12 Suppl 2:S10–516.

40 Pirotte B, de Tullio P, Lebrun P et al. 3-(Alkylamino)-4H-pyrido[4,3-e]-1,2,4-thiadiazine 1,1-dioxides as powerful inhibitors of insulin release from rat pancreatic B-cells: a new class of potassium channel openers? *J Med Chem* 1993; 36(21):3211–3213.

41 Zunkler BJ, Lenzen S, Mauer K, Panten U, Trube G. Concentration-dependent effects of tolbutamide, meglitinide, glipizide, glibenclamide and diazoxide on ATP-regulated K$^+$ currents in pancreatic B-cells. *Naunyn Schmiedebergs Arch Pharmacol* 1988; 337(2):225–230.

42 Quast U, Cook NS. *In vitro* and *in vivo* comparison of two K$^+$ channel openers, diazoxide and cromakalim, and their inhibition by glibenclamide. *J Pharmacol Exp Ther* 1989; 250(1):261–271.

43 Olesen SP, Munch E, Watjen F, Drejer J. NS 004 – an activator of Ca^{2+}-dependent K$^+$ channels in cerebellar granule cells. *Neuroreport* 1994; 5(8):1001–1004.

44 Macmillan S, Sheridan RD, Chilvers ER, Patmore L. A comparison of the effects of SCA40, NS 004 and NS 1619 on large conductance Ca^{2+}-activated K$^+$ channels in bovine tracheal smooth muscle cells in culture. *Br J Pharmacol* 1995; 116(1):1656–1660.

45 Holland M, Langton PD, Standen NB, Boyle JP. Effects of the BK_{Ca} channel activator, NS1619, on rat cerebral artery smooth muscle. *Br J Pharmacol* 1996; 117(1):119–129.

46 Edwards G, Weston AH. The role of potassium channels in excitable cells. *Diabetes Res Clin Pract* 1995; 28 Suppl:S57–S66.

47 Edwards G, Weston AH. Pharmacology of the potassium channel openers. *Cardiovasc Drugs Ther* 1995; 9(2):185–193.

48 McManus OB, Harris GH, Giangiacomo KM et al. An activator of calcium-dependent potassium channels isolated from a medicinal herb. *Biochemistry* 1993; 32(24):6128–6133.

49 Small RC, Berry JL, Foster RW. Potassium channel opening drugs and the airways. *Braz J Med Biol Res* 1992; 25(10):983–998.

50 Macmillan S, Sheridan RD, Chilvers ER, Patmore L. A comparison of the effects of SCA40, NS 004 and NS 1619 on large conductance Ca^{2+} activated K^+ channels in bovine tracheal smooth muscle cells in culture. *Br J Pharmacol* 1995; 116(1):1656–1660.

51 Mikawa K, Kume H, Takagi K. Effects of BK_{Ca} channels on the reduction of cytosolic Ca2 + in cGMP-induced relaxation of guinea-pig trachea. *Clin Exp Pharmacol Physiol* 1997; 24(2):175–181.

52 Buchheit KH, Hofmann A, Manley P, Pfannkuche HJ, Quast U. Atypical effect of minoxidil sulphate on guinea pig airways. *Naunyn Schmiedebergs Arch Pharmacol* 2000; 361(4):418–424.

53 Miura M, Belvisi MG, Ward JK, Tadjkarimi S, Yacoub MH, Barnes PJ. Bronchodilating effects of the novel potassium channel opener HOE 234 in human airways *in vitro*. *Br J Clin Pharmacol* 1993; 35(3):318–320.

54 Cooper J and MacLagan J. The effect of potassium channel opening drugs on guinea-pigs' pulmonary nerves. *Br J Pharmacol* 1990; 101:591P.

55 Burka JF, Berry JL, Foster RW, Small RC, Watt, AJ. Effect of cromakalim on neurally-mediated responses of guinea-pig tracheal muscle. *Br J Pharmacol* 1991; 104:263–269.

56 McCaig DJ, De Jonckheere B. Effect of cromakalim on bronchoconstriction evoked by cholinergic nerve stimulation in guinea-pig isolated trachea. *Br J Pharmacol* 1989; 98(2):662–668.

57 Hall AK, MacLagan J. Effect of cromakalim on cholinergic neurotransmission in the guinea-pig trachea. *Br J Pharmacol* 1988; 95:792P.

58 Ichinose M, Barnes PJ. A potassium channel activator modulates both excitatory noncholinergic and cholinergic neurotransmission in guinea pig airways. *J Pharmacol Exp Ther* 1990; 252(3):1207–1212.

59 Good DM, Hamilton TC. Effect of BRL 38227 on neurally-mediated responses in guinea-pig isolated bronchus. *Br J Pharmacol* 1991; 102:336P.

60 Miura M, Belvisi MG, Stretton CD, Yacoub MH, Barnes PJ. Role of K^+ channels in the modulation of cholinergic neural responses in guinea-pig and human airways. *J Physiol (Lond)* 1992; 455:1–15.

61 Patel HJ, Giembycz MA, Keeling JE, Barnes PJ, Belvisi MG. Inhibition of cholinergic neurotransmission in guinea pig trachea by NS1619, a putative activator of large-conductance, calcium-activated potassium channels. *J Pharmacol Exp Ther* 1998; 286(2):952–958.

62 Baird A, Hamilton T, Richards D, Tasker T, Williams AJ. Cromakalim, a potassium channel activator inhibits histamine induced bronchoconstriction in healthy volunteers (Abstract). *Br J Clin Pharm* 1988; 25:114P.

63 Williams AJ, Lee TH, Cochrane GM et al. Attenuation of nocturnal asthma by cromakalim. *Lancet* 1990; 336(8711):334–336.

64 Kidney JC, Fuller RW, Worsdell YM, Lavender EA, Chung KF, Barnes PJ. Effect of an oral potassium channel activator, BRL 38227, on airway function and responsiveness in asthmatic patients: comparison with oral salbutamol. *Thorax* 1993; 48(2):130–133.

65 Faurschou P, Mikkelsen KL, Steffensen I, Franke B. The lack of bronchodilator effect and the short-term safety of cumulative single doses of an inhaled potassium channel opener (bimakalim) in adult patients with mild to moderate bronchial asthma. *Pulm Pharmacol* 1994; 7(5):293–297.

66 Chapman ID, Mazzoni L, Morley J. Actions of SDZ PCO 400 and cromakalim on airway smooth muscle *in vivo*. *Agents Actions* Suppl. 1991; 34:53–62.

67 Chapman ID, Kristersson A, Mathelin G et al. Effects of a potassium channel opener (SDZ PCO 400) on guinea-pig and human pulmonary airways. *Br J Pharmacol* 1992; 106(2):423–429.

68 Mazzoni L, Chapman ID, Morley J. Changes in airway sensitivity to histamine are not necessarily paralleled by changed sensitivity to acetylcholine. *Agents Actions* Suppl. 1991; 34:257–266.

69 Buchheit KH, Hofmann A. KATP channel openers reverse immune complex-induced airways hyperreactivity independently of smooth muscle relaxation. *Naunyn Schmiedebergs Arch Pharmacol* 1996; 354(3):355–361.

70 Buchheit KH, Fozard JR. K^{ATP} channel openers for the treatment of airways hyperreactivity. *Pulm Pharmacol Ther* 1999; 12(2):103–105.

71 Spina D. Airway sensory nerves: a burning issue in asthma? *Thorax* 1996; 51(3):335–337.

72 Herd CM, Gozzard N, Page CP. Capsaicin pre-treatment prevents the development of antigen-induced airway hyperresponsiveness in neonatally immunised rabbits. *Eur J Pharmacol* 1995; 282(1–2):111–119.

73 Spina D, McKenniff MG, Coyle AJ et al. Effect of capsaicin on PAF-induced bronchial hyperresponsiveness and pulmonary cell accumulation in the rabbit. *Br J Pharmacol* 1991; 103(1):1268–1274.

74 Sanjar S, Kristersson A, Mazzoni L, Morley J, Schaeublin E. Increased airway reactivity in the guinea-pig follows exposure to intravenous isoprenaline. *J Physiol (Lond)* 1990; 425:43–54.

75 Rogers, DF. Neural control of airway secretions. In Barnes, PJ ed. *Autonomic Control of the Respiratory System.* The Netherlands: Harwood Academic Publishers GmbH; 1997: 201–227.

76 Ramnarine SI, Hirayama Y, Barnes PJ, Rogers DF. Sensory-efferent neural control of mucus secretion: characterization using tachykinin receptor antagonists in ferret trachea in vitro. *Br J Pharmacol* 1994; 113(4):1183–1190.

77 Ramnarine SI, Liu YC, Rogers DF. Neuroregulation of mucus secretion by opioid receptors and K(ATP) and BK(Ca) channels in ferret trachea in vitro. *Br J Pharmacol* 1998; 123(8):1631–1638.

78 Liu YC, Patel HJ, Khawaja AM, Belvisi MG, Rogers DF. Neuroregulation by vasoactive intestinal peptide (VIP) of mucus secretion in ferret trachea: activation of BK(Ca) channels and inhibition of neurotransmitter release. *Br J Pharmacol* 1999; 126(1):147–158.

79 Kamei J, Iwamoto Y, Narita M, Suzuki T, Misawa M, Kasuya Y. The antitussive effect of cromakalim in rats is not associated with adenosine triphosphate sensitive K$^+$ channels. *Res Commun Chem Pathol Pharmacol* 1993; 80(2):201–210.

80 Poggioli R, Benelli A, Arletti R, Cavazzuti E, Bertolini A. Antitussive effect of K$^+$ channel openers. *Eur J Pharmacol* 1999; 371(1):39–42.

9

Tachykinin and kinin antagonists

Pierangelo Geppetti

Department of Experimental and Clinical Medicine, Pharmacology Unit, University of Ferrara, Ferrara, Italy

Tachykinin, CGRP and their receptors

Substance P (SP), a major peptide neurotransmitter, was first found in the gut, and after two decades from its discovery it was proposed as a mediator of pain at the spinal level[1]. SP belongs to the tachykinin, a family of peptides that share a common C-terminus amino-acid sequence (Phe–X–Gly–Leu– Met–NH_2). In mammals the tachykinin are substantially confined to the central and peripheral nervous system. Three main tachykinin peptides have been described: SP, neurokinin A (NKA) and neurokinin B (NKB). SP and NKA are products of the preprotachykinin gene-I that via alternative splicing of the mRNA generates three different precursor proteins from which SP and NKA are produced at different ratios[2]. The sole biologically active product of the preprotachykinin gene-II is NKB[2]. NKB expression is apparently limited to the central nervous system, whereas SP and NKA are also found in a subpopulation of intrinsic neurones of the gut and in a subset of primary sensory neurones, including those of the trigeminal and dorsal root ganglia[3]. Of particular interest for this review is the notion that vagal (nodose and jugular) sensory ganglia are made up of a large proportion of neurones that contain and release tachykinin. Metabolism by membrane-bound peptidases, including neutral endopeptidase (NEP, EC 24.11) and angiotensin converting enzyme (ACE, EC 14.1), is one of the major factors that limit the biological effects of tachykinin[4,5]. Genetic disruption of NEP revealed the key role of this peptidase in the hitherto unrecognized control of baseline amounts of tachykinin and of baseline level of neurogenic plasma extravasation in mice[6].

The biological actions of tachykinin are mediated by three receptor subtypes, that belong to the seven transmembrane domain G protein-coupled receptor superfamily: these are the NK_1, NK_2 and NK_3 receptors. The existence of an NK_4 receptor subtype has been proposed[7], although molecular and pharmacological confirmation of its identity and biological role is lacking. All three tachykinin exhibit a similar high affinity for NK_1 receptors which is apparently the phylogenetically older tachykinin receptor subtype[8], whereas NKA and NKB have a better affinity for NK_2 and NK_3 receptors, respectively[8,9].

Calcitonin gene-related peptide (CGRP) is the product of an alternative splicing of the calcitonin gene that occurs in the nervous system, but not in the thyroid gland[10]. CGRP is co-stored in and co-released from, primary sensory neurones along with tachykinin[1]. The biological actions of CGRP are mediated via the activation of operationally defined receptors, the $CGRP_1$ and $CGRP_2$ receptors. These receptors, which are apparently regulated by the recently discovered receptor-activity-modifying protein(s) (RAMP)[11], are mainly localized at the vascular level where they induce vasodilatation, and contribute to neurogenic inflammatory responses (see below). Additional extravascular effects of CGRP include chronotropic and inotropic effects in the heart and dilatation of urinary tract smooth muscle.

Kinin and kinin receptors

Bradykinin is the best-known member of a family of short peptides produced by the action of proteases (kallikreins) that cleave larger precursor proteins, the kininogens. Plasma kallikriens cleave high molecular weight kininogen (HMWK), whereas glandular or other tissue kallikreins cleave low molecular weight kininogen (HMWK). The nonapeptide bradykinin is derived from the proteolytic cleavage of HMWK, whereas the extended form of bradykinin, lys-bradykinin (also called kallidin) originates from LMWK. Activation of kallikreins from inactive precursors, the pro-kallicreins, is produced by activation of the blood clotting cascade, lowering of the pH of the medium, inflammatory insults and other types of injury. The endopeptidases ACE (kininase II) and NEP are the main enzymes involved in the catabolism of kinin to inactive fragments. Cleavage of the C-terminus arginine from bradykinin and kallidin by an esopeptidase, the kininase I, is the origin for the des-arg[9] derivatives of kinin. Kinin receptors have been originally classified according to pharmacological criteria as B_1 and B_2 receptors[12]. In the last 10 years molecular cloning has confirmed the existence of these two receptors[13,14], whereas the proposal of additional receptor subtypes has not been proved yet. des-Arg[9] derivatives of bradykinin and kallidin selectively stimulate B_1 receptors[12,15]. The B_1 receptor has the unique feature of being inducible either after a few hours of incubation in vitro, or in vivo following exposure to a series of inflammatory stimuli and cytokines[15]. A few studies have been reported on the role of B_1 receptors in the airways to date. However, recent evidence that B_1 receptor is induced and exerts a motor response in the mouse trachea[16] suggests that this receptor may play a role in airway pathophysiological mechanisms.

B_2 receptors, as for B_1 receptors, belong to the G protein-coupled receptor superfamily, and they are distributed in a large variety of cells and tissues. The pleitropic, and often opposing, biological actions of bradykinin reflect the wide distribution of B_2 receptors. B_2 receptors have been documented by functional, histological and biochemical means in fibroblasts, endothelial and smooth muscle vascular cells, bronchial smooth muscle cells, epithelial and glandular cells as well as on sensory nerves of the airways. Localization of B_2 receptors on sensory nerves[17] is of particular relevance for bradykinin action in the airways because most of the responses caused by local application of bradykinin in this tissue are mediated indirectly by neurogenic mechanisms[18]. Bradykinin, along with its well-known pro-algesic property, due to its ability to initiate the afferent impulse that conveys nociceptive/painful information, induces the release of peptide neurotransmitters from peripheral terminals of sensory neurones, thus causing neurogenic inflammatory responses[1,18,19].

Neurogenic inflammation and biological responses to tachykinin

Neurogenic inflammation consists of inflammatory responses produced by neuropeptides (SP, NKA and CGRP) released from peripheral endings of primary sensory neurones. Neurogenic inflammation is particularly prominent at the vascular level where it causes vasodilatation of arterioles, plasma protein extravasation in post-capillary venules, and leukocyte adhesion to endothelial cells of venules. Non-vascular (urinary bladder, ureter, iris) smooth muscle relaxation/contraction, inotropic and chronotropic effect of the heart, and other effects are also tissue-specific neurogenic inflammatory responses. In the airways prominent extravascular actions mediated by neurogenic mechanisms are bronchoconstriction and in certain instances bronchorelaxation[20,21], secretion from seromucous glands[22], and release of mediators (including prostaglandins and nitric oxide, NO) from the airway epithelium. The sensory neuropeptide CGRP appears to be involved solely in the vasodilatation of bronchial arterioles in certain species[23]. Tachykinin and their receptors mediate all the other neurogenic inflammatory responses in the airways (Fig. 9.1 and Table 9.1). NK_2 receptors mediate bronchoconstriction in

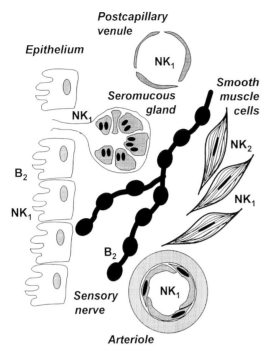

Fig. 9.1 Schematic representation of the localization of tachykinin and kinin receptors on different cells of the airways. NK_3 receptors have been involved in the cough response and hyperresponsiveness. However, their localization in the airways is not known. The localization of NK_1 and NK_2 receptors proposed to play a role in the cough response is also unclear. Representation of bradykinin B_2 receptors is limited to the role of these receptors in neurogenic inflammation.

Table 9.1. Tachykinin NK_1, NK_2 and NK_3 receptor antagonists and kinin B_2 receptor antagonists

NK_1	NK_3
CP-96345	SR 142801 (Osanetant)
CP-99994	SB 218795
CP-122721	**Dual NK_1/NK_2**
SR 140333 (Nolpitantium)	MDL 105,172
FK-888	FK-224
RP 67580	S 16474
MK-869	**B_2**
SDZ NKT 343	Hoe 140
LY 303870	WIN 64338
NK_2	FR-173657
SR 48968 (Saredutant)	**B_1**
MEN 11420 (Nepadutant)	[Leu^8-des-Arg^9]-bradykinin
GR 159897	R-715

Note:
This is a partial list of all the antagonists discovered and published.

lion level by tachykinin appears to be mediated by NK_1 receptors[24].

Modulation of neurogenic inflammation

Peptide-containing primary sensory neurones are characterized by their unique sensitivity to capsaicin, the pungent principal contained in the plants of the genus *Capsicum*[33]. The molecular basis of the selective action of capsaicin on sensory neurones has been recently clarified by the cloning of the channel operated by capsaicin[34]. This 6 transmembrane domain protein, that allows the influx of cations non-selectively, is physiologically stimulated by heat ($>43\ °C$) and by protons[35,36]. Capsaicin selectively stimulates primary sensory neurones and causes the release of sensory neuropeptide, thus promoting neurogenic inflammation. At higher concentrations capsaicin destroys the neurones thus, after a first excitatory phase, it blocks neurogenic inflammation[33]. These unique features of capsaicin have greatly contributed to the pathophysiological role of peptide-containing primary sensory neu-

most species[24,25]. However, in pig[26], guinea pig[27] and in human small[28] and medium size (Amadesi and P. Geppetti, unpublished observation) bronchi, NK_1 receptors appear to contribute to bronchoconstriction. NK_1 receptors mediate the increase in airway blood flow, plasma extravasation and leukocyte adhesion in postcapillary venules[29–31] and secretion from seromucous glands in the ferret and man[22,32]. NK_1 receptor stimulation in the tracheal epithelium promotes the secretion of bronchorelaxant NO in the guinea pig[21] and prostaglandins in the rat and mouse[20]. NK_2 receptors potentiate tachykinin-induced neurotransmission on postganglionic nerve terminals, whereas potentiation at the gang-

rones, which for this reason, have been defined as 'capsaicin-sensitive'[37].

Activation of inhibitory receptors on sensory nerves may limit neurogenic inflammatory responses[19]. These receptors include NPY[19], adenosine[38], 5-HT_{1D}[39], histamine H_3[40], dopamine D_2[41] receptors, to name but a few. Agonists for these receptors may thus be considered as anti-inflammatory agents. Likewise, tachykinin receptor antagonists are regarded as potential anti-inflammatory drugs.

A number of studies and review articles[1,18,19,42] have described the large variety of agents that stimulate sensory nerves, activating both their afferent and 'efferent' (neurogenic inflammation) functions. These stimuli include either autacoids like prostanoids, leukotrienes, histamine and serotonin[19], changes in the milieu, like lowering of the pH[35], increased osmolarity[43] and variations of the temperature or inflammatory or tissue injury conditions like anaphylaxis[44]. Among the stimulators of sensory nerves, kinin play a special role because kinin and tachykinin have been shown to share a final common pathway to produce inflammation in several important models of tissue injury in the airways[18]. Three examples of this assumption will be given in the next paragraphs.

Inflammatory models in the airways: role of kinin and tachykinin

A long series of mediators cause plasma extravasation and bronchoconstriction in the airways in vivo by releasing tachykinin: from the early studies showing that part of histamine- and serotonin-induced plasma extravasation was abolished by capsaicin pretreatment[45,46] to more recent evidence that tryptase, the major protease released from mast cells, releases tachykinin[47] and causes bronchoconstriction[48] by stimulating proteinase-activated receptor 2 (PAR-2) on sensory nerves. In addition to the large body of evidence that mediators may cause inflammation via neurogenic mechanisms, the involvement of sensory neuropeptides in airway inflammation has been obtained in more complex models of disease.

Tachykinin have been shown to mediate the dramatic increase in plasma extravasation caused by cigarette smoke inhalation in rats [49,50]. IgG-mediated alveolitis was reduced in mice in which the NK_1 receptor gene was deleted by homologous recombination and gene targeting[51]. Kinin levels have been shown to increase in the bronchoalveolar lavage of sensitized guinea pigs and asthmatic patients after antigen challenge[52]. Kinin antagonists have been shown to afford protection against inflammation in models of asthma in the sheep[46].

The cascade of inflammatory responses initiated by kinin and brought about by tachykinin is, however, described better in the following examples. Inhalation of cold air in guinea pigs' airways was found to increase plasma protein extravasation and total lung resistance[53,54]. Tachykinin NK_1 (plasma extravasation) or an NK_2 (bronchoconstriction) receptor antagonist or a B_2 receptor antagonist (both effects)[53,54] reduced or abolished these effects of cold air. Because exposure to cold air can trigger attacks of asthma and is known to worsen the disease, these findings are of relevance. Reflux of acid material from the stomach to the airways has been proposed as a mechanism of nocturnal asthma[55]. As mentioned before, acidic media possibly via direct stimulation of the capsaicin-activated channel[35,36], are powerful stimulants of sensory neurones. A combination of NK_2 and NK_1 receptor antagonists, abolished and a bradykinin B_2 receptor antagonist reduced[56] bronchoconstriction induced by citric acid inhalation in guinea pigs. Finally, in guinea pigs sensitized to and challenged with ovalbumin, an NK_1 receptor antagonist or a combination of NK_1/NK_2 receptor antagonists markedly reduced plasma extravasation and bronchoconstriction, respectively[44,57–59]. When tachykinin metabolism was blocked by the NEP inhibitor, phosphoramidon, the role of kinin/tachykinin was emphasized[44,57–59].

The inflammatory pathway described above and involving the ability of kinin to promote inflammation, releasing tachykinin from sensory nerves is well documented in guinea pigs[44]. As reported in the

Table 9.2. Effects inhibited or blocked by tachykinin, NK_1, NK_2 and NK_3 receptor antagonists in the airways of experimental animals and humans

(*a*) **Experimental animals**

Effect	*Stimulus*	*Receptor*
Plasma extravasation	Cigarette smoke, allergen, cold air	NK_1
Arterial vasodilatation	Capsaicin	NK_1
Bronchoconstriction	Capsaicin, allergen	NK_1, NK_2
Bronchodilatation	$[Sar^9, Met(O_2)^{11}]$-SP	NK_1
Leukocyte adhesion	Cigarette smoke, capsaicin	NK_1
Eosinophil accumulation	Allergen	NK_1, NK_2
Hyperresponsiveness	Allergen, citric acid, Toluene diisocyanate	NK_1, NK_2, NK_3
Cough	Capsaicin, Allergen, citric acid, mechanical stimulation	NK_1, NK_2, NK_3
Gland secretion	Substance P	NK_1

(*b*) **Humans**

Effect	*Stimulus*	*Receptor*
Bronchoconstriction in vivo	NKA, exercise, bradykinin	NK_2, NK_1 (?)
Bronchoconstriction in vitro	NKA, $[Sar^9, Met(O_2)^{11}]$-SP	NK_2, NK_1
Vasodilatation in vitro	$[Sar^9, Met(O_2)^{11}]$-SP	NK_1

Note:
This is a partial list of the airway effects inhibited by tachykinin receptor antagonists. Bradykinin B_2 receptor antagonists were shown to inhibit most of the responses in experimental animals listed above.

guinea pigs[60], bronchoconstriction induced by bradykinin in asthmatics is reduced by a dual NK_1/NK_2 receptor antagonist[61] and is markedly increased after inhibition of the L-Arg/NO synthase pathway[62]. However, to date there is no conclusive proof that kinin, either on their own or by stimulating tachykinin release, play a major role in asthma or in chronic obstructive pulmonary disease (COPD).

Tachykinin and kinin receptor antagonists

The search for high affinity, orally available and metabolically stable tachykinin and kinin antagonists has progressed through three main steps in the last 20 years. A first generation of peptide compounds originated from the substitution of critical amino acids on the backbone of naturally occurring peptides[9,63]. Although these molecules often retained agonist properties, they were useful for the in vitro characterization of receptor subtypes in specific tissues and gave a first impetus for the understanding of the physiological and pathophysiological role of kinin and tachykinin. Selectivity and affinity for respective receptors was markedly increased and in certain instances pharmacokinetic features were optimized in a second generation of peptide antagonists. Hoe 140 (Icatibant)[64], MEN 11420[65] or GR 159897[66] are examples of this improvement. Although these compounds have been used for a number of in vivo studies in experimental animals, and have been tested in man by local routes of administration, their poor oral bioavailability because of the peptide nature, limits their further exploitation in human studies.

The discovery of the first non-peptide antagonist for NK_1 receptors, CP-96,345, was reported in 1991[67]. Soon after a number of antagonists for NK_1, NK_2 and eventually NK_3 receptors appeared. Some of these drugs exhibit non-specific effects, including Ca^{2+}-channel antagonism[68] which reduced interest for further development. However, changes in lead molecules, or new molecules often obtained by the powerful combinatorial chemistry and high-throughput screening, rapidly offered new compounds that combined high affinity and selectivity with excellent pharmacokinetic profiles. A list of tachykinin and kinin antagonists is given in Table 9.2, and recent review articles[9,69] have described in detail the properties of tachykinin antagonists. Here, attention will be focused on those compounds that have been used in airway studies and those for which studies in man may be envisaged.

The use of CP-96,345 and CP-99,994[70] demonstrated unequivocally that neurogenic plasma protein extravasation in rodent trachea caused by a variety of stimuli, including cigarette smoke, is mediated by NK_1 receptors[50]. Another NK_1 selective antagonist, SR 140333[71], merits being mentioned because of its large use in experimental animals[6] and because it is derived from the chemical structure of the selective NK_2 antagonist, SR 48968[72]. It is worth mentioning that from the same chemical structure the first high affinity non-peptide antagonist for NK_3 receptors was discovered[73].

A random screening approach has also been the strategy for the discovery of non-peptide B_2 receptor antagonists. WIN 64338[74] was the first compound showing a reasonable affinity for the B_2 guinea pig receptor. However, it exhibited low affinity for the human receptor. A few years later FR-173657[75] overcame the drawbacks of WIN 64338, because of its high affinity and selectivity for B_2 receptors in most mammal species, including man. FR-173657 and other compounds derived from its structure, because of their non-peptide nature, have marked advantages over Icatibant. However, only a few studies have been performed with FR-173657 in the airways to date[76].

Tachykinin and kinin receptor antagonists in the airways

CP-96,345, CP-99,994 and SR 48968 were of critical value to discover the role of tachykinin and NK_1 and

NK_2 receptors in airway anaphylaxis in guinea pigs and monkeys[44,58,59,77,78]. These observations were confirmed with a dual antagonist for NK_1 and NK_2 receptors[79]. The use of these antagonists have contributed to show the role of tachykinin in cold air and low pH-induced airway inflammation[54,56].

The role of NK_3 receptors in airway pathophysiology is still unclear. First, the preferred agonist of NK_3 receptor, NKB, is not present in and released by peripheral neurones or by other cells in the airways. However, SR 142801 has revealed that NK_3 receptors contribute to the development of hyperresponsiveness after exposure to SP[80]. SB 218795[81], an additional NK_3 receptor antagonist, may further contribute to the discovery of new roles of NK_3 receptors in models of airway diseases.

The hypothesis that a drug with both bronchodilator and anti-inflammatory properties could result from the combination of NK_1 and NK_2 antagonism is derived from the observation that bronchial smooth muscle contraction is mainly due to NK_2 receptor[25,72], and proinflammatory vascular functions[82] and secretion from seromucous glands[22] are due to NK_1 receptor activation. Thus, a series of dual antagonists have been developed, including FK-224[83], MDL 105172[79] and S 16474[84].

Hoe 140 has markedly contributed in clarifying the role of kinin in a large array of pathophysiological models of respiratory diseases. These models include airway anaphylaxis[44,57], exposure to cold air[53,54], citric acid inhalation, and the release of NO from airway epithelium[62]. Similar studies with non-peptide B_2 receptor antagonists have not been performed yet.

Cough is a common symptom of most airway diseases that results from the activation of a complex reflex pathway in which $A\delta$- and C-fibres play a major initiating role. Possible involvement of kinin in cough is suggested by the epidemiological observation that cough is the most frequent adverse effect in patients in whom ACE (kininase II), the peptidase that cleaves bradykinin, is inhibited[85]. Studies in guinea pigs[86] and mice[87] showing that ACE inhibitors produced Icatibant-reversible proinflammatory effects in the airways and sensitization of the cough reflex, added further support to the hypothesis that kinin play a major role in causing the protective cough reflex.

The role of tachykinin and tachykinin receptors in cough seems to be more complex. Early evidence for the involvement of SP in cough has been reported[88]. Involvement of NK_2 receptors in the cough reflex is suggested by the finding that NK_2 receptor antagonists reduced or ablated citric acid-, cigarette smoke- and allergen-induced cough[89]. Involvement of NK_1 and NK_3 receptors has been also shown in the cough induced by different stimuli[90,91]. NK_1 and NK_2 antagonists revealed a dual (both peripheral and central) antitussive site of action for tachykinin antagonists in guinea pigs, whereas in the cat the antitussive site of action of tachykinin antagonists was only at the central level[92]. The multiple receptors involved in the cough response at diverse sites in different species underline the caution in extrapolating data from experimental animals to man.

Tachykinin and kinin receptor antagonists in the human airways

Clinical studies with tachykinin and kinin receptor antagonists in human airways are not abundant. This paucity may be the result of either conflicting findings obtained with early, peptide antagonists, poor outcome in studies whose endpoints were not the most appropriate or poor choice of the type of disease under investigation. Studies performed with FK-224, a dual NK_1 and NK_2 receptor antagonist are an example of the first case. Reduced bronchoconstriction in response to inhaled bradykinin was obtained after pretreatment with FK-224, given via a metered-dose inhaler in moderate asthmatic patients[61]. However, these results could not be reproduced[93], and FK-224 (4 mg q.i.d, administered over 4 weeks) did not ameliorate asthma symptoms of patients with mild to moderate asthma[94]. The finding that FK-224 failed to inhibit NKA-induced bronchoconstriction in moderate asthmatics whereas another NK_2 receptor antagonist, SR 48968, was effective[95] underlines the critical importance of the antagonist under investigation.

An example of the second case is offered by a study with the selective non-peptide NK_1 receptor antagonist CP-99,994. This drug, given intravenously (250 µg/kg) was ineffective in reducing bronchoconstriction and cough induced by inhalation of hypertonic saline in moderate asthmatics[96]. However, the fact that bronchoconstriction in man is mainly mediated by NK_2 receptor activation and the multiple tachykinin receptors involved in the tussive response in experimental animals suggest that the study endpoints were not the most suitable to investigate the role of a highly selective NK_1 antagonist.

The NK_1 receptor antagonist, FK-888, did not significantly attenuate the maximal fall in specific airway conductance; however, it did improve the recovery time from exercise-induced airway narrowing in asthmatics[97], thus suggesting that NK_1 receptors have a role in the recovery phase of exercise-induced airway narrowing. Whereas it is unlikely that tachykinin and their receptors play a major role in the majority of asthma patients the possibility exists that selected types of asthma might be a good target for unravelling the role of tachykinin in this disease: asthma with cough and nocturnal asthma induced by gastroesophageal reflux may be appropriate subtypes. COPD, a disease characterized by cough, sputum and progression of non-reversible airway obstruction might also be a suitable target for drugs that inhibit cough, seromucous gland secretion and bronchoconstriction.

The presence of B_2 receptors has been shown in a large number of airway cells, including epithelial cells[98]. In asthmatic patients in vivo the airways respond to aerosolized bradykinin with minor or exaggerated bronchoconstriction according to the status of the disease: the more severe the asthma, the more pronounced the bronchoconstriction[99,100]. In guinea pigs, bronchoconstriction by bradykinin is limited by NO release from the epithelium[57,62]. There is indirect evidence that exaggerated bradykinin-induced bronchoconstriction in severe asthma, a condition characterized by prominent epithelial shedding, results from the failure of bradykinin to release bronchoprotective NO from a damaged epithelium[99,100]. This hypothesis implies that in severe asthma, which is characterized by the loss of epithelium-dependent protective role of bradykinin, B_2 receptor antagonists may give better protection by blocking the remaining neurogenic detrimental role of bradykinin. Aerosolized Hoe 140 was found to give some protection in moderate asthma in a 4-week study[101]. The type of protection offered by Icatibant suggested that this drug possesses a more anti-inflammatory than bronchodilator property. However, the effect of bradykinin B_2 receptor antagonists has not been investigated in severe asthma.

REFERENCES

1 Holzer P. Local effector functions of capsaicin-sensitive sensory nerves endings: involvement of tachykinin, calcitonin gene-related peptide and other neuropeptides. *Neuroscience* 1988; 24:739–768.

2 Nakanishi S. Substance P precursor and kininogen:their structures, gene organization and regulation. *Physiol Rev* 1987; 67:117–1142.

3 Otsuka M, Yoshioka K. Neurotransmitter functions of mammalian tachykinin. *Physiol Rev* 1993; 73:229–308.

4 Di Maria GU, Bellofiore S, Geppetti P. Regulation of airway neurogenic inflammation by neutral endopeptidase [In Process Citation]. *Eur Respir J* 1998; 12:1454–62.

5 Nadel JA. Neutral endopeptidase modulates neurogenic inflammation. *Eur Respir J* 1991; 4:745–754.

6 Lu B, Figini M, Emanueli C, et al. The control of microvascular permeability and blood pressure by neutral endopeptidase. *Nat Med* 1997; 3:904–907.

7 Donaldson LF, Haskell CA, Hanley MR. Functional characterization by heterologous expression of a novel cloned tachykinin peptide receptor. *Biochem J* 1996; 320:1–5.

8 Maggi CA, Schwatz TW. The dual nature of the tachykinin NK_1 receptor. *Trends Pharmacol Sci* 1997; 18:351–55.

9 Regoli D, Boudon A, Fauchere J-L. Receptors and antagonists for substance P and related peptides. *Pharmacol Rev* 1994; 46:551–599.

10 Amara SG, Jonas V, Rosenfeld MG, Ong ES, Evans RM. Alternative RNA processing in calcitonin gene expression generates mRNAs encoding different polypeptide products. *Nature* 1982; 298:240–244.

11 McLatchie LM, Fraser NJ, Main MJ, et al. RAMPs regulate the transport and ligand specificity of the calcitonin-receptor-like receptor. *Nature* 1998; 393:333–339.

12 Regoli D, Barabe J. Pharmacology of bradykinin and related kinin. *Pharmacol Rev* 1980; 32:1–46.

13 Menke JG, Borkowski JA, Bierilo KK, et al. Expression cloning of a human B1 bradykinin receptor. *J Biol Chem* 1994; 269:21583–21586.

14 Hess JF, Borkowski JA, Young GS, Strader CD, Ransom RW. Cloning and pharmacological characterization of a human bradykinin (BK- 2) receptor. *Biochem Biophys Res Commun* 1992; 184:260–8.

15 Marceau F, Hess JF, Bacharov DR. The B1 receptors for kinin. *Pharmacol Rev* 1998; 50:357–386.

16 Trevisani M, Schmidlin F, Tognetto M, et al. Evidence for in vitro expression of B1 receptor in the mouse trachea and urinary bladder. *Br J Pharmacol* 1999; 126:1293–1300.

17 Steranka L, Manning D, DeHaas C, et al. Bradykinin as a pain mediator: receptors are localized to sensory neurons, and antagonists have analgesic actions. *Proc Natl Acad Sci USA* 1988; 85:3245–3249.

18 Geppetti P. Sensory neuropeptide release by bradykinin: mechanisms and pathophysiological implications. *Regu Pept* 1993; 47:1–23.

19 Maggi C. The pharmacology of the efferent function of sensory nerves. *J Auton Pharmacol* 1991; 11:173–208.

20 Frossard N, Rhoden KJ, Barnes PJ. Influence of epithelium on guinea pig airway responses to tachykinin: role of endopeptidase and cyclooxygenase. *J Pharmacol Exp Ther* 1989; 248:292–298.

21 Figini M, Emanueli C, Bertrand C, Javdan P, Geppetti P. Evidence that tachykinin relax the guinea-pig trachea *via* nitric oxide release and by stimulation of a septide-insensitive NK_1 receptor. *Br J Pharmacol* 1996; 115:128–132.

22 Geppetti P, Betrand C, Bacci E, Huber O, Nadel JA. Characterization of tachykinin receptors in the ferret trachea by peptide agonists and non-peptide antagonists. *Am J Physiol* 1993; 265:L164-L169.

23 Lundberg JM. Tachykinin, sensory nerves, and asthma – an overview. *Can J Physiol Pharmacol* 1995; 73:908–914.

24 Advenier C, Lagente V, Boichot E. The role of tachykinin receptor antagonists in the prevention of bronchial hyper-responsiveness, airway inflammation and cough. *Eur Respir J* 1997; 10:1892–1906.

25 Advenier C, Naline E, Toty L, et al. Effects on the isolated human bronchus of SR 48968, a potent and selective non-peptide antagonist of the neurokinin A (NK2) receptors. *Am Rev Respir Dis* 1992; 146:1177–81.

26 Scheldrick RLG, Ball DI, Coleman RA. Characterization of the neurokinin receptor mediating contraction of isolated tracheal preparations from a variety of species. *Agents Actions* 1990; Suppl, 31:205–210.

27 Bertrand C, Nadel JA, Graf PD, Geppetti P. Capsaicin

increases airflow resistance in guinea pigs in vivo by activating both NK_2 and NK_1 tachykinin receptors. *Am Rev Respir Dis* 1993; 148:909–914.

28 Naline E, Molimard M, Regoli D, Emonds-Alt X, Bellamy JF, Advenier C. Evidence for functional tachykinin NK1 receptors on human isolated small bronchi. *Am J Physiol* 1996; 271:L763–7.

29 Piedimonte G, Hoffman JI, Husseini WK, Snider RM, Desai MC, Nadel JA. NK1 receptors mediate neurogenic inflammatory increase in blood flow in rat airways. *J Appl Physiol* 1993; 74:2462–8.

30 Baluk P, Bertrand C, Geppetti P, McDonald DM, Nadel JA. NK1 receptors mediate leukocyte adhesion in neurogenic inflammation in the rat trachea. *Am J Physiol* 1995; 268:L263-L269.

31 Corboz MR, Rivelli MA, Ramos SI, Rizzo CA, Hey JA. Tachykinin NK1 receptor-mediated vasorelaxation in human pulmonary arteries. *Eur J Pharmacol* 1998; 350:R1–3.

32 Rogers DF, Aursudkij B, Barnes PJ. Effects of tachykinin on mucus secretion in human bronchi in vitro. *Eur J Pharmacol* 1989; 174:283–286.

33 Szallasi A, Blumberg PM. Vanilloid (capsaicin) receptors and mechanisms. *Pharmacol Rev* 1999; 51:159–211.

34 Caterina MJ, Schumacher MA, Tominaga M, Rosen TA, Levine JD, Julius D. The capsaicin receptor: a heat-activated ion channel in the pain pathway. *Nature* 1997; 389:816–824.

35 Bevan S, Geppetti P. Protons, small stimulants of capsaicin-sensitive sensory nerves. *Trends Neurosci* 1994; 17:509–512.

36 Tominaga M, Caterina MJ, Malmberg AB, et al. The cloned capsaicin receptor integrates multiple pain-producing stimuli. *Neuron* 1998; 21:531–543.

37 Szolcsanyi J. Capsaicin-sensitive chemoceptive neural system with dual sensory-efferent function. In *Antidromic Vasodilatation and Neurogenic Inflammation*. Budapest: Akademiai Kiado; 1984.

38 Rubino A, Mantelli L, Amerini S, Ledda F. Adenosine modulation of non-adrenergic non-cholinergic neurotransmission in isolated guinea-pig atria. *Naunyn Schmiedebergs Arch Pharmacol* 1990; 342:520–522.

39 Buzzi MG, Moskowitz MA, Peroutka SJ, Byun B. Further characterization of the putative 5-HT receptor which mediates blockade of neurogenic plasma extravasation in rat dura mater. *Br J Pharmacol* 1991; 103:1421–1428.

40 Imamura M, Smith NC, Garbarg M, Levi R. Histamine H3-receptor-mediated inhibition of calcitonin gene-related peptide release from cardiac C fibers. A regulatory negative-feedback loop. *Circ Res* 1996; 78:863–869.

41 Young A, Dougall IG, Blackham A, et al. AR -68397AA: the first dual D2-receptor and ß2-adrenoceptor agonist. *Am J Respir Crit Care Med* 1999; 12:A576.

42 Geppetti P, Holzer P. *Neurogenic Inflammation*. Boca Raton: CRC Press, 1996.

43 Umeno E, McDonald DM, Nadel JA. Hypertonic saline increases vascular permeability in the rat trachea by producing neurogenic inflammation. *J Clin Invest* 1990; 85:1905–1908.

44 Bertrand C, Geppetti P. Tachykinin and kinin receptor antagonists: therapeutic perspectives in allergic disease. *Trends Pharmacol Sci* 1996; 17:255–259.

45 Saria A, Lundberg J, Skofitsch G, Lembeck F. Vascular protein leakage in various tissues induced by substance P, capsaicin, bradykinin, serotonin and by histamine challenge. *Naunyn Schmideberg's Arch Pharmacol* 1983; 324:212–218.

46 Abraham WM, Burch RM, Farmer SG, Sielczak MW, Ahmed A, Cortes A. A bradykinin antagonist modifies allergen-induced mediator release and late bronchial responses in sheep. *Am Rev Respir Dis* 1991; 143:787–796.

47 Steinhoff M, Vergnolle N, Young SH, et al. Agonists of proteinase-activated receptor 2 induce inflammation by a neurogenic mechanism. *Nature Med* 2000; 6:151–158.

48 Ricciardolo FLM, Steinhoff M, Amadesi S, et al. Presence and bronchomotor activity of proteinase activated receptor-2 (PAR-2) in guinea-pig airways. *Am J Respir Crit Care Med* 2000; 161:1672–1680.

49 Lundberg J, Saria A. Capsaicin induced desensitization of the airway mucosa to cigarette smoke, mechanical and chemical irritants. *Nature* 1983; 302:251–253.

50 Delay-Goyet P, Lundberg JM. Cigarette smoke-induced airway oedema is blocked by the NK1 antagonist, CP-96,345. *Eur J Pharmacol* 1991; 203:157–158.

51 Bozic CR, Lu B, Hopken UE, Gerard C, Gerard NP. Neurogenic amplification of immune complex inflammation. *Science* 1996; 273:1722–1725.

52 Proud D, Kaplan AP. Kinin formation: mechanisms and role in inflammatory disorders. *Ann Rev Immunol* 1998; 6:49–84.

53 Yoshihara S, Geppetti P, Hara M, et al. Cold air-induced bronchoconstriction is mediated by tachykinin and kinin release in guinea pigs. *Eur J Pharmacol* 1996; 296:291–6.

54 Yoshihara S, Chan B, Yamawaki I, et al. Plasma extravasation in the rat trachea induced by cold air is mediated by tachykinin release from sensory nerves. *Am J Respir Crit Care Med* 1995; 151:1011–1017.

55 Sontag SJ. Gastroesophageal reflux and asthma. *Am J Med* 1997; 103:84S–90S.

56 Ricciardolo FLM, Rado V, Fabbri LM, Sterk PJ, Di Maria GU,

Geppetti P. Bronchoconstriction induced by citric acid inhalation in guinea pigs: role of tachykinin, bradykinin, and nitric oxide. *Am J Respir Crit Care Med* 1999; 159:557–562.

57 Ricciardolo FML, Nadel JA, Yoshihara S, Geppetti P. Evidence that bradykinin-induced bronchoconstriction in guinea-pigs is reduced by release of nitric oxide. *Br J Pharmacol* 1994; 113:1147–1152.

58 Bertrand C, Geppetti P, Baker J, Yamawaki I, Nadel JA. Role of neurogenic inflammation in antigen-induced vascular extravasation in guinea pig trachea. *J Immunol* 1993; 150:1479–1485.

59 Bertrand C, Geppetti P, Graf PD, Nadel JA. Involvement of neurogenic inflammation in antigen-induced broncho-constriction in guinea pigs. *Am J Physiol* 1993; 265:L507–L511.

60 Ichinose M, Belvisi MG, Barnes PJ. Bradykinin-induced bronchoconstriction in guinea pig in vivo: role of neural mechanisms. *J Pharmacol Exp Ther* 1990; 253:594–599.

61 Ichinose M, Nakajima N, Takahashi T, Yamauchi H, Inoue H, Takashima T. Protection against bradykinin-induced bronchoconstriction in asthmatic patients by neurokinin receptor antagonist. *Lancet* 1992; 340:1248–1251.

62 Figini M, Ricciardolo FLM, Javdan P, et al. Evidence that epithelium-derived relaxing factor released by bradykinin in the guinea-pig trachea is nitric oxide. *Am J Respir Crit Care Med* 1996; 153:918–923.

63 Stewart JM, Gera L, York EJ, Chan DC, Bunn P. Bradykinin antagonists: present progress and future prospects [In Process Citation]. *Immunopharmacology* 1999; 43:155–61.

64 Hock F, Wirth K, Albus U, et al. HOE 140 a new potent and long acting bradykinin-antagonist: *in vitro* studies. *Br J Pharmacol* 1991; 102:769–773.

65 Catalioto RM, Criscuoli M, Cucchi P, et al. MEN 11420 (Nepadutant), a novel glycosylated bicyclic peptide tachy-kinin NK2 receptor antagonist. *Br J Pharmacol* 1998; 123:81–91.

66 McElroy AB, Clegg SP, Deal MJ, et al. Highly potent and selective heptapeptide antagonists of the neurokinin NK-2 receptor. *J Med Chem* 1992; 35:2582–2591.

67 Snider R, Constantine J, Lowe I, et al. A potent nonpeptide antagonist of the substance P (NK$_1$) receptor. *Science* 1991; 251:435–437.

68 Schmidt AW, McLean S, Heym J. The substance P receptor antagonist CP-96,345 interacts with Ca^{2+} channels [corrected and republished article originally printed in *Eur J Pharmacol* 1992 May 14;215(2–3):351–2]. *Eur J Pharmacol* 1992; 219:491–2.

69 Geppetti P, Tognetto M, Trevisani M, Amadesi S, Bertrand

C. Tachykinin and kinin in airway allergy. *Exp Opin Invest Drug*s 1999; 8:947–956.

70 McLean S, Ganong A, Seymour PA, et al. Pharmacology of CP-99,994; a nonpeptide antagonist of the tachykinin neu-rokinin-1 receptor. *J Pharmacol Exp Ther* 1993; 267:472–479.

71 Emonds-Alt X, Doutremepuich JD, Heaulme M, et al. In vitro and in vivo biological activities of SR140333, a novel potent non-peptide tachykinin NK1 receptor antagonist. *Eur J Pharmacol* 1993; 250:403–413.

72 Emonds-Alt X, Vilain P, Goulaouic P, et al. A potent and selective non-peptide antagonist of the neurokinin A (NK2) receptor. *Life Sci* 1992; 50:L101–106.

73 Emonds-Alt X, Bichon D, Ducoux JP, et al. SR 142801, the first potent non-peptide antagonist of the tachykinin NK3 receptor. *Life Sci* 1995; 56:L27–32.

74 Sawutz DG, Salvino JM, Dolle RE, et al. The nonpeptide WIN 64338 is a bradykinin B2 receptor antagonist. *Proc Natl Acad Sci USA* 1994; 91:4693–4697.

75 Asano M, Inamura N, Hatori C, et al. The identification of an orally active, nonpeptide bradykinin B2 receptor antag-onist, FR173657. *Br J Pharmacol* 1997; 120:617–624.

76 Griesbacher T, Legat FJ. Effects of FR173657, a non-peptide B2 antagonist, on kinin-induced hypotension, visceral and peripheral oedema formation and bronchoconstriction. *Br J Pharmacol* 1997; 120:933–939.

77 Ricciardolo FLM, Nadel JA, Bertrand C, Yamawaki I, Chan B, Geppetti P. Tachykinin and kinin in antigen-evoked plasma extravasation in guinea-pig nasal mucosa. *Eur J Pharmacol* 1994; 261:127–132.

78 Turner CR, Andresen CJ, Patterson DK. Dual antagonism of NK1 and NK2 receptors by CP 99,994 and SR 48968 pre-vents airway hyperresponsiveness in primates. *Am J Respir Crit Care Med* 1996; 153:A160.

79 Kudlacz EM, Knippenberg RW, Logan DE, Burkholder TP. The effect of MDL 105,172A, a nonpeptide NK1/NK2 receptor antagonist in an allergic guinea pig model. *J Pharmacol Exp Ther* 1996; 279:732–739.

80 Daoui S, Cognon C, Naline E, Emonds-Alt X, Advenier C. Involvement of tachykinin NK3 receptors in citric acid-induced cough and bronchial responses in guinea pigs. *Am J Respir Crit Care Med* 1998; 158:42–48.

81 Giardina GA, Sarau HM, Farina C, et al. Discovery of a novel class of selective non-peptide antagonists for the human neurokinin-3 receptor. 1. Identification of the 4-quinoline-carboxamide framework. *J Med Chem* 1997; 40:1794–1807.

82 Bowden JJ, Garland AM, Baluk P, et al. Direct observation of substance P-induced internalization of neurokinin 1 (NK1) receptors at sites of inflammation. *Proc Natl Acad Sci USA* 1994; 91:8964–8968.

83 Murai M, Morimoto H, Maeda Y, Kiyotoh S, Nishikawa M, Fujii T. Effects of FK224, a novel compound NK1 and NK2 receptor antagonist, on airway constriction and airway edema induced by neurokinin and sensory nerve stimulation in guinea pigs. *J Pharmacol Exp Ther* 1992; 262:403–408.

84 Robineau P, Lonchampt M, Kucharczyk N, et al. In vitro and in vivo pharmacology of S 16474, a novel dual tachykinin NK1 and NK2 receptor antagonist. *Eur J Pharmacol* 1995; 294:677–684.

85 Aronow WS. The ELITE Study. What are its implications for the drug treatment of heart failure? Evaluation of losartan in the elderly study. *Drugs Aging* 1998; 12:423–428.

86 Fox AJ, Umesh GL, Belvisi M, Bernareggi M, Chung KF, Barnes PJ. Bradykinin-evoked sensitization of airways sensory nerves: a mechanism for ACE-inhibitor cough. *Nat Med* 1996; 2:814–817.

87 Emanueli C, Grady F.F, Madeddu P, et al. Acute ACE inhibition causes plasma extravasation in mice that is mediated by bradykinin and substance P. *Hypertension* 1998; 31:1299–1304.

88 Koroghi H, Graf PD, Sekizawa K, Borson DB, Nadel JA. Netral endopeptidase inhibitors potentiate substance P and capsaicin-induced cough in awake guinea-pigs. *J Clin Invest* 1988; 82:2063–2068.

89 Girard V, Naline E, Vilain P, Emonds Alt X, Advenier C. Effect of the two tachykinin antagonists, SR 48968 and SR 140333, on cough induced by citric acid in the unanaesthetized guinea pig. *Eur Respir J* 1995; 8:1110–1114.

90 Ujiie Y, Sekizawa K, Aikawa T, Sasaki H. Evidence for substance P as an endogenous substance causing cough in guinea pigs. *Am Rev Respir Dis* 1993; 148:1628–1632.

91 Advenier C, Daoui S, Cui YY, Lagente V, Emonds-Alt X. Inhibition by the tachykinin NK$_3$ receptor antagonist, SR 142801, of substance P-induced microvascular leakage hypersensitivity and airway hyperresponsiveness in guinea-pigs. *Am J Respir Crit Care Med* 1996; 153:A163.

92 Bolser DC, DeGennaro FC, O'Reilly S, McLeod RL, Hey JA. Central antitussive activity of the NK1 and NK2 tachykinin receptor antagonists, CP-99,994 and SR 48968, in the guinea-pig and cat. *Br J Pharmacol* 1997; 121:165–170.

93 Joos G, Scoor JV, Kips JC, Pauwels RA. The effect of inhaled FK224, a tachykinin NK-1 and NK-2 receptor antagonist, on neurokinin A-induced bronchoconstriction in asthmatics. *Am J Respir Crit Care Med* 1996; 153:1781–1784.

94 Lunde H, Hedner J, Svedmir N. Lack of efficacy of 4 weeks treatment with the neurokinin receptor antagonist FK244 in mild to moderate asthma. *Eur Respir J* 1994; 7(Suppl. 18):248s.

95 Van Schoor J, Joos GF, Chasson B, Brouard RJ, Pauwels RA. The effect of SR 48968, a nonpeptide neurokinin-2 receptor antagonist on neurokinin A-induced bronchoconstriction in asthmatics. *Eur Respir J* 1996; 9:289s.

96 Fahy JV, Wong HH, Geppetti P, et al. Effect of an NK-1 receptor antagonist (CP-99,994) on hypertonic saline-induced bronchoconstriction and cough in male asthmatic subjects. *Am J Respir Crit Care Med* 1995; 152:879–884.

97 Ichinose M, Miura M, Yamauchi H, et al. A neurokinin 1-receptor antagonist improves exercise-induced airway narrowing in asthmatic patients. *Am J Respir Crit Care Med* 1996; 153:936–941.

98 Ricciardolo FL, Lovett M, Halliday DA, et al. Bradykinin increases intracellular calcium levels in a human bronchial epithelial cell line via the B2 receptor subtype. *Inflamm Res* 1998; 47:231–235.

99 Ricciardolo FL, Geppetti P, Mistretta A, et al. Randomised double-blind placebo-controlled study of the effect of inhibition of nitric oxide synthesis in bradykinin-induced asthma. *Lancet* 1996; 348:374–377.

100 Ricciardolo FLM, Di Maria GU, Sapienza MA, Mistretta A, Geppetti P. Impairment of bronchoprotection by NO in severe asthma. *Lancet* 1997; 350:1297–1298.

101 Akbary AM, Wirth KJ, Scholkens BA. Efficacy and tolerability of Icatibant (Hoe 140) in patients with moderately severe chronic bronchial asthma. *Immunopharmacology* 1996; 33:238–242.

10

Drugs affecting IgE (synthesis inhibitors and monoclonal antibodies)

Lawrence G. Garland and Alan G. Lamont

Acambis PLC, Cambridge, UK

It is now well recognized that IgE plays a key role in the sequence of cellular events leading to an allergic reaction such as occurs in allergic rhinitis and asthma. Various strategies have been attempted to interfere with the IgE-dependent activation of mast cells and basophils, including trying to find antagonists to block the interaction between IgE and its high affinity receptor FcεRI. However, the affinity of IgE for FcεRI is extremely high, of the order of 10^{10}–10^{12}/mol/l[1,2]. For any drug to compete with IgE it would have to interact with FcεRI with comparable affinity: it is not surprising that this has been difficult to achieve and no such drugs have yet been described.

An alternative approach would be to decrease the level of IgE available to interact with FcεRI. This rationale is supported by evidence that serum levels of IgE have been reported to correlate with the severity of allergic symptoms, including in allergic asthma[3–5]. At the cellular level, the amount of IgE bound to FcεRI on human basophils correlates closely with serum levels of IgE. However, cell sensitivity to receptor cross-linking is influenced also by intracellular pathways such that in vitro the extent of mediator release appears to be independent of the number of IgE molecules per basophil[6]. Also, cross-linking of only a small number of IgE receptors (relative to the total available) is sufficient to stimulate secretion[7,8]. Thus, it is arguable that it would be very difficult to inhibit mast cell/basophil responses by decreasing the plasma level of IgE, as a decrease of > 99% would be required. Nevertheless, it is becoming clear, particularly from clinical studies with

rhuMAb-25 (see later), that decreasing plasma IgE has an antiallergic outcome. Critical to understanding the mechanism by which this occurs are recent observations that the expression of FcεRI on basophils and mast cells is regulated by levels of circulating IgE. A decrease in plasma IgE leads to a marked down-regulation of FcεRI on basophils and a substantial inhibition of the response of these cells to specific antigen[9–12]. Hence, the decrease in FcεRI density amplifies the antiallergic effect obtained. These observations give great impetus to therapeutic strategies designed to decrease plasma levels of IgE by drugs which act at the level of T or B lymphocytes, or by antibodies that deplete circulating IgE or by immunization to actively generate antibodies which block the interaction between IgE and its receptors.

In this chapter, we describe the progress which has been made with various strategies designed to decrease both IgE production and activity. Before this, however, we provide a brief description of how IgE synthesis is regulated, and how cytokines act to increase or decrease synthesis.

Regulation of IgE synthesis

The nature of the heavy chain carried by an immunoglobulin (Ig) molecule largely determines its effector function. In humans, five broad classes of heavy chain exist, giving rise to the different isotypes IgM, IgG, IgD, IgA, and IgE. It is one of the defining features of the immune system, and in particular the

B lymphocyte, that the cell can produce antibodies (Ab) which retain the original antigen (Ag) specificity, yet can express different heavy chain isotypes throughout the course of an immune response, thus altering the effector function attributed to a single specificity. This process, termed class switching, occurs in a predetermined manner within distinct sites in lymphoid tissue, and is driven both by intrinsic factors (e.g. related to cell cycle progression) and by extrinsic factors (e.g. influence of cytokines and cell–cell contact). Thus, early in the immune response to Ag, the dominant isotype is IgM. As the response progresses, IgG isotypes predominate, with some IgA observed particularly at mucosal sites. In normal individuals, IgE is rarely detected. In atopic individuals, however, high levels of IgE are observed, and these are associated with the development of hypersensitivities to common allergens. The process by which Ab class switching occurs is increasingly understood, and, in the case of switching to the epsilon (ε) isotype, has long been a favoured process, targeted by those seeking to selectively prevent IgE production. To understand how a B-cell becomes committed to IgE production, it is first necessary to appreciate the structure and arrangement of the Ig genes within the heavy chain locus, and the DNA rearrangement process by which the variable segment is juxtaposed beside the Cε locus. (For a more complete description of Ig gene organization and the process of isotype switching, the reader is referred to recent reviews[13,14].)

Nature of B cell gene rearrangement

The Ig heavy chain locus is located on chromosome 14 in humans and the organization of the heavy chain genes in the germline is shown in Fig. 10.1. To produce functional heavy chain, two sets of rearrangement are required:

(i) The variable region of the Ig heavy chain is encoded by the V, D, and J segments which recombine during B cell ontogeny to form a contiguous segment which defines the antigen binding site of the Ig. This segment lies upstream of the genes encoding the μ and δ heavy chains.

Transcription at this stage can produce RNA molecules containing the VDJ region together with the Cμ and Cδ gene segments, and the production of mature IgM and IgD molecules results from differential splicing of the RNA transcript.

(ii) Rearrangement of the VDJ segment to lie beside a gene encoding an alternative heavy chain can occur through a mechanism known as deletional switch recombination. Taking the example of a B cell which is switching to produce IgE from IgM[15], the switch regions upstream of the Cμ and Cε gene segments can ligate and join, promoting circularization of the intervening DNA. Once these circles are excised, RNA transcription from VDJ through to Cε, and splicing of the message to remove the switch regions, will result in the production of a mature heavy chain mRNA encoding antigen-specific IgE.

Although many of the overall details of the gene rearrangement process are understood in broad terms, specific molecular details regarding how the process is directed remain unresolved. For example, the recombination event is catalysed by an enzyme termed the 'switch recombinase'. The nature and activity of this complex remain the subject of current studies[16,17]. Similarly, switching is preceded by transcription of the germline heavy chain gene segment from the I exon through to the end of the C exons to which the cell is switching[18]. This produces a germline transcript, which is not translated due to the presence of a stop codon within the I exon. Transcription through this region may be required to signal accessibility to switch recombination, although how this occurs is still largely unknown[19].

It is the nature of these processes as a whole, and the extracellular signals which promote and control their activity to which this chapter will now turn.

Signals required for IgE production

A large body of evidence has accumulated to indicate that two signals are required to promote isotype switching of B-cells to IgE production[14,20,21]. The initial signal, delivered by IL-4 and IL-13, can induce the production of the germline Cε

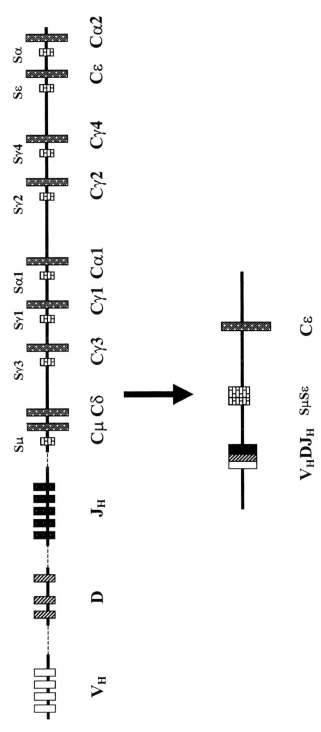

Fig. 10.1 Ig heavy chain gene organization and DNA rearrangement events which occur during B-cell ontogeny and isotype switching. Differentiation into a B-cell capable of synthesising IgE requires recombination of the variable (V), diversity (D) and joining (J) genes, and the rearrangement of the heavy chain genes by deletional switch recombination. The switch regions (Sμ and Sε) can ligate and the intervening DNA is excised to allow juxtaposition of the appropriate constant (Cε) region to the specificity defining VDJ segment. For further details, see text.

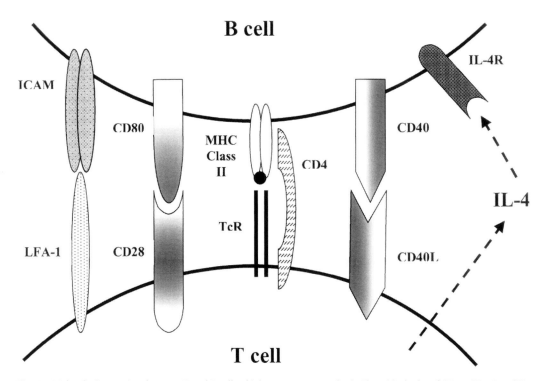

Fig. 10.2 Molecular interactions between T- and B-cells which promote IgE synthesis. The critical roles of CD40 : CD40L and IL-4 release are discussed in the text.

transcript, while the second signal, delivered following binding of B cell CD40 to its cognate ligand CD40L (CD154), will drive the isotype switching process. Both signals are delivered following the interaction of antigen-specific B-cells with T-cells, which occurs through a series of interactions between ligand : receptor pairs expressed on the surface of these cells (Fig. 10.2).

The process is initiated when antigen is captured by surface Ig expressed on the B cell. This complex is internalized and transported through a series of endosomal and lysosomal compartments in which antigen is first denatured, and subsequently proteolysed into peptidic fragments[22]. Selected fragments can bind with high affinity to MHC Class II molecules, which are then transported back to the cell surface for presentation to T-cells. Recognition of

the peptide/MHC complex by a T-cell bearing the appropriate specificity will promote activation of the cell, and in conjunction, up-regulation of CD40L expression on the T-cell surface occurs[23]. Ligation of CD40 on the B-cell by its cognate ligand will, in turn, induce expression of CD80, which through its engagement of CD28 back on the T-cell, will deliver the costimulatory signal to the T-cell necessary to promote production of various cytokines, including IL-4. The secreted IL-4 will bind to the IL-4 receptor (IL-4R) on the surface of B cells, and, together with the signal delivered by CD40, will drive IgE isotype switching and synthesis.

Binding of IL-4 to its receptor will initiate transcription of the Iε–Cε germline transcript. IL-13 also fulfils this function; however, it is considered less potent than IL-4[24,25]. The receptors used by these cytokines share many features, although critical differences exist which may in part explain the difference in potencies[26]. The IL-4R is composed of an α chain and the common γ_c chain, shared by many cytokine receptor complexes (e.g. IL-2, IL-7, IL-9, and IL-15). The IL-4R α chain also forms part of the IL-13 receptor, together with a unique IL-13R α chain. The configuration of receptor chains in hematopoietic cells underlies the observation that IL-4 can bind and signal through IL-13R, while IL-13 is unable to bind IL-4R. Cytokine-induced dimerization of adjacent receptors results in the activation of tyrosine kinases, and the initiation of intracellular signalling cascades. None of the receptors mentioned previously has endogenous kinase activity encoded within its sequence; therefore, a family of receptor associated tyrosine kinases termed JAKs (Janus family kinases) are critical for the signalling process. Three members of this family have been proposed to be associated with the IL-4R complex[27]; JAK-1 and JAK-2 with the IL-4R α chain, and JAK-3 with the γ_c chain. In the case of JAK-2, this kinase has been shown to be of importance in IL-13 signalling, in conjunction with another member of the Janus family, Tyk 2. Activation of the kinases following receptor engagement by IL-4 or IL-13 results in phosphorylation of specific residues within the intracellular domains of the IL-4R α chain[28], which in turn, act as binding sites for another important molecule in the signalling cascade, STAT-6 (signal transducer and activation of transcription)[29–32]. Once phosphorylated, STAT-6 disengages from the IL-4R α cytoplasmic tail, dimerizes, and then translocates to the nucleus, where it interacts with the promoter regions of IL-4 responsive genes[33]. A STAT-6 binding site is situated upstream of the Iε exon, and this transcription factor is of critical importance in the activation and/or enhancement of germline Cε transcription.

The signals delivered by cytokine, however, are not sufficient to drive isotype switching and IgE production, and additional signals, primarily provided by CD40, are required[34–36]. This molecule is a member of the tumour necrosis factor receptor (TNF-R) superfamily of receptors, which includes TNF-R1, TNF-R2, CD30, CD27, Fas and several others. Although CD40 is expressed on a number of cell types, including macrophages, monocytes, dendritic cells, endothelial cells and mast cells, it is its pivotal role in promoting activation of deletional switch recombination which characterizes its role in B-cells[23].

The process is activated when cell to cell contact between T- and B-cells allows the interaction of CD40 with CD40L, and the signals which are transduced ultimately result in the targeting of a transcriptionally active Cε gene. Exemplification of this mechanism comes from studies using mice in which the gene for CD40 has been deleted[37]. In this example, for a response to a nominal thymus-dependent antigen, germinal centre formation was poor and IgM was the predominant antibody isotype generated, suggesting that switching did not occur. In addition, a condition in humans termed X-linked Hyper IgM syndrome has been observed in which a deficiency of serum IgA , IgG and IgE is attributable to a lack of functional CD40L[38,39].

Several studies have identified signalling molecules which associate with the intracellular domain of B cell CD40. For example, the TNF receptor associated family (TRAF) members TRAF-2, TRAF-3, TRAF-5 and TRAF-6 have all been demonstrated to bind to CD40 and are hypothesized to play a role in isotype switching[40,41]. Interaction of CD40L with CD40 has been shown to promote rapid tyrosine phosphorylation of a number of intracellular substrates, possibly through the activities of the Lyn and Syk kinases[42]. Nevertheless, significant difficulties have been encountered in the resolution of CD40 signalling cascades in B-cells (e.g. anti-CD40, antibodies; Abs, stimulate poor tyrosine phosphorylation in vitro), and these have meant that the precise nature of the control of switch recombination by CD40 has yet to be understood.

Cytokine/cytokine receptor modulation

The advances in the understanding of the mechanisms by which IgE synthesis is regulated has correspondingly led to an increase in the perceived therapeutic opportunities available to block IgE production. Many of these are targeted at inhibiting the production and/or activity of IL-4 and IL-13, as these cytokines have been shown to play a critical role in the induction of an IgE response (both IL-4 and IL-13 gene knockout mice have much reduced IgE responses to antigen)[43,44].

Antibodies to both cytokines have been used to block production of IgE in vitro and in vivo. Thus, anti-IL-4 Abs can act synergistically with anti-IL-13 Abs to block IgE production in vitro using cells taken from atopic individuals[45]. When administered to mice, anti-IL-4 Abs can prevent the induction of an IgE response to the sensitizing antigen[46], and when given together with anti-IL-5 Abs, can block the antigen induced airway hyperresponsiveness in a murine model of bronchial asthma[47].

Another promising approach to IL-4 : IL-4R antagonism has been described by scientists at Immunex. They have produced a soluble form of the receptor α chain, which in preclinical studies in mice, has been shown to inhibit production of IgE stimulated by endogenous IL-4[48]. The human version of this receptor has been produced and has entered Phase II clinical studies in mild to moderate asthmatics. Recent data from these initial studies has suggested that a single dose of this drug given by inhalation has stabilized disease symptoms and has resulted in a decrease in β_2-agonist use.

Further series of antagonists have been produced by introducing selected mutations into the sequence of IL-4. For example, replacement of a tyrosine residue with an aspartic acid at position 124 results in an IL-4 mutant protein which retains high binding affinity for the receptor, yet prevents IgE synthesis in vitro driven by both IL-4 and IL-13[49,50]. A similar IL-4 mutant protein (BAY 16–9996) has recently entered clinical trials for an asthma indication. In addition, a novel isoform of IL-4 has been described (IL-4δ2) which results from alternative splicing of IL-4 mRNA. This molecule is a potent antagonist of both IL-4 and IL-13, and prevents cytokine induced synthesis of IgE and CD23 expression[29,51]. Finally, a molecule that binds with high affinity to IL-13 has recently been isolated from mouse serum and urine (IL-13BP)[52], and the possibility exists that this could be used to modulate the effects of IL-13. A human version of this molecule, however, has yet to be identified.

In addition to the approaches aimed at directly antagonizing the cytokines themselves, alternative methods targeted at modulating the effects of the pro-allergic cytokines have been suggested. Thus, prototypical Type 1 cytokines such as IL-12, IL-18 and IFNγ have all been demonstrated to inhibit either the production or activity of IL-4 in a number of assay systems[53–56]. Other cytokines have also been active in reducing the function of IL-4. For example, both IL-8 and IL-10 are active in inhibiting IL-4-induced IgE production from human B cells[57–59]. Despite these data, however, the therapeutic opportunities afforded by cytokine therapy are limited, due, for the most part, to the short half lives of many of the cytokines when administered exogenously, and to the pleiotropic nature of the cytokines' activities in vivo.

To circumvent this problem, several approaches have been examined in which administration of agents that promote type 1 cytokine production, rather than the delivery of the cytokines themselves, have been attempted. These have the potential advantage in inducing sustained production of endogenous cytokines at the site at which the development of the allergic response occurs, i.e. regional lymph nodes. Many of these agents are derived from bacteria, and have been examined either separately, or when given in conjunction with specific allergen immunotherapy. For example, preclinical studies using the micro-organism *Mycobacterium vaccae* have shown that administration of this bacteria to allergen-sensitized animals can suppress a Th2 immune response, and decrease IgE levels in the serum[60]. This therapy has entered clinical trials in the UK for the treatment of seasonal pollen rhinitis. A product derived from *Streptococcus* bacteria

(OK432) has previously shown promise as an immunopotentiator in oncology therapy. Due to its ability to promote release of type 1 cytokines[61], it may also prove useful for allergy treatment. A more recent discovery concerns the immunomodulatory effects of bacterial DNA. This material, containing a high proportion of unmethylated CpG dinucleotide motifs, has been found to be a potent inducer of B cell activation[62] and type 1 cytokine production[63]. In vitro, CpG motifs induce IL-12, IL-18 and IFNγ production in cells taken from allergic individuals, and can inhibit IgE synthesis[64]. In vivo, CpG can both prevent and treat allergen induced airway inflammation[65]. First clinical trials for this agent have been initiated, and it is anticipated that it may enter the clinic for the treatment of allergic disorders within the next 2 years.

Finally, the role of the cell surface low affinity IgE receptor (CD23) in regulating IgE production is relevant to this discussion. Originally identified as a B cell activation marker[66], subsequent studies have identified its presence on a number of hematopoietic cell types, e.g. follicular dendritic cells, eosinophils, macrophages and some T cells[67,68]. A significant body of evidence now exists to demonstrate that the expression of this molecule is regulated by factors which can increase or decrease IgE synthesis. It maintains a dual role in IgE regulation. A membrane anchored form of this molecule (mCD23) can bind IgE-containing immune complexes, resulting in downregulation of IgE synthesis[69,70]. By contrast, a soluble version of the extracellular portion of this molecule (sCD23) acts to increase synthesis of IgE[71,72]. It is logical to propose, therefore, that agents which can prevent the generation of sCD23, or can promote the expression and/or the binding of IgE:Ag complexes to mCD23 will have a negative effect on IgE production.

Drugs which affect IgE synthesis

Increased understanding about the natural control of B cell function and the process of antibody class-switching has raised the possibility that drugs might be found which inhibit the production of IgE as a strategy towards decreasing atopic disease. Drugs that are already in clinical use have activity on this process and novel agents have been reported which may have therapeutic value in the future because of their effects on B cell function.

Drugs in clinical use

Selective β_2 adrenoceptor agonists such as salbutamol are important drugs for treatment of allergic asthma, principally through their bronchodilator effects. They also have antiallergic activity by suppressing IgE-mediated release of mediators from lung mast cells and basophils. It has also been suggested that long acting drugs such as salmeterol have additional anti-inflammatory actions by suppressing migration and activation of leukocytes in vivo. It is interesting to note, therefore, that not all activities of β_2 adrenoceptor agonists tend towards an antiallergic outcome. For example, salbutamol and fenoterol have been shown to increase IL-4 induced production of IgE from human PBMC in vitro, an effect accompanied by the increased expression of CD23, the increased release of soluble CD23 and a decreased release of IFN-γ[73–75]. Furthermore, the proinflammatory effects of CD23 ligation with IgE/antiIgE complexes were potentiated by salbutamol. These effects on human PBMC required low concentrations of drug acting through stimulation of β- adrenoceptors (blocked by butoxamine and D,L-propranolol) and probably involved a PKA-dependent intracellular pathway, being associated with an increase in cAMP and blocked by protein kinase inhibitors such as H8 and Rp-AMP[76]. Similar effects have been reported with murine B-lymphocytes in vitro and have been extended to in vivo studies where daily injections of salbutamol led to an increase in antigen-specific IgE. This was associated with an increased production of Th2-type cytokines from murine splenocytes stimulated ex vivo with conconavalin A[77]. However, the importance of all these observations to the clinical use of β_2 agonists is uncertain since the regular administration of oral salbutamol to atopic volunteers in a double-blind, placebo-controlled trial led to no increase in serum IgE levels, compared to controls, whilst the drug significantly decreased both vascular and non-vascular symptoms of rhinitis brought about by seasonal exposure to grass pollen[78].

Glucocorticoids block allergic responses in several ways but have been shown to substantially increase IgE synthesis by human PBMC in vitro. This probably reflects an immunomodulatory effect on T lymphocytes and is not confined to IgE, secretion of IgG_1, IgG_2 and IgG_3 (but not IgG_4) also being increased[79,80]. This has raised the concern that such an effect on IgE production might also occur clinically. However, several studies have shown that when given either systemically (prednisone) or topically (beclomethasone; fluticasone) glucocorticoids did not increase either systemic or local levels of IgE in allergic subjects[79,81,82]. Rather, they decreased levels of IgE, consistent with their suppressive effect on T-cell function.

Cyclosporin A is a powerful immunosuppressant with its principal effect being to suppress T-cell function. Its main clinical use is to limit rejection of transplanted tissue but it has recently been shown to be effective in relieving chronic severe corticosteroid-dependent asthma[83,84]. The anti-inflammatory action of cyclosporin A in asthma is consistent with an effect on T-lymphocytes to decrease eosinophil-active cytokines, rather than the weaker suppressant effect on mast cell responses[85]. Like corticosteroids, cyclosporin A also greatly increases IgE synthesis by human PBMC in vitro, by up to 40-fold in one study[86]. A similar effect has been observed in mice where cyclosporin A and FK506 have both been shown to increase antigen-specific and total IgE in the serum[87]. This was consistent with the drugs selectively suppressing Th1 rather than Th2 lymphocytes under the conditions of these experiments. However, these experimental observations may also have little relevance clinically as even small doses of cyclosporin A have been shown to decrease significantly levels of serum IgE[88]. The cephalosporin, cefadroxil, has also been shown to substantially reduce IgE levels and improve the condition of a child with atopic asthma and dermatitis[89].

Disodium cromoglycate and nedocromil are antiallergic agents which have clinical efficacy (especially prophylactically) in mild–moderate atopic asthma, rhinitis, conjunctivitis and other IgE-mediated conditions. The mechanism of action of these drugs is unclear but, at least in asthma, their mast cell stabilizing properties are not sufficient to explain their efficacy and other actions have been sought[90]. It has recently been shown that in vitro both drugs inhibit IgE synthesis by human B-cells. For example, nedocromil acts on highly purified B-cells to inhibit IgE synthesis induced by anti-CD40 and IL-4. It had no effect on the induction of E-germline transcripts by IL-4 but strongly inhibited CD40-mediated $s\mu \rightarrow s\varepsilon$ deletional switch recombination[91]. The effect of nedocromil extended also to inhibition of CD40/IL-4 induced synthesis of IgG4 by B-cells, and so was not specific for IgE. It caused only moderate inhibition of spontaneous synthesis of IgE by B-cells with hyper-IgE syndrome, suggesting it has little effect on B-cells that have already undergone isotype switching. These results strongly suggest that nedocromil inhibits IgE isotype switching by inhibiting deletional switch recombination[91]. Very similar effects have been reported for cromoglycate[92] and both studies support the original observation of Kimata and Mikawa[93] that nedocromil inhibits IgE and IgG4 production without affecting synthesis of other IgE isotypes or classes of immunoglobulin by IL-4 stimulated monocytes from non-atopic donors. It is possible, therefore, that the clinical effect of these drugs is due to a combination of antiallergic activities, including a decrease in IgE synthesis. This effect is likely to be manifest locally in allergically inflamed tissues, especially when the drugs are applied topically (which includes inhalation), and so may not result in a marked decrease in circulating IgE. This suggestion is consistent with observations in food allergic subjects where oral challenge with specific food allergens led to symptoms of urticaria and wheezing, and an increase in IgE levels in faecal extracts. Patients treated orally with cromoglycate showed no increase in faecal IgE levels and exhibited decreased symptoms compared to controls[94].

New drugs and investigational agents

Suplatast tosilate (IPD-11517)

This is an antiallergic/immunomodulatory drug introduced into Japan in the last few years and its activities have been extensively described in a number of studies[95–102]. It is orally active and has a class-specific effect to suppress the primary IgE antibody response in immunized BALB/C mice, without affecting the IgG antibody response. When studied in vitro, the drug inhibited production of IL-4 by the Th 2 cell line D1OG4.1 but did not suppress production of IgE or IgG$_1$ by normal splenic B-cells stimulated with lipopolysaccharide and IL-4. Furthermore, IL-4 induced expression of FcεRII on normal spleen cells was not inhibited. These observations suggest that suppression of IgE synthesis is a consequence of the action of suplatast on T-cells to inhibit IL-4 production. This interpretation was supported by results of experiments with an allergen-specific helper T-cell line (SN-4) from a patient allergic to Japanese cedar pollen. Suplatast blocked allergen-dependent IgE synthesis in autologous B-cells cocultured with SN-4 T-cells, but did not significantly block IgG synthesis. It has no antagonistic effect on IL-4 receptors but did inhibit IL-4 production by allergen-stimulated (SN-4) T-cells, as well as IL-4 production by PHA-stimulated PBMC isolated from normal donors. The agent appears to act at the level of IL-4 gene transcription, blocking PHA-induced expression of IL-4 mRNA in normal PBMCs. It also blocked IL-5 production (by conalbumin-stimulated D10 cells in vitro) but in contrast, it had no inhibitory effect on IFN-γ production by either allergen-stimulated (SN-4) T-cells or those from a normal donor stimulated with an anti CD-3 monoclonal antibody. The overall effect of this agent would, thus, appear to be to shift the balance from the Th2 phenotype towards the Th1 by inhibiting IL-4 and IL-5 production by T-cells. Further experiments illustrate the sequelae of this activity since suplatast has been shown to block eosinophil recruitment and proliferation of mast cell progenitor cells (but not of splenocytes or mature mast cells) both of which require IL-4 and/or IL-5.

Furthermore, this drug inhibited antigen-induced infiltration of CD4 + T-cells, eosinophils and macrophages into lung tissue of sensitized guinea pigs following bronchial challenge. The airway hyperreactivity that accompanies lung inflammation was also inhibited. In rats, suplatast has been shown to decrease IgE production in vivo and bring about a commensurate decrease in airway responses provoked by exposure to antigen. This interesting drug has also been tested clinically in patients with perennial allergic rhinitis to *Dermatophagoides farinae*. Oral administration of 300 mg/day for up to 6 months significantly decreased serum levels of IL-4 and allergen-specific IgE, the rate of decrease of specific IgE correlated significantly with the rate of decrease in IL-4. The drug was effective alone but more effective when administered concomitantly with allergen immunotherapy. In addition, suplatast has been reported to prevent the 'rebound' increase in Th2 cytokines observed when atopic subjects discontinue treatment with topical steroids such as dexamethasone. These results indicate that the modulatory effect of suplatast extends beyond IL-4 and IL-5, to include also IL-10 and IL-13. In conclusion, suplatast has a novel pharmacological profile, modulating the allergic phenotype at the Th 2 cell level, and has the potential to control allergic disease in a fundamental way.

M50367

This is another agent, chemically distinct from suplatast, which has been discovered by screening to modulate the Th1/Th2 balance and suppress IgE synthesis in experimental models[103]. When splenocytes were prepared from mice treated orally with M50367 (10 or 30 mg/kg/day for 9 days) the compound was found to change the cytokine profile induced by conconavalin A, increasing IFNγ but decreasing IL-4 and IL-5. However, the active metabolite M50354 had no direct effect on cytokine production by splenocytes in vitro. The authors suggest M50367 may act on either antigen presenting cells or Th progenitor cells, but the exact mechanism of action in vivo still has to be elucidated. Alterations in Th1/Th2 cytokine production in vivo were accompanied by suppression of plasma levels of IgE, inhibition of allergen-induced increase in airway hyperreactivity and pulmonary eosinophilia. Unlike prednisolone or cyclosporin A, M50367 had no cytoxicity to splenocytes in vitro and no influence on body weight gain in vivo. Hence, its activity is distinguishable from these immunosuppressants and may be the prototype of yet another class of Th1/Th2 modulatory drugs.

Leflunomide

This is a new immunosuppressive agent with anti-inflammatory activity. It has shown high tolerability and efficacy in Phase II trials and is currently in Phase III clinical trial for the treatment of rheumatoid arthritis. A substantial body of evidence has emerged during the past few years to describe the actions of this compound in both in vitro and in vivo models[104–112]. The activity of leflunomide is attributed to its primary metabolite A77 1726, a malononitrilamide, which inhibits T- and B-cell proliferation, suppresses immunoglobulin production and interferes with cell adhesion. It acts on the enzyme dehydroorotate dehydrogenase to inhibit *de novo* synthesis of pyrimidines, but may also inhibit a number of protein kinases. Thus, while the addition of uridine-restored proliferation and IgM secretion to leflunomide treated, LPS-stimulated, B-cells, it did not restore secretion of IgG antibody. Leflunomide also decreased tyrosine phosphorylation of JAK3 and STAT6 in the absence or presence of uridine, and also decreased binding of STAT6 to the STAT6 DNA binding site in the IgG_1 promoter. These data led to the suggestion that leflunomide blocks IgG_1 production by inhibiting tyrosine kinases. In sensitized animals, leflunomide has been shown to significantly reduce antigen-specific IgE as well as IgG. As a consequence mast cell FcεRI have become depleted of IgE, resulting in a significant reduction of bronchospasm and infiltration of eosinophils and neutrophils following pulmonary antigen challenge. T-cells from sensitized, leflunomide treated animals failed to proliferate when stimulated with specific antigen but were able to respond to conconavalin A. Down-regulation of immunoglobulin production

was not restricted to IgE since levels of allergen-specific IgG1 and IgG2 and IgM were also reduced. This indicates that leflunomide does not act to inhibit immunoglobulin class switching; the general decrease in immunoglobulin levels may be due to a loss in production of the T-helper cell-derived B-cell differentiation factor IL-5. Taken together, these observations position leflunomide more as an alternative to cyclosporin A for treatment of severe allergy/asthma than as a truly novel immunomodulator for treatment of a broader range of allergic diseases.

Protease inhibitors

These may also be the source of novel drugs to control the synthesis of IgE. The low affinity receptor for IgE present on B-cells (FcεRII; also called CD23) is involved in the regulation of IgE synthesis, and is part of a feedback loop whereby occupancy of CD23 by IgE acts to stop further synthesis of IgE. However, this feed back control tends to be offset by other concomitant events. First, the amounts of CD23 on B-cells is increased by cytokines such as IL-4 which stimulate IgE synthesis. Secondly, protease(s) present on B-cell membranes cleave CD23, which not only removes the low affinity receptor for IgE but also yields the soluble sCD23 which acts as a cytokine to amplify IgE synthesis. Furthermore, many allergens have proteolytic activities with the potential to amplify allergen-specific IgE production through cleavage of CD23. Hence, such proteases, but more importantly those present endogenously on B cell membranes, are possible targets for drugs to diminish IgE synthesis by protecting CD23 from proteolytic cleavage. The precise nature of the protease(s) involved in this process is currently the subject of much work. Several studies with standard protease inhibitors have implicated a zinc-dependent metalloproteinase rather than cysteine-, serine- or acid-proteases. Hence, CD23-cleaving activity found in an enriched fraction of plasma membranes from B-cells was inhibited by standard inhibitors of metalloproteinases (1,10-phenanthroline, imidazole and batimastat) but not inhibitors of the other classes of proteinase[113,114]. Limited structure-activity studies amongst a series of hydroxamic acids related to batimastat suggested that the B-cell enzyme(s) were distinguishable from collagenase[115,116]. Consistent with its effect to block CD23 processing to sCD23 on B-cells and monocytes, batimastat inhibited IgE production from human and murine B-cells stimulated in vitro with IL-4 anti CD40. Furthermore, batimastat inhibited IgE production in vivo in mice sensitized with ovalbumin. These observations with batimastat have been confirmed and extended by experiments with another hydroxamate-type inhibitor of zinc-metalloproteinases, GI 129471[117]. This compound also blocked release of sCD23 from human B-cells in vitro and potently inhibited production of IgE ($IC_{50} = 250$ nM). This effect was selective for IgE as concentrations up to 10 μM had no effect on production of IgG1 or IgG4. These observations are sufficient to encourage further research to characterize the B-cell metalloproteinase(s) and identify selective, non-toxic inhibitors with in vivo activity.

Type 4 phosphodiesterase inhibitors

These have been shown to modulate the activity of virtually all cells involved in the inflammatory process. So-called second generation, selective PDE4 inhibitors (e.g. Cilomilast; SB 207499) which display a more reduced side effect profile than the first-generation of this class of compound (e.g. rolipram) are now beginning to appear and have been shown to have broad anti-inflammatory/antiasthmatic activity[118]. Coqueret et al.[119] reported the effect of first-generation PDE4 inhibitors on IgE production by human PBMC and purified B lymphocytes from non-allergic donors. Selective PDE4 inhibitors, rolipram and Ro 20–1724 inhibited IL-4 included IgE production by PBMC but not by purified B lymphocytes. Inhibitors of other phosphodiesterase isoenzymes (PDE3; PDE5) had no effect. The PDE4 inhibitors did not suppress lymphocyte proliferation induced by PHA and did not affect cell surface expression of the IL-4 receptor. However, incubation of monocytes alone with the PDE4 inhibitor did bring about a significant reduction of IL-4 induced synthesis of IgE. These results suggest that PDE4 inhibitors act on monocytes to suppress the costimulating signals required to evoke IgE production by B lymphocytes.

Anti-IgE therapeutic antibodies

Preclinical

The discovery of novel drugs which suppress IgE production is clearly ongoing, and discrete molecular targets are becoming identified. In advance of such agents, the present method of choice for depleting circulating IgE is the use of specific antibodies. Such therapeutic antibodies have several clear advantages. These are:

(i) Exquisite specificity: the selection of antibody to bind to a specific antigen is based on a theoretical repertoire size of 10^{11-12}.

(ii) High intrinsic affinity: for the most part, affinity constants for Ab. binding to its target Ag. range from 10^{-9}–10^{-11}M.

(iii) Favourable pharmacokinetics: appropriately humanized Abs have very low rates of clearance from the systemic circulation compared with most drugs.

Against this background, several groups have produced novel monoclonal antibodies (Mabs) to human IgE, and this section will describe the nature and characterization of some of these. This list is not exhaustive; rather it will focus on those where the potential for antiallergic therapy has been indicated.

MAb MAE11/huMAb-E25

The antibody MAE11 and its humanized counterpart E25 were developed by Genentech and are the furthest advanced in terms of clinical development (see below). A panel of MAbs were raised against human IgE, and the screening strategy employed was based on the selection of Abs which recognized IgE at the same site as that which is critical in determining binding to the high affinity receptor FcεRIα. Therefore, by design, the Abs will not bind to IgE present on mast cells and will not be capable of degranulation (anaphylactogenicity). Several clones were isolated, the best of which was termed MAE11.

Humanization produced a version of the antibody (E25) which retained the affinity and properties of the original molecule, but is suitable for in vivo administration to allergic individuals[120]. The MAb binds to free IgE, and IgE present on isotype-committed B cells, but does not recognize other isotypes (IgM, IgG, or IgA). It can block binding of IgE to basophils, but is unable to recognize IgE once it has bound to FcεRI[121,122]. When used during in vitro sensitization with antigen-specific IgE, MAE11/E25 can abolish antigen-dependent mast cell histamine release from human and monkey tissues[123,124]. No evidence was obtained indicating that the antibody could induce histamine release from passively sensitized tissues[125]. This antibody can also prevent IgE synthesis when added to in vitro culture, and can block IgE binding to the low affinity FcεRII (CD23). In summary, the evidence indicated that MAE11/E25 should have significant therapeutic benefits for the treatment of IgE-mediated diseases, and later sections will go on to describe in detail the results from clinical studies with this molecule.

CGP51901/Hu-901

Although it has originated from a different source (Tanox/Novartis), the antihuman IgE MAb CGP51901 demonstrates the same properties in vitro as E25, and was also being processed as a clinical candidate for atopy. With an agreement to co-develop between the three parties, E25 is currently being advanced for the treatment of allergic rhinitis and atopic asthma, while CGP51901 is being pursued separately for the niche market of peanut allergy.

BSW17

A panel of antihuman IgE MAbs has been described from the laboratory of Stadler[126,127], with one in particular, BSW17, revealing an interesting phenotype. Despite the fact that this MAb can recognize receptor-bound IgE, it is not anaphylactogenic[128]. Furthermore, it is capable of preventing IgE association with both FcεRIα and FcεRII[129], and can promote a net loss in receptor-bound IgE. The antibody can also inhibit IgE synthesis in vitro[130]. The

data thus indicate that BSW17 has a number of properties which suggest it may have value as a therapeutic antibody. However, there is little evidence to suggest that a humanized version of this MAb is being pursued, with recent publications suggesting it is being used to define mimotopes for use as novel vaccine candidates in the generation of an anti-human IgE response[131,132].

PTMAb0005 and 0011

We have recently identified two MAbs which recognize human IgE both free and receptor bound, and which can prevent IgE binding to FcεRIα. In contrast to BSW17, however, the MAbs can promote binding of IgE to FcεRII, a property which may enhance the CD23 mediated down-regulation of an IgE response. In cell based assay systems, both MAbs are non-anaphylactogenic across a range of donors and can prevent basophil sensitization when coincubated with antigen-specific IgE. Perhaps the most interesting property of these MAbs, however, is their ability to inhibit the responses of presensitized basophils (Fig. 10.3). Thus, basophils are removed from atopic individuals, and incubated with specific allergen and either PTMAb0005, PTMAb0011 or isotype matched controls. Under these circumstances, basophil histamine release is abolished by the anti-IgE Abs, but not by the isotype matched controls. To our knowledge, these are the first antihuman IgE MAbs described which have a stabilizing effect on allergic basophil degranulation, and thus may represent a novel class of antibodies for allergy treatment. A subclass of natural autoantibodies against IgE which can down-regulate basophil mediator release has been demonstrated in the sera of certain atopics[133], and PTMAb0005 and 0011 may represent a monoclonal version of these.

migis Antibodies

An alternative approach to inhibiting IgE in allergic individuals is to specifically target the IgE committed B-cells, and so remove the source of production. Following the identification of unique epitopes exposed on the membrane-proximal regions of Ig expressed on B-cells, the feasibility of this approach

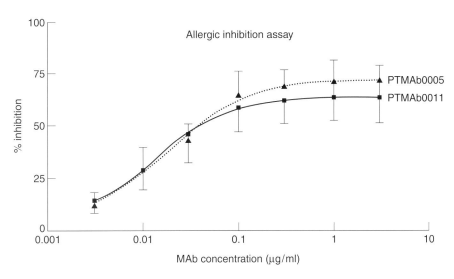

Fig. 10.3 The effect of PTMAb0005 and 0011 on allergen-induced histamine release from peripheral blood basophils. PBMC from Lolp1-sensitive donors were prepared by Ficoll–Paque separation and incubated with varying concentrations of antihuman IgE monoclonal antibodies for 30 min at 37 °C. Cells were then triggered with Lolp1 for a further 30 min at 37 °C. Reactions were terminated by centrifugation (500 g, 5 min) and supernatants were collected. Histamine in supernatants was determined by Histamine EIA (Immunotech). Data are mean from three separate experiments from different donors.

has been examined. These regions, termed *migis* (membrane-bound immunoglobulin isotype specific) epitopes are distinct across isotypes[134,135], and consist of a segment of 13–32 amino acids comprising a high proportion of acidic and polar residues. In one example, monoclonal antibodies have been raised to the *εmigis* sequence, and have been shown to preferentially target IgE⁺B-cells. This approach may be amenable to either a passive strategy (the use of humanized antibodies) or an active strategy (immunization with *εmigis* epitope linked to a protein carrier).

Clinical

Early clinical trials of rhuMAb-E25 included at least four Phase I studies to establish detailed pharmacokinetics, dose-ranging, acceptability of the product and preliminary assessment of efficacy in allergic subjects. These have been followed by at least six Phase II multicentre, double-blind, placebo-controlled, parallel group trials; three in allergic rhinitis patients and three in allergic asthma patients. In addition, results of a Phase III trial in seasonal allergic rhinitis were recently reported.

In summary, pharmacokinetics and early clinical studies show that intravenous rhuMAb-E25 causes an immediate fall in serum free IgE. Peak serum concentrations of the therapeutic antibody are achieved between 3 and 14 days after subcutaneous administration and it is slowly cleared from the circulation with a terminal half-life of 1–4 weeks after either intravenous or subcutaneous administration[136–139].

An important observation from the study of Casale et al.[137] was that the impact of rhuMAb-E25 on serum free IgE levels was not only dependent on the dose but also the baseline level of IgE before treatment: the higher the baseline IgE, the lower the effect of a particular dose of rhuMAb-E25. The concept that arose from this study concerned the pharmacodynamic relationship between rhuMAb-E25 and both free and complexed IgE. Consistent suppression of serum free IgE to the lowest level of detection required the ratio of rhuMAb: total IgE (i.e.

free IgE plus complex of IgE/rhuMAb-E25) to be in the range of 10:1 to 15:1. Thus, the efficacy of rhuMAb-E25 will be influenced not only by body weight but also individual baseline IgE levels among patients. A dose of approximately 0.005 mg/kg/week for each IU per ml of baseline IgE was estimated as being required to suppress free IgE to a steady state level at the limit of detection. From this and other studies it has been estimated that serum free IgE needs to be decreased below 40 ng/ml for $Fc\varepsilon RI$ receptor-bound IgE to become depleted (as a result of the shift in equilibrium towards free IgE) and a therapeutic effect to be obtained.

This pharmacodynamic interpretation was consistent with the overall failure of rhuMAb-E25 in this early trial[137] to decrease symptoms during the ragweed pollen rhinitis season. After the trial it was judged that only 11 patients in the highest dose group received sufficient treatment (with repeated doses of 0.5 mg/kg i.v.) to suppress free IgE enough to deplete cell-fixed IgE. Because of these observations, subsequent studies in seasonal allergic rhinitis patients used higher doses of rhuMAb-E25 adjusted for basal levels of serum-free IgE. In randomized, double-blind, placebo-controlled trials involving several hundred patients; the effect of rhuMAb-25 on primary outcome measures of symptom/medication scores and quality of life questionnaire was examined[140]. The doses of rhuMAb-E25 were 300, 150 or 50 mg administered subcutaneously every 3 or 4 weeks, based on total serum IgE levels (151–700 and 30–150 IU/ml, respectively) for 12 weeks. In both studies, significant clinical improvement was observed with the two higher doses (300 and 150 mg s.c.) whereas the 50 mg dose was not different from placebo.

A Phase III trial was presented at the 20th Annual Nordic Congress on Allergology by Sandstrom (May 1999). This was a randomized, placebo-controlled, multicentre trial which examined symptoms of rhinoconjunctivitis and rescue medication usage in 251 adult patients in Scandinavia with a history of birch pollen allergy. Patients were treated with either 300 mg rhuMAb-E25 or placebo given subcutaneously, two injections given 3 or 4 weeks apart during the 1998 birch tree pollen season in Scandinavia. Rescue medications, such as antihistamines, were used when patients determined that their symptoms were severe enough to require additional medication. Using a scale of 0 for no symptoms and 3 for severe symptoms, rhuMAb-E25 compared to placebo led to a decrease in patient nasal and ocular symptoms of 0.23 and 0.09, respectively. Results show that patients receiving the anti-IgE treatment used on average 0.5 antihistamine tablets per day vs. 1.3 tablets per day in the placebo group, and used allergy medication on less than half as many days. The treatment was well tolerated during this trial. No antibodies against anti-IgE were detected and no serum sickness, immune complex disease, anaphylactic reactions, systemic urticaria or other allergy-related side effects were reported.

Studies with rhuMAb-E25 in patients with allergic asthma initially were designed to assess safety and tolerance of the product and also responses to inhaled allergens by subjects with stable mild disease (baseline $FEV_1 \geq 70\%$ predicted, requiring only inhaled β_2-agonist on demand, no corticosteroids). In all asthma trials reported so far, rhuMAb-E25 has been administered intravenously. Fahy et al.[138] reported a randomized, double-blind, placebo-controlled, parallel-group trial in which the dosing regimen of rhuMAb-E25 was chosen to produce trough serum concentrations of the therapeutic antibody of 14 μg/ml at steady state. This required a dose of 0.5 mg/kg to be given as an i.v. infusion over 5 minutes, every week for 9 weeks. Nineteen subjects were characterized by spirometry, methacholine reactivity and skin tests to allergens, they were also taught to record in diaries peak flow, asthma symptoms, bronchodilator use and nocturnal asthma. They then underwent airway challenge tests, with allergen and methacoline, and sputum induction. After the first intravenous infusion of rhuMAb-E25 to nine subjects serum free IgE fell from a baseline level of ≤ 500 IU/ml to below the limit of detection (10 IU/ml) and remained low for the duration of the study: by 6 weeks until the end of the study six of nine subjects had consistently undetectable free serum IgE while in three subjects it was between 12 and 33 IU/ml. Treatment with rhuMAb-E25 significantly attenuated both the early and late phase responses to airway challenge with allergen. Changes in the early phase response included both a smaller fall in FEV_1 and a larger concentration of allergen required to cause bronchospasm. No differences were observed in responses of the placebo group to allergen challenge. The late phase bronchospasm and eosinophilia in induced sputum after allergen challenge were significantly decreased as was methacholine sensitivity (but this was not significant). These observations implicate IgE-dependent events in the inflammatory responses that underlie airway hyperreactivity of asthma. In contrast to responses to allergen challenge, measures of asthma symptoms and brochodilator usage did not change significantly. It is possible that the dose of therapeutic antibody was not sufficient, as suggested by incomplete blockade of the early phase response to allergen challenge. Higher doses may have improved asthma symptoms. However, the authors also emphasize that the study involved patients with very mild asthma, in whom it would be difficult to demonstrate improvement.

In a parallel study[139] in mild atopic asthmatics, allergen sensitivity was assessed by measuring FEV_1 responses provoked by inhaling increasing amounts of allergen, in doubling concentrations, at 10-minute intervals until a 15% fall in FEV_1 was achieved. This is referred to as the PC_{15}. Non-specific airway hyperreactivity was assessed in a similar manner by inhaling increasing concentrations of methacholine to achieve the PC_{20}. The therapeutic antibody was given intravenously (over 5 min) as an initial loading dose (2 mg/kg) followed by six subsequent doses (1 mg/kg) initially weekly (2 doses) and then 2 weekly (4 doses). The mean serum concentration of total rhuMAb-E25 reached approximately 31 μg/ml at day 77 of the study. Geometric mean values (± s.e.) for serum free IgE decreased from 288 ± 124 ng/ml to 30 ± 11 ng/ml at day 77. In seven out of ten subjects free IgE was below the limit of detection. During treatment, the amount of allergen tolerated increased significantly, the PC_{15} increasing by 2.3–2.7 doubling doses on days 27–77; the metha-

choline PC_{20} also improved slightly but was only significant towards the end of the trial (day 76). No changes were seen in the placebo group. The authors emphasized that changes in the allergen PC_{15} seen in this study were large, comparable to what has been reported with inhaled corticosteroids, and may have been underestimated since several subjects did not bronchoconstrict with an increase in allergen of three doubling doses which was the upper limit imposed for safety reasons. Despite blocking responses to inhaled allergen, rhuMAb-E25 did not change respiratory symptoms or medication usage during the treatment period. As in the study of Fahy et al.[138] the authors conclude that it would be difficult to observe improvement in these measures in such mild disease.

In a further trial, Milgrom et al.[141] investigated the effect of the therapeutic antibody on exacerbations of asthma following corticosteroid withdrawal in subjects who had received 12 weeks of inhaled/oral corticosteroid and $β$-agonists plus placebo-controlled rhuMAb-E25. The doses of rhuMAb-E25 were adjusted according to body weight and basal-free IgE, as discussed earlier: they were 0.006 and 0.014 mg/kg/IU/ml administered intravenously every 2 weeks. This treatment significantly decreased exacerbations of asthma and also decreased daily symptom scores and $β_2$-agonist rescue medication, whilst also allowing a decrease in use of corticosteroid. Hence, it is becoming apparent that with an appropriate dosing regimen, the depletion of circulating free IgE by rhuMAb-E25 exerts an anti-inflammatory effect in allergic asthmatics sufficient to allow reduction in concomitant therapy.

A second humanized anti-IgE therapeutic antibody has also been investigated in clinical trials. This is Hu-901 which is a non-anaphylactogenic mouse/human chimeric antibody (previously known as CGP-51901) that binds to free IgE and surface IgE of IgE-expressing B cells but not to IgE bound to FcεRI on mast cells or basophils or FcεRII on other cells. A Phase I single dose study was conducted double-blind, placebo-controlled in 33 male volunteers sensitive to mixed grass pollens[142]. Mean baseline levels of serum free IgE ranged between 239 and 395 IU/ml. Doses of Hu-901 of 3, 10, 30 or 100 mg were administered by intravenous infusion over 30 min. The therapeutic antibody was well tolerated and brought about a rapid and dose-related fall in free IgE, being more than 96% depleted after the highest dose. Total IgE, composed of free and complexed IgE increased. Complexed IgE was eliminated at a rate comparable with the terminal half-life of free Hu-901 which was between 11 and 13 days. The time of recovery to 50% of baseline IgE was also dose dependent, ranging from 1.3 days to 39 days for the 3 mg and 100 mg doses, respectively. This antibody was further studied in a randomized, placebo-controlled trial involving 153 patients with seasonal allergic rhinitis and treated with placebo or Hu-901 at doses of 15, 30 or 60 mg, given intravenously 6 times at 2-weekly intervals[143]. This study provided valuable pharmacokinetic and pharmacodynamic profiles which indicated that repeat-dosing was safe and a concentration of about 5 µg/ml would be required to decrease serum free IgE by 85%: this would be obtained with the highest dose given. In addition, patients appeared to benefit from the anti-IgE treatment during the pollen season, especially the high dose group in whom symptoms were fewer and less medication was needed. Having established safety and pharmacodynamic efficacy, Hu-901 is now undergoing trials in patients with severe peanut allergy.

There are a number of potential safety issues which have been assessed during early clinical trials. The first has been to ensure that the inability of anti-IgE therapeutic antibodies to stimulate mast cells and basophils, which has been observed with human blood cells in vitro[125], also occurs when the antibody is introduced into the body. There have been a small number of subjects in whom they have caused a generalized urticarial rash which required treatment and at least one subject in whom it appeared to provoke a mild asthma attack. However, the general experience, with more than a thousand subjects having been exposed, is that such therapeutic antibodies appear to be quite free of anaphylactogenic properties.

There is a theoretical risk that immune complex formation between serum free IgE and anti-IgE will occur, and that its subsequent deposition in organs such as the kidney will lead to significant immune pathology. However, the complexes rhuMAb-E25 formed are very small and no clinical problem has arisen. Also, because of the isotype of IgG chosen as the template for humanization of the mouse monoclonal E-25, activation of complement does not occur. Furthermore, there are no reports of immune responses to the humanized form of the antibody after repeated injection into allergic subjects.

Questions have also been raised, theoretically, about the possible impact on safety of a therapeutic strategy which interferes with IgE-dependent processes, particularly concerning the role of mast cells in host defence.

The presence of high affinity IgE receptors on mast cells and eosinophils, the prominence of the IgE response against parasites, and the lack of IgE negative mutants in the human population argue for a biological function for IgE in recent evolutionary history: probably in defence against parasite infestation. However, available evidence is not wholly supportive. There are several lines of argument to suggest that the IgE/FcεRI interaction is not involved in protective immune responses and does not seem to be essential for normal immunological function.

(i)   Individuals who have either no detectable or very low levels of IgE in their blood[144], or mice rendered IgE deficient by immunological[145,146] or genetic[43] treatments live normally without impaired immune function.

(ii) IgE appears very late in evolution and is presumed to be teleologically justified for its protective role in immunity to chronic infection with parasites such as gut helminths. This concept arises from observations of strongly elevated levels of IgE after parasite infections in man and animals[147] and expulsion of parasites is believed to involve mediator release from gut mast cells sensitized through the high affinity IgE receptor (FcεRI).

However, while serum IgE increases in response to parasitic infections[148,149], it is not clear that the IgE/mast cell system is entirely beneficial[150].

(i) Mice infected with *Leishmania* showed a high mortality in BALB/c mice that gave high IgE responses but no mortality in C57/BL/6 mice that gave only low IgE responses to the parasite[151].

(ii) Treatment of high IgE responder mice with anti IL-4 antibody, which inhibits IgE responses[152], converted a parasitic infection from a lethal into a non-lethal outcome.

(iii) The presence of mast cells significantly augmented the size of cutaneous lesions during *Leishmania major* infection in mice, but did not significantly influence either the parasite burden or ultimate resolution of the infection[153].

(iv) Depletion of mast cells with antistem cell-factor significantly decreased parasite egg production during *N. brasiliensis* infection[154].

This indicates that the IgE/mast cell response to parasitic infection in mice has no protective role but, instead, may contribute to a detrimental course of the disease process. In addition to IgE, other immune mechanisms are implicated in the host defence response against parasites, including eosinophil-dependent killing mediated by IgA and IgG antibodies[155–160]. Thus, not only is there little need for protection against parasitic infections in developed countries, but the protective role of IgE is not entirely clear. Furthermore, it is evident that several mechanisms contribute to the immune protective response against parasites.

Recent evidence[161,162] has identified an important new role for the mast cell in natural immunity against bacteria. However, this involves an antibody-independent mechanism quite distinct from IgE-dependent processes involved in allergy.

Conclusions

Therapeutic agents which decrease levels of IgE in the circulation have a beneficial effect in treating allergic asthma and rhinitis which is independent of the sensitizing allergen. Evidence from Phase II trials with rhuMAb-E25 has been particularly important in illustrating that circulating IgE must be depleted substantially before an antiallergic effect is obtained. This is consistent with the high affinity and slow off-rate shown by IgE for FcεRI, although down-regulation of FcεRI expression probably amplifies the mast cell/basophil blockade obtained. A number of drugs, such as suplatast, are now beginning to appear which decrease IgE synthesis and have an antiallergic/anti-asthmatic effect. Bearing in mind the extent to which levels of IgE must be decreased by rhuMAb-E25 before a therapeutic effect is seen, the clinical effect of suplatast may be the result of several properties (mast cell stabilization; decreased IL-4; decreased IgE) acting in concert.

The critical importance of IgE as an initiator of acute allergic inflammation is well supported by these clinical findings; but what, if any, is the associated risk? The important role of the mast cell in host defence is becoming clear. However, the role of the IgE/FcεRI interaction on mast cells in host defence is uncertain; there is almost certainly redundancy in the immune mechanisms involved and these may have little importance in populations who are not exposed to intestinal parasites. Thus, safety issues associated with even profound decreases in IgE appear to be negligible, and drugs or vaccines designed to have this effect will probably play an important future role in controlling allergic disease.

REFERENCES

1 Ishizaka T, Dvorak AM, Conrad DH, Niebyl JR, Marquette JP, Ishizaka K. Morphologic and immunologic characterization of human basophils developed in cultures of cord blood mononuclear cells. *J Immunol* 1985; 134:532–540.

2 Rossi G, Newman SA, Metzger H. Assay and partial characterization of the solubilized cell surface receptor for immunoglobulin E. *J Biol Chem* 1977; 252:704–711.

3 Bahna SL. The 1988 Bela Schick memorial lecture. A 21-year salute to IgE. *Ann Allergy* 1989; 62:471–478.

4 Mascia A, Frank S, Berkman A et al. Mortality versus

improvement in severe chronic asthma: physiologic and psychologic factors. *Ann Allergy* 1989; 62:311–317.

5 Platts-Mills TA. Mechanisms of bronchial reactivity: the role of immunoglobulin E. *Am Rev Respir Dis* 1992; 145:S44-S47.

6 Conroy MC, Adkinson NF, Jr., Lichtenstein LM. Measurement of IgE on human basophils: relation to serum IgE and anti-IgE-induced histamine release. *J Immunol* 1977; 118:1317–1321.

7 MacGlashan DW, Jr., Peters SP, Warner J, Lichtenstein LM. Characteristics of human basophil sulfidopeptide leukotriene release: releasability defined as the ability of the basophil to respond to dimeric cross-links. *J Immunol* 1986; 136:2231–2239.

8 MacGlashan DW, Jr. Releasability of human basophils: cellular sensitivity and maximal histamine release are independent variables. *J Allergy Clin Immunol* 1993; 91:605–615.

9 MacGlashan DW, Jr., Bochner BS, Adelman DC et al. Downregulation of Fc(epsilon)RI expression on human basophils during in vivo treatment of atopic patients with anti-IgE antibody. *J Immunol* 1997; 158:1438–1445.

10 MacGlashan D, Jr., McKenzie-White J, Chichester K et al. In vitro regulation of FcepsilonRIalpha expression on human basophils by IgE antibody. *Blood* 1998; 91:1633–1643.

11 Saini SS, MacGlashan DW, Jr., Sterbinsky SA et al. Downregulation of human basophil IgE and FC epsilon RI alpha surface densities and mediator release by anti-IgE-infusions is reversible in vitro and in vivo. *J Immunol* 1999; 162:5624–5630.

12 Yamaguchi M, Lantz CS, Oettgen HC et al. IgE enhances mouse mast cell Fc(epsilon)RI expression in vitro and in vivo: evidence for a novel amplification mechanism in IgE-dependent reactions. *J Exp Med* 1997; 185:663–672.

13 Harriman W, Volk H, Defranoux N, Wabl M. Immunoglobulin class switch recombination. *Annu Rev Immunol* 1993; 11:361–384.

14 Bacharier LB, Geha RS. Regulation of IgE synthesis: the molecular basis and implications for clinical modulation. *Allergy Asthma Proc* 1999; 20:1–8.

15 Shapira SK, Jabara HH, Thienes CP et al. Deletional switch recombination occurs in interleukin-4-induced isotype switching to IgE expression by human B cells. *Proc Natl Acad Sci USA* 1991; 88:7528–7532.

16 Volk H, Wabl M. A protein binding specifically to the IgG2b switch region. *Dev Immunol* 1997; 5:105–114.

17 Borggrefe T, Wabl M, Akhmedov AT, Jessberger R. A B-cell-specific DNA recombination complex. *J Biol Chem* 1998; 273:17025–17035.

18 Gauchat JF, Lebman DA, Coffman RL, Gascan H, de Vries JE. Structure and expression of germline epsilon transcripts in human B cells induced by interleukin 4 to switch to IgE production. *J Exp Med* 1990; 172:463–473.

19 Snapper CM, Marcu KB, Zelazowski P. The immunoglobulin class switch: beyond 'accessibility'. *Immunity* 1997; 6:217–223.

20 Clark EA, Ledbetter JA. How B and T cells talk to each other. *Nature* 1994; 367:425–428.

21 Warren WD, Berton MT. Induction of germ-line gamma 1 and epsilon Ig gene expression in murine B cells. IL-4 and the CD40 ligand-CD40 interaction provide distinct but synergistic signals. *J Immunol* 1995; 155:5637–5646.

22 Watts C. Capture and processing of exogenous antigens for presentation on MHC molecules. *Annu Rev Immunol* 1997; 15:821–850.

23 Foy TM, Aruffo A, Bajorath J, Buhlmann JE, Noelle RJ. Immune regulation by CD40 and its ligand GP39. *Annu Rev Immunol* 1996; 14:591–617.

24 Keegan AD, Nelms K, Wang LM, Pierce JH, Paul WE. Interleukin 4 receptor: signaling mechanisms. *Immunol Today* 1994; 15:423–432.

25 Ezernieks J, Schnarr B, Metz K, Duschl A. The human IgE germline promoter is regulated by interleukin-4, interleukin-13, interferon-alpha and interferon-gamma via an interferon-gamma-activated site and its flanking regions. *Eur J Biochem* 1996; 240:667–673.

26 Welham MJ, Learmonth L, Bone H, Schrader JW. Interleukin-13 signal transduction in lymphohemopoietic cells. Similarities and differences in signal transduction with interleukin-4 and insulin. *J Biol Chem* 1995; 270:12286–12296.

27 Nelms K, Keegan AD, Zamorano J, Ryan JJ, Paul WE. The IL-4 receptor: signaling mechanisms and biologic functions. *Annu Rev Immunol* 1999; 17:701–738.

28 Smerz-Bertling C, Duschl A. Both interleukin 4 and interleukin 13 induce tyrosine phosphorylation of the 140-kDa subunit of the interleukin 4 receptor. *J Biol Chem* 1995; 270:966–970.

29 Atamas SP, Choi J, Yurovsky VV, White B. An alternative splice variant of human IL-4, IL-4 delta 2, inhibits IL-4-stimulated T cell proliferation. *J Immunol* 1996; 156:435–441.

30 Darnell JE, Jr. STATs and gene regulation. *Science* 1997; 277:1630–1635.

31 Linehan LA, Warren WD, Thompson PA, Grusby MJ, Berton MT. STAT6 is required for IL-4-induced germline Ig gene transcription and switch recombination. *J Immunol* 1998; 161:302–310.

32 Patel BK, Pierce JH, LaRochelle WJ. Regulation of interleukin 4-mediated signaling by naturally occurring dominant negative and attenuated forms of human Stat6. *Proc Natl Acad Sci USA* 1998; 95:172–177.

33 Mikita T, Campbell D, Wu P, Williamson K, Schindler U. Requirements for interleukin-4-induced gene expression and functional characterization of Stat6. *Mol Cell Biol* 1996; 16:5811–5820.

34 Cerutti A, Zan H, Schaffer A et al. CD40 ligand and appropriate cytokines induce switching to IgG, IgA, and IgE and coordinated germinal center and plasmacytoid phenotypic differentiation in a human monoclonal IgM + IgD + B cell line. *J Immunol* 1998; 160:2145–2157.

35 Iciek LA, Delphin SA, Stavnezer J. CD40 cross-linking induces Ig epsilon germline transcripts in B cells via activation of NF-kappaB: synergy with IL-4 induction. *J Immunol* 1997; 158:4769–4779.

36 Splawski JB, Fu SM, Lipsky PE. Immunoregulatory role of CD40 in human B cell differentiation. *J Immunol* 1993; 150:1276–1285.

37 Kawabe T, Naka T, Yoshida K et al. The immune responses in CD40-deficient mice: impaired immunoglobulin class switching and germinal center formation. *Immunity* 1994; 1:167–178.

38 Korthauer U, Graf D, Mages HW et al. Defective expression of T-cell CD40 ligand causes X-linked immunodeficiency with hyper-IgM. *Nature* 1993; 361:539–541.

39 Allen RC, Armitage RJ, Conley ME et al. CD40 ligand gene defects responsible for X-linked hyper-IgM syndrome. *Science* 1993; 259:990–993.

40 Ishida T, Mizushima S, Azuma S et al. Identification of TRAF6, a novel tumor necrosis factor receptor-associated factor protein that mediates signaling from an amino-terminal domain of the CD40 cytoplasmic region. *J Biol Chem* 1996; 271:28745–28748.

41 Ishida TK, Tojo T, Aoki T et al. TRAF5, a novel tumor necrosis factor receptor-associated factor family protein, mediates CD40 signaling. *Proc Natl Acad Sci USA* 1996; 93:9437–9442.

42 Ren CL, Morio T, Fu SM, Geha RS. Signal transduction via CD40 involves activation of lyn kinase and phosphatidylinositol-3-kinase, and phosphorylation of phospholipase C gamma 2. *J Exp Med* 1994; 179:673–680.

43 Kuhn R, Rajewsky K, Muller W. Generation and analysis of interleukin-4 deficient mice. *Science* 1991; 254:707–710.

44 McKenzie GJ, Emson CL, Bell SE et al. Impaired development of Th2 cells in IL-13-deficient mice. *Immunity* 1998; 9:423–432.

45 Levy F, Kristofic C, Heusser C, Brinkmann V. Role of IL-13 in CD4 T cell-dependent IgE production in atopy. *Int Arch Allergy Immunol* 1997; 112:49–58.

46 Zhou CY, Crocker IC, Koenig G, Romero FA, Townley RG. Anti-interleukin-4 inhibits immunoglobulin E production in a murine model of atopic asthma. *J Asthma* 1997; 34:195–201.

47 Tanaka H, Nagai H, Maeda Y. Effect of anti-IL-4 and anti-IL-5 antibodies on allergic airway hyperresponsiveness in mice. *Life Sci* 1998; 62:L169-L174.

48 Sato TA, Widmer MB, Finkelman FD et al. Recombinant soluble murine IL-4 receptor can inhibit or enhance IgE responses in vivo. *J Immunol* 1993; 150:2717–2723.

49 Carballido JM, Aversa G, Schols D, Punnonen J, de Vries JE. Inhibition of human IgE synthesis in vitro and in SCID-hu mice by an interleukin-4 receptor antagonist. *Int Arch Allergy Immunol* 1995; 107:304–307.

50 Carballido JM, Schols D, Namikawa R et al. IL-4 induces human B cell maturation and IgE synthesis in SCID-hu mice. Inhibition of ongoing IgE production by in vivo treatment with an IL-4/IL-13 receptor antagonist. *J Immunol* 1995; 155:4162–4170.

51 Arinobu Y, Atamas SP, Otsuka T et al. Antagonistic effects of an alternative splice variant of human IL-4, IL-4delta2, on IL-4 activities in human monocytes and B cells. *Cell Immunol* 1999; 191:161–167.

52 Zhang JG, Hilton DJ, Willson TA et al. Identification, purification, and characterization of a soluble interleukin (IL)-13-binding protein. Evidence that it is distinct from the cloned Il-13 receptor and Il-4 receptor alpha-chains. *J Biol Chem* 1997; 272:9474–9480.

53 Xu L, Rothman P. IFN-gamma represses epsilon germline transcription and subsequently down-regulates switch recombination to epsilon. *Int Immunol* 1994; 6:515–521.

54 Yoshimoto T, Okamura H, Tagawa YI, Iwakura Y, Nakanishi K. Interleukin 18 together with interleukin 12 inhibits IgE production by induction of interferon-gamma production from activated B cells. *Proc Natl Acad Sci USA* 1997; 94:3948–3953.

55 Hofstra CL, Van AI, Hofman G, Kool M, Nijkamp FP, Van Oosterhout AJ. Prevention of Th2-like cell responses by coadministration of IL-12 and IL-18 is associated with inhibition of antigen-induced airway hyperresponsiveness, eosinophilia, and serum IgE levels. *J Immunol* 1998; 161:5054–5060.

56 Okamura H, Kashiwamura S, Tsutsui H, Yoshimoto T, Nakanishi K. Regulation of interferon-gamma production by IL-12 and IL-18. *Curr Opin Immunol* 1998; 10:259–264.

57 Kimata H, Yoshida A, Ishioka C, Lindley I, Mikawa H. Interleukin 8 (IL-8) selectively inhibits immunoglobulin E

production induced by IL-4 in human B cells. *J Exp Med* 1992; 176:1227–1231.

58 Punnonen J, de Waal MR, van Vlasselaer P, Gauchat JF, de Vries JE. IL-10 and viral IL-10 prevent IL-4-induced IgE synthesis by inhibiting the accessory cell function of monocytes. *J Immunol* 1993; 151:1280–1289.

59 Jeannin P, Lecoanet S, Delneste Y, Gauchat JF, Bonnefoy JY. IgE versus IgG4 production can be differentially regulated by IL-10. *J Immunol* 1998; 160:3555–3561.

60 Wang CC, Rook GA. Inhibition of an established allergic response to ovalbumin in BALB/c mice by killed Mycobacterium vaccae. *Immunology* 1998; 93:307–313.

61 Katano M, Morisaki T. The past, the present and future of the OK-432 therapy for patients with malignant effusions. *Anticancer Res* 1998; 18:3917–3925.

62 Krieg AM, Yi AK, Matson S et al. CpG motifs in bacterial DNA trigger direct B-cell activation. *Nature* 1995; 374:546–549.

63 Klinman DM, Yi AK, Beaucage SL, Conover J, Krieg AM. CpG motifs present in bacteria DNA rapidly induce lymphocytes to secrete interleukin 6, interleukin 12, and interferon gamma. *Proc Natl Acad Sci USA* 1996; 93:2879–2883.

64 Bohle B, Jahn-Schmid B, Maurer D, Kraft D, Ebner C. Oligodeoxynucleotides containing CpG motifs induce IL-12, IL-18 and IFN-gamma production in cells from allergic individuals and inhibit IgE synthesis in vitro. *Eur J Immunol* 1999; 29:2344–2353.

65 Kline JN, Waldschmidt TJ, Businga TR et al. Modulation of airway inflammation by CpG oligodeoxynucleotides in a murine model of asthma. *J Immunol* 1998; 160:2555–2559.

66 Meinke GC, Magro AM, Lawrence DA, Spiegelberg HL. Characterization of an IgE receptor isolated from cultured B-type lymphoblastoid cells. *J Immunol* 1978; 121:1321–1328.

67 Nonaka M, Hsu DK, Hanson CM, Aosai F, Katz DH. Cloning of cDNA coding for low-affinity Fc receptors for IgE on human T lymphocytes. *Int Immunol* 1989; 1:254–259.

68 Gordon J, Flores-Romo L, Cairns JA et al. CD23: a multi-functional receptor/lymphokine? *Immunol Today* 1989; 10:153–157.

69 Yu P, Kosco-Vilbois M, Richards M, Kohler G, Lamers MC. Negative feedback regulation of IgE synthesis by murine CD23. *Nature* 1994; 369:753–756.

70 Luo HY, Hofstetter H, Banchereau J, Delespesse G. Cross-linking of CD23 antigen by its natural ligand (IgE) or by anti-CD23 antibody prevents B lymphocyte proliferation and differentiation. *J Immunol* 1991; 146:2122–2129.

71 Pene J, Chretien I, Rousset F, Briere F, Bonnefoy JY, de Vries JE. Modulation of IL-4-induced human IgE production in

vitro by IFN-gamma and IL-5: the role of soluble CD23 (s-CD23). *J Cell Biochem* 1989; 39:253–264.

72 Saxon A, Ke Z, Bahati L, Stevens RH. Soluble CD23 containing B cell supernatants induce IgE from peripheral blood B-lymphocytes and costimulate with interleukin-4 in induction of IgE. *J Allergy Clin Immunol* 1990; 86:333–344.

73 Paul-Eugene N, Kolb JP, Calenda A et al. Functional interaction between beta 2-adrenoceptor agonists and interleukin-4 in the regulation of CD23 expression and release and IgE production in human. *Mol Immunol* 1993; 30:157–164.

74 Paul-Eugene N, Kolb JP, Damais C et al. Beta 2-adrenoceptor agonists regulate the IL-4-induced phenotypical changes and IgE-dependent functions in normal human monocytes. *J Leukoc Biol* 1994; 55:313–320.

75 Coqueret O, Dugas B, Mencia-Huerta JM, Braquet P. Regulation of IgE production from human mononuclear cells by beta 2-adrenoceptor agonists. *Clin Exp Allergy* 1995; 25:304–311.

76 Coqueret O, Demarquay D, Lagente V. Role of cyclic AMP in the modulation of IgE production by the beta 2-adrenoceptor agonist, fenoterol. *Eur Respir J* 1996; 9:220–225.

77 Coqueret O, Petit-Frere C, Lagente V, Moumen M, Mencia-Huerta JM, Braquet P. Modulation of IgE production in the mouse by beta 2-adrenoceptor agonist. *Int Arch Allergy Immunol* 1994; 105:171–176.

78 Corne JM, Linaker CH, Howarth PH et al. Effect of systemic beta-agonist therapy on IgE production in allergic subjects in vivo. *J Allergy Clin Immunol* 1998; 102:727–731.

79 Klebl FH, Weber G, Kalden JR, Nusslein HG. In vitro and in vivo effect of glucocorticoids on IgE and IgG subclass secretion. *Clin Exp Allergy* 1994; 24:1022–1029.

80 Akdis CA, Blesken T, Akdis M, Alkan SS, Heusser CH, Blaser K. Glucocorticoids inhibit human antigen-specific and enhance total IgE and IgG4 production due to differential effects on T and B cells in vitro. *Eur J Immunol* 1997; 27:2351–2357.

81 Zieg G, Lack G, Harbeck RJ, Gelfand EW, Leung DY. In vivo effects of glucocorticoids on IgE production. *J Allergy Clin Immunol* 1994; 94:222–230.

82 Pullerits T, Praks L, Sjostrand M, Rak S, Skoogh BE, Lotvall J. An intranasal glucocorticoid inhibits the increase of specific IgE initiated during birch pollen season. *J Allergy Clin Immunol* 1997; 100:601–605.

83 Alexander AG, Barnes NC, Kay AB, Corrigan CJ. Clinical response to cyclosporin in chronic severe asthma is associated with reduction in serum soluble interleukin-2 receptor concentrations. *Eur Respir J* 1995; 8:574–578.

84 Lock SH, Kay AB, Barnes NC. Double-blind, placebo-

controlled study of cyclosporin A as a corticosteroid-sparing agent in corticosteroid-dependent asthma. *Am J Respir Crit Care Med* 1996; 153:509–514.

85 Sihra BS, Kon OM, Durham SR, Walker S, Barnes NC, Kay AB. Effect of cyclosporin A on the allergen-induced late asthmatic reaction. *Thorax* 1997; 52:447–452.

86 Wheeler DJ, Robins A, Pritchard DI, Bundick RV, Shakib F. Potentiation of in vitro synthesis of human IgE by cyclosporin A (CsA). *Clin Exp Immunol* 1995; 102:85–90.

87 Nagai H, Hiyama H, Matsuo A, Ueda Y, Inagaki N, Kawada K. FK-506 and cyclosporin A potentiate the IgE antibody production by contact sensitization with hapten in mice. *J Pharmacol Exp Ther* 1997; 283:321–327.

88 Etzioni A, Shehadeh N, Brecher A, Yorman S, Pollack S. Cyclosporin A in hyperimmunoglobulin E syndrome. *Ann Allergy Asthma Immunol* 1997; 78:413–414.

89 Tang AT, Lau YL, Jones B, Halpern GM, Yeung CY. Cefadroxil reduces the production of IgE in a 3 year old asthmatic with juvenile rheumatoid arthritis. *Allergol Immunopathol (Madr)* 1993; 21:131–135.

90 Garland LG. Pharmacology of prophylactic anti-asthma drugs. In: Page CP, Barnes PJ, eds. *Pharmacology of Asthma.* Basel: Springer Verlag; 1991: 261–290.

91 Loh RK, Jabara HH, Geha RS. Mechanisms of inhibition of IgE synthesis by nedocromil sodium: nedocromil sodium inhibits deletional switch recombination in human B cells. *J Allergy Clin Immunol* 1996; 97:1141–1150.

92 Loh RK, Jabara HH, Geha RS. Disodium cromoglycate inhibits S mu – >S epsilon deletional switch recombination and IgE synthesis in human B cells. *J Exp Med* 1994; 180:663–671.

93 Kimata H, Mikawa H. Nedocromil sodium selectively inhibits IgE and IgG4 production in human B cells stimulated with IL-4. *J Immunol* 1993; 151:6723–6732.

94 Sasai K, Furukawa S, Sugawara T, Kaneko K, Baba M, Yabuta K. IgE levels in faecal extracts of patients with food allergy. *Allergy* 1992; 47:594–598.

95 Yanagihara Y, Kiniwa M, Ikizawa K, Shida T, Matsuura N, Koda A. Suppression of IgE production by IPD-1151T (suplatast tosilate), a new dimethylsulfonium agent: (2). Regulation of human IgE response. *Jpn J Pharmacol* 1993; 61:31–39.

96 Yanagihara Y, Kiniwa M, Ikizawa K, Shida T, Matsuura N, Koda A. Suppression of IgE production by IPD-1151T (suplatast tosilate), a new dimethylsulfonium agent: (2). Regulation of human IgE response. *Jpn J Pharmacol* 1993; 61:31–39.

97 Yamaya H, Basaki Y, Togawa M, Kojima M, Kiniwa M, Matsuura N. Down-regulation of Th2 cell-mediated murine peritoneal eosinophilia by antiallergic agents. *Life Sci* 1995; 56:1647–1654.

98 Konno S, Adachi M, Asano K et al. Suppressive effects of IPD-1151T (suplatast-tosilate) on induction of mast cells from normal mouse splenocytes. *Eur J Pharmacol* 1994; 259:15–20.

99 Taniguchi H, Togawa M, Ohwada K et al. Suplatast tosilate, a new type of antiallergic agent, prevents the expression of airway hyperresponsiveness in guinea pigs. *Eur J Pharmacol* 1996; 318:447–454.

100 Hanashiro K, Tamaki N, Koga T, Nakamura M, Kinjoh K, Kosugi T. Inhibitory effect of azelastine hydrochloride and suplatast tosilate on airway responses in sensitized rats following exposure to antigen. *Int J Tissue React* 1997; 19:163–169.

101 Washio Y, Ohashi Y, Tanaka A et al. Suplatast tosilate affects the initial increase in specific IgE and interleukin-4 during immunotherapy for perennial allergic rhinitis. *Acta Otolaryngol* Suppl 1998; 538:126–132.

102 Kimata H. Selective enhancement of production of IgE, IgG4, and Th2-cell cytokine during the rebound phenomenon in atopic dermatitis and prevention by suplatast tosilate. *Ann Allergy Asthma Immunol* 1999; 82:293–295.

103 Kato Y, Manabe T, Tanaka Y, Mochizuki H. Effect of an orally active Th1/Th2 balance modulator, M50367, on IgE production, eosinophilia, and airway hyperresponsiveness in mice. *J Immunol* 1999; 162:7470–7479.

104 Chong AS, Finnegan A, Jiang X et al. Leflunomide, a novel immunosuppressive agent. The mechanism of inhibition of T cell proliferation. *Transplantation* 1993; 55:1361–1366.

105 Halloran PF. Molecular mechanisms of new immunosuppressants. *Clin Transplant* 1996; 10:118–123.

106 Silva Junior HT, Morris RE. Leflunomide and malononitrilamides. *Am J Med Sci* 1997; 313:289–301.

107 Uhlig T, Cooper D, Eber E, McMenamin C, Wildhaber JH, Sly PD. Effects of long-term oral treatment with leflunomide on allergic sensitization, lymphocyte activation, and airway inflammation in a rat model of asthma. *Clin Exp Allergy* 1998; 28:758–764.

108 Eber E, Uhlig T, McMenamin C, Sly PD. Leflunomide, a novel immunomodulating agent, prevents the development of allergic sensitization in an animal model of allergic asthma. *Clin Exp Allergy* 1998; 28:376–384.

109 Bruneau JM, Yea CM, Spinella-Jaegle S et al. Purification of human dihydro-orotate dehydrogenase and its inhibition by A77 1726, the active metabolite of leflunomide. *Biochem J* 1998; 336 (2):299–303.

110 Siemasko K, Chong AS, Jack HM, Gong H, Williams JW, Finnegan A. Inhibition of JAK3 and STAT6 tyrosine phos-

phorylation by the immunosuppressive drug leflunomide leads to a block in IgG1 production. *J Immunol* 1998; 160:1581–1588.

111 Jarman ER, Kuba A, Montermann E, Bartlett RR, Reske-Kunz AB. Inhibition of murine IgE and immediate cutaneous hypersensitivity responses to ovalbumin by the immunomodulatory agent leflunomide. *Clin Exp Immunol* 1999; 115:221–228.

112 Mizushima Y, Amano Y, Kitagawa H, Ogata K. Oral administration of leflunomide (HWA486) results in prominent suppression of immunoglobulin E formation in a rat type 1 allergy model. *J Pharmacol Exp Ther* 1999; 288:849–857.

113 Christie G, Barton A, Bolognese B et al. IgE secretion is attenuated by an inhibitor of proteolytic processing of CD23 (Fc epsilonRII). *Eur J Immunol* 1997; 27:3228–3235.

114 Marolewski AE, Buckle DR, Christie G. CD23 (FcepsilonRII) release from cell membranes is mediated by a membrane-bound metalloprotease. *Biochem J* 1998; 333 (3):573–579.

115 Bailey S, Bolognese B, Buckle DR et al. Selective inhibition of low affinity IgE receptor (CD23) processing. *Bioorg Med Chem Lett* 1998; 8:29–34.

116 Bailey S, Bolognese B, Buckle DR et al. Hydroxamate-based inhibitors of low affinity IgE receptor (CD23) processing. *Bioorg Med Chem Lett* 1998; 8:23–28.

117 Wheeler DJ, Parveen S, Pollock K, Williams RJ. Inhibition of sCD23 and immunoglobulin E release from human B cells by a metalloproteinase inhibitor, GI 129471. *Immunology* 1998; 95:105–110.

118 Underwood DC, Bochnowicz S, Osborn RR et al. Antiasthmatic activity of the second-generation phosphodiesterase 4 (PDE4) inhibitor SB 207499 (Ariflo) in the guinea pig. *J Pharmacol Exp Ther* 1998; 287:988–995.

119 Coqueret O, Boichot E, Lagente V. Selective type IV phosphodiesterase inhibitors prevent IL-4-induced IgE production by human peripheral blood mononuclear cells. *Clin Exp Allergy* 1997; 27:816–823.

120 Presta LG, Lahr SJ, Shields RL et al. Humanization of an antibody directed against IgE. *J Immunol* 1993; 151:2623–2632.

121 Shields RL, Whether WR, Zioncheck K et al. Inhibition of allergic reactions with antibodies to IgE. *Int Arch Allergy Immunol* 1995; 107:308–312.

122 Shields RL, Werther WR, Zioncheck K et al. Anti-IgE monoclonal antibodies that inhibit allergen-specific histamine release. *Int Arch Allergy Immunol* 1995; 107:412–413.

123 Saban R, Haak-Frendscho M, Zine M et al. Human FcERI-IgG and humanized anti-IgE monoclonal antibody MaE11 block passive sensitization of human and rhesus monkey lung. *J Allergy Clin Immunol* 1994; 94:836–843.

124 Saban R, Haak-Frendscho M, Zine M, Presta LG, Bjorling DE, Jardieu P. Human anti-IgE monoclonal antibody blocks passive sensitization of human and rhesus monkey bladder. *J Urol* 1997; 157:689–693.

125 Fei DT, Lowe J, Jardieu P. A novel bioactivity assay for monoclonal antibodies directed against IgE. *J Immunol Methods* 1994; 171:189–199.

126 Kings MA, Conroy MC, Stadler BM, Magnusson CG, Skvaril F, de Weck AL. Histamine release from human leukocytes by anti-IgE antibodies: influence of multiple or single epitope recognition. *Diagn Immunol* 1986; 4:89–96.

127 Grassi J, Didierlaurent A, Stadler BM. Quantitative determination of total and specific human IgE with the use of monoclonal antibodies. *J Allergy Clin Immunol* 1986; 77:808–822.

128 Rudolf MP, Furukawa K, Miescher S, Vogel M, Kricek F, Stadler BM. Effect of anti-IgE antibodies on Fc epsilonRI-bound IgE. *J Immunol* 1996; 157:5646–5652.

129 Miescher S, Vogel M, Stampfli MR et al. Domain-specific anti-IgE antibodies interfere with IgE binding to Fc epsilon RII. *Int Arch Allergy Immunol* 1994; 105:75–82.

130 Stampfli MR, Miescher S, Aebischer I, Zurcher AW, Stadler BM. Inhibition of human IgE synthesis by anti-IgE antibodies requires divalent recognition. *Eur J Immunol* 1994; 24:2161–2167.

131 Rudolf MP, Vogel M, Kricek F et al. Epitope-specific antibody response to IgE by mimotope immunization. *J Immunol* 1998; 160:3315–3321.

132 Kricek F, Ruf C, Rudolf MP, Effenberger F, Mayer P, Stadler BM. IgE-related peptide mimotopes. Basic structures for anti-allergy vaccine development. *Int Arch Allergy Immunol* 1999; 118:222–223.

133 Shakib F, Smith SJ. In vitro basophil histamine-releasing activity of circulating IgG1 and IgG4 autoanti-IgE antibodies from asthma patients and the demonstration that anti-IgE modulates allergen-induced basophil activation. *Clin Exp Allergy* 1994; 24:270–275.

134 Chang TW, Davis FM, Sun NC, Sun CR, MacGlashan DW, Jr., Hamilton RG. Monoclonal antibodies specific for human IgE-producing B cells: a potential therapeutic for IgE-mediated allergic diseases. *Biotechnology (NY)* 1990; 8:122–126.

135 Davis FM, Gossett LA, Chang TW. An epitope on membrane-bound but not secreted IgE: implications in isotype-specific regulation. *Biotechnology (NY)* 1991; 9:53–56.

136 Fox JA, Hotaling TE, Struble C, Ruppel J, Bates DJ, Schoenhoff MB. Tissue distribution and complex formation with IgE of an anti-IgE antibody after intravenous administration in cynomolgus monkeys. *J Pharmacol Exp Ther* 1996; 279:1000–1008.

137 Casale TB, Bernstein IL, Busse WW et al. Use of an anti-IgE humanized monoclonal antibody in ragweed-induced allergic rhinitis. *J Allergy Clin Immunol* 1997; 100:110–121.

138 Fahy JV, Fleming HE, Wong HH et al. The effect of an anti-IgE monoclonal antibody on the early- and late-phase responses to allergen inhalation in asthmatic subjects. *Am J Respir Crit Care Med* 1997; 155:1828–1834.

139 Boulet LP, Chapman KR, Cote J et al. Inhibitory effects of an anti-IgE antibody E25 on allergen-induced early asthmatic response. *Am J Respir Crit Care Med* 1997; 155:1835–1840.

140 Casale TB, Condemi J, LaForce C et al. Effect of omalizumab on symptoms of seasonal allergic rhinitis: a randomized controlled trial. *J Am Med Assoc* 2001; 286:2956–2967.

141 Milgrom H, Fick RB, Jr., Su JQ et al. Treatment of allergic asthma with monoclonal anti-IgE antibody. rhuMAb-E25 Study Group. *N Engl J Med* 1999; 341:1966–1973.

142 Corne J, Djukanovic R, Thomas L et al. The effect of intravenous administration of a chimeric anti-IgE antibody on serum IgE levels in atopic subjects: efficacy, safety, and pharmacokinetics. *J Clin Invest* 1997; 99:879–887.

143 Racine-Poon A, Botta L, Chang TW et al. Efficacy, pharmacodynamics, and pharmacokinetics of CGP 51901, an anti-immunoglobulin E chimeric monoclonal antibody, in patients with seasonal allergic rhinitis. *Clin Pharmacol Ther* 1997; 62:675–690.

144 Levy DA, Chen J. Healthy IgE-deficient person. *N Engl J Med* 1970; 283:541–542.

145 Haba S, Nisonoff A. Inhibition of IgE synthesis by anti-IgE: role in long-term inhibition of IgE synthesis by neonatally administered soluble IgE. *Proc Natl Acad Sci USA* 1990; 87:3363–3367.

146 Marshall JS, Bell EB. Induction of an auto-anti-IgE response in rats I. Effects on serum IgE concentrations. *Eur J Immunol* 1985; 15:272–277.

147 Ishizaka T, Urban J, Jr., Takatsu K, Ishizaka K. Immunoglobulin E synthesis in parasite infection. *J Allergy Clin Immunol* 1976; 58:523–538.

148 Eisen HN. Antibody-mediated (immediate-type) hypersensitivity. In: Davis BD, Dulbecco R, Eisen HN, Ginsberg HS, eds. *Microbiology*. Philadelphia: Harper & Row; 1980: 468–492.

149 Rocklin RE, David J. Immediate hypersensitivity. In: Rubenstein E, Federman DD, eds. *Scientific American Medicine*. New York: Scientific American, 1991: 33–35.

150 Moqbel R, Pritchard DI. Parasites and allergy: evidence for a 'cause and effect' relationship. *Clin Exp Allergy* 1990; 20:611–618.

151 Sadick MD, Heinzel FP, Holaday BJ, Pu RT, Dawkins RS, Locksley RM. Cure of murine leishmaniasis with anti-interleukin 4 monoclonal antibody. Evidence for a T cell-dependent, interferon gamma-independent mechanism. *J Exp Med* 1990; 171:115–127.

152 Finkelman FD, Holmes J, Katona IM et al. Lymphokine control of in vivo immunoglobulin isotype selection. *Annu Rev Immunol* 1990; 8:303–333.

153 Wershil BK, Theodos CM, Galli SJ, Titus RG. Mast cells augment lesion size and persistence during experimental *Leishmania* major infection in the mouse. *J Immunol* 1994; 152:4563–4571.

154 Newlands GF, Miller HR, MacKellar A, Galli SJ. Stem cell factor contributes to intestinal mucosal mast cell hyperplasia in rats infected with *Nippostrongylus brasiliensis* or *Trichinella spiralis*, but anti-stem cell factor treatment decreases parasite egg production during *N. brasiliensis* infection. *Blood* 1995; 86:1968–1976.

155 Abu-Ghazaleh RI, Fujisawa T, Mestecky J, Kyle RA, Gleich GJ. IgA-induced eosinophil degranulation. *J Immunol* 1989; 142:2393–2400.

156 Chandrashekar R, Rao UR, Subrahmanyam D. Antibody-mediated cytotoxic effects in vitro and in vivo of rat cells on infective larvae of *Brugia malayi*. *Int J Parasitol* 1990; 20:725–730.

157 De Simone C, Salvi MC, Ferrarelli G, De Santis G, Mango G, Sorice F. Human eosinophils and parasitic diseases – III. Beta-interferon increases eosinophil IgG-Fc receptor expression and capacity. *Int J Immunopharmacol* 1986; 8:479–485.

158 Dunne DW, Richardson BA, Jones FM, Clark M, Thorne KJ, Butterworth AE. The use of mouse/human chimaeric antibodies to investigate the roles of different antibody isotypes, including IgA2, in the killing of *Schistosoma mansoni* schistosomula by eosinophils. *Parasite Immunol* 1993; 15:181–185.

159 Hamada A, Greene BM. Clq enhancement of IgG-dependent eosinophil-mediated killing of schistosomula in vitro. *J Immunol* 1987; 138:1240–1245.

160 Smith PD, Keister DB, Elson CO. Human host response to Giardia lamblia. II. Antibody-dependent killing in vitro. *Cell Immunol* 1983; 82:308–315.

161 Echtenacher B, Mannel DN, Hultner L. Critical protective role of mast cells in a model of acute septic peritonitis. *Nature* 1996; 381:75–77.

162 Malaviya R, Ikeda T, Ross E, Abraham SN. Mast cell modulation of neutrophil influx and bacterial clearance at sites of infection through TNF-alpha. *Nature* 1996; 381:77–80.

11

Drugs targeting cell signalling

Brydon L. Bennett, Yoshitaka Satoh and Alan J. Lewis

Signal Research Division, Celgene Corporation, San Diego, CA, USA

Introduction

Cellular responses to external stimuli are coordinated by intracellular transducers, which rapidly relay a chemical signal from the cell membrane to specific effector sites inside the cell. The transducers are typically enzymes and adaptor proteins, such as kinases, phosphatases, lipases, and G-proteins, while the signal is frequently an allosteric activator such as Ca^{2+}, cAMP, phospholipid, and phosphate. Response to external signals may occur in seconds, e.g. changes in ion channels and membrane structure, to minutes, e.g. trafficking of proteins to cell surface, to hours, e.g. changes in protein levels due to gene expression. The diversity and detail of these signalling pathways is both remarkable and only partly understood[1]. The discovery of numerous proteins within decipherable biochemical pathways has provided novel approaches to controlling specific cell responses[2]. For instance, the overexpression of multiple genes encoding inflammatory enzymes, cytokines, adhesion molecules, and proteases is responsible for diseases such as asthma, chronic obstructive pulmonary disease (COPD), rheumatoid arthritis, inflammatory bowel disease psoriasis and colitis[3]. By targeting key signalling components of these pathways for therapeutic intervention, it is believed that a new generation of drugs will attack the underlying cause of disease and not just the disease symptoms[4].

A sufficient description of all of the molecular drug targets available in cell signalling pathways is not possible within the confines of this chapter, when it is estimated that there are between 400 and 600 protein kinases alone encoded in the human genome[1]. Instead, this chapter focuses on an emerging subset of protein kinases for which first generation inhibitors are starting to enter - pre-clinical development and clinical trials. Serine–threonine kinases play an important role in cell growth, differentiation, apoptosis, cell mobility and mitogenesis. Over the past decade, five serine–threonine protein kinase cascades, critical for regulating inflammatory gene expression, have been described. The challenges faced in identifying potent small molecule inhibitors with kinase and isoform selectivity, known mechanism of action, and efficacy in disease models, are well illustrated with these drug targets.

p38 kinase pathway

The mitogen activated protein kinase, p38, is the human homologue of the yeast HOG1 protein kinase, and has retained a name based on its molecular weight of 38 000 Daltons. While both kinases are activated in response to osmotic shock[5], mammalian p38s are also induced by inflammatory cytokines, bacterial endotoxin, hypoxia, UV, heat shock, and other cell stresses[6]. Activation occurs by serial phosphorylation of tyrosine and threonine residues in a TGY motif present in the activation loop (the related MAPKs, ERK and JNK, contain TEY and TPY motifs, respectively) and is mediated by the MAPKKs, MKK3, MKK6 and MKK4 (Fig. 11.1). Four p38 isoforms have been identified, each the product of a unique gene. p38α was originally identified as a

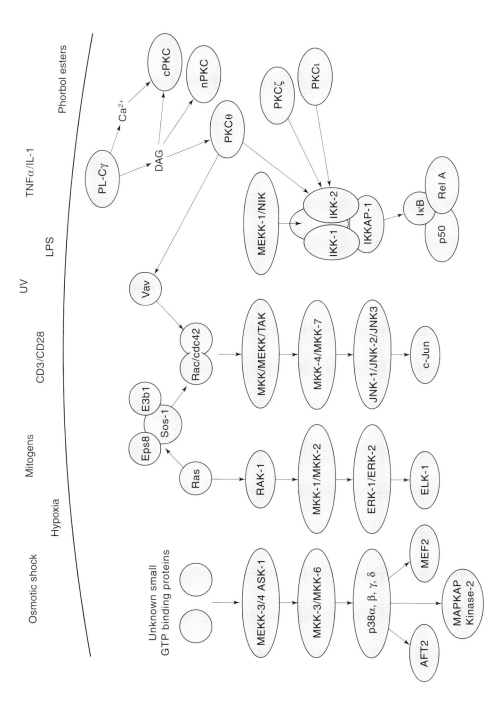

Fig. 11.1 Serine–threonine protein kinase cascades in inflammatory disease. Five major serine–threonine protein kinase cascades that modulate inflammatory gene expression have been identified. A plethora of external stimuli may induce proinflammatory responses by activating one or more of these pathways. Typically these stimuli activate cell surface receptors that transduce signal across the membrane and activate receptor associated tyrosine kinases (not shown)[181] and GTP binding proteins[182]. Protein kinases are highlighted in bold, and the major signalling pathways connected by arrows.

LPS-inducible kinase activity[5,7] and as a protein that bound to a class of small molecule cytokine inhibitors[8]. It has a broad tissue distribution that includes the lung, trachea and hematopoietic cells. p38β (p38–2) has 72% amino acid identity to p38α, and has highest expression in the brain and major organs[9]. It is not expressed in hematopoietic cells, spleen, bone marrow, placenta or lung. Kinetic analyses indicate p38β has a two-fold higher substrate affinity and 100-fold greater catalytic activity than p38α for the substrate, ATF2. p38γ, originally identified as ERK6, has 60% amino acid identity to p38α[10]. It has a restricted tissue distribution with high levels observed only in skeletal muscle, and low levels in brain. p38δ has 57% amino acid homology to p38α[11]. It is expressed predominantly in glandular–epithelial tissues with lower levels in hematopoietic cells. p38δ does not phosphorylate the p38α substrate, MAPKAP kinase-2. Therefore, p38 isoforms exhibit differences in both tissue distribution and substrate selectivity. The important isoforms in the lung are likely to be p38α and p38δ.

Many proteins have been proposed as putative substrates for p38, although confirmation of their physiological relevance has been less forthcoming. Candidate substrates include the transcription factors ATF2, GADD153, Elk-1, MEF2A, MEF2C, and kinases MAPKAP kinase-2, -3, Mnk1 and 2, Msk1 and PRAK[12]. The best validated of these targets are MEF2 and MAPKAP kinase-2. Myocyte-enhancer factor 2 (MEF2) was isolated as a potential target of p38 following stringent binding in a yeast two-hybrid screen[13], and has been identified as an essential regulator of myocardial growth[14]. Both MEF2A and MEF2C, but not MEF2B or MEF2D, are p38 substrates, and are activated by phosphorylation of dual threonine residues in the activation domain[15]. A docking domain (D) on MEF2 is sufficient for p38 binding even if the domain is fused to non-p38 substrates[16]. Mitogen activated protein kinase activated protein kinase-2 (MAPKAP kinase-2) is an essential post-transcriptional regulator of TNFα synthesis. Treatment of LPS stimulated monocytes with the p38 kinase inhibitor, SB 203580 (see below), blocked p38 activity, MAPKAP kinase-2 activity, and TNFα

secretion but not the increase in TNFα mRNA[17]. This observation was confirmed when mice deficient in MAPKAP kinase-2 were found to express normal levels of TNFα mRNA following LPS stimulation, but showed a 90% reduction in TNFα protein levels[18]. Targeted disruption of p38α causes developmental failure in utero[19]. Experiments with heterozygous (-/ +) and homozygous null (-/-) embryonic fibroblasts demonstrate that p38α is essential for IL-1 induced IL-6 synthesis, and the phosphorylation of MAPKAP kinase-2. Therefore, p38 clearly mediates effects at both the transcriptional and post-transcriptional levels.

Two upstream MAPKKs have been identified as key activators of p38[20]. Experiments using over-expression of MKK3 and MKK6 suggest that MKK6 may play a more dominant role in activating p38[20], perhaps in part because, while MKK6 can activate all p38 isoforms, MKK3 appears to selectively activate p38α[21]. Mkk6-/- mice have not yet been described but Mkk3-/- mice are viable and display no morphological defects. Murine embryonic fibroblasts and macrophages from Mkk3-/- mice exhibit a selective defect in p38 activation following TNFα and LPS stimulation[12,22]. p38 activation by IL-1, osmotic shock, and UV radiation are normal. A striking observation was the loss of IL-12 expression in macrophages and dendritic cells stimulated with LPS or CD40L respectively[12]. This suggests Mkk3-/- animals may fail to mount a viable Th1 type immune response.

The kinetic mechanism of p38 phosphorylation of ATF2 has been described[23]. Data indicate that catalysis follows an ordered sequential mechanism with binding of substrate (GST-ATF2) an essential prerequisite for ATP binding. Such a binding mechanism is atypical of MAPKs and indicates a high affinity for substrate. Furthermore, the K_m for ATP is unusually high, being in the vicinity of 20–150 μM[24,25], compared to values of 2 μM and 0.2 μM for JNK2 and IKK2, respectively. Our understanding of the binding mode for ATP, as well as for p38 inhibitors, has been enhanced by the crystallization of p38[26]. Structural information has been critical in the design of novel inhibitors as well as optimization of the original pyridinyl-imidazole compounds first described as inhibitors of TNF-α and IL-1 in vitro and in vivo[27]. This compound class was subsequently called CSAIDs (cytokine-suppressive anti-inflammatory drugs, Fig. 11.2). In 1994, with the aid of radiolabelled compound, scientists from SmithKline Beecham reported the isolation of a protein that bound these inhibitors (cytokine-suppressor binding protein, CSBP), and established that the target protein was identical to murine p38[8]. SB 203580[28], an early pyridinyl-imidazole p38 inhibitor, emerged as a potent, orally active inhibitor of p38 with a spectrum of anti-inflammatory activity in animal pharmacology models, and remains the most extensively studied inhibitor of p38. Many patent applications for SB 203580-like inhibitors have appeared and have been reviewed elsewhere[29].

Enzymology studies show that SB 203580 is an ATP competitive, reversible inhibitor with a K_i value of 21 nM[30]. Using a CSBP/p38 binding assay with ^{3}H-SB 202190 as the radioligand, SB 203580 had an IC$_{50}$ value of 42 nM[31]. The X-ray crystallography studies[32] of a close analogue of SB 203580 bound to p38 clearly show that the nitrogen atom of the 4-pyridyl group of SB 203580 forms an essential interaction with methionine 109 while the fluorophenyl group provides a critical hydrophobic binding in a lipophilic pocket in the active site. The p38 crystal structure with a similar p38 inhibitor, VK-19911, has also been published[33]. In monocyte assays, SB 203580 inhibited LPS stimulated production of IL-1β and TNF-α at 0.05 and 0.1 μM, respectively. SB 203580 inhibited TNF-α induced IL-6 and GM-CSF production in murine L929 cells, human U937 cells, and HeLa cells. No effect of SB 203580 on the TNF-α-induced NF-κB DNA binding in L929 cells was observed. SB 203580 inhibited IL-1 stimulated p38 kinase activity in bovine cartilage-derived chondrocytes, an in vitro model of rheumatoid arthritis, with an IC$_{50}$ value of 1.0 μM.

SB 203580 was extensively evaluated in a series of animal pharmacology models of inflammation[34]. SB 203580 was shown to be a potent inhibitor of cytokine production in mice and rats at ED$_{50}$ = 15–25 mg/kg p.o., and had therapeutic activity in collagen-

induced arthritis at 50 mg/kg p.o., b.i.d. in DBA/LACJ mice. In the adjuvant-induced arthritis models in Lewis rats, SB 203580 administered at 30 and 60 mg/kg p.o., improved both bone mineral density and histological scores. SB 203580 reduced mortality in a murine model of endotoxin-induced shock in a dose-dependent manner at 25 – 100 mg/kg p.o. In order to determine whether chronic administration of CSAIDs leads to immunosuppression, ovalbumin-sensitized BALB/c mice were treated for 2 weeks with SB 203580 at 60 mg/kg i.p. Although the ovalbumin antibody titre was marginally suppressed, ex vivo lymphocytic responses were unaffected.

Increased liver weight and significant elevations of hepatic P-450 enzymes observed with SB 203580 in 10-day dose-ranging toxicological studies in rats were attributed to potent inhibition of cytochrome P-450s by this pyridine-based compound. A search for a surrogate functionality for the pyridine group yielded potent p38 inhibitors based on 2-aminopyrimidines including SB 220025[35], SB 216385[36], and SB 226882[37], which inhibited p38 at 0.060, 0.48, and 0.032 μM, respectively. These compounds showed much less affinity toward a variety of P-450 isozymes, and therefore are presumed to be more suitable for clinical development. SB 220025, at 30 mg/kg b.i.d. p.o., inhibited inflammatory angiogenesis by 40% in the murine air pouch granuloma model. SB 220025 reduced LPS-induced TNFα production with an ED$_{50}$ value of 7.5 mg/kg p.o. in mice. In the mouse collagen-induced arthritis model, SB 220025 inhibited the progression of arthritis. SB 226882 showed inhibition of LPS-induced TNF-α production at 3.0 and 5.7 mg/kg p.o. in the mouse and rat, and was effective in both the rat adjuvant- and mice collagen-induced arthritis models.

SB 239063, is a second-generation p38 inhibitor (IC$_{50}$ = 44 nM)[24]. In the LPS-induced human peripheral blood mononuclear cells (PBMC), SB 239063 blocked IL-1 and TNFα with an IC$_{50}$ of 120 and 350 nM, respectively. The ED$_{50}$ (TNFα) value in vivo was 5.8 mg/kg p.o. In ovalbumin sensitized mice, airway eosinophilia measured 96 hrs after ovalbumin challenge was reduced by 93% when the animals were treated with SB 239063 at 12 mg/kg p.o., while total

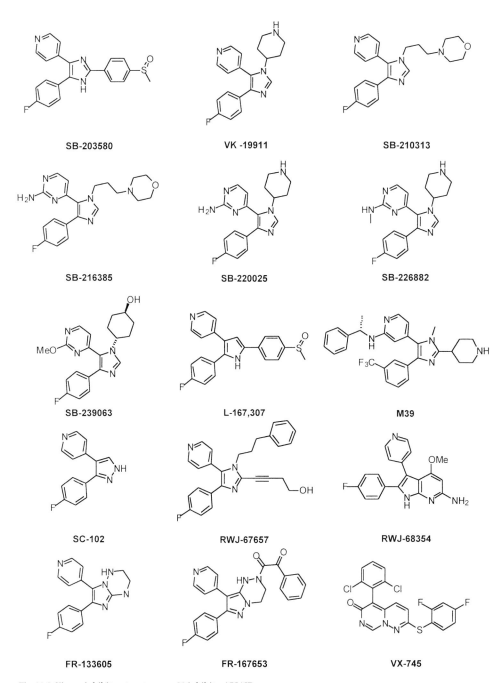

Fig. 11.2 Kinase inhibitor structures: p. 38 inhibitor/CSAID.

leukocyte accumulation in the bronchoalveolar lavage fluid was reduced by 47%. In similar experiments using guinea pigs, 50% reduction in airway eosinophilia was observed at 10 and 30 mg/kg p.o. Bronchoconstriction and airway resistance were not resolved in this model, suggesting that SB 239063 may have efficacy in reducing the inflammatory component of asthma.

A number of 1-(4-pyridyl)-2-arylheterocycles have been identified as potent inhibitors of p38 kinase. L-167,307[38] a pyrrole analogue of SB 203580, was shown to inhibit p38α and p38β with the IC$_{50}$ values of 5.0 and 8.1 nM, respectively. This compound is also a modest inhibitor of Raf kinase (0.47 μM). LPS-induced TNF-α release was inhibited in human monocytes with an IC$_{50}$ of 65 nM. It is interesting to note that upon i.v. or p.o. administration to the rat, L-167,307 is readily metabolized to the corresponding sulfone which shows much longer $t_{1/2}$ than the sulfoxide precursor. L-167,307 reduced paw edema in the rat adjuvant arthritis model with an ED$_{50}$ of 7.4 mg/kg p.o. b.i.d. At 20 mg/kg, radiographic examination of the hind paws showed reduced joint destruction.

An aminopyridine-based inhibitor, M39[39], was shown to be a highly potent (0.19 nM) inhibitor of p38 with >5000-fold selectivity against JNK2, p56Lck, EGF receptor tyrosine kinase, MEK, PKA and PKC. Raf kinase was inhibited at 810 nM. No P-450 liability was found when this compound was tested in a battery of rat and human P-450 assays. LPS-induced TNFα production in human whole blood was blocked with an IC$_{50}$ of 2.8 nM. M39 shows greatly improved in vivo activity over the first-generation derivative. Introduction of the N-methyl group resulted in significant improvement of plasma half-life. Oral bioavailability in rat and rhesus monkey were 85 and 86% respectively. In vivo TNFα production was inhibited with an ED$_{50}$ of 0.6 mg/kg p.o. in the mouse model of endotoxin shock. In the 21-day rat adjuvant arthritis model, oral administration of M39 reduced joint destruction with an ED$_{50}$ of 17.5 mg/kg b.i.d. M39 was also evaluated in the in vitro and in vivo mouse models of pulmonary inflammation[40]. TNFα and MIP-2 production were inhibited by M39 at a concentration <0.1 nM when murine neutrophils were treated with LPS, although much higher (0.1–1 μM) concentrations of M39 were necessary to achieve similar results in mouse alveolar macrophages. In both assays, KC chemokine levels were not affected. M39 administered at 3 mg/kg p.o. decreased neutrophil accumulation, and TNFα release in mice intratracheally administered LPS. However, recruitment of monocytes and macrophages were not affected by M39 in the same model. These results suggest involvement of p38 MAP kinase in early responses in endotoxin challenged lung inflammation.

Analogue synthesis of indole and pyrrolopyridine templates has yielded a series of CSAIDs/p38 inhibitors[41,42]. RWJ-68354[43,44] inhibits immunoprecipitated human monocyte p38 at 150 nM, suppresses LPS-induced production of TNFα and IL-1β at 6.3 and 26 nM, respectively, and inhibits *Staphylococcus* enterotoxin B-induced TNFα generation at 23 nM. In female BALB/c mice and male Lewis rats, RWJ-68354 prevented LPS-induced TNFα production in a dose-dependent manner upon oral administration. In the adjuvant arthritis model in male Lewis rats, RWJ-68354 reduced the size of hind paw edema by 50% at 50 mg/kg/day. An imidazole-based compound, RWJ-67657[45], blocked p38 with an IC$_{50}$ value of 3 nM and reduced TNF-α levels in LPS-treated mice and rats at the ED$_{50}$ value of 25 and 10 mg/kg p.o., respectively.

A pyridinylpyrazole, SC-102[46], inhibits p38 at the IC$_{50}$ value of 50 nM, and blocks TNF-α, IL-1 and IL-6 production in LPS-stimulated mice at ED$_{50}$ = 1–10 mg/kg p.o.

Two Fujisawa CSAIDs, FR-133605 and FR-167653, have structural features very similar to the pyridinylimidazole p38 inhibitors, although no information on their MAP kinase inhibitory selectivity and activity is currently available. These compounds are worth mentioning since rather extensive pharmacological studies were performed which may help understand the role of CSAID/p38 inhibitors in a variety of disease states[47,48]. FR-133605 showed inhibition of LPS-induced IL-1 and TNFα production at 0.52 and 1.0 μM in human monocytes, and reduced the production of LPS-stimulated serum IL-1 and TNFα at the ED$_{50}$ of 4.3 and 2.0 mg/kg in the mice. In the adjuvant arthritis model in rats, FR-133605 reduced paw swelling and destruction of bone and cartilage. In LPS-treated human monocytes, FR-167653 inhibited IL-1α, IL-1β, and TNF-α at 0.84, 0.088, and 1.1 μM, respectively, and TNF-α at 0.072 μM in lymphocytes stimulated with phytohemagglutinin-M. In the LPS-induced disseminated intravascular coagulation model in the rat, FR-167653 markedly improved thrombocytopenia and plasma coagulation. Complete suppression of IL-1 and TNFα was observed. In the rabbit model of septic shock, FR-167653 reduced mortality, attenuated the hypotensive response and returned mean arterial blood pressure to control levels[49]. In the dog model of liver resection with ischemia, FR-167653 improved liver function and survival[50] and dose-dependently reduced the size of myocardial infarct size in the rat model of ischemia–reperfusion[51]. TNF-α and IL-1β mRNA levels were also reduced in this study. FR-167653 at 30 mg/kg reduced the accumulation of exudate by 50% in the rat carrageenan-induced pleurisy model[52]. Chronic infusion of LPS at 150 μg/kg/h in conscious male Long Evans rats caused hypotension and damage to kidney and liver. Coinfusion of FR-167653 at 0.32 mg/kg/h normalized mean arterial pressure, but did not improve kidney and liver function[53]. Acute pancreatitis induced by infusion of caerulein at 5 μg/kg/h[54] or by surgical closure of duodenal loop[55] was prevented by FR-167653. In a model of cerebral ischemia–reperfusion in mongrel dogs, FR-167653 given continuously at 1.0 mg/kg/h i.v. improved cerebral blood flow and cerebral glucose metabolism rate, while cerebral oxygen metabolism and carbon dioxide excretion were not affected[56].

VX-745, a pyrimidinopyridazinone based p38 inhibitor, has an IC$_{50}$ value of 10 and 220 nM in the p38α and p38β assay, respectively[57]. This compound is highly selective toward these two isoforms of p38, showing no inhibition of p38δ, p38γ, Erk2, JNK1/2, p56Lck, Src, and MAPKAP kinase-2. In the in vitro LPS-induced cytokine production models, VX-745 inhibited Il-1β and TNFα production at 56 and 52 nM, respectively. Oral anti-inflammatory efficacy was demonstrated in the CIA and adjuvant arthritis

models. The potential of VX-745 for the treatment of rheumatoid arthritis is currently being evaluated in the Phase 2 clinical trials.

In summary, dramatic progress has been made in the past decade in identifying potent, orally active inhibitors of p38. The pharmacological effects of such inhibitors are actively being investigated, and being profiled in a variety of animal models of acute and chronic inflammatory diseases, septic shock, bone loss and ischemia–reperfusion. Moreover, a structurally related CSAID, FR-167653, is efficacious in additional disease models of cardiac and liver ischemia, and stroke. However, the full scope of the usefulness of p38 inhibitors as therapeutic agents is far from being understood. Currently two compounds are known to be in clinical trials: VX-745 (Vertex, for inflammation) and HEP-689 (SB-235699, Leo Pharmaceuticals, for psoriasis). Clinical trial data, which will undoubtedly become available in the near future, should provide further insight in this regard.

Extracellular regulated kinase (ERK) pathway

The extracellular regulated kinases, ERK1 and ERK2, were the first mammalian MAPK family members identified[58]. Like other MAPK family enzymes, they are activated by dual phosphorylation on tyrosine and threonine residues present in the activation loop. The characteristic amino acid triplet for ERK is TEY (see first paragraph of p38 kinase). Enzymatic studies suggest a 'two-collision distributive method' whereby the upstream kinase preferentially phosphorylates tyrosine, while the subsequent phosphorylation of threonine requires an independent binding/catalytic event[59]. Phosphorylation of both tyrosine and threonine residues is required for activation. Crystallographic data has positioned the activation loop as a 'phosphorylation lip' present at the mouth of the active site. In the inactive state, the lip blocks binding of substrate (ATP). Upon phosphorylation, a major conformational shift is effected which rotates the N- and C-domains of the enzyme and opens the active site for substrate docking[60]. An additional consequence of the active conformation is the ability to form homodimers[61] (Fig. 11.1). This dimerization is essential for regulating activity both by altering substrate binding and promoting nuclear localization[61]. Translocation of ERK to the nucleus is critical because this is the location of the most well characterized substrate for ERK, the transcription factor Elk-1[62]. Elk-1 is an essential component of the serum responsive transcriptional complex that regulates *c-fos* gene expression. Two other genes induced by ERK are the MAPK phosphatases, MKP-1 and MKP-2[63]. MKP levels are induced by serum, overexpression of Raf or ERK, and can be blocked by the MEK inhibitor, PD 98059. This observation is compelling, because MKP-1, -2 can dephosphorylate ERK to effect a negative feed-back loop to switch-off ERK activity. Recently an ERK specific MKP family member has been identified which is constitutively expressed, tyrosine specific, and localized to the nucleus[64]. This phosphatase may play a role in acute inactivation of ERK in contrast to MKP-1, which requires *de novo* synthesis.

Phosphorylation of ERK is mediated by two ERK selective MAPKK enzymes, MEK1 and MEK2 (Fig. 11.1). Interestingly, although MEK is predominantly cytoplasmic, it contains a nuclear export signal suggesting there are circumstances where MEK may be nuclear and act in competition with nuclear phosphatases to prolong ERK activity[65]. Identification of MEK as the MAPKK in the ERK pathway occurred relatively early on since it was identified as a major protein in complexes containing both Ras and Raf[66]. Like its upstream regulators, the role of MEK in the ERK pathway is validated by its ability to promote neurite outgrowth in PC12 cells (differentiation) and transform fibroblasts[67]. *Mek1-/-* mice die in utero from apparent failure to fully vascularize the placenta indicating MEK1 is essential for angiogenesis and endothelial migration[68]. Indeed, extensive literature indicates that the ERK pathway is predominantly activated by mitogens and is essential for cell proliferation, differentiation and tumourogenesis. However, supporting data also indicate that the ERK pathway plays a critical role in certain inflammatory responses. This is because the transcription factor, AP-1, which is a heterodimer of c-Fos and c-Jun is a key regulator of

many inflammatory genes. The structural interactions of Fos/Jun heterodimers with DNA has been reported[69,70]. A key example is the regulation of interleukin-2 (IL-2), an autocrine growth factor for T-cells. IL-2 gene transcription is regulated by essential AP-1, NF-AT and NF-κB promoter elements[71]. Inhibition by the MEK inhibitor, U-0126 blocks T-cell proliferation by down-regulating IL-2 mRNA levels[72]. ERK may also regulate inflammatory signalling pathways such as phosphorylating STAT proteins thereby modulating gene expression induced by interferons[73].

Surprisingly little is known about small molecule ERK inhibitors. A report describing a substrate docking motif in ERK[74] may lead to new inhibitors using structure based drug design. A recently published patent describes pyrimidinylimidazoles to be inhibitors of ERK, although no biological data was reported[75]. Instead, it is MEK that has been the target of the most significant ERK pathway inhibitors so far reported.

PD 98059 inhibits MEK at low micromolar concentrations without significant effects on ERKs[76]. Inhibition of MEK by PD 98059 was shown to prevent downstream activation of ERK and subsequent phosphorylation of ERK substrates in vitro. PD 98059 prevented stimulation of cell growth and reversed phenotype of ras-transformed mouse 3T3 fibroblast cells and rat kidney cells. PD 98059 appears to preferentially bind the non-phosphorylated form of MEK, and is highly selective among related serine/threonine kinases[77]. PD 98059 has been extensively used as a research tool to identify the role of the MEK cascade in a variety of pharmacological assays.

U-0126 is a dual inhibitor of MEK-1 and -2 with IC_{50} values of 72 and 58 nM, respectively for phosphorylation of ERK. This compound is selective against other closely related kinases[78]. The inhibition is reversible and non-competitive with respect to both ATP and ERK. This compound prevents T-cell proliferation induced by concanavalin A and anti-CD3 cross-linking, and blocks PMA/ionomycin-stimulated up-regulation of IL-2 mRNA in peripheral blood leukocytes[72]. Anti-inflammatory activity of U-0126 was demonstrated in the

TPA-induced ear edema model ($ED_{50} = 64$ μg/ear) and a carrageenan-induced paw edema model ($ED_{30} = 10$ mg/kg i.p.)[79].

Screening of fermentation broths for inhibitors of T cell activation yielded Ro 09–2210[80], a macrocyclic lactam from *Curvularia* sp. Ro 09–2110 inhibits anti-CD3- and ionomycin-induced T cell activation at 58–139 nM, and anti-CD3-stimulated IL-2 release in Jurkat T cells at 16 nM. Rabbit skeletal muscle MEK and human recombinant MEK1 were potently inhibited by Ro 09–2110 at 59 and 140 nM, respectively, while no or little inhibition was observed with ERK, PKC, ZAP-70 and p56Lck. In contrast to PD 98059, Ro 09–2110 is able to bind both phosphorylated and unphosphorylated MEK.

L-783,277[81], a structurally related natural product isolated from *Phoma* sp. was recently reported to be a potent MEK1 inhibitor with an IC_{50} value of 4 nM. PKC, PKA and RAF were not inhibited by L-783,277, while modest ($IC_{50} = 750$ nM) inhibition was observed in the p56Lck assay. Detailed enzyme kinetic studies showed that L-783,277 is an ATP-competitive, irreversible inhibitor of MEK. SAR also supports this observation since the α,β-unsaturated ketone moiety appears to be essential for the inhibition. Paradoxically, inhibition of p56Lck by L-783 277 was shown to be fully reversible. This compound was found to be active in cellular and animal models of tumour growth, although no experimental data has been reported at this time (Fig. 11.3).

Jun-N-terminal kinase (JNK) pathway

The Jun-N-terminal kinases (JNK), also known as stress activated protein kinases (SAPK), are members of the mitogen activated protein kinase (MAPK) family[82,83]. JNKs are encoded by three separate genes, *Jnk1, Jnk2 and Jnk3*, although alternative splicing results in a total of 10 isoforms[84]. The most well-characterized role for JNK is the phosphorylation of serines 63 and 73 on c-Jun, a component of the transcription factor, activator protein-1 (AP-1)[85,86]. JNK can also phosphorylate and activate the transcription factors ATF2[87] and Elk-1[88]. Activation

of Elk-1 may in part mediate the proliferative activity of JNK. AP-1 and ATF2 are implicated in a host of inflammatory diseases including asthma, and in the transcriptional regulation of multiple genes, particularly in synergy with the transcription factor NF-κB[89]. Acute lung inflammation is associated with elevated leukocytes in bronchoalveolar lavage and these cells exhibit high levels of AP-1 DNA binding activity[90]. Lung epithelial cells exposed to particulate matter as a model of air pollution showed increased c-Jun phosphorylation, AP-1 activity, and cell proliferation[91]. Examination of clinical cases of steroid-resistant asthma revealed increased levels of activated JNK and phosphorylated c-Jun[92]. Finally, emerging evidence indicates that AP-1 is critical for the transcriptional regulation of several matrix metalloproteinase family members and thus may have special significance for COPD[92]. Together, this experimental evidence suggests that inhibition of JNK may provide significant therapeutic benefit to patients with inflammatory lung disease.

JNK is the terminal kinase in a MAPK signalling cascade comprised of MAPK kinase kinases (MAPKKK; e.g. MEKK-1, 2, 3, MLK-3, ASK1, TAK1, Tpl2), MAPK kinases (MAPKK; MKK4 and MKK7) and MAPK (JNK1, 2, 3) (Fig. 11.1). JNK is activated by dual phosphorylation of a threonine and tyrosine residue present in a T-P-Y triplet motif in the kinase domain. JNK can be deactivated by MAPK phosphatases (MKP), specifically MKP-1, 2, and 5[93]. Many of these phosphatases are activated by the kinases they deactivate, and MKP gene transcription is induced by the transcription factors downstream of the MAPK. Together, these systems provide feedback loops that tightly regulate the activity of JNK and other MAPKs.

Additional regulation of the JNK pathway has been revealed in the discovery of scaffold proteins that enable specificity and efficiency in signalling, coupling distinct stimuli to specific components of the cascade. The JNK-interacting protein, JIP-1 has binding domains for a MAPK, MAPKK and MAPKKK. Specificity studies show JIP-1 can bind either JNK1, 2, or 3, MKK7 but not MKK4, and MLK but not MEKK family members. Therefore JIP-1 coordinates a sig-

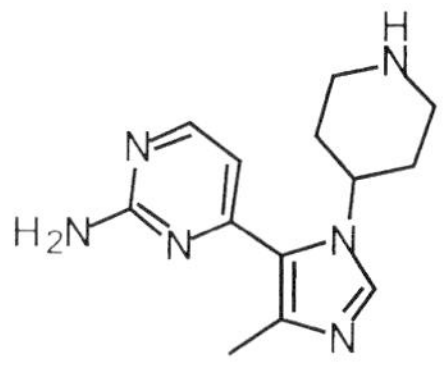

WO-9961440 (SKB)

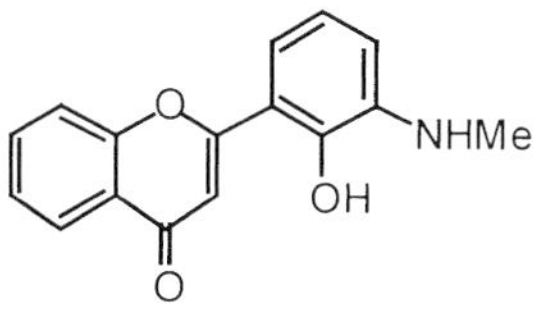

PD-98059

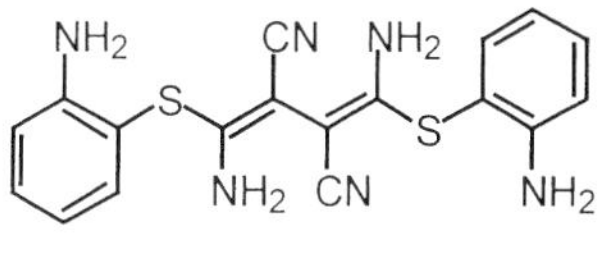

U-0126

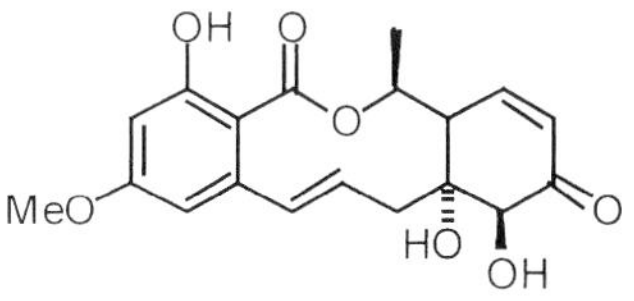

Ro 09-2110

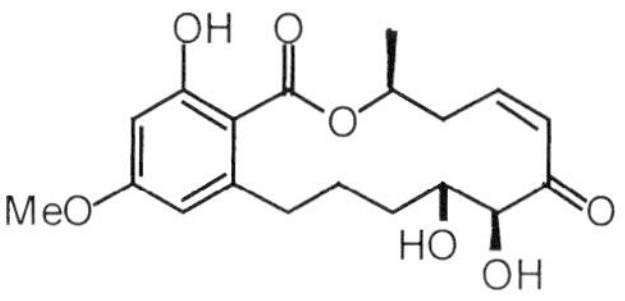

L-783,277

Fig. 11.3 ERK and MEK inhibitors.

nalling module composed of MLK-3, MKK-7, and JNK[94]. Additional JNK scaffold proteins have been identified including JIP-2[95], JIP3[96], and JSAP-1[97]. JIP3 is notable in being highly expressed in the brain in common with JNK3. JSAP1 appears to bind a distinct signalling module containing MEKK-1, MKK4 and JNK.

The identification of multiple upstream kinases that lead to JNK activation is a likely reflection of the multiple stimuli that can activate this pathway. Additional research is required to fully delineate the role of all the MAPKKK enzymes in JNK activation. The most well characterized MAPKKK is MEKK-1,

which has a validated role in JNK activation following stimulation with TNF, osmotic shock and cold stress[98,99]. However, genetic deletion of MEKK-1 does not block JNK activation following heat shock or UV irradiation. ASK1 is also activated by TNF and potentially drives JNK mediated apoptosis[100]. In contrast, MLK-3 is not activated by TNF but is strongly induced following CD3/CD28 co-stimulation in T-cells[101] and by over-expression of the small GTP binding proteins Rac1 and Cdc42[102]. TAK1–JNK signalling is activated by transforming growth factor β[103]. Therefore, preliminary studies of these kinases suggest a degree of stimulus specific activation and/or specificity for downstream substrates MKK4 or MKK7.

Our understanding of the roles of MKK4 and MKK7 is more established. Homozygous deletion of *Mkk4* results in a loss of anisomycin and heat shock induced JNK activation, while stimulation by UV, osmotic shock and cytokine was retained[104]. This led to a search for a second JNK activating kinase identified as MKK7[105] that when deleted in embryonic stem cells resulted in the additional loss of JNK activity following UV irradiation and osmotic shock[106]. Therefore MKK4 and MKK7 fulfil non-redundant roles in the regulation of JNK and may represent an opportunity for selectively inhibiting the JNK signalling cascade.

JNK1 and JNK2 are widely expressed in human tissues, while JNK3 is restricted to the brain, heart and testis. JNK3 has not been observed in the lung. Mice deficient in JNK3 are viable, but exhibit resistance to kainate-induced seizures and to neuronal apoptosis in the hippocampus[107]. JNK1 or JNK2 knockout animals are also viable, although both display defects in T-cell differentiation. Effects on lung morphology and function have not been reported. *Jnk1-/-* CD4+ cells skew to a Th2 phenotype when activated by CD3/CD28 co-stimulation and cells hyper-proliferate and exhibit reduced cell death[108]. Similarly, *Jnk2-/-* CD4+ cells fail to differentiate into a Th1 population upon exposure to IL-12[109]. Although the phenotypes of *Jnk1* and *Jnk2* deletion appear similar, the mechanistic deficits appear distinct. In *Jnk1-/-* cells, it has been proposed that failure to phosphorylate, and translocate the Th2 transcription factor NF-ATc out of the nucleus leads to unregulated transcription of Th2 cytokine genes. In contrast, *Jnk2-/-* cells fail to polarize to a Th1 phenotype following IL-12 stimulation, at least in part by failing to produce the Th1 cytokine, interferon-gamma (IFN-γ). Interestingly, CD4+ cells deficient in both JNK1 and JNK2 show no defect in IL-2 expression despite earlier reports linking JNK and AP-1 activity to IL-2 gene expression[106,110]. Consistent with the single knockout experiments, these cells also preferentially polarize to a Th2-like phenotype. It is not yet clear if inhibition of JNK will

benefit or exacerbate lung inflammation, which frequently follows a Th2 type immune response. One could hypothesize that inhibiting the ability of T-cells to differentiate to the Th1 subset will only amplify the Th2 response. It will be of interest whether *Jnk1-/- or Jnk2-/-* animals exhibit altered leukocyte or Th1:Th2 ratios in models of lung inflammation. Furthermore, inhibition of JNK in alveolar eosinophils and macrophages may provide significant anti-inflammatory benefit. As well as promoting Th1 differentiation, JNK1 and JNK2 appear to regulate apoptosis by promoting mitochondrial permeability and cytochrome c release[111]. *Jnk1-/-Jnk2-/-* embryonic fibroblasts are resistant to UV-C, mitomycin C, and anisomycin induced apoptosis as measured by DNA fragmentation. Additional studies are required on the role of JNK in ischemic injury but JNK inhibitors hold significant promise in myocardial infarction and stroke. As these genetic models are used in additional clinical models of disease it is likely that new roles for JNK will be identified.

Recently, a small molecule inhibitor of JNK has been disclosed by Celgene Corporation's Signal Research Division[183]. SP600125 is an anthrapyrazolone, MW 220.2, with a K_i of 190 nM vs. JNK2. The compound showed no selectivity to other JNK isoforms but exhibited a minimum 20-fold selectivity to 16 other kinases examined. SP600125 was ATP competitive and the binding was fully reversible. Based on these kinetic properties, limited SAR, and the structure of other kinase inhibitors, it can be hypothesized that the pyrazole moiety is required for hydrogen bonding to the ATP binding site of JNK. SP600125 showed both in vitro and in vivo activity. The IC50 in cells for inhibition of c-Jun phosphorylation, TNFa and IL-2 expression was approximately 5 μM. In an animal model of adjuvant-induced arthritis, SP600125 suppressed the destruction of bone and cartilage in the joint[184] and the expression of matrix metalloproteinase enzymes known to be transcriptionally regulated by AP-1/c-Jun.

The only JNK pathway inhibitor that has completed preclinical development is CEP-1347 (Cephalon). Although efficacy has not been reported in models of lung inflammation, its effects in neuronal disease is enlightening. CEP 1347, also known as KT 7515, was reported as a JNK pathway inhibitor as early as 1998[112]. CEP 1347 inhibits JNK-1 activity with an IC_{50} of 30 nM with little or no inhibition observed for trk and PKC. MAPKAP kinase-2 activity in Cos7 cells was not affected by CEP 1347, indicating that the p38 pathway was not significantly inhibited. CEP 1347 prevents cell death in a number of neuronal cell lines supporting a role for JNK in apoptosis. Most recently, CEP 1347 was specifically identified as a potent inhibitor of mixed-lineage kinases (MLKs), which are MAPKKK upstream kinases of JNKs[113]. In human recombinant MLK assays, CEP 1347 inhibited MLK1, MLK2, and MLK3 at 23, 64, and 23 nM respectively. Neuroprotective effects of CEP 1347 have been demonstrated in a series of animal models. Peripheral administration of 0.5 and 1.0 mg/kg CEP 1347 reduced death of motor neurons of the spinal nucleus of the bulbocavernosus in postnatal female rats[114]. Reduction in choline acetyltransferase activity in cortex and the number of cortically projecting neurons in the nucleus basalis induced by infusion of ibotenate into the nucleus basalis magnocellularis of rats was attenuated by CEP 1347[115]. Further behavioural examination[116] of the animals used in the ibotenatic acid-induced lesion model revealed that CEP 1347-treated rats committed fewer errors in a memory retention test. CEP 1347 treated animals showed 40% recovery as compared to the control animals in choline acetyltransferase activity in the frontal cortex when tested 3 months after cessation of the drug treatment. In the MPTP-mediated dopaminergic neurotoxicity model in rats, an animal model of Parkinson's disease, administration of 0.3 mg/kg/day of CEP 1347 reduced the loss of dopaminergic cell bodies and terminals[117]. These results clearly demonstrate clinical potential of JNK and JNK pathway inhibitors for the treatment of neurodegenerative diseases such as epilepsy, traumatic brain damage, Alzheimer's disease and Parkinson's disease.

In a noise-trauma model in guinea pigs, subcutaneous administration of CEP 1347 attenuated noise-induced hearing loss and hair cell death in cochleas.

In vitro in the cochlear cultures, CEP 1347 prevented neomycin-induced hair cell death[118]. In a similar manner observed with FR-167653, CEP 1347 ameliorated caerulein-induced pancreatic edema formation and reduced histological severity of pancreatitis[119].

Encouraging pharmacological success with CEP 1347 in a variety of animal models provides ample evidence that intervention of the JNK pathway will provide highly attractive therapeutic opportunities for many diseases with unmet medical needs. CEP 1347 is currently under evaluation in Phase 2 clinical trials for neurodegenerative diseases.

IκB kinase (IKK) pathway

Since its initial description in 1986, the transcription factor NF-κB has been implicated in multiple inflammatory and immune diseases[120]. The expression of more than 70 known proteins is transcriptionally regulated by the binding of NF-κB to specific sequence elements in the promoter region of these genes[121]. In non-activated cells, NF-κB is retained in the cytoplasm by an inhibitory molecule, IκB, which binds to NF-κB and masks its nuclear localization signal[122]. Following an inflammatory insult, IκBα is phosphorylated on serines 32 and 36 to form a unique recognition motif that is specifically bound by the IκBα E3 ubiquitin ligase, βTRcP, in association with other proteins[123]. Ubiquitin is covalently attached to IκBα at lysine 21 or 22 thereby targeting IκBα for degradation by the 26S proteosome. In the absence of IκB, free NF-κB translocates to the nucleus to promote the transcription of immune genes.

The dominant role of NF-κB in inflammatory diseases such as asthma has focused attention on identifying NF-κB regulatory proteins for targeted therapeutic intervention. The current frontline treatment for severe asthma, glucocorticoids, suppress the expression of multiple NF-κB regulated genes. The mechanism of action of steroid drugs is unresolved, but may include up-regulation of IκB[124] or disruption of histone acetylation and DNA

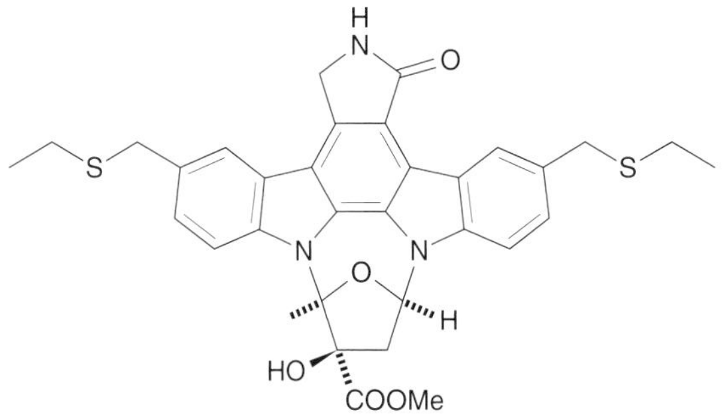

CEP-1347 (KT-7515)
MLK inhibitor

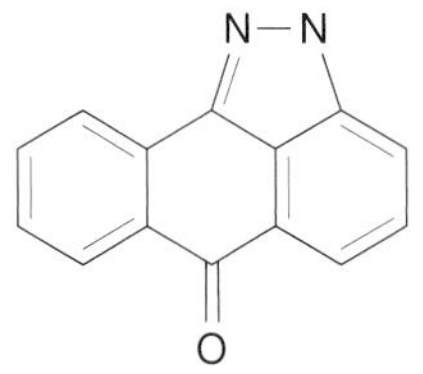

SP600125
JNK inhibitor

Fig. 11.4 JNK pathway inhibitors.

re-arrangement necessary for gene transcription[125]. These observations suggest that a selective inhibitor of NF-κB could have efficacy comparable to steroids without the unwanted side effects (Fig. 11.4).

A focus of current drug discovery efforts is the IκB kinase (IKK), which appears to be the central integrator of diverse inflammatory signals leading to the phosphorylation of IκB. Two kinases, IKK-1/IKKα and IKK-2/IKKβ, and a regulatory protein IKK-γ/IKKAP-1, have been identified as part of a large multiprotein complex called the 'Signalsome'[126,127]. Although both kinases can phosphorylate IκB in vitro, early studies using genetic mutants indicated that IKK-2, but not IKK-1, was essential for activation of NF-κB by proinflammatory stimuli such as IL-1β and TNFα[126]. Furthermore, only catalytically inactive mutants of IKK-2 blocked the expression of NF-κB regulated genes such as monocyte chemotactic protein (MCP-1) and intercellular adhesion molecule (ICAM-1)[25]. These data were confirmed by *Ikk-1* and *Ikk-2* knock-out mice. *Ikk-2 -/-* mice display an embryonic lethal phenotype with striking similarity to the IκBα and RelA knockout animals[128–132]. Embryonic fibroblasts from *Ikk-2* deleted animals, stimulated with IL-1β or TNFα, show defective activation of NF-κB, and reduced expression of NF-κB regulated genes such as IL-6. This is consistent with experiments using dominant negative mutants of IKK-2 delivered by adenovirus[25]. In contrast, *Ikk-1 -/-* mice are born viable but die

within hours. These animals exhibit skeletal and limb defects along with dysregulated proliferation of epidermal keratinocytes[132].

Therefore, cell and animal experiments indicate that IKK-2 plays a central role in the immune response. IKK-2 is activated in response to multiple inflammatory stimuli and signalling pathways, many of which play an important role in respiratory disease including IL-1β, LPS, TNFα, CD3/CD28 (antigen presentation), CD40L, viral infection, and oxidative stress. The ubiquitous expression of NF-κB, along with its response to multiple stimuli means that almost all cell types present in the lung are potential targets for anti-NF-κB/IKK-2 therapy. This includes alveolar epithelium, mast cells, fibroblasts, vascular endothelium, and infiltrating leukocytes; neutrophils, macrophages, lymphocytes, eosinophils and basophils. By inhibiting the expression of genes such as cyclooxygenase-2 and 12-lipoxygenase (synthesis of inflammatory mediators), TAP-1 peptide transporter (antigen processing), MHC class I H-2K and class II Ii invariant chains (antigen presentation), E-selectin and vascular cell adhesion molecule (leukocyte recruitment), interleukins-1, 2, 6, 8 (cytokines), RANTES, eotaxin, GM-CSF (chemokines), and superoxide dismutase and NADPH quinone oxidoreductase (reactive oxygen species), inhibitors of IKK-2 should display broad anti-inflammatory activity.

Recently, two new kinases with sequence similarity to IKK-1 and IKK-2 have been reported. Despite apparent structural homology, both kinases are components of unique high molecular weight signalling complexes, and under in vivo conditions may not phosphorylate IκB directly. The first kinase, IKK-i/IKKε is transcriptionally induced by LPS, TNF and IL-1, and is expressed predominantly in immune cells[133,134]. Although its activity is inducible by PMA, its precise role remains unknown. The second kinase, TBK1/NAK, was found to associate with the adaptor proteins TRAF-2 and TANK that lead to the phosphorylation and activation of IKK-2[135,136]. Preliminary evidence indicates TBK1/NAK may play a role in signalling from PKC isozymes and/or CD40. Both IKK-i/IKKε and TBK1/NAK represent new targets that may provide a stimulus selective means for modulating NF-κB activity.

Initial studies characterizing the physicochemical properties of IKK-2 have been published. Understanding both the mechanisms of catalysis and structural motifs that characterize IKK-2 will provide key insights into the discovery and design of selective pharmacologic inhibitors. This is especially true since the IKK enzymes show relatively low sequence homologies with other kinases, and early profiles with known kinase inhibitors have not identified compounds with striking potency[25,137]. Kinetic analysis shows that IKK-2 binds to and phosphorylates IκBα, IκBβ, and IκBε with high and relatively equal affinities[138]. Recombinant IKK-2 phosphorylates IκBα peptide 26–42 with near equal affinity to full length IκBα; however, the native IKK 'Signalsome' phosphorylates full-length IκBα 25 000-fold more efficiently, suggesting important regulatory sequences in the C-terminal region of IκBα, or additional regulatory proteins in the IKK 'Signalsome' that accelerate the rate of catalysis[139]. Both variables provide important insights for the design of compound screens. Phosphorylation of IκBα occurs via a random sequential kinetic mechanism, meaning either ATP or IκBα may bind first to IKK-2, but that both must be bound before phosphorylation of IκBα can take place[137]. IKK-2 binds ATP with uniquely high affinity ($K_i = 130$ nM) compared to other serine-threonine kinases such as p38

and JNK, perhaps indicating a unique ATP binding pocket that reflects the relatively poor activity of many broad specificity kinase inhibitors when tested against IKK-2.

To date, no crystal structure of IKK-2 has been reported. However, homology modelling has identified 3 structural domains including an N-terminal kinase domain with an activation loop, a leucine zipper domain that likely mediates the formation of IKK-1 and IKK-2 homo/heterodimers, and a C-terminal helix–loop–helix with serine-rich tail. Activation of IKK-2 is critically dependent upon phosphorylation of serine 177 and 181 in the activation or T loop. Alanine mutations abolish activity, while glutamate mutations result in a constitutively active enzyme[126]. Several kinases appear to be physiologically relevant in this activation process. Mitogen activated protein kinase kinase kinase-1 (MEKK-1) has been identified in IKK immunoprecipitates from activated cells[126]. MEKK-1 preferentially phosphorylates IKK-2 with high efficiency, while a dominant negative mutant of MEKK-1 significantly blocks IKK activity and the expression of NF-κB regulated genes[140]. Note that MEKK-1 is also a key upstream activator of the JNK pathway. A novel kinase, NF-κB inducing kinase (NIK) was identified by two-hybrid screening, and found to phosphorylate both IKK-1 and IKK-2. Dominant negative mutants of NIK block TNFα, CD95 (Fas) and IL-1 mediated activation of NF-κB[141]. NIK deficient mice exhibit a pathology distinct from IKK-2 deficient animals, suggesting that NIK is not essential for IKK-2 activation[142]. Recently a third candidate IKK-kinase has been reported. It has been known for several years that the atypical protein kinase C (aPKC) isoforms (PKC λ/ι, ζ) can promote the phosphorylation of IκBα and the transcriptional activity of NF-κB. With the cloning of IKK-1 and IKK-2, direct association experiments have been performed and it appears that these PKC isoforms are part of an IKK immunoprecipitable complex. Furthermore, PKCζ can directly phosphorylate IKK-2 on serines[143,177]. The novel PKC isoform, θ, is an important mediator of CD3/CD28 activation in T-cells, and has been recently identified as an upstream activator of

IKK-2[144,145]. Therefore MEKK-1, NIK and PKC all appear to be able to activate IKK-2 directly. Their specific roles will likely be found to depend on both the inflammatory stimulus and the cell type.

The helix–loop–helix domain has been proposed to interact directly with the kinase domain to stabilize the active conformation, and/or with IKKAP-1, to stabilize the multiprotein complex. Mutations or deletions in this region abolish enzyme activity[146]. These observations suggest that disruption of the leucine zipper or helix–loop–helix may provide a route of inhibition distinct from the kinase active site.

No selective inhibitors of IKK have been reported to be in preclinical development although many pharmaceutical companies are actively working in this area. Several known kinase inhibitors have been reported to inhibit IKK and we briefly describe these here. Staurosporine is a ubiquitous ATP competitive inhibitor of kinases and blocks IKK-2 with a $K_i = 172$ nM[137]. However, this activity is much less potent than its inhibition of PKC, $K_i = 10$ nM. Similarly, quercetin inhibits many kinases and is only a micromolar inhibitor of IKK[137]. The anti-inflammatory effects of aspirin (salicylate) are known to be due at least in part to the inhibition of cyclooxygenase activity and prostaglandin synthesis. It has also been reported that aspirin inhibits IKK-2 activity in an ATP competitive manner with an IC50 of 50–100 μM in vitro, although at low nM ATP concentrations. In vivo, the IC50 for TNFα inhibition is also 50 μM[147]. Because high dose treatment can result in serum levels of 1–5 mM, it has been postulated that inhibition of IKK-2 may contribute to the anti-inflammatory effects observed with aspirin. Recently, the mechanism of aspirin mediated inhibition of IKK-2 in vivo has been questioned. Instead it is proposed that aspirin leads to activation of MKK3 and p38 which in turn interferes with NF-κB signalling stimulated by TNF, but not by IL-1[147]. Potential biological inhibitors of IKK-2 are the A- and J-type cyclopentenone prostaglandins, and their mechanism of inhibition is informative for drug discovery efforts. It has been known for several years that prostaglandin A1 can inhibit the activation of NF-κB by

TNF or PMA with an IC50 of 5 μM[148]. Recently the mechanism of inhibition has been identified as direct covalent binding to cysteine 179 on IKK-2 that leads to irreversible inactivation of the enzyme[149]. This data indicates that compounds with strong Michael acceptors will be reactive to IKK-2.

Protein kinase C (PKC)

Protein kinase C (PKC) describes a family of 11 structurally related serine-threonine kinase isoenzymes[150–152]. These signalling enzymes are critical mediators of receptor activation events that release phospholipid second messengers. PKC isoenzymes are important for a diversity of physiologic effects ranging from the regulation of ion channels and secretion, cell–cell communication and substrate adherence, cell proliferation, differentiation, tumorogenesis and apoptosis. PKC enzymes are divided into three classes based on their cofactor requirements for activation. The conventional PKCs (cPKC), α, βI, βII, γ, are regulated by diacylglycerol (DAG), phosphatidylserine (PS) and calcium ion (Ca^{2+}). The novel PKCs (nPKC), δ, ε, η, θ, μ, lack a Ca^{2+} binding domain and are regulated by DAG and PS. The atypical PKCs (aPKC), ζ, λ/ι (mouse/human), do not respond to Ca^{2+} or DAG but can be regulated by PS and other acidic phospholipids.

PKCs are single polypeptide enzymes with a N-terminal regulatory half containing the C1 and C2 domains, and a C-terminal catalytic half containing the C3 and C4 domains. The constant domains (C) are separated by five variable (V) regions. The C1 domain is cysteine rich and coordinates two Zn^{2+} atoms forming dual Zn finger motifs. This domain binds DAG and the synthetic DAG mimic, phorbol ester. In the aPKC isoenzymes, there is only one Zn finger motif and these enzymes do not bind DAG. The C2 domain is responsible for binding of Ca^{2+} and PS. The nPKC and aPKC isoenzymes lack key aspartate residues necessary for Ca^{2+} binding. The C3 and C4 domains constitute the kinase portion of the enzyme. The C3 domain binds ATP and is highly conserved across isoenzymes. However, despite this high sequence similarity, isoenzyme selective small molecule inhibitors that target the ATP binding site have been reported[153]. The C4 domain in combination with V4 and V5 forms the substrate binding domain and the site for phosphate transfer.

PKC activity is regulated by trans- and cis-phosphorylation at three sites in the catalytic half of the enzyme. One site in the activation loop (threonine 500 in PKC βII) is phosphorylated by upstream kinases. For cPKC isoenzymes, the phosphatidylinositide dependent kinase (PDK) is a candidate upstream activator. PDK-1 phosphorylates a highly analogous site on protein kinase B (PKB) and has been shown to associate directly with PKC in vivo. This phosphorylation event is independent of either the phosphorylation state of the C-terminus or binding of the cofactors, DAG, Ca^{2+} and PS[154]. The nPKCs and aPKCs appear to be phosphorylated at the activation loop by phosphoinositide 3-kinase (PI3K). At least two sites in the carboxyl terminus must be phosphorylated for maximum activity. These sites (threonine 641 and serine 660 in PKC βII) are phosphorylated only after the activation loop site is phosphorylated, and appear to be due to autophosphorylating activity of PKC.

The phospholipid second messengers/cofactors that maximally activate PKC are released following ligand engagement of hormone and growth factor receptors and associated G-proteins and tyrosine kinases. Briefly, receptor binding leads to activation of a family of PI3K enzymes and phospholipases, probably in part by SH2 domain association with receptor adaptor molecules like the insulin receptor substrate, IRS[155]. PI3K phosphorylates the membrane lipid, phosphatidylinositide (PI) to give PI 4-phosphate (PIP) and PI 4,5-bisphosphate (PIP2). PIP2 is then hydrolysed to DAG and inositol 1,4,5-triphosphate (IP3) by phospholipase C (PLC). IP3 is released into the cytoplasm where it binds to a specific receptor on the endoplasmic reticulum, depolarizing the membrane to release Ca^{2+}. It is via this abbreviated scheme that two key cofactors of PKC are produced. A more prolonged activation of PKC may occur when DAG is produced by hydrolysis of phosphatidylcholine (PC) via specialized isoforms of PLC and PLD. This is because PC derived DAGs contain variable acyl linkages that are poor substrates for the enzymes that convert DAG back to PI.

The precise order of events leading to PKC activation remain uncertain and is probably in part a reflection of the different isoenzymes, cell types and stimuli used in experimental studies. Newly translated PKC contains a pseudosubstrate domain at the N-terminus (not found in isoenzyme μ) that masks both the activation loop and the substrate-binding domain. Structural studies indicate that the pseudosubstrate must be displaced prior to phosphorylation of the activation loop. This change in pseudosubstrate conformation renders it highly susceptible to proteolytic degradation by endogenous proteases. Other studies report that the pseudosubstrate is displaced following binding of DAG. A majority of the PKC isolated from non-stimulated cells is already phosphorylated and experimental evidence indicates that phosphorylation must occur before PKC can bind DAG and acidic phospholipids. Therefore, phosphorylation is most likely an event associated with post-translational modification rather than acute stimulation, and may occur during or when the enzyme is initially transported to its subcellular address. Following cell stimulation, the activity of the upstream kinase activators PDK and PI3K is up-regulated, thereby increasing the proportion of activated PKC in the cell. Coordinately, PI3K and PLC drive the synthesis of lipid cofactors necessary for complete and maximal activation of PKC.

PKCs have been shown to associate with, and phosphorylate a host of substrates. Because PKCs localize to the plasma membrane as well as nuclear and intracellular membranes, many of these substrates are membrane- and cytoskeleton-associated proteins. These include the myristolated alanine rich C kinase substrate (MARCKS) and MacMARCKS proteins, ribosomal proteins (e.g. S6), cytoskeletal proteins (e.g. troponin, synapsin, annexin), histones (e.g. histone H1), metabolic enzymes (e.g. pyruvate kinase, glycogen synthase) and signalling proteins (e.g. IKK-2, GTPases)[156]. This promiscuity for substrates necessitates the tight regulation of these enzymes. We have already described regulation of PKC via selective binding of cofactors, activation by phosphorylation, structural variations in the substrate binding domain, and cell specific expression of different isoenzymes. Additional regulatory mechanisms include scaffold proteins that stabilize PKC and enforce subcellular localization, proteolytic degradation of PKC, and binding of inhibitory phospholipids. Together these have been referred to as the 'sevenfold way of PKC regulation'[157]. Scaffold proteins include the receptors for activated C-kinases (RACKs), perinuclear binding protein (PICK) and PKA anchoring proteins (AKAPs). The most well-studied inhibitory phospholipid is sphingosine, which binds to the C1 domain in competition with DAG and PS.

The complexity of PKC isoenzyme expression and activity holds true when examined in the lung. A major reason is the diversity of cell types that constitute this tissue. Studies in human airway smooth muscle identified PKC α, βI, βII, ε, η, μ, ζ[158]. A similar pattern was observed in canine airway smooth muscle although PKC α and η were not detected[159]. Increased activity of PKCζ and PI3K may be associated with smooth muscle cell proliferation, cyclin D1 and DNA synthesis. Analysis of human lung revealed PKC α, βII, ε, η, ζ, while more selective analysis has revealed that epithelial cells are the exclusive site of PKCη expression[160] so that this isoform has been called the lung-type PKC. Stimulation of airway epithelium with phorbol ester leads to PKC activation and increased chloride secretion[161]. PKCη is highly expressed in the differentiated secretory epithelium of the mammary gland, giving rise to an interesting parallel and potential role for PKCη in secretory lung epithelium and mucus production[162]. Studies of lung vascular endothelium have not been reported, although experiments with human umbilical vein endothelial cells identified PKC α, ε, ζ. Stimulation with phorbol ester, bradykinin or TNFα resulted in activation and translocation of PKC α and ε, and subsequent increase in microvascular permeability[163]. Respiratory disease is associated with a marked increase in leukocyte infiltrate into the lung tissue and airways. Several studies have identified the PKC isoenzymes in lung leukocytes including basophils (PKC βI, βII, δ), eosinophils (PKC α, βI, βII, ζ), alveolar macrophages (PKC α, βI, βII, ε, η, γ, ζ), and lymphocytes (PKC α, βI, βII, δ, ε, θ, ζ)[164–167]. One key isoenzyme that is the focus of efforts to down-regulate the immune response is PKCθ. Mention has already been made in the section on IKK2 of the role that PKCθ plays in regulating the NF-κB pathway by phosphorylating IKK-2[144]. This isoenzyme appears to show marked tissue selectivity for hematopoietic cells, particularly T lymphocytes. Immuno-fluorescent studies have revealed that of the six isoforms identified in T-cells, only one, PKCθ, translocated to the site of cell contact following antigen presentation[168]. Following costimulation of the CD3 and CD28 receptors on T cells, PKCθ has been shown to activate JNK and IL-2 gene expression[169] and to synergize with Vav to promote IL-4 gene expression[170]. Both IL-2 and IL-4 are critical T cell growth and differentiation factors. PKCθ does not appear to be important for T-cell activation via NF-κB in immature lymphocytes suggesting a selective inhibitor of this isoenzyme will target mature T-cells and not developing thymocytes[171].

A number of PKC inhibitors based on the indolocarbazole and bisindolylmaleimide template have been synthesized and profiled pharmacologically. Due to the fact that the parent inhibitors for this class of compounds, staurosporine and K252a, are notoriously ubiquitous inhibitors of protein kinases, it would appear unlikely that the pharmacological profiles of so-called indolecarbazole PKC inhibitors can be fully rationalized solely based on PKC isoenzyme selectivity. Despite these challenges, many PKC inhibitors have advanced to the clinical stages. Among the forerunners are midostaurin, LY-333531, and Ro-31–8425. Studies in models of lung inflammation are not yet available.

Midostaurin (CGP-41251, Novartis), the N-benzoyl derivative of staurosporine, is a potent PKC inhibitor currently in Phase 2 clinical trials for the treatment of a variety of tumours. An extensive review of midostaurin is available[172]. In vitro, midostaurin inhibited PKC-α, γ, and δ at 30, 21, and 265 nM, respectively, but failed to block PKC-ε and ζ

activity. This observation is in marked contrast to staurosporine, which inhibited all the isoenzymes tested at 4 – 70 nM, except for PKC-ζ ($>$1 μM)[173]. It should be noted that PDGF receptor tyrosine auto-phosphorylation was potently ($<$0.1 μM) inhibited by midostaurin while no inhibition up to 1 μM was observed in the EGF receptor tyrosine kinase assay[174].

LY-333531, a macrocyclic bisindolylmaleimide is a PKC-β selective inhibitor currently at phase 3 clinical trial for diabetic retinopathy. PKC-βI,II were selectively inhibited by LY-333531 with IC$_{50}$ values of approximately 5 nM[153]. Selectivity against the other PKCs were $>$50-fold. Oral administration of LY-333531 at 0.1–10 mg/kg dose dependently improved glomerular filteration rate, albumin excretion rate, and retinal circulation in diabetic rats. Transgenic mice overexpressing PKC-βII exhibited severe vascular dysfunction including left ventricular hypertrophy, necrosis of cardiomyocytes, multifocal fibrosis, and decreased left ventricular performance. Treatment of PKC-βII transgenic mice with LY-333531 markedly improved both vascular histology and function[153].

Ro 31–8425 (Roche) represents a PKC inhibitor under clinical development for inflammatory indications. This compound shows little selectivity between the PKC isoenzymes, inhibiting all isoenzymes at 32–45 nM[175]. Ro 32–0432, the S-enantiomer of Ro 31–8425, appears to be more selective against PKCε[176] and inhibits PMA/PHA-induced IL-2 production in human peripheral blood T-lymphocytes at 30 nM[177]. Oral administration of Ro 32–0432 reduced PMA-induced paw edema and graft-induced increase of popliteal lymph node wet weight in rats. In rat adjuvant arthritis, Ro 32–0432 reduced paw swelling and improved joint lesion scores.

Obtaining PKC isoenzyme selectivity, as well as understanding the pharmacological effects of such compounds remains a tough challenge for those involved in drug discovery efforts. However, as already demonstrated, PKCs clearly play essential roles in a number of disease conditions and potent inhibitors are emerging. This area is expected to remain highly competitive for years to come (Fig. 11.5).

Conclusions

Protein kinase signal-transduction cascades provide a rich source of targets for small-molecule drugs with potential to control both multiple and individual inflammatory protein expression and activity. Issues that remain unanswered include the preferred level for targeted intervention of the kinase cascades. For example, is it better to develop a MEKK inhibitor or a MAPK inhibitor? There are reasons to suggest that inhibitors of each step of the cascade might provide a different profile of activity based on the cellular environment, activation and amplification steps.

Likewise, protein kinases are challenging drug targets. Inhibitors directed at the ATP binding site initially seemed unlikely since the binding site for ATP in different kinases should be similar and consequently selectivity would be impossible to achieve. The very high intracellular ATP concentration (approximately 1 to 5 mM) suggested that inhibitors competing for binding with ATP would have to be highly potent to demonstrate efficacy. Furthermore, the large number of kinases in the human genome suggested that inhibitors directed to the ATP binding site could be associated with unwanted side effects. Despite the conventional dogma that the catalytic site inhibitors are nonspecific, the identification of several very selective kinase inhibitors has created considerable optimism for the future. There is also the promise that protein substrate binding sites will provide additional opportunities for kinase inhibitor design.

Protein kinases form tight complexes with their substrates. These complexes are bridged by a third protein such as a scaffold or involve a direct high-affinity interaction between the kinase and a short substrate sequence, known as a docking site[178]. Several docking sites can exist for a single substrate increasing the affinity for a kinase. For example, c-Jun contains a distinct docking sequence, known as the delta domain, which is essential for specific phosphorylation of JNK. These docking sites may be used to generate competitive inhibitors of protein phosphorylation. Unfortunately, the structural

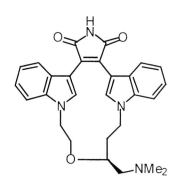

Midostaurin (CGP-41251)

LY-333531

Ro-31-8425

Ro-32-0432

Fig. 11.5 PKC inhibitors.

details of how docking sites bind to protein kinases is lacking in most cases.

Specificity of signalling pathways may be achieved, in part, by the use of scaffolding or anchoring proteins[179,180]. For example the MAPK scaffold protein JIP-1 (JNK interacting protein-1) is a cytoplasmic protein which functions as a scaffolding protein for specific component kinases in the JNK pathway. JIP-1 binds a MAPKKK, MKKK, and MKK for selective regulation of JNK activation[94]. These scaffolds may also provide novel drug targets to selectively modulate signalling pathways in inflammatory cells.

Finally, the rapid progress made in the production of crystal structures of a number of serine/threonine and tyrosine-specific protein kinases has identified the catalytic core of these important enzymes. In particular, recent X-ray crystallographic and protein mutagenesis experiments have provided a basis for understanding the selectivity of p38 MAP kinase inhibitors. As greater knowledge of active site inhibitors for kinases emerges, it is becoming clearer how to modify compounds to create greater potency and specificity.

A debate also exists as to the benefits of developing reversible inhibitors that block the enzyme for only a few hours, in contrast to irreversible inhibitors that provide greater duration of inhibition. Because protein kinases are intracellular enzymes, issues related to cell penetration, selectivity and in vivo efficacy and safety remain the challenge for the medicinal chemist. In this age of increased chemical diversity, it is anticipated that to address these issues, new kinase inhibitor templates will emerge from chemical libraries and natural product screening, as well as from the availability of massive combinatorial libraries. Biologically enhanced screening capacities resulting from HTS together with the availability of multiple recombinant human kinases is expediting selective kinase inhibitor identification. There are numerous kinases within the cell and, consequently, rapid and broad profiling remains an important goal. Understanding of the secondary and tertiary events that are modified by selective kinase inhibition will be greatly facilitated by gene microarray methodologies that will allow transcript profiles to be obtained. Such profiles will be extremely useful in evaluating the selectivity of drug candidates.

It is anticipated that multiple kinase inhibitors will be developed in a variety of immuno-inflammatory and proliferative diseases and it is hoped that our capability to generate kinase inhibitors will allow the rapid transition from novel kinase to validated target to clinical application and the marketplace. As more kinases are discovered and their activities identified, it can be anticipated that this large gene family will provide numerous therapeutic opportunities in multiple major diseases including asthma.

REFERENCES

1 Hunter T. Signaling – 2000 and beyond. *Cell* 2000; 100:113–127.

2 Huang C-Y and Ferrell J. Ultrasensitivity in the Mitogen-Activated Protein Kinase Cascade. *Proc Nat Acad Sci, USA* 1996; 93:10078–10083.

3 Barnes PJ. Therapeutic strategies for allergic diseases. *Nature* 1999; 402:B31–B38.

4 Druker B and Lydon N. Lessons learned from the development of an Abl tyrosine kinase inhibitor for chronic myelogenous leukemia. *J Clin Investig* 2000; 105:3–7.

5 Han J, Lee J, Bibbs L, Ulevitch R. A MAP Kinase targeted by endotoxin and hyperosmolarity in mammalian cells. *Science* 1994; 265:808–811.

6 Raingeaud J, Gupta S, Rogers J et al. Pro-inflammatory cytokines and environmental stress cause p38 mitogen-activated protein kinase activation by dual phosphorylation on tyrosine and threonine. *J Biol Chem* 1995; 270:7420–7426.

7 Han J, Richter B, Li Z, Kravchenko VV, Ulevitch RJ. Molecular cloning of human p38 MAP kinase. *Biochim et Biophys Acta* 1995; 1265:224–227.

8 Lee J, Laydon J, McDonnell P et al. A protein kinase involved in the regulation of inflammatory cytokine biosynthesis. *Nature* 1994; 372:739–746.

9 Stein B, Yang M, Young D et al. p38–2, a Novel mitogen-activated protein kinase with distinct properties. *J Biol Chem* 1997; 272:19509–19517.

10 Lechner C, Zahalka M, Giot J, Moller N, Ullrich A. ERK6, a mitogen-activated protein kinase involved in C2C12 myoblast differentiation. *Proc Nat Acad Sci, USA* 1996; 93:4355–4359.

11 Wang X, Diener K, Manthey C et al. Molecular cloning and characterization of a novel p38 mitogen-activated protein kinase. *J Biol Chem* 1997; 272:23668–23674.

12 Lu H, Yang D, Wysk M et al. Defective IL-12 production in mitogen-activated protein (MAP) kinase kinase 3 (Mkk3)-deficient mice. *Embo J* 1999; 18:1845–1857.

13 Han J, Jiang Y, Li Z, Kravchenko V, Ulevitch R. Activation of the transcription factor MEF2C by the MAP kinase p38 in inflammation. *Nature* 1997; 386:297–297.

14 Kolodziejczyk S, Wang L, Balazsi K, DeRepentigny Y, Kothary R, Megeney L. MEF2 is upregulated during cardiac hypertrophy and is required for normal post-natal growth of the myocardium. *Curr Biol* 1999; 9:1203–1206.

15 Zhao M, New L, Kravchenko V et al. Regulation of the MEF2 family of transcription factors by p38. *Molecular and Cellular Biology* 1999; 19:21–20.

16 Yang S, Galanis A, Sharrocks A. Targeting of p38 mitogen-activated protein kinases to MEF2 transcription factors. *Mol Cell Biol* 1999; 19:4028–4038.

17 Baldassare J, Bi Y, Bellone C. The role of p38 mitogen-acti-

vated protein kinase in IL-1 beta transcription. *J Immunol* 1999; 162:5367–5373.

18 Kotlyarov A, Neininger A, Schubert C et al. MAPKAP kinase 2 is essential for LPS-induced TNF-alpha biosynthesis. *Nat Cell Biol* 1999; 1:94–97.

19 Allen M, Svensson S, Roach M, Hambor J, McNeish J, Gabel C. Deficiency of the stress kinase p38alpha results in embryonic lethality: characterization of the kinase dependence of stress responses of enzyme-deficient embryonic stem cells. *J Exp Med* 2000; 191:859–870.

20 Raingeaud J, Whitmarsh A, Barrett T, Derijard B, Davis R. MKK3- and MKK6-regulated gene expression is mediated by the p38 mitogen-activated protein kinase signal transduction pathway. *Mol Cell Biol* 1996; 16:1247–1255.

21 Enslen H, Raingeaud J, Davis R. Selective activation of p38 mitogen-activated protein (MAP) kinase isoforms by the MAP kinase kinases MKK3 and MKK6. *J Biol Chem* 1998; 273:1741–1748.

22 Wysk M, Yang D, Lu H, Flavell R, Davis R. Requirement of mitogen-activated protein kinase kinase 3 (MKK3) for tumor necrosis factor induced cytokine expression. *Proc Nat Acad Sci, USA* 1999; 96:3763–3768.

23 LoGrasso P, Frantz B, Rolando A, O'Keefe S, Hermes J, O'Neill E. Kinetic mechanism for p38 MAP kinase. *Biochemistry* 1997; 36:10422–10427.

24 Underwood D, Osborn R, Kotzer C et al. SB 239063, a potent p38 MAP kinase inhibitor, reduces inflammatory cytokine production, airways eosinophil infiltration, and persistence. *J Pharmacol Exp Therap*, 2000; 293:281–288.

25 Bennett B L. Personal communication 2000.

26 Tong L, Pav S, White D et al. A highly specific inhibitor of human p38 MAP kinase binds in the ATP pocket. *Nat Struct Biol* 1997; 4:311–216.

27 Lee J, Badger AM, Griswold D et al. Bicyclic imidazoles as a novel class of cytokine biosynthesis inhibitors. *Ann NY Acad Sci* 1993; 696:149–170.

28 Gallagher TF, Seibel GL, Kassis S. Regulation of stress-induced cytokine production by pyridinylimidazoles; inhibition of CSBP kinase. *Bioorg Med Chem* 1997; 5:49–64.

29 Hanson G, Gunner J. Inhibitors of p38 kinase. *Expert Opin Therap Patents* 1997; 7:729–733.

30 Young P, McLaughlin M, Kumar S et al. Pyridinyl imidazole inhibitors of p38 mitogen-activated protein kinase bind in the ATP site. *J Biol Chem* 1997; 272:12116–12121.

31 Boehm J, Smietana J, Sorenson M et al. 1-substituted 4-aryl-5-pyridinylimidazoles: a new class of cytokine suppressive drugs with low 5-lipoxygenase and cyclooxygenase inhibitory potency. *J Med Chem* 1996; 39:3929–3937.

32 Tong L, Pav S, White D et al. A highly specific inhibitor of human p38 MAP kinase binds in the ATP pocket. *Nat Struct Biol* 1997; 4:311–216.

33 Wilson K, McCaffrey P, Hsiao K et al. The structural basis for the specificity of pyridinylimidazole inhibitors of p38 MAP kinase. *Chem Biol*, 1997; 4:423–431.

34 Badger AM, Bradbeer J, Votta B, Lee J, Adams J, Griswold D. Pharmacological profile of SB 203580, a selective inhibitor of cytokine suppressive binding protein/p38 kinase, in animal models of arthritis, bone resorption, endotoxin shock and immune function. *J Pharmaceut Exp Therap* 1996; 279:1453–1461.

35 Jackson J, Bolognese B, Hillegass L et al. Pharmacological effects of SB 220025, a selective inhibitor of P38 mitogen-activated protein kinase, in angiogenesis and chronic inflammatory disease models. *J Pharmacol Exp Therap* 1998; 284:687–692.

36 Adams J, Boehm J, Kassis S et al. Pyrimidinylimidazole inhibitors of CSBP/p38 kinase demonstrating decreased inhibition of hepatic cytochrome P450 enzymes. *Bioorg Med Chem Lett* 1998; 8:3111–2116.

37 Adams J. p38/CSBP MAP kinase inhibitors: structural basis of pyridinylimidazole specificity and therapeutic potential. *XVth EFMC International Symposium on Medicinal Chemistry* 1998.

38 de Laszlo S, Visco D, Agarwal L et al. Pyrroles and other heterocycles as inhibitors of P38 kinase. *Bioorg Med Chem Lett* 1998; 8:2689–2694.

39 Liverton N, Butcher J, Claiborne C et al. Design and synthesis of potent, selective, and orally bioavailable tetrasubstituted imidazole inhibitors of p38 mitogen-activated protein kinase. *J Med Chem* 1999; 42:2180–2190.

40 Nick J, Young S, Brown K et al. Role of p38 mitogen-activated protein kinase in a murine model of pulmonary inflammation. *J Immunol* 2000; 164:2151–2159.

41 Zablocki J. Aryl and heteroaryl substituted fused pyrrole antiinflammatory agents. *Patent WO 9822457*.

42 Dodd J, Henry J, Rupert K. Preparation of substituted pyrrolopyridines for the treatment of inflammatory diseases. *Patent WO 9847899* 1988.

43 Henry J, Rupert K, Dodd J et al. 6-Amino-2-(4-fluorophenyl)-4-methoxy-3- (4-pyridyl)-[1]H-pyrrolo[2, 3-b]pyridine (RWJ 68354): a potent and selective p38 kinase inhibitor. *J Med Chem* 1998; 41:4196–4198.

44 Henry J, Rupert K, Dodd J et al. Potent inhibitors of the MAP kinase p38. *Bioorg Med Chem Lett* 1998; 8:3335–3340.

45 Wadsworth S, Cavender D, Beers S et al. RWJ 67657, a potent, orally active inhibitor of p38 mitogen-activated protein kinase. *J Pharmacol Exp Therap*, 1999; 291:680–291.

46 Mourey R. Development of p38 kinase inhibitors as novel anti-inflammatory drugs. *Inflammation Research Association Ninth International Conference* 1998.

47 Yamamoto N, Sakai F, Yamazaki H, Nakahara K, Okuhara M. Effect of FR167653, a cytokine suppressive agent, on endotoxin-induced disseminated intravascular coagulation. *Eur J Pharmacol* 1996; 314:137–142.

48 Yamamoto N, Sakai F, Yamazaki H, Kawai Y, Nakahara K, Okuhara M. Effect of FR133605, a novel cytokine suppressive agent, on bone and cartilage destruction in adjuvant arthritic rats. *J Rheumatol* 1996; 23:1778–1783.

49 Yamamoto N, Sakai A, Yamazaki H, Sato N, Nakahara K, Okuhara M. FR167653, a dual inhibitor of interleukin-1 and tumor necrosis factor-alpha, ameliorates endotoxin-induced shock. *Eur J Pharmacol* 1997; 327:169–174.

50 Kobayashi J, Takeyoshi I, Ohwada S et al. The effects of FR167653 in extended liver resection with ischemia in dogs. *Hepatology* 1998; 28:459–465.

51 Hoshida S, Tanouchi J, Yamada Y, Kuzuya T, Hori M. The effect of FR-167653 in an extended liver resection with ischemia. *J Amer Coll Cardiol* 1998; 31:279A.

52 Kawamura M, Hatanaka K, Harada Y. Suppression of COX-2 expression by FR167653 in rat carrageenin-induced pleurisy. *71st Annual Meeting of Japan Pharmaceutical Society* 1998.

53 Gardiner S, Kemp P, March J, Bennett T. Influence of FR 167653, an inhibitor of TNF-alpha and IL-1, on the cardiovascular responses to chronic infusion of lipopolysaccharide in conscious rats. *J Cardiovasc Pharmacol* 1999; 34:64–69.

54 Hirano T, Hirano K. Effect of a cytokine suppressive agent on the exocrine pancreas in rats with caerulein-induced acute pancreatitis. *Med Sci Res* 1999; 27:523–526.

55 Hirano T. Cytokine suppressive agent improves survival rate in rats with acute pancreatitis of closed duodenal loop. *J Surg Res* 1999; 81:224–229.

56 Oshima KSY, Takeyoshi I, Yamagishi T, Mohara J, Ishikawa S, Morishita Y. The effect of FR 167653 on cerebral ischemic-reperfusion injury during and after retrograde cerebral perfusion. *Nippon Teitaion Kenkyukai Kaishi* 1999; 19:20–23.

57 Salituro FG, Bemis GW, Germann RA et al. Discovery of VX-745: a novel, orally bioavailable and selective p38 MAP kinase inhibitor. *27th National Medicinal Chemistry Symposium* 2000.

58 Boulton T, Yancopoulos G, Gregory J et al. An insulin-stimulated protein kinase similar to yeast kinases involved in cell cycle control. *Science* 1990; 249:64–67.

59 Ferrell Jr J, Bhatt R. Mechanistic studies of the dual phosphorylation of mitogen-activated protein kinase. *J Biol Chem* 1997; 272:19008–19016.

60 Cobb M, Goldsmith E. How MAP kinases are regulated. *J Biol Chem* 1995; 270:14843–14846.

61 Cobb M, Goldsmith E. Dimerization in MAP-kinase signaling. *Trends in Biochem Sci* 2000; 25:7–9.

62 Gille H, Sharrocks A, Shaw P. Phosphorylation of transcription factor p62TCF by MAP kinase stimulates ternary complex formation at c-fos promoter. *Nature*, 1992 358:414–417.

63 Brondello J, Brunet A, Pouyssegur J, McKenzie F. The dual specificity mitogen-activated protein kinase phosphatase-1 and -2 are induced by the p42/p44^{Mapk} cascade. *J Biol Chem* 1997; 272:1368–1376.

64 Todd J, Tanner K, Denu J. Extracellular regulated kinases (ERK) 1 and ERK2 are authentic substrates for the dual-specificity protein-tyrosine phosphatase VHR. A novel role in down-regulating the ERK pathway. *J Biol Chem* 1999; 274:13271–13280.

65 Jaaro H, Rubinfeld H, Hanoch T, Seger R. Nuclear translocation of mitogen-activated protein kinase kinase (MEK1) in response to mitogenic stimulation. *Proc Nat Acad Sci, USA* 1997; 94:3742–3747.

66 Moodie S, Willumsen B, Weber M, Wolfman A. Complexes of Ras.GTP with Raf-1 and mitogen-activated protein kinase kinase. *Science* 1993; 260:1658–1661.

67 Cowley S, Paterson H, Kemo P, Marshall C. Activation of MAP kinase kinase is necessary and sufficient for PC12 differentiation and for transformation of NIH 3T3 cells. *Cell* 1994; 77:841–852.

68 Giroux S, Tremblay M, Bernard D et al. Embryonic death of Mek1-deficient mice reveals a role for this kinase in angiogenesis in the labyrinthine region of the placenta. *Curr Biol* 1999; 9:369–372.

69 Kerppola, T and Curran T. Transcription. Zen and the art of Fos and Jun [news and views]. *Nature* 1995; 373:199–200.

70 Chen L, Glover J, Hogan P, Rao A, Harrison S. Structure of the DNA-binding domains from NFAT, Fos and Jun bound specifically to DNA. *Nature* 1998; 392:42–48.

71 Whitehurst C, Geppert T. MEK1 and the extracellular signal-regulated kinases are required for the stimulation of IL-2 gene transcription in T cells. *J Immunol* 1996; 156:1020–1029.

72 DeSilva D, Jones E, Favata M et al. Inhibition of mitogen-activated protein kinase kinase blocks T cell proliferation but does not induce or prevent anergy. *J Immunol* 160:4175–4181.

73 David M, Petricoin III E, Benjamin C, Pine R, Weber M, Larner A. Requirement for MAP kinase (ERK2) activity in interferon alpha- and interferon beta-stimulated gene expression through STAT proteins. *Science* 1995; 269:1721–1723.

74 Tanoue T, Adachi O, Moriguchi T, Nishida E. A conserved docking motif in MAP kinases common to substrates, activators and regulators. *Nat Cell Biol* 2000; 2:110–116.

75 Adams Novel 1,4,5-substituted imidazole compounds useful as ERK/MAP kinase inhibitors. *Patent WO-09961440* 1999.

76 Dudley D, Pang L, Decker S, Bridges A, Saltiel A. A synthetic inhibitor of the mitogen-activated protein kinase cascade. *Proc Nat Acad Sci, USA* 1995; 92:7686–7689.

77 Alessi D, Cuenda A, Cohen P, Dudley D, Saltiel A. PD 098059 is a specific inhibitor of the activation of mitogen-activated protein kinase kinase *in vitro* and *in vivo*. *J Biol Chem* 1995; 270:27489–27494.

78 Cohen P, Goedert M. Engineering protein kinases with distinct nucleotide specificities and inhibitor sensitivities by mutation of a single amino acid. *Chem Biol* 1998; 5:R161–R164.

79 Trzaskos. Blockade of AP-1-driven gene transcription by U0126: a MAP kinase kinase inhibitor. *3rd World Congress of Inflammation* 1998.

80 Williams D, Wilkinson S, Purton T, Lamont A, Flotow H, Murray E. Ro 09–2210 exhibits potent anti-proliferative effects on activated T cells by selectively blocking MKK activity. *Biochemistry* 1998; 37:9579–9585.

81 Zhao A, Lee S, Mojena M et al. Resorcylic acid lactones: naturally occurring potent and selective inhibitors of MEK. *J Antibiotics (Tokyo)* 1999; 52:1086–1094.

82 Ip YT, Davis RJ. Signal transduction by the c-Jun N-terminal kinase (JNK) – from inflammation to development. *Curr Opin Cell Biol* 1998; 10:205–219.

83 Minden A, Karin M. Regulation and function of the JNK subgroup of MAP kinases. *Biochim Biophys Acta* 1997; 1333:F85–F104.

84 Gupta S, Barrett T, Whitmarsh AJ et al. Selective interaction of JNK protein kinase isoforms with transcription factors. *Embo J* 1996; 15:2760–2770.

85 Karin M. The regulation of AP-1 activity by mitogen-activated protein kinases. *J Biol Chem* 1995; 270:16483–16486.

86 Claret F-X, Hibi M, Dhut S, Toda T, Karin M. A new group of conserved coactivators that increase the specificity of AP-1 transcription factors. *Nature* 1996; 383:453–457.

87 Gupta S, Campbell D, Derijard B, Davis RJ. Transcription factor ATF2 regulation by the JNK signal transduction pathway. *Science* 1995; 267:389–393.

88 Yang SH, Whitmarsh AJ, Davis RJ, Sharrocks AD. Differential targeting of MAP kinases to the ETS-domain transcription factor Elk-1. *Embo J* 1998; 17:1740–1749.

89 Barnes PJ, Adcock IM. Transcription factors and asthma. *Eur Respir J* 1998; 12:221–234.

90 Manning AM, Bell FP, Rosenbloom CL et al. NF-kappa B is activated during acute inflammation in vivo in association with elevated endothelial cell adhesion molecule gene expression and leukocyte recruitment. *J Inflammation* 1995; 45:283–296.

91 Driscoll K, BeruBe K, Churg A et al. Ambient particulate matter causes activation of the c-jun kinase/stress-activated protein kinase cascade and DNA synthesis in lung epithelial cells. *Cancer Res* 1998; 58:4543–4547.

92 Benbow U, Brinckerhoff CE. The AP-1 site and MMP gene regulation: what is all the fuss about? *Matrix Biol* 1997; 15:519–526.

93 Tanoue T, Moriguchi T, Nishida E. Molecular cloning and characterization of a novel dual specificity phosphatase, MKP-5. *J Biol Chem* 1999; 274:19949–19956.

94 Whitmarsh AJ, Cavanagh J, Tournier C, Yasuda J, Davis RJ. A mammalian scaffold complex that selectively mediates MAP kinase activation. *Science* 1998; 281:1671–1674.

95 Yasuda J, Whitmarsh AJ, Cavanagh J, Sharma M, Davis RJ. The JIP group of mitogen-activated protein kinase scaffold proteins. *Mol Cell Biol* 1999; 19:7245–7254.

96 Kelkar N, Gupta S, Dickens M, Davis RJ. Interaction of a mitogen activated protein kinase signaling module with the neuronal JIP3. *Mol Cell Biol* 2000; 20:1030–1043.

97 Itoh M, Yoshioka K, Akechi M et al. JSAP1, a novel jun N-terminal protein kinase (JNK)-binding protein that functions as a scaffold factor in the JNK signaling pathway. *Mol Cell Biol* 1999; 19:7539–7548.

98 Karin M, Delhase M. JNK or IKK, AP-1 or NF-kappaB, which are the targets for MEK kinase 1 action? *Proc Nat Acad Sci, USA* 1998; 95:9067–9069.

99 Yujiri T, Sather S, Fanger GR, Johnson GL. Role of MEKK1 in cell survival and activation of JNK and ERK pathways defined by targeted gene disruption. *Science* 1998; 282:1911–1914.

100 Ichijo H, Nishida E, Irie K et al. Induction of apoptosis by ASK1, a mammalian MAPKKK that activates SAPK/JNK and p38 signaling pathways. *Science* 1997; 275:90–94.

101 Hehner SP, Hofmann TG, Ushmorov A et al. Mixed-lineage kinase 3 delivers CD3/CD28-derived signals into the IkappaB kinase complex. *Mol Cell Biol* 2000; 20:2556–2568.

102 Teramoto H, Coso OA, Miyata H, Igishi T, Miki T, Gutkind JS. Signaling from the small GTP-binding proteins Rac1 and Cdc42 to the c-Jun N-terminal kinase/stress-activated protein kinase pathway. *J Biol Chem* 1996; 271:27225–27228.

103 Wang W, Zhou G, Hu MCT, Yao Z, Tan TH. Activation of the hematopoietic progenitor kinase-1 (HPK1)-dependent, stress-activated c-Jun N-terminal kinase (JNK) pathway by transforming growth factor beta (TGF-beta)-activated kinase (TAK1), a kinase mediator of TGF beta signal transduction. *J Biol Chem* 1997; 272:22771–22775.

104 Yang D, Tournier C, Wysk M et al. Targeted disruption of the MKK4 gene causes embryonic death, inhibition of c-Jun NH_2-terminal kinase activation, and defects in AP-1 transcriptional activity. *Proc Nat Acad Sci, USA* 1997; 94:3004–3009.

105 Tournier C, Whitmarsh A, Cavanagh J, Barrett T, Davis R. Mitogen-activated protein kinase kinase 7 is an activator of the c-Jun NH_2-terminal kinase. *Proc Nat Acad Sci* 1997; 94:7337–7342.

106 Dong C, Yang DD, Tournier C et al. JNK is required for effector T-cell function but not for T-cell activation. *Nature* 2000; 405:91–94.

107 Yang D, Kuan C, Whitmarsh A et al. Absence of excitotoxicity-induced apoptosis in the hippocampus of mice lacking the Jnk3 gene. *Nature* 1997; 389:865–870.

108 Dong C, Yang D, Wysk M, Whitmarsh A, Davis R, Flavell R. Defective T cell differentiation in the absence of Jnk1. *Science* 1998; 282:2092-2095.

109 Yang D, Whitmarsh A, Conze D et al. Differentiation of CD4 + T cells to Th1 cells requires MAP kinase JNK2. *Immunity* 1998; 9:575–585.

110 Sabapathy K, Hu Y, Kallunki T et al. JNK2 is required for efficient T-cell activation and apoptosis but not for normal lymphocyte development. *Curr Biol* 1999; 9:116–125.

111 Tournier C, Hess P, Yang DD et al. Requirement of JNK for stress-induced activation of the cytochrome c-mediated death pathway. *Science* 2000; 288:870–874.

112 Maroney AC, Glicksman MA, Basma AN et al. Motoneuron apoptosis is blocked by CEP-1347 (KT 7515), a novel inhibitor of the JNK signaling pathway. *J Neurosci* 1998; 18:104–111.

113 Potential of CEP-1347 for the treatment of Parkinson's disease. 4th International Symposium on Medicinal Chemistry of Neurodegenerative Diseases. 2000. Cancun, Mexico. 2000.

114 Glicksman MA, Murakata C, Dionne CA et al. CEP-1347/KT7515 prevents motor neuronal programmed cell death and injury-induced dedifferentiation in vivo. *J Neurobiol* 1998; 35:361–270.

115 Saporito MS, Brown ER, Carswell S et al. Preservation of cholinergic activity and prevention of neuron death by CEP-1347/KT-7515 following excitotoxic injury of the nucleus basalis magnocellularis. *Neuroscience* 1998; 86:461–472.

116 DiCamillo AM, Neff NT, Carswell S, Haun FA. Chronic sparing of delayed alternation performance and choline acetyltransferase activity by CEP-1347/KT-7515 in rats with lesions of nucleus basalis magnocellularis. *Neuroscience* 1998; 86:473–483.

117 Saporito MS, Brown EM, Miller MS, Carswell S. CEP-1347/KT-7515, an inhibitor of c-jun N-terminal kinase activation, attenuates the 1-methyl-4-phenyl tetrahydropyridine-mediated loss of nigrostriatal dopaminergic neurons *in vivo*. *J Pharmacol Exp Therap* 1999; 288:421–427.

118 Pirvola U. Rescue of hearing, auditory hair cells, and neurons by CEP-1347/KT7515, an inhibitor of c-Jun N-terminal kinase activation. *J Neurosci* 2000; 20:43–50.

119 Wagner AC. CEP-1347 inhibits caerulein-induced rat pancreatic JNK activation and ameliorates caerulein pancreatitis. *Am J Physiol* 2000; 278:G165-G172.

120 Sen R, Baltimore D. Inducibility of kappa immunoglobulin enhancer-binding protein Nf-kappa B by a posttranslational mechanism. *Cell* 1986; 47:921–928.

121 Baeuerle PA, Baichwal V. NF-kappa B as a frequent target for immunosuppressive and anti-inflammatory molecules. *Adv Immunol* 1997; 65:111–137.

122 Alkalay I, Yaron A, Hatzubai A, Orian A, Ciechanover A, Ben-Neriah Y. Stimulation-dependent IkBα phosphorylation marks the NF-kB inhibitor for degradation via the ubiquitin–proteasome pathway. *Proc Nat Acad Sci, USA* 1995; 92:10599–10603.

123 Yaron A, Hatzubai A, Davis M. Identification of the receptor component of the IkappaBalpha – ubiquitin ligase. *Nature* 1998; 396:590–594.

124 Scheinman R, Cogswell P, Lofquist A, Baldwin Jr A. Role of transcriptional activation of I*k*Bα in mediation of immunosuppression by glucocorticoids. *Science* 1995; 270:283–299.

125 Barnes PJ. Anti-inflammatory actions of glucocorticoids: molecular mechanisms. *Clin Sci (Colch)* 1998; 94:557–572.

126 Mercurio F, Zhu H, Murray B et al. IKK-1 and IKK-2: cytokine-activated IkappaB kinases essential for NF-kappaB activation. *Science* 1997; 278:860–866.

127 Mercurio F, Murray B, Shevchenko A et al. IkappaB kinase

(IKK)-associated protein 1, a common component of the heterogeneous IKK complex. *Molec Cell Biol* 1999; 19:1526–1538.

128 Li Q, Lu Q, Hwang J et al. IKK1-deficient mice exhibit abnormal development of skin and skeleton. *Genes Dev* 1999; 13:1322–1328.

129 Tanaka M, Fuentes M, Yamaguchi K et al. Embryonic lethality, liver degeneration, and impaired NF-kappa B activation in IKK-beta-deficient mice. *Immunity* 1999; 10:421–429.

130 Li Q, Van Antwerp D, Mercurio F, Lee K, Verma I. Severe liver degeneration in mice lacking the IkappaB kinase 2 gene. *Science* 1999; 284:321–225.

131 Hu Y, Baud V, Delhase M et al. Abnormal morphogenesis but intact IKK activation in mice lacking the IKK alpha subunit of I kappa B kinase. *Science* 1999; 284:316–320.

132 Takeda K, Takeuchi O, Tsujimura T et al. Limb and skin abnormalities in mice lacking IKK alpha. *Science* 1999; 284:313–316.

133 Shimada T, Kawai T, Takeda K et al. IKK-i, a novel lipopolysaccharide-inducible kinase that is related to IKB kinases. *Int Immunol* 1999; 11:1357–1362.

134 Peters R, Liao S-M, Maniatis T. IKKepsilon is a part of a novel PMA-inducible kinase complex. *Molec Cell* 2000; 5:513–522.

135 Tojima Y, Fujimoto A, Delhase M et al. NAK is an IkappaB kinase-activating kinase. *Nature* 2000; 404:782.

136 Pomerantz J, Baltimore D. NF-kappaB activation by a signaling complex containing TRAF2, TANK and TBK1, a novel IKK-related kinase. *Embo J* 1999; 18:6694–6704.

137 Peet G, Li J. IkB kinases alpha and beta show a random sequential kinetic mechanism and are inhibited by staurosporine and quercetin. *J Biol Chem* 1999; 274:32655–32661.

138 Heilker R, Freuler F, Vanek M et al. The kinetics of association and phosphorylation of IkappaB isoforms by IkappaB kinase 2 correlate with their cellular regulation in human endothelial cells. *Biochem* 1999; 38:6231–6238.

139 Burke J, Wood M, Ryseck R, Walther S, Meyers C. Peptides corresponding to the N and C termini of IκB-α, -β, and -ε as probes of the two catalytic subunits of IκB kinase, IKK-1 and IKK-2. *J Biol Chem* 1999; 274:36146–36152.

140 Nemoto S, Didonato JA, Lin A. Coordinate regulation of IkappaB kinases by mitogen-activated protein kinase kinase kinase 1 and NF-kappaB-inducing kinase. *Mol Cell Biol* 1998; 18:7336–7343.

141 Malinin N, Boldin M, Kovalenko A, Wallach D. MAP3K-related kinase involved in NF-kB Induction by TNF, CD95 and IL-1. *Nature* 1997; 385:540–544.

142 Shinkura R, Kitada K, Matsuda F et al. Alymphoplasia is caused by a point mutation in the mouse gene encoding Nf-kappa b-inducing kinase. *Nat Genet* 1999; 22:74–77.

143 Lallena M, Diaz-Meco M, Bren G, Paya C, Moscat J. Activation of IkappaB kinase beta by protein kinase C isoforms. *Mol Cell Biol* 1999; 19:2180–2188.

144 Lin X, O'Mahony A, Mu Y, Geleziunas R, Greene WC. Protein kinase C-theta participates in NF-kappaB activation induced by CD3-CD28 costimulation through selective activation of IkappaB kinase beta. *Mol Cell Biol* 2000; 20:2933–2940.

145 Coudronniere N, Villalba M, Englund N, Altman A. NF-kappa B activation induced by T cell receptor/CD28 costimulation is mediated by protein kinase C-theta. *Proc Nat Acad Sci, USA* 2000; 97:3394–3399.

146 Delhase M, Hayakawa M, Karin M. Positive and negative regulation of IkB kinase activity through IKKB subunit phosphorylation. *Science* 1999; 284:309–313.

147 Yin M, Yamamoto Y, Gaynor R. The anti-inflammatory agents aspirin and salicylate inhibit the activity of I(kappa)B kinase-beta. *Nature* 1998; 396:77–80.

148 Rossi A, Elia G, Santoro M. Inhibition of nuclear factor kB by prostaglandin A$_1$: an effect associated with heat shock transcription factor activation. *Proc Nat Acad, USA* 1997; 94:746–750.

149 Rossi A, Kapahi P, Natoli G et al. Anti-inflammatory cyclopentenone prostaglandins are direct inhibitors of IκB kinase. *Nature* 2000; 403:103–108.

150 Newton regulation of protein kinase C. *Curr Opin Cell Biol* 1997; 9:161–167.

151 Kanashiro C, Khalil R. Signal transduction by protein kinase C in mammalian cells *Clin Exp Pharmacol Physiol*, 1998; 25:974–985.

152 Mellor H, Parker P. The extended protein kinase C superfamily. *Biochem J*, 1998; 332:281–292.

153 Ishii H, Jirousek M, Koya D et al. Amelioration of vascular dysfunctions in diabetic rats by an oral PKC beta inhibitor. *Science* 1996; 272:728–731.

154 Dutil E, Toker A, Newton A. Regulation of conventional protein kinase C isozymes by phosphoinositide-dependent kinase 1 (PDK-1). *Curr Biol* 1998; 8:1366–1375.

155 Vanhaesebroeck B, Leevers S, Panayotou G, Waterfield M. Phosphoinositide 3-kinases: a conserved family of signal transducers. *Trends Biochem Sci* 1997; 22:267–272.

156 Hofmann J. The potential for isoenzyme-selective modulation of protein kinase C. *FASEB J* 1997; 11:649–669.

157 Liu W, Heckman A. The sevenfold way of PKC regulation. *Cell Signaling* 1998; 10:529–542.

158 Webb B, Lindsay M, Barnes PJ, Giembycz M. Protein kinase C isoenzymes in airway smooth muscle. *Biochem J* 1997; 324:167–175.

159 Donnelly R, Yang K, Omary M, Azhar S, Black J. Expression of multiple isoenzymes of protein kinase C in airway smooth muscle. *Am J Respir Cell Mol Biol* 1995; 13:253–256.

160 Osada S, Hashimoto Y, Nomura S et al. Predominant expression of nPKC eta, a Ca(2+)-independent isoform of protein kinase C in epithelial tissues, in association with epithelial differentiation. *Cell Growth Differentiation* 1993; 4:167–175.

161 Cloutier M, Guernsey L. Tannin inhibition of protein kinase C in airway epithelium. *Lung* 1995; 173:307–319.

162 Masso-Welch P, Verstovsek G, Darcy K, Tagliarino C, Ip M. Protein kinase C eta upregulation and secretion during postnatal rat mammary gland differentiation. *Eur J Cell Biol* 1998; 77:48–59.

163 Ross D, Joyner W. Resting distribution and stimulated translocation of protein kinase C isoforms alpha, epsilon and zeta in response to bradykinin and TNF in human endothelial cells. *Endothelium* 1997; 5:321–232.

164 Miura K, MacGlashan D. Expression of protein kinase C isozymes in human basophils: regulation by physiological and nonphysiological stimuli. *Blood* 1998; 92:1206–1218.

165 Evans D, Lindsay M, Webb B et al. Expression and activation of protein kinase C-zeta in eosinophils after allergen challenge. *Am J Physiol* 1999; 277:L233–L239.

166 Monick M, Carter A, Gudundsson G, Geist L, Hunninghake G. Changes in PKC isoforms in human alveolar macrophages compared with blood monocytes. *Am J Physiol* 1998; 275:L389–L397.

167 Baier-Bitterlich G, Uberall F, Bauer B et al. Protein kinase C-theta isoenzyme selective stimulation of the transcription factor complex AP-1 in T lymphocytes. *Mol Cell Biol* 1996; 16:1842–1850.

168 Monks C, Kupfer H, Tamir I, Barlow A, Kupfer A. Selective modulation of protein kinase C-theta during T-cell activation. *Nature* 1997; 385:83–86.

169 Werlen G, Jacinto E, Xia Y, Karin M. Calcineurin preferentially synergizes with PKC-theta to activate JNK and IL-2 promoter in T lymphocytes. *Embo J* 1998; 17:3101–2111.

170 Hehner SP, Li-Weber M, Giaisi M, Droge W, Krammer P, Schmitz M. Vav synergizes with protein kinase C theta to mediate IL-4 gene expression in response to CD28 costimulation in T cells. *J Immunol* 2000; 164:389–3836.

171 Sun Z, Arendt C, Ellmeier W et al. PKC-theta is required for

172 Fabbro D, Buchdunger E, Wood J et al. Inhibitors of protein kinases: CGP 41251, a protein kinase inhibitor with potential as an anticancer agent. *Pharmacol Therap* 82:293–301.

173 Geiges D, Meyer T, Marte B et al. Activation of protein kinase C subtypes alpha, gamma, delta, epsilon, zeta, and eta by tumor-promoting and nontumor-promoting agents. *Biochem Pharmacol* 1997; 53:865–875.

174 Andrejauskas-Buchdunger E, Regenass U. Differential inhibition of the epidermal growth factor-, platelet-derived growth factor-, and protein kinase C-mediated signal transduction pathways by the staurosporine derivative CGP 41251. *Cancer Res* 1992; 52:5353–5358.

175 Bit R, Davis P, Elliot L et al. Inhibitors of protein kinase C. 3. Potent and highly selective bisindolylmaleimides by conformational restriction. *J Med Chem* 1993; 36:21–29.

176 Wilkinson S, Parker P, Nixon J. Isoenzyme specificity of bisindolylmaleimides, selective inhibitors of protein kinase C. *Biochem J* 1993; 294:335–337.

177 Birchall A, Bishop J, Bradshaw D et al. Ro 32–0432, a selective and orally active inhibitor of protein kinase C prevents T-cell activation. *J Pharmacol Exp Therap* 1994; 268:922–929.

178 Holland P, Cooper J. Protein modification: docking sites for kinases. *Curr Biol* 1999; 9:R329–R331.

179 Fanning A, Anderson J. Protein modules as organizers of membrane structure. *Curr Opin Cell Biol* 1999; 11:432–439.

180 Pawson T, Scott J. Signaling through scaffold, anchoring, and adaptor proteins. *Science* 1997; 278:2075–2080.

181 Levitzki A, Gazit A. Tyrosine kinase inhibition: an approach to drug development. *Science* 1995; 267:1782–1788.

182 Lopez-Ilasaca M. Signaling from G-protein-coupled receptors to mitogen-activated protein (MAP)-kinase cascades. *Biochem Pharmacol* 1998; 56:269–277.

TCR-induced NF-kappaB activation in mature but not immature T lymphocytes. *Nature* 2000; 404:402–407.

REFERENCES ADDED IN PROOF

183 Bennett BL, Sasaki D, Murray B et al. SP600125, an anthrapyrazolone inhibitor of Jun-N-terminal kinase (JNK). *PNAS 98* 2001; 13681–13686.

184 Han H, Boyle D, Chang L. c-Jun N-terminal kinase is required for metalloproteinases expression and joint destruction in inflammatory arthritis. *J Clin Inv* 2001; 108:73–81.

Part II

Diffuse parenchymal lung disease

12

Current approaches to the treatment of parenchymal lung diseases

Joseph P. Lynch, III and Michael Keane

Division of Pulmonary and Critical Care Medicine, Department of Internal Medicine,
University of Michigan Medical Center, Ann Arbor, MI, USA

Interstitial lung diseases (ILDs) are a heterogeneous group of disorders characterized by a spectrum of inflammatory and fibrotic changes affecting alveolar walls and airspaces[1–7]. Clinical manifestations are protean, but progressive cough, dyspnea, parenchymal infiltrates on chest radiographs, and loss of pulmonary function are characteristic. More than 150 causes of ILD are known and include disorders due to specific agents or antigens (e.g. pneumoconioses, asbestosis, silicosis, berylliosis, granulomatous infections, hypersensitivity pneumonia) as well as myriad disorders in which the etiological factors have not been identified (e.g., cryptogenic fibrosing alveolitis, sarcoidosis, etc.)[1–6,8,9]. Before discussing specific diseases, we review diagnostic strategies to differentiate these diverse ILDs (Table 12.1).

Pulmonary function tests (PFTs) are useful to assess extent of impairment and follow the course of the disease (natural history or response to therapy)[1,2]. Initial testing for patients with suspected ILD should include spirometry, lung volumes, single breath diffusing capacity for carbon monoxide (DL_{CO}), and oxygen saturation[10]. Characteristic physiological aberrations in ILDs include: reductions in DL_{CO} and lung volumes (e.g. vital capacity (VC), total lung capacity (TLC)), and impaired oxygenation (either at rest or with exercise)[1,10]. Formal cardiopulmonary exercise tests (CPET) are more sensitive than resting physiological testing to detect aberrations[11] but are expensive, require significant technical support, are modestly uncomfortable, and are logistically difficult (particularly in elderly or debilitated patients). Oximetry is less accurate than direct measurement of arterial blood gases, but is non-invasive and well tolerated. A 6-minute walk test with oximetry is adequate to assess the need for supplemental oxygen or evolution of disease over time[12]. Physiological tests (PFTs or CPET) cannot reliably predict prognosis or therapeutic responsiveness[13–15] but serial PFTs are invaluable to monitor the course and assess response to therapy[1,2].

Chest radiographs are often the first clue to the presence of ILD[3,5,6,16]. Parenchymal infiltrates, cystic radiolucencies or nodules are present in most patients with ILD. The distribution and pattern of radiographic lesions suggest specific ILDs[3–7,16]. Upper lobe predominance is characteristic of sarcoidosis, granulomatous infections, silicosis, pulmonary eosinophilic granuloma (EG), chronic eosinophilic pneumonia, cystic fibrosis, or ankylosing spondylitis[2–6,17]. By contrast, lower lobe predominance is highly characteristic of fibrosing alveolitis (cryptogenic or associated with collagen vascular disease) or asbestosis[2,3,5,6,17]. Although chest radiographs are non-specific, serial radiographs are invaluable in assessing chronicity or evolution of ILDs. Review of old films is critical in patients with newly diagnosed ILD.

High resolution computed tomographic scanning (HRCT), employing 1–2 mm thin sections of the lung parenchyma, is far superior to conventional chest radiographs in depicting fine parenchymal details and demarcating honeycombing, cystic changes, alveolar opacities, or interstitial disease[3,5,6]. HRCT is

Table 12.1. Diagnostic evaluation of interstitial lung disease[a]

Careful occupational, exposure, drugs, family history, risk factors
Conventional chest radiographs
    (compare with old films)
Pulmonary function tests
    Spirometry, flow-volume loop, lung volumes, DLCO, oximetry (rest, exercise)
    Formal cardiopulmonary exercise tests (arterial cannulation) (selected patients)
Serologies (selected patients)
    (e.g. collagen vascular disease profile, complement fixation for fungi, serum angiotensin converting enzyme, hypersensitivity pneumonitis screen)
High resolution thin section computed tomographic scan (HRCT)
Lung biopsy (selected patients)*
    Fibreoptic bronchoscopy (FB) with transbronchial lung biopsies and BAL
    Video-assisted thoracoscopic (VATS) lung biopsy (when FB non-diagnostic and no contraindications to surgical biopsy exist)

[a] The need for lung biopsy depends upon extent, severity, chronicity, and nature of the disease; risk/benefit of biopsy and therapeutic options available must be carefully assessed. In most patients, transbronchial lung biopsies and BAL are performed prior to considering VATS since a specific diagnosis can sometimes be made by TBBs (e.g. sarcoidosis, pulmonary alveolar proteinosis, malignancy, granulomatous infections, etc.), averting the need for surgical biopsies.
Reprinted with permission[8].

non-invasive, does not require contrast, and is useful to assess the extent and nature of the disease and prognosis[1,3,5,6,14]. The pattern of HRCT aberrations may be highly characteristic of specific etiological diagnoses (e.g. lymphangioleiomyomatosis, pulmonary EG, lymphangitic carcinomatosis)[1,3,5–7,17]. HRCT also discriminates end-stage fibrosis from potentially reversible disease[14,16,18–23]. HRCT should be part of the initial diagnostic evaluation for most patients with suspected ILD[3,6].

Radionuclide scans (e.g. gallium-[67] citrate or tech-netium-99) or positron-emission tomographic (PET) scans were used as surrogate markers of alveolitis in ILDs (e.g. sarcoidosis, IPF), but are expensive, inconvenient, non-specific, and lack prognostic value[1,17]. We see no practical role for radionuclide scans in either the diagnosis or follow-up of ILDs.

Since clinical, radiographic, and physiological manifestations of chronic ILDs overlap, lung biopsy is required to substantiate a precise diagnosis, and assess the extent and nature of the disease[5,7,24,25]. Fibreoptic bronchoscopy with transbronchial lung biopsies (TBBs), which can be done as an outpatient with light sedation, is usually performed prior to surgical lung biopsy. For some ILDs, TBBs often establishes the diagnosis (e.g. sarcoidosis, hypersensitivity pneumonitis, pulmonary alveolar proteinosis, pulmonary EG, malignancy, etc.), provided adequate parenchyma is sampled[3,4,26]. However, because of the small size (2–5 mm), TBBs cannot substantiate the diagnosis of idiopathic interstitial pneumonias (discussed in detail later) or assess the degree of inflammation or fibrosis[1,15]. When TBBs are not definitive, and the diagnosis remains uncertain, surgical lung biopsy is warranted (unless specific contraindications exist). Video-assisted thoracoscopic (VATS) lung biopsy has less morbidity than open lung biopsy, and is the preferred surgical technique[1,3]. At least two sites should be sampled (from the upper and lower lobes), to provide a representative analysis. Biopsies are obtained from apparently normal lung as well as grossly abnormal areas[1,3]. Surgical lung biopsy achieves three purposes: (*a*) alternative etiologies are definitely excluded; (*b*) the extent of inflammatory and fibrotic lesions is directly assessed; (*c*) a histopathological pattern is discerned[27–29]. Histopathological classification schema allow a precise histopathological diagnosis and have prognostic value[28,29]. Given the expense and morbidity associated with surgical lung biopsies, the decision to perform lung biopsy needs to be individualized[7]. We favour VATS lung biopsy in patients with suspected idiopathic interstitial pneumonias when clinical features, HRCT, and TBBs are equivocal provided no specific contraindications to biopsy exist. The risks of VATS are excessive in elderly or extremely debilitated patients. In such patients, we rely upon less invasive diagnostic studies, e.g. HRCT, clinical features, PFTs, TBBs. It should be emphasized that HRCT features are highly characteristic or even pathognomonic for some disorders[4–7,30]. When HRCT scans are classical for a specific diagnosis, lung biopsy is not required[3,4,7,31–23].

BAL has contributed significant insights into the pathogenesis of diverse ILDs[1,34–36], but its clinical value is limited. Characterization of cell profiles narrow the differential diagnosis in patients with ILDs. Marked lymphocytosis on BAL (>30%) is characteristic of sarcoidosis or hypersensitivity pneumonia, but is rare in cryptogenic fibrosing alveolitis (CFA)[2,17,35,36]. BAL neutrophilia is characteristic of idiopathic or collagen-vascular disease-associated FA (noted in more than 80% of patients)[1,2,17,26] but is rare in sarcoidosis[37,38]. Striking BAL eosinophilia suggests chronic or acute eosinophilic pneumonia or infectious etiologies (particularly parasitic)[39–41]. However, BAL cell profiles are not specific, and do not predict prognosis. BAL has an important role in identifying infectious organisms (particularly in immunocompromised hosts). Furthermore, specific cytological features in BAL fluid (sometimes with immunohistochemical stains) are diagnostic for specific ILDs, e.g. pulmonary EG[42]; pulmonary alveolar proteinosis[43,44].

Corticosteroids and immunosuppressive or cytotoxic agents are the mainstay of therapy for some ILDs, but have significant toxicities[1,45]. Lung transplantation is an option for severe, life-threatening chronic ILD refractory to medical therapy[46–48]. Due to a shortage of donor organs, waiting time for donor organs may be prolonged (often exceeding 2 years); patients may die while awaiting transplantation[46–48]. Contraindications to lung transplantation include: age >60 years, coronary artery disease, extrapulmonary organ failure (e.g. liver, renal, cardiac), or unstable or inadequate psychosocial profile/stability[46,48]. In the following sections, we review clinical, radiographic, and histological features of specific ILDs, and discuss therapeutic options.

Idiopathic interstitial pneumonias

Classification schema for idiopathic interstitial pneumonias recently evolved[25,29]. An initial schema defined five groups of idiopathic interstitial pneumonias based on histopathological features[49]. These five entities included: usual interstitial pneumonia (UIP); desquamative interstitial pneumonia (DIP); bronchiolitis obliterans with interstitial pneumonia (BIP); giant cell interstitial pneumonia (GIP); and lymphoid interstitial pneumonia (LIP)[49]. It was later recognized that GIP was the histopathological manifestation of hard metal pneumoconiosis[25]. BIP is primarily a disease of small airways and is now termed bronchiolitis obliterans organizing pneumonia (BOOP) or cryptogenic organizing pneumonia[25,31,50]. Subsequently, additional histopathological variants were described including: acute interstitial pneumonia (AIP)[51]; non-specific interstitial pneumonia (NSIP)[52]; and respiratory bronchiolitis interstitial lung disease (RBILD)[53,54]. In a recent review, Katzenstein and Myers proposed subdividing idiopathic interstitial pneumonias into 4 categories: UIP, DIP/RBILD, AIP, and NSIP[25]. Lymphoid interstitial pneumonia (LIP) was dropped from the schema, as this is a lymphoproliferative disorder[55]. Most experts now agree that the terms cryptogenic fibrosing alveolitis (CFA) or idiopathic pulmonary fibrosis (IPF) should be restricted to the histopathological entity UIP[1,25]. The literature continues to evolve, and the value of these histopathological classifications[25,29] is controversial. Each of these pathological entities is discussed below.

Cryptogenic fibrosing alveolitis/(idiopathic pulmonary fibrosis)

Cryptogenic fibrosing alveolitis (CFA), also termed idiopathic pulmonary fibrosis (IPF), is synonymous with the pathological variant usual interstitial pneumonia (UIP)[1,25,27]. The literature is confusing, as older published series of CFA/IPF included patients with diverse histological entities including UIP, DIP,

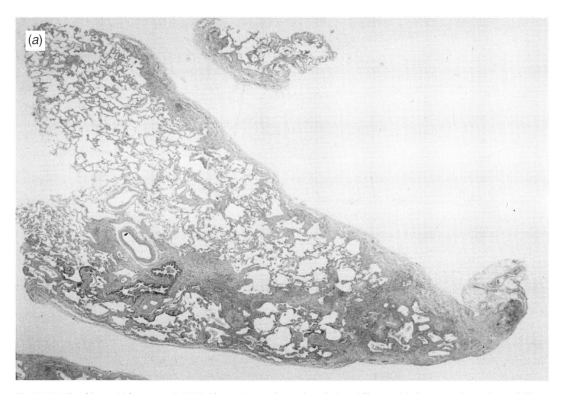

Fig. 12.1(a) Usual interstitial pneumonia (UIP). Photomicrograph: patchy subpleural fibrosis with dense scarring and remodelling of lung architecture. The fibrosis is heterogeneous with areas of relatively unaffected adjacent lung (hematoxylin–eosin). (Reproduced with permission.)[68]

RB-ILD, NSIP, and AIP[25]. These entities are distinct from UIP and the clinical syndrome CFA/IPF, and differ widely in prognosis and responsiveness to therapy. Surgical lung biopsies are required to distinguish these histopathological disorders. Cardinal histological features of UIP include: patchy, non-uniform (heterogeneous) involvement; a proclivity for bibasilar and subpleural regions; 'fibroblastic foci'; honeycomb cysts; distortion of the alveolar architecture[25,56] (Fig. 12.1(a) and 12.1(b)). Temporal heterogeneity, which can be appreciated at low power magnification, distinguishes UIP from other idiopathic interstitial pneumonias, e.g. DIP, NSIP, and AIP[25,29,31,33,56]. Aggregates of proliferating myofibroblasts and fibroblasts (termed 'fibroblastic foci') are invariably present in UIP[25]. Zones of acellular collagen bundles ('old' fibrosis), normal lung, and honeycomb change are present concomi-

tantly[25,56]. A mononuclear inflammatory cell infiltrate is present within the alveolar interstitium, but is not severe[25]. Intra-alveolar inflammation is not prominent[25,29]. Granulomas, vasculitis, microorganisms, or minerals (e.g. silica crystals, ferruginous bodies, etc.) are absent[15,25].

The estimated prevalence of CFA/UIP ranges from 5 to 29 cases per 100 000[1,15,57,58]. CFA/UIP is distinctly more common in older adults. In one study, the prevalence of CFA (per 100 000) was 2.7 among adults between the ages of 35 and 44 years but rose to 175 per 100,000 in adults older than 74 years[58]. CFA does not occur in children. While the etiology is unknown, exposure to or inhalation of minerals, dusts, organic solvents, urban pollution, or cigarette smoke is associated with an increased risk[1,59–61]. No genetic basis has been found, but familial forms exist[1,62].

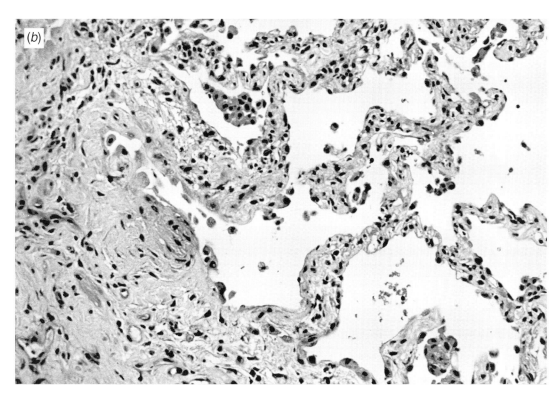

Fig. 12.1(b) Usual interstitial pneumonia (UIP). Photomicrograph: Areas of fibrosis. Fibrosis shows heterogeneity with dense eosinophilic collagen and a fibroblastic focus (hematoxylin–eosin). (Reproduced with permission.)[68]

Clinical features include cough, dyspnea, end-inspiratory velcro rales, diffuse parenchymal infiltrates on chest radiographs, honeycombing on HRCT scans, hypoxemia, and a restrictive ventilatory defect on PFTs[15,31,33,63]. Crackles are present on chest auscultation in >90% of patients; digital clubbing, in 20 to 50%[1,15,31–23,63]. Extrapulmonary involvement does not occur. Laboratory aberrations are non-specific[1,15,31,33,63].

Chest radiographs are abnormal in 95% of patients with CFA/UIP[1,15,63] (Fig. 12.2). Bilateral interstitial or reticulonodular infiltrates, with a predilection for basilar and subpleural regions, are characteristic[1]. As the disease progresses, lung volumes shrink. Similar features are found in asbestosis and collagen vascular disease-associated pulmonary fibrosis[5,6]. Intrathoracic lymphadenopathy or pleural thickening are not evident on chest radio-

graphs, but may be noted on HRCT scans[5,6]. Chest radiographs cannot predict functional impairment or responsiveness to therapy[1,15], but serial radiographs provide insight into the rate of progression of the disease[32]. HRCT scans are superior to conventional chest radiographs in depicting the salient aberrations and demarcating the extent and distribution of the disease[14,18,20,64–68]. HRCT scans in UIP reveal heterogeneity (alternating zones of normal and abnormal lung), subpleural, bibasilar predominance, honeycomb cysts, and coarse reticular lines; ground glass opacities (hazy zones of increased alveolar attenuation) are rare or absent[31,33,64] (Fig. 12.3 and 12.4). Specific HRCT *patterns* have prognostic value[14,21,64,65,69]. Ground glass opacities reflect either inflammation, i.e. alveolitis, or fibrosis[18–20,66,69–71] and sometimes regress with therapy[21,72]. Reticular or linear lines do not improve

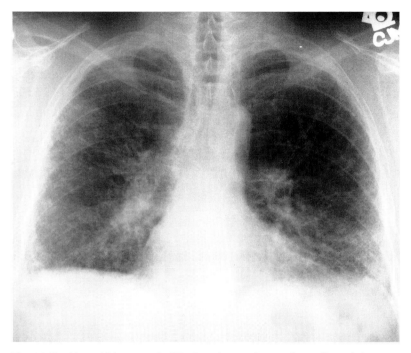

Fig. 12.2 Usual interstitial pneumonia (UIP). Posterior-anterior (PA) chest radiograph demonstrates diffuse interstitial infiltrates and areas of cystic radiolucencies. Note the peripheral predominance. VATS lung biopsy demonstrated UIP. (Reproduced with permission.)[67]

with therapy[21,72.]. Honeycomb cysts, traction bronchiectasis, or bronchioloectasis indicate irreversible destruction of alveolar walls and fibrosis[19,21,64,66,70,72]. HRCT is often used in lieu of surgical lung biopsies to diagnose UIP[32,33,56,73,74]. When HRCT scans are 'typical' or 'definite' of UIP, specificity exceeds 90%[32,33]. HRCT scans 'typical of UIP' predict a poor prognosis and low rate of response to therapy[33,56,73]. Radionuclide scans, e.g. gallium-67 citrate or positron emission tomography, have no role in the management of CFA/UIP[1].

Physiological aberrations in CFA include: reduced DL_{CO} and lung volumes; preserved expiratory flow rates (except in smokers); impaired oxygenation (at rest or with exercise)[13,15,75]. With exercise, the alveolar-arterial (A-aD02) gradient widens[1]. When concomitant emphysema is present, expiratory flow rates are reduced and lung volumes are preserved[13,20,75]. Not surprisingly, severe impairment in VC, DL_{CO}, or oxygenation are associated with worse

survival[13,15,32,57]. However, static or exercise PFTs cannot discriminate alveolitis from fibrosis or predict therapeutic responsiveness[13,14,76]. Sequential PFTs (often combined with 6-minute walk or cardiopulmonary exercise tests (CPET) are used to monitor the course of the disease. Stability or improvement in VC or DL_{CO} with corticosteroid therapy is associated with an improved prognosis and survival[14,15,76].

Bronchoalveolar lavage (BAL) fluid in CFA reveals increased numbers and percent neutrophils in >80% of patients (increases in eosinophils or lymphocytes may occur, but are less common)[1,35,36]. BAL cell profiles do not predict prognosis or therapeutic responsiveness[1].

The cause or pathogenetic mechanisms responsible for IPF are unknown. The fibrotic process involves complex interactions between inflammatory and mesenchymal cell populations[1,15]. Injury to alveolar epithelial cells, followed by an inflamma-

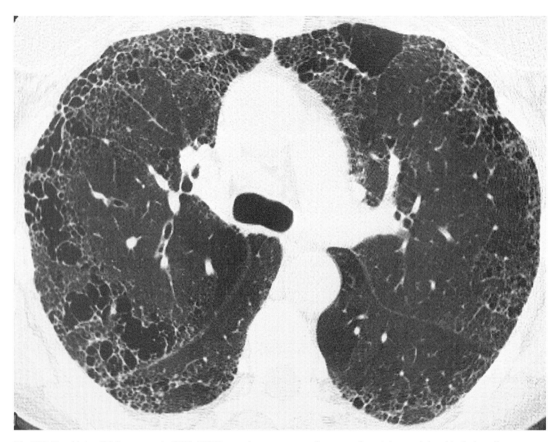

Fig. 12.3 Usual interstitial pneumonia (UIP). HRCT scan shows numerous honeycomb cysts in a peripheral (subpleural) distribution. Ground glass opacities are absent. (Reproduced with permission.)[67]

tory and reparative response, plays a central role. The factors responsible for initiation, evolution, and perpetuation of the process are not known.

CFA is a frustrating disorder to manage, since treatment is largely ineffective[31,32,57,77]. The disease progresses inexorably over months to years. Spontaneous remissions do not occur, but some patients stabilize after an initial decline[1]. Median survival from the onset of symptoms is 2.7 to 3.2 years[32,56,57]; 10-year survival, only 10 to 20%[27,29,33,56]. Response to therapy (corticosteroids or immuno-suppressive agents) is dismal (response rates, 0 to 16%)[27,29,31–23,56,66]. Earlier studies of patients with CFA/IPF cited higher response rates (10 to 28%), but included a mix of histopathological categories, e.g. UIP, NSIP, RBILD[35,36,78–81]. Survival among patients

with UIP is distinctly worse than other histological subgroups[27,29,31,33,56].

Corticosteroids have been the mainstay of therapy for CFA[15,57,77], but randomized, placebo-controlled trials are lacking, and the value of corticosteroids is debated[32,57,73,77]. Optimal dose or duration of therapy has not been studied. Some investigators initiate treatment with high dose prednisone (1.0 mg/kg/day) for 4 to 6 weeks, with gradual taper[36,81]. Lower doses have been used in Europe[2,80]. Responses to corticosteroids are achieved in fewer than 20% of patients and are incomplete[1,31,32,73,77]. Recent studies which analysed UIP as a distinct entity from NSIP or RBILD cited low rates of response to therapy (all forms)[31–23,73]. In three studies comprising 56 patients with UIP treated with

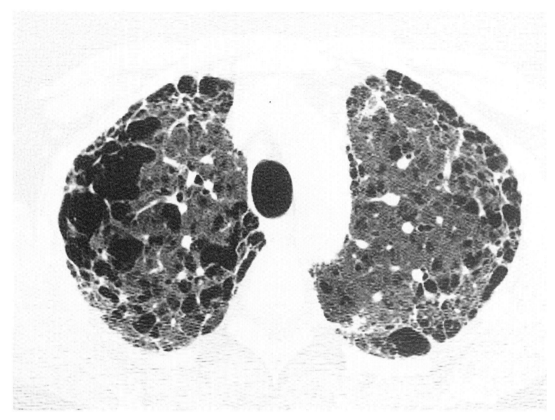

Fig. 12.4 Usual interstitial pneumonia (UIP). HRCT scan demonstrates numerous honeycomb cysts with greater involvement in peripheral (subpleural) regions. Extensive distortion and destruction of the lung parenchyma is evident. Ground glass opacities are not seen. (Reproduced with permission.)[67]

corticosteroids (alone or combined with immuno-suppressive agents), only one patient improved; >80% worsened[31,33,73]. A retrospective study of 487 patients with CFA/UIP seen at the Mayo Clinic from 1994–1996 noted that survival rates (by multivariate analysis) with prednisone, colchicine, oxygen, or immunosuppressive agents were no different than no therapy[32]. Toxicities associated with high dose corticosteroids are appreciable[15,73,77]. Two recent international consensus statements[1,2] advocate an individualized approach to therapy of CFA. Treatment is reserved for patients with significant impairment or declining lung function. The risks of treatment are balanced by potential benefits. Both consensus statements[1,2] recommend combining

prednisone or prednisolone (0.5 mg/kg/day) with either azathioprine (AZA) or cyclophosphamide (CP) as initial therapy for CFA/IPF[1,2]. These recommendations are reasonable, but published studies employing these regimens are lacking.

Importantly, therapy has *not* been shown to improve survival in CFA[1,32,57]. Anecdotal successes were cited with AZA or CP[15,33,80–82], but long-term efficacy is not established. No studies have compared AZA with CP as therapy for CFA. Published data evaluating AZA are limited to anecdotal cases and two prospective studies (only one of which was randomized)[81,82]. In both prospective studies, azathioprine (2–3 mg/kg/day) was combined with high dose prednisone. Favourable responses were noted, but the independent effect of AZA is impossible to ascertain. Despite the paucity of data, AZA may be used as initial primary therapy, as adjunctive therapy (to achieve a steroid-sparing effect), or for patients failing or experiencing adverse effects from corticosteroids.

Data evaluating cyclophosphamide (CP) are limited to several retrospective studies[32,35,57,78,83–87], one prospective, but non-randomized trial[88], and two randomized studies[80,89]. In one randomized study, 28 patients with 'mid-course IPF' were randomized to prednisone alone, CP (1.5 mg/kg/day) alone or CP plus prednisone[89]. At 6 months, BAL neutrophil counts declined among CP-treated patients but PFTs did not improve in any cohort. In a controlled trial in England, 43 patients with untreated IPF were randomized to oral CP (1 mg/kg/day) plus low dose prednisolone (20 mg every other day) or high dose prednisolone alone[80]. Patients failing therapy were crossed over to the other arm at the investigators' discretion. At one year, 5 of 21 patients receiving CP improved (defined as >10% improvement above baseline PFT); 7 of 22 in the prednisolone arm improved. By 3 years, 3 of 21 CP-treated patients had died compared to 10 of 22 deaths in the prednisone group. The apparent survival benefit with CP likely reflected differences in severity of disease between groups at the time of randomization. Among 12 patients with initial (pre-therapy) TLC below 60% of predicted, 9 were randomized to prednisolone; only 3 were randomized to CP. All 12 failed therapy. Several retrospective studies failed to demonstrate efficacy of CP[32,57,86,87,90]. In a retrospective study of 244 cases of CFA from England, the use of either CP or corticosteroids was associated with worse survival[57]. A study from the University of Iowa cited a greater rate of decline in PFTs among patients receiving CP[90]. These negative results[57,90] likely reflect selection bias, since treated patients likely had more severe disease. Others cited low response rates in CFA patients failing corticosteroids[15,86–88]. In three studies, only one of 38 patients failing >3 months of corticosteroid therapy subsequently responded to CP[86–88]. High-dose intravenous 'pulse' CP was used

to treat corticosteroid-recalcitrant CFA, but results are unimpressive[83–85]. Immunosuppressive and cytotoxic drugs have myriad potential adverse effects[45], and the appropriate use of these agents needs to be clarified. Favourable responses to cyclosporine A were cited in retrospective studies[91–93], but data are sparse. Cyclosporine A is exceptionally expensive and causes a plethora of adverse effects[45]. Currently, we see little role for cyclosporine A as therapy for CFA. Other cytotoxic drugs such as methotrexate or mycophenolate mofetil have not been studied in CFA.

Agents with potential antifibrotic activity have been tried as therapy for CFA, but are of unproven value. D-Penicillamine was tried, but data affirming benefit are lacking[2,94]. Given its toxicities, we see no role for this agent in IPF. Colchicine, which suppresses fibroblast growth factors in vitro and inhibits collagen deposition in animal models, was tried in retrospective[32,95] and prospective trials[73]. Colchicine is safer than prednisone, but its value is unproven. In summary, the prognosis of CFA/UIP is poor, with a low rate of response to existing therapies.

Improved survival in CFA/UIP awaits the development of novel therapies. Recently, investigators from Austria cited beneficial responses with interferon gamma-1b (γ-IFN-1b) plus low dose corticosteroids in an open, randomized trial of 18 CFA patients failing therapy with corticosteroids or immunosuppressive agents[96]. These data are intriguing, but additional studies are required to determine the role of γ-IFN to treat CFA. A multicentre randomized study in the United States evaluating γ-IFN is planned. Recently, a multicentre, placebo-controlled trial assessing β-interferon (*Avonex*) (Biogen, Cambridge, MA) for CFA patients failing conventional therapy, i.e. corticosteroids or immunosuppressive therapy, was completed in the United States; results are not yet published. Possible future therapies include: perfenidone[7], lovastatin[97], proline inhibitors[98], antioxidants[99], inhibitors of leukocyte integrins, cytokines and proteases[100].

Single lung transplantation is the preferred option for patients with severe CFA failing medical

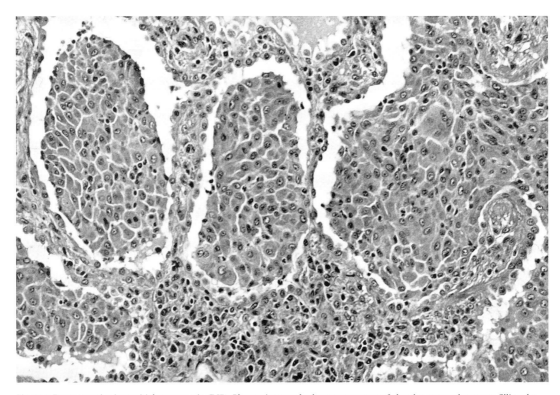

Fig. 12.5 Desquamative interstitial pneumonia (DIP). Photomicrograph: dense aggregates of alveolar macrophages are filling the airspaces. The process is extensive and diffuse. The alveolar architecture is preserved. Fibrosis or honeycomb cysts are absent. (Hematoxylin–eosin). (Reproduced with permission.)[68]

therapy[46–48]. Patients with severe functional impairment (FVC<60% predicted or DLCO<40% predicted), oxygen dependency, and deteriorating status should be listed promptly since waiting time for transplantation may exceed 2 or even 3 years[48]. Two- and 5-year survival rates following single lung transplantation approximate 70% and 50%, respectively[46,47].

Desquamative interstitial pneumonia (DIP) and respiratory bronchiolitis interstitial lung disease (RBILD)

Desquamative interstitial pneumonia (DIP) lacks the heterogeneity of UIP noted on surgical lung biopsies; the alveolar architecture is preserved and fibrosis is mild or absent[25,27,56]. Fibroblastic foci, a cardinal feature of UIP, are not found in DIP[25]. The most striking feature of DIP is filling of alveolar spaces with macrophages containing finely granular, yellow–brown pigment derived from complex phagolysosomes[25,27,56] (Fig. 12.5). Bronchiolar inflammation and lymphoid aggregates may be present[29] but interstitial inflammation or honeycomb cysts are absent or minimal[25].

DIP is much less common than UIP[25,29,56]. In retrospective reviews of surgical lung biopsies performed for diffuse lung disease, DIP was found in 8 to 18% of biopsies; UIP was found in 27 to 62%[29,56,74]. UIP and DIP differ strikingly in HRCT features, therapeutic responsiveness, and prognosis[31,64,65,69]. Compared to UIP, patients with DIP are younger[27,29,56], exhibit dense ground-glass opacities with minimal or no honeycombing on HRCT scans

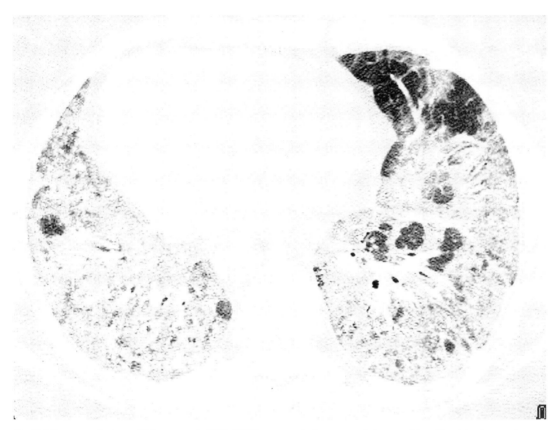

Fig. 12.6 Desquamative interstitial pneumonia (DIP). HRCT scan reveals dense ground glass opacities with minimal areas of normal lung parenchyma. Honeycomb cysts are not seen. (Hematoxylin–eosin). (Reproduced with permission.) [68]

(Fig. 12.6), and usually respond to corticosteroids[27,54,65,66,69,70,74]. Long-term prognosis of DIP is excellent. Improvement can occur spontaneously[27], following cessation of cigarette smoking[54], or with corticosteroid therapy[27,29,66]. Corticosteroids are warranted for patients with symptoms or progressive disease following cessation of smoking[27,29,56]. Five-year survival exceeds 90%[27,29,56]. Progression to severe honeycombing is rare[66].

Another histological variant, termed respiratory bronchiolitis interstitial lung disease (RBILD), is characterized by dense collections of pigmented alveolar macrophages within respiratory bronchioles; the distal lung parenchyma is spared[25,53,54,101]. Honeycombing is minimal or absent[25,53,54]. Microscopic centrilobular emphysema is common[102]. The

pathological lesion respiratory bronchiolitis (RB) was originally described in 1974 in an autopsy series of young cigarette smokers who died of non-pulmonary causes[103]. The lesions were subsequently termed 'small airways disease'[104] or 'smoker's bronchiolitis'[101] or 'respiratory bronchiolitis-associated interstitial lung disease' (RBILD)[25,54]. Histological features overlap with DIP, but DIP is more uniform and extensive than RBILD and exhibits a striking intra-alveolar component[25,54].

More than 90% of cases of RBILD occur in smokers[53,54,102], but some cases are ascribed to noxious or occupational exposures[102]. Most experts believe that RBILD and DIP share a common pathogenesis and are responses to constituents in cigarette smoke or inhaled noxious agents[25]. Patients are

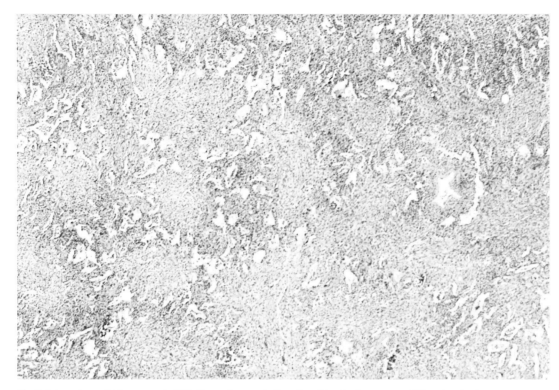

Fig. 12.7 Acute interstitial pneumonia (AIP). Photomicrograph: Open lung biopsies demonstrate diffuse alveolar damage, organizing phase. The process is extensive and diffuse. Honeycomb cysts are absent. (Hematoxylin-eosin). (Reproduced with permission.)[68]

relatively young (mean age 36 years)[53,54] with mild symptoms of cough, dyspnea, or sputum production[53,54,102]. Chest radiographs show small irregular opacities ('dirty lungs')[101] or reticular or reticulonodular infiltrates[54] but are normal in up to 28% of patients with RBILD [54]. HRCT scans reveal numerous, 2 to 3 mm irregular peribronchiolar nodules; ground glass opacities or emphysema may also be present[102,105].

The prognosis of RB or RBILD is excellent[25,53,54] but data are limited. Smoking cessation is the mainstay of therapy. Following cessation of smoking, symptoms improve or resolve in >90% of patients[53,54]. Corticosteroids were used in a minority of patients[53,54]. Severe pulmonary fibrosis is rare[101], but patients may deteriorate[102]. British investigators identified 10 patients of RBILD from 1980 to 1998; 6 had previously been classified as 'cryptogenic fibrosing alveolitis'[102]. Seven were treated with prednisolone (combined with AZA or CP in 6)[102]. Three deteriorated despite treatment *and* cessation of smoking. The spectrum of RBILD is broader than in the original descriptions[53,54]; additional studies are required to elucidate the long-term prognosis.

Acute interstitial pneumonia (Hamman–Rich syndrome)

Acute interstitial pneumonia (formerly Hamman–Rich syndrome) is the most fulminant of the idiopathic interstitial pneumonias, progressing to fatal respiratory failure within 1 to 6 months (often within a few days)[25,51,56,106–109]. Histologically, AIP is characterized by acute and organizing diffuse alveolar damage (DAD) with hyaline membranes, fibrinous exudates, and epithelial cell necrosis[51] (Fig. 12.7).

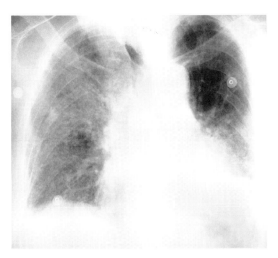

Fig. 12.8 Acute interstitial pneumonia. PA chest radiograph in a 71-year-old male with known UIP (for >2 years) who presented with acute decompensation, severe hypoxemia requiring mechanical ventilatory support. Note confluent alveolar opacification in the right upper lobe. Bibasilar infiltrates are also present. The left hemidiaphragm is elevated consistent with prior phrenic nerve injury. Open lung biopsy demonstrated AIP with diffuse alveolar damage (DAD). No infectious cause was identified. Following high dose i.v. methylprednisolone, he improved dramatically and the right upper lobe infiltrate resolved completely.

Additional features include: intra-alveolar hemorrhage; interstitial and intra-alveolar edema; proliferating type II alveolar cells; interstitial mononuclear cell infiltrates; fibroblasts and myofibroblasts[25,29,51]. The changes are temporally uniform and relatively acute[25]. Proliferating fibroblasts are numerous but collagen deposition (a marker of old fibrosis) is minimal[25,106]. As the process heals, hyaline membranes are resorbed and connective tissue proliferates within the interstitium and airspaces[51,106]. The histological features of AIP are non-specific, and are found with myriad disorders including acute respiratory distress syndrome (ARDS), inhalation or drug-induced injury[25,106], collagen vascular diseases[110–112], vasculitis[113,114], or infections[25,106]. In addition, a subset of patients with CFA develop an accelerated course, often as a terminal event, with features of DAD on lung biopsy or necropsy[107,109,115] (Fig. 12.8).

The factors responsible for this accelerated phase of CFA are unknown, but viral infections, high concentrations of oxygen, or drug reactions are plausible etiological factors[109].

The clinical presentation and course of AIP is similar to ARDS[107,109,116]. The onset is acute (1–2 weeks), with cough, dyspnea, bilateral alveolar infiltrates, hypoxemia, and progressive respiratory failure requiring mechanical ventilation[107,109,116]. Fever and an antecedent viral illness are present in 50% of patients[25,106,109,116]. Mean age at onset is 49 years (range 7 to 83 years); there is no gender predominance[109]. HRCT scans reveal extensive, homogeneous ground glass opacities with consolidation; in the acute phases, honeycombing is absent[107,109,116–118] (Fig. 12.9). In later phases (>7 days after the onset), foci of honeycombing, traction bronchiectasis, and distortion may be observed[109,116–118]. Data are limited, but BAL neutrophilia has been noted[109,115].

Initial treatment is supportive, with supplemental oxygen and mechanical ventilation (often with positive end-expiratory pressure)[106,109,116]. Most patients die within 1 month; >70% die within 6 months[51,106,109,116,118]. Although data regarding therapy are sparse, some patients respond dramatically to high dose corticosteroids[51,106–108]. We advocate high dose intravenous methylprednisolone (250 to 1000 mg/day, for 3–4 days), with subsequent taper. The roles of cytotoxic agents, surfactant, anticytokine antibodies, or inhaled nitric oxide are not known[109]. Patients surviving the initial episode of AIP may heal with no sequelae or with variable degrees of fibrosis[51,106,109]. Survivors do not develop progressive disease and do not evolve to CFA[106,109].

Non-specific interstitial pneumonitis/fibrosis (NSIP)

The term non-specific interstitial pneumonitis/fibrosis (NSIP) was proposed in 1994 for cases of idiopathic interstitial pneumonias that do not fit histopathological criteria for the other categories (i.e. UIP, DIP/RBILD, AID)[25,52]. Since clinical, physio-

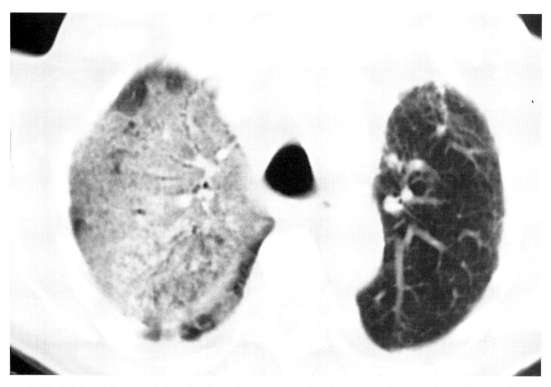

Fig. 12.9 Acute interstitial pneumonia (AIP). HRCT scan from the same patient demonstrates dense alveolar opacification of the right upper lobe. Honeycombing is absent. The left lung demonstrates a few thick septal lines but is relatively unaffected.

logical, and radiographic features of NSIP overlap with UIP and DIP, examples of NSIP prior to 1994 were included in series of CFA or IPF. Several recent studies[29,31,33,56,119], after re-reviewing open lung biopsies previously labelled as CFA or IPF, identified a significant proportion (10 to 15%) of patients with histological features consistent with NSIP. Other terms previously used to refer to NSIP include 'unclassified pneumonia'[120] or 'cellular interstitial pneumonia'[25,110]. NSIP may complicate collagen vascular disease (CVD)[110,119] and is a stereotypic response to diverse lung injuries or toxins[25,121]. The term NSIP is confusing, since this previously referred to a non-specific histological lesion in immunocompromised hosts (HIV-infected patients or bone marrow transplant recipients)[122–124]. Currently, the term idiopathic NSIP is reserved for a specific histological lesion in immunocompetent

hosts with clinical and radiographic features mimicking CFA/UIP[52].

Although NSIP resembles UIP and DIP clinically, these entities are distinguished by histopathological criteria. The cardinal feature differentiating NSIP from UIP is the temporal homogeneity seen in NSIP[25,52] (Fig. 12.10). In NSIP, the lesions are of similar age; in UIP both recent and old lesions are present concomitantly[8,25,31,52,56]. Inflammation and fibrosis are observed in both NSIP and UIP, but honeycombing is rarely severe in NSIP[25,29,31,33,56]. Compared to UIP, NSIP is associated with less fibrosis and less destruction of the alveolar architecture[25,27]. Foci of BOOP, bronchiolocentricity, germinal centres, and granulomas are often noted in NSIP, but are not found in UIP[29,31,33,52,119] (Fig. 12.11). Compared to UIP, patients with NSIP are younger[29,33,56] and there is a slight female predomi-

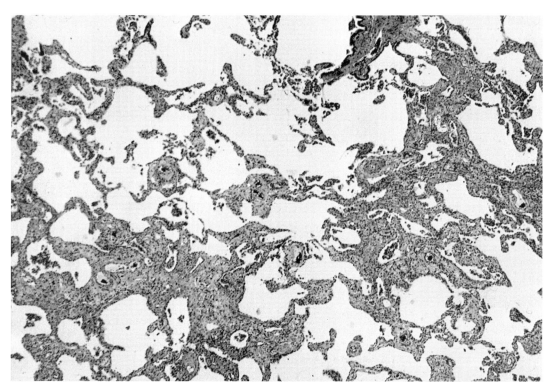

Fig. 12.10 Non-specific interstitial pneumonia (NSIP). Photomicrograph demonstrates patchy interstitial fibrosis that lacks the subpleural distribution and temporal heterogeneity of UIP. (Reproduced with permission.)[68]

nance[25,31,125]. The clinical course is subacute in NSIP (1 to 4 months), but insidious in UIP (>1–2 years)[31]. Fever, noted in one third of patients with NSIP, is never seen in UIP[31]. Chest radiographic and HRCT features differ between NSIP and UIP. Bilateral patchy alveolar or ground glass opacities are a prominent feature of NSIP but are rare in UIP[31,33,125,126] (Fig. 12.12). Honeycombing, a cardinal feature of UIP, is rare in NSIP[31,33,125]. BAL lymphocytosis is common in NSIP, but rare in UIP[31,119].

Most importantly, the prognosis of NSIP is better than UIP. More than two thirds of patients with NSIP improve (with or without therapy)[31,52]. Three year survival exceeds 80%[29,31,33,56]. Prognosis is influenced by the degree of fibrosis or cellularity on surgical lung biopsies[29,31,52,119]. Patients with 'cellular' NSIP have a better prognosis (fatalities, <10%) compared to 'fibrotic' NSIP (fatalities, 13–65%)[29,31,33]. The designa-

tion NSIP is excessively broad, and should be replaced by categories of 'cellular' or 'fibrotic' forms[29]. All of these studies were retrospective, so conclusions are limited. Prospective studies are required to elucidate the long-term prognosis of NSIP.

Collagen vascular diseases

Pulmonary complications of collagen vascular disorders (CVDs) are protean, and are important causes of morbidity and mortality[127]. Fibrosing alveolitis (FA) complicates diverse CVDs, and can be the presenting feature[26]. The spectrum of histopathological changes of CVD-FA includes: UIP; NSIP; cellular or follicular bronchiolitis; bronchiolitis obliterans (with or without organizing pneumonia)[25,26,110,128]. Progressive pulmonary fibrosis, indistinguishable

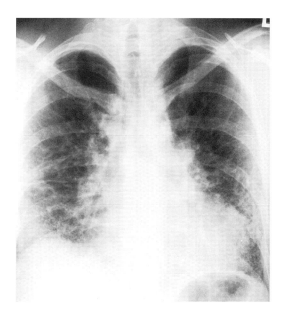

Fig. 12.11 Non-specific interstitial pneumonia (NSIP). PA chest radiograph demonstrates diffuse interstitial infiltrates. Note the peripheral predominance. VATS lung biopsy demonstrated NSIP.

clinically, physiologically, and radiographically from CFA, can occur[26,129]. However, the course of CVD-FA is more indolent than CFA[26,129]. Symptoms of non-productive cough or dyspnea progress slowly over years[26]. End-inspiratory (velcro) bibasilar rales are typical[26]. Bibasilar reticular infiltrates, shrinking lung volumes, and honeycombing on chest radiographs evolve over months or years[26,129]. PFTs demonstrate reduced lung volumes and/or DLCO[26,129]. Chest radiographs or PFTs cannot assess the extent of alveolitis or fibrosis, but serial studies are invaluable to follow the course of the disease. Historically, the approach to CVD-FA was nihilistic, owing to the chronicity of the process, low rate of response to therapy, and need for long-term (potentially toxic) therapy. Optimal therapy of CVD-FA is controversial, but corticosteroids and immunosuppressive or cytotoxic agents may ablate any inflammatory component. Therapy should be stratified according to acuity and severity of disease, to identify patients at greatest risk for disease progression who may benefit from therapy.

Progressive systemic sclerosis (PSSc)

Pulmonary complications of PSSc include: fibrosing alveolitis, pulmonary hypertension, recurrent aspiration pneumonia (among patients with severe esophageal dysfunction), and rarely, bronchiolitis obliterans, pulmonary hemorrhage, or bronchioloalveolar cell carcinoma[26]. In this chapter, we discuss only FA, which affects most patients with PSSc at some point during the course of the disease. Chronic FA is the most common cause of death from PSSc[18,129,130]. More than 80% of patients with PSS exhibit FA at necropsy[26]. Chest radiographs demonstrate reticular or reticulonodular infiltrates consistent with FA in 20 to 45% of patients with PSSc[26]. Dilatation of the esophagus (reflecting aperistalsis) or pulmonary hypertension are sometimes present[26]. Pulmonary function tests are similar to CFA, except 15 to 30% of PSSc-FA patients exhibit an obstructive component (likely reflecting peribronchiolar fibrosis)[26]. The course of PSSc-FA is heterogenous[26] but most patients deteriorate gradually over many years[18,127,129]. The course is less severe than IPF, even when HRCT scans and PFTs are comparable at presentation[18,129]. In a recent study, 5-year survival from the onset of dyspnea was 86% in patients with PSSc-FA compared to only 50% with CFA[129]. Neither the duration of PSSc nor the extent of extrapulmonary involvement correlate with the extent of FA[131]. Histological features of PSSc-FA are similar to IPF/CFA[26]. Additional features include follicular bronchiolitis and small airway disease[18]. Increases in inflammatory cells (e.g., neutrophils, eosinophils, or lymphocytes) were found in most patients with PSSc, even when PFTs and HRCT were normal[18,131,132]. Factors associated with a deteriorating course and likelihood of developing pulmonary hypertension include: peripheral vascular involvement, digital pitting or ulcerations, severe Raynaud's phenomenon, and a history of smoking[26,133]. Pulmonary hypertension or DLCO less than 40% predict an increased mortality[26,133].

Because of the indolent course of PSSc-FA, and potential adverse effects with therapy, the historical approach has been nihilistic. However, a subset of

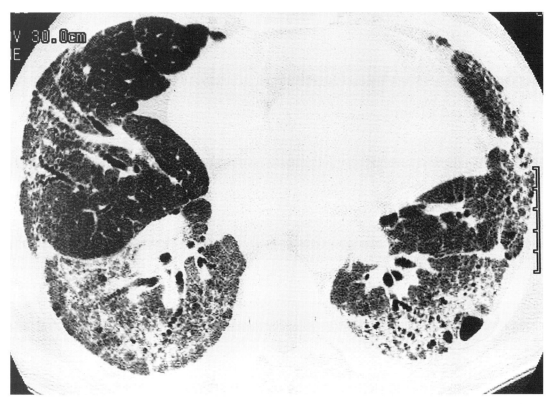

Fig. 12.12 Non-specific interstitial pneumonia (NSIP). HRCT scan reveals areas of ground glass opacities and small honeycomb cysts. Note the focal, peripheral (subpleural) predominance. VATS lung biopsy demonstrated NSIP.

patients with PSSc manifest active alveolitis[127,131,132,134] and may benefit from treatment. Although controlled, randomized therapeutic trials are lacking, anecdotal responses were achieved with corticosteroids or immunosuppressive agents[127,134–136]. Several studies cited favourable responses with CP (oral or i.v. pulse) for PSSc, even in patients failing corticosteroids[134–136]. In one retrospective study, improvement in VC was greatest among PSSc-FA patients treated with CP compared to D-penicillamine, corticosteroids, other immunosuppressive agents, or no therapy[136]. A prospective, non-randomized trial cited improvement in PFTs in 14 of 18 patients treated with oral CP (2–2.5 mg/kg/day) plus prednisone[135]. In a recent study, monthly i.v. pulse CP (750 mg/m²) for 12 months was as effective as daily oral CP (2–2.5 mg/kg) for the same period[137]. All patients received concurrent cor-

ticosteroids (10 mg/day)[137]. Neither regimen was effective when a reticular appearance predominated on HRCT[137]. Rates of response are likely highest if active alveolitis is present[135,136]. Although CP is the best studied agent for PSSc-FA, potential long term sequelae (including neoplasia) make CP less attractive for long-term use[45]. Data evaluating other agents are limited. In two uncontrolled studies, D-penicillamine was of equivocal benefit compared to corticosteroids[138] or no treatment[139]. In a non-randomized trial, cyclosporin did not affect pulmonary or cardiac involvement in 10 patients with PSSc[140]. Chlorambucil was ineffective in one three-year randomized, prospective study[141]. Published data employing azathioprine (AZA) for PSSc-FA are lacking. A recent international consensus panel[2] suggested using CP plus low dose prednisolone for patients with PSSc-FA requiring therapy. We do not believe treatment is indicated for most patients with PSSc-FA, but an empirical trial of therapy is reasonable in patients with an acute or subacute course, particularly if ancillary evidence for alveolitis, e.g. ground glass opacities on HRCT; lymphocytosis on BAL, are present. In this context, CP, AZA, or corticosteroids (alone or in combination) can be considered.

Rheumatoid arthritis (RA)

Pleuropulmonary manifestations of rheumatoid arthritis (RA) are protean and include: pleural effusions; fibrosing alveolitis; obliterative bronchiolitis (with or without organizing pneumonia); lymphocytic infiltration of the walls of small airways; rheumatoid pulmonary nodules; Caplan's syndrome; pulmonary vasculitis; bronchiectasis; pulmonary hypertension[26]. Complications related to pharmacological therapy of RA include opportunistic infections[142] or toxic or hypersensitivity pneumonias[26,45,143,144]. In this chapter, we limit our discussion to FA complicating RA (also termed 'rheumatoid lung').

The prevalence of FA in RA varies widely (3 to 41%) among published studies, which reflects heterogeneous patient populations and different methods to detect disease[26]. The presence of FA does not correlate with extent, duration, or activity of the articular or systemic components[26]. Risk factors for RA-FA include: male gender; age >60 years; history of smoking; high titres of circulating rheumatoid factor; variant α-1-antitrypsin phenotypes, and HLA-B40[26]. Aberrations in chest radiographs or PFTs are common, even in asymptomatic patients. Aberrations in HRCT scan were noted in 29 to 52% of patients with RA, even in the absence of pulmonary symptoms[16,145–147]. Pulmonary function tests reveal restrictive defects or reduced DLCO in 10 to 40% of patients with RA, even without pulmonary symptoms. Histological features of 'rheumatoid lung' are similar to CFA, but additional features may be observed, e.g. lymphoid hyperplasia, LIP; follicular bronchiolitis; rheumatoid nodules[26].

The course of FA complicating RA is usually indolent, but 1 to 4% of patients with RA develop severe, disabling FA[26]. The natural history of asymptomatic rheumatoid lung disease is not known. However, among symptomatic patients with RA-FA, 5-year mortality exceeds 30%[26,148]. In an autopsy series of 81 patients with RA, pulmonary fibrosis was present in 35%; 8 patients died of respiratory failure[149]. Optimal therapy is not clear, as controlled therapeutic trials have not been done. Treatment of rheumatoid lung disease is similar to FA complicating other CVDs. Corticosteroids are most often used as initial therapy[26]. Immunosuppressive or cytotoxic agents are reserved for patients failing or intolerant of corticosteroids[26,148,150,151].

Polymyositis and dermatomyositis

Pulmonary complications of polymyositis (PM) or dermatomyositis (DM) include: respiratory failure due to severe neuromuscular weakness; aspiration pneumonia due to weakness of the pharyngeal musculature; diaphragmatic paresis or dysfunction; fibrosing alveolitis; bronchiolitis obliterans (with or without organizing pneumonia); opportunistic infections[26,110,128]. We limit our discussion to FA which complicates PM/DM in 3 to 10% of patients[26]. Clinical, radiographic, physiological, and histopathological features are similar to FA complicating other CVDs[16,26]. The course is usually gradual and insidious, but acute, fatal respiratory insufficiency can occur[26]. Fibrosing alveolitis occurs at any point in the course of PM or DM, and may be the presenting feature[110]. The severity of FA does not correlate with the course of the muscle disease, muscle enzymes, or systemic features[26,110]. Serological markers identify patients at greatest risk for FA. Circulating autoantibodies to the enzyme histidyl-tRNA-synthetase (anti-Jo1, anti-PL7, and anti-PL-12) or KJ are present in a majority of patients with PM or DM *with* FA but in <20% of patients with PM or DM *without* FA[26,152]. These autoantibodies are rarely present in other CVDs[26,152,153]. Long-term prognosis of FA is poor, with 3 year fatality rates exceeding 30% in some studies[26,110].

Corticosteroids are the cornerstone of therapy for myopathic and systemic manifestations of PM or DM, but data evaluating FA are sparse[153]. Corticosteroids are most likely to be efficacious in patients with active alveolitis and before irreversible damage has been incurred[26,110]. Immunosuppressive or cytotoxic agents are reserved for patients failing or intolerant of corticosteroids. Anecdotal successes have been cited with methotrexate, azathioprine, cyclophosphamide, or cyclosporine A[153]. In a recent study, six patients with rapidly progressive FA complicating diverse CVDs were treated with monthly i.v. pulse CP plus prednisone for 6 to 9 months[154]. All 6 improved (based on PFTs, exercise capacity, HRCT, and BAL cell counts)[154]. Remissions were then maintained with hydroxychloroquine, azathioprine or cyclosporine A[154]. Others cited response to i.v. pulse CP, followed by oral azathioprine, in a patient with corticosteroid-recalcitrant FA[155]. In a separate study, cyclosporine A was effective in all 5 patients with FA complicating PM or DM who had failed corticosteroids[156]. Patients without elevated creatine phosphokinase (CPK) levels were more likely to be resistant to corticosteroids[156]. These reports are encouraging, but data are sparse and the optimal agent for FA complicating PM or DM has not been elucidated.

Systemic lupus erythematosus

Pleuropulmonary complications of systemic lupus erythematosus (SLE) are protean[157–159]. Pleuritis is the most common thoracic manifestation, affecting 45 to 60% of patients during the course of the disease[157,158]. Pulmonary complications of SLE included acute lupus pneumonitis, fibrosing alveolitis, alveolar hemorrhage (capillaritis); pulmonary embolism (often due to circulating anticardiolipin antibodies); bronchiolitis obliterans (with or without organizing pneumonia)[128,160]; cavitating pulmonary nodules; pulmonary vasculitis; diaphragmatic dysfunction; opportunistic infections or drug toxicity from immunosuppressive therapy[45,142].

Pulmonary hemorrhage is a rare and potentially

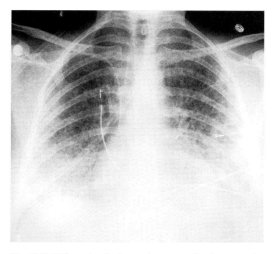

Fig. 12.13 Diffuse alveolar hemorrhage complicating systemic lupus erythematosus (SLE). PA chest radiograph demonstrating bilateral alveolar infiltrates in a 22-year-old female with SLE, hemoptysis, anemia, and acute renal failure. Bronchoscopy demonstrated fresh blood, serosanguinous BAL fluid, and hemosiderin-laden macrophages.

fatal complication of SLE[161]. Diffuse alveolar hemorrhage (DAH) presents with bilateral alveolar infiltrates, hypoxemia, dyspnea, and anemia[158,161] (Fig. 12.13). DAH usually occurs in patients with a known history of SLE, high titres of circulating anti-DNA antibody, and active extrapulmonary disease[158,161]. Glomerulonephritis is often present[158,159,161]. The diagnosis can be assumed in the appropriate clinical context by bronchoscopy with BAL[157]. The presence of gross blood in the airways, serosanguinous BAL fluid, hemosiderin-laden macrophages, absence of purulent sputum, and lack of infectious organisms by appropriate stains strongly support the diagnosis of DAH. Open lung biopsy has potential morbidity in patients with life-threatening DAH and is rarely warranted. Although randomized trials are lacking, high dose intravenous pulse methylprednisolone is recommended[157]. Cyclophosphamide is reserved for corticosteroid failures. Plasmapheresis has been used, with anecdotal successes, but is reserved for severe DAH refractory to corticosteroids and cytotoxic agents[162,163].

Acute lupus pneumonitis, presenting as cough,

dyspnea, hypoxemia, and fever, occurs in 1–4% of patients with SLE[157,158,164]. This entity as controversial, as features overlap with DAH and myriad other causes (including infection). Lung biopsies are obtained infrequently. Histological features overlap with acute DAH; inflammatory cellular infiltrates, edema, hemorrhage, hyaline membranes, and capillaritis may be present[157]. Data evaluating therapy are spare. Corticosteroids are recommended for patients with a fulminant course, provided infectious etiologies are excluded. Immunosuppressive or cytotoxic agents are reserved for corticosteroid-recalcitrant patients.

Clinically significant FA complicates SLE in 3 to 13% of patients, but is rarely severe[127,157,158]. Asymptomatic FA is common. Chest radiographic abnormalities consistent with FA are present in 6 to 24% of patients in unselected patients with SLE[157,165]; abnormalities in PFTs are noted in up to two-thirds of patients[158,165]. In a recent prospective study of 34 patients with SLE who had HRCT scans, features consistent with FA were present in 11 patients (9 had pulmonary symptoms)[165]. PFTs were abnormal in 7 of these 11 patients. Mild or asymptomatic FA is common, but severe pulmonary fibrosis is rare[127,157,158]. A review of 120 necropsies in SLE patients detected moderate or severe pulmonary fibrosis in only 4 patients[166]. Histological features of FA complicating SLE are non-specific and include: varying degrees of chronic inflammatory cell infiltrates; peribronchial lymphoid hyperplasia; interstitial fibrosis; hyperplasia of type II pneumocytes[157,158]. The presence of scleroderma-like traits (e.g. Raynaud's phenomenon, swollen fingers, sclerodactyly, telangiectasia, dyspnea, nailfold capillary abnormalities) among patients with SLE was associated with a higher prevalence of restrictive defects or reduced DLCO[167]. Progressive, severe FA rarely complicates SLE, but may be seen in a subset of patients with SLE in the context of overlap syndrome[157] (Fig. 12.14). Data evaluating therapy are sparse. Corticosteroids, immunosuppressive or cytotoxic agents may be efficacious, but therapeutic trials are lacking[157,158].

Overlap syndrome and mixed connective tissue disease (MCTD)

Overlap syndrome is characterized by clinical manifestations overlapping with two or more of the five major CVDs (e.g., PSSc, RA, PM, DM, or SLE)[26]. Features of two or more CVDs may occur concurrently, or the disease may evolve from one CVD to another. Early manifestations include arthralgias, Raynaud's phenomenon, myalgias, esophageal dysfunction, and circulating antinuclear antibodies[26]. Mixed Connective Tissue Disease (MCTD) displays overlapping features of SLE, PSSc, or PM; high titre circulating antibodies (anti-RNP) to a ribonuclease-sensitive extractable nuclear antigen (ENA) and a speckled antinuclear antibody (ANA) are present; antibodies to Sm are absent[168]. The designation of MCTD as a distinct clinical syndrome is controversial. Pulmonary manifestations occur in up to 85% of patients with MCTD. Of these, fibrosing alveolitis[168] and pulmonary hypertension[169] are the most common and important. Rare pulmonary complications include: recurrent aspiration pneumonias (in patients with esophageal dysmotility); BOOP; pulmonary hemorrhage[26]. Fibrosing alveolitis develops in 25 to 85% of patients with MCTD during the course of the disease[26,168,170]. The clinical expression of FA complicating MCTD is variable. Treatment is similar to FA complicating other CVDs.

Sjogren's syndrome (SS)

Sjogren's syndrome (SS) is characterized by lymphocytic infiltration and destruction of exocrine glands and symptoms of xerostomia and/or xerophthalmia (sicca syndrome)[26]. Sjogren's syndrome may occur as a primary syndrome (pSS) or as a secondary syndrome (sSS) in the context of a specific autoimmune disorder, e.g. RA, SLE, PM/DM, PSSc[26]. The incidence of pSS is 1 in 2500; sSS is more common (up to 0.5% of the population)[26,171]. Pulmonary manifestations of primary or secondary SS are protean and include: FA; LIP; lymphoproliferative disorders (pseudolymphoma and lymphoma), xerotrachea; BOOP; pleural effusions or fibrosis[26]. Fibrosing

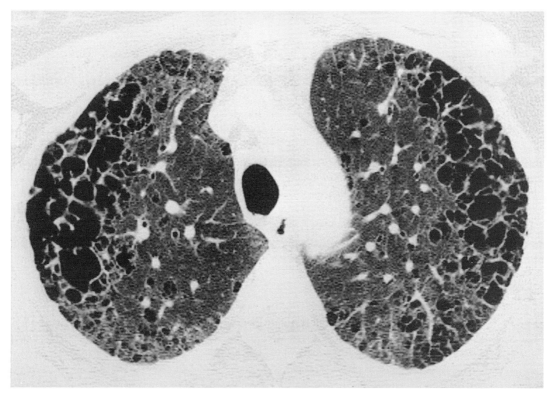

Fig. 12.14 Usual interstitial pneumonia (UIP) complicating overlap syndrome. HRCT scan demonstrates extensive honeycomb cysts which a predilection for the peripheral (subpleural) regions in a patient with overlapping features of PSSc and SLE.

alveolitis complicating SS is indistinguishable from FA complicating other CVDs[26]. The reported incidence of FA in SS ranges from 9 to 55%[26,172–175], reflecting variations in diagnostic testing and populations studied. Chest radiographs are abnormal in 25 to 62% of patients with SS; PFTs are abnormal in 25 to 44%[172–175]. Several studies detected alveolitis (as assessed by BAL, gallium-67 scans, or HRCT) in approximately 50% of patients with SS, even in asymptomatic patients[26,171,174]. Overall, pulmonary complications are more common in sSS, but FA is more common in pSS[26,171]. Clinical or serological features fail to identify patients with SS most likely to develop pulmonary disease[171,173,174]. Histopathological features are similar to FA complicating other CVDs[26,171,176].

The course of FA complicating SS is variable, and treatment is not well defined. Favourable responses were cited with corticosteroids, AZA or CP[171,177], but controlled treatment trials have not been done. In one study, 11 patients with SS-FA were treated with AZA (6 received corticosteroids concomitantly)[171]. Vital capacity improved by at least 10% in 7 patients (66%). None of 5 untreated patients improved. Others cited favourable responses to low dose cyclosporine A (1 mg/kg), even in corticosteroid-refractory FA complicating SS[178–180].

Occupational lung disease

Materials inhaled at the workplace can induce upper or lower airway injury[181–183]. The spectrum of illness is broad, and ranges from rhinitis, laryngitis, tracheitis, bronchitis, bronchiolitis, asthma, pneumonitis, or even life-threatening respiratory failure[181–184]. Isocyanates, widely used in polyurethane foams and paints, cause occupational asthma[181] but >250 substances evoke similar responses[181,183,185]. Diverse occupational substances produce industrial bronchitis, e.g. welding, noxious chemicals, mining, storage and processing of grains and feeds, cotton textile milling, etc.[181,184,186,187]. Severe bronchiolitis obliterans or constrictive bronchiolitis may follow exposure to nitrogen dioxide (silo filler's disease), chlorine, or noxious chemicals[181,188]. Several occupational dusts cause or contribute to chronic obstructive lung disease or emphysema[181,187,189,190]. Beryllium dust, silica, and hard metals, e.g. cadmium, cobalt, manganese, aluminium, cause severe, progressive pneumoconiosis[181,191–195]. The link between exposure to an offending noxious agent, irritant, or allergen may not be obvious, since only a small proportion of exposed individuals develop clinical symptoms. Differences in host and genetic susceptibility are marked[181,196]. Several substances in the workplace can cause lung cancer in humans, e.g. asbestos, radon, silica, chromium, cadmium, nickel, arsenic, and beryllium[181]. Discussion of these myriad occupational respiratory illnesses is beyond the scope of this chapter and is reviewed elsewhere[181–183].

Interstitial lung disease caused by workplace exposures may be due to direct injury, allergic responses, e.g. hypersensitivity pneumonia, or diverse unknown mechanisms[181–183]. Most cases of severe fibrotic lung disease due to occupational exposures are attributed to coal worker's pneumoconiosis, silicosis, and asbestosis, but cobalt, talc, and kaolin are important[181,197]. It is highly likely that many cases of 'idiopathic' pulmonary fibrosis are non-specific reactions to diverse occupational or environmental exposures which are not recognized by the treating physicians[60,198]. The link between occupational exposure and lung injury may not be obvious, particularly when a long latent period exists between exposure and development of symptoms. Workplace environments with high levels of irritants, dust, smoke, or chemicals are often suspected,

but even low-grade exposures to solvents, paints, oils, or chemicals can elicit immune or injurious responses. Treatment for occupational lung disease primarily involves removing patients from the offending environment. Corticosteroids are used for patients with fulminant or severe injury, but data supporting their efficacy are lacking.

Recent reports of previously unrecognized occupational lung diseases, e.g. chronic non-granulomatous interstitial lung disease among workers in the nylon flocking industry[199–201] and hypersensitivity pneumonia among workers in a peat moss packaging plant[202] underscore the fact that myriad other toxins/allergens in the environment are likely (albeit unrecognized) causes of idiopathic interstitial pneumonias.

Drug-induced interstitial lung disease

A variety of drugs and exogenous agents elicit lung injury or fibrosis, resulting in acute or chronic pneumonitis, acute alveolar hemorrhage, or non-cardiac pulmonary edema[203–206]. The clinical course of drug-induced pneumonitis/fibrosis is variable, ranging from acute, fulminant respiratory failure to a chronic, indolent course, with progressive dyspnea over months or even years. Multiple mechanisms and agents/drugs induce lung injury.

Cytotoxic drugs, e.g. cyclophosphamide, chlorambucil, busulfan, bleomycin, nitrosoureas, mitomycin, cause direct lung injury via oxygen radicals, DNA intercalation, or direct cytotoxicity[45,203,206]. The risk is highest with carmustine (BCNU) (>30%)[207,208,209]; intermediate with busulfan, bleomycin, and mitomycin (2 to 10%)[203,206]; uncommon with cyclophosphamide (<1%)[210]. Prior chemotherapy or radiation therapy amplifies the risk. For BCNU and bleomycin, the risk of lung injury is dose dependent[203,208]. Pulmonary toxicity develops in 50% of patients[203] when the cumulative dose of BCNU exceeds 1500 mg/m^2. Risk factors for bleomycin-induced lung injury include: cumulative dose >450 units; age >70 years; use of supplemental oxygen[203]. Histopathological features of cytotoxic drug-induced lung injury include: type II cell proliferation and cellular atypia; inflammatory cell infiltrates in the alveolar septae or spaces; varying degrees of fibrosis[206,209]. Prognosis of alkylating agent-induced lung disease is poor. Prompt cessation of therapy is mandatory, but the disease may still progress; mortality exceeds 10% in severe cases[204,206,209]. Corticosteroids are warranted for severe or progressive cases, but are often ineffectual. Responses may occur if treatment is initiated early[208,209,211].

Aggressive multiagent chemotherapeutic regimens with autologous bone marrow transplantation (ABMT) and/or peripheral blood progenitor cell support are increasingly used to treat high risk primary breast cancer with extensive lymph node involvement[207–209,211]. Delayed pulmonary toxicity syndrome (DPTS), due to drug-induced interstitial pneumonia, may occur following high dose chemotherapy or ABMT in this population[207]. Standard dose induction chemotherapy adversely affects lung function, and induces an inflammatory cellular response (even in asymptomatic patients)[211]. Subsequent high dose consolidation chemotherapy or stem cell transplantation amplifies the injury[211]. Delayed pulmonary toxicity syndrome developed in 72% of breast cancer patients who received *both* initial and consolidation high dose chemotherapy compared to only 4% among patients receiving standard dose chemotherapy[211]. The risk of DPTS did not correlate with age, smoking history, or prior lung disease[211]. Early treatment with prednisone substantially attenuates injury in symptomatic patients with declining PFTs following chemotherapy[211].

Methotrexate, sulfasalazine, and gold salts evoke a T-suppressor cell (CD8+) predominant alveolitis consistent with hypersensitivity pneumonia (HP)[203,212]. The risk is highest with methotrexate (2 to 7%)[45,212] and rare (<1%) with other agents[203]. Lung biopsies reveal dense infiltrates with lymphocytes and plasma cells, foamy macrophages, and scattered non-necrotizing granulomata[206,212]. BAL reveals CD8(+)-predominant lymphocytosis[203]. Hypersensitivity pneumonia may complicate use of hydroxy-methylglutaryl coenzyme A (HMG-CoA) reductase inhibitors[213] or cabergoline, a dopaminer-

gic anti-Parkinson drug[214]. Other dopamine agonists, e.g. ergotamine, mesulergine, lisuride, bromocriptine, and methysergide, can cause pleuropulmonary disease and mediastinal and retroperitoneal fibrosis[215]. Pharmacological agents or drugs may elicit acute eosinophilic pneumonia, which sometimes progresses to hypoxemic respiratory failure[216–220]. The prognosis of drug-induced HP or eosinophilic pneumonia is usually favourable following withdrawal of the offending agent[203,214,216–220]. Corticosteroids hasten resolution and are recommended for severe or progressive cases.

Amiodarone, an iodinated anti-arrhythmic agent, causes pulmonary toxicity in 5 to 10% of patients[221,222]. Pulmonary toxicity is rare with other anti-arrhythmics. The incidence is highest with tocainide (0.3%) and rare (<0.01%) with mexiletine or flecainide[203]. Amiodarone can cause acute or chronic pneumonitis. Acute amiodarone pneumonitis presents with fever, mixed alveolar–interstitial infiltrates on chest radiographs, and leukocytosis, mimicking pneumonia[221,222]. Rarely, the course is fulminant, progressing to ARDS[222]. Chronic pneumonitis presents with dry cough; progressive dyspnea, interstitial infiltrates on chest radiographs; and a restrictive defect on PFTs[222]. HRCT scans reveal localized or diffuse areas of very high attenuation, corresponding to accumulations of 'foamy macrophages' containing iodine[222]. These features may be observed even in asymptomatic patients receiving amiodarone. Histopathological features of amiodarone toxicity include: abundant, intraalveolar macrophages; chronic mononuclear infiltrates; foci of fibrosis[221,206]. With fulminant forms, diffuse alveolar damage (DAD), hyaline membranes, and intra-alveolar hemorrhage may be seen[206]. Foamy macrophages may be present in BAL fluid or lung biopsy even in asymptomatic patients receiving amiodarone[221]. Risk factors for amiodarone toxicity are not well defined. Total cumulative dose, serum levels, or prior pulmonary disease do not predict toxicity[222]. Treatment involves discontinuing amiodarone and switching to an alternative antiarrhythmic agent. Corticosteroids are warranted for severe or progressive disease.

Nitrofurantoin causes acute or chronic interstitial pneumonitis in <1% of treated patients[203,206]. Acute pneumonitis may present within the first month of therapy, with fever, dry cough, and dyspnea; myalgias, arthralgias, or skin rash are present in up to 30%[203,205]. Mild cases often resolve promptly with discontinuation of nitrofurantoin. Severe cases require treatment with corticosteroids. Chronic interstitial pneumonia, indistinguishable from CFA, may also occur[203,205]. Prognosis is less favourable, as fibrosis may be significant by the time the relationship between the drug and pulmonary disease is recognized.

Non-cardiac pulmonary edema (NPE) rarely complicates the use of salicylates, thiazide diuretics, narcotics, and cytarabine (a chemotherapeutic agent)[203,206]. Mechanisms are varied. Some agents cause damage to alveolar endothelium and epithelium, resulting in capillary leak syndrome[203,206]. Narcotics cause acute pulmonary hypertension. Acute pulmonary hemorrhage is a rare complication of trimellitic anhydrides, isocyanates, D-penicillamine, prophylthiouracil, and cocaine[223]. Irrespective of implicated agent, NPE usually resolves following withdrawal of the drug.

Acute or chronic eosinophilic pneumonias rarely complicate the use of sulfonamides, β-lactam antibiotics, isoniazid, pyrimethamine-dapsone, and other antimicrobials[203,205,206]. Hydralazine, procainamide, quinine, and isoniazid can cause a lupus-like syndrome with pleural effusions, fever, arthritis, pericarditis, and positive antinuclear antibodies, but pulmonary parenchymal infiltrates are rarely observed[157].

Genetic disorders associated with pulmonary fibrosis

Hermansky–Pudlak syndrome

Pulmonary fibrosis may complicate Hermansky–Pudlak syndrome (HPS), a rare autosomal recessive disorder characterized by lysosomal accumulation of ceroid lipofuscin, a platelet storage pool deficiency, and oculocutaneous albinism[224]. Clinical manifestations include: bruising, prolonged bleeding time, hypopigmentation of skin and hair, congenital nystagmus, iris transillumination, and, in some patients, granulomatous colitis or pulmonary fibrosis[225]. HPS occurs worldwide, but is most common in Puerto Rico, where the incidence is 1:800[225]. Pulmonary fibrosis develops in the fourth or fifth decade of life, but time of onset and clinical severity is variable[225–227]. Cough and dyspnea progress insidiously; PFTs reveal a restrictive defect with low DLCO[225,226]. HRCT features resemble CFA[225,226] but upper lobe bullae and bronchiectasis also occur[228]. Lung biopsies demonstrate fibrosis, honeycomb cysts, and a chronic inflammatory infiltrate with macrophages containing lipofuscin[227]. These macrophages stain positively with periodic acid-Schiff (PAS) and fluoresce intensely orange–red under ultraviolent light due to the engulfed ceroid[228]. Progressive, fatal respiratory insufficiency can occur[227], but the course is variable. No therapy is of proven benefit[228].

Neurofibromatosis

Pulmonary fibrosis occurs in 7 to 20% of patients with neurofibromatosis (NF), an autosomal dominant disease with primarily neurological and cutaneous manifestations[228,229]. The incidence is 1:3000 births; nearly half of cases arise by spontaneous mutation[228]. Extrapulmonary features include: multiple neurofibromas; café au lait spots; axillary freckling; Lisch nodules (hamartomatous formations of the iris); meningiomas or gliomas[228,229]. The incidence and onset of pulmonary disease are variable. Pulmonary symptoms usually appear after age 35[228]. Radiographic features include diffuse interstitial infiltrates or bullous disease; intercostal neuromas; intrathoracic meningomyelocoeles; vertebral defects; scoliosis[228]. Pulmonary function tests reveal restrictive or obstructive defects[228]. The pathology of pulmonary fibrosis complicating NF is similar to CFA[228]. Data are limited; the natural history is not known. Some patients progress to pulmonary hypertension, cor pulmonale, or fatal respiratory failure[230]. No therapy is of proven benefit[228].

Gaucher's disease

Gaucher's disease (GD), a lysosomal storage disease resulting from deficiency of glucocerebrosidase, is inherited as an autosomal recessive trait[228]. Clinical manifestations are caused by accumulation of glucocerebroside in cells of the reticuloendothelial system[228,231,232]. Identification of Gaucher cells, which autofluoresce and stain positively with PAS, is diagnostic[231]. Pulmonary involvement, due to infiltrating Gaucher cells in the alveolar interstitium, spaces, or capillaries, is common in infantile GD, but is rare in the adult form[228,231,232]. Infantile and adult GD differ strikingly in clinical presentation and prognosis. Infantile GD is usually fatal within the first two years of life (due to progressive neurological impairment)[228]. Primary manifestations of GD in adults include hepatosplenomegaly, pancytopenia, bone pain and fractures due to bone marrow replacement with Gaucher cells[228]. Neurological lesions are rare in adults[228,231,232]. Laboratory features of GD include pancytopenia, elevated liver enzymes, and increased acid phosphatase[228]. Pulmonary manifestations include: reduced lung volumes; low DLCO; diffuse interstitial or miliary infiltrates on chest radiographs[228,231,232]. Gaucher cells may be found in sputum or BAL[228]. Obliteration of pulmonary capillaries may cause pulmonary hypertension and cor pulmonale[232]. Pulmonary fibrosis or alveolar inflammation are absent[231,232]. Treatment options are limited and include enzyme (glucocerebrosidase) replacement therapy[233] or bone marrow transplantation[228].

Niemann–Pick disease

Niemann–Pick disease is a rare lipid storage disease characterized by accumulation of sphingomyelin in the CNS and reticuloendothelial system[228]. Inheritance is autosomal recessive[228]. Infiltration of alveolar spaces and interstitium with reticuloendothelial cells filled with sphingomyelin cause reticulonodular or miliary infiltrates; progression to honeycombing and fibrosis may occur[228]. No treatment is available.

Hypocalciuric hypercalcemia and interstitial lung disease

Hypocalciuric hypercalcemia and interstitial lung disease is a rare inherited disorder characterized by hypocalciuric hypercalcemia, pulmonary fibrosis, granulocyte dysfunction and recurrent respiratory tract infections[234]. The disease presents after age 30, with reticulonodular infiltrates, reduced DLCO, a restrictive defect on PFTs, hypercalcemia and hypocalciuria[234]. Granulocytes are deficient in myeloperoxidase and exhibit impaired phagocytosis and killing of *Staphylococcus aureus*[234]. Lung biopsies demonstrate poorly defined granulomas, multinucleated giant cells, varying degrees of fibrosis, and alveolar macrophages containing dark cytoplasmic inclusions of unknown nature[234]. Progressive pulmonary fibrosis, with honeycombing, and decline in lung function over several years is the rule[234]. Owing to the rarity of this disorder, optimal treatment is not known. Anecdotal responses to corticosteroids have been cited[234].

Pulmonary lymphoproliferative disorders

Lymphoid interstitial pneumonia (LIP), diffuse lymphoid hyperplasia, pseudolymphoma, and follicular bronchitis/bronchiolitis (FB) are rare lymphoproliferative disorders which share common clinical and histological features[55,235–239]. These are polyclonal 'reactive' disorders primarily involving B lymphocytes, usually associated with autoimmune disorders or immunodeficiency states[55,235,237,239]. Some cases are linked to Epstein–Barr (EB) virus infection[55,235,237,239]. In some patients, LIP and FB coexist, without predominance of either histological lesion[235]. In addition to these 'reactive' lymphoproliferative disorders, malignant neoplastic disorders arising primarily in the lung have clinical and histological features which overlap with LIP or FB. These include: primary pulmonary lymphomas originating from bronchus-associated lymphoid tissue (BALT)[55,235,237,240], and lymphomatoid granulomatosis[241–244]. Each of these 'reactive' or neoplastic lymphoid disorders will be discussed below.

Lymphoid interstitial pneumonia (LIP)

Lymphoid interstitial pneumonia (LIP) is a rare disorder primarily observed in patients with connective tissue disorders (particularly Sjogren's syndrome), chronic liver disease, EB virus infection, myasthenia gravis, or diverse autoimmune disorders or immunodeficiency states including acquired immunodeficiency syndrome (AIDS) and common variable immune deficiency (CVID)[49,55,239,245–248]. In children, LIP is usually linked to AIDS[122,246,247,249] whereas most cases in adults occur in non-HIV infected patients[239,244]. Liebow initially described LIP in 1966; and outlined the salient features in a series of 18 cases gleaned from a large pulmonary pathology consultation file[49]. Apart from sporadic case reports, data over the next decade were limited to two series from major referral centres[237,245]. In 1978, Strimlan reported 13 patients with LIP seen at the Mayo Clinic from 1966 to 1976[245]. A review of pathological files from the Armed Forces Institute of Pathology identified 18 cases of LIP over 35 years (from 1949 to 1983)[237]. By the mid-1980s, LIP in HIV-infected children was recognized[122,246,247,250]. In HIV-negative patients, LIP typically affects adults older than 40 years of age; women are affected twice as often as men[49,55,251]. Nine to 25% of adults with LIP have Sjogren's syndrome (SS); 1% of patients with SS have LIP[55].

Clinical presentation of LIP is indolent, with progressive cough, dyspnea, and pulmonary infiltrates[246,247,251–253]. In non-HIV infected patients, extrapulmonary symptoms are rare[55,245,252]. Fever, constitutional symptoms, weight loss, lymphadenopathy, hepatosplenomegaly, and salivary gland enlargement are common in HIV-infected children with LIP[122,247,250]. Dysproteinemia is characteristic in both HIV (−) and HIV (+) patients[55,239,247,251,252]. Polyclonal hypergammaglobulinemia occurs in 70 to 80% of patients; hypogammaglobulinemia, in 10 to 20%[55,251,252].

Chest radiographs demonstrate bilateral reticular or reticulonodular infiltrates, dense alveolar infiltrates, or focal nodules[55,245–247,252,253]. Pleural effusions or mediastinal lymphadenopathy are usually absent[55,239,245,251]. HRCT scans reveal 2 to 4 mm interstitial or peribronchovascular nodules; thickened bronchovascular bundles, interlobular septal thickening, or diffuse ground glass opacities[246,247,254]. Honeycomb cysts are uncommon[254,255]. Pulmonary function tests demonstrate a restrictive pattern, with reduced DLCO[55,239,245].

In LIP, dense infiltrates of small lymphocytes and plasma cells are found in the alveolar septae and along lymphatics[55,123,237,247,251–253]. Germinal centres are prominent; the terms 'pulmonary lymphoid hyperplasia' or 'diffuse hyperplasia of BALT' are also used[55,235]. Scattered multinucleated giant cells or loose non-necrotizing granulomas are present in up to 50 to 72% of cases of LIP[55,235,237,252]. Fibrosis and honeycomb cysts are not prominent. Distinguishing LIP from low-grade pulmonary lymphomas is difficult, as histological features overlap[55,237,252]. Immunohistochemical stains and/or gene rearrangement studies discriminate lymphomas from benign disorders. Lymphomas exhibit a monoclonal population of plasma cells[237,253]; LIP is polyclonal[55,235]. Rare cases of LIP evolve to malignant lymphoma[55,245,251,252].

The pathogenesis of LIP is not clear, but may represent response to retroviruses[123,239] or EB virus[55]. In HIV-infected patients with LIP, HIV antigens are present in BAL fluid and lung tissue macrophages[55,123]. EB viruses are activated by HIV and produce polyclonal B cell hyperplasia[55]. In sheep, LIP-like lesions, consisting of T cytotoxic/suppressor cells, are induced by ovine lentivirus[55].

The natural history of LIP ranges from spontaneous resolution to fatal respiratory failure[55,121,122,245,251,252]. The course is indolent, with progressive cough, dyspnea, and deteriorating PFTs over months or even years[55,121,122,245,251,252]. Among HIV-infected patients, fatalities are due to opportunistic infections or advanced HIV infection rather than LIP[122,247,249,250]. Owing to the rarity of LIP, optimal therapy is not known. Favourable responses to corticosteroids were cited in both HIV-infected and non-infected patients[55,235,237,245,247]. Immunosuppressive[55,235,239] or cytotoxic agents[245,252], and antiviral agents, e.g. zidovudine[247], have been tried; their efficacy is unproven. A recent report cited response to low dose cyclosporine and prednisone in a woman with common variable immunodeficiency (CVID) syndrome[248].

Follicular bronchitis/bronchiolitis (FB)

Follicular bronchitis/bronchiolitis (also termed hyperplasia of bronchus associated lymphoid tissue (BALT)), is characterized by polyclonal lymphoid follicles along bronchioles with a minor alveolar interstitial inflammatory component[54,55,235,256]. Reactive germinal centers are present along bronchioles, and to a lesser extent, bronchi[54,55,235,256]. FB differs from LIP by its bronchiolocentricity and lack of diffuse alveolar septal involvement[54,55,257]. Both LIP and FB may be present in individual patients, and pathogenetic mechanisms appear to be similar. Primary and secondary forms of FB exist. Primary FB is associated with collagen vascular diseases, hypersensitivity reactions, or immunodeficiency states (including AIDS)[54,55,235,257]. Secondary FB occurs as a complication of cystic fibrosis, bronchiectasis, obstructive pneumonias, or chronic inflammatory disorders of the airways[257]. Clinical symptoms attributable to FB are mild, and include cough and dyspnea. Chest radiographs demonstrate reticular or reticulonodular infiltrates[257]. Cardinal features of FB on HRCT scans include: bilateral centrilobular and peribronchial nodules (<3 mm in diameter) and focal ground glass opacities[256]. Data regarding treatment are limited. Corticosteroids have been used, with anecdotal successes, but are reserved for patients with significant pulmonary symptoms.

Pseudolymphoma (nodular lymphoid hyperplasia)

Pseudolymphomas of the lung are reactive polymorphous lymphoid proliferations containing numerous germinal centres; the term 'nodular lymphoid hyperplasia' is synonymous[55,236,257]. Immunohistochemical stains demonstrate a mixed population of CD4 and CD8 lymphocytes[55]. The literature is confusing, as some published examples of pseudolymphomas (prior to availability of immunohistochemical stains) undoubtedly were low-grade lymphomas[55,236,257]. Pseudolymphomas are exceptionally rare, and the diagnosis can be accepted only after immunohistochemical studies exclude low-grade BALT lymphomas[257]. Pseudolymphomas typically present as asymptomatic, solitary nodular lesions on chest radiographs (2 to 5 cm in diameter)[55,236,257]. Intrathoracic lymph node enlargement does not occur[55,236,257]. Surgical resection is usually curative, but the disease recurs in 10 to 15% of patients[55,236]. Fatalities are rare.

Primary pulmonary lymphoma

Primary pulmonary lymphomas are low grade BALT lymphomas but histological features overlap with LIP[257]. Germinal centres are present in 20 to 69% of BALT lymphomas[55]. Multinucleated giant cells or granulomas are found in up to 50% of patients[55]. In contrast to LIP, BALT lymphomas obliterate the lung architecture and invade pleura and bronchial cartilage[55,236]. Confluent lymphoid cells stain for B-cell markers and exhibit monoclonality (light chain restriction), and clonal rearrangement of the joining region of the Ig heavy chain gene[55]. BALT lymphomas usually present as mass lesions on chest radiographs, with air-bronchograms[257], but a nodular interstitial pattern can occur[55]. Pleural effusions or intrathoracic adenopathy are uncommon[257]. Cough, dyspnea, or chest pain may be present, but up to 50% of patients are asymptomatic at the time of diagnosis[257]. The prognosis is related to histological stage. Seventy per cent of pulmonary BALT lymphomas are stage I at presentation[258]; hilar lymph node enlargement is present in 0 to 30%[55,236]. Surgical resection is usually curative for localized lesions, with 5-year survival rates exceeding 85%[55,257,258]. Evolution to aggressive immunoblastic lymphoma occurs in 5% of cases[55,258]. Prognosis is poor with advanced stage (> stage 2) or when extrapulmonary spread has occurred[55,258].

Lymphomatoid granulomatosis

Lymphomatoid granulomatosis (LYG) is a rare lymphoproliferative disorder characterized by multiple pulmonary nodules (with a vasculitic component), and prominent extrapulmonary manifestations involving the CNS (30%), skin (>40%), kidney (30%), or other organs[242,257,259,260]. Although LYG was originally classified as a pulmonary vasculitis, LYG actually represents a spectrum of angiocentric lymphomas, either of B-cell[243], T-cell, or natural killer (NK) cell origin[241,242,251]. The term 'angioimmunoproliferative lesion/angiocentric lymphoma' (AIL) is suggested in lieu of LYG[55,260]. Solitary involvement of the CNS or other organs can be the presenting feature; involvement of lymph nodes or bone marrow is unusual[261]. LYG is more common in immunocompromised patients (including AIDS)[244,251,260,261]. Most patients with pulmonary LYG have cough, chest pain, or dyspnea[261]. Chest radiographs typically reveal bilateral pulmonary nodules (25% cavitate) (Fig. 12.15); other features include focal mass lesions, diffuse or localized reticulonodular or alveolar infiltrates[55,261]. Hilar lymphadenopathy is absent.

Histological features of LYG include nodules with angiocentric, polymorphous, and atypical lymphoreticular infiltrates, and necrosis[55,244,260]. Epithelioid granulomas or giant cells are uncommon; hence the term 'granulomatosis' is misleading. A histological grading system for AIL/LYG distinguishes lesions by degree of cytological atypia, extent of necrosis, and retention of a polymorphous cellular infiltrate[262]. Grade 1 lesions are polymorphous, with little or no atypia, and lack necrosis. Grade 2 lesions are polymorphous, have atypical cells, and foci of necrosis. Grade 3 lesions exhibit monomorphism, severe cellular atypia and necrosis and are considered malig-

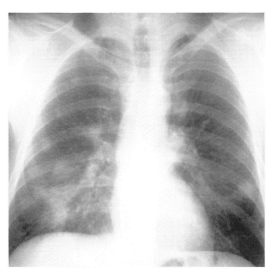

Fig. 12.15 Lymphomatoid granulomatosis (LYG). PA chest radiograph reveals multiple bilateral pulmonary nodules. Open lung biopsy revealed a polymorphic lymphohistiocytic infiltrate and vasculitis, consistent with LYG.

nant 'angiocentric' lymphomas[262]. One third of grade 1 lesions and two thirds of grade 2 lesions progress to malignant lymphoma[55]. Early studies suggested a T cell origin[251], but recent studies suggest that most cases of LYG are EB-virus associated B-cell lymphoproliferative disorders[241,243,244]. Most background lymphocytes are T cells, but the cytologically atypical lymphoid cells stain positively for B-cell markers (CD20 or L26), express EB virus genome[241–244,259,260], and proliferate at a rapid rate[242]. LYG is more common in immunocompromised patients[241,244,259,260], suggesting that deficient regulation of EB virus is critical to the pathogenesis.

The clinical course of LYG is variable. The disease usually progresses relentlessly, eventuating in death; however, spontaneous remissions can occur[260,261]. Given the rarity of LYG, optimal therapy for LYG is not clear. Initial studies employed corticosteroids and cyclophosphamide, with anecdotal remissions, but malignant lymphomas developed in most of the surviving patients[263]. Current therapeutic regimens include multiagent chemotherapy or radiation therapy; results are variable[55,260]. Anecdotal successes with interferon α-2b were cited in a few cases[259].

Post-transplant lymphoproliferative disorder

A spectrum of EB virus-associated lymphoproliferative lesions arise in allogeneic organ transplant recipients receiving aggressive immunosuppression[257,264]. Post-transplant lymphoproliferative disorders (PTLD) develop within weeks or months of initiation of immunosuppressive therapy[257,264]. The incidence of PTLD ranges from 0.6 to 4% in most organ transplant recipients, but higher rates were cited among heart transplant recipients[264]. Lung involvement can occur in isolation or with multiple extrapulmonary sites[257,264]. Pulmonary PTLD typically presents as multiple nodules; necrosis may be prominent[257,264]. Histological features are variable (ranging from non-specific reactive hyperplasia to high-grade immunoblastic lymphoma)[257,264]. Dense infiltrates of lymphocytes, plasma cells, and immunoblasts are present, often with angioinvasion or angiodestruction[257,264]. EB virus can be identified by *in situ* hybridization or polymerase chain reaction[257,264]. Categorizing lesions based on the nature of the lymphoid infiltrate as 'polymorphous' (heterogeneous) or 'monomorphous' (homogeneous) is helpful, but histology does not reliably predict prognosis[257,264]. Polymorphous lesions are usually polyclonal, and may regress after reducing the level of immunosuppression[257,264]. In contrast, monomorphic lesions resemble malignant immunoblastic lymphomas, are often monoclonal, and respond poorly to therapy (even conventional chemotherapy)[257,264].

Sarcoidosis

Sarcoidosis, a multisystemic granulomatous disease of uncertain etiology, involves the lung or intrathoracic lymph nodes in more than 90% of patients[37,38,265,266]. The clinical spectrum of sarcoidosis is protean, but pulmonary manifestations predominate[37,38,265,267]. Cough or dyspnea reflect endobronchial or pulmonary involvement, but 30 to 60% of patients with pulmonary sarcoidosis are asymptomatic, with incidental findings on chest radiographs[37,38,265,267]. Physical examination of the chest is often unimpressive, even when extensive parenchymal infiltrates are present[38]. Crackles are present in fewer than 20% of patients with sarcoidosis; clubbing is rare[268]. Extrapulmonary involvement is common, and may be the presenting or dominant feature[265,267]. Skin, eye, and peripheral lymph nodes are each involved in 20 to 30% of patients[37,265,267]. Clinically significant involvement of liver, spleen, heart, central nervous system, bone, or kidney occurs in 2 to 7% of patients[37,265,267]. Virtually any organ can be affected[37,38,265,267].

Sarcoidosis is worldwide in distribution, but the prevalence varies among countries, geographic locales, and ethnic groups[37,269–272]. Sarcoidosis is 4 to 8 times more common in blacks than whites[37,269,270]. The incidence among Caucasians in North America and Northern Europe is 6 to 20 cases per 100 000[37,269,270], but exceeds 60 per 100 000 in certain parts of the British Isles[271,272]. The incidence is much lower (<2 per 100 000) in southern Europe[271,273,274]. Sarcoidosis is rarely diagnosed in Africa or South America, but whether this represents under-recognition or reduced prevalence of the disease is not known. Sarcoidosis is slightly more common in women (1.4/1.0 female to male ratio)[269,270]. More than two-thirds of patients present between age 20 and 40 years[37,270]. Familial sarcoidosis (defined as having a first- or second-degree relative with sarcoidosis) occurs in 17% of African–American patients with sarcoidosis compared to 6% among Caucasian cases[269]. However, a specific genetic defect has not been identified[270].

The histological hallmark of sarcoidosis is non-necrotizing (non-caseating) granulomata, characterized by multinucleated giant cells, epithelioid cells, and mononuclear phagocytes in the central core, surrounded by a cuff of lymphocytes[37] (Figs. 12.16 and 12.17). Varying degrees of fibrosis and destruction or distortion of parenchyma may be present. In the lung, granulomata are distributed along bronchovascular bundles and lymphatics[37]. Coalescent granulomata give rise to confluent mass

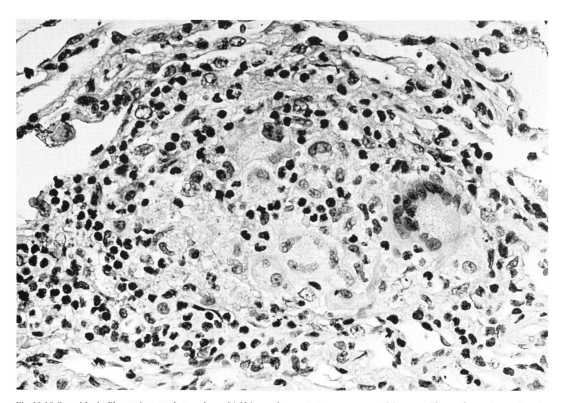

Fig. 12.16 Sarcoidosis. Photomicrograph: transbronchial biopsy demonstrates a non-necrotizing sarcoid granuloma. A prominent multinucleated giant cell is present with scattered epithelioid cells and lymphocytes (hematoxylin–eosin). (Reproduced with permission.)[551]

lesions, nodules or consolidation of lung parenchyma. Bronchiectasis, bronchioloectasis, alveolar septal fibrosis, and honeycomb cysts reflect end-stage disease[37,38]. Fibreoptic bronchoscopy with TBBs is the preferred technique to substantiate the diagnosis of sarcoidosis in patients with bilateral hilar lymphadenopathy (BHL) and/or parenchymal infiltrates. The yield of TBBs ranges from 60 to 97%[38]. Mediastinoscopic lymph node biopsies or surgical (open or VATS) lung biopsies have higher yields, but are expensive and have increased morbidity[275]. Biopsy of extrapulmonary sites is appropriate when specific lesions or abnormalities are identified, e.g. peripheral lymphadenopathy, skin lesions, abnormal liver enzymes, etc[267].

Interactions between activated mononuclear phagocytes and helper/inducer (CD4+) lymphocytes are instrumental in driving the granulomatous response in sarcoidosis[276]. At sites of disease activity, increases in activated CD4+ cells, increased CD4/CD8 ratio, and diverse cytokines are observed[276–278]. The signals responsible for inciting or driving the sarcoid granulomatous response are not known. Exposure to beryllium, hard metals, or infectious agents elicit granulomatous responses, suggesting that infections and/or environmental agents may be involved[195]. Genetic factors are likely instrumental in determining the clinical expression of the disease.

Laboratory features are non-specific. Elevations in serum calcium occur in 1 to 4% of patients; hypercalciuria, in 15 to 40%[37,267,279]. These derangements in calcium metabolism reflect enhanced production of 1,2-dihydroxycalciferol by mononuclear phagocytes from sarcoid granulomas[279]. Polyclonal hyper-

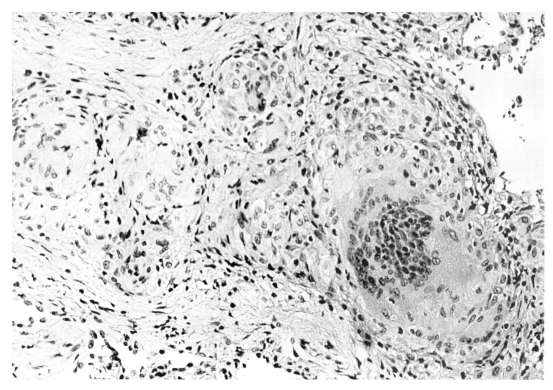

Fig. 12.17 Sarcoidosis. Photomicrograph: Transbronchial lung biopsy demonstrating granulomatous inflammation with a prominent multinucleated giant cell and scattered lymphocytes, fibroblasts, and epithelioid cells in a patient with pulmonary sarcoidosis (hematoxylin-eosin). (Reproduced with permission.)[551]

gammaglobulinemia occurs in 30 to 80% of patients with chronic sarcoidosis[267,280]. Serum angiotensin converting enzyme (ACE) levels are increased in 30 to 80% of patients with sarcoidosis[281]. Changes in serum ACE often parallel disease activity, but do not predict response to therapy[281].

Chest radiographs are abnormal in more than 90% of patients with sarcoidosis[37,38]. The most characteristic finding is BHL, with or without concomitant right paratracheal node enlargement[38,282] (Fig. 12.18). Parenchymal infiltrates are present in 25 to 55% of patients[37,38]. Reticulonodular, interstitial shadows or conglomerate alveolar infiltrates may be observed; these infiltrates have a predilection for

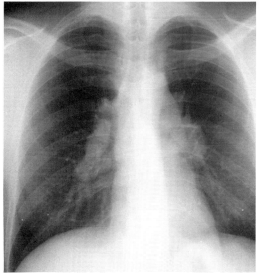

Fig. 12.18 Stage I sarcoidosis. Chest radiograph from a 35-year-old male demonstrating bilateral hilar lymphadenopathy. Lymph nodes in the left para-aortic region and aortopulmonary window are also enlarged.

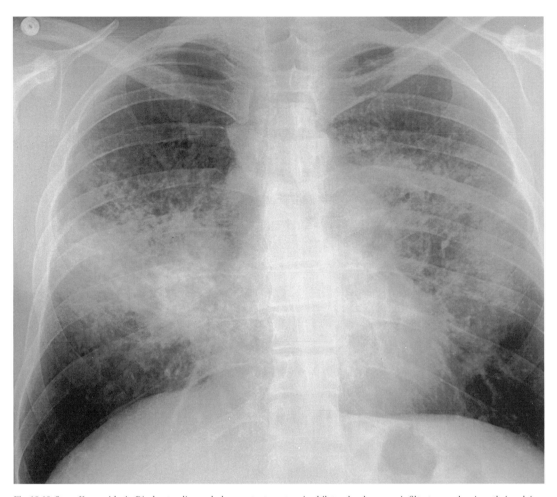

Fig. 12.19 Stage II sarcoidosis. PA chest radiograph demonstrates extensive bilateral pulmonary infiltrates predominantly involving perihilar, mid and upper lung zones. Numerous small nodules are present throughout both lungs. Bilateral hilar lymphadenopathy is present.

upper and mid lung zones[37,38] (Fig. 12.19). Multiple, well-circumscribed pulmonary nodules >1 cm in size, known as nodular or nummular sarcoid, occurs in 2 to 4% of patients[38,283]. Pleural effusions are rare (<2%)[38]. Destruction of lung parenchyma may cause bullae, distortion, honeycomb cysts, broad septal bands, volume loss, or upward retraction of the hilae[38] (Fig. 12.20). Late features include: mycetomas (fungus balls), pleural thickening, calcified hilar or mediastinal lymph nodes, and secondary pulmonary hypertensive changes[38].

Characteristic features on HRCT scans include: parenchymal opacities or nodules in the mid or upper lung zones; patchy involvement; distribution along central bronchovascular bundles; focal or confluent alveolar opacities with consolidation; ground glass opacities; thickened intra- and inter-lobular septae; fibrosis, distortion, cysts[22] (Fig. 12.21(*a*) (*b*)). Nodules, ground glass opacities or alveolar opacities represent conglomerate granulomas[22] (Fig. 12.22). Distortion, cysts, bullae, or traction bronchiectasis reflect end-stage disease[22,38]

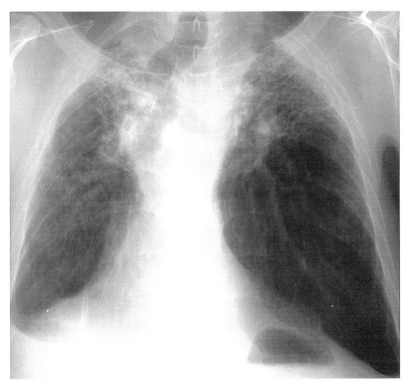

Fig. 12.20 Stage IV sarcoidosis. PA chest radiograph from a 57-year-old man demonstrates extensive pulmonary parenchymal infiltrates involving the upper lobes, with volume loss and deviation of the trachea to the right. Extensive emphysematous changes are noted in the lower lobes, particularly on the left. Thirty-two years earlier, he had bilateral hilar lymphadenopathy and erythema nodosum consistent with stage I sarcoidosis. (Reproduced with permission.)[38]

(Fig. 12.23). Routine HRCT is not necessary to stage or follow the course of the disease, but may be prognostically useful in selected patients with persistent parenchymal infiltrates. Honeycombing, distortion, bullae, or thick septal lines indicate fibrosis and predict unresponsiveness to corticosteroid therapy[16,22,23]. By contrast, focal alveolar opacities, ground glass attenuation, or nodules are associated with an inflammatory component and predict a higher rate of response to therapy[16,22,23].

Pulmonary function tests are abnormal in 40 to 70% of patients with parenchymal infiltrates (radiographic stage II or III) and in 10 to 20% of patients with stage I[16,38,284]. Reduced lung volumes (e.g. VC or TLC) are characteristic[38]. The DLCO is usually preserved, but is reduced with advanced disease[38]. Up to one third of patients with pulmonary sarcoidosis exhibit concomitant obstructive defects[38]. Airflow obstruction may reflect submucosal or endobronchial inflammation, parenchymal distortion, bronchostenosis, or exaggerated bronchial reactivity[38]. Cardiopulmonary exercise tests (CPET) are abnormal in up to 50% of patients with sarcoidosis, even when static PFTs are normal [284]. However, CPET are logistically cumbersome, and have limited practical value. Spirometry is the most useful test to follow the course of the disease (or assess response to therapy). More complex studies (e.g. lung volumes, DLCO) are reserved for selected patients.

Bronchoalveolar lavage in active pulmonary sarcoidosis reveals increased numbers of lymphocytes,

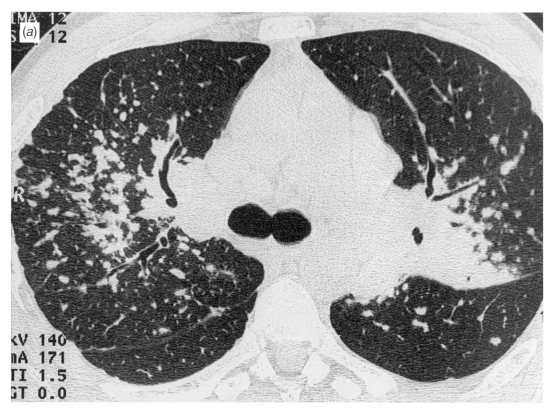

Fig. 12.21(a) Stage II sarcoidosis. HRCT demonstrates bilateral hilar lymphadenopathy, perihilar infiltrates, with areas of coalescent alveolar opacities. Multiple nodules, representing coalescent granulomas are present in both lungs.

T helper lymphocytes (CD4+), increased CD4/CD8 ratios, activated alveolar macrophages, diverse lymphokines, monokines, and biochemical markers[276,278]. BAL provides invaluable insights into the pathogenesis of sarcoidosis, but has marginal clinical or prognostic value[38,285]. Initial BAL CD4/CD8 ratios do not predict outcome or responsiveness to corticosteroid therapy[37,286,287]. BAL is expensive and invasive, and we see no role for BAL in gauging the need for therapeutic intervention. Radionuclide scans are of unproven value. Increased uptake of gallium-67 citrate in lung, hilar and mediastinal lymph glands, salivary, lacrimal and parotid glands is characteristic of sarcoidosis but does not predict prognosis or responsiveness to therapy[288,289]. Radionuclide scans are expensive, inconvenient (scanning is performed 48 hours after injection of

the radioisotope), and have no role in the management of sarcoidosis.

The clinical course of sarcoidosis is variable. Spontaneous remissions occur in nearly two thirds of patients but the course is chronic in 10 to 30%[37,38,265,267,290]. Chronic granulomatous inflammation may cause fibrosis and irreversible dysfunction of affected organs[37,38,265,267,290]. Chronic sarcoidosis involving lungs, heart, skin, bones, CNS, or other organs may be debilitating[37,38,267,280]. Fatalities occur in 1 to 4% of patients with sarcoidosis, typically due to progressive respiratory insufficiency, CNS or myocardial involvement[37,38,265,267,291,292].

Certain clinical syndromes have prognostic value. The constellation of fever, BHL, erythema nodosum, and polyarthritis (Lofgren's syndrome) portends an excellent prognosis, with a high rate (80–95%) of

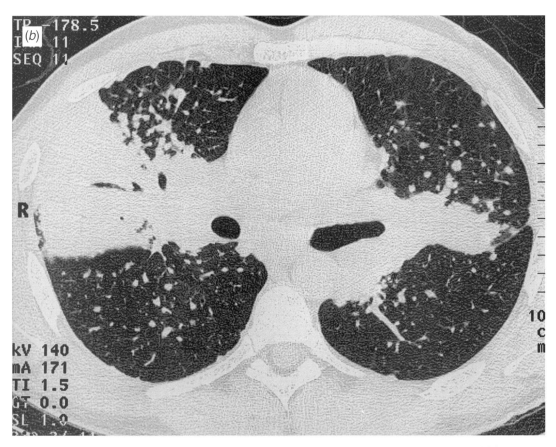

Fig. 12.21(b) Stage II sarcoidosis. HRCT from the same patient demonstrates conglomerate masses arising from both hilae, representing conglomerate granulomata. Air-bronchograms are visible in the right perihilar mass. Multiple nodules are scattered throughout both lungs.

spontaneous remissions; late sequelae are rare[38,280,293,294]. By contrast, several clinical features predict a chronic or relapsing course (e.g. chronic uveitis, chronic hypercalcemia, nephrocalcinosis, lupus pernio, involvement of nasal mucosa, central nervous system, or bone)[267,280]. The clinical course and prognosis of sarcoidosis are influenced by genetic and ethnic factors. Black race is associated with a higher rate of extrapulmonary involvement, chronic progressive disease, worse long-term prognosis, and higher rate of relapses[265,280,290,295]. The influence of human leukocyte antigen (HLA) markers and prognosis is controversial[265,296]. The chest radiographic schema espoused more than 40

years ago is prognostically useful. In that schema, stages are defined as follows: stage 0 (normal chest radiograph); stage I (BHL without parenchymal infiltrates); stage II (BHL plus parenchymal infiltrates); stage III (parenchymal infiltrates without BHL); stage IV (extensive fibrosis with architectural distortion and/or bullae)[38]. Prognosis is best with stage I and worst with stage III or IV disease. Spontaneous remissions occur in 60 to 90% of patients with stage I disease; in 40 to 70% with stage II; 10 to 20% with stage III[38,272,297]. By definition, stage IV indicates irreversibility. Serious sequelae are rare with stage I sarcoidosis, but may be appreciable in patients with stage II, III, or IV. The course of sarcoidosis is usually

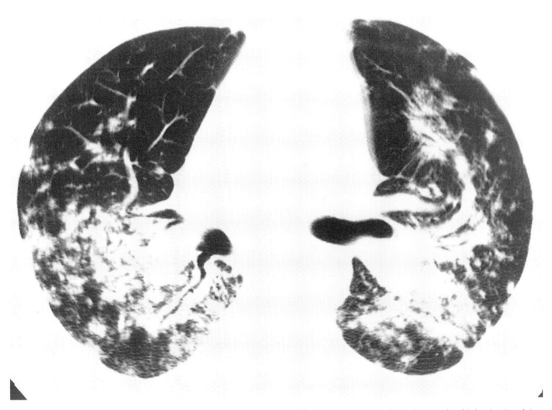

Fig. 12.22 Sarcoidosis. HRCT image (1.5 mm collimation) of a 36-year-old man demonstrates bronchovascular thickening involving the axial interstitium and multiple nodules in both lungs. Confluent disease is present in the central portion of the lung. Air-bronchograms are also apparent within the consolidated mass lesions. (Reproduced with permission.)[38]

evident within the first 2 years after diagnosis. Spontaneous remissions occur in up to 40% of patients within the first 6 months[298,299]. More than 85% of remissions occur within the first 2 years[300]. Failure to remit during that time frame predicts a low rate of subsequent resolution. Late relapses or permanent sequelae are uncommon (<10%) in patients who spontaneously remit[295,298,299].

Treatment of sarcoidosis is controversial[301]. Corticosteroids are recommended for patients with persistent or progressive sarcoidosis (pulmonary or extrapulmonary), but efficacy is controversial[297,301]. Indications for treatment should be focused and circumscribed. Toxicities of corticosteroids argue against the routine use for patients with minimal symptoms. Given the variable natural history, and

the potential for spontaneous remissions, the influence of therapeutic interventions is difficult to ascertain. Several prospective randomized trials failed to show benefit from early institution of corticosteroids[302–306]. However, patients with severe or progressive disease were excluded from the randomized trials, and were treated with corticosteroids. In most studies, patients were asymptomatic and had normal or near normal PFTs; few patients with radiographic stage III disease were included[302]. Interpretation of efficacy of therapy is clouded by heterogeneous patient populations, different doses or duration of therapy, lack of objective markers of disease activity, and inability to discriminate the effects of corticosteroids from the natural history of the disease. Failure to respond to corticosteroids

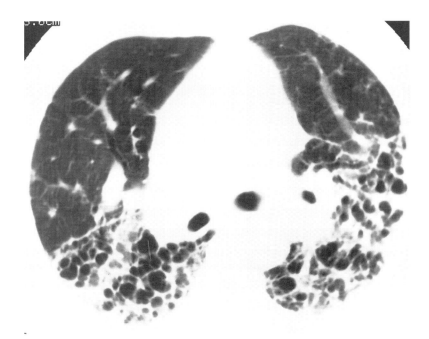

Fig. 12.23 Stage IV sarcoidosis. CT image (5-mm collimation) in a 55-year-old woman demonstrates extensive cystic destruction and honeycomb formation that predominantly affected the posterior aspects of the upper lobes. (Reproduced with permission.)[38]

may reflect irreversible fibrosis, inadequate dose or duration of therapy, noncompliance, or intrinsic corticosteroid resistance. The paucity of placebo-controlled therapeutic trials reflects the belief that corticosteroids are warranted for patients with severe, persistent, or progressive symptoms.

There is little doubt that corticosteroids are efficacious in some patients with sarcoidosis. Short-term responses are often dramatic[290,297,299,301]. In uncontrolled studies, 50 to 90% respond favourably to corticosteroids[290,297,299,301]. A recent multicentre trial by the British Thoracic Society[298] supports the use of corticosteroids for patients with chronic, persistent radiographic infiltrates. In that study, 158 patients with stage II or III sarcoidosis were observed for 6 months prior to randomization. By 6 months, spontaneous remission had occurred in 58 (39%) of patients; 33 (22%) were treated with corticosteroids for clinical indications and were never randomized. The remaining 58 patients (39%) had persistent radiographic infiltrates after 6 months and were randomized to prednisolone (30 mg daily for 1 month,

tapered to 10 mg by 3 months) or placebo. However, even in the placebo cohort, patients could receive corticosteroids if deemed necessary by their attending physician. Both groups were followed for a mean of 5 years. At long-term follow-up, chest radiographs and pulmonary function tests were significantly improved in the corticosteroid-treated cohort. Long-term impact is less clear, as relapses occur in one-third to one-half of patients after taper or discontinuation of corticosteroids[290,295,297,301].

Corticosteroids have myriad adverse effects, and their routine use in asymptomatic or minimally symptomatic patients should be discouraged. A trial of therapy should be offered to patients with severe, progressive, or persistent symptoms or organ dysfunction (pulmonary or extrapulmonary). In patients with mild impairment, the decision to treat can be delayed for up to 12 months to determine if spontaneous resolution ensues. Patients with chronic symptoms lasting >1 year should be treated, as spontaneous remissions are uncommon in this context. Therapy is rarely efficacious in patients with far-advanced fibrosis, honeycombing, or bullae (radiographic stage IV)[38,301]. In this context, treatment is reserved for patients with a progressive course or ancillary evidence for alveolitis. Optimal dose or duration of corticosteroid therapy has not been studied. Doses as high as 1 mg/kg/day prednisone have been used[299], but lower doses (e.g., prednisone 40 mg/day for 4 weeks, with a taper) are often efficacious and are less toxic. We reserve higher doses (1 mg/kg/day) for CNS or cardiac involvement. Patients responding to therapy are maintained on a tapering dose for a total course of 12 to 18 months. The dose and rate of taper is guided by the response and presence or absence of side effects. Patients exhibiting a proclivity to relapse require long term (sometimes indefinite) therapy with low dose alternate day prednisone (e.g., 10 to 20 mg every other day).

Inhaled corticosteroids suppress endobronchial or alveolar inflammation, and have been used with anecdotal successes in patients with sarcoidosis[307,308]. However, two recent randomized double-blind trials failed to show benefit with inhaled corticosteroids for pulmonary sarcoidosis[309,310]. Inhaled corticosteroids have a limited role for treating endobronchial sarcoidosis, but are not adequate for severe pulmonary parenchymal involvement.

Immunosuppressive or cytotoxic agents have been used to treat sarcoidosis, with anecdotal successes. Randomized trials comparing these agents are lacking. Methotrexate (MTX), administered once weekly orally or intramuscularly[45] has been used to treat sarcoidosis, with anecdotal successes[311]. In three studies by investigators from the University of Cincinnati comprising more than 230 patients, favourable responses to MTX were cited in 52 to 66%[311–213]. Relapses were frequent upon discontinuation of therapy, but responded to reintroduction of MTX[311]. These studies were not blinded or controlled. These investigators recently published a double-blind, randomized study of 24 patients with new onset, symptomatic sarcoidosis[314]. Following initial treatment with prednisone for 4 weeks, patients were randomized to MTX or placebo for 6 months. Prednisone was tapered according to a predetermined schedule. Only 15 of 24 patients enrolled received at least 6 months of therapy. Among patients receiving >6 months of MTX, a steroid sparing-effect was suggested. However, MTX was no better than placebo when all patients were considered. While these various studies are not definitive, oral MTX (10 to 20 mg once weekly) has a role for patients failing or intolerant of corticosteroids. Because of potential hepatotoxicity with prolonged use[45], we prefer azathioprine when more than 2 years of therapy is contemplated.

Azathioprine (dose 2–3 mg/kg/day), has been used in patients with sarcoidosis, with anecdotal responses[45,315–317]. Data are limited to anecdotal cases[301,318] and a few small series[315–317]; randomized trials have not been done. In two early studies, 10 of 20 patients failing corticosteroids responded to AZA[315,316]. Another retrospective study cited reponses in 8 of 14 patients treated with AZA for neurosarcoidosis[319]. Diab et al. cited favorable responses in all 7 patients treated with a combination of AZA and prednisone[320]. In contrast, AZA was marginally effective in a retrospective study of 10 patients with chronic pulmonary sarcoidosis[317]. All had only partial or no response to corticosteroids. Sustained improvement in PFTs was achieved in only two patients with AZA; 2 others transiently improved. Although data are limited, we believe azathioprine is useful as a steroid-sparing agent or in selected patients with severe or progressive sarcoidosis refractory to corticosteroids.

Cytotoxic alkylating agents (e.g. cyclophosphamide and chlorambucil) have been used to treat corticosteroid-recalcitrant sarcoidosis, but data are limited to anecdotal cases and a few small non-randomized series[301,313,321,322]. Favourable responses were cited in 20 of 31 patients (64%) treated with chlorambucil[322]. Only 5 had failed corticosteroid therapy; the remaining patients required unacceptably high doses of corticosteroids. Because chlorambucil is oncogenic and has myriad toxicities[45], we do not recommend this agent for sarcoidosis. Data regarding cyclophosphamide (CP) are limited to a few case reports and one small series[313]. Favourable responses were achieved in 8 of 10 patients with neurosarcoidosis treated with 'pulse' intravenous CP[313]. All had failed corticosteroids; 8 had failed methotrexate. Cyclophosphamide is oncogenic and has numerous potential toxicities[45]. We reserve pulse CP for patients with severe CNS sarcoidosis refractory to corticosteroids and other immunosuppressive agents (e.g. azathioprine, methotrexate, and/or hydroxychloroquine).

Antimalarial drugs (e.g. chloroquine, hydroxychloroquine) inhibit several facets of immune responses, including antigen presentation and cytokine production[301]. Antimalarials concentrate in cells of the reticuloendothelial system and melanin-containing tissues (e.g. skin, spleen, leukocytes, kidney) and are preferentially concentrated in epithelioid, mononuclear, and giant cells comprising sarcoid granulomata[301]. Anecdotal successes were cited with antimalarials for treating sarcoid-induced hypercalcemia[279,323,324], cutaneous[325–328], central nervous system[329] or osseous lesions[330]. In one uncontrolled[328] and two randomized trials[331,332], favourable responses were cited with chloroquine (CQ) for pulmonary sarcoidosis. A recent randomized trial of 23 patients with symptomatic pulmonary sarcoidosis (stage II or III) suggested benefit with CQ[332]. Unfortunately, irreversible retinopathy and blindness are potential, albeit rare, complications of prolonged CQ use. For this reason, CQ has been used sparingly. Hydroxychloroquine (hydroxyCQ) is much less toxic than CQ; retinal toxicity with this agent occurs in <1% of patients, even with prolonged use[301]. Although hydroxychloroquine is less potent than CQ, we use hydroxyCQ (dose 200 mg once or twice daily) as a steroid-sparing agent or as adjunctive therapy in patients failing corticosteroids or immunosuppressive agents. Combining hydroxyCQ with corticosteroids or immunosuppressive agents may enhance immunomodulatory effects[333]. The half-life of hydroxyCQ is prolonged; responses may be delayed for 2 to 6 months. A six-month trial is recommended before abandoning this agent. For chronic maintenance therapy, a dose of 200 mg daily may be adequate. The major toxicities of antimalarials include: gastrointestinal symptoms (nausea, diarrhea, bloating); cutaneous effects (rash, urticaria, pruritus, discoloration of skin); headache, nervousness, insomnia, dizzyness; retinopathy; corneal deposits affecting colour vision[332]. Ophthalmological examinations should be performed every 6 months to monitor for ocular toxicity. Retinal changes mandate discontinuation of therapy.

Cyclosporin A (CsA), which inhibits T lymphocyte activation, proliferation, and lymphokine release[45], has been used to treat sarcoidosis, with anecdotal successes[317,319,334]. However, overall clinical experience is disappointing[334,335]. In a recent randomized, controlled trial, oral CsA plus prednisone was no more effective than prednisone alone in patients with progressive pulmonary sarcoidosis[336]. Given its expense and potential for myriad adverse effects[45], CsA has at best a marginal role as salvage therapy for patients with severe, progressive sarcoidosis refractory to other agents.

Anecdotal successes were cited with pentoxifylline, an immunomodulatory agent[337] which inhibits the synthesis of tumour necrosis factor-α (TNF-α) and γ-interferon in vitro[338]. In one study, 23 patients with untreated sarcoidosis and progressive disease were treated with oral pentoxifylline (25 mg/kg/day) for 6 months[339]. Among 18 evaluable patients, 11 improved; 7 remained stable; none deteriorated. Three additional patients with corticosteroid-refractory disease improved when pentoxifylline was added to prednisone. Additional studies are required to determine the role (if any) of pentoxifylline. Anecdotal responses were claimed with thalidomide, an agent with antifibrotic and immunomodulatory effects[340,341] in a few patients with cutaneous[342] or pulmonary sarcoidosis[343]. These data are sparse, and efficacy of thalidomide is unproven. Principal side effects associated with thalidomide include: teratogenicity, somnolence, and neuropathy[340].

Lung transplantation is an option for patients with end-stage pulmonary sarcoidosis[160,344,345]. Overall survival is comparable to non-sarcoid transplant recipients[344]. Recurrence of granulomata in the lung allograft(s) is common, cited in 5 of 8 patients[344]. Clinically significant granulomata, with pulmonary dysfunction, is rare[160,344].

Hypersensitivity pneumonia (extrinsic allergic alveolitis)

Hypersensitivity pneumonia (HP) (also termed extrinisic allergic alveolitis) is a cell-mediated response to a variety of inhaled organic dusts or inorganic chemicals[346,347]. Exposure in the workplace environs (e.g. agricultural or textile occupations), hobbies (e.g. raising birds), or home (e.g. humidifers) elicits the syndrome. More than 50 different occupational and environmental sources of antigen associated with HP are known[347]. The prototype of HP is 'farmer's lung', caused by inhalation of thermophilic actinomycetes spores from moldy hay[347,348]. Exposure evokes the clinical syndrome in only 1 to 8% of[347,348]. Other syndromes elicited by thermophilic actinomycetes in occupational settings include air conditioner (humidifer) lung[349], mushroom worker's lung[350], and bagassosis (from exposure to sugar cane). In Mexico, domestic exposure to pigeon antigens (pigeon breeder's lung) is the most common cause of HP[351]. Six to 15% of pigeon breeders develop HP[347,351]. In Japan, summer-type HP results from contamination of homes with *Trichosporon cutaneum*[352] or *Cryptococcus albidus*[353]. Several antigens are implicated in humidifier lung including thermophilic *Actinomyces*, *Sphaeropsidales*, *Penicillium* sp., protozoa, and *Klebsiella oxytoca*[354]. Other causes of HP included contaminated heated swimming pools[355], composting waste at home[356]; *Pseudomonas fluorescens* in machine operator's lung[357]; *Mycobacterium avium* (in hot tubs)[354]; *Klebsiella oxytoca* (in hot tubs)[358]; *Pezizia domiciliana* (home contamination)[359]. A recent report cited 2 cases of HP in peat moss processing plant workers[202]. High levels of molds (i.e., *Monocillium* spp and *Penicillium citreonigrum*) were found in peat moss in the packaging plant; serum antibodies

to these microorganisms were identified in both patients with HP. A few specific syndromes due to HP related to antigenic exposures are listed in Table 12.2.

Irrespective of etiological agents, the clinical presentations of HP are similar. Acute HP presents with fever, dyspnea, cough, peripheral leukocytosis, and pulmonary infiltrates, 2 to 12 hours following exposure to the offending antigen[346,347,360]. Basilar crackles, and occasionally cyanosis, may be present[202,346]. Chest radiographs in acute HP usually reveal bilateral alveolar or interstitial infiltrates, but may be normal[361–263]. In subacute and chronic HP, fine linear or nodular shadows and cystic radiolucencies predominate[351,364]. Hilar lymphadenopathy or pleural effusions are not features of HP[347,362,363]. HRCT scans in acute or subacute HP reveal micronodules, ground glass opacities, a peribronchiolar distribution, a predilection for mid or upper lung zones, and variable areas of attenuation[19,362–364] (Fig. 12.24). Patchy areas of hyperlucency in a lobular distribution reflect bronchial obstruction[19,362,363]. With end-stage disease, fibrosis or emphysema are observed[348,364]. Pulmonary function tests demonstrate restrictive, obstructive, or mixed defects[347,348,361], with reduced DLCO[346]. In severe cases, hypoxemia is prominent[346]. Following removal of the offending antigen, symptoms abate or resolve within 12 to 48 hours[346,347]. Repeated acute exposures to relevant antigen(s) lead to recurrent episodes of acute HP[346,365] or chronic HP[351,364].

Chronic, low dose exposure to sensitizing antigens causes chronic HP, which evolves over months or years. Cardinal features of chronic HP are progressive cough, dyspnea, crackles, a restrictive defect on PFTs, hypoxemia, and basilar interstitial infiltrates on chest radiographs[351,364]. These features mimic CFA/UIP. Repetitive damage may cause airways obstruction, emphysema[348,366] and even fatal respiratory insufficiency or cor pulmonale[367]. Although CT features of chronic HP and CFA/UIP overlap, HRCT is helpful to distinguish these entities[364]. Micronodules and extensive ground glass opacities are present in 32 to 42% of patients with chronic HP, but in only 6 to 12% of patients with

Table 12.2. Selected causes of hypersensitivity pneumonitis (HP)[a]

Disease syndrome	Source	Offending antigen
	Plant products	
Farmer's lung	Mouldy hay or corn	Thermophilic actinomycetes
Ventilator lung	Air conditioner, humidifier	Thermophilic actinomycetes
Bagassosis	Mouldy sugar cane	Thermophilic actinomycetes
Mushroom worker's lung	Mouldy compost	Thermophilic actinomycetes
Hot tub lung	Mould on ceiling	*Cladosporium* sp.
Suberosis	Mouldy cork	*Penicillium* sp.
Maple bark stripper's disease	Contaminated maple	*Cryptostroma corticale*
Malt worker's lung	Contaminated barley	*Aspergillus clavatus*
Tobacco worker's lung	Mould on tobacco	*Aspergillus* spp
Wine grower's disease	Mould on grapes	*Aspergillus* spp
Wood pulp worker's disease	Wood pulp	*Alternaria* spp
Japanese summer house HP	House dust	*Trichosporon cutaneum*
	Animal products	
Pigeon breeder's disease	Excreta or feathers	Avian antigens
Laboratory worker's lung	Rat fur	Rat urine protein
Pituitary snuff	Pituitary powder	Vasopressin
Miller's lung	Grain weevils in wheat flour	*Sitophilius granarius* proteins
	Reactive chemicals	
TDI HP	Toluene diisocyanate	Altered proteins
TMA HP	Trimellitic anhydride	Altered proteins

[a] Reprinted with permission[8].

IPF[364]. Honeycombing, lower lobe predominance, and subpleural location are cardinal features of CFA/UIP (noted in >80% of patients) but are evident in a minority of patients with chronic HP[364].

Surgical lung biopsies in acute HP demonstrate intense lymphocytic infiltration, a bronchocentric distribution, foam cells, scattered loosely formed granulomata, and foci of bronchiolitis obliterans[346,361]. These features may be lacking on TBBs, due to the small sample size[361]. Chronic HP causes severe fibrosis and end-stage honeycomb lung (indistinguishable from CFA)[351,364]. Surgical biopsy is not always necessary, provided the clinical scenario is classic. Bronchoalveolar lavage in HP reveals striking lymphocytosis (>40%) with CD8+ predominance and high levels of immunoglobulins (IgG and IgM); BAL neutrophilia may coexist[202,347]. These features are non-specific, as BAL lymphocytosis occurs in exposed individuals without symptoms or clinical disease[202,347,361]. Rare patients manifest CD4 predominant forms of HP, which may progress to fibrosis[368].

Serum precipitating antibodies to the offending antigen(s) are present in more than 90% of patients with HP, but are non-specific, as circulating antibodies are present in up to 50% of exposed individuals without clinical disease[347,351,360]. Many hospitals or research laboratories screen for HP by a panel of precipitating antibodies to the most commonly implicated antigens (e.g. thermophilic *actinomyces, aspergillus* spp., *Micropolyspora faenii,* avian antigens). These 'hypersensitivity pneumonia screens' are highly sensitive (provided the offending antigen is implicated), but miss less common antigens[202,346,359]. A diagnosis of HP is assumed in the appropriate clinical context if the

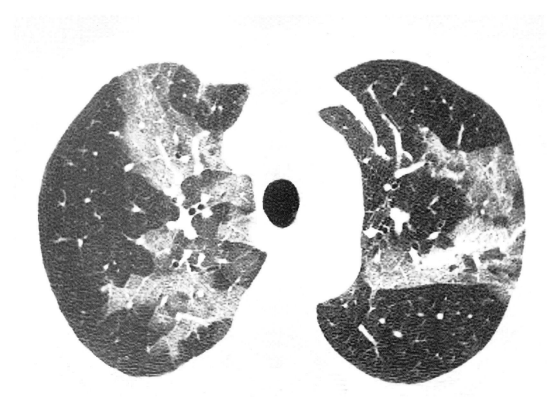

Fig. 12.24 Hypersensitivity pneumonia. HRCT scan from a 59-year-old woman with fever, cough, and dyspnea demonstrating dense focal alveolar (ground glass) opacities in a peribronchiolar distribution. Transbronchial lung biopsies demonstrated lymphocytic infiltrates, foamy macrophages, and non-caseating granulomas, consistent with HP. The disease cleared completely following institution of corticosteroids and avoidance of further exposure to moulds.(Reproduced with permission.)[9]

following criteria are present; a sensitizing agent is implicated by environmental or occupational history; serum antibodies to the presumed sensitizing agent are demonstrable; BAL lymphocytosis (particularly if CD8+ is predominant) is present; symptoms resolve following removal of the offending agent[346,347,360].

Avoidance of the offending agent is the mainstay of treatment for HP. In some cases, inspection of the home for unrecognized causes detects the etiological agent[359]. For example, an unusual fungus, *Pezizia domiciliana*, was implicated as a cause of HP on the basis of detection of fungal spores in the home, high titre precipitating antibodies to *P. domiciliana* in the serum, a compatible open lung biopsy,

resolution of HP following prednisone therapy, and eradication of the fungus from the home[359]. Prognosis of HP depends upon the chronicity, duration and extent of antigen exposure, and extent of fibrosis, honeycombing, or emphysema. Prognosis of Farmer's Lung Disease (FLD) is excellent (<1% fatalities), provided farmers are removed from exposure before significant fibrosis develops[367]. Emphysema is a late complication[348,366]. In early studies (antedating HRCT scans), interstitial fibrosis was believed to be the most common long-term consequence of chronic FLD. More recent studies using HRCT found that emphysema is a more common sequelae (even in non-smokers) and correlates with recurrent episodes of FLD[348,366]. Similarly, among patients with chronic bird breeder's lung, emphysematous changes were demonstrated by HRCT in 11 of 24 (44%) patients[369]. Pigeon breeder's disease in the United States and Europe is rarely disabling or fatal. However, in Mexico, 5-year fatality rate among 78 patients with chronic pigeon breeder's lung was 29%[351]. The role of corticosteroids to treat HP is controversial, but short term responses occur[347,359,365]. Corticosteroids are recommended for severe or progressive cases[347,365,370]. Corticosteroids accelerate improvement in acute farmer's lung disease, but long term impact is less clear[365]. In one study, corticosteroids were ineffective for chronic pigeon breeder's lung[351]. Data on immunosuppressive or cytotoxic agents are limited to anecdotal cases; efficacy is unproven.

Chronic eosinophilic pneumonia

Chronic eosinophilic pneumonia (CEP) is characterized by cough, dyspnea, wheezing, migratory alveolar infiltrates, constitutional symptoms, blood eosinophilia, and dense pulmonary infiltration with eosinophils[39–41,371]. Extrapulmonary involvement is lacking. Symptoms develop over several weeks or months[39,371]; rarely, the course is more fulminant[41,372,373]. Atopy or clinical asthma often precede CEP, and parallel the course of the radiographic infiltrates[39,40]. Blood eosinophil counts and ESR are increased in >80% of patients with CEP, and correlate with disease activity[39,40,371]. PFTs demonstrate obstructive or restrictive patterns, reduced DLCO, or hypoxemia[39,40]. Chest radiographs reveal patchy, subpleural alveolar infiltrates, with a predilection for the upper lobes[39,40] (Fig. 12.25). The peripheral distribution of alveolar infiltrates, with central sparing, is termed 'the photographic negative of pulmonary edema'[39,40]. Less common patterns include focal lobar consolidation or patchy or diffuse reticulonodular infiltrates[39,40,371]. HRCT scans depict the alveolar nature and peripheral distribution of CEP, but are non-specific, expensive, and of doubtful clinical value[40].

Histopathological features include: dense aggregates of eosinophils, histiocytes and multinucleated giant cells within alveolar spaces, septae, and bron-

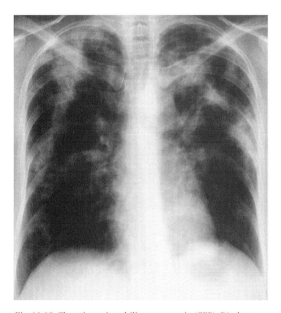

Fig. 12.25 Chronic eosinophilic pneumonia (CEP). PA chest radiograph from a 35-year-old woman with fever, cough, and wheezing demonstrates multiple, focal dense alveolar infiltrates in the upper lobes and axillary regions. BAL demonstrated marked eosinophilia. Transbronchial lung biopsies demonstrated eosinophilic abscesses consistent with CEP. The infiltrates resolved following institution of corticosteroid therapy.

chioles; eosinophilic abscesses; degenerating, necrotic eosinophils; Charcot-Leyden crystals; alveolar macrophages containing eosinophilic fragments; foci of bronchiolitis obliterans; scattered lymphocytes and plasma cells[39,40] (Fig. 12.26). Extensive fibrosis or parenchymal necrosis are rare. Surgical lung biopsy is usually not necessary, as the diagnosis of CEP can be affirmed by bronchoscopic techniques (TBBs or BAL eosinophilia) (provided the clinical context is appropriate)[39,40,371].

Corticosteroid therapy is highly efficacious[39,40,371]. An initial dose of prednisone 40 to 60 mg per day is usually adequate; higher doses are reserved for more severe cases[40]. Responses to corticosteroids are often dramatic. Fever, blood eosinophilia, and symptoms abate within 24 to 48 hours[39,40]. Chest radiographs normalize within 2 to 3 weeks[39,40,371]

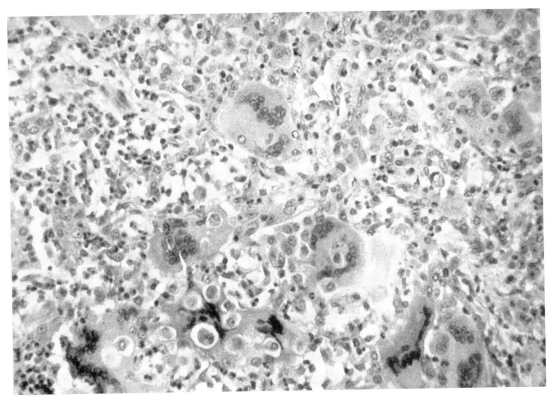

Fig. 12.26 Chronic eosinophilic pneumonia (CEP). Photomicrograph from open lung biopsy from a patient with CEP demonstrating numerous Touton-type multinucleated giant cells within alveolar spaces. Eosinophils are also interspersed within the pulmonary interstitium and alveolar spaces. (Reproduced with permission.)[552]

(Fig. 12.27(*a*) (*b*)). This rapidity of response is distinctive and affirms the diagnosis even when histological confirmation is lacking[39,40,371]. The dose of corticosteroid and rate of taper is guided by clinical, radiographic, and laboratory parameters (e.g. blood eosinophil counts or erythrocytic sedimentation rate (ESR). Relapses occur in 80% of patients upon discontinuation of corticosteroids[39,40,371]. Corticosteroids should be continued for a minimum of 12 months. Indefinite therapy with low dose prednisone (e.g. 10 to 20 mg every other day) is warranted in some patients with repetitive relapses.

Acute eosinophilic pneumonia

Idiopathic 'acute eosinophilic pneumonia' is an acute febrile illness (1 to 21 days' duration), with cough, chest pain, dyspnea, diffuse infiltrates on chest radiographs, severe hypoxemic respiratory failure, striking BAL eosinophilia (>25% eosinophils), and histological features consistent with CEP[40,41,372–375]. Diffuse alveolar damage (DAD) with hyaline membranes may be prominent on open lung biopsy[373]. The course is abrupt, often progressing to severe hypoxemic respiratory failure. Peripheral blood eosinophilia is sometimes present[41,372–374]. A careful history of drug ingestion is mandatory, as several medications or drugs cause eosinophilic pneumonia[216–220]. Acute eosinophilic pneumonia is potentially life-threatening, but responds dramatically to corticosteroids[40,41,372–375]. Because infections can evoke similar responses[376], appropriate special stains and cultures of BAL fluid or lung tissue should be done prior to initiating cor-

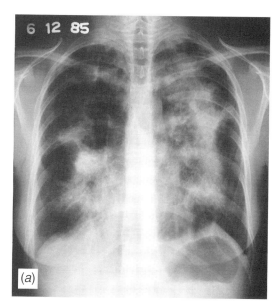

Fig. 12.27(a) Chronic eosinophilic pneumonia. PA chest radiograph demonstrating widespread but focal alveolar opacities with a ground glass appearance in a 28-year-old woman with fever, wheezing, and dyspnea. Transbronchial lung biopsies were compatible with CEP. (Reproduced with permission.)[40]

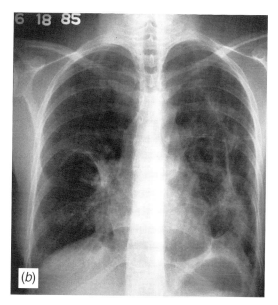

Fig. 12.27(b) Follow-up chest radiograph 5 days after institution of prednisone therapy demonstrating marked, albeit partial, resolution of infiltrates. (Reproduced with permission.)[40]

ticosteroid therapy. For fulminant cases, high dose intravenous corticosteroids should be given empirically, while awaiting microbiological results. Among responding patients, oral prednisone (1 mg/kg/day, with a gradual taper), is substituted. Symptoms improve within hours to days; chest radiographs normalize within 1 to 2 weeks[41,372-374]. A brief (2 to 3 month) course of therapy may be adequate, as late relapses are uncommon[41,372-374].

Cryptogenic organizing pneumonia (COP)

Cryptogenic organizing pneumonia (COP), also termed bronchiolitis obliterans organizing pneumonia (BOOP), is a rare disease of unknown cause characterized by a subacute course, cough, dyspnea, crackles, and focal infiltrates on chest radiographs[50,377-379]. Secondary causes include: connective tissue diseases[128]; inflammatory bowel disease[380]; Wegener's granulomatosis[381]; autoim-

mune disorders[378]; drugs[378]; radiation therapy[382,383]; chemotherapy[384]; infections[378]; bone marrow[380,385] or lung transplant[386] recipients. Extrapulmonary involvement does not occur. However, a viral syndrome within the previous 1–2 months is noted in more than one third of patients[50,377,378]. Fever and constitutional symptoms may be prominent, either at presentation or during relapses[378,387]. Most cases of COP are in adults between 50 and 60; there is no gender predominance[378].

Rapidly progressive COP, with severe hypoxemia and ARDS, has been described, but is rare[388,389]. Lung biopsies demonstrated features consistent with COP, but diffuse alveolar damage, severe fibrosis, and honeycombing were also present[388]. Despite aggressive therapy with corticosteroids (often combined with immunosuppressive agents), most patients died. Such cases may represent an unusual subset of COP, but are more likely to be either acute interstitial pneumonia (AIP) or organizing ARDS[378].

Chest radiographs in COP reveal focal, alveolar opacities (mimicking pneumonia) in 67 to 85% of

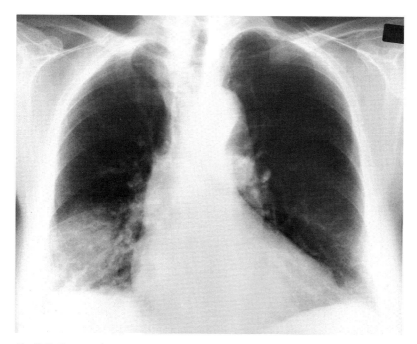

Fig. 12.28 Cryptogenic organizing pneumonia. PA chest radiograph demonstrates dense alveolar infiltrate in the right lower lobe. Three months earlier, a dense alveolar infiltrate in the right upper lobe was noted. Transbronchial lung biopsies confirmed the diagnosis of COP. Prednisone (40 mg every other day) was instituted, with rapid and prompt clearing.

patients; a reticulonodular pattern is found in 15 to 30%[50,378,387] (Fig. 12.28). HRCT scans show focal peripheral alveolar opacities with striking air-bronchograms[378,383] (Fig. 12.29(*a*) (*b*)). Less commonly, diffuse interstitial or small nodular opacities are present[377,378]. Pulmonary function tests demonstrate a restrictive defect with reduced DLCO; mild hypoxemia is common[50,377,378,383]. Airflow obstruction is noted only in smokers[50,378]. Laboratory features are non-specific. Increases in ESR and C-reactive protein (CRP) are common[378,383,387].

Lung biopsies reveal plugs of granulation tissue plugging terminal bronchioles and extending into alveolar ducts and spaces (the organizing pneumonia component)[50,378] (Fig. 12.30). The alveolar walls are infiltrated by mononuclear cells; foam cells may be observed[50,378]. The alveolar architecture is preserved; necrosis or fibrosis are absent. Open lung biopsy was the diagnostic method of choice in initial studies[50]. However, TBBs may substantiate the diagnosis, provided clinical and radiographic features are consistent and infectious etiologies are excluded[238,378,379,383,387,390,391]. Bronchoalveolar lavage often shows increases in neutrophils, lymphocytes, and/or eosinophils; CD4/CD8 ratio is decreased[378,383].

The pathogenesis of COP is not known, but COP likely represents a stereotypic host response to diverse injurious or inflammatory stimuli[378]. The frequent association of antecedent viral or respiratory tract infections in COP suggests that inhaled antigens induce bronchiolar or alveolar injury. Immune complex deposition and recruitment of inflammatory cells may elicit the pathological response.

Corticosteroids are the cornerstone of therapy for COP (either idiopathic or associated with an underlying disease)[50,377,378,383]. Responses to corticosteroid therapy are usually excellent and often dra-

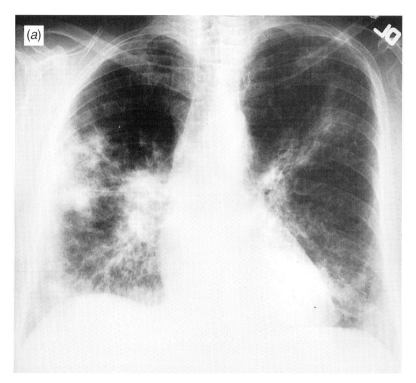

Fig. 12.29(a) Cryptogenic organizing pneumonia. PA chest radiograph from a 67-year-old woman demonstrates patchy bilateral infiltrates. She had been given three courses of antibiotics by her personal physician during the preceding 7 weeks because of persistant cough, fever, and dyspnea, with no improvement. Changes revealed by transbronchial lung biopsy were consistent with COP, and corticosteroids (1 mg of prednisone per kilogram of body weight per day) were initiated. (Reproduced with permission.)[4]

matic[377,378,383] (Fig. 12.31(*a*)–(*c*)). The optimal dose and duration of therapy has not been studied. Some investigators initiate treatment with prednisone (1 mg/kg/day, followed by a gradual taper)[50] but lower doses (0.75 mg/kg/day) are usually efficacious[378]. Relapses may occur as the corticosteroid is tapered or discontinued[377,378,387,392]. Rates of clinical failures or relapses are higher in secondary forms compared to idiopathic COP[379,387]. Other factors associated with a worse prognosis include: predominantly interstitial pattern on chest radiographs or HRCT[378]; lack of lymphocytosis on BAL[393]. Data on immuno-suppressive or cytotoxic drugs are limited to anec-dotal cases[378,394]. We reserve these agents for patients with severe or progressive disease refractory to cor-ticosteroids.

Obliterative bronchiolitis (OB)

Obliterative bronchiolitis (also termed constrictive bronchiolitis) is a stereotypic response to diverse insults affecting terminal bronchioles which results in severe and progressive air flow obstruction[238,395]. Most cases occur in the context of a specific disease or risk factor. Obliterative bronchiolitis complicates heart–lung or lung transplantation in 30 to 50% of patients, and represents chronic allograft rejec-tion[396–399]. Obliterative bronchiolitis may complicate bone marrow transplantation (BMT), principally in allogeneic recipients manifesting chronic graft-vs.-host disease (GVHD) in skin, mucous membranes, liver, or extrapulmonary sites[398]. The prevalence of OB is 10 to 12% among long-term survivors with

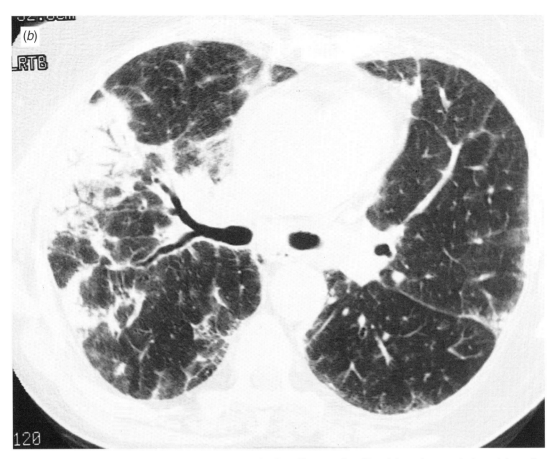

Fig. 12.29(b) CT from the same patient demonstrates dense alveolar infiltrates with striking air bronchograms in the periphery of the right lung. (Reproduced with permission.)[4]

GVHD but is rare (<1%) in allogeneic BMT recipients without GVHD or autologous recipients[238,398]. Other rare conditions associated with OB include: collagen vascular diseases (particularly rheumatoid arthritis)[128], exposure to or inhalation of toxic fumes, metals, dusts, or drugs; respiratory tract infections[238]. When no cause is identified, the term idiopathic OB is used. Idiopathic OB is distinctly rare. In one series, Turton and colleagues detected 10 patients with OB among 2094 cases of airflow obstruction[400].

Clinically, OB differs markedly from COP in clinical features, prognosis, and responsiveness to therapy. Patients with OB present with cough,

dyspnea, and severe airflow obstruction, which progresses relentlessly over weeks to months[238,395]. In late phases, recurrent infections due to *Pseudomonas aeruginosa* or *Staphylococcus aureus* are common, and accelerate the process[238,395]. Severe reductions in FEV1 and FEV1/FVC ratio are characteristic[401]. Air-trapping (increased residual volume) or hyperinflation (increased TLC) are common[400]. Reduction in DLCO is seen with severe impairment (FEV1 < 1.0 l)[401]. Physical examination reveals diminished breath sounds, rhonchi, or midinspiratory squeaks; rales are present in fewer than 20%[238,395,400]. Chest radiographs are usually normal or demonstrate hyperflation[401,402]. Diffuse reticular

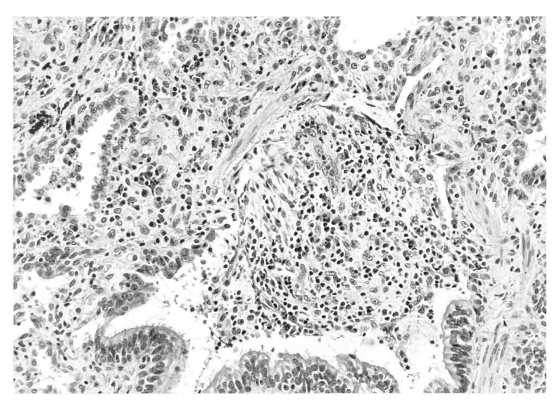

Fig. 12.30 Cryptogenic organizing pneumonia. Photomicrograph of open lung biopsy specimen demonstrating a plug of granulation tissue within a respiratory bronchiole. A peribronchiolar mononuclear inflammatory cell infiltrate is also evident (hematoxylin-eosin stain). (Reproduced with permission.)[553]

or micronodular shadows are present in a minority of patients[401,402]. With advanced disease, ring shadows and bronchiectasis develop. The cardinal HRCT feature in OB is patchy lobular or segmental regions of decreased lung attenuation, accentuated by expiration (a mosaic pattern)[401] (Fig. 12.32). These low attenuation lesions are due to air-trapping distal to obstructed bronchioles and are interspersed with areas of normal or increased attenuation[401]. Dynamic expiratory CT scans are superior to inspiratory scans in detecting air trapping[401,403]. Additional CT features (noted in more than two thirds of patients) include: peribronchiolar nodules; dilated bronchioles and bronchi; bronchiectasis or bronchioloectasis[401,402].

Obliterative (constrictive) bronchiolitis is centred on terminal and respiratory bronchioles[238,395,404].

Bronchioles are concentrically narrowed by this fibrotic/inflammatory process; lumens are effaced or obliterated[238,395,404]. The lesions are patchy and may be missed, even on open lung biopsy, unless serial sections and trichrome stains are scrutinized. Remnants of destroyed bronchioles are surrounded by normal lung parenchyma. In contrast to COP, alveolar ducts and lung parenchyma are spared[238,395,404]. In late phases, distortion of bronchiolar lumens, bronchiolar dilatation, mucostasis, and bronchiectasis are present[404].

Irrespective of etiology, prognosis of OB is poor. Progressive airflow obstruction, resulting in fatal respiratory failure, is characteristic[128,238,395,404]. Spontaneous remissions do not occur. Corticosteroids, immunosuppressive or cytotoxic agents are often tried, but are usually ineffectual[238,395–398].

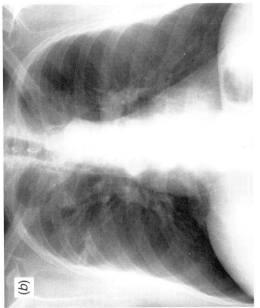

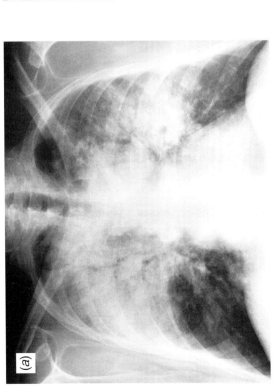

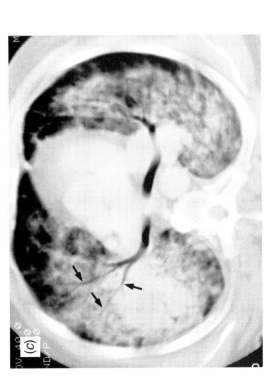

Fig. 12.31(a) Cryptogenic organizing pneumonia. PA chest radiograph from a 62-year-old man demonstrates confluent alveolar infiltrates in both upper lobes with extensive air bronchograms. He had been treated with broad-spectrum parenteral antibiotics for 2 weeks without improvement and with worsening findings on chest radiographs. (Reproduced with permission.)[4]

(b) PA chest radiograph from the same patient 3 weeks after institution of corticosteroid therapy demonstrates nearly complete resolution of alveolar infiltrates. (Reproduced with permission.)[4]

(c) Cryptogenic organizing pneumonia (COP). High-resolution CT from the same patient demonstrates confluent alveolar infiltrates and striking air bronchograms (arrows). Transbronchial lung biopsies demonstrated typical features of COP. Corticosteroids were initiated, and the process resolved during the next few weeks. (Reproduced with permission.)[4]

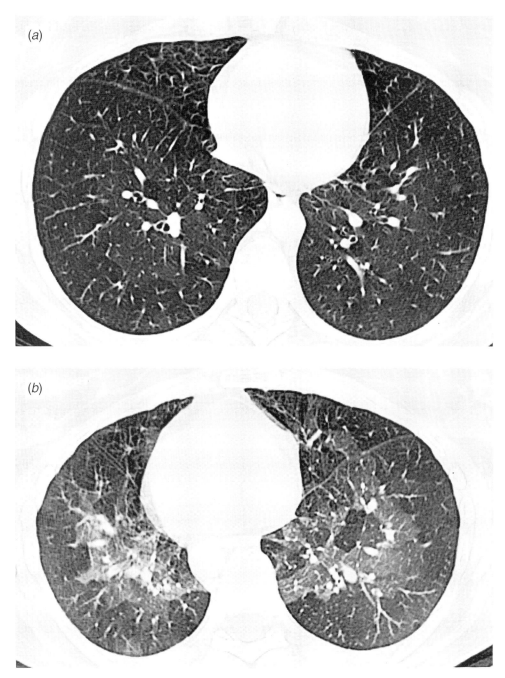

Fig. 12.32(a) Obliterative (constrictive) bronchiolitis (OB). Inspiratory CT scan in a 43-year-old female with systemic lupus erythematosus and OB (confirmed by thoracoscopic lung biopsy). Faint areas of ground glass opacity are present. (Reproduced with permission.)[128]

(b) Obliterative (constrictive) bronchiolitis (OB). Expiratory CT scan in the same individual with an accentuation of a mosaic pattern of ground-glass opacity. (Reproduced with permission.)[128]

Secondary bacterial or viral infections accelerate the course. Antibiotic therapy for secondary suppurative infections is critical. Lung transplantation is a viable option for patients with severe OB refractory to medical therapy.

Diffuse panbronchiolitis

Diffuse panbronchiolitis (DPB) is a chronic bronchiolar inflammatory process primarily seen in Japan and Korea which resembles cystic fibrosis[405,406]. Cardinal features of DPB include: chronic sinusitis, cough, sputum production, bronchiectasis, repetitive suppurative infections of the upper and lower respiratory tract, and progressive respiratory insufficiency[405]. The disease begins with sinusitis in the second or third decade of life followed by chronic cough, sputum production, and bronchiectasis 10 or more years later[405,407]. The cause is not known, but a strong genetic predisposition exists[406,408]. DPB is more common in men[407] and primarily occurs in Japanese and Koreans[405,406,408,409]. More than 60% of Japanese patients with DPB express HLA B-54, an antigen restricted to Asians[405,406,408,409]. In Koreans, a strong association between HLA-A11 and DPB was noted[406]. Only a few patients with DPB have been recognized in the United States or Europe[410]. It is likely that the candidate gene involved in DPB is located within the HLA region, between HLA-A and HLA-B loci[406].

Chest radiographs reveal hyperinflation and diffuse micronodules (1 to 4 mm in diameter), with a predilection for the lung bases; tram lines, ring-shadows, and dilated bronchioles reflect cystic bronchiectasis[405,407]. HRCT scans demonstrate diffuse micronodules, with a centrilobular distribution, thickened bronchial walls, bronchioloectasis, mosaic perfusion, air-trapping, and bronchial dilatation[405,407,411]. Obstructive defects, hypoxemia, and air-trapping are present on PFTs[405,407]. Laboratory tests reveal elevations in the ESR, C-reactive protein, and serum immunoglobulins[407]. The most distinctive feature is elevated cold agglutinins[407]. Serum antibodies against *Mycoplasma pneumoniae* are not found[405,407].

The cardinal histological feature of DPB is small nodules centred on respiratory bronchioles (bronchiolocentric), extending into peribronchiolar tissue[407]. These nodules correspond to dense peribronchiolar and intraluminal infiltrates of acute and chronic inflammatory cells[412]. Additional features include: aggregates of lipid-laden macrophages in the walls of respiratory bronchioles and alveolar ducts; intrabronchial mucus; narrowing or obliteration of respiratory bronchioles; bronchioloectasis and bronchiectasis; an alveolar component is lacking or minimal[405,412]. BAL shows intense neutrophilia (>50% of cells)[405,407].

Repetitive lower respiratory tract infections over many years lead to progressive respiratory failure and cor pulmonale[405,407]. Colonization of the lower respiratory tract with *Pseudomonas aeruginosa* (often mucoid strains), is associated with an accelerated course. Low dose erythromycin (600 mg/day) is the treatment of choice. Following the introduction of erythromycin as therapy for DPB in Japan, 5-year survival from the onset of respiratory symptoms improved from 63% to 91%[405,407]. Other macrolide antibodies (e.g. clarithromycin, roxithromycin, and azithromycin) also appear to be effective[407]. The mechanism of action of macrolides may reflect anti-inflammatory or immunomodulatory effects rather than direct antimicrobial effects[407,414]. Optimal duration of therapy is not known; a minimum of 6 to 12 months is advised[414]. Corticosteroids or immunosuppressive agents are of no value and may exacerbate infections. Interestingly, DPB recurred in the lung allograft in an African–American patient within 10 weeks of bilateral lung transplantation[415].

ANCA-associated vasculitides

Systemic necrotizing vasculitis may involve the lung, either as focal or cavitary infiltrative lesions, diffuse capillaritis (manifest as alveolar hemorrhage), or pulmonary aneurysms. Diffuse alveolar hemorrhage (due to capillaritis) may occur in the context of a pulmonary–renal syndrome (e.g. microscopic polyangiitis (MPA) or pauci-immune glomerulonephritis)[416,417], systemic necrotizing vasculitis (particularly Wegener's granulomatosis (WG))[223,418], Behçet's syndrome[419–421], Takayasu's disease[419], Henoch-Schonlein purpura[419], or connective tissue disease[161,422,423]. Classical polyarteritis nodosa (PAN) rarely involves the lung[424]. Pulmonary arterial aneurysms may complicate Takayasu's disease or Behçet's syndrome[425], and cause severe, even fatal, hemorrhage. In this chapter, we limit our discussion to pulmonary vasculitides associated with circulating autoantibodies directed against cytoplasmic components of neutrophils (ANCA)[426,427]. ANCAs are frequently present in necrotizing vasculitic syndromes affecting the lung[426–428]. ANCAs with different antigenic specificities have differing clinical and prognostic significance. Antibodies with a cytoplasmic pattern on immunofluorescence (c-ANCA) and antigenic specificity for proteinase-3 (PR-3-ANCA) are >70% sensitive and >90% specific for Wegener's granulomatosis but are found in a minority of patients with MPA or Churg–Strauss syndrome (CSS)[426–431]. In contrast, autoantibodies with a perinuclear pattern (p-ANCA) and antigenic specificity for myeloperoxidase (MPO) are uncommon in WG but are found in myriad disorders including MPA, CSS, pauci-immune glomerulonephritis, and diverse non-vasculitic inflammatory disorders (e.g. collagen vascular disease; inflammatory bowel disease)[426–431].

Wegener's granulomatosis (WG)

Wegener's granulomatosis (WG), the most common of the pulmonary granulomatous vasculitides, typically involves the upper respiratory tract (e.g. sinuses, ears, nasopharynx, oropharynx, trachea); lower respiratory tract (e.g. bronchi and lungs), and kidneys, with varying degrees of disseminated vasculitis[432–436]. The cardinal histopathological features of WG are: necrotizing vasculitis involving capillaries, venules, and arterioles; granulomatous inflammation; geographic necrosis; mixed inflammatory infiltrate; varying degrees of fibrosis[432,433,435]. These features may be lacking when small or non-representative biopsy specimens are obtained[435,437,438]. Estimated prevalence ranges from 1.3 to 3 cases per

100 000 persons per 5-year period[439]. The peak incidence is in the fourth through sixth decades of life; the disease is rare in children[432–435].

Clinical manifestations are protean; virtually any organ can be involved. Generalized WG may involve multiple organs, but limited variants (involving only 1 or 2 organs) exist[435]. The upper respiratory tract is involved in >85% of patients; chronic sinusitis, epistaxis, or otitis media are often the presenting symptoms[432–434]. Nasal manifestations occur in 60 to 80% of patients, and include epistaxis, rhinorrhea, nasal crusting, mucosal ulcers, or septal perforation[432–434]. Saddle nose deformity, resulting from destroyed nasal cartilage, occurs in 10 to 25% of patients[432–435]. Otological involvement occurs in 30 to 50%; symptoms include otalgia, chronic otitis media, chronic mastoiditis, tinnitus, and deafness[432–435]. Ocular involvement occurs in 20 to 50% of patients with WG[432–435]. Manifestations are diverse and include uveitis, conjunctivitis, episcleritis, proptosis, and blindness[432–435].

Granulomatous inflammation causes stenosis of the trachea or major bronchi in 10 to 30% of patients with WG[433,440–442]. Stenosis of the large airways may develop years after the initial diagnosis of WG[440,441]. Concomitant involvement of the nose or paranasal sinuses is nearly invariably present[433,441]. Subglottic stenosis can cause life-threatening upper airway obstruction (UAO), and can develop while the disease is quiescent at other sites[440,441]. Mucosal biopsies of trachea or bronchi are usually non-diagnostic, even with clinically significant involvement[440,441]. Truncation of the inspiratory limb of the flow-volume is a clue to UAO[441]. Fibreoptic bronchoscopy confirms the extent and site of stenosis. Subglottic stenosis may require dilatation, intralesional depo-corticosteroid injections, tracheostomy, or reconstructive surgery[435,441]. Spiral CT scans are useful to follow the course of the disease and response to therapy[443].

Lung involvement occurs in more than two-thirds of patients with WG[433–435,442]. Chest radiographs typically demonstrate multiple nodular infiltrates, with or without cavitation[433–435,442] (Fig. 12.33). Other features include focal pneumonic infiltrates; mass

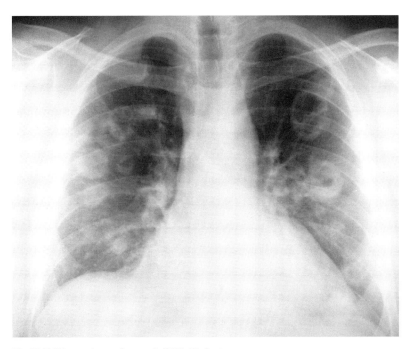

Fig. 12.33 Wegener's granulomatosis (WG). PA chest radiograph from a 40-year-old male demonstrates thin-walled cavitary pulmonary nodules. Open lung biopsy demonstrated a necrotizing granulomatous vasculitis, consistent with WG. (Reproduced with permission.)[135]

lesions (Fig. 12.34); diffuse reticulonodular infiltrates[433–435,442]. CT scans are more sensitive than chest radiographs in depicting parenchymal lesions[442,444] (Fig. 12.35). Surgical (open or VATS) lung biopsy is usually required to substantiate the diagnosis of pulmonary WG[438,445]. Among patients with pulmonary involvement, the triad of necrosis, vasculitis, and granulomatous inflammation is found in 90% of surgical lung biopsies, but in only 3 to 18% of endobronchial or transbronchial lung biopsies[438,442,445]. Massive diffuse alveolar hemorrhage (DAH), reflecting capillaritis, is a rare but life-threatening complication of WG[223,433–435,442,446] (Fig. 12.36). Rapidly progressive glomerulonephritis (RPGN), an uncommon early finding in WG, is present in >90% of patients with DAH[223,435,446]. In contrast, upper airway symptoms are present in a

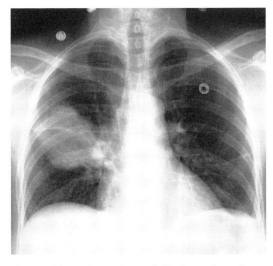

Fig. 12.34 Wegener's granulomatosis. PA chest radiograph demonstrates right upper lobe mass in a 36-year-old woman with leukocytoclastic vasculitis, fever, sinusitis, and cough. Transbronchial lung biopsies demonstrated granulomatous vasculitis with extensive necrosis and a polymorphous inflammatory cell infiltrate consistent with WG. (Reproduced with permission.)[135]

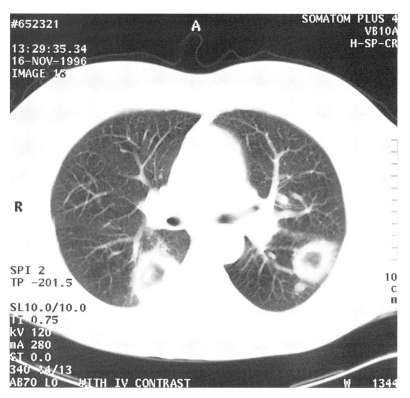

Fig. 12.35 Wegener's granulomatosis. CT scan from a patient with Wegener's granulomatosis demonstrates thick-walled cavitary nodules. Thoracoscopic lung biopsy demonstrated WG.

minority of patients with DAH[435]. Chest radiographs in DAH demonstrate bilateral alveolar infiltrates; the classic nodular or cavitary lesions of WG are lacking[435]. In contrast to patients with localized nodules or infiltrates, we do not advise surgical lung biopsy for patients with massive DAH. The diagnosis of DAH can be assumed by high titre circulating c-ANCA, compatible clinical and radiographic features, and bronchoscopy showing serosanguinous BAL fluid and large numbers of hemosiderin-laden macrophages[223,418]. Surgical lung biopsy is hazardous in the setting of massive DAH, and reveals non-specific findings of hemorrhage and capillaritis[446]. Granulomatous vasculitis or extensive parenchymal necrosis are lacking[435,446]. Massive DAH is a medical emergency. Immediate treatment with pulse intravenous methylprednisolone (1 g daily for 3 days) is recommended[223]. This is followed by conventional therapy with prednisone and cyclophosphamide[432,433] (discussed in greater detail below).

Glomerulonephritis (pauci-immune) occurs in 70 to 85% of patients with WG during the course of the disease[432–435]. The cardinal histological lesion on renal biopsy is focal, segmental, glomerulonephritis (GN)[432–435,442]. With more fulminant forms, a necrotizing, crescentic GN is observed[433,435]. Granulomatous vasculitis is present in fewer than 10% of patients undergoing renal biopsy[433–435,442]. Microscopic hematuria or proteinuria precede abnormalities in renal function[433,435]. Renal insufficiency is evident at the time of presentation in fewer than 20% of patients with WG[432–435]. Once renal failure is present, rapid progression ensues within days to weeks. Aggressive and prompt therapy with cyclophosphamide and corticosteroids[432,433] (discussed below) is essential to avoid irreversible renal

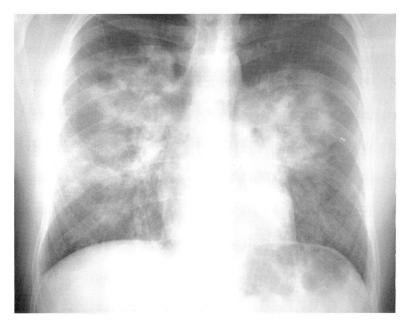

Fig. 12.36 Alveolar hemorrhage complicating Wegener's granulomatosis. PA chest radiograph demonstrated bilateral alveolar infiltrates in a 54-year-old male with hemoptysis, rapidly progressive renal failure, and high titre circulating c-ANCA.

damage. Chronic renal failure requiring dialysis occurs in 10 to 30% of patients with WG[433,435].

Central or peripheral nervous system involvement occurs in <4% of patients at presentation, but develops in 10 to 34% during the course of the disease[433,435,447]. Mononeuritis multiplex is most common, but cerebral infarction or mass lesions may be catastrophic[433,435,447]. Other features of WG include: constitutional symptoms (30 to 60%); cutaneous lesions (40–50%); cardiac involvement (5 to 15%); GI tract involvement (<10%)[432–435].

Striking elevations in ESR (often >100 mm/h) or C-reactive protein are characteristic of active, generalized WG[432–435]. Circulating c-ANCA (PR-3) are present in 60 to 97% of patients with WG, and are highly specific (>90%) for WG[428,435,448]. Changes in c-ANCA titres often correlate with disease activity, but c-ANCA persists in one third or more of patients even after complete clinical remissions are achieved[426,428,430,449]. Treatment decisions should not rest on c-ANCA titres alone[430,431,449]. However, sequential ANCA assays have an adjunctive role

(along with clinical criteria) to assess activity of the disease[426,428,430,449].

Prior to the availability of therapy, >80% of patients with WG died within 3 years of onset of symptoms, usually due to progressive renal failure[435]. Corticosteroids improved survival modestly. In the early 1970s, Fauci and colleagues combined oral cyclophosphamide (CP) (1–2 mg/kg/day) with prednisone (1 mg/kg/day, with gradual taper) as therapy for WG[432,433,435]. With this regimen, survival improved dramatically. Remissions are achieved in 80 to 93% of patients; early mortality rates are <15%[432–435]. Late mortality rates are higher, due to sequelae of vasculitis or complications of immunosuppressive or cytotoxic therapy[45,432,433,435,450]. Relapses occur in 50 to 75% of patients upon cessation or tapering of therapy[432,433,435]. A minimum of 12 to 18 months of therapy is advised.

Complications associated with chronic corticosteroid or CP use are appreciable[435,451]. Toxicities of CP include: bone marrow suppression; opportunistic infections; pulmonary toxicity; infertility; stomatitis; GI toxicities; hemorrhagic cystitis; bladder cancer; hematological malignancies[45,433,450]. Hemorrhagic cystic occurs in 5 to 50% of patients receiving chronic oral CP therapy[45,433] and is a precursor to bladder cancer[450]. Intravenous (i.v.) pulse CP is comparable to oral CP in inducing remissions in patients with WG, but remissions are not as durable[451–455]. Sustained remissions were achieved with i.v. pulse CP in only 21 to 48% of patients in five studies[451–455]. Daily oral CP/prednisone remains the gold standard for WG. Anecdotal successes were cited with chlorambucil, another alkylating agent, as therapy for WG[435,456]. Chlorambucil is oncogenic, and we prefer methotrexate or azathioprine for patients experiencing adverse effects from CP.

Oral methotrexate plus prednisone is an option for limited or non-fulminant WG[435,457]. In a non-randomized trial from the N.I.H., 42 patients with WG were treated with oral MTX plus prednisone[457]. Remissions were achieved in 71%; survival was 92%. Relapses occurred in 11 of 30 patients (36%), but reintroduction of MTX/prednisone led to remissions in 6 of 8. Data regarding MTX/prednisone for severe, generalized WG are lacking. Azathioprine was used in early studies of WG, but is less effective than CP and should not be used as initial therapy[432,435]. Azathioprine has a role to *maintain* remissions in patients responding to but experiencing adverse effects from CP[435].

Trimethoprim/sulfamethoxazole (T/S) reduces relapse rates in patients with WG[458] and has a role in limited, initial phase WG[459–461]. However, T/S is of doubtful value for severe or fulminant WG[435] and should not supplant conventional therapy with CP and corticosteroids. Anecdotal responses were cited in patients with systemic vasculitis (including WG) with high dose intravenous immunoglobulin G[462] or monoclonal antibodies targeted against T-cells[463]. Interpretation of efficacy is clouded by the concomitant use of CP or corticosteroids in many patients.

Microscopic polyangiitis (MPA)

Microscopic polyangiitis (previously termed overlap polyangiitis syndrome) exhibits clinical and serological features which overlap with WG and CSS[424,448,464–467]. Renal involvement is an invariable feature[424,448,464,468]. Renal biopsies reveal necrotizing crescentic glomerulonephritis with few or no immune complexes (pauci-immune)[424,448,464,468]. Other prominent features include: circulating ANCA (40 to 80%) and pulmonary capillaritis (20 to 40%)[424,448,464,468]. Diffuse alveolar hemorrhage may be life-threatening[424,464,466,468]. Other sites of involvement include: skin (leukocytoclastic vasculitis) (40–60%); GI tract (20–50%); peripheral neuropathy, (10–20%); oropharynx or nasopharynx (5 to 15%); heart (3–15%)[448,464,466,468]. A prodromal respiratory illness precedes the onset of vasculitis in one third of patients[448,464,466,468]. Arthralgias and myalgias may be prominent[468]. Renal infarcts or visceral aneurysms, cardinal features of PAN, are rarely found in MPA[424,468].

Microscopic polyangiitis is rare, with an estimated prevalence of 2.4 cases per million[439]. As the name implies, small vessels (e.g. capillaries, venules, arterioles) are invariably involved in MPA; these are spared in classical PAN[424]. Circulating ANCA are present in 40 to 80% of patients with MPA (usually p-ANCA-MPO but occasionally anti-PR3)[424,468]. In classic PAN, ANCA are uncommon (<20%)[424,468]. Further, glomerulonephritis or DAH are rarely observed in PAN[424,448,464]. Clinical and serological features of MPA overlap with WG and CSS. However, a granulomatous component (common to both WG and CSS), is lacking in MPA[424]. Asthma or eosinophilia, cardinal features of CSS, are not found in MPA[424].

Because of the rarity of MPA, optimal therapy is not known. Diverse treatment regimens employing prednisone, azathioprine, cyclophosphamide, and plasmapheresis, alone or in combination, are used[448,464,466,468,469]. Most investigators employ oral CP and corticosteroids, similar to the regimen advocated for WG[433,451,466,468]. Favourable responses are cited in >80%; ten year survival exceeds 70%[448,464,466,468]. Intravenous immunoglobulins (IVIg) were tried in a few patients with corticosteroid-recalcitrant MPA; 40% responded[468].

Churg–Strauss syndrome

Churg–Strauss syndrome (CSS), also termed allergic angiitis and granulomatosis, is a rare syndrome characterized by necrotizing vasculitis, asthma, hypereosinophilia, and extravascular eosinophilic granulomas[467,468,470]. CSS is rare, with an estimated incidence of 2.4 to 3.3 cases/million/year[439,471]. The incidence is higher in asthmatics (up to 64 cases/million/year)[472]. Asthma *precedes* the diagnosis of CSS in >90% of patients, and is usually the presenting feature[467,470]. A second phase of peripheral blood and tissue eosinophilia ensues[467,468,470]. The third phase, vasculitis, develops years after these earlier phases[467,468,470]. Manifestations of vasculitis are protean. Mononeuritis multiplex or CNS involvement occurs in 60 to 75% of patients with CSS[467,468,470,473]. Weight loss, fever, and constitutional features are usually present; 50% experience myalgias or polyarthralgias[467,470]. Cutaneous lesions occur in 50–60% (e.g. palpable purpura; skin nodules; urticaria; livedo; papules)[467,468,470]. Abdominal involvement occurs in 30 to 62%; abdominal pain may reflect perforation, ischemia, or vasculitis of mesenteric arteries[467,468,470]. Pulmonary infiltrates are present in 30 to 70 % of patients; alveolar hemorrhage is rare (<5%)[467,468,470]. Frequencies of other organ involvement are: renal (16–49%); cardiac (15–59%); ocular (<5%)[448,467,468,473]. In contrast to WG or MPA, severe glomerulonephritis rarely complicates CSS[448,467,473].

The ESR, CRP, and blood eosinophil counts are elevated in 80 to 91% of patients during the acute vasculitic phase or exacerbations[448,467,468,470]. Serum IgE is increased in three quarters of patients[467,468]. Circulating ANCAs (typically pANCA MPO) are present in two thirds of patients with CSS[424,448,467,468].

Cardinal histopathological features of CSS include: small vessel vasculitis (involving arterioles, venules, and capillaries); necrosis; eosinophilic infiltrates; a granulomatous component[424,467]. The pronounced eosinophilic and granulomatous components distinguish CSS from other vasculitides[424]. Major diagnostic criteria for CSS include: asthma; eosinophilia >10%; pulmonary infiltrate; paranasal sinusitis, histological proof of vasculitis; mononeuritis multiplex[474].

Although data on therapy are limited, corticosteroids (with or without cytotoxic or immunosuppressive agents) are the mainstay of therapy[467,468,470]. Choice of therapy depends upon the extent and severity of the disease. Renal insufficiency, severe GI tract involvement or involvement of the heart or CNS are associated with a worse prognosis[467]. For mild to moderate CSS, corticosteroids alone may be adequate (>80% of patients improve)[467,470]. For severe or multisystemic disease, corticosteroids are combined with CP (oral or pulse)[448,466–468]. Plasmapheresis is reserved for fulminant disease refractory to corticosteroids and CP[468]. With these diverse regimens, survival rates were comparable (3 year survival, 80–90%; 10-year survival, 72–78%[466–468]. Relapses occur in 20–30% of patients, often as the dose of corticosteroid or cytotoxic drug is reduced[467,468]. Fatalities reflect refractory vasculitis or complications of therapy[467,468]. Despite control of the vasculitis with therapy, asthma persists[467,468]. Anecdotal responses were cited with α-interferon (IFN α) in a few patients failing corticosteroid or cytotoxic therapy[448,475], but data are sparse.

Recently, cases of CSS have been noted in patients receiving cysteinyl leukotriene type 1 receptor antagonists (LTRAs) (e.g. zafirlukast, montelukast, pranlucast)[472,476–479]. A causal relationship between the use of LTRAs and CSS is unlikely. The occurrence of CSS likely reflects unmasking of the underlying vasculitic syndrome in patients with severe asthma and atopy rather than a direct effect of the drug[472,477].

Pulmonary eosinophilic granuloma (EG)

Langerhans' cell histiocytosis (LCH), also termed Langerhans' cell granulomatosis, pulmonary histiocytosis X, or pulmonary eosinophilic granuloma, is a rare disease of unknown etiology occurring almost exclusively in cigarette smokers[480–484]. Predominant symptoms include cough, dyspnea, or pneumothorax[481,484,485]. Symptoms develop insidiously, over weeks or months, but the onset is abrupt when pneumothorax is the presenting feature. Con-

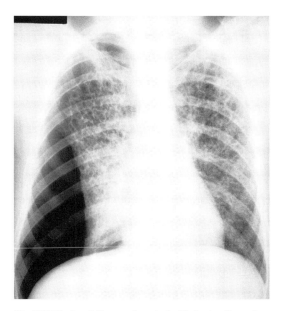

Fig. 12.37 Eosinophilic granulomatosis. PA chest radiograph demonstrates far-advanced cystic changes throughout lung parenchyma and bilateral pneumothoraces in a patient with pulmonary EG. (Reproduced with permission.)[4]

stitutional symptoms (e.g. low-grade fever, malaise, weight loss, or anorexia) are present in 15 to 30% of patients with pulmonary EG; extrapulmonary involvement (e.g. osteolytic bone lesions or diabetes insipidus) occurs in 15 to 20%[481,483–485]. Ten to 25% of patients with pulmonary EG are asymptomatic, with incidental findings on chest radiographs[484,485]. Physical examination is usually unremarkable, but rales, rhonchi, or wheezes may be present. There are no distinctive blood or serological aberrations. Peripheral blood eosinophilia is not a feature[481,484]. Some studies cited a high incidence of bronchogenic cancer (2 to 6%) in patients with pulmonary EG[486–488] but none of 48 patients in a series from the National Institutes of Health had lung cancer[484].

Chest radiographs reveal diffuse reticular, reticulonodular, or cystic lesions (primarily affecting the upper lobes); the costophrenic angles are spared[480,481,484,485]. Pleural effusions or intrathoracic lymphadenopathy are not found. Pneumothorax occurs in 6 to 20% of patients[483–485] (Fig. 12.37).

HRCT features in pulmonary EG are distinctive[489]. HRCT reveals numerous thin-walled cysts, preferentially involving the upper and mid lung zones[489] (Fig. 12.38). Peribronchiolar nodules (2 to 5 mm in size), reflecting cellular granulomatous lesions, are present in 60 to 80% of patients (Fig. 12.38(*b*) (*c*)). As the disease progresses, nodules are replaced by cysts, which coalesce, reaching sizes exceeding 2 to 3 cm in diameter. Cystic radiolucences are observed in other lung diseases (e.g. lymphangioleiomyomatosis, UIP, emphysema, etc.)[6,17], but the proclivity for upper and mid lung zones and nodular component distinguishes EG from these entities.

Pulmonary function tests typically reveal reduced DLCO and lung volumes (VC or TLC); normal or increased FEV1/FVC; impaired gas exchange[480,481,484,490]. Pure restrictive or mixed obstructive-restrictive patterns may be observed; hyperinflation (TLC > 110% predicted) is rare[490]. PFTs are normal in 15 to 20% of patients[484]

Pulmonary EG is almost exclusively seen in Caucasians, suggesting a genetic predisposition[483]. There is a slight male predominance[491] but some studies cite a female predominance[483,484]. Pulmonary EG typically affects adults between ages 20 and 50 and is rare in children[484,491].

Histologically, pulmonary EG is characterized by inflammatory, cystic, nodular, and fibrotic lesions distributed in a bronchocentric fashion[484] (Fig. 12.39). Langerhans cells (also termed histiocytosis X cells) are the cornerstone of the diagnosis. Langerhans cells (LC cells) are large ovoid histiocytes with pale eosinophilic cytoplasm, indented (grooved or 'coffee-bean') nuclei, and inconspicuous nucleoli[484,492] (Fig. 12.40). In equivocal cases, immunohistochemical stains [e.g., S100 protein or common thymocyte antigen (OKT6)] are used to substantiate the identity of LC cells[484,492]. LC cells may be found in small numbers in normal lung, but rarely constitute >3% of cells. Large aggregates of LC cells within stellate nodules or granulomatous lesions[484] or >3% of OKT6 or S100 (+) cells on BAL[42] are virtually pathognomonic of pulmonary EG. Recently, positive immunohistochemical staining to a mouse monoclonal CD1a antibody (Mab O10) was

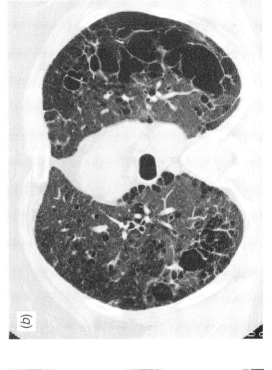

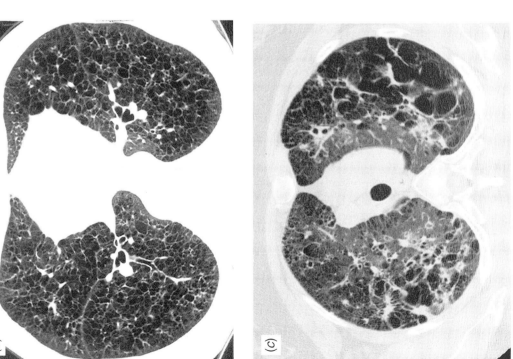

Fig. 12.38(a) Eosinophilic granulomatosis. CT demonstrates multiple, well-defined cystic spaces with walls measuring 1 to 2 cm in size. A few ill-defined, scattered interstitial nodules are also present but are subtle. (Reproduced with permission.)[4] *(b)* Eosinophilic granulomatosis. CT from another patient demonstrates marked destruction of lung parenchyma by cysts, some of which have coalesced and assumed bizarre shapes. A few faint nodules are visible. *(c)* Eosinophilic granulomatosis. CT from the same point demonstrates extensive cystic radiolucencies. Marked peribronchiolar thickening and scattered dense nodules are present, consistent with an active inflammatory component.

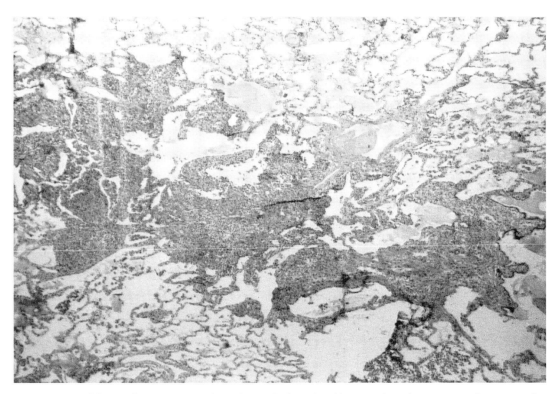

Fig. 12.39 Eosinophilic granuloma. Low-power photomicrograph of open lung biopsy specimen demonstrates stellate pattern of fibrosis. H&E stain. (Reproduced with permission.)[34]

demonstrated in 33 of 34 paraffin-embedded LCH samples[492].

The diagnosis of pulmonary EG can be inferred on open lung biopsy by the pattern and distribution of lesions on low-power light microscopy. Characteristic features include: a stellate pattern of fibrosis (noted in >80% of patients); peribronchiolar nodules; areas of intervening normal lung[483,484]. Under high power light microscopy, the peribronchiolar nodules are comprised of cellular, granulomatous lesions, with LC cells and a polymorphous inflammatory cellular infiltrate[484]. In late phases, the inflammatory component is sparse or absent. These cases resemble end-stage honeycomb lung[484]. Retention of a stellate pattern of fibrosis is a clue to the diagnosis[484]. Surgical (open or thoracoscopic) lung biopsies are often required to substantiate the diagnosis. In some patients, TBBs are definitive[484].

When basing the diagnosis on TBBs, ancillary techniques such as immunohistochemical stains (OKT6 or S100 protein) and HRCT should be supportive.

Although the pathogenesis of pulmonary EG is unknown, an uncontrolled immune response initiated or regulated by Langerhans cells appears to be critical. Since the vast majority (>90%) of cases are in smokers[480–484,491], components of cigarette smoke initiate a dysregulated or exuberant immune response[18,493,494,495].

The prognosis and natural history of pulmonary EG is variable. Spontaneous resolution may occur. Stabilization or improvement occurs in more than two-thirds of patients, within 6 to 24 months of onset of symptoms[484,485]. In 15 to 31% of patients, the disease progresses, destroying lung parenchyma and causing irrevocable loss of pulmonary function[481,483–485]. Fatalities rates range from 6 to 27%[481,483–485,491]. Factors

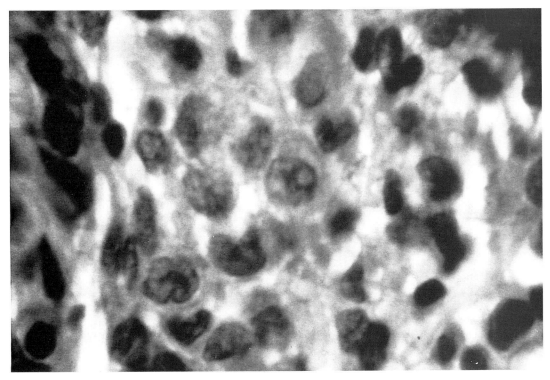

Fig. 12.40 Eosinophilic granulomatosis. Photomicrograph of open lung biopsy specimen demonstrates an intense cellular infiltrate with multiple Langerhans' cells exhibiting the characteristically clefted nuclei. H&E, high power. (Reproduced with permisson.)[4]

associated with an adverse prognosis include: advanced age at diagnosis; numerous cysts on HRCT; multisystem generalized disease; severe impairment in DLCO or VC; continuation of tobacco use[480,481,483,491].

Due to its rarity and variable natural history, therapy for pulmonary EG is controversial. Cessation of cigarette smoking is mandatory. In three small series, radiographic resolution occurred in 6 of 6 patients following smoking cessation[496–498]. The disease also spontaneously regressed in two patients who continued to smoke[498]. Anecdotal responses have been claimed with corticosteroids, vinca alkaloids (vinblastine or vincristine), D-penicillamine, and immunosuppressive and cytotoxic drugs[480,481,484,485,491,499], but data affirming efficacy are lacking. Given the paucity of data, we reserve corticosteroids for patients with severe or progressive disease, particularly when HRCT or biopsy features suggest an active granulomatous phase. Unless the acuity of illness is severe, we observe for several weeks to see if spontaneous remission occurs following smoking cessation. Immunosuppressive or cytotoxic agents are of unproven benefit but may be tried for severe corticosteroid-refractory disease. Lung transplantation is an option for patients with end-stage pulmonary EG[500]. Disease may recur in the transplanted lung allograft upon resumption of smoking[500].

Lymphangioleiomyomatosis (LAM)

Lymphangioleiomyomatosis (LAM) is a rare disease of unknown etiology affecting only women (primarily premenopausal)[501–505]. Predominant symptoms include: dyspnea (>80%); pneumothorax (50 to 80%); hemoptysis (28 to 40%); chylothorax or

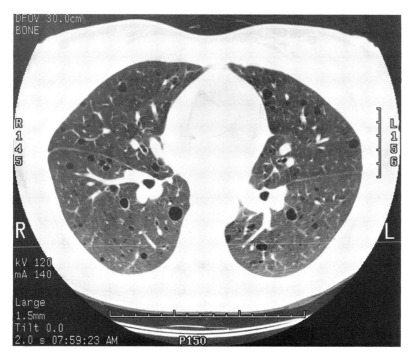

Fig. 12.41 Lymphangioleiomyomatosis. HRCT scan from a 28-year-old female with a history of recurring pneumothoraces. Multiple, well circumscribed cysts are present bilaterally, with large areas of intervening lung parenchyma.

chylous ascites (7 to 39%)[501,504,506]. Mean age at the onset of symptoms is 30 to 36 years old[501,504,506].

Chest radiographs in LAM demonstrate cystic or reticular shadows, pneumothoraces, and hyperinflation in 60 to 80%; chylous pleural effusions, in 11 to 29%[504,506]. HRCT scans are far superior to chest radiographs, and are virtually pathognomonic[30]. HRCT scans reveal numerous thin-walled cysts involving all lung fields, without predilection for any particular lobe[501,505]. The cysts range in size from a few millimetres to >6 cm; the intervening lung parenchyma is normal[30,501,507] (Figs. 12.41 and 12.42). Nodules are not found[30,507]. The severity of quantitative HRCT scores correlates inversely with DLCO and FEV1/FVC[502]. Other CT abnormalities found in a minority of patients include: retrocrural adenopathy; pleural or pericardial effusions; dilated thoracic duct; pneumothorax[501]. Ventilation lung scans demonstrate a 'speckled' pattern in 97% of patients with LAM[501]; these findings are non-specific. PFTs demonstrate: reduced DLCO in 83 to 100% of patients; airflow limitation, in 51 to 67%[490,501,502,504,506]. Lung volumes are normal or increased[490,501,502,504,506]. Worsening airflow obstruction progresses inexorably over years[504,506].

Extrapulmonary involvement is common. Abdominal CT scans reveal cysts or angiomyolipomas in kidney, spleen, abdominal or retroperitoneal lymph nodes, uterus, and ovaries in up to 60% of patients with LAM[501,508–510]. Angiomyolipomas exhibit fat attenuation on CT and hyperechogenicity on ultrasonography[501]. The major complication of angiomyolipomas is massive bleeding[501]. Smooth muscle cells in angiomyolipomas and LAM lesions are immunoreactive with melanoma-related marker (HMB45) antibody[501]. Pulmonary LAM complicates tuberous sclerosis complex (TSC), an autosomal dominant disorder associated with mental retardation and cutaneous manifestations, in 1% of patients[508]. Renal angiomyolipomas are observed in

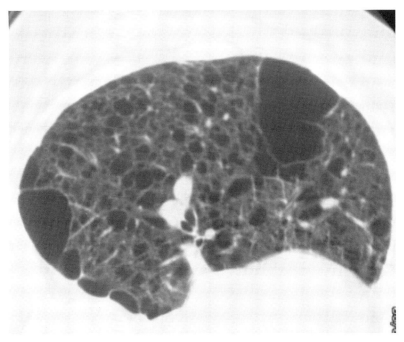

Fig. 12.42 Lymphangioleiomyomatosis. CT in a 44-year-old woman with LAM demonstrates multiple, thin-walled cystic radiolucencies bilaterally. Note the two large lesions, representing confluent cysts. (Reproduced with permission.)[4]

up to 80% of patients with TSC; renal cysts, in 20%[501]. Tuberous sclerosis differs from LAM, as neurological or cutaneous manifestations are not observed in LAM[508].

Histopathological features of pulmonary LAM include: innumerable small cysts (ranging from 2 to >30 mm); proliferations of atypical/immature smooth muscle cells (LAM cells; dilated pulmonary lymphatics)[502,506]. Predominantly cystic lesions on open lung biopsy suggest a worse survival; the extent of smooth muscle proliferation or hemosiderosis do not correlate with survival[506]. The atypical smooth muscle cells in LAM stain positively for muscle-specific actin, desmin, and HMB-45 antibody[501,505,506]. Historically, open lung biopsy was used to substantiate the diagnosis of pulmonary LAM[502]. In some patients, TBBs with immuno-histochemical stains (HMB45) may confirm the diagnosis, provided clinical features are compatible[501,502,505]. More importantly, the diagnosis of LAM can be assumed without histological confirmation,

provided HRCT features are classical and clinical features are compatible[501,502,505].

The course of LAM (with or without therapy) is poor, with inexorable progression over 5 to 15 years[504–506,511]. Ten-year survival ranges from 23% to 78%; most deaths are due to progressive respiratory failure[504–506,511]. Controlled therapeutic trials have not been done, and optimal therapy is controversial. LAM is exacerbated by estrogens; exogenous estrogens and pregnancy are contraindicated[505]. Treatment strategies are designed to ablate the effects of estrogen and include: surgical oophorectomy and/or anti-estrogen regimens (e.g. progesterone, tamoxifen, androgens, luteinizing hormone-releasing agonists)[501,502,504–506]. Tamoxifen has partial estrogen-agonist activity, and should not be used. Improvement is rare with oophorectomy or medical therapy alone[502,504–506]. In one review, only 2 of 40 LAM patients treated with diverse therapies improved; 9 stabilized; 29 deteriorated[506]. A retrospective survey of 50 patients with LAM cited lower rates of decline in FEV1 and DLCO among patients treated with progesterone[505]. Among premenopausal patients, mean declines in FEV1 were 47 ml/h and 170 ml/y among treated and untreated patients, respectively[505]. Similar trends were found among postmenopausal women (mean rates of decline of 18 ml/y and 86 ml/y, respectively). These trends did not achieve statistical significance, but suggest that progesterone slows the course of the disease. Optimal dose and route of administration of progesterone varies. Most investigators use a mean dose of >10 mg progesterone daily[505,506,512]. Given the poor prognosis of untreated LAM, we believe a trial of intramuscular medroxyprogesterone acetate (400 to 800 mg i.m. monthly), oophorectomy, or both, is reasonable. Patients should be strongly counselled to avoid pregnancy or exogenous estrogens. Bronchodilators improved symptoms in one study[501]. Single or bilateral lung transplantation is reserved for patients with incapacitating disease and severe airflow obstruction (e.g. FEV1 < 30% predicted) or other complications (e.g. refractory, recurrent pneumothoraces)[509]. Pneumothorax in the native lung may occur after lung transplantation[509]. A retrospective analysis of 34 patients with LAM cited one- and two-year survival rates following lung transplantation of 69% and 58%, respectively[509]. Recurrent LAM in the lung allograft occurs in fewer than <5% of patients[509,513].

Pulmonary alveolar proteinosis

Pulmonary alveolar proteinosis (PAP), also termed alveolar phospholipidosis, is a rare disease of unknown etiology in which alveolar spaces are filled with granular, eosinophilic material composed of surfactant apoproteins[43,44]. The disease is usually idiopathic, but secondary forms complicate opportunistic infections, acquired immunodeficiency syndrome, and hematological malignancies[43,44,514]. Secondary PAP is usually mild, and regresses with successful treatment of the underlying disease[43]. A genetic basis for primary PAP has not been found, but rare cases of familial PAP occur in infants and children[43,515]. The estimated incidence of primary

PAP is one in two million people[43]. PAP is 2.5 times more common in men; over 80% of cases occur in the third or fourth decade of life[43,516].

Dyspnea is the most common presenting symptom[43,44]. Cough, hypoxemia, and worsening dyspnea evolve over weeks to months[43,44,516]. Extrapulmonary involvement does not occur. In early reports, opportunistic infections due to *Nocardia* spp., *Staphylococcus aureus, Mycobacteria,* and fungi were cited in up to 20% of patients with PAP[44]. In recent series, infections are absent or rare[44,516,517]. Chest auscultation may be normal or reveal inspiratory crackles; clubbing is noted in one third of cases[43]. Serum lactate dehydrogenase (LDH) is elevated in 80% of patients[43,44,516]. Hypoxemia, due to intrapulmonary shunting, is the cardinal physiological aberration[43,44]. PFTs demonstrate reductions in DLCO and lung volumes; expiratory flow rates are normal [43,44].

Chest radiographs reveal symmetrical, fluffy, perihilar alveolar infiltrates (a batwing appearance)[43,44] (Fig. 12.43). Asymmetrical or unilateral involvement occurs in 20%[43,44]. HRCT scans more clearly depict the alveolar pattern, with air bronchograms[43,516] (Fig. 12.44). Thickened interlobular septae, clearly visible within the affected lung, produce what is termed 'crazy paving' pattern[43] (Fig. 12.45). These CT features may also be seen in bronchioloalveolar cell carcinoma or lipoid pneumonia[43].

Historically, the diagnosis of PAP required open lung biopsy[44]. The alveolar spaces and respiratory bronchioles are filled with granular acidophilic material on hematoxylin/eosin stains, which stains bright pink with PAS and negative with alcian blue[43,44] (Fig. 12.46). Interstitial inflammation or fibrosis does not occur. The major constituent of intraalveolar material is lecithin, the main component of surfactant[43]. Electron microscopy (performed for research purposes) reveals lamellar bodies within the alveolar lumen, identical to phospholipid inclusions found in normal type II pneumocytes[43]. Alveolar macrophages contain complex phospholipoprotein inclusions[43]. Fibreoptic bronchoscopy with BAL or TBBs is distinctive [43,44,516,518]. BAL fluid is opaque and milky, and sediments into

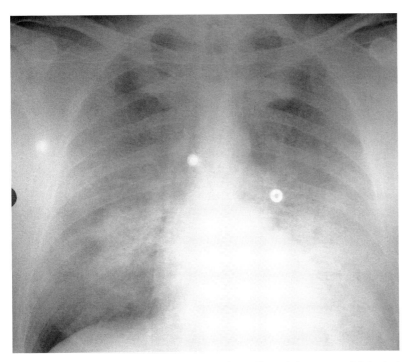

Fig. 12.43 Pulmonary alveolar proteinosis (PAP). PA chest radiograph demonstrates bilateral extensive ground glass opacities in a 58-year-old male with hypoxemia and dyspnea. Bronchoscopy with BAL confirmed the diagnosis of PAP.

multiple layers upon standing[43,44]. Microscopic features reveal diffuse eosinophilic staining, large eosinophilic bodies, and few alveolar macrophages[43,44,516]. Positive PAS and negative alcian blue stains of the foamy BAL fluid confirm the diagnosis[43]. When bronchoscopy is non-diagnostic, surgical (VATS) lung biopsy should be performed.

Research investigations noted elevations in tumour markers[519], mucin-like glycoprotein (KL-6)[520], surfactant proteins A[43,521] and D[522] and monocyte chemoattractant protein-1 (MCP-1)[523] in serum and BAL fluid in patients with PAP. The pathogenesis of PAP is not known. Defects in clearance or excessive production of surfactant by type II pneumocytes is postulated. Alveolar macrophages in PAP exhibit defects in chemotaxis, phagocytosis, and phagolysosomal fusion[43]. Inciting stimuli for PAP are not known, but exposures to hydrocarbons, chemicals, fibreglass, aluminium, cadmium, metals, dusts, or solvents can be elicited in 50% of cases[43,44]. In

animal models, inhalation of fine dust particles elicit a PAP-like syndrome[43,44].

The natural history of PAP is variable. Spontaneous resolution occurs in up to 40% of patients[516,524]. Prior to the availability of therapy, one-third of patients died of respiratory failure or infectious complications. Whole lung lavage is the treatment of choice, and is recommended for patients with severe or progressive symptoms[43,44]. Patients with mild symptoms may not require treatment[516]. Whole lung lavage involves instilling large volumes of sterile saline (20 to 50 litres) over a 3 to 5 hour period into each lung (usually at separate times)[43,44]. Some centres perform bilateral sequential lung lavage in one treatment session[43]. This process physically removes the copious, thick viscid material, allowing the alveolar spaces to re-expand and participate in gas exchange. Whole lung lavage is usually efficacious, and fatalities are now rare [43,44,516]. Relapses occur in 15 to 30% of treated

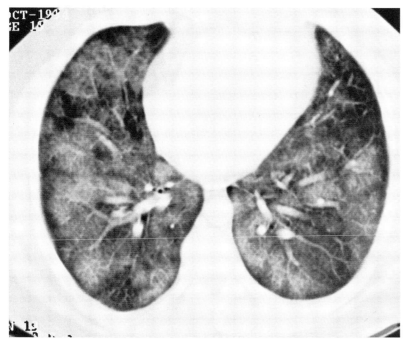

Fig. 12.44 Pulmonary alveolar proteinosis. CT scan demonstrates multiple foci of ground-glass opacification throughout parenchyma. Open lung biopsy demonstrated classic features of PAP. (Reproduced with permission.)[4]

patients, and require retreatment[43,44,516]. When occupational exposure to solvents, chemicals, or dust is suspected as the etiology, withdrawal from that occupation is advised.

Pharmacological alternatives to whole lung lavage have been proposed, but data are sparse. In a murine model, mice deficient in granulocyte monocyte colony-stimulating factor (GM-CSF) or the CM-CSF/interleukin-3/IL-5 receptor develop a pulmonary lesion closely resembling PAP histologically[525–527]. In humans, defects in the GM-CSF receptor were detected in 4 out of 8 pediatric patients with PAP[528] but were not found in adults with PAP[527]. Reconstituting the gene for GM-CSF to the respiratory epithelia of CM-CSF deficient mice corrected the PAP lesion[529]. Bone marrow transplantation and hematopoietic reconstitution of GM-CSF-deficient mice reverses this abnormality[530] A case report cited physiological improvement in a patient with PAP following administration of GM-

CSF[531]. The authors hypothesized that GM-CSF activates alveolar macrophages and increases the rate of surfactant clearance. Three other cases were treated with GM-CSF; only one responded[43].

Relapsing polychondritis

Relapsing polychondritis (RP), a rare disease of unknown cause, is characterized by episodic inflammation and destruction of cartilage of the ears, nose, larynx, trachea, and peripheral joints[532,533]. Other proteoglycan-rich structures (e.g. eye, heart, blood vessels, inner ear) can be affected[532]. The course of RP typically evolves over years[532,533]. Fever, sweats, weight loss, and lethargy are common[532,533]. Cardiovascular manifestations (e.g. aortitis, vasculitis, valvular insufficiency, aneurysms) occur in up to 30% of patients[532,533] and may be lethal. Renal involvement was cited in 8% of patients[532]. Otolaryngological manifestations predominate. The

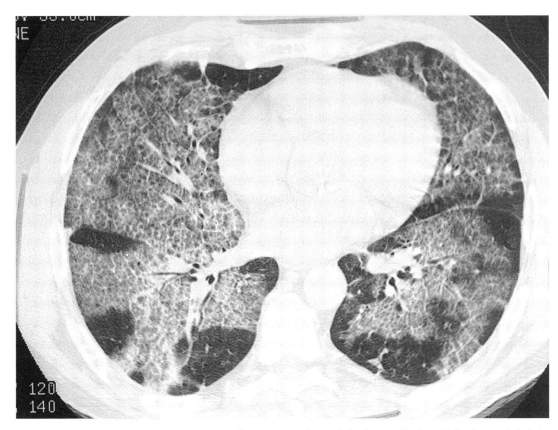

Fig. 12.45 Pulmonary alveolar proteinosis. HRCT scan demonstrates widespread alveolar opacification with focal areas of relatively uninvolved lung parenchyma. Thickened interlobular septae, clearly visible within the affected lung, produce what has been termed a 'crazy paving' pattern.

ears are involved in >80% of patients; chondritis may cause deformities of the external ear[533]. Nasal manifestations are present in two-thirds; saddle nose deformity is common[533]. Laryngeal or tracheal manifestations (e.g. hoarseness, laryngeal tenderness, aphonia, stridor) are evident in 14 to 38% of patients at presentation, but develop in 56 to 68% of patients during the course of the disease[532–535]. Inflammation of bronchial or tracheal cartilage causes dyspnea, stridor, or wheezing. Upper airway obstruction (UAO) can result from subglottic edema, cicatricial contraction of the tracheal lumen, or dissolution of the cartilaginous supporting sructure of the trachea, causing dynamic collapse of the airway[533–535].

Chest CT scans demonstrate diffuse or focal tracheal or bronchial stenosis, with thickening and calcification of airway walls[532,536]. Peripheral bronchi can be affected[537]. Computed tomography (CT) with multiplanar reformations (MPRs) are useful to measure the length of strictures and detect dynamic inspiratory and expiratory collapse[443,537]. A flow-volume loop is a sensitive measure of dynamic airway collapse. Tracheal stenosis causes truncation of inspiratory and expiratory limbs of the flow-volume loop[532]. Fibreoptic bronchoscopy is warranted when UAO is suspected. Bronchoscopy reveals inflammation in the trachea, with or without stenosis[532]. Patients with severe tracheal stenosis refractory to medical

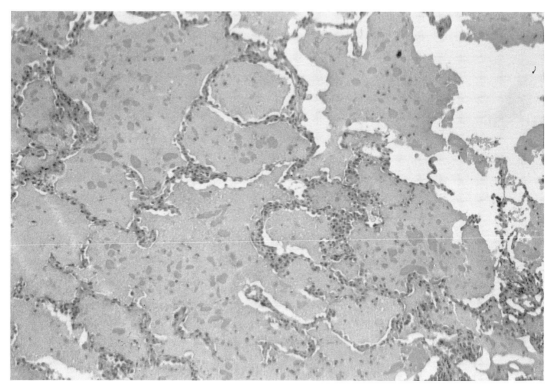

Fig. 12.46 Pulmonary alveolar proteinosis. Photomicrograph: open lung biopsy demonstrates filling of alveolar spaces with viscid, lipoproteinaceous material.

therapy require tracheostomy[534,535]. Ten to 15% of patients with RP die of respiratory failure (most often due to tracheal stenosis or collapse)[533,538]. Pulmonary infections result from impaired drainage, ineffective cough, and airway collapse and contribute to mortality[532].

No biopsy finding is specific for RP[532]. Histological features include: perichondral inflammation; loss of basophilic staining of cartilage; capillary endothelial cell proliferation; perivascular inflammatory cell; necrotic, vacuolated chondrocytes[532]. Biopsies are often non-specific, and create additional cosmetic deformity[532]. The diagnosis of RP is often made on clinical grounds. Major defining criteria include: bilateral auricular chondritis; non-erosive seronegative inflammatory arthritis; nasal chondritis; ocular inflammation; respiratory tract chondritis; audiovestibular damage[533]. The episodic nature of the disease, indolent progression over months to years, and response to corticosteroids or dapsone support the diagnosis when histological criteria are lacking[532].

The cause of RP is unknown. Serum antibodies to type II collagen and immune complexes are found during acute attacks[532]. In 10 to 25% of patients, RP is associated with connective tissue or autoimmune disorders[532]. The efficacy of high dose corticosteroids supports an immune-mediated mechanism.

Treatment of RP involves agents which ablate the inflammatory response (e.g. corticosteroids or dapsone)[532]. Corticosteroids are the mainstay of therapy. Because RP is episodic, corticosteroids are often reserved for acute flares. For acute or severe respiratory tract involvement, high dose corticosteroids are required. Non-steroidal anti-inflammatory drugs (NSAIDs) have an adjunctive role. Dapsone, an agent that inhibits lysosomal enzymes, is often used, but data affirming benefit are lacking[532]. Chronic use of dapsone may cause methemoglobinemia and anemia[532]. Alternative cytotoxic or immunosuppressive agents (e.g. cyclophosphamide, methotrexate, azathioprine) are reserved for corticosteroid-recalcitrant cases[532]. Five-year survival ranges from 70 to 94%[532]. Tracheostomy[539] or tracheal stents[540] may be required for patients with severe laryngeal or tracheal involvement failing medical therapy. Tracheal reconstruction is considered as a last resort[539]. Patients with cardiac valvular insufficiency require valve replacement

Amyloidosis

Amyloidosis is a group of diseases characterized by deposition of insoluble β-pleated fibrillar protein in the extracellular matrix of involved tissues[541]. Primary amyloidosis, the most common variant, is associated with deposition of the immunoglobulin light chain fragment (amyloid AL), and can be idiopathic or associated with plasma cell dyscrasias (e.g. multiple myeloma)[541]. Secondary amyloidosis (amyloid AA) complicates bronchiectasis and diverse chronic inflammatory disorders (e.g. tuberculosis, chronic infections, collagen vascular or autoimmune diseases, etc.)[541]. Familial transthyretin-associated amyloidosis (ATTR) also exists[541]. Amyloidosis is rare. Only 1275 to 3200 new cases of primary (AL) amyloidosis are diagnosed annually in the United States[541]; familial amyloidosis (ATTR) is 5 to 10 times less common than AL[541]. With the marked reduction in chronic infectious diseases such as tuberculosis, osteomyelitis, and bronchiectasis in the Western Hemisphere, secondary (AA) amyloidosis is rare, but may complicate untreated familial Mediterranean fever, inflammatory bowel disease, or rheumatoid arthritis[541].

Clinical manifestations of AL amyloidosis are protean. Amyloidosis can involve any organ, but predominant sites of amyloid deposition include the tongue, heart, joints, kidney, gastrointestinal tract, spleen, liver, skin, nervous system, and upper and lower respiratory tracts[541–544]. Clinically significant lung involvement occurs in 10 to 30% of patients with primary (AL) amyloidosis, but is rare in secondary forms[541–545]. Prognosis of AL amyloidosis is dictated by cardiac or extrapulmonary organ involvement. Mean survival is less than two years[542,544]. Most deaths are due to cardiac, renal, or non-pulmonary causes[542,544].

Pulmonary manifestations of amyloidosis include: focal mass lesions; diffuse reticulonodular or micronodular amyloid lesions; hemorrhagic pleural effusions; hemoptysis; mediastinal or hilar lymphadenopathy; pulmonary hypertension[542,543,545,546]. Rare manifestations include: sleep apnea (secondary to involvement of the tongue) and respiratory muscle weakness (due to amyloid infiltrating the diaphragm)[541,542].

'Primary' pulmonary amyloidosis also occurs[543,545,547]. In this entity, amyloid deposits are present only in the lungs or associated structures (i.e. tracheobronchial tree, pleura, and hilar or mediastinal lymph nodes)[543,547]. Multiple focal nodules or plaques are characteristic[543,547]. Depending on the site and extent of involvement, patients may be asymptomatic or have cough, wheezing, dyspnea, hemoptysis, atelectasis, or recurrent pneumonias[543]. Fewer than 100 cases of tracheobronchial amyloidosis have been published[547]. Virtually all such cases are localized amyloidosis. The largest series was 10 patients with tracheobronchial amyloidosis seen at a single medical centre over a 15-year period[547]. Tracheobronchial amyloidosis was never seen in 685 patients with AL amyloidosis seen during that time frame.[547]. Tracheobronchial amyloidosis may cause inflammation or stenosis of trachea, bronchi, or larynx, causing stridor, dyspnea, wheezing, or hoarseness[543,547]. Amyloidosis involving the trachea may cause severe (even fatal) airflow obstruction[547]. Calcification of amyloid deposits causes tracheobronchopathia osteoplastica, characterized by calcified or cartilagenous submucosal nodules within the tracheobronchial tree[547,548]. Bronchoscopy (rigid or fibreoptic) is most useful to establish the diagnosis of localized amyloidosis[547]. CT scans are used to quantitatively assess the degree and sites of airway narrowing, and follow the course of the disease[547].

The diagnosis of amyloidosis is confirmed by demonstrating amyloid fibrils in involved tissue(s). Amyloid protein stains pink with hematoxylin–eosin, but Congo red dyes are more specific. Amyloid takes up Congo red and exhibits apple green birefringence under polarized microscopy[541,542].

Optimal therapy for primary amyloidosis is not clear. Colchicine has been used for both primary and secondary amyloidosis; its value is doubtful[544]. Alkylating agents are efficacious in amyloidosis due to multiple myeloma, and improve survival modestly in idiopathic AL amyloidosis[544,549]. In secondary forms of amyloidosis, aggressive treatment of the underlying disease delays or reverses deposition of amyloid protein[541]. Interferon-α is ineffective[550]. Optimal treatment of diffuse amyloid infiltrating lung or tracheobronchial tree is not known. For localized endobronchial disease, dilatation with rigid bronchoscopy or laser resection may be useful[547]. Resection of localized amyloid deposits surgically or by laser is beneficial in some patients[547]. In rare cases, laryngeal dilatation or tracheostomy are required[547].

Acknowledgement

Supported in part by National Institutes of Health grant IP50HL46487.

REFERENCES

1 American Thoracic Society, and European Respiratory Society. Idiopathic Pulmonary Fibrosis: Diagnosis and Treatment. International consensus statement. *Am J Respir Crit Care Med* 2000; 161:646–664.

2 British Thoracic Society, and Standards of Care Committee. The diagnosis, assessment and treatment of diffuse parenchymal lung disease in adults. *Thorax* 1999; 54 (Suppl. 1):S1–S30.

3 Raghu G. Interstitial lung disease: a diagnostic approach. Are CT scan and lung biopsy indicated in every patient? *Am J Respir Crit Care Med* 1995; 151:909–914.

4 Lynch JP III, Raghu G. Major disease syndromes of unknown etiology. In: Baum G, Crapo J, eds. *Textbook of Pulmonary Disease*, 6th edn. Boston, MA: Little, Brown and Company; 1998; 431–476.

5 Colby TV, Swensen SJ. Anatomic distribution and histopathologic patterns in diffuse lung disease: correlation with HRCT. *J Thorac Imaging* 1996:11:1–26.

6 Grenier P, Chevret S, Beigelman C et al. Chronic diffuse infiltrative lung disease: determination of the diagnostic value of clinical data, chest radiography, and CT and Bayesian analysis. *Radiology* 1994; 191:383–390.

7 Raghu G, Mageto Y. N, Lockhart D et al. The accuracy of the clinical diagnosis of new-onset idiopathic pulmonary fibrosis and other interstitial lung disease: a prospective study. *Chest* 1999; 116:1168–1174.

8 Lynch J-P III, Myers JL. Interstitial lung discases. In: Bone RC, Campbell GD Jr, Payne DK, eds. *Bone's Atlas of Pulmonary and Critical Care Medicine*. Baltimore, MD: Williams & Wilkins; 1999; Chapter 18:1–12.

9 Kuru T, Lynch JP, III. Nonresolving or slowly resolving pneumonia. *Clin Chest Med* 1999; 20:623–651.

10 Robertson H. Clinical application of pulmonary function and exercise tests in the management of patients with interstitial lung disease. *Semin Respir Crit Care Med* 1994:15:1–9.

11 Martinez FJ. Cardiopulmonary exercise testing: practical and clinical concepts. *Semin Respir Crit Care Med* 1998; 19:393–402.

12 Sciurba FC, Slivka WA. Six-minute walk testing. *Semin Respir Crit Care Med* 1998; 19:383–392.

13 Erbes R, Schaberg T, Loddenkemper R. Lung function tests in patients with idiopathic pulmonary fibrosis. Are they helpful for predicting outcome? *Chest* 1997:111:51–57.

14 Gay SE, Kazerooni EA, Toews GB et al. Idiopathic pulmonary fibrosis: predicting response to therapy and survival. *Am J Respir Crit Care Med* 1998; 157:1063–1072.

15 Lynch JP III, Toews GB. Idiopathic pulmonary fibrosis. In: Fishman A, ed. *Textbook of Pulmonary Diseases and Disorders*, 3rd edn. New York: McGraw-Hill; 1997; 1193–1210.

16 Remy-Jardin M, Remy J, Cortet B et al. Lung changes in rheumatoid arthritis: CT findings. *Radiology* 1994; 193:375–382.

17 Lynch JP III, Raghu G. Major disease syndromes of unknown etiology. In: Baum GAC, ed. *Textbook of Pulmonary Diseases*, 6th edn. Boston, MA: Little, Brown and Co.: 1997.

18 Wells AU, Cullinan P, Hansell DM et al. Fibrosing alveolitis associated with systemic sclerosis has a better prognosis

than lone cryptogenic fibrosing alveolitis. *Am J Respir Crit Care Med* 1994; 149:1583–1590.

19 Remy-Jardin M, Giraud F, Remy J et al. Importance of ground-glass attenuation in chronic diffuse infiltrative lung disease: pathologic–CT correlation. *Radiology* 1993; 189:693–698.

20 Wells AU, King AD, Rubens MB et al. Lone cryptogenic fibrosing alveolitis: a functional-morphologic correlation based on extent of disease on thin-section computed tomography. *Am J Respir Crit Care Med* 1997; 155:1367–1375.

21 Wells A, Hansell D, Haslam P et al. Bronchoalveolar lavage cellularity: long cryptogenic fibrosing alveolitis compared with the fibrosing alveolitis of systemic sclerosis. *Am J Respir Crit Care Med* 1998; 157:1474–1482.

22 Wells A. High resolution computed tomography in sarcoidosis: a clinical perspective. *Sarcoidosis Vasc Diffuse Lung Dis* 1998; 15:140–146.

23 Brauner MW, Lenoir S, Grenier P et al. Pulmonary sarcoidosis: CT assessment of lesion reversibility. *Radiology* 1992; 182:349–354.

24 Corrin B. Pathology of interstitial lung disease. *Semin Respir Crit Care Med* 1994; 15:61–76.

25 Katzenstein A, Myers J. Idiopathic pulmonary fibrosis. Clinical relevance of pathological classification. *Am J Respir Crit Care Med* 1998; 157:1301–1315.

26 Lynch JP III, Orens J, Kazerooni EA. Collagen vascular diseases. In: Sperber M, ed. *Diffuse Lung Diseases: A Comprehensive Clinical-Radiological Overview.* London: Springer-Verlag; 1999:325–355.

27 Carrington CB, Gaensler EA, Coutu R. E et al. Natural history and treated course of usual and desquamative interstitial pneumonia. *N Engl J Med* 1978; 298:801–809.

28 Katzenstein AL, Myers JL. Idiopathic pulmonary fibrosis: clinical relevance of pathologic classification. *Am J Respir Crit Care Med* 1998; 157:1301–1315.

29 Travis WD, Matsui K, Moss J et al. Idiopathic nonspecific interstitial pneumonia: prognostic significance of cellular and fibrosing patterns: survival comparison with usual interstitial pneumonia and desquamative interstitial pneumonia. *Am J Surg Pathol* 2000; 24:19–33.

30 Lenoir S, Grenier P, Brauner MW et al. Pulmonary lymphangiomyomatosis and tuberous sclerosis: comparison of radiographic and thin-section CT findings. *Radiology* 1990; 175:329–334.

31 Nagai S, Kitaichi M, Itoh H et al. Idiopathic nonspecific interstitial pneumonia/fibrosis: camparison with idiopathic pulmonary fibrosis and BOOP. *Eur Respir J* 1998; 12:1010–1019.

32 Douglas WW, Ryu JH, Schroeder DR. Idiopathic pulmonary fibrosis: impact of oxygen and colchicine, prednisone, or no therapy on survival. *Am J Respir Crit Care Med* 2000; 161:1172–1178.

33 Daniil ZD, Gilchrist FC, Nicholson AG et al. A histologic pattern of nonspecific interstitial pneumonia is associated with a better prognosis than usual interstitial pneumonia in patients with cryptogenic fibrosing alveolitis. *Am J Respir Crit Care Med* 1999; 160:899–905.

34 Lynch JP III, Chavis AD. Chronic interstitial pulmonary disorders. In: Lu V, ed. *Clinical Pulmonary Disorders.* Boston, MA: Little, Brown, and Co.; 1992:193–264.

35 Turner-Warwick M, Haslam PL. The value of serial bronchoalveolar lavages in assessing the clinical progress of patients with cryptogenic fibrosing alveolitis. *Am Rev Respir Dis* 1987; 135:26–34.

36 Watters LC, Schwarz MI, Cherniack RM et al. Idiopathic pulmonary fibrosis. Pretreatment bronchoalveolar lavage cellular constituents and their relationships with lung histopathology and clinical response to therapy. *Am Rev Respir Dis* 1987; 135:696–704.

37 American Thoracic Society. Statement on Sarcoidosis. *Am J Respir Crit Care Med* 1999; 160:736–755.

38 Lynch JP III, Kazerooni EA, Gay SE. Pulmonary sarcoidosis. *Clin Chest Med* 1997; 18:755–85.

39 Jederlinic PJ, Sicilian L, Gaensler EA. Chronic eosinophilic pneumonia. A report of 19 cases and a review of the literature. *Medicine (Baltimore)* 1988; 67:154–162.

40 Shannon J, Lynch JP, III. Eosinophilic pulmonary syndromes. *Clin Pulm Med* 1995; 2:19–38.

41 Allen JN, Davis WB. Eosinophilic lung diseases. *Am J Respir Crit Care Med* 1994; 150:1423–1438.

42 Chollet S, Soler P, Dournovo P et al. Diagnosis of pulmonary histiocytosis X by immunodetection of Langerhans cells in bronchoalveolar lavage fluid. *Am J Pathol* 1984; 115:225–232.

43 Shah PL, Hansell D, Lawson PR et al. Pulmonary alveolar proteinosis: clinical aspects and current concepts on pathogenesis. *Thorax* 2000; 55:67–77.

44 Prakash UB, Barham SS, Carpenter HA et al. Pulmonary alveolar phospholipoproteinosis: experience with 34 cases and a review. *Mayo Clin Proc* 1987; 62:499–518.

45 Lynch JP III, McCune WJ. Immunosuppressive and cytotoxic pharmacotherapy for pulmonary disorders. *Am J Respir Crit Care Med* 1997; 155:395–420.

46 Trulock EP. Lung transplantation. *Am J Respir Crit Care Med* 1997; 155:789–818.

47 Arcasoy S, Kotloff R. Lung transplantation. *N Engl J Med* 1999; 340:1081–1091.

48 Maurer J, Frost A, Estenne M et al. International Guidelines for the Selection of Lung Transplant Candidates. *J Heart Lung Transplant* 1998; 17:703–709.

49 Liebow AA, Carrington CB. Diffuse pulmonary lymphoreticular infiltrations associated with dysproteinemia. *Med Clin North Am* 1973; 57:809–843.

50 Epler GR, Colby TV, McLoud TC et al. Bronchiolitis obliterans organizing pneumonia. *N Engl J Med* 1985; 312:152–158.

51 Katzenstein AL, Myers JL, Mazur MT. Acute interstitial pneumonia. A clinicopathologic, ultrastructural, and cell kinetic study. *Am J Surg Pathol* 1986; 10:256–267.

52 Katzenstein AL, Fiorelli RF. Nonspecific interstitial pneumonia/fibrosis. Histologic features and clinical significance. *Am J Surg Pathol* 1994; 18:136–147.

53 Myers JL, Veal CF Jr, Shin MS et al. Respiratory bronchiolitis causing interstitial lung disease. A clinicopathologic study of six cases. *Am Rev Respir Dis* 1987; 135:880–884.

54 Yousem SA, Colby TV, Carrington CB. Follicular bronchitis/bronchiolitis. *Hum Pathol* 1985; 16:700–706.

55 Koss MN. Pulmonary lymphoid disorders. *Semin Diagn Pathol* 1995; 12:158–171.

56 Bjoraker JA, Ryu JH, Edwin MK et al. Prognostic significance of histopathologic subsets in idiopathic pulmonary fibrosis. *Am J Respir Crit Care Med* 1998; 157:199–203.

57 Hubbard R, Johnston I, Britton J. Survival in patients with cryptogenic fibrosing alveolitis. A population-based cohort study. *Chest* 1998; 113:396–400.

58 Coultas DB, Zumwalt RE, Black WC et al. The epidemiology of interstitial lung diseases. *Am J Respir Crit Care Med* 1994; 150:967–972.

59 Baumgartner KB, Samet JM, Stidley CA et al. Cigarette smoking: a risk factor for idiopathic pulmonary fibrosis. *Am J Respir Crit Care Med* 1997; 155:242–248.

60 Hubbard R, Lewis S, Richards K et al. Occupational exposure to metal or wood dust and aetiology of cryptogenic fibrosing alveolitis. *Lancet* 1996; 347:284–289.

61 Iwai K, Mori T, Yamada N et al. Idiopathic pulmonary fibrosis. Epidemiologic approaches to occupational exposure. *Am J Respir Crit Care Med* 1994; 150:670–675.

62 Bitterman PB, Rennard SI, Keogh BA et al. Familial idiopathic pulmonary fibrosis. Evidence of lung inflammation in unaffected family members. *N Engl J Med* 1986; 314:1343–1347.

63 Johnston ID, Prescott RJ, Chalmers JC et al. British Thoracic Society study of cryptogenic fibrosing alveolitis: current presentation and initial management. Fibrosing Alveolitis Subcommittee of the Research Committee of the British Thoracic Society. *Thorax* 1997; 52:38–44.

64 Nishimura K, Itoh H. High-resolution computed tomographic features of bronchiolitis obliterans organizing pneumonia. *Chest* 1992; 102:26S–31S.

65 Lee JS, Im JG, Ahn JM et al. Fibrosing alveolitis: prognostic implication of ground-glass attenuation at high-resolution CT. *Radiology* 1992; 184:451–454.

66 Hartman TE, Primack SL, Kang EY et al. Disease progression in usual interstitial pneumonia compared with desquamative interstitial pneumonia. Assessment with serial CT. *Chest* 1996; 110:378–382.

67 Lynch JP III, Martinez FJ, Travis W. Idiopathic pulmonary fibrosis: diagnosis and staging. *J Respir Dis* 1999; 20:614–628.

68 Lynch JP III, Martinez JJ, Travis W. Idiopathic pulmonary fibrosis: is lung biopsy essential? *J Respir Dis* 2000; 21:197–214.

69 Hartman TE, Primack SL, Swensen SJ et al. Desquamative interstitial pneumonia: thin-section CT findings in 22 patients. *Radiology* 1993; 187:787–790.

70 Akira M, Sakatani M, and Ueda E. Idiopathic pulmonary fibrosis: progression of honeycombing at thin-section CT. *Radiology* 1993; 189:687–691.

71 Kazerooni EA, Martinez FJ, Flint A et al. Thin-section CT obtained at 10-mm increments versus limited three-level thin-section CT for idiopathic pulmonary fibrosis: correlation with pathologic scoring. *Am J Roentgenol* 1997; 169:977–983.

72 Xaubet A, Agusti C, Luburich P et al. Pulmonary function tests and CT scan in the management of idiopathic pulmonary fibrosis. *Am J Respir Crit Care Med* 1998; 158:431–436.

73 Douglas W, Ryu J, Swensen S et al. Colchicine versus prednisone in the treatment of idiopathic pulmonary fibrosis: a randomized prospective study. *Am J Respir Crit Care Med* 1998; 158:220–225.

74 Johkoh T, Muller NL, Cartier Y et al. Idiopathic interstitial pneumonias: diagnostic accuracy of thin-section CT in 129 patients. *Radiology* 1999; 211:555–560.

75 Doherty MJ, Pearson MG, O'Grady EA et al. Cryptogenic fibrosing alveolitis with preserved lung volumes. *Thorax* 1997; 52:998–1002.

76 Hanson D, Winterbauer RH, Kirtland SH et al. Changes in pulmonary function test results after 1 year of therapy as predictors of survival in patients with idiopathic pulmonary fibrosis. *Chest* 1995; 108:305–310.

77 Mapel DW, Samet JM, Coultas DB. Corticosteroids and the treatment of idiopathic pulmonary fibrosis. Past, present, and future. *Chest* 1996; 110:1058–1067.

78 Turner-Warwick M, Burrows B, Johnson A. Cryptogenic

fibrosing alveolitis: response to corticosteroid treatment and its effect on survival. *Thorax* 1980; 35:593–599.

79 Tukiainen P, Taskineu E, Holsti P et al. Prognosis of cryptogenic fibrosing alveolitis. *Thorax* 1983; 38:349–355.

80 Johnson MA, Kwan S, Snell NJ et al. Randomised controlled trial comparing prednisolone alone with cyclophosphamide and low dose prednisolone in combination in cryptogenic fibrosing alveolitis. *Thorax* 1989; 44:280–288.

81 Raghu G, Depaso WJ, Cain K et al. Azathioprine combined with prednisone in the treatment of idiopathic pulmonary fibrosis: a prospective double-blind, randomized, placebo-controlled clinical trial. *Am Rev Respir Dis* 1991; 144:291–296.

82 Winterbauer RH, Hammar SP, Hallman KO et al. Diffuse interstitial pneumonitis. Clinicopathologic correlations in 20 patients treated with prednisone/azathioprine. *Am J Med* 1978; 65:661–672.

83 Dayton CS, Schwartz DA, Helmers RA et al. Outcome of subjects with idiopathic pulmonary fibrosis who fail corticosteroid therapy. Implications for further studies. *Chest* 1993; 103:69–73.

84 Baughman RP, Lower EE. Use of intermittent, intravenous cyclophosphamide for idiopathic pulmonary fibrosis. *Chest* 1992; 102:1090–1094.

85 Kolb M, Kirschner J, Riedel W et al. Cyclophosphamide pulse therapy in idiopathic pulmonary fibrosis. *Eur Respir J* 1988; 12:1409–1414.

86 van Oortegem K, Wallaert B, Marquette CH et al. Determinants of response to immunosuppressive therapy in idiopathic pulmonary fibrosis. *Eur Respir J* 1994; 7:1950–1957.

87 Eliasson O, Cole S, Degragff A. Adverse effects of cyclophosphamide in idiopathic pulmonary fibrosis. *Conn Med* 1985; 49:286–289.

88 Zisman D, Lynch III J, Toews G et al. Cyclophosphamide in the treatment of idiopathic pulmonary fibrosis. A prospective study in patients with failed corticosteroids. *Chest* 2000; 117:1619–1626.

89 O'Donnell K, Keogh B, Cantin A et al. Pharmacologic suppression of the neutrophil component of the alveolitis in idiopathic pulmonary fibrosis. *Am Rev Respir Dis* 1987; 136:288–292.

90 Schwartz DA, Van Fossen DS, Davis CS et al. Determinants of progression in idiopathic pulmonary fibrosis. *Am J Respir Crit Care Med* 1994; 149:444–449.

91 Moolman J, Bardin P, Rossouw D et al. Cyclosporin as a treatment for interstitial lung disease of unknown etiology. *Thorax* 1991; 46:592–595.

92 Alton E, Johnson M, Turner-Warwick M. 1989. Advanced cryptogenic fibrosing alveolitis: preliminary report on treatment with cyclosporin A. *Respir Med* 1989; 83:277–279.

93 Venuta F, Rendina E, Ciriaco P et al. Efficacy of cyclosporine to reduce steroids in patients with idiopathic pulmonary fibrosis before lung transplantation. *J Heart Lung Transplant* 1993; 12:909–914.

94 Selman M, Carrillo G, Salas J et al. Colchicine, D-penicillamine, and prednisone in the treatment of idiopathic pulmonary fibrosis. A controlled clinical trial. *Chest* 1998; 114:507–512.

95 Peters SG, McDougall JC, Douglas WW et al. Colchicine in the treatment of pulmonary fibrosis. *Chest* 1993; 103:101–104.

96 Ziesche R, Hofbauer E, Wittmann K et al. A preliminary study of long-term treatment with interferon gamma-1b and low-dose prednisolone in patients with idiopathic pulmonary fibrosis. *N Engl J Med* 1999; 341:1264–1269.

97 Tan AH, Levrey C, Dahm V. A et al. Lovastatin induces fibroblast apoptosis *in vitro* and *in vivo*: a possible therapy for fibroproliferative disorders. *Am J Respir Crit Care Med* 1999; 159:220–227.

98 Greco MJ, Kemnitzer JE, Fox JD et al. Polymer of proline analogue with sustained antifibrotic activity in lung fibrosis. *Am J Respir Crit Care Med* 1997; 155:1391–1397.

99 Behr J, Maier K, Degenkolb B et al. Antioxidative and clinical effects of high-dose *N*-acetylcysteine in fibrosing alveolitis. Adjunctive therapy to maintenance immunosuppression. *Am J Respir Crit Care Med* 1997; 156:1897–1901.

100 Mason RJ, Schwarz MI, Hunninghake GW et al. NHLBI Workshop Summary. Pharmacological therapy for idiopathic pulmonary fibrosis. Past, present, and future. *Am J Respir Crit Care Med* 1999; 160:1771–1777.

101 King TE Jr. Respiratory bronchiolitis-associated interstitial lung disease. *Clin Chest Med* 1993; 14:693–698.

102 Moon J, du Bois RM, Colby TV et al. Clinical significance of respiratory bronchiolitis on open lung biopsy and its relationship to smoking related interstitial lung disease. *Thorax* 1999; 54:1009–1014.

103 Niewoehner DE, Kleinerman J, Rice DB. Pathologic changes in the peripheral airways of young cigarette smokers. *N Engl J Med* 1974; 291:755–758.

104 Wright JL, Cagle P, Churg A et al. Diseases of the small airways. *Am Rev Respir Dis* 1992; 146:240–262.

105 Holt RM, Schmidt RA, Godwin JD et al. High resolution CT in respiratory bronchiolitis-associated interstitial lung disease. *J Comput Assist Tomogr* 1993; 17:46–50.

106 Olson J, Colby TV, Elliott CG. Hamman–Rich syndrome revisited. *Mayo Clin Proc* 1990; 65:1538–1548.

107 Akira M, Hamada H, Sakatani M et al. CT findings during phase of accelerated deterioration in patients with idiopathic pulmonary fibrosis. *Am J Roentgenol* 1997; 168:79–83.

108 Yokoyama A, Kohno N, Hamada H et al. Circulating KL-6 predicts the outcome of rapidly progressive idiopathic pulmonary fibrosis. *Am J Respir Crit Care Med* 1998; 158:1680–1684.

109 Bouros D, Nicholson AC, Polychronopoulos V et al. Acute interstitial pneumonia. *Eur Respir J* 2000; 15:412–418.

110 Tazelaar HD, Viggiano RW, Pickersgill J et al. Interstitial lung disease in polymyositis and dermatomyositis. Clinical features and prognosis as correlated with histologic findings. *Am Rev Respir Dis* 1990; 141:727–733.

111 Muir TE, Tazelaar HD, Colby TV et al. Organizing diffuse alveolar damage associated with progressive systemic sclerosis. *Mayo Clin Proc* 1997; 72:639–642.

112 Nobutoh T, Kohda M, Doi Y et al. An autopsy case of dermatomyositis with rapidly progressive diffuse alveolar damage. *J Dermatol* 1998; 25:32–36.

113 Akikusa B, Kondo Y, Irabu N et al. Six cases of microscopic polyarteritis exhibiting acute interstitial pneumonia. *Pathol Int* 1995; 45:580–588.

114 Kreidstein SH, Lytwyn A, Keystone EC. Takayasu arteritis with acute interstitial pneumonia and coronary vasculitis: expanding the spectrum. Report of a case. *Arthritis Rheum* 1993; 36:1175–1178.

115 Kondoh Y, Taniguchi H, Kawabata Y et al. Acute exacerbation in idiopathic pulmonary fibrosis. Analysis of clinical and pathologic findings in three cases. *Chest* 1993; 103:1808–1812.

116 Primack SL, Hartman TE, Ikezoe J et al. Acute interstitial pneumonia: radiographic and CT findings in nine patients. *Radiology* 1993; 188:817–820.

117 Akira M, Hara H, Sakatani M. Interstitial lung disease in association with polymyositis – dermatomyositis: long-term follow-up CT evaluation in seven patients. *Radiology* 1999; 210:333–338.

118 Ichikado K, Johkoh T, Ikezoe J et al. Acute interstitial pneumonia: high-resolution CT findings correlated with pathology. *Am J Roentgenol* 1997; 168:333–338.

119 Cottin V, Donsbeck A-V, Revel D et al. Nonspecific interstitial pneumonia. Individualization of a clinicopathologic entity in a series of 12 patients. *Am J Respir Crit Care Med* 1998; 158:1286–1293.

120 Kitaichi M. Pathologic features and the classification of interstitial pneumonia of unknown etiology. *Bull Chest Dis Res Inst Kyoto Univ* 1990; 23:1–18.

121 Colby T, Carrington C. Infiltrative lung disease. In:

Thurlbeck W, ed. *Pathology of the Lung*, 2nd edn. New York: Thieme Medical; 1995:589–738.

122 Griffiths MH, Miller RF, Semple SJ. Interstitial pneumonitis in patients infected with the human immunodeficiency virus. *Thorax* 1995; 50:1141–1146.

123 Travis WD, Fox CH, Devaney KO et al. Lymphoid pneumonitis in 50 adult patients infected with the human immunodeficiency virus: lymphocytic interstitial pneumonitis versus nonspecific interstitial pneumonitis. *Hum Pathol* 1992; 23:529–541.

124 Sattler F, Nichols L, Hirano L et al. Nonspecific interstitial pneumonitis mimicking Pneumocystis carinii pneumonia. *Am J Respir Crit Care Med* 1997; 156:912–917.

125 Kim T, Lee K, Chung M et al. Nonspecific interstitial pneumonia with fibrosis: High resolution CT and pathologic findings. *Am J Roentgenol* 1998; 171:1645–1650.

126 Park JS, Lee KS, Kim JS et al. Nonspecific interstitial pneumonia with fibrosis: radiographic and CT findings in seven patients. *Radiology* 1995; 195:645–648.

127 Todd NW, Wise RA. Respiratory complications in the collagen vascular diseases. *Clin Pulm Med* 1996; 3:101–112.

128 Lynch JP III, Belperio J, Flilnt A et al. Bronchiolar complications of connective tissue disorders. *Semin Respir Crit Care Med* 1999; 20:149–168.

129 Wells AU, Hansell DM, Rubens MB et al. Fibrosing alveolitis in systemic sclerosis. Bronchoalveolar lavage findings in relation to computed tomographic appearance. *Am J Respir Crit Care Med* 1994; 150:462–468.

130 Wells AU, Hansell DM, Rubens MB et al. Functional impairment in lone cryptogenic fibrosing alveolitis and fibrosing alveolitis associated with systemic sclerosis: a comparison. *Am J Respir Crit Care Med* 1997; 155:1657–1664.

131 Remy-Jardin M, Remy J, Wallaert B et al. Pulmonary involvement in progressive systemic sclerosis: sequential evaluation with CT, pulmonary function tests, and bronchoalveolar lavage. *Radiology* 1993; 188:499–506.

132 Silver RM, Miller KS, Kinsella MB et al. Evaluation and management of scleroderma lung disease using bronchoalveolar lavage. *Am J Med* 1990; 18:470–476.

133 Groen H, Wichers G, ter Borg E. J et al. Pulmonary diffusing capacity disturbances are related to nailfold capillary changes in patients with Raynaud's phenomenon with and without an underlying connective tissue disease. *Am J Med* 1990; 89:34–41.

134 Silver RM, Warrick JH, Kinsella MB et al. Cyclophosphamide and low-dose prednisone therapy in patients with systemic sclerosis (scleroderma) with interstitial lung disease. *J Rheumatol* 1993; 20:838–844.

135 Akesson A, Scheja A, Lundin A et al. Improved pulmonary

function in systemic sclerosis after treatment with cyclo-phosphamide. *Arthritis Rheum* 1994; 37:729–735.

136 Steen VD, Lanz JK Jr, Conte C et al. Therapy for severe inter-stitial lung disease in systemic sclerosis. A retrospective study. *Arthritis Rheum* 1994; 37:1290–1296.

137 Davas EM, Peppas C, Maragou M et al. Intravenous cyclo-phosphamide pulse therapy for the treatment of lung disease associated with scleroderma. *Clin Rheumatol* 1999; 18:455–461.

138 de Clerck LS, Dequeker J, Francx L et al. D-penicillamine therapy and interstitial lung disease in scleroderma. A long-term followup study. *Arthritis Rheum* 1987; 30:643–650.

139 Steen VD, Owens GR, Redmond C et al. The effect of D-penicillamine on pulmonary findings in systemic sclerosis. *Arthritis Rheum* 1985; 28:882–888.

140 Clements PJ, Lachenbruch PA, Sterz M et al. Cyclosporine in systemic sclerosis. Results of a forty-eight-week open safety study in ten patients. *Arthritis Rheum* 1993; 36:75–83.

141 Furst DE, Clements PJ, Hillis S et al. Immunosuppression with chlorambucil, versus placebo, for scleroderma. Results of a three-year, parallel, randomized, double-blind study. *Arthritis Rheum* 1989; 32:584–593.

142 Toews GB, Lynch JP, III. Pathogenesis and clinical features of pulmonary infections in patients with rheumatic disease. In: Cannon GW, Zimmerman GA, eds, *The Lung in Rheumatic Diseases, Lung Biology in Health and Disease.* New York: 4Marcel Dekker, Inc.; 1990; 5:179–226.

143 Tomioka R, King TE Jr. Gold-induced pulmonary disease: clinical features, outcome, and differentiation from rheu-matoid lung disease. *Am J Respir Crit Care Med* 1997; 155:1011–1020.

144 Zitnik RJ, Cooper JA Jr. Pulmonary disease due to antirheu-matic agents. *Clin Chest Med* 1990; 11:139–150.

145 Gabbay E, Tarala R, Will R et al. Interstitial lung disease in recent onset rheumatoid arthritis. *Am J Respir Crit Care Med* 1997; 156:528–535.

146 Fujii M, Adachi S, Shimizu T et al. Interstitial lung disease in rheumatoid arthritis: assessment with high-resolution computed tomography. *J Thorac Imaging* 1993; 8:54–62.

147 McDonagh J, Greaves M, Wright AR et al. High resolution computed tomography of the lungs in patients with rheu-matoid arthritis and interstitial lung disease. *Br J Rheumatol* 1994; 33:118–122.

148 Gilligan DM, O'Connor CM, Ward K et al. Bronchoalveolar lavage in patients with mild and severe rheumatoid lung disease. *Thorax* 1990; 45:591–596.

149 Suzuki A, Ohosone Y, Obana M et al. Cause of death in 81 autopsied patients with rheumatoid arthritis. *J Rheumatol* 1994; 21:33–36.

150 Hakala M. Poor prognosis in patients with rheumatoid arthritis hospitalized for interstitial lung fibrosis. *Chest* 1988; 93:114–118.

151 Roschmann RA, Rothenberg RJ. Pulmonary fibrosis in rheumatoid arthritis: a review of clinical features and therapy. *Semin Arthritis Rheum* 1987; 16:174–185.

152 Marguerie C, Bunn CC, Beynon HL et al. Polymyositis, pul-monary fibrosis and autoantibodies to aminoacyl-tRNA synthetase enzymes. *Q J Med* 1990; 77:1019–1038.

153 Adams-Gandhi LB, Boyd AS, and King LE Jr. Diagnosis and management of dermatomyositis. *Compr Ther* 1996; 22:156–164.

154 Schnabel A, Reuter M, Gross WL. Intravenous pulse cyclo-phosphamide in the treatment of interstitial lung disease due to collagen vascular diseases. *Arthritis Rheum* 1998; 41:1215–1220.

155 Yoshida T, Koga H, Saitoh F et al. Pulse intravenous cyclo-phosphamide treatment for steroid-resistant interstitial pneumonitis associated with polymyositis. *Intern Med* 1999; 38:733–738.

156 Nawata Y, Kurasawa K, Takabayashi K et al. Corticosteroid resistant interstitial pneumonitis in dermatomyo-sitis/polymyositis: prediction and treatment with cyclo-sporine. *J Rheumatol* 1999; 26:1527–1533.

157 Keane MP, Lynch JP, III. Pleuropulmonary manifestations of systemic lupus erythematosus. *Thorax* 2000; 55:159–166.

158 Orens JB, Martinez FJ, Lynch JP III. Pleuropulmonary man-ifestations of systemic lupus erythematosus. *Rheum Dis Clin North Am* 1994; 20:159–193.

159 de Andrade J, Kennedy JIJ. The lung in systemic lupus ery-thematosus. *Semin Respir Crit Care Med* 1999; 20:169–177.

160 Martinez FM, Lynch JP III. Collagen vascular disease-asso-ciated bronchiolitis obliterans organizing pneumonia. In: Epler GR, ed, *Diseases of the Bronchoiles*. New York: Raven Press; 1994:347–366.

161 Zamora MR, Warner ML, Tuder R et al. Diffuse alveolar hemorrhage and systemic lupus erythematosus. Clinical presentation, histology, survival, and outcome. *Medicine (Baltimore)* 1997; 76:192–202.

162 Keane MP, Van De Ven CJ, Lynch JP III et al. Systemic lupus during pregnancy with refractory alveolar haemorrhage: recovery following termination of pregnancy. *Lupus* 1997; 6:730–733.

163 Erickson RW, Franklin WA, Emlen W. Treatment of hemor-rhagic lupus pneumonitis with plasmapheresis. *Semin Arthritis Rheum* 1994; 24:114–123.

164 Matthay RA, Schwarz MI, Petty TL et al. Pulmonary mani-

festations of systemic lupus erythematosus: review of twelve cases of acute lupus pneumonitis. *Medicine (Baltimore)* 1975; 54:397–409.

165 Fenlon HM, Doran M, Sant SM et al. High-resolution chest CT in systemic lupus erythematosus. *Am J Roentgenol* 1996; 166:301–307.

166 Haupt HM, Moore GW, Hutchins GM. The lung in systemic lupus erythematosus. Analysis of the pathologic changes in 120 patients. *Am J Med* 1981; 71:791–798.

167 Groen H, ter Borg EJ, Postma DS et al. Pulmonary function in systemic lupus erythematosus is related to distinct clinical, serologic, and nailfold capillary patterns. *Am J Med* 1992; 93:619–627.

168 Sullivan WD, Hurst DJ, Harmon CE et al. A prospective evaluation emphasizing pulmonary involvement in patients with mixed connective tissue disease. *Medicine (Baltimore)* 1984; 63:92–107.

169 Jolliet P, Thorens JB, Chevrolet JC. Pulmonary vascular reactivity in severe pulmonary hypertension associated with mixed connective tissue disease. *Thorax* 1995; 50:96–97.

170 Lazaro MA, Maldonado Cocco JA, Catoggio LJ et al. Clinical and serologic characteristics of patients with overlap syndrome: is mixed connective tissue disease a distinct clinical entity? *Medicine (Baltimore)* 1989; 68:58–65.

171 Deheinzelin D, Capelozzi VL, Kairalla RA et al. Interstitial lung disease in primary Sjogren's syndrome. Clinical–pathological evaluation and response to treatment. *Am J Respir Crit Care Med* 1996; 154:794–799.

172 Papathanasiou MP, Constantopoulos SH, Tsampoulas C et al. Reappraisal of respiratory abnormalities in primary and secondary Sjogren's syndrome. A controlled study. *Chest* 1986; 90:370–374.

173 Constantopoulos SH, Papadimitriou CS, Moutsopoulos HM. Respiratory manifestations in primary Sjogren's syndrome. A clinical, functional, and histologic study. *Chest* 1985; 88:226–229.

174 Dalavanga YA, Constantopoulos SH, Galanopoulou V et al. Alveolitis correlates with clinical pulmonary involvement in primary Sjogren's syndrome. *Chest* 1991; 99:1394–1397.

175 Kelly C, Gardiner P, Pal B et al. Lung function in primary Sjogren's syndrome: a cross sectional and longitudinal study. *Thorax* 1991; 46:180–183.

176 Kadota J, Kusano S, Kawakami K et al. Usual interstitial pneumonia associated with primary Sjogren's syndrome. *Chest* 1995; 108:1756–1758.

177 Tsuzaka K, Ogasawara T, Tojo T et al. Relationship between autoantibodies and clinical parameters in Sjogren's syndrome. *Scand J Rheumatol* 1993; 22:1–9.

178 Ogasawara H, Murashima A, Kaneko H et al. Effect of low-dose cyclosporin treatment on interstitial pneumonitis associated with Sjogren's syndrome [letter]. *Br J Rheumatol* 1998; 37:348–349.

179 Ogasawara H, Sekiya M, Murashima A et al. Very low-dose cyclosporin treatment of steroid-resistant interstitial pneumonitis associated with Sjogren's syndrome. *Clin Rheumatol* 1998; 17:160–162.

180 Sekigawa I, Ogasawara H, Sugiyama M et al. Extremely low dose treatment of cyclosporine for autoimmune diseases [letter]. *Clin Exp Rheumatol* 1998; 16:352.

181 Beckett WS. Occupational respiratory diseases. *N Engl J Med* 2000; 342:406–413.

182 Newman LS. Occupational illness. *N Engl J Med* 1995; 333:1128–1134.

183 Chan-Yeung M, Malo JL. Occupational asthma. *N Engl J Med* 1995; 333:107–112.

184 Fishwick D, Bradshaw LM, D'Souza W et al. Chronic bronchitis, shortness of breath, and airway obstruction by occupation in New Zealand. *Am J Respir Crit Care Med* 1997; 156:1440–1446.

185 Chan-Yeung M. Assessment of asthma in the workplace. ACCP consensus statement. American College of Chest Physicians. *Chest* 1995; 108:1084–1117.

186 Barker RD, van Tongeren MJ, Harris JM et al. Risk factors for sensitisation and respiratory symptoms among workers exposed to acid anhydrides: a cohort study. *Occup Environ Med* 1998; 55:684–691.

187 Kennedy SM, Demers PA. Occupational airways disease from chronic low level exposure to mineral dusts, and mixed exposures. *Semin Respir Crit Care Med* 1999; 20:541–550.

188 Wright JL. Inhalational lung injury causing bronchiolitis. *Clin Chest Med* 1993; 14:635–644.

189 Sunyer J, Kogevinas M, Kromhout H et al. Pulmonary ventilatory defects and occupational exposures in a population-based study in Spain. Spanish Group of the European Community Respiratory Health Survey. *Am J Respir Crit Care Med* 1998; 157:512–517.

190 Hendrick DJ. Occupational and chronic obstructive pulmonary disease (COPD). *Thorax* 1996; 51:947–955.

191 Kreiss K, Mroz MM, Zhen B et al. Risks of beryllium disease related to work processes at a metal, alloy, and oxide production plant. *Occup Environ Med* 1997; 54:605–612.

192 Newman LS, Lloyd J, Daniloff E. The natural history of beryllium sensitization and chronic beryllium disease. *Environ Health Perspect* 1996; 104 Suppl 5:937–943.

193 Cugell DW, Morgan WK, Perkins DG et al. The respiratory effects of cobalt. *Arch Intern Med* 1990; 150:177–183.

194 Figueroa S, Gerstenhaber B, Welch L et al. Hard metal interstitial pulmonary disease associated with a form of welding in a metal parts coating plant. *Am J Ind Med* 1992; 21:363–373.

195 Newman LS. Metals that cause sarcoidosis. *Semin Respir Infect* 1998; 13:212–220.

196 Cowden JD, Will JG, Schwartz DA. Genetics of environmental lung disease. *Semin Respir Crit Care Med* 1999; 20:531–540.

197 Auchincloss JH, Abraham JL, Gilbert R et al. Health hazard of poorly regulated exposure during manufacture of cemented tungsten carbides and cobalt. *Br J Ind Med* 1992; 49:832–836.

198 Mapel DW, Coultas DB. The enviromental epidemiology of idiopathic interstitial lung disease including sarcoidosis. *Semin Respir Crit Care Med* 1999; 20:521–530.

199 Eschenbacher WL, Kreiss K, Lougheed MD et al. Nylon flock-associated interstitial lung disease. *Am J Respir Crit Care Med* 1999; 159:2003–2008.

200 Kern DG, Crausman RS, Durand KT et al. Flock worker's lung: chronic interstitial lung disease in the nylon flocking industry. *Ann Intern Med* 1998; 129:261–272.

201 Kern DG, Kuhn C, 3rd, Ely EW et al. Flock worker's lung: broadening the spectrum of clinicopathology, narrowing the spectrum of suspected etiologies. *Chest* 2000; 117:251–259.

202 Cormier Y, Israel-Assayag E, Bedard G et al. Hypersensitivity pneumonitis in peat moss processing plant workers. *Am J Respir Crit Care Med* 1998; 158:412–417.

203 Rosenow EC III, Limper AH. Drug-induced pulmonary disease. *Semin Respir Infect* 1995; 10:86–95.

204 Cooper JA Jr, White DA, Matthay RA. Drug-induced pulmonary disease. Part 1: Cytotoxic drugs. *Am Rev Respir Dis* 1986; 133:321–340.

205 Cooper JA Jr, White DA, Matthay RA. Drug-induced pulmonary disease. Part 2: Noncytotoxic drugs. *Am Rev Respir Dis* 1986; 133:488–505.

206 Smith GJ. The histopathology of pulmonary reactions to drugs. *Clin Chest Med* 1990; 11:95–117.

207 Wilczynski SW, Erasmus JJ, Petros WP et al. Delayed pulmonary toxicity syndrome following high-dose chemotherapy and bone marrow transplantation for breast cancer. *Am J Respir Crit Care Med* 1998; 157:565–573.

208 Chap L, Shpiner R, Levine M et al. Pulmonary toxicity of high-dose chemotherapy for breast cancer: a non- invasive approach to diagnosis and treatment. *Bone Marrow Transplant* 1997; 20:1063–1067.

209 Todd NW, Peters WP, Ost AH et al. Pulmonary drug toxicity in patients with primary breast cancer treated with high-dose combination chemotherapy and autologous bone marrow transplantation. *Am Rev Respir Dis* 1993; 147:1264–1270.

210 Malik SW, Myers JL, DeRemee RA et al. Lung toxicity associated with cyclophosphamide use. Two distinct patterns. *Am J Respir Crit Care Med* 1996; 154:1851–1856.

211 Bhalla KS, Wilczynski SW, Abushamaa AM et al. Pulmonary toxicity of induction chemotherapy prior to standard or high-dose chemotherapy with autologous hematopoietic support. *Am J Respir Crit Care Med* 2000; 161:17–25.

212 Imokawa S, Colby TV, Leslie KO et al. Methotrexate pneumonitis: review of the literature and histopathological findings in nine patients. *Eur Respir J* 2000; 15:373–381.

213 Liebhaber MI, Wright RS, Gelberg HJ et al. Polymyalgia, hypersensitivity pneumonitis and other reactions in patients receiving HMG-CoA reductase inhibitors: a report of ten cases. *Chest* 1999; 115:886–889.

214 Frank W, Moritz R, Becke B et al. Low dose cabergoline induced interstitial pneumonitis. *Eur Respir J* 1999; 14:968–970.

215 Pfitzenmeyer P, Foucher P, Dennewald G et al. Pleuropulmonary changes induced by ergoline drugs. *Eur Respir J* 1996; 9:1013–1019.

216 Salerno SM, Strong JS, Roth BJ et al. Eosinophilic pneumonia and respiratory failure associated with a trazodone overdose. *Am J Respir Crit Care Med* 1995; 152:2170–2172.

217 Kondo K, Inoue Y, Hamada H et al. Acetaminophen-induced eosinophilic pneumonia. *Chest* 1993; 104:291–292.

218 De Vriese AS, Philippe J, Van Renterghem DM et al. Carbamazepine hypersensitivity syndrome: report of 4 cases and review of the literature. *Medicine (Baltimore)* 1995; 74:144–151.

219 Seebach J, Speich R, Fehr J et al. GM-CSF-induced acute eosinophilic pneumonia. *Br J Haematol* 1995; 90:963–965.

220 Fleisch MC, Blauer F, Gubler JG et al. Eosinophilic pneumonia and respiratory failure associated with venlafaxine treatment. *Eur Respir J* 2000; 15:205–208.

221 Coudert B, Bailly F, Lombard JN et al. Amiodarone pneumonitis. Bronchoalveolar lavage findings in 15 patients and review of the literature. *Chest* 1992; 102:1005–1012.

222 Martin WJ II. Amiodarone pulmonary toxicity. Recognition and pathogenesis. *Chest* 1988; 93:1067–1075; 1242–1248.

223 Lynch JP III, Leatherman JW. Alveolar hemorrhage syndromes. In: Fishman AP, ed, *Fishman's Pulmonary Diseases and Disorders*, 3rd edn. New York: McGraw-Hill; 1998;1193–1210.

224 Gahl WA, Brantly M, Kaiser-Kupfer MI et al. Genetic defects and clinical characteristics of patients with a form of ocu-

locutaneous albinism (Hermansky–Pudlak syndrome). *N Engl J Med* 1998; 338:1258–1264.

225 Brantly M, Avila NA, Shotelersuk V et al. Pulmonary function and high-resolution CT findings in patients with an inherited form of pulmonary fibrosis, Hermansky–Pudlak syndrome, due to mutations in HPS-1. *Chest* 2000; 117:129–136.

226 Shimizu K, Matsumoto T, Miura G et al. Hermansky–Pudlak syndrome with diffuse pulmonary fibrosis: radiologic-pathologic correlation. *J Comput Assist Tomogr* 1998; 22:249–251.

227 Reynolds SP, Davies BH, Gibbs AR. Diffuse pulmonary fibrosis and the Hermansky–Pudlak syndrome: clinical course and postmortem findings. *Thorax* 1994; 49:617–618.

228 Raghu G, Hert R. Interstitial lung diseases: genetic predisposition and inherited interstitial lung diseases. *Semin Respir Med* 1993; 14:323–332.

229 Riccardi VM. Von Recklinghausen neurofibromatosis. *N Engl J Med* 1981; 305:1617–1627.

230 Porterfield JK, Pyeritz RE, Traill TA. Pulmonary hypertension and interstitial fibrosis in von Recklinghausen neurofibromatosis. *Am J Med Genet* 1986; 25:531–535.

231 Smith RL, Hutchins GM, Sack GH Jr et al. Unusual cardiac, renal and pulmonary involvement in Gaucher's disease. Interstitial glucocerebroside accumulation, pulmonary hypertension and fatal bone marrow embolization. *Am J Med* 1978; 65:352–360.

232 Schneider EL, Epstein CJ, Kaback MJ et al. Severe pulmonary involvement in adult Gaucher's disease. Report of three cases and review of the literature. *Am J Med* 1977; 63:475–480.

233 Beutler E, Kay A, Saven A et al. Enzyme replacement therapy for Gaucher disease. *Blood* 1991; 78:1183–1189.

234 Demedts M, Auwerx J, Goddeeris P et al. The inherited association of interstitial lung disease, hypocalciuric hypercalcemia, and defective granulocyte function. *Am Rev Respir Dis* 1985; 131:470–475.

235 Nicholson AG, Wotherspoon AC, Diss TC et al. Reactive pulmonary lymphoid disorders. *Histopathology* 1995; 26:405–412.

236 Koss MN, Hochholzer L, Nichols PW et al. Primary non-Hodgkin's lymphoma and pseudolymphoma of lung: a study of 161 patients. *Hum Pathol* 1983; 14:1024–1038.

237 Koss MN, Hochholzer L, Langloss JM et al. Lymphoid interstitial pneumonia: clinicopathological and immunopathological findings in 18 cases. *Pathology* 1987; 19:178–185.

238 Poletti V, Zompatori M, Cancellieri A. Clinical spectrum of adult chronic bronchiolitis. *Sarcoidosis Vasc Diffuse Lung Dis* 1999; 16:183–196.

239 Fishback N, Koss M. Update on lymphoid interstitial pneumonitis. *Curr Opin Pulm Med* 1996; 2:429–433.

240 Cordier JF. Cryptogenic organizing pneumonitis. Bronchiolitis obliterans organizing pneumonia. *Clin Chest Med* 1993; 14:677–692.

241 Guinee D Jr, Jaffe E, Kingma D et al. Pulmonary lymphomatoid granulomatosis. Evidence for a proliferation of Epstein–Barr virus infected B-lymphocytes with a prominent T-cell component and vasculitis. *Am J Surg Pathol* 1994; 18:753–764.

242 Guinee DG Jr, Perkins SL, Travis WD et al. Proliferation and cellular phenotype in lymphomatoid granulomatosis: implications of a higher proliferation index in B cells. *Am J Surg Pathol* 1998; 22:1093–1100.

243 Taniere P, Thivolet-Bejui F, Vitrey D et al. Lymphomatoid granulomatosis – a report on four cases: evidence for B phenotype of the tumoral cells. *Eur Respir J* 1998; 12:102–106.

244 Haque AK, Myers JL, Hudnall SD et al. Pulmonary lymphomatoid granulomatosis in acquired immunodeficiency syndrome: lesions with Epstein–Barr virus infection. *Mod Pathol* 1998; 11:347–356.

245 Strimlan CV, Rosenow ECD, Weiland LH et al. Lymphocytic interstitial pneumonitis. Review of 13 cases. *Ann Intern Med* 1978; 88:616–621.

246 McGuinness G, Scholes JV, Jagirdar JS et al. Unusual lymphoproliferative disorders in nine adults with HIV or AIDS: CT and pathologic findings. *Radiology* 1995; 197:59–65.

247 Schneider R. Lymphocytic interstitial pneumonitis and nonspecific interstitial pneumonitis. *Clin Chest Med* 1996; 17:763–766.

248 Davies CW, Juniper MC, Gray W et al. Lymphoid interstitial pneumonitis associated with common variable hypogammaglobulinaemia treated with cyclosporin A. *Thorax* 2000; 55:88–90.

249 Prosper M, Omene JA, Ledlie et al. Clinical significance of resolution of chest X-ray findings in HIV- infected children with lymphocytic interstitial pneumonitis (LIP). *Pediatr Radiol* 1995; 25(Suppl 1):S243–S246.

250 Grieco MH, Chinoy-Acharya P. Lymphocytic interstitial pneumonia associated with the acquired immune deficiency syndrome. *Am Rev Respir Dis* 1985; 131:952–955.

251 Myers JL, Kurtin PJ, Katzenstein AL et al. Lymphomatoid granulomatosis. Evidence of immunophenotypic diversity and relationship to Epstein–Barr virus infection. *Am J Surg Pathol* 1995; 19:1300–1312.

252 Liebow AA. The J. Burns Amberson lecture – pulmonary angiitis and granulomatosis. *Am Rev Respir Dis* 1973; 108:1–18.

253 Kurosu K, Yumoto N, Furukawa M et al. Third complementarity-determining-region sequence analysis of lymphocytic interstitial pneumonia: most cases demonstrate a minor monoclonal population hidden among normal lymphocyte clones. *Am J Respir Crit Care Med* 1997; 155:1453–1460.

254 Johkoh T, Muller NL, Pickford HA et al. Lymphocytic interstitial pneumonia: thin-section CT findings in 22 patients. *Radiology* 1999; 212:567–572.

255 Ichikawa Y, Kinoshita M, Koga T et al. Lung cyst formation in lymphocytic interstitial pneumonia: CT features. *J Comput Assist Tomogr* 1994; 18:745–748.

256 Howling SJ, Hansell DM, Wells AU et al. Follicular bronchiolitis: thin-section CT and histologic findings. *Radiology* 199; 212:637–642.

257 Myers J, Kurtin P. Lymphoproliferative disorders of the Lung. In: Thurlbeck W, Churg A, eds, *Pathology of the Lung*, 2nd edn. New York: Thieme; 1995.

258 Li G, Hansmann ML, Zwingers T et al. Primary lymphomas of the lung: morphological, immunohistochemical and clinical features. *Histopathology* 1990; 16:519–531.

259 Wilson WH, Kingma DW, Raffeld M et al. Association of lymphomatoid granulomatosis with Epstein–Barr viral infection of B lymphocytes and response to interferon-alpha 2b. *Blood* 1996; 87:4531–4537.

260 Jaffe ES, Wilson WH. Lymphomatoid granulomatosis: pathogenesis, pathology and clinical implications. *Cancer Surv* 1997; 30:233–248.

261 Katzenstein AL, Carrington CB, Liebow AA. Lymphomatoid granulomatosis: a clinicopathologic study of 152 cases. *Cancer* 1979; 43:360–373.

262 Lipford EH Jr, Margolick JB, Longo DL et al. Angiocentric immunoproliferative lesions: a clinicopathologic spectrum of post-thymic T-cell proliferations. *Blood* 1988; 72:1674–1681.

263 Fauci AS, Haynes BF, Costa J et al. Lymphomatoid granulomatosis. Prospective clinical and therapeutic experience over 10 years. *N Engl J Med* 1982; 306:68–74.

264 Craig FE, Gulley ML, Banks PM. Posttransplantation lymphoproliferative disorders. *Am J Clin Pathol* 1993; 99:265–276.

265 Newman LS, Rose CS, Maier LA. Sarcoidosis. *N Engl J Med* 1997; 336:1224–1234.

266 Lynch JP III, Fantone JC III. Other pulmonary granulomatous vasculitis syndromes. In: Lynch JP III, DeRemee RA, eds, *Immunologically Mediated Pulmonary Diseases*. Philadelphia, PA: Lippincott Co.; 1991:302–319.

267 Lynch JP III, Baughman RP, Sharma O. Extrapulmonary sarcoidosis. *Semin Respir Infect* 1998; 13:229–254.

268 Sharma O, Badr A. Sarcoidosis: diagnosis, staging, and newer diagnostic modalities. *Clin Pulm Med* 1994; 1:18–26.

269 Rybicki BA, Major M, Popovich J Jr et al. Racial differences in sarcoidosis incidence: a 5-year study in a health maintenance organization. *Am J Epidemiol* 1997; 145:234–241.

270 Rybicki BA, Maliarik MJ, Major M et al. Epidemiology, demographics, and genetics of sarcoidosis. *Semin Respir Infect* 1998; 13:166–173.

271 Hosoda Y, Yamaguchi M, Hiraga Y. Global epidemiology of sarcoidosis. What story do prevalence and incidence tell us? *Clin Chest Med* 1997; 18:681–694.

272 Hillerdal G, Nou E, Osterman K et al. Sarcoidosis: epidemiology and prognosis. A 15-year European study. *Am Rev Respir Dis* 1984; 130:29–32.

273 Mana J, Badrinas F, Morera J et al. Sarcoidosis in Spain. *Sarcoidosis* 1992; 9:118–122.

274 Fazzi P, Solfanelli S, Di Pede F et al. Sarcoidosis in Tuscany. A preliminary report. *Sarcoidosis* 1992; 9:123–126.

275 Reich JM, Brouns MC, O'Connor EA et al. Mediastinoscopy in patients with presumptive stage I sarcoidosis: a risk/benefit, cost/benefit analysis. *Chest* 1998; 113:147–153.

276 Muller-Quernheim J. Sarcoidosis: immunopathogenetic concepts and their clinical application. *Eur Respir J* 1998; 12:716–738.

277 Agostini C, Semenzato G. Cytokines in sarcoidosis. *Semin Respir Infect* 1998; 13:184–196.

278 Moller DR. Etiology of sarcoidosis. *Clin Chest Med* 1997; 18:695–706.

279 Sharma OP. Vitamin D, calcium, and sarcoidosis. *Chest* 1996; 109:535–539.

280 Neville E, Walker AN, James DG. Prognostic factors predicting the outcome of sarcoidosis: an analysis of 818 patients. *Q J Med* 1983; 52:525–533.

281 Costabel U. CD4/CD8 ratios in bronchoalveolar lavage fluid: of value for diagnosing sarcoidosis? *Eur Respir J* 1997; 10:2699–2700.

282 Winterbauer RH, Belic N, Moores KD. Clinical interpretation of bilateral hilar adenopathy. *Ann Intern Med* 1973; 78:65–71.

283 Onal E, Lopata M, Lourenco RV. Nodular pulmonary sarcoidosis. Clinical, roentgenographic, and physiologic course in five patients. *Chest* 1977; 72:296–300.

284 Miller A, Brown LK, Sloane MF et al. Cardiorespiratory responses to incremental exercise in sarcoidosis patients with normal spirometry. *Chest* 1995; 107:323–329.

285 Laviolette M, La Forge J, Tennina S et al. Prognostic value of bronchoalveolar lavage lymphocyte count in recently diagnosed pulmonary sarcoidosis. *Chest* 1991; 100:380–384.

286 Ward K, O'Connor C, Odlum C et al. Prognostic value of bronchoalveolar lavage in sarcoidosis: the critical influence of disease presentation. *Thorax* 1989; 44:6–12.

287 Drent M, Jacobs JA, de Vries J et al. Does the cellular bronchoalveolar lavage fluid profile reflect the severity of sarcoidosis? *Eur Respir J* 1999; 13:1338–1344.

288 Sulavik SB, Spencer RP, Palestro CJ et al. Specificity and sensitivity of distinctive chest radiographic and/or 67Ga images in the noninvasive diagnosis of sarcoidosis. *Chest* 1993; 103:403–409.

289 Mana J. Sarcoidosis, imaging N [67]galliium, [201]thallium, [18]flabeled fluoro2-deoxy-D-glucose positron emission tomography. *Clin Chest Med* 1997; 18:799–811.

290 Johns CJ, Michele TM. The clinical management of sarcoidosis. A 50-year experience at the Johns Hopkins Hospital. *Medicine (Baltimore)* 1999; 78:65–111.

291 Gideon NM, Mannino DM. Sarcoidosis mortality in the United States 1979–1991: an analysis of multiple-cause mortality data. *Am J Med* 1996; 100:423–427.

292 Perry A, Vuitch F. Causes of death in patients with sarcoidosis. A morphologic study of 38 autopsies with clinicopathologic correlations. *Arch Pathol Lab Med* 1995; 119:167–172.

293 Mana J, Gomez-Vaquero C, Montero A et al. Lofgren's syndrome revisited: a study of 186 patients. *Am J Med* 1999; 107:240–245.

294 Gran JT, Bohmer E. Acute sarcoid arthritis: A favorable outcome? A retrospective survey of 49 patients with review of the literature. *Scand J Rheumatol* 1996; 25:70–73.

295 Gottlieb JE, Israel HL, Steiner RM et al. Outcome in sarcoidosis. The relationship of relapse to corticosteroid therapy. *Chest* 1997; 111:623–631.

296 Pasturenzi L, Martinetti M, Cuccia M et al. HLA class I, II, and III polymorphism in Italian patients with sarcoidosis. The Pavia–Padova Sarcoidosis Study Group. *Chest* 1993; 104:1170–1175.

297 Sharma OP. Pulmonary sarcoidosis and corticosteroids. *Am Rev Respir Dis* 1993; 147:1598–1600.

298 Gibson GJ, Prescott RJ, Muers MF et al. British Thoracic Society Sarcoidosis study: effects of long term corticosteroid treatment. *Thorax* 1996; 51:238–247.

299 Hunninghake GW, Gilbert S, Pueringer R et al. Outcome of the treatment for sarcoidosis. *Am J Respir Crit Care Med* 1994; 149:893–898.

300 Romer FK. Presentation of sarcoidosis and outcome of pulmonary changes. *Dan Med Bull* 1982; 29:27–32.

301 Baughman RP, Sharma OP, Lynch JP III. Sarcoidosis: is therapy effective? *Semin Respir Infect* 1998; 13:255–273.

302 Eule H, Weinecke A, Roth I et al. The possible influence of corticosteroid therapy on the natural course of pulmonary sarcoidosis. Late results of a continuing clinical study. *Ann N Y Acad Sci* 1986; 465:695–701.

303 Israel HL, Fouts DW, Beggs RA. A controlled trial of prednisone treatment of sarcoidosis. *Am Rev Respir Dis* 1973; 107:609–614.

304 Zaki MH, Lyons HA, Leilop L et al. Corticosteroid therapy in sarcoidosis. A five-year, controlled follow-up study. *N Y State J Med* 1987; 87:496–499.

305 Yamamoto M, Saito N, Tachibana T. Effects of an 18 month corticosteroid therapy to stage I and stage II sarcoidosis patients (control trial). In: Chreitien J, Marsac J, Saltiel , eds, *Sarcoidosis and Other Granulomatous Disorders.* Paris: Pergamon; 1980:470–474.

306 Young RL, Harkleroad LE, Lordon RE et al. Pulmonary sarcoidosis: a prospective evaluation of glucocorticoid therapy. *Ann Intern Med* 1970; 73:207–212.

307 Alberts C, van der Mark TW, Jansen HM. Inhaled budesonide in pulmonary sarcoidosis: a double-blind, placebo-controlled study. Dutch Study Group on Pulmonary Sarcoidosis. *Eur Respir J* 1995; 8:682–688.

308 Spiteri M. Inhaled corticosteroids in pulmonary sarcoidosis. *Postgrad Med* 1991; 67:237–329.

309 du Bois RM, Greenhalgh PM, Southcott AM et al. Randomized trial of inhaled fluticasone propionate in chronic stable pulmonary sarcoidosis: a pilot study. *Eur Respir J* 1999; 13:1345–1350.

310 Pietinalho A, Tukiainen P, Haahtela T et al. Oral prednisolone followed by inhaled budesonide in newly diagnosed pulmonary sarcoidosis: a double-blind, placebo-controlled multicenter study. Finnish Pulmonary Sarcoidosis Study Group. *Chest* 1999; 116:424–431.

311 Lower EE, Baughman RP. Prolonged use of methotrexate for sarcoidosis. *Arch Intern Med* 1995; 155:846–851.

312 Baughman RP, Lower EE. Steroid-sparing alternative treatments for sarcoidosis. *Clin Chest Med* 1997; 18:853–864.

313 Lower EE, Broderick JP, Brott TG et al. Diagnosis and management of neurological sarcoidosis. *Arch Intern Med* 1997; 157:1864–1868.

314 Baughman RP, Winget DB, Lower EE. Methotrexate is steroid sparing in acute sarcoidosis: results of a double blind, randomized trial. *Sarcoidosis Vasc Diffuse Lung Dis* 2000; 17:60–66.

315 Pacheco Y, Marechal C, Marechal F et al. Azathioprine treatment of chronic pulmonary sarcoidosis. *Sarcoidosis* 1985; 2:107–113.

316 Sharma O, Hughs DTD, James DG et al. Immunosuppressive therapy with azathioprine in sarcoidosis. In: Levnisky L, Macholoa F, eds, *Fifth International Conference*

on Sarcoidosis and Other Granulomatous Disorders. Prague; 1971:635–637.

317 Lewis SJ, Ainslie GM, Bateman ED. Efficacy of azathioprine as second-line treatment in pulmonary sarcoidosis. *Sarcoidosis Vasc Diffuse Lung Dis* 1999; 16:87–92.

318 Chapelon C, Ziza JM, Piette JC et al. Neurosarcoidosis: signs, course and treatment in 35 confirmed cases. *Medicine (Baltimore)* 1990; 69:261–276.

319 Agbogu BN, Stern BJ, Sewell C et al. Therapeutic considerations in patients with refractory neurosarcoidosis. *Arch Neurol* 1995; 52:875–879.

320 Diab SM, Karnik AM, Ouda B. A et al. Sarcoidosis in Arabs: the clinical profile of 20 patients and review of the literature. *Sarcoidosis* 1991; 8:56–62.

321 Kataria YP. Chlorambucil in sarcoidosis. *Chest* 1980; 78:36–43.

322 Israel HL, McComb BL. Chlorambucil treatment of sarcoidosis. *Sarcoidosis* 1991; 8:35–41.

323 Adams JS, Diz MM, Sharma OP. Effective reduction in the serum 1,25-dihydroxyvitamin D and calcium concentration in sarcoidosis-associated hypercalcemia with short-course chloroquine therapy. *Ann Intern Med* 1989; 111:437–438.

324 O'Leary TJ, Jones G, Yip A et al. The effects of chloroquine on serum 1,25-dihydroxyvitamin D and calcium metabolism in sarcoidosis. *N Engl J Med* 1986; 315:727–730.

325 Johns CJ, Schonfeld SA, Scott PP et al. Longitudinal study of chronic sarcoidosis with low-dose maintenance corticosteroid therapy. Outcome and complications. *Ann N Y Acad Sci* 1986; 465:702–712.

326 Jones E, Callen JP. Hydroxychloroquine is effective therapy for control of cutaneous sarcoidal granulomas. *J Am Acad Dermatol* 1990; 23:487–489.

327 Zic JA, Horowitz DH, Arzubiaga C et al. Treatment of cutaneous sarcoidosis with chloroquine. Review of the literature. *Arch Dermatol* 1991; 127:1034–1040.

328 Siltzbach LE, Teirstein AS. Chloroquine therapy in 43 patients with intrathoracic and cutaneous sarcoidosis. *Acta Med Scand Suppl* 1964; 425:302–308.

329 Sharma OP. Neurosarcoidosis: a personal perspective based on the study of 37 patients. *Chest* 1997; 112:220–228.

330 Rahbar M, Sharma OP. Hypertrophic osteoarthropathy in sarcoidosis. *Sarcoidosis* 1990; 7:125–127.

331 British Tuberculosis Association. Chloroquine in the treatment of sarcoidosis. *Tubercle* 1967; 48:257–272.

332 Baltzan M, Mehta S, Kirkham TH et al. Randomized trial of prolonged chloroquine therapy in advanced pulmonary sarcoidosis. *Am J Respir Crit Care Med* 1999; 160:192–197.

333 O'Dell JR, Haire CE, Erikson N et al. Treatment of rheumatoid arthritis with methotrexate alone, sulfasalazine and hydroxychloroquine, or a combination of all three medications. *N Engl J Med* 1996; 334:1287–1291.

334 Stern EJ, Webb WR, Golden JA et al. Cystic lung disease associated with eosinophilic granuloma and tuberous sclerosis: air trapping at dynamic ultrafast high-resolution CT. *Radiology* 1992; 182:325–329.

335 Martinet Y, Pinkston P, Saltini C et al. Evaluation of the in vitro and in vivo effects of cyclosporine on the lung T-lymphocyte alveolitis of active pulmonary sarcoidosis. *Am Rev Respir Dis* 1988; 138:1242–1248.

336 Wyser CP, van Schalkwyk EM, Alheit B et al. Treatment of progressive pulmonary sarcoidosis with cyclosporin A. A randomized controlled trial. *Am J Respir Crit Care Med* 1997; 156:1371–1376.

337 Funk JO, Ernst M, Schonharting MM et al. Pentoxifylline exerts synergistic immunomodulatory effects in combination with dexamethasone or cyclosporin A. *Int J Immunopharmacol* 1995; 17:1007–1016.

338 Rieneck K, Diamant M, Haahr PM et al. In vitro immunomodulatory effects of pentoxifylline. *Immunol Lett* 1993; 37:131–138.

339 Zabel P, Entzian P, Dalhoff K et al. Pentoxifylline in treatment of sarcoidosis. *Am J Respir Crit Care Med* 1997; 155:1665–1669.

340 Raje N, Anderson K. Thalidomide – a revival story. *N Engl J Med* 1999; 341:1606–1609.

341 Singhal S, Mehta J, Desikan R et al. Antitumor activity of thalidomide in refractory multiple myeloma. *N Engl J Med* 1999; 341:1565–1571.

342 Barriere H. [Cutaneous sarcoidosis. Treatment with thalidomide]. *Presse Med* 1983; 12:963.

343 Carlesimo M, Giustini S, Rossi A et al. Treatment of cutaneous and pulmonary sarcoidosis with thalidomide. *J Am Acad Dermatol* 1995; 32:866–869.

344 Nunley DR, Hattler B, Keenan RJ et al. Lung transplantation for end-stage pulmonary sarcoidosis. *Sarcoidosis Vasc Diffuse Lung Dis* 1999; 16:93–100.

345 Johnson BA, Duncan SR, Ohori NP et al. Recurrence of sarcoidosis in pulmonary allograft recipients. *Am Rev Respir Dis* 1993; 148:1373–1377.

346 Schuyler M, Cormier Y. The diagnosis of hypersensitivity pneumonitis. *Chest* 1997; 111:534–536.

347 Sharma OP, Fujimura N. Hypersensitivity pneumonitis: a noninfectious granulomatosis. *Semin Respir Infect* 1995; 10:96–106.

348 Lalancette M, Carrier G, Laviolette M et al. Farmer's lung.

Long-term outcome and lack of predictive value of bronchoalveolar lavage fibrosing factors. *Am Rev Respir Dis* 1993; 148:216–221.

349 Suda T, Sato A, Ida M et al. Hypersensitivity pneumonitis associated with home ultrasonic humidifiers. *Chest* 1995; 107:711–717.

350 Van den Bogart HG, Van den Ende G, Van Loon PC et al. Mushroom worker's lung: serologic reactions to thermophilic actinomycetes present in the air of compost tunnels. *Mycopathologia* 1993; 122:21–28.

351 Perez-Padilla R, Salas J, Chapela R et al. Mortality in Mexican patients with chronic pigeon breeder's lung compared with those with usual interstitial pneumonia. *Am Rev Respir Dis* 1993; 148:49–53.

352 Ando M, Arima K, Yoneda R et al. Japanese summer-type hypersensitivity pneumonitis. Geographic distribution, home environment, and clinical characteristics of 621 cases. *Am Rev Respir Dis* 1991; 144:765–769.

353 Miyagawa T, Hamagami S, Tanigawa N. Cryptococcus albidus-induced summer-type hypersensitivity pneumonitis. *Am J Respir Crit Care Med* 2000; 161:961–966.

354 Embil J, Warren P, Yakrus M et al. Pulmonary illness associated with exposure to Mycobacterium-avium complex in hot tub water. Hypersensitivity pneumonitis or infection? *Chest* 1997; 111:813–816.

355 Moreno-Ancillo A, Vicente J, Gomez L et al. Hypersensitivity pneumonitis related to a covered and heated swimming pool environment. *Int Arch Allergy Immunol* 1997; 114:205–206.

356 Brown JE, Masood D, Couser JI et al. Hypersensitivity pneumonitis from residential composting: residential composter's lung. *Ann Allergy Asthma Immunol* 1995; 74:45–47.

357 Bernstein DI, Lummus ZL, Santilli G et al. Machine operator's lung. A hypersensitivity pneumonitis disorder associated with exposure to metalworking fluid aerosols. *Chest* 1995; 108:636–641.

358 Kane GC, Marx JJ, Prince DS. Hypersensitivity pneumonitis secondary to Klebsiella oxytoca. A new cause of humidifier lung. *Chest* 1993; 104:627–629.

359 Wright RS, Dyer Z, Liebhaber MI et al. Hypersensitivity pneumonitis from *Pezizia domiciliana*. A case of el nino lung. *Am J Respir Crit Care Med* 199; 160:1758–1761.

360 Gurney JW. Hypersensitivity pneumonitis. *Radiol Clin North Am* 1992; 30:1219–1230.

361 Lacasse Y, Fraser RS, Fournier M et al. Diagnostic accuracy of transbronchial biopsy in acute farmer's lung disease. *Chest* 1997; 112:1459–1465.

362 Adler BD, Padley SP, Muller NL et al. Chronic hypersensitivity pneumonitis: high-resolution CT and radiographic features in 16 patients. *Radiology* 1992; 185:91–95.

363 Akira M, Kita N, Higashihara T et al. Summer-type hypersensitivity pneumonitis: comparison of high-resolution CT and plain radiographic findings. *Am J Roentgenol* 1992; 158:1223–1228.

364 Lynch DA, Newell JD, Logan PM et al. Can CT distinguish hypersensitivity pneumonitis from idiopathic pulmonary fibrosis? *Am J Roentgenol* 1995; 165:807–811.

365 Kokkarinen JI, Tukiainen HO, Terho EO. Effect of corticosteroid treatment on the recovery of pulmonary function in farmer's lung. *Am Rev Respir Dis* 1992; 145:3–5.

366 Erkinjuntti-Pekkanen R, Rytkonen H, Kokkarinen JI et al. Long-term risk of emphysema in patients with farmer's lung and matched control farmers. *Am J Respir Crit Care Med* 1998; 158:662–665.

367 Kokkarinen J, Tukiainen H, Terho EO. Mortality due to farmer's lung in Finland. *Chest* 1994; 106:509–512.

368 Murayama J, Yoshizawa Y, Ohtsuka M et al. Lung fibrosis in hypersensitivity pneumonitis. Association with CD4+ but not CD8+ cell dominant alveolitis and insidious onset. *Chest* 1993; 104:38–43.

369 Remy-Jardin M, Remy J, Wallaert B et al. Subacute and chronic bird breeder hypersensitivity pneumonitis: sequential evaluation with CT and correlation with lung function tests and bronchoalveolar lavage. *Radiology* 1993; 189:111–118.

370 Kokkarinen JI, Tukiainen HO, Terho EO. Recovery of pulmonary function in farmer's lung. A five-year follow-up study. *Am Rev Respir Dis* 1993; 147:793–796.

371 Naughton M, Fahy J, FitzGerald MX. Chronic eosinophilic pneumonia. A long-term follow-up of 12 patients. *Chest* 1993; 103:162–165.

372 Allen JN, Pacht ER, Gadek JE et al. Acute eosinophilic pneumonia as a reversible cause of noninfectious respiratory failure. *N Engl J Med* 1989; 321:569–574.

373 Tazelaar HD, Linz LJ, Colby TV et al. Acute eosinophilic pneumonia: histopathologic findings in nine patients. *Am J Respir Crit Care Med* 1997; 155:296–302.

374 Pope-Harman AL, Davis WB, Allen ED et al. Acute eosinophilic pneumonia. A summary of 15 cases and review of the literature. *Medicine (Baltimore)* 1996; 75:334–342.

375 Buchheit J, Eid N, Rodgers G Jr et al. Acute eosinophilic pneumonia with respiratory failure: a new syndrome? *Am Rev Respir Dis* 1992; 145:716–718.

376 Lombard CM, Tazelaar HD, Krasne DL. Pulmonary eosinophilia in coccidioidal infections. *Chest* 1987; 91:734–736.

377 Alasaly K, Muller N, Ostrow DN et al. Cryptogenic organizing pneumonia. A report of 25 cases and a review of the literature. *Medicine (Baltimore)* 1995; 74:201–211.

378 Cordier JF. Organising pneumonia. *Thorax* 2000; 55:318–328.

379 Lohr RH, Boland BJ, Douglas WW et al. Organizing pneumonia. Features and prognosis of cryptogenic, secondary, and focal variants. *Arch Intern Med* 1997; 157:1323–1329.

380 Baron FA, Hermanne JP, Dowlati A et al. Bronchiolitis obliterans organizing pneumonia and ulcerative colitis after allogeneic bone marrow transplantation. *Bone Marrow Transplant* 1998; 21:951–954.

381 Uner AH, Rozum-Slota B, Katzenstein AL. Bronchiolitis obliterans-organizing pneumonia (BOOP)-like variant of Wegener's granulomatosis. A clinicopathologic study of 16 cases. *Am J Surg Pathol* 1996; 20:794–801.

382 Bayle JY, Nesme P, Bejui-Thivolet F et al. Migratory organizing pneumonitis 'primed' by radiation therapy. *Eur Respir J* 1995; 8:322–326.

383 Crestani B, Valeyre D, Roden S et al. Bronchiolitis obliterans organizing pneumonia syndrome primed by radiation therapy to the breast. The Groupe d'Etudes et de Recherche sur les Maladies Orphelines Pulmonaires (GERM'O'P). *Am J Respir Crit Care Med* 1998; 158:1929–1935.

384 Battistini E, Dini G, Savioli C et al. Bronchiolitis obliterans organizing pneumonia in three children with acute leukaemias treated with cytosine arabinoside and anthracyclines. *Eur Respir J* 1997; 10:1187–1190.

385 Mathew P, Bozeman P, Krance R. A et al. Bronchiolitis obliterans organizing pneumonia (BOOP) in children after allogeneic bone marrow transplantation. *Bone Marrow Transplant* 1994; 13:221–222.

386 Chaparro C, Chamberlain D, Maurer J et al. 1996. Bronchiolitis obliterans organizing pneumonia (BOOP) in lung transplant recipients. *Chest* 110:1150–4.

387 Watanabe K, Senju S, Wen FQ et al. Factors related to the relapse of bronchiolitis obliterans organizing pneumonia. *Chest* 1998; 114:1599–606.

388 Cohen AJ, King TE Jr, Downey GP. Rapidly progressive bronchiolitis obliterans with organizing pneumonia. *Am J Respir Crit Care Med* 1994; 149:1670–1675.

389 Perez de Llano LA, Soilan JL, Garcia Pais MJ et al. Idiopathic bronchiolitis obliterans with organizing pneumonia presenting with adult respiratory distress syndrome. *Respir Med* 1998; 92:884–886.

390 Bartter T, Irwin RS, Nash G et al. Idiopathic bronchiolitis obliterans organizing pneumonia with peripheral infiltrates on chest roentgenogram. *Arch Intern Med* 1989; 49:273–279.

391 Dina R, Sheppard MN. The histological diagnosis of clinically documented cases of cryptogenic organizing pneumonia: diagnostic features in transbronchial biopsies. *Histopathology* 1993; 23:541–545.

392 Davison AG, Heard BE, McAllister WA et al. Cryptogenic organizing pneumonitis. *Q J Med* 1983; 52:382–394.

393 Costabel U, Guzman J, Teschler H. Bronchiolitis obliterans with organizing pneumonia: outcome. *Thorax* 1995; 50(Suppl 1):559–564.

394 Purcell IF, Bourke SJ, Marshall SM. Cyclophosphamide in severe steroid-resistant bronchiolitis obliterans organizing pneumonia. *Respir Med* 1997; 91:175–177.

395 Ezri T, Kunichezky S, Eliraz A et al. Bronchiolitis obliterans: Current concepts. *QJ Med* 1994; 87:1–10.

396 Snell GI, Esmore DS, Williams TJ. Cytolytic therapy for the bronchiolitis obliterans syndrome complicating lung transplantation. *Chest* 1996; 109:874–878.

397 Ross DJ, Jordan SC, Nathan SD et al. Delayed development of obliterative bronchiolitis syndrome with OKT3 after unilateral lung transplantation. A plea for multicenter immunosuppressive trials. *Chest* 1996; 109:870–873.

398 Kelly KJ, Hertz MI. Obliterative bronchiolitis. *Clin Chest Med* 1997; 18:319–338.

399 Zheng L, Haydn Walters E, Ward C et al. Airway neutrophilia in stable and bronchiolitis obliterans syndrome patients following lung transplantation. *Thorax* 2000; 55:53–59.

400 Turton CW, Williams G, Green M. Cryptogenic obliterative bronchiolitis in adults. *Thorax* 1981; 36:805–810.

401 Hansell DM, Rubens MB, Padley SP et al. Obliterative bronchiolitis; individual CT signs of small airways disease and functional correlation. *Radiology* 1997; 203:721–726.

402 Muller NL, Miller RR. Diseases of the bronchioles: CT and histopathologic findings. *Radiology* 1995; 196:3–12.

403 Aquino SL, Webb WR, Golden J. Bronchiolitis obliterans associated with rheumatoid arthritis: Findings on HRCT and dynamic expiratory CT. *J Comput Assist Tomogr* 1994; 18:555–558.

404 Colby TV. Bronchiolitis pathologic considerations. *Am J Clin Pathol* 1998; 109:101–109.

405 Homma H, Yamanaka A, Tanimoto S et al. Diffuse panbronchiolitis. A disease of the transitional zone of the lung. *Chest* 1983; 83:63–69.

406 Park MH, Kim YW, Yoon HI et al. Association of HLA class I antigens with diffuse panbronchiolitis in Korean patients. *Am J Respir Crit Care Med* 1999; 159:526–529.

407 Koyama H, Geddes DM. Erythromycin and diffuse panbronchiolitis. *Thorax* 1997; 52:915–918.

408 Keicho N, Tokunaga K, Nakata K et al. Contribution of HLA

genes to genetic predisposition in diffuse panbronchiolitis. *Am J Respir Crit Care Med* 1998; 158:846–850.

409 Sugiyama Y, Kudoh S, Maeda H et al. Analysis of HLA antigens in patients with diffuse panbronchiolitis. *Am Rev Respir Dis* 1990; 141:1459–1462.

410 Fitzgerald JE, King TE Jr, Lynch DA et al. Diffuse panbronchiolitis in the United States. *Am J Respir Crit Care Med* 1996; 154:497–503.

411 Nishimura K, Kitaichi M, Izumi T et al. Diffuse panbronchiolitis: correlation of high-resolution CT and pathologic findings. *Radiology* 1992; 184:779–785.

412 Iwata M, Colby TV, Kitaichi M. Diffuse panbronchiolitis: diagnosis and distinction from various pulmonary diseases with centrilobular interstitial foam cell accumulations. *Hum Pathol* 1994; 25:357–363.

413 Nagai H, Shishido H, Yoneda R et al. Long-term low-dose administration of erythromycin to patients with diffuse panbronchiolitis. *Respiration* 1991; 58:145–149.

414 Kadota J, Sakito O, Kohno S et al. A mechanism of erythromycin treatment in patients with diffuse panbronchiolitis. *Am Rev Respir Dis* 1993; 147:153–159.

415 Baz MA, Kussin PS, Van Trigt P et al. Recurrence of diffuse panbronchiolitis after lung transplantation. *Am J Respir Crit Care Med* 1995; 151:895–898.

416 Jayne D. Pulmonary–renal syndrome. *Semin Respir Crit Care Med* 1996; 19:69–78.

417 Niles JL, Bottinger EP, Saurina GR et al. The syndrome of lung hemorrhage and nephritis is usually an ANCA-associated condition. *Arch Intern Med* 1996; 156:440–445.

418 Schnabel A, Reuter M, Csernok E et al. Subclinical alveolar bleeding in pulmonary vasculitides: correlation with indices of disease activity. *Eur Respir J* 1999; 14:118–124.

419 Schwarz MI. The nongranulomatous vasculitides of the lung. *Semin Respir Crit Care Med* 1998; 19:47–56.

420 Raz I, Okon E, Chajek-Shaul T. Pulmonary manifestations in Behcet's syndrome. *Chest* 1989; 95:585–589.

421 Efthimiou J, Johnston C, Spiro SG et al. Pulmonary disease in Behcet's syndrome. *Q J Med* 1986; 58:259–280.

422 Schwarz MI, Zamora MR, Hodges TN et al. Isolated pulmonary capillaritis and diffuse alveolar hemorrhage in rheumatoid arthritis and mixed connective tissue disease. *Chest* 1998; 113:1609–1615.

423 Schwarz MI, Sutarik JM, Nick JA et al. Pulmonary capillaritis and diffuse alveolar hemorrhage. A primary manifestation of polymyositis. *Am J Respir Crit Care Med* 1995; 151:2037–2040.

424 Jennette JC, Falk RJ, Andrassy K et al. Nomenclature of systemic vasculitides. Proposal of an international consensus conference. *Arthritis Rheum* 1994; 37:187–92.

425 Stricker H, Malinverni R. Multiple, large aneurysms of pulmonary arteries in Behcet's disease. Clinical remission and radiologic resolution after corticosteroid therapy. *Arch Intern Med* 1989; 149:925–927.

426 Hoffman GS, Specks U. Antineutrophil cytoplasmic antibodies. *Bull Rheum Dis* 1998; 47:5–8.

427 Gaudin PB, Askin FB, Falk RJ et al. The pathologic spectrum of pulmonary lesions in patients with anti-neutrophil cytoplasmic autoantibodies specific for anti-proteinase 3 and anti-myeloperoxidase. *Am J Clin Pathol* 1995; 104:7–16.

428 Rao JK, Weinberger M, Oddone EZ et al. The role of anti-neutrophil cytoplasmic antibody (c-ANCA) testing in the diagnosis of Wegener granulomatosis. A literature review and meta- analysis. *Ann Intern Med* 1995; 123:925–932.

429 Hogan SL, Nachman PH, Wilkman AS et al. Prognostic markers in patients with antineutrophil cytoplasmic autoantibody-associated microscopic polyangiitis and glomerulonephritis. *J Am Soc Nephrol* 1996; 7:23–32.

430 Cohen Tervaert JW. The value of serial ANCA testing during follow-up studies in patients with ANCA-associated vasculitides. *J Nephrol* 1996; 9:232–240.

431 Kyndt X, Reumaux D, Bridoux F et al. Serial measurements of antineutrophil cytoplasmic autoantibodies in patients with systemic vasculitis. *Am J Med* 1999; 106:527–533.

432 Fauci AS, Haynes BF, Katz P et al. Wegener's granulomatosis: prospective clinical and therapeutic experience with 85 patients for 21 years. *Ann Intern Med* 1983; 98:76–85.

433 Hoffman GS, Kerr GS, Leavitt RY et al. Wegener granulomatosis: an analysis of 158 patients. *Ann Intern Med* 1992; 116:488–498.

434 Sullivan EJ, Hoffman GS. Wegener's granulomatosis. *Semin Respir Crit Care Med* 1998; 19:13–25.

435 Lynch JP III, Hoffman GS. Wegener's granulomatosis: controversies and current concepts. *Compr Ther* 1998; 24:421–440.

436 Langford CA, Hoffman GS. Rare diseases.3: Wegener's granulomatosis. *Thorax* 1999; 54:629–637.

437 Devaney KO, Travis WD, Hoffman G et al. Interpretation of head and neck biopsies in Wegener's granulomatosis. A pathologic study of 126 biopsies in 70 patients. *Am J Surg Pathol* 1990; 14:555–564.

438 Travis WD, Hoffman GS, Leavitt RY et al. Surgical pathology of the lung in Wegener's granulomatosis. Review of 87 open lung biopsies from 67 patients. *Am J Surg Pathol* 1991; 15:315–333.

439 Watts RA, Carruthers DM, Scott DG. Epidemiology of systemic vasculitis: changing incidence or definition? *Semin Arthritis Rheum* 1995; 25:28–34.

440 Daum TE, Specks U, Colby TV et al. Tracheobronchial involvement in Wegener's granulomatosis. *Am J Respir Crit Care Med* 1995; 151:522–526.

441 Langford CA, Sneller MC, Hallahan CW et al. Clinical features and therapeutic management of subglottic stenosis in patients with Wegener's granulomatosis. *Arthritis Rheum* 1996; 39:1754–1760.

442 Cordier JF, Valeyre D, Guillevin L et al. Pulmonary Wegener's granulomatosis. A clinical and imaging study of 77 cases. *Chest* 1990; 97:906–912.

443 Quint LE, Whyte RI, Kazerooni EA et al. Stenosis of the central airways: evaluation by using helical CT with multiplanar reconstructions. *Radiology* 1995; 194:871–877.

444 Papiris SA, Manoussakis MN, Drosos AA et al. Imaging of thoracic Wegener's granulomatosis: the computed tomographic appearance. *Am J Med* 1992; 93:529–536.

445 Lombard C. M, Duncan S. R, Rizk N. W et al. The diagnosis of Wegener's granulomatosis from transbronchial biopsy specimens. *Hum Pathol* 1990; 21:838–42.

446 Travis WD, Colby TV, Lombard C et al. A clinicopathologic study of 34 cases of diffuse pulmonary hemorrhage with lung biopsy confirmation. *Am J Surg Pathol* 1990; 14:1112–1125.

447 Nishino H, Rubino FA, DeRemee RA et al. Neurological involvement in Wegener's granulomatosis: an analysis of 324 consecutive patients at the Mayo Clinic. *Ann Neurol* 1993; 33:4–9.

448 Gross WL, Schnabel A, Trabandt A. New perspectives in pulmonary angiitis: From pulmonary angiitis and granulomatosis to ANCA associated vasculitis. *Sarcoidosis Vascul Diffuse Lung Dis* 2000; 17:33–52.

449 Kerr GS, Fleisher TA, Hallahan CW et al. Limited prognostic value of changes in antineutrophil cytoplasmic antibody titer in patients with Wegener's granulomatosis. *Arthritis Rheum* 1993; 36:365–371.

450 Talar-Williams C, Hijazi YM, Walther MM et al. Cyclophosphamide-induced cystitis and bladder cancer in patients with Wegener granulomatosis. *Ann Intern Med* 1996; 124:477–484.

451 Guillevin L, Cordier JF, Lhote F et al. A prospective, multicenter, randomized trial comparing steroids and pulse cyclophosphamide versus steroids and oral cyclophosphamide in the treatment of generalized Wegener's granulomatosis. *Arthritis Rheum* 1997; 40:2187–2198.

452 Hoffman GS, Leavitt RY, Fleisher TA et al. Treatment of Wegener's granulomatosis with intermittent high-dose intravenous cyclophosphamide. *Am J Med* 1990; 89:403–410.

453 Drosos AA, Sakkas LI, Goussia A et al. Pulse cyclophospha-
mide therapy in Wegener's granulomatosis: a pilot study. *J Intern Med* 1992; 232:279–282.

454 Haubitz M, Frei U, Rother U et al. Cyclophosphamide pulse therapy in Wegener's granulomatosis. *Nephrol Dial Transplant* 1991; 6:531–535.

455 Reinhold-Keller E, Kekow J, Schnabel A et al. Influence of disease manifestation and antineutrophil cytoplasmic antibody titer on the response to pulse cyclophosphamide therapy in patients with Wegener's granulomatosis. *Arthritis Rheum* 1994; 37:919–924.

456 Israel HL, Patchefsky AS, Saldana MJ. Wegener's granulomatosis, lymphomatoid granulomatosis, and benign lymphocytic angiitis and granulomatosis of lung. Recognition and treatment. *Ann Intern Med* 1977; 87:691–699.

457 Sneller MC, Hoffman GS, Talar-Williams C et al. An analysis of forty-two Wegener's granulomatosis patients treated with methotrexate and prednisone. *Arthritis Rheum* 1995; 38:608–613.

458 Stegeman CA, Tervaert JWC, de Jong PE et al. Trimethoprim-sulfamethoxazole (co-trimoxazole) for the prevention of relapses of Wegener's granulomatosis. *N Engl J Med* 1996; 335:16–20.

459 DeRemee RA. The treatment of Wegener's granulomatosis with trimethoprim/sulfamethoxazole: illusion or vision? *Arthritis Rheum* 1988; 31:1068–1074.

460 Georgi J, Ulmer M, Gross WL. Cotrimoxazole in Wegener's granulomatosis – a prospective study. *Immun Infekt* 1991; 19:97–98.

461 Reinhold-Keller E, De Groot K, Rudert H et al. Response to trimethoprim/sulfamethoxazole in Wegener's granulomatosis depends on the phase of disease. *Q J Med* 1996; 89:15–23.

462 Jayne DR, Esnault VL, Lockwood CM. ANCA anti-idiotype antibodies and the treatment of systemic vasculitis with intravenous immunoglobulin. *J Autoimmun* 1993; 6:207–219.

463 Lockwood CM, Thiru S, Isaacs JD et al. Long-term remission of intractable systemic vasculitis with monoclonal antibody therapy. *Lancet* 1993; 341:1620–1622.

464 Savage COS, Winearls CG, Evans DJ et al. Microscopic polyarteritis: presentation, pathology, and prognosis. *Q J Med* 1985; 56:467–483.

465 Guillevin L, Lhote F, Cohen P et al. Corticosteroids plus pulse cyclophosphamide and plasma exchanges versus corticosteroids plus pulse cyclophosphamide alone in the treatment of polyarteritis nodosa and Churg–Strauss syndrome patients with factors predicting poor prognosis. A prospective, randomized trial in sixty-two patients. *Arthritis Rheum* 1995; 38:1638–1645.

466 Guillevin L, Lhote F, Gayraud M et al. Prognostic factors in polyarteritis nodosa and Churg–Strauss syndrome. A prospective study in 342 patients. *Medicine (Baltimore)* 1996; 75:17–28.

467 Guillevin L, Cohen P, Gayraud M et al. Churg–Strauss syndrome. Clinical study and long-term follow-up of 96 patients. *Medicine (Baltimore)* 1999; 78:26–37.

468 Lhote F, Guillevin L. Polyarteritis nodosa, microscopic polyangiitis, and Churg–Strauss syndrome. *Semin Respir Crit Care Med* 1998; 19:27–45.

469 Calabrese LH, Hoffman GS, Guillevin L. Therapy of resistant systemic necrotizing vasculitis. Polyarteritis, Churg–Strauss syndrome, Wegener's granulomatosis, and hypersensitivity vasculitis group disorders. *Rheum Dis Clin North Am* 1995; 21:41–57.

470 Lanham JG, Elkon KB, Pusey CD et al. Systemic vasculitis with asthma and eosinophilia: a clinical approach to the Churg–Strauss syndrome. *Medicine (Baltimore)* 1984; 63:65–81.

471 Reid AJ, Harrison BD, Watts RA et al. Churg–Strauss syndrome in a district hospital. *Q J Med* 1998; 91:219–229.

472 Wechsler ME, Finn D, Gunawardena D et al. Churg–Strauss syndrome in patients receiving montelukast as treatment for asthma. *Chest* 2000; 117:708–713.

473 Sehgal M, Swanson JW, DeRemee RA et al. Neurologic manifestations of Churg–Strauss syndrome. *Mayo Clin Proc* 1995; 70:337–341.

474 Masi AT, Hunder GG, Lie JT et al. The American College of Rheumatology 1990 criteria for the classification of Churg–Strauss syndrome (allergic granulomatosis and angiitis). *Arthritis Rheum* 1990; 33:1094–1100.

475 Tatsis E, Schnabel A, Gross WL. Interferon-alpha treatment of four patients with the Churg–Strauss syndrome. *Ann Intern Med* 1998; 129:370–374.

476 Wechsler ME, Garpestad E, Flier SR et al. Pulmonary infiltrates, eosinophilia, and cardiomyopathy following corticosteroid withdrawal in patients with asthma receiving zafirlukast. *JAMA* 1998; 279:455–457.

477 Stirling RG, Chung KF. Leukotriene antagonists and Churg–Strauss syndrome: the smoking gun. *Thorax* 1999; 54:865–866.

478 Franco J, Artes MJ. Pulmonary eosinophilia associated with montelukast. *Thorax* 1999; 54:558–560.

479 Kinoshita M, Shiraishi T, Koga T et al. Churg–Strauss syndrome after corticosteroid withdrawal in an asthmatic patient treated with pranlukast. *J Allergy Clin Immunol* 1999; 103:534–535.

480 Schonfeld N, Frank W, Wenig S et al. Clinical and radiologic features, lung function and therapeutic results in pulmonary histiocytosis X. *Respiration* 1993; 60:38–44.

481 Basset F, Corrin B, Spencer H et al. Pulmonary histiocytosis X. *Am Rev Respir Dis* 1978; 118:811–820.

482 Colby TV, Lombard C. Histiocytosis X in the lung. *Hum Pathol* 1983; 14:847–856.

483 Friedman PJ, Liebow AA, Sokoloff J. Eosinophilic granuloma of lung. Clinical aspects of primary histiocytosis in the adult. *Medicine (Baltimore)* 1981; 60:385–396.

484 Travis WD, Borok Z, Roum JH et al. Pulmonary Langerhans cell granulomatosis (histiocytosis X). A clinicopathologic study of 48 cases. *Am J Surg Pathol* 1993; 17:971–986.

485 Selman M, Carillo G, Gaxiola M et al. Pulmonary histiocytosis X (eosinophilic granuloma): clinical behavior, pathogenesis, and therapeutic strategies of an unusual interstitial lung disease. *Clin Pulm Med* 1996; 3:191–198.

486 Sadoun D, Vaylet F, Valeyre D et al. Bronchogenic carcinoma in patients with pulmonary histiocytosis X. *Chest* 1992; 101:1610–1613.

487 Lombard CM, Medeiros LJ, Colby TV. Pulmonary histiocytosis X and carcinoma. *Arch Pathol Lab Med* 1987; 111:339–341.

488 Egeler RM, Neglia JP, Puccetti DM et al. Association of Langerhans cell histiocytosis with malignant neoplasms. *Cancer* 1993; 71:865–873.

489 Brauner MW, Grenier P, Mouelhi MM et al. Pulmonary histiocytosis X: evaluation with high-resolution CT. *Radiology* 1989; 172:255–258.

490 Crausman RS, Jennings CA, Tuder RM et al. Pulmonary histiocytosis X: pulmonary function and exercise pathophysiology. *Am J Respir Crit Care Med* 1996; 153:426–435.

491 Delobbe A, Durieu J, Duhamel A et al. Determinants of survival in pulmonary Langerhans' cell granulomatosis (histiocytosis X). Groupe d'Etude en Pathologie Interstitielle de la Societe de Pathologie Thoracique du Nord. *Eur Respir J* 1996; 9:2002–2006.

492 Emile JF, Wechsler J, Brousse N et al. Langerhans' cell histiocytosis. Definitive diagnosis with the use of monoclonal antibody O10 on routinely paraffin-embedded samples. *Am J Surg Pathol* 1995; 19:636–641.

493 Youkeles LH, Grizzanti JN, Liao Z et al. Decreased tobacco-glycoprotein-induced lymphocyte proliferation in vitro in pulmonary eosinophilic granuloma. *Am J Respir Crit Care Med* 1995; 151:145–50.

494 Aguayo SM, King TE Jr, Waldron JA Jr et al. Increased pulmonary neuroendocrine cells with bombesin-like immunoreactivity in adult patients with eosinophilic granuloma. *J Clin Invest* 1990; 86:838–844.

495 Aguayo SM. Determinants of susceptibility to cigarette smoke. Potential roles for neuroendocrine cells and neuropeptides in airway inflammation, airway wall

remodeling, and chronic airflow obstruction. *Am J Respir Crit Care Med* 1994; 149:1692–1698.

496 Igarashi T, Nakagawa A, Nishino M et al. Improvement of pulmonary eosinophilic granuloma after smoking cessation in two patients. *Nihon Kyobu Shikkan Gakkai Zasshi* 1995; 33:1125–1129.

497 Mogulkoc N, Veral A, Bishop P. W et al. Pulmonary Langerhans' cell histiocytosis: radiologic resolution following smoking cessation. *Chest* 1999; 115:1452–1455.

498 Tazi A, Montcelly L, Bergeron A et al. Relapsing nodular lesions in the course of adult pulmonary Langerhans cell histiocytosis. *Am J Respir Crit Care Med* 1998; 157:2007–2010.

499 Ladisch S, Gadner H. Treatment of Langerhans cell histiocytosis – evolution and current approaches. *Br J Cancer Suppl* 1994; 23:S41–S46.

500 Etienne B, Bertocchi M, Gamondes JP et al. Relapsing pulmonary Langerhans cell histiocytosis after lung transplantation. *Am J Respir Crit Care Med* 1998; 157:288–291.

501 Chu SC, Horiba K, Usuki J et al. Comprehensive evaluation of 35 patients with lymphangioleiomyomatosis. *Chest* 1999; 115:1041–1052.

502 Oh YM, Mo EK, Jang SH et al. Pulmonary lymphangioleiomyomatosis in Korea. *Thorax* 1999; 54:618–621.

503 Kalassian KG, Doyle R, Kao P et al. Lymphangioleiomyomatosis: new insights. *Am J Respir Crit Care Med* 1997; 155:1183–1186.

504 Taylor JR, Ryu J, Colby TV et al. Lymphangioleiomyomatosis. Clinical course in 32 patients. *N Engl J Med* 1990; 323:1254–1260.

505 Johnson SR, Tattersfield AE. Decline in lung function in lymphangioleiomyomatosis: relation to menopause and progesterone treatment. *Am J Respir Crit Care Med* 1999; 160:628–633.

506 Kitaichi M, Nishimura K, Itoh H et al. Pulmonary lymphangioleiomyomatosis: a report of 46 patients including a clinicopathologic study of prognostic factors. *Am J Respir Crit Care Med* 1995; 151:527–533.

507 Crausman RS, Lynch DA, Mortenson RL et al. Quantitative CT predicts the severity of physiologic dysfunction in patients with lymphangioleiomyomatosis. *Chest* 1996; 109:131–137.

508 Torres VE, Bjornsson J, King BF et al. Extrapulmonary lymphangioleiomyomatosis and lymphangiomatous cysts in tuberous sclerosis complex. *Mayo Clin Proc* 1995; 70:641–648.

509 Boehler A, Speich R, Russi E. W et al. Lung transplantation for lymphangioleiomyomatosis. *N Engl J Med* 1996; 335:1275–1280.

510 Bernstein SM, Newell JD Jr, Adamczyk D et al. How common are renal angiomyolipomas in patients with pulmonary lymphangiomyomatosis? *Am J Respir Crit Care Med* 1995; 152:2138–2143.

511 Silverstein EF, Ellis K, Wolff M et al. Pulmonary lymphangiomyomatosis. *Am J Roentgenol Radium Ther Nucl Med* 1974; 120:832–850.

512 Eliasson AH, Phillips YY, Tenholder MF. Treatment of lymphangioleiomyomatosis. A meta-analysis. *Chest* 1989; 96:1352–1355.

513 Curtis J, Schuyler M. Immunologicallly mediated lung diseases. In: Baum G, Crapo R, Celli B, Karlinsky J, eds. *Textbook of Pulmonary Diseases*. Philadelphia: Lippincott-Raven; 1998: 1:367–406.

514 Cordonnier C, Fleury-Feith J, Escudier E et al. Secondary alveolar proteinosis is a reversible cause of respiratory failure in leukemic patients. *Am J Respir Crit Care Med* 1994; 149:788–794.

515 Teja K, Cooper PH, Squires JE et al. Pulmonary alveolar proteinosis in four siblings. *N Engl J Med* 1981; 305:1390–1392.

516 Goldstein LS, Kavuru MS, Curtis-McCarthy P et al. Pulmonary alveolar proteinosis: clinical features and outcomes. *Chest* 1998; 114:1357–1362.

517 Claypool WD, Rogers RM, Matuschak GM. Update on the clinical diagnosis, management, and pathogenesis of pulmonary alveolar proteinosis (phospholipidosis). *Chest* 1984; 85:550–558.

518 Crocker HL, Pfitzner J, Doyle IR et al. Pulmonary alveolar proteinosis: two contrasting cases. *Eur Respir J* 2000; 15:426–429.

519 Hirakata Y, Kobayashi J, Sugama Y et al. Elevation of tumour markers in serum and bronchoalveolar lavage fluid in pulmonary alveolar proteinosis. *Eur Respir J* 1995; 8:689–696.

520 Nakajima M, Manabe T, Niki Y et al. Serum KL-6 level as a monitoring marker in a patient with pulmonary alveolar proteinosis. *Thorax* 1998; 53:809–811.

521 Kuroki Y, Tsutahara S, Shijubo N et al. Elevated levels of lung surfactant protein A in sera from patients with idiopathic pulmonary fibrosis and pulmonary alveolar proteinosis. *Am Rev Respir Dis* 1993; 147:723–729.

522 Honda Y, Kuroki Y, Matsuura E et al. Pulmonary surfactant protein D in sera and bronchoalveolar lavage fluids. *Am J Respir Crit Care Med* 1995; 152:1860–1866.

523 Iyonaga K, Suga M, Yamamoto T et al. Elevated bronchoalveolar concentrations of MCP-1 in patients with pulmonary alveolar proteinosis. *Eur Respir J* 1999; 14:383–389.

524 Singh G, Katyal SL, Bedrossian CW et al. Pulmonary alveolar proteinosis. Staining for surfactant apoprotein in alveo-

lar proteinosis and in conditions simulating it. *Chest* 1983; 83:82–86.

525 Stanley E, Lieschke GJ, Grail D et al. Granulocyte/macrophage colony-stimulating factor-deficient mice show no major perturbation of hematopoiesis but develop a characteristic pulmonary pathology. *Proc Natl Acad Sci USA* 1994; 91:5592–5596.

526 Dranoff G, Crawford AD, Sadelain M et al. Involvement of granulocyte–macrophage colony-stimulating factor in pulmonary homeostasis. *Science* 1994; 264:713–716.

527 Bewig B, Wang XD, Kirsten D et al. GM-CSF and GM-CSF beta c receptor in adult patients with pulmonary alveolar proteinosis. *Eur Respir J* 2000; 15:350–357.

528 Dirksen U, Nishinakamura R, Groneck P et al. Human pulmonary alveolar proteinosis associated with a defect in GM-CSF/IL-3/IL-5 receptor common beta chain expression. *J Clin Invest* 1997; 100:2211–2217.

529 Huffman JA, Hull WM, Dranoff G et al. Pulmonary epithelial cell expression of GM-CSF corrects the alveolar proteinosis in GM-CSF-deficient mice. *J Clin Invest* 1996; 97:649–655.

530 Nishinakamura R, Wiler R, Dirksen U et al. The pulmonary alveolar proteinosis in granulocyte macrophage colony-stimulating factor/interleukins 3/5 beta c receptor-deficient mice is reversed by bone marrow transplantation. *J Exp Med* 1996; 183:2657–2662.

531 Seymour JF, Dunn AR, Vincent JM et al. Efficacy of granulocyte-macrophage colony-stimulating factor in acquired alveolar proteinosis. *N Engl J Med* 1996; 335:1924–1925.

532 Tillie-Leblond I, Wallaert B, Leblond D et al. Respiratory involvement in relapsing polychondritis. Clinical, functional, endoscopic, and radiographic evaluations. *Medicine (Baltimore)* 1998; 77:168–176.

533 McAdam LP, O'Hanlan MA, Bluestone R et al. Relapsing polychondritis: prospective study of 23 patients and a review of the literature. *Medicine (Baltimore)* 1976; 55:193–215.

534 Clark LJ, Wakeel RA, Ormerod AD. Relapsing polychondritis – two cases with tracheal stenosis and inner ear involvement. *J Laryngol Otol* 1992; 106:841–844.

535 Eng J, Sabanathan S. Airway complications in relapsing polychondritis. *Ann Thorac Surg* 1991; 51:686–692.

536 Im JG, Chung JW, Han SK et al. CT manifestations of tracheobronchial involvement in relapsing polychondritis. *J Comput Assist Tomogr* 1988; 12:792–793.

537 Davis SD, Berkmen YM, King T. Peripheral bronchial involvement in relapsing polychondritis: demonstration by thin-section CT. *Am J Roentgenol* 1989; 153:953–954.

538 Sheffield E, Corrin B. Fatal bronchial stenosis due to isolated relapsing chondritis. *Histopathology* 1992; 20:442–443.

539 Lynch JP III, Quint L. Tracheobronchial and esophageal manifestations of systemic diseases. In: Cummings CW, ed, *Otoloaryngology – Head and Neck Surgery*, 3rd edn. St. Louis, MO: Mosby Year Book; 1998:2343–2367.

540 Dunne JA, Sabanathan S. Use of metallic stents in relapsing polychondritis. *Chest* 1994; 105:864–867.

541 Falk RH, Comenzo RL, Skinner M. The systemic amyloidoses. *N Engl J Med* 1997; 337:898–909.

542 Utz JP, Swensen SJ, Gertz MA. Pulmonary amyloidosis. The Mayo Clinic experience from 1980 to 1993. *Ann Intern Med* 1996; 124:407–413.

543 Thompson PJ, Citron KM. Amyloid and the lower respiratory tract. *Thorax* 1983; 38:84–87.

544 Kyle RA, Gertz MA, Greipp PR et al. A trial of three regimens for primary amyloidosis: colchicine alone, melphalan and prednisone, and melphalan, prednisone, and colchicine. *N Engl J Med* 1997; 336:1202–1207.

545 Cordier JF, Loire R, Brune J. Amyloidosis of the lower respiratory tract. Clinical and pathologic features in a series of 21 patients. *Chest* 1986; 90:827–831.

546 Hui AN, Koss MN, Hochholzer L et al. Amyloidosis presenting in the lower respiratory tract. Clinicopathologic, radiologic, immunohistochemical, and histochemical studies on 48 cases. *Arch Pathol Lab Med* 1986; 110:212–218.

547 O'Regan A, Fenlon HM, Beamis JF Jr et al. Tracheobronchial amyloidosis: the Boston University Experience from 1984 to 1999. *Medicine* 2000; 79:69–79.

548 Nienhuis DM, Prakash UB, Edell ES. Tracheobronchopathia osteochondroplastica. *Ann Otol Rhinol Laryngol* 1990; 99:689–964.

549 Skinner M, Anderson J, Simms R et al. Treatment of 100 patients with primary amyloidosis: a randomized trial of melphalan, prednisone, and colchicine versus colchicine only. *Am J Med* 1996; 100:290–298.

550 Gertz MA, Kyle RA. Phase II trial of recombinant interferon alfa-2 in the treatment of primary systemic amyloidosis. *Am J Hematol* 1993; 44:125–128.

551 Lynch JP III. Pulmonary sarcoidosis: current concepts and controversies. *Compr Ther* 1997; 23:197–210.

552 Lynch JP III, Flint A. Sorting out the pulmonary eosinophilic syndrome. *J Respir Dis* 1984; 5:61–78.

553 Neagos GR, Lynch JP III. Making sense out of bronchiolitis obliterans. *J Respir Dis* 1991; 12:801.

13

Drug treatments of the future in fibrotic lung disease

Athol U. Wells

Interstitial Lung Disease Unit, Departments of Radiology, Pathology and Physiology, Royal Brompton Hospital, Sydney Street, London, UK

Introduction

In diffuse fibrotic lung disease, open and blinded therapeutic trials have largely been confined to patients with idiopathic pulmonary fibrosis (IPF, synonymous with cryptogenic fibrosing alveolitis). The results of these studies and the anecdotal experience of chest physicians throughout the world have demonstrated that current treatments do not prevent the progression of IPF in most cases. However, in the last 5 years, there has been a major change in the overall conceptual approach to therapy. Previously, it had been argued in IPF (and other diffuse fibrotic lung diseases) that inflammation precedes and leads to fibrosis). Thus, current treatments, which are largely ineffective, are based upon the suppression of inflammation (usually by means of corticosteroid and immunosuppressive therapy). The notion of a histopathological continuum in IPF, in which inflammation and fibrosis are seen as closely inter-related, was reinforced by the use of the terms 'desquamative interstitial pneumonia' (DIP) and 'usual interstitial pneumonia' (UIP)[1,2]. This terminology, coined in the 1970s, was thought by many to denote the early inflammatory phase of disease and the later irreversible fibrotic form, respectively[3,4].

More recently, the view that inflammation infallibly leads to fibrosis has been challenged. As discussed later, it is now widely accepted that DIP and UIP are separate disorders, and that there is no evidence that DIP progresses to UIP. It is increasingly proposed that the major histopathological process leading to progression of pulmonary fibrosis is fibroblastic activity; although it is possible that chronic inflammation plays an important modulatory role, it is equally possible that inflammatory cell infiltration is an epiphenomenon, which plays only a minor role in fibrogenesis in UIP. This new view of the pathogenesis of IPF is likely to explain the lack of effectiveness of agents that suppress inflammation but have little effect on other mechanisms. The result of this radical conceptual change has been an increasing interest in a number of interventions which might have direct or indirect effects upon fibroblast activity (based upon in vitro work and animal studies).

In this chapter, the problems of evaluating new pharmacological therapies are detailed. Potentially important pathogenetic mechanisms are outlined. Individual agents are then discussed.

The problem of demonstrating benefit in a rare irreversible disease

Although not a rare disease, IPF is infrequently encountered in routine secondary respiratory practice. A mortality rate in excess of 1400 patients per year in the UK[5] indicates that IPF has a significant impact upon community and hospital resources. However, it is difficult for any single medical practitioner to accumulate worthwhile numbers of patients for entry in a definitive controlled study: until recently, no completed therapeutic trial has contained more than 50 patients. The small number of suitable patients, even when accumulated at tertiary units, requires a multicentre approach. Until recently, this has been unattainable. Multicentre studies usually require a very major input from pharmaceutical companies, who may be reluctant to invest the considerable required resources without the reasonable likelihood of a worthwhile outcome. The relative rarity of IPF, compared to asthma or chronic obstructive pulmonary disease, has been a powerful disincentive to pharmaceutical investment.

Recently, pessimism about the lack of research into new treatments of IPF has been alleviated by the realization that antifibrotic treatments might be applicable to a wide variety of pulmonary and non-pulmonary disorders. A number of multicentre studies are now under way, evaluating agents discussed later in this chapter. However, the small number of patients suitable for clinical studies remains a major constraint. The enrolment of the pool of eligible patients into large multicentre studies necessarily prevents therapeutic research into other new agents at the centres taking part. Thus, the decision whether a novel intervention is sufficiently promising to justify a major investment in time and resources is a considerable dilemma for clinicians. In theory, this problem can be overcome by the use of pilot studies in small groups of patients at single centres. In this way, a number of new agents can be evaluated at different centres, with the intention to proceed to a definitive multicentre study when pilot results are encouraging. However, the construction and interpretation of pilot studies poses a number of major problems.

First, the irreversible nature of pulmonary fibrosis is a major difficulty. Patients with evidence of significant reversible inflammatory cell infiltration at biopsy[6,7] or on high resolution computed tomography (CT)[8,9] are likely to respond to current treatments and are not usually deemed appropriate for novel interventions. Thus, for most patients taking part in clinical trials, a significant improvement is not a realistic goal. In the context of relentlessly advancing fibrosis, long-term stability can be viewed as a radical improvement in the natural course of disease; a significant slowing in the pro-gression of disease amounts to success. In small groups with progressive IPF, a period of pilot treatment with a novel agent for 3 to 6 months is unlikely to disclose a reduction in disease progression, unless the therapeutic benefit is striking. This difficulty is especially problematic in the patient populations commonly chosen for pilot intervention.

The problem of selection bias

By definition, pilot studies are speculative. IPF has had a 5-year survival of 50% or less from the onset of dyspnea throughout the last three decades[6,7,10], and many patients present late in the course of disease, long after dyspnea has developed. In smokers, dysp-noea is often wrongly ascribed to chronic obstruc-tive pulmonary disease, and in other patients a confident diagnosis of IPF proves elusive. The outlook is often poor if a final diagnosis is made only when pulmonary fibrosis is advanced. Historically, clinicians have found it necessary to initiate conven-tional agents (corticosteroid and immunosuppres-sive agents) as first-line therapy. Pilot studies of other treatments have tended to be reserved for patients with pre-terminal disease, who have been clearly seen to progress despite standard treatment. Thus, a major selection bias has resulted. The extrapolation of those with very advanced disease to a larger IPF population with less extensive disease is highly questionable. In other chronic diseases, inter-vention in the hope of changing natural history has been more successful when instituted early in disease. A good example is the use of angiotensin-converting-enzyme inhibition immediately after myocardial infarction in patients without evidence of left ventricular impairment, resulting in a striking reduction in the prevalence of heart failure a year later[11]. Thus, the finding in a pilot study performed in the 1980s that cyclosporin therapy did not have an obvious benefit in IPF in a handful of severely com-promised patients[12] does not necessarily exclude a major benefit in those with less advanced disease.

A second subgroup often considered suitable for speculative treatments consists of patients in whom the course is unusually benign, who progress insidi-ously despite traditional therapy, and are enrolled in pilot interventions before disease is disabling. The interpretation of outcomes in this context poses an entirely different problem. Disease that is inherently slowly progressive requires a lengthy period of treat-ment before an apparent therapeutic benefit becomes apparent. Moreover, a good outcome with treatment may not be applicable to patients with typical progressive IPF. A recurring difficulty with pilot studies is the possibility that the treated popu-lations may not be representative of typical IPF to two standard deviations of disease behaviour. A recently published study of gamma-interferon[13], discussed in detail later, excited a good deal of inter-est because the outcome was substantially better in treated patients than in control subjects. The results were very much better than reported in any previous therapeutic trial in IPF. However, strikingly, the mor-tality was extremely low in all patients, including those receiving placebo gamma-interferon; a sub-group requiring supplemental oxygen therapy at entry were all alive 12 months later, and serial lung function indices in patients in the placebo arm showed a surprising lack of deterioration. Thus, the patients enrolled in this study did not have the entity of relentlessly progressive IPF encountered in routine practice. The findings caused some to ques-tion whether the studied patients in that study all had IPF, or whether the population was partially composed of less aggressive diffuse lung diseases, including the recently characterized entity of non-specific interstitial pneumonia (NSIP).

The problem of diagnostic contamination

Diagnostic contamination is a major consideration in diffuse lung disease, in pilot studies and definitive clinical trials alike. The attainment of a secure diag-nosis of IPF has been complicated by the recent defi-nition of NSIP, which makes up a significant subgroup of patients in recent histological series[14–17]. The definition of NSIP resulted indirectly from the recent realization that the histological

appearances of DIP and UIP are likely to represent separate clinical entities. This, in turn, underlined the importance of reclassifying histological sub-groups and led to an international consensus on a new histological and clinical classification for the idiopathic interstitial pneumonias, of which UIP (thought traditionally to correspond to the clinical entity of IPF) and NSIP are the most prevalent vari-ants. Early studies indicate that NSIP has a signifi-cantly better prognosis than UIP, with a good outcome in the majority of cases[14–17]. However, many patients with the histological appearance of NSIP do not have the clinical entity of IPF, but more closely resemble relatively benign conditions such as cryptogenic organizing pneumonia[18,19] or sub-acute extrinsic allergic alveolitis[19], clinically and/or radiologically. It should be stressed that, when patients with a clinical and radiographical picture of IPF are evaluated, a histological diagnosis of fibrotic NSIP is more likely to be associated with progressive pulmonary fibrosis than in other clinical contexts[17]. However, even allowing for this caveat, the outcome of NSIP is clearly better than the outcome of UIP, and a significant proportion of patients with NSIP survive for 10 years or longer after presentation.

Thus, in pilot studies performed on patients with the clinical features of IPF and slowly progressive disease, NSIP is likely to be over-represented. It is not clear whether antifibrotic agents might be less (or even more) effective in NSIP than in UIP and this poses an important dilemma in the design of trials of new agents. Ideally, a histological diagnosis of NSIP or UIP should be secured before patients are entered in a therapeutic study. The performance of a lung biopsy gives the investigator greater confidence in evaluating the efficacy of intervention; in a con-trolled study, equal proportions of NSIP and UIP can be assigned to all subgroups, or entry can be restricted to UIP or NSIP alone. However, thoraco-scopic biopsies are increasingly reserved for the minority of patients with atypical clinical or CT fea-tures, and it is seldom practicable or acceptable to patients to perform biopsies solely for the purposes of a clinical study. In routine clinical practice in the UK, less than 10% of patients with IPF undergo open or thoracoscopic biopsy[20]. Thus, series composed entirely of biopsied patients are subject to a major selection bias. Patients undergoing biopsy tend to be younger and have less functional impairment.[21] The large subgroup of patients who are unfit for biopsy, either because of loss of pulmonary reserve or due to significant comorbidity, are excluded. Moreover, the recruitment rate is necessarily low if a histological diagnosis is required and the large numbers of patients required in order to complete definitive controlled studies are probably unattainable.

The problem of diagnostic contamination is lessened by the careful use of CT. There are now a large number of diagnostic studies which have shown that CT is acceptably accurate in predicting a histological diagnosis in interstitial lung disease, especially if the radiological diagnosis is confident[22–26]. Because NSIP has been defined relatively recently, the CT appearances of NSIP have yet to be definitively documented in patients with the clinical features of IPF. However, it is increasingly accepted that a coarse reticular pattern on CT, in association with a predominantly basal subpleural distribution, denotes a high likelihood of a histological diagnosis of UIP, especially if there is overt honeycombing[19]. Recent experience indicates that many patients with NSIP are characterized by prominent ground-glass attenuation on CT and finer fibrosis, without extensive honeycombing[27]. In this context, a ground-glass pattern on CT may be indicative of fine fibrosis, rather than reversible inflammatory cell infiltration. In IPF series published before the prognostic importance of NSIP had been established, prominent ground-glass attenuation on CT was associated with a good outcome, whereas the predominance of a reticular pattern was a malignant prognostic determinant[8,9]. These findings probably reflected the NSIP/UIP dichotomy, at least in part. Thus, it can be argued that in pilot studies, entry should be restricted to the majority of IPF patients with frank honeycombing on CT, to ensure that the studied population is largely composed of UIP. In larger definitive studies, there is a strong case for stratifying entry, based upon the presence or absence of significant ground-glass attenuation, and these CT features need to be taken into account in analyses of outcome.

The problem of selection of end-points

In pilot studies and in major multicentre studies alike, the selection of end-points in fibrotic lung disease remains problematic. In a disease which is often fatal within 2 years of presentation (especially if there are significant delays in making the diagnosis after the onset of dyspnea), the most robust method is analysis of survival. In a definitive study, the ideal design would be placebo controlled and double blind; patients would remain on treatment until death, without knowledge of whether the agent was active. In trials of oncological drugs, this problem can be overcome by comparing a new treatment with the best current management. However, this approach is weakened in IPF by the fact that the efficacy of present treatments in preventing progression of fibrosis has never been quantified. A double-blind placebo-controlled design, continued indefinitely, places unacceptable demands upon patients and clinicians. Patients are unlikely to accept a blinded treatment which may be inactive, once it becomes obvious that disease has progressed; for the same reasons, physicians may be reluctant to refer patients to participate in such a trial, and may insist upon open 'rescue therapy', once deterioration has been demonstrated.

Moreover, death is not always directly due to progression of lung disease in IPF; in many series, cardiac disease is a major source of mortality, and lung cancer has a greatly increased incidence in patients with established pulmonary fibrosis[28]. Cardiac problems are often disclosed by progression of IPF, and may not become apparent in patients with stable disease; thus, a new agent which is able to prevent or slow deterioration may delay death from cardiac causes. However, this will not invariably be the case; current or previous smokers in their seventh decade (the typical patient with IPF), are likely to be at greatly increased risk of myocardial infarction, irrespective of pulmonary disease. Thus, analyses of survival will be partially confounded by non-respiratory mortality; this, in turn, increases the number of patients required to demonstrate a change in survival with intervention.

These constraints are likely to account for the fact that no definitive long-term placebo controlled study has ever been performed in IPF. For the most part, pilot assessment has consisted of a period of observation, sometimes for a standardized period such as 1 year. Change in disease severity has been evaluated, often in isolation, although sometimes by comparison with untreated patients. However, even in this apparently simple framework, the selection of end-points has not been straightforward. It is widely accepted that lung function tests are a more reliable reflection of the underlying disease severity than symptoms or findings on chest radiography[29]. Despite this consensus, there is no overall agreement amongst clinicians as to which of a wide variety of lung function tests should be the cardinal measure of disease severity. In most serial analyses of patients with IPF, the forced vital capacity (FVC) and total gas transfer (Dlco) have been chosen as primary indices. It is now known that Dlco levels have a closer correlation with the extent of IPF on CT than any other lung function measure[30,31], and it can be argued that change in Dlco might be the most reliable indicator of change in underlying disease severity. However, the prevailing difficulty with interpreting lung function tests precisely is their sensitivity to other disease processes, especially smoking-related damage. Emphysema is evident on CT in over 20% of patients with IPF; the combination of emphysema and fibrosis results in a spurious preservation of lung volumes and a devastating reduction in measures of gas transfer[31,32]. Similarly, functional decline in IPF may result from infection or supervening cardiac failure, especially in individuals with significant hypoxia. Thus, the interpretation of changes in lung function indices is often difficult.

It is likely that serial CT examination will play an increasing role in refining the evaluation of new treatments. The major theoretical advantage of CT is that changes in the extent of IPF can be quantified, independent of the presence of emphysema or other confounding disorders. The difficulty with this use of CT is technical. Currently, CT sections are interspaced; data are acquired at 10 mm or 20 mm intervals, with sampling widths of 1–2 mm. Thus, at follow-up, most CT sections are not anatomically comparable: a difference of 2 or 3 mm between sections results in apparently significant changes in disease extent which are spurious. This difficulty has seriously limited the role of CT in evaluating the evolution of pulmonary fibrosis. However, the problem is likely to be solved within 2 to 3 years by the increasing application of spiral CT, which captures all the morphological data from the lung apices to the bases. It will eventually be possible to ensure strict anatomical comparability with the initial examination at follow-up CT; thus it is highly likely that serial CT will ultimately supersede other investigative modalities in the evaluation of new treatments in diffuse lung disease.

For all the reasons listed above, the evaluation of new treatments in IPF and other fibrotic lung diseases will remain problematic in the foreseeable future. Clinicians will need to overcome or interpret bias due to the selection of patients with advanced disease or intrinsically less progressive disease. The methods used to diagnose IPF, and especially to exclude NSIP, will remain a subject of scrutiny and contention. The quantification of change in disease severity with and without treatment will be a vexing difficulty in the intermediate future. The design of therapeutic trials in IPF and in other less common diffuse lung diseases will require meticulous attention to detail if the results are to be robust.

Pathogenesis

Current models of the pathogenesis of IPF are largely autoimmune. It has been widely surmised that following initial damage, an influx of acute and chronic inflammatory cells resulted in continuing immunologically mediated damage and was primarily responsible for disease progression[33–37]. Circumstantial support for an immunopathogenetic mechanism include the presence of abundant activated antigen-primed memory T-cells in the lung interstitium, in patients with pulmonary fibrosis associated with scleroderma[38], and the prominence of lymphoid germinal centres in idiopathic pulmonary fibrosis[39]. Macrophages have also been believed to play an important role, by production of tumour necrosis factor α, interleukin-1, interleukin-6, chemokines enhancing inflammatory cell traffic (interleukin-8, MCP-1, MCP-1α, MIP1β, MIP-2), and fibrogenetic factors (TGF-β, IGF-1, PDGF)[40]. Tissue damage has been ascribed to generation of oxygen radicals and proteolytic enzymes by neutrophils[41]. It has also been suggested that eosinophils and mast cells might damage the lung by releasing eosinophilic cationic products and vasoactive amines[42,43]. Thus, using lung involvement in connective tissue disease as a prototype, it has been argued that the pathogenesis of fibrotic lung disease involves amplification of lung injury and the immune response by environmental trigger factors in genetically susceptible individuals[44,45].

However, the validity of the traditional view, that in fibrotic lung diseases, irrespective of cause, inflammatory cell infiltration precedes and leads to fibrosis, is now increasingly questioned. It had been widely argued, during the last two decades, that desquamative interstitial pneumonia (DIP) was the early form of usual interstitial pneumonia, based, in part, on the presence of variably intense intra-alveolar macrophage accumulation in the latter disease[46]. However, many patients with UIP are current or former smokers and it is now accepted that DIP and the closely related airway-centred macrophage accumulation disorder, respiratory bronchiolitis with associated interstitial lung disease, represent a response to cigarette smoke[47]. Thus, the presence of intra-alveolar macrophage accumulation in UIP is not necessarily a primary pathogenetic feature.

Importantly, there is no good evidence in fibrotic lung disease in general, and in UIP in particular, that end-stage fibrosis is necessarily preceded by prominent inflammation. In cases of early UIP, the inflammatory component is generally minor and occurs in areas of collagen deposition, not involving otherwise normal lung parenchyma[48]. Moreover, in both sarcoidosis and hypersensitivity pneumonitis, many patients exhibit marked interstitial inflammation early in the course of disease, but in many cases these disorders do not evolve to severe fibrosis. In principle, if inflammation precedes and leads to fibrosis in UIP, suppression of inflammation by anti-inflammatory and immunosuppressive agents should be associated with a good outcome. However, it is now increasingly accepted that high dose corticosteroid therapy is not effective in UIP[49], even in combination with immunosuppressive treatment. Furthermore, clinical markers of inflammation bear little relationship to outcome in UIP. Lung gallium-67 uptake has a good correlation with inflammatory cell content in lung tissue but high gallium uptake does not equate with a good response to treatment[50]. Similarly, increased bronchoalveolar lavage cellularity is not a consistent guide to outcome[51]. In support of these observations, serial CT evaluation in patients with UIP has not demonstrated an evolution from areas of isolated or predominant ground-glass attenuation, denoting increased cellularity, to a fixed reticular pattern, indicating established fibrosis[52], although ground-glass attenuation admixed with fibrotic abnormalities, denoting fine fibrosis, may coarsen to a fibrotic reticular pattern in time[53,54]. Moreover, there is evidence in animal models that the inflammatory and fibrotic responses can be dissociated. Transgenic animals have been shown to exhibit inflammation without the development of pulmonary fibrosis (e.g. mice deficient in the integrin avb6 exposed to bleomycin[55], mice deficient in interleukin-10 instilled with silica)[56]. Pulmonary fibrosis has been demonstrated in a mouse model of 95% hyperoxia, despite the absence of blood components and a paucity of macrophages in lung explant tissue[57]. In this model, fibroblast growth was particularly prominent in areas exhibiting severe epithelial damage, indicating that inflammation is not an essential prerequisite for pulmonary fibrosis associated with epithelial damage.

Thus, the concept of DIP and UIP as a histological

continuum has probably seriously retarded the understanding of pathogenetic mechanisms in UIP. It remains unclear to what extent increased cellularity promotes disease progression in established fibrotic disease, given the ability of macrophages and other inflammatory cells to stimulate fibroblasts, through a wide variety of growth factors. Thus, it remains possible that proinflammatory cytokines play a major ancillary role in recruiting inflammatory cells and amplifying lung damage and fibrosis. This consideration is important because of the possibility that the new antifibrotic agents currently under evaluation may be more efficacious when given in combination with anti-inflammatory agents. However, there is no good evidence that interstitial or intra-alveolar inflammation is associated with the development of fibroblastic foci, the cardinal histological feature of early UIP.

Fibroblastic foci are made up of an interstitial aggregation of fibroblasts and myofibroblasts; on immunohistologic and electron microscopy evaluation, these appearances are compatible with microscopic foci of acute lung injury, characterized also by destruction of alveolar epithelial cells and disruption of the basement membrane. The characteristic secondary fibroblast proliferation and subsequent collagen deposition can be regarded as a failed healing process; even at this stage, cellular infiltration is not prominent. Thus, it has been elegantly argued by Selman and colleagues, in a seminal review, that UIP represents a model of abnormal wound healing, with epithelial injury as the early lesion, and inadequate re-epithelialization, associated with myofibroblast abnormalities[58]. There is an increasing body of support for the central importance of fibroblast foci and associated abnormalities in the pathogenesis of progressive fibrotic lung disease[48,59,60]. Recently, Travis and colleagues reported that on multivariate analysis, the profusion of fibroblastic foci was the sole histopathological feature linked to subsequent progression of disease in UIP[16] and this conclusion is strongly supported by analyses of biopsies of UIP patients recently undertaken by the author and colleagues. However, it is not yet clear which of several associated abnormalities – fibroblast and myofibroblast activity within fibroblast foci, epithelial injury and disruption of the basement membrane – is the most important pathogenetic feature in progressive lung fibrosis.

One possible explanation for on-going epithelial damage in UIP is fibroblast activity. Fibroblasts and myofibroblasts from patients with UIP have been shown to induce epithelial cell death in vitro[61]. More compellingly, apoptotic alveolar epithelial cells, identified by in situ end labelling and electron microscopy, appear to be concentrated adjacent to foci of myofibroblasts[62]. It is now known that angiotensinogen mediates myofibroblast apoptotic activity[63], and it has also been suggested that tumour suppressor protein up-regulation in alveolar epithelial cells may play an important contributory role[64]. Thus, fibroblastic foci may be primarily responsible for progression of fibrotic lung disease, with alveolar epithelial damage serving an ancillary role. It is highly likely that myofibroblast proliferation within fibroblastic foci results in architectural distortion[59]. Moreover, fibroblasts from patients with UIP are deficient in cyclooxygenase-2 expression and prostaglandin E2 synthesis (which has an antifibrogenic effect)[65].

However, it is equally plausible that the cardinal pathogenetic event is alveolar epithelial damage, resulting in the production of a number of profibrogenic cytokines and growth factors. Failure to heal epithelial injury appears to be a consistent feature of UIP, judging from loss of type I cells, type II cell hyperplasia and changes in the expression of adhesion molecules[66–68]. Alveolar epithelial cells from UIP patients, especially hyperplastic type 2 cells, synthesize transforming growth factor-β1[69,70], tumour necrosis factor[70,71] and platelet-derived growth factor[72]. In advanced fibrotic lung disease, the main source of transforming growth factor-β1 is alveolar epithelial cells, as opposed to macrophages in earlier disease[73], and it argued that epithelial expression of transforming growth factor-β1 is a key determinant of progressive fibrosis[58]. In addition, alveolar epithelial cells may be responsible for the local procoagulant and antifibrinolytic activity observed in UIP, by virtue of expression of tissue factor and plasminogen activator inhibitor-1 and -2.[74–76] Failure to remove extravasated blood constituents (an initial feature of tissue injury) may seriously retard healing by limiting cell movement through the extracellular matrix[58].

Based upon current knowledge, it is unrealistic to assign a primary pathogenetic role to either alveolar epithelial damage or fibroblast activity in isolation. It is likely that these and other features are synergistic and virtually certain that they interact with each other to promote progression of disease. The same reservations apply to assigning pathogenetic significance to basement membrane disruption, a prominent feature of fibrotic lung disease. Fibroblasts and myofibroblasts migrate into alveolar spaces through damaged epithelial basement membranes[60,77]. Furthermore, it is likely that basement membrane damage contributes to disruption of repair of damaged type I alveolar epithelial cells. However, little is known about the dynamics of basement membrane turnover. In UIP, myofibroblasts adjacent to denuded basement membrane have been shown to secrete gelatineses A and B, which are known to degrade type IV collagen within the basement membrane[78–81]. Thus, it has been argued that subepithelial myofibroblasts may be primarily responsible for basement membrane damage, enhancing their ability to migrate into epithelial spaces[58].

The end result of the pathogenetic mechanisms discussed above is accumulation of connective tissue matrix cells and proteins, including collagen, fibronectin, elastic fibres and proteoglycans, resulting in extensive structural disruption. Fibroblasts from patients with lung disease exhibit dysregulated type 1 collagen biosynthesis and impaired mRNA down-regulation; control mechanisms for collagen deposition are poorly understood and may become autonomous[82]. Connective tissue growth factor (up-regulated by TGF-β) is a powerful stimulant of collagen production[40,83,84]. However, failure of collagen degradation may be equally important or more so, and it appears likely that an imbalance between collagenases and tissue inhibitors of matrix metalloproteinases (TIMPs) may be important.

Collagenase-1 and –3 levels appear to be deficient in the lung interstitium in idiopathic pulmonary fibrosis, whereas TIMP expression may be increased[85]. In addition to inhibiting metalloproteinases (which participate in extracellular matrix remodelling), TIMPs act to promote mesenchymal cell proliferation and survival[86].

The difficulty in designing new treatments in IPF is the large number of possible pathogenetic mechanisms. It is hoped that a few pathways might turn out to be central in IPF, a necessary assumption if monotherapy is eventually to be successful in most patients. However, it is equally possible that the common histological appearance of UIP results from a diversity of mechanisms, or highly variable contributions from several pathways in individual patients. Thus, agents that act to inhibit a multiplicity of pathways are intrinsically attractive.

New agents theoretically of benefit in fibrotic lung disease

Pirfenidone

Pirfenidone has been shown to reduce the toxic pulmonary fibrotic effects induced by bleomycin in hamsters, preventing bleomycin-induced increases in lung hydroxyproline levels, malondialdehyde equivalent levels, prolyl hydroxylase activity and myeloperoxidase activity, both when given with a single dose of bleomycin[87], and after the second of three doses, administered at weekly intervals[88]. Pirfenidone also has a direct anti-inflammatory effect in the hamster model, suppressing the bleomycin-induced increased pulmonary vascular permeability and influx of inflammatory cells, as judged by bronchoalveolar lavage cellularity and protein levels[89]. These effects are mirrored by a protective effect by pirfenidone against bleomycin-induced reductions in pulmonary function indices in hamsters[90]. In a mouse model of cyclophosphamide-induced lung fibrosis, pirfenidone attenuated increases in total lung hydroxyproline content and reduced the incidence of lung fibrosis[91]. It has an in vitro inhibitory effect upon lung fibroblasts cultured from patients with IPF, blocking the mitogenic effect of profibrotic cytokines[92]. Pirfenidone also has an inhibitory effect upon collagen synthesis in the hamster model by several mechanisms. It down-regulates the bleomycin-induced overexpression of lung procollagen I and III genes[93] and suppresses the bleomycin-induced overexpression of the trans-forming growth factor-beta (TGF-β) gene[94]. It inhibits the bleomycin-induced synthesis of plate-let-derived growth factor (PDGF) and reduces mito-genic activity in bronchoalveolar fluid, following bleomycin exposure, suggesting that the protective effects of pirfenidone against lung fibrosis might be partially mediated by a reduction in PDGF isoforms produced by lung macrophages[95].

Pirfenidone was first evaluated clinically in IPF by Raghu and colleagues in a large non-blinded study [96]. Mortality and changes in lung function indices were evaluated in 54 patients who had deteriorated despite standard anti-inflammatory treatment or were unwilling to accept conventional therapy. No control arm was included; the authors contrasted the course of disease in treated patients with histor-ical experience of IPF. The use of pirfenidone was associated with a slower progression of disease than is generally reported. One- and two-year survival rates of 78% and 63%, respectively, were reported: the authors commented that most patients were considered to be terminally ill, based upon evidence of progression before entry and an estimated life expectancy of 18 months, judging from previous therapeutic studies in IPF. Importantly, a significant subgroup of patients exhibited stability or improve-ment in lung function indices: after one year of follow-up, improvement or stability was docu-mented in the forced vital capacity in 22 patients (41%), compared to 21 patients who had died or exhibited decline in the forced vital capacity (39%). Similar proportions were observed when changes in the total gas transfer were evaluated, although a further significant subgroup were unable to repeat pulmonary function tests due to severe dyspnea. Thus, approximately 40% could be classified as having apparent stability of disease. Furthermore,

conventional treatment was withdrawn within 2 months of starting pirfenidone in most cases (all 32 patients using immunosuppressive agents, 38 of 46 patients receiving corticosteroid therapy). Improve-ments in chest radiographic abnormalities were not observed. Pirfenidone treatment was associated with little toxicity.

Despite apparently encouraging results, this study must be viewed as inconclusive. The problems in interpreting the results are typical of those encoun-tered in therapeutic trials in IPF, discussed earlier. Selection bias was a particular difficulty. The lengthy duration of symptoms at entry was striking. The mean duration of symptoms was 4.6 years, with an upper limit of 15 years, and thus the population con-sisted of a disproportionate number of survivors, compared to the entity of IPF encountered in routine clinical practice. In one large recent study of patients with a clinical presentation of IPF, drawn from secondary centres, the average survival from the onset of dyspnoea was less than two years[97]. Thus, it must be concluded that the population studied by Raghu had unusually slowly progressive IPF; the absence of a control arm can be construed as a serious flaw. The authors observed a high prev-alence of stabilization of pulmonary function indices following deterioration immediately before entry. However, this observation is also difficult to interpret; step-wise decline is often observed in IPF and, thus, lung function decline is often followed by temporary stability, irrespective of therapeutic inter-vention. Diagnostic contamination is also an impor-tant consideration. The great majority of patients (42 of 54) had undergone surgical lung biopsy; diagno-sis in the remaining 12 patients was based upon typical clinical and CT features of IPF, and the absence of granulomatous disease on transbron-chial biopsy. However, the proportion of patients with fibrotic NSIP, rather than UIP, is uncertain: the prognostic importance of a histological diagnosis of NSIP has become increasingly evident since the study was completed.

Despite these important caveats, the outcome of the study was viewed as promising in the recent report of an NHLBI workshop[98], held to review opportunities to develop novel treatments for IPF. The important conclusion was reached that the results justified the investment of resources in a larger prospective double-blind study. Thus, the pirfenidone study of Raghu can be viewed essentially as a pilot study.

Interferon-beta

Interferon-beta has been used extensively for its anti-inflammatory effects in a number of chronic inflammatory disorders, including hepatitis C[99] and multiple sclerosis[100]. The only evidence of a pulmonary effect was disclosed in an animal study; interferon-beta protected against radiation-induced pulmonary fibrosis in mice[101]. However, interferon-beta has been shown to reduce the migration and proliferation of human skin fibroblasts[102], and to reduce collagen synthesis by palatal granulation fibroblasts, without affecting protein synthesis by normal fibroblasts[103]). Because this agent is already used clinically in non-pulmonary disorders and the side-effect profile has been largely acceptable, it was relatively straightforward to construct a large prospective clinical study, in which 167 patients with IPF were enrolled[104]. The results were presented orally at the 2001 American Thoracic Society meeting (but are not published at the date of writing); interferon-beta was not efficacious compared to placebo. However, this study is noteworthy because it establishes, for the first time, that large multicentre placebo-controlled studies of new therapies are feasible in IPF.

Interferon-gamma

In theory, interferon-gamma is a very attractive candidate as an antifibrotic agent because it has effects upon a multiplicity of mechanisms relevant to the pathogenesis of IPF. Interferon-gamma modulates macrophage and fibroblast function[105,106]. It directly suppresses the proliferation of fibroblasts in a dose-dependent manner, reduces fibroblast protein synthesis and has a number of potentially important indirect effects on fibroblast function[107,108]. It inhib-

its a fibrogenic growth factor secreted by mast cells (fibroblast growth factor-2)[109] and reduces the expression of a second fibrogenic growth factor produced by macrophages (insulin-like growth factor-1)[110]. In a mouse model of bleomycin-induced pulmonary fibrosis, exogenous interferon-gamma was found to down-regulate gene transcription for TGF-beta mRNA (known to cause pulmonary fibrosis in rats when administered by means of an adenovirus vector) and procollagen mRNA, leading to a decreased collagen content[111]. There is in vitro and in vivo evidence that in fibrosing lung disease, including IPF, interferon-gamma production is sometimes impaired[112,113], reflecting a shift from type 1 (Th1) to type 2 (Th2) immunological responses. Opposing effects on lung fibroblasts by interferon-gamma and interleukin-4 have been demonstrated with a marked increase in total collagen production and types I and III procollagen mRNA on IL-4 stimulation, but a marked reduction in collagen production on interferon-gamma stimulation[114]. Thus, IL-4 and interferon-gamma can be viewed as fibrogenic and antifibrogenic cytokines, respectively. In patients with IPF, a type 2 (Th2) pattern of cytokines predominates; although there is evidence for a type 1 response, there is a paucity of interferon-gamma[115], compared to levels in biopsy tissue in patients with fibrosing alveolitis associated with systemic sclerosis, extrinsic allergic alveolitis and sarcoidosis[116,117]. Interferon-gamma modulates the expression of a number of neutrophil-derived chemokines[118]. It has also been shown to upregulate c-Met/hepatocyte growth factor receptor expression in alveolar epithelial cells; hepatocyte growth factor is a powerful mitogen for alveolar epithelial cells and has shown antifibrotic activity[119].

Interferon-gamma was administered to patients with IPF by Ziesche and colleagues[13]. The results, recently published in the *New England Journal of Medicine*, have excited enormous interest and a great deal of controversy. The findings suggest a greater therapeutic benefit than ever previously reported in IPF with any other agent. Following encouraging preliminary findings in patients with IPF, sarcoidosis and pulmonary fibrosis associated with scleroderma, the authors constructed an open randomized trial containing 18 patients with IPF, nine in each treatment arm. All were considered to have histological findings and appearances on high resolution computed tomography compatible with IPF. The cardinal entry criterion was a deterioration of 10% in lung function indices over the preceding year, despite at least six months of continuous corticosteroid and/or immunosuppressive treatment. Severe pulmonary fibrosis was an exclusion criterion (total lung capacity less than 45%). All patients were treated initially with 50 mg of oral prednisolone daily for four weeks, tapering to the maintenance dose over the next fortnight. Nine patients were treated for 12 months with interferon-gamma (200 µg three times weekly subcutaneously), in combination with prednisolone 7.5 mg daily; the remaining nine patients received prednisolone 7.5 mg daily for 12 months. Lung function indices at entry were virtually identical in the two groups, and all 18 patients reported exertional dyspnoea.

Serial lung function trends over the year of treatment differed strikingly between the two subgroups. Patients receiving prednisolone alone exhibited a decline in lung function indices, although the deterioration was insidious and failed to reach statistical significance. By contrast, interferon-γ was associated with increased total lung capacity (an average rise of 9% of predicted and 14% of baseline values) and arterial oxygen pressure at rest in all cases, and reduced oxygen desaturation on maximal exercise in all but two instances. Exertional dyspnea resolved in eight of nine patients receiving interferon-γ but never regressed in the remaining subjects. Side effects ascribable to interferon-γ (fevers, chills, bone pain, muscle aches) resolved within 3 months in all cases.

At evaluation of tissue taken at transbronchial biopsy, performed after initial high dose steroid therapy, gene transcription of transforming growth factor-β and connective tissue growth factor were strikingly increased, compared to normal subjects, and were significantly suppressed after 6 months of interferon-γ treatment, but not in patients receiving prednisolone alone. Gene transcription for interferon-γ was not detected in any instance.

On the face of it, these results must be viewed as extremely encouraging. An improvement in lung function indices with treatment in all cases is unprecedented in IPF and the bronchoscopic findings provide a logical explanation for the outcome, which is wholly compatible with previous in vitro and in vivo work. It has even been argued that this study justifies the immediate use of interferon-γ in clinical practice[120]. However, most clinicians have significant and, in some cases, major reservations. The number of patients treated is not, in itself, a major statistical problem, with the application of appropriate analyses. The greater difficulty, which clearly applies in this instance, is that very small groups are often unrepresentative of the larger unselected population with the disease in question. The population had unusually slowly progressive disease. Patients were followed for at least 1 year before entry (median follow-up not stated) and did not have end-stage disease. The course of disease was unusually benign in the control group; extraordinarily, two oxygen-dependent patients who did not receive interferon-γ were alive 2 years later, and a striking deterioration was never observed. Thus, the studied population, including the control subjects, exhibited a treated course which was not at all typical of IPF in general, even to within one standard deviation of disease behaviour. It has been suggested that fibrotic NSIP might have been greatly over-represented, but this concern was allayed by a recent review of the histological appearances; after exclusion of several patients with NSIP, the results remained statistically significant (personal communication, TE King Jr).

Thus, the possibility that any therapeutic benefit with interferon-gamma applies solely to a small subgroup of IPF patients with very slowly progressive disease cannot be excluded. Equally, it may transpire that patients with total non-expression of interferon-γ are a special case and were grossly over-represented in the therapeutic trial, by chance, or by association with a relatively benign course. It is to be hoped that these hypotheses will be explored further in carefully selected subgroups if a major multicentre study currently in progress turns out to be disappointing. A rise in lung function indices in a group with reticular disease on CT (denoting morphological abnormalities previously considered irreversible) raises the intriguing possibility of partial regression of pulmonary fibrosis, which, in itself, is unprecedented in IPF. None the less, the interferon-gamma trial should be viewed solely as pilot work, which may or may not be ground-breaking, and justifies a definitive study. Routine interferon-gamma therapy in IPF is not yet warranted but remains a treatment of the future.

Eicosanoids

There is increasing evidence that the antifibrotic and anti-inflammatory prostaglandin PGE2, which can be administered orally as a PGE2 analogue, merits therapeutic evaluation. In a mouse model of bleomycin-induced lung fibrosis, lung fibroblastic production of PGE2 was significantly reduced in bleomycin-treated animals[121]. Compared to control tissue, lung fibroblasts isolated from patients with IPF exhibit a marked reduction in PGE2 synthesis, ascribable to diminished basal and stimulated cyclooxygenase-2 protein activity[122]. In GM-CSF deficient mice, bleomycin treatment has resulted in enhanced fibrogenesis in association with reduced levels of PGE2, compared to findings in wild-type mice[123]. Exogenous GM-CSF reversed the PGE2 synthesis defect but administration of indomethacin (a prostaglandin synthesis inhibitor) after bleomycin worsened the severity of pulmonary fibrosis; thus, it is likely that impaired production of PGE2 enhances bleomycin-induced fibrosis[123]. Normal human lung fibroblasts down-regulate the production of tumour necrosis factor (TNF)-alpha. By contrast, fibroblasts from fibrotic lung tissue exhibit reduced down-regulation of TNF-alpha in association with reduced PGE2 production; moreover, PGE2 induction by TNF-alpha is reduced (with reduced expression of cyclooxygenase-2)[124]. Thus, impaired production of PGE2 by fibrotic cells may allow a markedly increased release of TNF-alpha from activated monocytes.

An alternative approach is inhibition of leukotriene production, which is immediately attractive because of the current availability of leukotriene blocking agents. Leukotrienes are, for the most part, pro-inflammatory, but also have a wide variety of other biological actions, including powerful stimulatory effects upon collagen synthesis and the facilitation of fibroblast chemotaxis and proliferation. There is circumstantial evidence to indicate a potential pathogenic role in IPF. Human leukotriene B4 (LTB4), a very potent neutrophil chemotactic factor, is consistently increased in bronchoalveolar lavage fluid and homogenates of lung tissue in patients with IPF[125,126]. LTB4 secretion by macrophages is higher in patients with IPF than in control subjects, and the frequency of a pattern of constitutive 5-lipoxygenase activation is increased in IPF lung tissue[125]. LTB4 may also play an important role in eosinophil recruitment into the lungs in bleomycin-induced pulmonary fibrosis; eosinophil chemotactic activity of human fibroblasts cultured in the presence of bleomycin was significantly reduced by an LTB4 receptor antagonist[127]. Similarly, an LTB_4 receptor antagonist inhibits both neutrophil and monocyte chemotactic activity release (in response to smoke extract) from human fetal lung fibroblasts[128]. Leukotriene C4 (LTC4) inhibition may also be fruitful in IPF. LTC4 is increased in bronchoalveolar lavage fluid of patients with IPF[125]; it has been shown to enhance collagenase m-RNA expression in normal and IPF-derived lung fibroblasts and may, thus, play a role in extracellular matrix remodelling[129].

Relaxin

This protein was shown to have a dose-dependent inhibitory effect on TGF-beta-mediated over-expression of interstitial collagen types I and III by human lung fibroblasts, but had no effect on basal collagen production, in the absence of TGF-beta stimulation[130]. Relaxin also reduced fibronectin production by human lung fibroblasts (by inhibiting TGF-beta), as well as increasing matrix metalloproteinase I (procollagenase) expression and suppressing the production of a metalloproteinase tissue inhibitor. In a bleomycin-induced murine model, relaxin inhibited bleomycin-induced alveolar wall thickening and prevented collagen accumulation[130].

Relaxin also has a powerful in vivo protective effect in animal studies, reducing pulmonary fibrosis induced by implanted polyvinyl sponges and by bleomycin[131].

Angiotensin-converting enzyme inhibitors and angiotensin II receptor antagonists

There is good evidence in animal studies that angiotensin-converting enzyme (ACE) inhibitors exert protective effects against radiation-induced pulmonary fibrosis. In a rat model, the ACE inhibitor CL 242817 was observed to attenuate increases in lung hydroxyproline content following irradiation [132]; in a subsequent study, this effect was reproducible and captopril was found to be equally protective[133]. In both studies, ACE inhibitors were also protective against radiation-induced pulmonary endothelial damage, as judged by lung ACE activity, plasminogen activator activity, and prostacyclin and thromboxane production. Recently, these protective effects were re-examined in rats using a single dose of irradiation and, in a separate experiment, using a model of irradiation for total bone marrow transplant[134]. Captopril, enalapril, two other ACE inhibitors (CL 24817, CGS 13945) and an angiotensin II type I receptor blocker, L-158,809, were evaluated. All agents were effective in preventing radiation-induced pneumonitis and subsequent lung fibrosis in both radiation models.

Captopril has been shown to produce a dose-dependent reduction in human lung fibroblast proliferation, both under basal conditions and, more strikingly, with fibroblast growth factor stimulation[135]. The cytostatic effect of captopril, a free-thiol compound, was partially reproduced by penicillamine, also a thiol compound, but not by lisinopril, a non-thiol ACE inhibitor; thus, this effect of captopril could be ascribed to a non-specific sulfhydryl effect, rather than to ACE inhibition. Recently, attention has focused upon inhibition of apoptosis as a possible mechanism of the anti-fibrotic effect of captopril. Lung epithelial cell apoptosis is likely to be involved in the pathogenesis of lung fibrosis.

Fibroblasts cultured from patients with IPF secrete soluble inducers of alveolar epithelial cell apoptosis[61], which have been identified (by Western blotting and by abrogation of apoptosis by an angiotensin II antagonist, saralasin, and by anti-angiotensin II antibodies) as angiotensin peptides[136]. Captopril has been shown to exert a concentration-dependent inhibition of apoptosis of human lung epithelial cells (induced by monoclonal antibodies that activate the Fas receptor)[137]; angiotensin converting enzyme is directly involved in apoptosis of alveolar epithelial cells[138]. In a rat model of bleomycin-induced epithelial apoptosis and lung fibrosis, rats receiving captopril or a capsase inhibitor exhibited a marked reduction in collagen accumulation and epithelial apoptosis detected by in situ end labelling[139]. Thus, there is ample preliminary evidence to justify therapeutic studies of ACE inhibitors in fibrotic lung disease. Because captopril and other related compounds are widely used in clinical practice, these agents should be relatively easy to evaluate in IPF; at the time of writing, a multicentre study is in the process of formulation.

Other fibroblast apoptotic agents

Lovastatin has been proposed as a potential therapy for patients with fibroproliferative disorders[140]. This agent is widely prescribed to lower serum cholesterol levels, acting by depleting cells of the cholesterol precursor, mevalonic acid (by inhibiting 3-hydroxy 3-methylglutaryl-coenzyme A reductase)[141]. Mevalonic acid is also a precursor for lipid moieties that are attached to isoprenylated proteins (which play an essential role in normal cell homeostasis)[142]. Lovastatin inhibits a number of molecules responsible for cellular viability and proliferation, including Ras. The active form of Ras, Ras-GTP, stimulates phosphoinositide-3 kinase, which is essential for cell survival (preventing oncoprotein-induced fibroblast apoptosis)[143], and mitogen-activated protein kinase, which is implicated in cell proliferation[144]. Lovastatin has induced apoptosis in malignant and transformed cell lines at clinically achievable concentrations[145,146]. Tan and colleagues found that lovastatin had a dose- and time-dependent apoptotic effect on normal and fibrotic lung fibroblasts[140]. Fibroblast apoptosis was associated with lower levels of mature Ras, and was blocked by exogenous mevalonic acid. In addition, in a guinea-pig model, lovastatin reduced wound granulation tissue formation, without inducing fibroblast apoptosis, ascribed by the authors to disruption of multiple cellular functions. Possible mechanisms, based upon observations in earlier studies, include inhibition of the growth factor signalling cascade[147,148], interruption of cell cycle progression[141,149], and inhibition of cell migration and adhesion[150,151]. Thus, lovastatin has the potential to inhibit multiple pathways in fibroproliferative disorders, in addition to the induction of apoptosis, which adds to its attractiveness as a potential antifibrotic agent.

Pulmonary surfactant protein A (SP-A) and surfactant lipids are known to modulate lymphocyte proliferation[152], inflammatory cytokine production, including tumour necrosis factor-alpha and interleukins[153], and the expression of cell surface markers on macrophages[154]; in general, SP-A has a stimulatory effect, whereas surfactant lipids are inhibitory. In addition, both synthetic and natural surfactant downregulate DNA synthesis and inhibit the release of IL-6 and prostaglandin E2 in normal human lung fibroblasts[155]. The effects of SP-A and Survanta (an exogenous surfactant replacement preparation) on human lung fibroblasts, harvested from patients undergoing resection of lung tumours, have recently been evaluated[156]. Survanta was found to cause fibroblast apoptosis, as well as inducing collagenase-1 expression and decreasing type I collagen synthesis; the use of a combination of Survanta and SP-A was associated with partial reversal of the effects of Survanta. The authors suggest that surfactant lipids may contribute to programmed fibroblast death, now considered to be largely responsible for the removal of intra-alveolar lung fibroblasts following acute lung injury[157]. In IPF, marked reductions in bronchoalveolar lavage phospholipid and phosphatidylglycerol have been observed, correlating with the severity of lung fibrosis[158] and probably ascribable to the presence of fibrinogen in alveolar fluid[159]. Thus, it can be argued that surfactant may have an important antifibrotic effect in vivo, which is attenuated in fibrotic lung disease, and that exogenous surfactant adminstration merits evaluation in patients with IPF[156].

Suramin

This sulfonated naphthylurea has been used to treat prostate cancer and onchocerciasis, as well as having antiretroviral activity in vitro. The potential of suramin as an antifibrotic agent was highlighted at a NHLBI workshop devoted to past, present and future pharmacological therapy for IPF[98]. Although there are no in vivo data showing that suramin has a modulatory effect in pulmonary fibrosis, there is one important argument in its favour: it binds a very wide variety of growth factors, to the extent that it delays wound healing. It is probably over-simplistic to imagine that any single growth factor consistently predominates in mediating collagen deposition and fibroblast proliferation; thus, it appears intuitively unlikely that an inhibitory agent specific to one growth factor will prove clinically beneficial. Suramin antagonizes a wide variety of growth factors in vitro, including TGF-β, insulin-like growth factor-1, PDGF, epidermal-like growth factor and fibroblast growth factor-2. However, it has recently been observed that suramin has no protective effect on bleomycin-induced lung injury in a mouse model and does not inhibit the TGF-beta-mediated increase of alpha-1 collagen mRNA in human lung fibroblasts[160].

Keratinocyte growth factor

Keratinocyte growth factor (KGF) has been advanced as a potential agent in IPF because it is potent in stimulating epithelial cells, inducing type 2 cell proliferation in vitro and in vivo, without acting on mesenchymal cells or fibroblasts[161,162]; the KGF receptor appears only on epithelial surfaces. Additional effects that are beneficial in modulating lung injury include pleiotrophic cytoprotection in pulmonary epithelial cells, increased sodium/potassium ATPase, and heightened surfactant protein gene expression[163,164]. In animals pretreated with KGF, there is a striking and reproducible protective effect from lung injury and subsequent fibrosis, induced by bleomycin, radiation, acid installation, oxygen toxicity and α-naphthylthiourea[165–172].

In all these scenarios, it is necessary to administer KGF before the induction of lung injury. KGF administered after intrabronchial acid installation in rats did not prevent lung damage; moreover, although KGF administered 72 hours before acid installation was protective, KGF administered 24 or 48 hours beforehand was not[167]. KGF pre-treatment was equally effective in preventing bleomycin-induced lung injury in rats when given 48 or 72 hours before bleomycin, but KGF given after bleomycin did not ameliorate pulmonary fibrosis[166]. Strikingly, pre-treatment with KGF remained effective in preventing lung damage in rats challenged with a lethal combination of bleomycin and bilateral thoracic irradiation[170]. It is entirely uncertain whether KGF would be similarly effective in preventing further progression of IPF, given the established and often severe nature of lung damage in that disorder. However, further exploration appears warranted. Disruption of epithelial permeability (as indicated by increased clearance of inhaled technetium-labelled diethylene triamine pentacetate) appears to be associated with more aggressive pulmonary fibrosis[173]. It has been argued that type II cell hyperplasia helps to reduce fibroblast migration, proliferation and matrix production[98], and thus a beneficial effect of KGF in IPF cannot be excluded. However, the argument for KGF as a therapeutic agent is not entirely straightforward. Type II epithelial cells may produce fibrogenic cytokines and growth factors; thus, it is theoretically possible that KGF might have a deleterious fibro-proliferative effect, which might outweigh its advantages[98].

Antioxidants (*N*-acetylcysteine)

It has been argued that an imbalance between oxidants and anti-oxidants is likely to play an important role in the pathogenesis of IPF. Excessive oxidative stress in the lower respiratory tract, a characteristic feature of IPF, may contribute to lung injury, and initial fibroblast activation. It has long been known that macrophages spontaneously release exaggerated amounts of hydrogen peroxide in patients with IPF, which acts with increased myeloperoxidase levels to cause increased epithelial cell injury[174]. Oxidant activity may also play an important role in progression of established disease. Glutathione (the major antioxidant in human lung tissue) is abundantly present in alveolar epithelial lining fluid of normal controls[175] but is markedly diminished in concentration in bronchoalveolar lavage fluid in IPF, suggesting that there is an alveolar oxidant–antioxidant imbalance[176,177], which is also reflected as systemic oxidative stress[177]. In part, this may reflect increased oxidative activity by bronchoalveolar lavage inflammatory cells in IPF, resulting in decreases in extracellular glutathione and corresponding increases in the metabolite, glutathione disulphide[178]. It has also been suggested that IPF patients have an impaired glutathione metabolism, based upon increased amounts of oxidized glutathione in the blood, indicating the possibility of impairment of the glutathione redox cycle[179]. Thus, there is compelling evidence of oxidative stress in IPF from bronchoalveolar cell, extracellular fluid and plasma data. In support of the pathogenetic significance of these findings, there is an inverse correlation between oxidative products and pulmonary function indices in IPF, as well as a positive correlation between oxidative products and bronchoalveolar lavage fluid cellularity[180].

As well as damaging lung tissue by direct action, intracellular oxidants may act indirectly to promote fibrosis by upregulating cytokine production. Depletion of glutathione within alveolar macrophages is associated with significantly increased production of tumour necrosis factor-alpha and interleukin-8; by contrast, glutathione reduces levels of tumour necrosis factor-alpha, interleukin-6 and interleukin-8, independently of glutathione metabolism[181]. The marked increase in fibroblast proliferation induced in vitro by exposure to bronchoalveolar lavage fluid from IPF patients is directly suppressed by extracellular glutathione[182]. *N*-acetylcysteine attenuates TGF-beta-1-induced IL6-gene expression and protein synthesis in human lung fibroblasts[183].

Thus, there is circumstantial support for the hypothesis that an increased oxidant load and/or decreased antioxidant defences are likely to act synergistically with proteases to promote injury and fibrogenesis. It appears logical to augment lung antioxidant levels with glutathione or the oxidant scavengers, *N*-acetylcysteine and ambroxol[184,185]. The administration of aerosolized glutathione to IPF patients has been shown to increase epithelial lining fluid glutathione concentrations, and to reduce spontaneous superoxide anion release by alveolar macrophages[186]. Attenuation of bleomycin lung by inhaled *N*-acetylcysteine has been demonstrated in a mouse model[187]. Meyer and coworkers demonstrated that oral *N*-acetylcysteine, administered for five days to 17 patients with IPF, increased glutathione levels in bronchoalveolar lavage fluid[188]. The same group found that intravenous *N*-acetylcysteine had a similar effect in IPF patients (but not controls) in increasing total glutathione concentrations in bronchoalveolar lavage and epithelial lining fluid[189]. Behr and colleagues treated 18 patients with IPF with oral *N*-acetylcysteine (600 mg three times daily) for 12 weeks[190]. An anti-oxidant effect was observed, with increased glutathione levels in bronchoalveolar lavage and epithelial lining fluid, and decreased methionine sulfoxide content of bronchoalveolar lavage proteins (an indicator of alveolar oxidative stress). There was minor but statistically significant increases in pulmonary function indices, although the clinical relevance of this finding is uncertain, due to the short duration of treatment.

Despite their implication in the amplification of lung injury, it has yet to be established that oxidants have a central role in the pathogenesis of IPF. It is highly unlikely that this question will be resolved, except by means of a definitive clinical trial of antioxidant therapy. A large multicentre European study (the 'Ifigenia' study) of the efficacy of *N*-acetylcysteine in IPF, now under way, may provide conclusive information in the near future.

Endothelin receptor antagonists

The biologically active endothelins are 21-amino-acid peptides, which are expressed in a variety of pulmonary pathological conditions, including pulmonary vascular disease, asthma and pulmonary fibrosis[191]. Most attention has focused on endothelin-1 (ET-1), which is produced by endothelial cells[192], epithelial cells[193], alveolar macrophages[194], polymorphonuclear leukocytes[195] and fibroblasts[196]. Although initially identified as a smooth-muscle spasmogen, ET-1 is now recognized as a pro-inflammatory cytokine, with the ability to stimulate elastase release from neutrophils[197] and interleukin-1β, -6, -8, tumour necrosis factor-alpha and transforming growth factor-beta from monocytes[198]. ET-1 also induces fibronectin production and release from human bronchial epithelial cells (thus contributing to extracellular matrix turnover)[199], as well as stimulating fibroblast proliferation and chemotaxis[200] and procollagen production[201].

There is accumulating evidence that ET-1 may contribute to pulmonary fibrogenesis, stimulating recent interest in the therapeutic potential of endothelin receptor antagonists. The expression of endothelin-1 is increased in endothelial cells, macrophages and epithelial cells (especially type II pneumocytes) of patients with IPF[202,203], and in epithelial cells and macrophages in the rat model of bleomycin lung[204,205], with ET1 localized in fibrotic lesions[204]. Endothelin receptor antagonists have been observed in vitro to inhibit the endothelin-1 stimulation of human lung fibroblast proliferation[206] and collagen synthesis[201]. In rat models the endothelin receptor antagonist, Bosentan, reduced extracellular matrix production in bleomycin-induced pulmonary fibrosis[205] and in hepatic fibrosis following the induction of liver injury[207]. However, conflicting findings were reported by Mutsaers and colleagues, who observed no attenuation of collagen deposition with the adminstration of selective and non-selective endothelin receptor antagonists in the rat model of bleomycin lung[208]. Thus, further preliminary studies are desirable before endothelin receptor antagonists are evaluated in a therapeutic study.

Interleukin-10

Recombinant human interleukin-10 (IL-10) is currently under evaluation in a number of chronic inflammatory diseases including rheumatoid arthritis[209], Crohn's disease[210], and psoriasis[211]. It has been proposed that IL-10 may eventually play a therapeutic role in chronic inflammation by virtue of inhibiting a wide variety of inflammatory cells and cytokines[212–214]. However, as discussed earlier, the long-term outcome with the use of anti-inflammatory and immunosuppressive agents in IPF is disappointing, suggesting that the antifibrotic effects of IL-10 may be more important therapeutically. IL-10 is known to down-regulate type 1 collagen gene expression, and to enhance collagenase and stromelysin gene expression in human skin fibroblasts[215]. Similarly, IL-10 mRNA expression is positively associated with collagenase expression and negatively associated with collagen-1 expression in activated hepatic stellate cells[216].

To date, there have been few studies evaluating the role of IL-10 in modulating the evolution of fibrotic lung disease. Interleukin-10 levels are reduced in concentration in the bronchoalveolar lavage fluid of patients with IPF, compared to normal controls, despite significantly increased expression of the IL-10 gene by alveolar macrophages[217]. Attenuation of bleomycin-induced lung injury in mice was observed with the introduction of the IL-10 gene before bleomycin administration[218]. By contrast, the transfection of normal human lung fibroblasts with human IL-10 DNA was not associated with significant changes in fibroblast proliferation, or fibronectin or type I procollagen production[219]. However, despite the paucity of experimental lung work and the difficulties in extrapolating these findings to therapy, a multicentre multinational double-blind placebo-controlled study in IPF, is currently under discussion. IL-10 has the advantage, not shared by some other potential antifibrotic agents, that it has been widely evaluated in human therapeutic studies and is known to have an acceptable side effect profile.

REFERENCES

1 Liebow AA. Definition and classification of interstitial pneumonias in human pathology. *Prog Respir Res* 1975; 8:1–23.

2 Liebow AA, Steer A, Billingsley JG. Desquamative interstitial pneumonitis. *Am J Med* 1965; 39:369–404.

3 Parchefsky AS, Israel HL, Hoch WS, Gordon G. Desquamative interstitial pneumonia: relationship to interstitial fibrosis. *Thorax* 1973; 28:680–693.

4 Tubbs RR, Benjamin SP, Reich NE, McCormack LJ, van Ordstrand HS. Desquamative interstitial pneumonitis: cellular phase of fibrosing alveolitis. *Chest* 1977; 72:159–165.

5 Johnston I, Britton J, Kinnear W, Logan R. Rising mortality from cryptogenic fribrosing alveolitis. *Br Med J* 1990; 301:1017–1021.

6 Carrington CB, Gaensler EA, Coutu RE, Fitzgerald MX, Gupta RG. Natural history and treated course of usual and desquamative interstitial pneumonia. *N Engl J Med* 1978; 298:801–809.

7 Turner-Warwick M, Burrows B, Johnson A. Cryptogenic fibrosing alveolitis: clinical features and their influence on survival. *Thorax* 1980; 35:171–180.

8 Wells AU, Hansell DM, Rubens MB, Cullinan P, Black CM, du Bois RM. The predictive value of thin-section computed tomography in fibrosing alveolitis. *Am Fev Respir Dis* 1993; 148:1076–1082.

9 Gay SE, Kazerooni EA, Toews GB. Idiopathic pulmonary fibrosis: predicting response to therapy and survival. *Am J Respir Crit Care Med* ????; 157:1063–1072.

10 Schwartz DA, Helmers RA, Galvin JR et al. Determinants of survival in idiopathic pulmonary fibrosis. *Am Rev Respir Dis* 1994; 149:450–454.

11 Sharpe N, Smith H, Murphy J, Greaves S, Hart H, Gamble G. Early prevention of left-ventricular dysfunction after myocardial infarction with angiotensin-converting-enzyme inhibition. *Lancet* 1991; 337:872–876.

12 Alton EW, Johnson M, Turner-Warwick M. Advanced cryptogenic fibrosing alveolitis: preliminary report on treatment with cyclosporin A. *Respir Med* 1989; 83:277–279.

13 Ziesche R, Hofbauer E, Wittmann K, Petkov V, Block LH. A preliminary study of long-term treatment with interferon gamma-1β and low-dose prednisolone in patients with idiopathic pulmonary fibrosis. *N Engl J Med* 1999; 341:1264–1269.

14 Bjoraker JA, Ryu JH, Edwin MK et al. Prognostic significance of histopathological subsets in idiopathic pulmonary fibrosis. *Am J Respir Crit Care Med* 1998; 157:199–203.

15 Daniil ZD, Gilchrist FC, Nicholson AG et al. A histologic pattern of nonspecific interstitial pneumonia is associated with a better prognosis than usual interstitial pneumonia in patients with cryptogenic fibrosing alveolitis. *Am J Respir Crit Care Med* 1999; 160:899–905.

16 Travis WD, Matsui K, Moss J, Ferrans VJ. Idiopathic non-specific interstitial pneumonia: prognostic significance of cellular and fibrosing patterns – survival comparison with usual interstitial pneumonia and desquamative interstitial pneumonia. *Am J Surg Pathol* 2000; 24:19–33.

17 Nicholson AG, Colby TV, du Bois RM, Hansell DM, Wells AU. The prognostic significance of the histologic pattern of interstitial pneumonia in patients presenting with the clinical entity of cryptogenic fibrosing alveolitis. *Am J Respir Crit Care Med* 2000; 162:2213–2217.

18 Nagai S, Kitaichi M, Itoh H et al. Idiopathic nonspecific interstitial pneumonia/fibrosis: comparison with idiopathic pulmonary fibrosis and BOOP. *Eur Respir J* 1998; 12:1010–1019.

19 Hartman TE, Swensen SJ, Hansell D et al. Nonspecific interstitial pneumonia: variable appearances at high resolution chest CT. *Radiology* 2000; 217:701–705.

20 Johnston IDA, Gomm SA, Kalra S, Woodcock AA, Evans CC, Hind CRC. The management of cryptogenic fibrosing alveolitis in three regions of the United Kingdom. *Eur Respir J* 1993; 6:891–903.

21 Wells AU, Cullinan P, Hansell DM et al. Fibrosing alveolitis associated with scleroderma has a better prognosis than lone cryptogenic fibrosing alveolitis. *Am J Respir Crit Care Med* 1994; 149:1583–1590.

22 Mathieson JR, Mayo JR, Staples CA, Muller NL. Chronic diffuse infiltrative lung disease: comparison of diagnostic accuracy of CT and chest radiography. *Radiology* 1989;171:111–116.

23 Padley SPG, Hansell DM, Flower CDR, Jennings P. Comparative accuracy of high resolution computed tomography and chest radiography in the diagnosis of chronic diffuse infiltrative lung disease. *Clin Radiol* 1991;44:222-226.

24 Grenier P, Valeyre D, Cluzel P, Brauner MW, Lenoir S, Chastang C. Chronic diffuse infiltrative lung disease: diagnostic value of chest radiography and high-resolution CT. *Radiology* 1991;178:123–132.

25 Grenier P, Chevret S, Beigelman C, Brauner MW, Chastang C, Valeyre D. Chronic diffuse infiltrative lung disease: determination of the diagnostic value of clinical data, chest radiography, and CT and bayesian analysis. *Radiology* 1994; 191:383–390.

26 Raghu G, Mageto YN, Lockhart D, Schmidt RA, Wood DE, Godwin JD. The accuracy of the clinical diagnosis of new-onset idiopathic pulmonary fibrosis and other interstitial lung disease. *Chest* 1999;116:1168–1174.

27 McDonald SLS, Rubens MB, Hansell DM et al. Nonspecific interstitial pneumonia and usual interstitial pneumonia: comparative appearances and diagnostic accuracy of high-resolution computed tomography. *Radiology* 2001; in press.

28 Turner-Warwick M, Lebowicz M, Burrows B, Johnson A. Cryptogenic fibrosing alveolitis and lung cancer. *Thorax* 1980; 35:496–499.

29 Keogh BA, Crystal RG. Pulmonary function testing in interstitial lung disease. What does it tell us? *Chest* 1980; 78:856–864.

30 Staples CA, Muller NL, Vedal S, Abboud R, Ostrow D, Miller RR. Usual interstitial pneumonia: correlation of CT with clinical, functional and radiologic findings. *Radiology* 1987; 162:377–381.

31 Wells AU, King AD, Rubens MB, Cramer D, du Bois RM, Hansell DM. Lone cryptogenic fibrosing alveolitis: a functional-morphologic study based on extent of disease on thin-section computed tomography. *Am J Respir Crit Care Med* 1997; 155:1367–1375.

32 Wiggins J, Strickland B, Turner-Warwick M. Combined cryptogenic fibrosing alveolitis and emphysema: the value of high resolution computed tomography in assessment. *Respir Med* 1990; 84:365–369.

33 Agostini C, Siverio M, Semenzato G. Immune effector cells in idiopathic pulmonary fibrosis. *Curr Opin Pulm Med* 1997; 3:348–355.

34 Keane MP, Standiford TJ, Strieter RM. Chemokines are important cytokines in the pathogenesis of interstitial lung disease. *Eur Respir J* 1997; 10:339–355.

35 Keane MP, Arenberg DA, Lynch JP et al. The CXC chemokines, IL-8 and IP-10, regulate angiogenic activity in idiopathic pulmonary fibrosis. *J Immunol* 1997; 159:1437–1443.

36 Kunkel SL, Lukacs NW, Strieter RM, Chensue SW. The role of chemokines in the immunopathology of pulmonary disease. *Forum (Genova)* 1999; 9:339–355.

37 Paine R III, Ward PA. Cell adhesion molecules and pulmonary fibrosis. *Am J Med* 1999; 107:268–279.

38 Wells AU, Lorimer S, Majumdar S et al. Fibrosing alveolitis in scleroderma: increase in memory T-cells in lung interstitium. *Eur Respir J* 1995; 8:266–271.

39 Campbell DA, Poulter LW, Janossy G, du Bois RM. Immunohistochemical analysis of lung tissue from patients with cryptogenic fibrosing alveolitis suggesting local expression of immune hypersensitivity. *Thorax* 1985; 40:405–411.

40 Gauldie J, Jordana M, Cox G. Cytokines and pulmonary fibrosis. *Thorax* 1993; 48:931–935.

41 Rahman I, Skwarska E, Henry M et al. Systemic and pulmonary oxidative stress in idiopathic pulmonary fibrosis. *Free Radic Biol Med* 1999; 27:60–68.

42 Allen JN, Davis WB. Eosinophilic lung diseases. *Am J Respir Crit Care Med* 1994; 150:1423–1438.

43 Davis WB, Sun XH, Gadek JE, Jaurand MC, Bignon J, Crystal RG. Cytotoxicity of eosinophils for lung parenchymal cells. *Am Rev Respir Dis* 1982; 125:178A.

44 Yurovsky VV, Wigley FM, Wise RA, White B. Skewing of the CD8 + T-cell repertoire in the lungs of patients with systemic sclerosis. *Hum Immunol* 1996; 48:84–97.

45 Yurovsky VV, White B. T cell repertoire in systemic sclerosis. *Int Rev Immunol* 1995; 12:97–105

46 Keogh BA, Crystal RG. Alevolitis: the key to the interstitial lung disorders [editorial]. *Thorax* 1982; 37:1–10.

47 Heyneman LE, Ward S, Lynch DA, Remy-Jardin M, Johkoh T, Muller NL. Respiratory bronchiolitis, respiratory bronchiolitis-associated interstitial lung disease, and desquamative interstitial pneumonia: different entities or part of the same disease process? *Am J Roentgenol* 1999; 173:1617–1622.

48 Katzenstein AL, Myers JL. Idiopathic pulmonary fibrosis. Clinical relevance of pathologic classification. *Am J Respir Crit Care Med* 1998; 157:1301–1315.

49 Collard HR, King TE. Treatment of idiopathic pulmonary fibrosis: the rise and fall of corticosteroids. *Am J Med* 2001; 110:326–328.

50 Panos RJ, Mortensen RL, Niccoli SA, King TE. Clinical deterioration in patients with idiopathic pulmonary fibrosis: causes and assessment. *Am J Med* 1990; 88:396–404.

51 Howard P. Clinical usefulness of bronchoalveolar lavage. *Eur Respir J* 1990; 3:377–378.

52 Wells AU, Rubens MB, du Bois RM, Hansell DM. Serial CT in fibrosing alveolitis: prognostic significance of the initial pattern. *Am J Radiol* 1993; 161:1159–1165.

53 Akira M, Sakatani M, Ueda E. Idiopathic pulmonary fibrosis: progression of honeycombing at thin section CT. *Radiology,* 189:687–691.

54 Terriff BA, Kwan SY, Chan-Yeung MM, Muller NL. Fibrosing alveolitis: chest radiology and CT as predictors of clinical and functional impairment at follow-up in 26 patients. *Radiology* 1992; 184:445–449.

55 Munger JS, Huang X, Kawakatsu H et al. The integrin avB6 binds and activates latent TGF β1: a mechanism for regulating pulmonary inflammation and fibrosis. *Cell* 1999; 96:319–328.

56 Huaux F, Louahed J, Hudspith B et al. Role of interleukin-10 in the lung response to silica in mice. *Am J Respir Cell Mol Biol* 1998; 18:51–59.

57 Adamson IY, Young L, Bowden DH. Relationship of alveolar epithelial injury and repair to the induction of pulmonary fibrosis. *Am J Pathol* 1988; 130:377–383.

58 Selman M, King TE, Pardo A. Idiopathic pulmonary fibrosis: prevailing and evolving hypotheses about its pathogenesis and implications for therapy. *Ann Intern Med* 2001; 134:136–151.

59 Kuhn C 3rd, McDonald JA. The roles of the myofibroblast in idiopathic pulmonary fibrosis: ultrastructural and immunohistochemical features of sites of active extracellular matrix synthesis. *Am J Pathol* 1991; 138:1257–1265.

60 Kuhn C 3rd, Boldt J, King TE Jr, Crouch E, Vartio T, McDonald JA. An immunohistochemical study of architectural remodelling and connective tissue synthesis in pulmonary fibrosis. *Am Rev Respir Dis* 1989; 140:1693–1703.

61 Uhal BD, Joshi I, True AL, Raza A, Pardo A, Selman M. Fibroblasts isolated after fibrotic lung injury induce apoptosis of alveolar epithelial cells in vitro. *Am J Physiol* 1995; 269:L819–828.

62 Uhal BD, Joshi I, Hughes WF, Ramos C, Pardo A, Selman M. Alveolar epithelial cells adjacent to underlying myofibroblasts in advanced fibrotic human lung. *Am J Physiol* 1998; 275:L1192–1199.

63 Wang R, Ramos C, Joshi I et al. Human lung myofibroblast-derived inducers of alveolar epithelial apoptosis identified as angiotensin peptides. *Am J Physiol* 1999; 277:L1158–1164.

64 Kuwano K, Kunitake R, Kawasaki M et al. P21Waf1/Cip1/Sdi1 and p53 expression in association with DNA strand breaks in idiopathic pulmonary fibrosis. *Am J Respir Crit Care Med* 1996; 154:477–483.

65 Wilborn J, Crofford LJ, Burdick MD, Kunkel SL, Strieter RM, Peters-Golden M. Cultured lung fibroblasts isolated from patients with idiopathic pulmonary fibrosis have a diminished capacity to synthesize prostaglandin E2 and to express cyclooxygenase-2. *J Clin Invest* 1995; 95:1861–1868.

66 Kasper M, Haroske G. Alterations in the alveolar epithelium after injury leading to pulmonary fibrosis. *Histol Histopathol* 1996; 11:463–483.

67 Kasper M, Koslowski R, Luther T, Schuh D, Muller M, Wenzel KW. Immunohistochemical evidence for loss of ICAM-1 by alveolar epithelial cells in pulmonary fibrosis. *Histochem Cell Biol* 1995; 104:397–405.

68 Kallenberg CG, Schilizzi BM, Beaumont F, De Leij L, Poppema S, The TH. Expression of class II major histocompatability complex antigens on alveolar epithelium in

interstitial lung disease: relevance to pathogenesis of idiopathic pulmonary fibrosis. *J Clin Pathol* 1987; 40:725–733.

69 Khalil N, O'Connor RN, Unruh HW et al. Increased production and immunochemical localisation of transforming growth factor-beta in idiopathic pulmonary fibrosis. *Am J Respir Cell Mol Biol* 1991; 5:155–162.

70 Kapanci Y, Desmouliere A, Pache JC, Redard M, Gabbiani G. Cytoskeletal protein modulation in pulmonary alveolar myofibroblasts during idiopathic pulmonary fibrosis. Possible role of transforming growth factor β and tumour necrosis factor A. *Am J Respir Crit Care Med* 1995; 152:2163–2169.

71 Nash JR, McLaughlin PJ, Butcher D, Corrin B. Expression of tumour necrosis factor α in cryptogenic fibrosing alveolitis. *Histopathology* 1993; 22:343–347.

72 Antoniades HN, Bravo MA, Avila RE, Galanopoulus T, Neville J, Selman M. Platelet-derived growth factor in idiopathic pulmonary fibrosis. *J Clin Invest* 1990; 86:1055–1064.

73 Khalil N, O'Connor RN, Flanders KC, Unruh H. TGF-β1, but not TGF-β2 or TGF-β3, is differentially present in epithelial cells of advanced pulmonary fibrosis: an immunohistochemical study. *Am J Respir Cell Mol Biol* 1996; 14:131–138.

74 Chapman HA, Allen CL, Stone OL. Abnormalities in pathways of alveolar fibrin turnover among patients with interstitial lung disease. *Am Rev Respir Dis* 1986; 133:437–443.

75 Kotani I, Sato A, Hayakawa H, Urano T, Takada Y, Takada A. Increased procoagulant and antifibrinolytic activities in the lungs with idiopathic pulmonary fibrosis. *Thromb Res* 1995; 77:493–504.

76 Imokawa S, Sato A, Hayakawa H, Kotani M, Urano T, Takada A. Tissue factor expression and fibrin deposition in the lungs of patients with idiopathic pulmonary fibrosis and systemic sclerosis. *Am J Respir Crit Care Med* 1997; 156:631–636.

77 Fukuda Y, Ishizaki M, Kudoh S, Kitaichi M, Yamanaka N. Localization of matrix metalloproteinases -1, -2, and -9 and tissue inhibitor of metalloproteinase-2 in interstitial lung diseases. *Lab Invest* 1998; 78:687–698.

78 Wilhelm SM, Collier IE, Marmer BL, Eisen AZ, Grant GA, Goldberg GI. SV40-transformed fibroblasts secrete a 92 kDa type IV collagenase which is identical to that secreted by normal macrophages. *J Biol Chem* 1989; 264:17213–17221.

79 Pardo A, Ridge K, Uhal B, Sznajder JI, Selman M. Lung alveolar epithelial cells synthesize interstitial collagenase and gelatinases A and B in vitro. *Int J Biochem Cell Biol* 1997; 29:901–910.

80 Selman M, Ruiz V, Cabrera S et al. Localization of tissue inhibitor of metalloproteinases (TIMPs) -1, -2, -3, and -4 in idiopathic pulmonary fibrosis. TIMPs/collagenases imbalance in the fibrotic lung microenvironment. *Am J Physiol* 2000; 279:L562–574.

81 Hayashi T, Stetler-Stevenson WG, Fleming MV et al. Immunohistochemical study of metalloproteinases and their tissue inhibitors in the lungs of patients with diffuse alveolar damage and idiopathic pulmonary fibrosis. *Am J Pathol* 1996; 149:1241–1256.

82 Jordana M, Ohno I, Xing Z, Gauldie J. Cytokines in lung and airway fibrosis. *Reg Immunol* 1993; 5:201–206.

83 Xing Z, Tramblay GM, Sime PJ, Gauldie J. Overexpression of granulocyte-macrophage colony-stimulating factor induces pulmonary granulation tissue formation and fibrosis by induction of transforming growth factor-beta 1 and myofibroblast accumulation. *Am J Pathol* 1997; 150:59–66.

84 Sime PJ, Xing Z, Graham FL, Csaky KG, Gauldie J. Adenovector-mediated gene transfer of active transforming growth factor-beta1 induces prolonged severe fibrosis in rat lung. *J Clin Invest* 1997; 100:768–776.

85 Selman N, Ruiz V, Cabrera S et al. Localization of tissue inhibitor of metalloproteinases (TIMPs) -1, -2, -3, -4 in idiopathic pulmonary fibrosis. TIMPs/collagenases imbalance in the fibrotic lung microenvironment. *Am J Physiol* 2000; 279:L562–574.

86 Brew K, Dinakarpandian D, Nagase H. Tissue inhibitors of metalloproteinases: evolution, structure and function. *Biochim Biophys Acta* 2000; 1477:267–283.

87 Iyer SN, Wild JS, Schiedt MJ, Hyde DM, Margolin SB, Giri SN. Dietary intake of pirfenidone ameliorates bleomycin-induced lung fibrosis in hamsters. *J Lab Clin Med* 1995; 125:779–785.

88 Iyer SN, Margolin SB, Hyde DM, Giri SN. Lung fibrosis is ameliorated by pirfenidone fed in diet after the second dose in a three-dose bleomycin-hamster model. *Exp Lung Res* 1998; 24:119–132.

89 Iyer SN, Hyde DM, Giri SN. Anti-inflammatory effect of pirfenidone in the bleomycin-hamster model of lung inflammation. *Inflammation* 2000; 24:477–491.

90 Schelegele ES, Mansoor JK, Giri S. Pirfenidone attenuates bleomycin-induced changes in pulmonary functions in hamsters. *Proc Soc Exp Biol Med* 1997; 216:392–397.

91 Kehrer JP, Margolin SP. Pirfenidone diminishes cyclophosphamide-induced lung fibrosis in mice. *Toxicol Lett* 1997; 90:125–132.

92 Lurton JM, Trejo T, Narayaman AS, Raghu G. Pirfenidone inhibits the stimulatory effects of profibrotic cytokines on

human lung fibroblasts in vitro. *Am J Respir Crit Care Med* 1996; 153:A403.

93 Iyer SN, Gurujeyalakshmi G, Giri SN. Effects of pirfenidone on procollagen gene expression at the transcriptional level in bleomycin hamster model of lung fibrosis. *J Pharmacol Exp Ther* 1999; 289:211–218.

94 Iyer SN, Gurujeyalakshmi G, Giri SN. Effects of pirfenidone on transforming growth factor-beta gene expression at the transcriptional level in bleomycin hamster model of lung fibrosis. *J Pharmacol Exp Ther* 1999; 291:367–373.

95 Gurujeyalakshmi G, Hollinger MA, Giri SN. Pirfenidone inhibits PDGF isoforms in bleomycin hamster model of lung fibrosis at the translational level. *Am J Physiol* 1999; 276:L311-L318.

96 Raghu G, Johnson C, Lockhart D, Mageto Y. Treatment of idiopathic pulmonary fibrosis with a new antifibrotic agent, pirfenidone: results of a prospective open label study. *Am J Respir Crit Care Med* 1999; 159:1061–1069.

97 Johnston ID, Prescott RJ, Chalmers JC, Rudd RM. British Thoracic Society study of cryptogenic fibrosing alveolitis: current presentation and initial management. *Thorax* 1997; 52:38–44.

98 Mason RJ, Schwarz MI, Hunninghake GW, Musson RA. Pharmacological therapy for idiopathic pulmonary fibrosis: past, present and future. *Am J Respir Crit Care Med* 1999; 160:1771–1777.

99 Everson GT. Maintenance interferon for chronic hepatitis C: more issues than answers. *Hepatology* 2000; 32:436–438.

100 Comi G, Colombo B, Martinelli V. Prognosis modifying therapy in multiple sclerosis. *Neurol Sci* 2000; 21:S83-S90.

101 McDonald S, Rubin P, Chang AY et al. Pulmonary changes induced by combined mouse beta-interferon (rMuIFN-beta) and irradiation in normal mice – toxic versus protective effects. *Radiother Oncol* 1993; 26:212-218.

102 Kondo H, Yonezawa Y, Ito H. Interferon-beta, an autocrine cytokine, suppresses human fetal skin fibroblast migration into a denuded area in a cell monolayer but is not involved in the age-related decline of cell migration. *Mech Ageing Dev* 1996; 87:141–153.

103 Cornelissen AM, Von den Hoff JW, Maltha JC, Kuijpers-Jagtman AM. Effects of interferons on proliferation and collagen synthesis of rat palatal wound fibroblasts. *Arch Oral Biol* 1999; 44:541–547.

104 Raghu G, Bozic CR, Brown K. Feasibility of a trial of interferon beta-1a in the treatment of idiopathic pulmonary fibrosis. *Am J Respir Crit Care Med* 2001; 5:A707.

105 Paulnock DM, Demick KP, Coller SP. Analysis of interferon-gamma-dependent and –independent pathways of macrophage activation. *J Leukoc Biol* 2000; 67:677–682.

106 Okada T, Sugie I, Aisaka K. Effects of gamma-interferon on collagen and histamine content in bleomycin-induced lung fibrosis in rats. *Lymphokine Cytokine Res* 1993; 12:87–91.

107 Elias JA, Freundlich B, Kern JA, Rosenbloom J. Cytokine networks in the regulation of inflammation and fibrosis in the lung. *Chest* 1990; 97:1439–1445.

108 Bienskowski RS, Gorkin MG. Control of collagen deposition in mammalian lung. *Proc Soc Exp Biol Med* 1995; 209:118–140.

109 Inoue Y, King TE Jr, Tinkle SS, Dockstader K, Newman LS. Human mast cell basic fibroblast growth factor in pulmonary fibrotic disorders. *Am J Pathol* 1996; 149:2037–2054.

110 Winston BW, Krein PM, Mowat C, Huang Y. Cytokine-induced macrophage differentiation: a tale of two genes. *Clin Invest Med* 1999; 22:236–255.

111 Gurujeyalakshmi G, Giri SN. Molecular mechanisms of antifibrotic effect of interferon gamma in bleomycin-mouse model of lung fibrosis: downregulation of TGF-beta and procollagen I and III gene expression. *Exp Lung Res* 1995; 21:791–808.

112 Prior C, Haslam PL. In vivo levels and in vitro production of interferon-gamma in fibrosing interstitial lung diseases. *Clin Exp Immunol* 1992; 88:280–287.

113 Lesur OJ, Mancini NM, Humbert JC, Chabot F, Polu JM. Interleukin-6, interferon-gamma, and phospholipid levels in the alveolar lining fluid of human lungs. Profiles in coal worker's pneumoconiosis and idiopathic pulmonary fibrosis. *Chest* 1994; 106:407–413.

114 Sempowski GD, Derdak S, Phipps PR. Interleukin-4 and interferon-gamma discordantly regulate collagen biosynthesis by functionally distinct lung fibroblast subsets. *J Cell Physiol* 1996; 167:290–296.

115 Wallace WA, Ramage EA, Lamb D, Howie SE. A type 2 (Th2-like) pattern of immune response predominates in the pulmonary interstitium of patients with cryptogenic fibrosing alveolitis. *Clin Exp Immunol* 1995; 101:436–441.

116 Majumdar S, Li D, Ansari T et al. Different cytokine profiles in cryptogenic fibrosing alveolitis and fibrosing alveolitis associated with systemic sclerosis: a quantitative study of open lung biopsies. *Eur Respir J* 1999; 14:251–257.

117 Wallace WA, Howie SE. Immunoreactive interleukin-4 and interferon-gamma expression by type II alveolar epithelial cells in interstitial lung disease. *J Pathol* 1999; 187:475–480.

118 Kasama T, Strieter RM, Lukacs NW, Lincoln PM, Burdick MD, Kunkel SL. Interferon-gamma modulates the expression of neutrophil-derived chemokines. *J Investig Med* 1995; 43:58–67.

119 Nagahori T, Dohi M, Matsumoto K et al. Interferon-

gamma upregulates the c-Met/hepatocyte growth factor receptor expression in alveolar epithelial cells. *Am J Respir Cell Mol Biol* 1999; 21:490–49.

120 Britton J. Interferon gamma-ib therapy for cryptogenic fibrosing alveolitis. *Thorax* 2000; 55:S37–40.

121 Ogushi F, Endo T, Tani K et al. Decreased prostaglandin E2 synthesis by lung fibroblasts isolated from rats with bleomycin-induced lung fibrosis. *Int J Exp Pathol* 1999; 80:41–49.

122 Wilborn J, Crofford LJ, Burdick MD, Kunkel SL, Strieter RM, Peters-Golden M. Cultured lung fibroblasts isolated from patients with idiopathic pulmonary fibrosis have a diminished capacity to synthesize prostaglandin E2 and to express cyclooxygenase-2. *J Clin Invest* 1995; 95:1861–1868.

123 Moore BB, Coffey MJ, Christensen P et al. GM-CSF regulates bleomycin-induced pulmonary fibrosis via a prostaglandin-dependent mechanism. *J Immunol* 2000; 165:4032–4039.

124 Vancheri C, Sortino MA, Tomaselli V et al. Different expression of TNF-alpha receptors and prostaglandin E(2) production in normal and fibrotic lung fibroblasts: potential implications for the evolution of the inflammatory process. *Am J Respir Cell Mol Biol* 2000; 22:628–634.

125 Wilborn J, Baille M, Coffey M, Burdick M, Strieter R, Peters-Golden M. Constitutive activation of 5-lipoxygenase in the lungs of patients with idiopathic pulmonary fibrosis. *J Clin Invest* 1996; 97:1827–1836.

126 Ozaki O, Hayashi H, Tani K, Ogushi F, Yasuoka U, Ogura T. Neutrophil chemotactic factor in the respiratory tract of patients with chronic airway diseases or idiopathic pulmonary fibrosis. *Am Rev Respir Dis* 1992; 145:85–91.

127 Sato E, Koyama S, Robbins RA. Bleomycin stimulates lung fibroblast and epithelial cell lines to release eosinophil chemotactic activity. *Eur Respir J* 2000; 16:951–958.

128 Sato E, Koyama S, Takamizawa A et al. Smoke extract stimulates lung fibroblasts to release neutrophil and monocyte chemotactic activities. *Am J Physiol* 1999; 277:1149–1157.

129 Medina L, Perez-Ramos J, Ramirez R, Selman M, Pardo A. Leukotriene C4 upregulates collagenase expression and synthesis in human lung fibroblasts. *Biochim Biophys Acta* 1994; 1224:168–174.

130 Unemori EN, Pickford LB, Salles AL et al. Relaxin induces an extracellular matrix-degrading phenotype in human lung fibroblasts in vitro and inhibits lung fibrosis in a murine model in vitro. *J Clin Invest* 1996; 98:2739–2745.

131 Unemori EN, Beck LS, Lee WP. Human relaxin decreases collagen accumulation in vivo in two rodent models of fibrosis. *J Invest Dermatol* 1993; 101:280–285.

132 Ward WF, Molteni A, Ts'ao CH. Radiation-induced endo-

thelial dysfunction and fibrosis in rat lung: modification by the angiotensin converting enzyme inhibitor CL242817. *Radiat Res* 1989; 117:342–350.

133 Ward WF, Molteni A, Ts'ao CH, Kim YT, Hinz JM. Radiation pneumotoxicity in rats: modification by inhibitors of angiotensin converting enzyme. *Int J Radiat Oncol Biol Phys* 1992; 22:623–625.

134 Molteni A, Moulder JE, Cohen EF et al. Control of radiation-induced pneumopathy and lung fibrosis by angiotensin-converting enzyme inhibitors and an angiotensin II type I receptor blocker. *Ont J Radiat Biol* 2000; 76:523–532.

135 Nguyen L, Ward WF, Ts'ao CH, Molteni A. Captopril inhibits proliferation of human lung fibroblasts in culture: a potential antifibrotic mechanism. *Proc Soc Exp Biol Med* 1994; 205:80–84.

136 Wang R, Ramos C, Joshi I et al. Human lung myofibroblast-derived inducers of alveolar epithelial apoptosis identified as angiotensin peptides. *Am J Physiol* 1999; 277:L1158-L1164.

137 Uhal BD, Gidea C, Bargout R et al. Captopril inhibits apoptosis in human lung epithelial cells: a potential antifibrotic mechanism. *Am J Physiol* 1998; 275:L1013-L1017.

138 Wang R, Zagariya A, Ang E, Ibarra-Sunga O, Ubal BD. Fas-induced apoptosis of alveolar epithelial cells requires ANG-II generation and receptor interaction. *Am J Physiol* 1999; 277:L1245-L1250.

139 Wang R, Ibarra-Sunga O, Verlinski L, Pick R, Uhal BD. Abrogation of bleomycin-induced epithelial apoptosis and lung fibrosis by captopril or by a capsase inhibitor. *Am J Physiol Lung Cell Mol Physiol* 2000; 279:L143-L151.

140 Tan A, Levrey H, Dahm C, Polunovsky VA, Rubins J, Bitterman PB. Lovastatin induces fibroblast apoptosis in vitro and in vivo. A possible therapy for fibroproliferative disorders. *Am J Respir Crit Care Med* 1999; 159:220–227.

141 Soma MR, Corsini A, Paoletti R. Cholesterol and mevalonic acid modulation in cell metabolism and multiplication. *Toxicol Lett* 1992; 64–65:1–15.

142 Maltese WA. Posttranslational modification of proteins by isoprenoids in mammalian cells. *FASEB J* 1990; 4:3319–3328.

143 Kauffman-Zeh A, Rodriguez-Viciana P, Ulrich E et al. Suppression of c-Myc-induced apoptosis by Ras signalling through PI(3)K and PKB. *Nature* 1997; 385:544–548.

144 Marshall CJ. Specificity of receptor tyrosine kinase signalling: transient versus sustained extracellular signal-regulated kinase activation. *Cell* 1995; 80:179–185.

145 Perez-Sala D, Mollinedo F. Inhibition of isoprenoid biosynthesis induces apoptosis in human promyelocytic HL-60 cells. *Biochem Biophys Res Commun* 1994; 199:1209–1215.

146 Padayatty SJ, Marcelli M, Shao TC, Cunningham GR. Lovastatin-induced apoptosis in prostate stromal cells. *J Clin Endocrin Metab* 1997; 82:1434–1439.

147 Vincent TS, Wulfert E, Merler E. Inhibition of growth factor signalling pathways by lovastatin. *Biochem Biophys Res Commun* 1991; 180:1284–1289.

148 Ortiz MB, Goin M, de Alzaga MBG, Hammarstrom S, de Asua LJ. Mevalonate dependency of the early cell cycle mitogenic response to epidermal growth factor and prostaglandin F2α in Swiss 3T3 cells. *J Cell Physiol* 1995; 162:139–146.

149 Hengst L, Dulic V, Slingerland JM, Lees E, Reed SI. A cell cycle-regulated inhibitor of cyclin-dependent kinases. *Proc Natl Acad Sci USA* 1994; 91:5291–5295.

150 Chong LD, Traynor-Kaplan A, Bokoch GM, Schwartz MA. The small GTP-binding protein Rho regulates a phosphatidyl-inositol-4-phosphate 5-kinase in mammalian cells. *Cell* 1994; 79:507–513.

151 Pietsch A, Erl W, Lorenz RL. Lovastatin reduces expression of the combined adhesion and scavenger receptor CD36 in human monocytic cells. *Biochem Pharmacol* 1996; 52:433–439.

152 Kremlev SG, Umstead TM, Phelps DS. Effects of surfactant protein A and surfactant lipids on lymphocyte proliferation in vitro. *Am J Physiol* 1994; 267:357–364.

153 Kremlev SG, Phelps DS. Surfactant protein A stimulation of inflammatory cytokine and immunoglobulin production. *Am J Physiol* 1994; 267:L712–719.

154 Kremlev SG, Phelps DS. Effect of SP-A and surfactant lipids on expression of cell surface markers in the THP-1 monocytic cell line. *Am J Physiol* 1997; 272:L1070–L1077.

155 Thomassen MJ, Antal JM, Barna BP, Divis LT, Meeker DP, Wiedemann HP. Surfactant downregulates synthesis of DNA and inflammatory mediators in normal human lung fibroblasts. *Am J Physiol* 1996; 270:L159-L163.

156 Vasquez de Lara L, Becerril C, Montano M et al. Surfactant components modulate fibroblast apoptosis and type I collagen and collagenase-1 expression. *Am J Physiol* 2000; 279:L950-L957.

157 Polunovsky VA, Chen B, Henke C et al. Role of mesenchymal cell death in lung remodelling after injury. *J Clin Invest* 1993; 92:221–239.

158 Robinson PC, Watters LC, King TE, Mason RJ. Idiopathic pulmonary fibrosis. Abnormalities in bronchoalveolar lavage fluid phospholipids. *Am Rev Respir Dis* 1988; 137:585–591.

159 Seeger W, Elssner A, Gunther A, Kramer HJ, Kalinowski HO. Lung surfactant phospholipids associate with polymerizing fibrin: loss of surface activity. *Am J Respir Cell Mol Biol* 1993; 9:213–220.

160 Lossos IS, Izbicki G, Or R, Goldstein RH, Breuer R. The effect of suramin on bleomycin-induced lung injury. *Life Sci* 2000; 67:2873–2881.

161 Ulich TR, Yi ES, Longmuir K et al. Keratinocyte growth factor is a growth factor for type II pneumoncytes in vivo. *J Clin Invest* 1994; 93:1298–1306.

162 Panos RJ, Rubin JS, Aaronson SA, Mason RJ. Keratinocyte growth factors and hepatocyte growth factor/scatter factor are heparin-binding growth factors for alveolar type II cells in fibroblast-conditioned medium. *J Clin Invest* 1993; 92:969–977.

163 Yano T, Deterding RR, Nielsen LD, Jacoby C, Shannon JM, Mason RJ. Surfactant protein and CC-10 expression in acute lung injury and in response to keratinocyte growth factor. *Chest* 1997; 111:137S-138S.

164 Sugahara K, Rubia JS, Mason RJ, Aronsen EL, Shannon JM. Keratinocyte growth factor increases mRNAs for SP-A and SP-B in adult rat alveolar type II cells in culture. *Am J Physiol* 1995; 269:L344-L350.

165 Panos R, Bak JP, Simonet WS, Aukerman SL, Rubin JS, Smith LJ. Keratinocyte growth factor (KGF) prevents hyperoxia-induced mortality in rats. *Am J Respir Crit Care Med* 1995; 151:A181.

166 Deterding RR, Havill AM, Yano T et al. Prevention of bleomycin-induced lung injury in rats by keratinocyte growth factor. *Proc Assoc Am Phys* 1997; 109:254–268.

167 Yano T, Deterding RR, Simonet WS, Shannon JM, Mason RJ. Keratinocyte growth factor reduces lung damage due to acid installation in rats. *Am J Respir Cell Mol Biol* 1996; 15:433–442.

168 Guo J, Yi ES, Havill AM, et al. Intravenous keratinocyte growth factor protects against experimental pulmonary injury. *Am J Physiol* 1998; 275:L800-L805.

169 Mason CM, Guery BPH, Summer WR, Nelson S. Keratinocyte growth factor protects attenuates lung leak induced by alpha-naphthylthiourea in rats. *Crit Care Med* 1996; 24:925–931.

170 Yi ES, Williams ST, Lee H et al. Keratinocyte growth factor ameliorates radiation- and bleomycin-induced lung injury and mortality. *Am J Pathol* 1996; 149:1963–1970.

171 Sugahara K, Iyama K, Kuroda MJ, Sano K. Double intratracheal instillation of keratinocyte growth factor prevents bleomycin-induced lung fibrosis in rats. *J Pathol* 1998; 186:90–98.

172 Yi ES, Salgado M, Williams S et al. Keratinocyte growth factor decreases pulmonary oedema, transforming growth factor-beta and platelet-derived growth factor-BB expression, and alveolar type II cell loss in bleomycin-induced lung injury. *Inflammation* 1998; 22:315–325.

173 Wells AU, Hansell DM, Lawrence R, Harrison NK, Black CM, du Bois RM. Clearance of inhaled ^{99m}Tc-DTPA predicts the clinical course of fibrosing alveolitis. *Eur Resp J* 1993: 6:797–802.

174 Cantin AM, North SL, Fells GA, Hubbard RC, Crystal RG. Oxidant-mediated epithelial cell injury in idiopathic pulmonary fibrosis. *J Clin Invest* 1987; 79:1665–1673.

175 Cantin AM, North SL, Hubbard RC, Crystal RG. Normal alveolar epithelial lining fluid contains high levels of glutathione. *J Appl Physiol* 1987; 63:152–157.

176 Cantin AM, Hubbard RC, Crystal RG. Glutathione deficiency in the epithelial lining fluid of the lower respiratory tract in idiopathic pulmonary fibrosis. *Am Rev Respir Dis* 1989; 139:370–372.

177 Rahman I, Skwarska E, Henry M et al. Systemic and pulmonary oxidative stress in idiopathic pulmonary fibrosis. *Free Radic Biol Med* 1999; 27:60–68.

178 Behr J, Degenkolb B, Maier K et al. Increased oxidation of extracellular glutathione by bronchoalveolar inflammatory cells in diffuse fibrosing alveolitis. *Eur Respir J* 1995; 8:1286–1292.

179 Teramoto S, Fukuchi Y, Uejima Y, Shu CY, Orimo H. Superoxide anion formation and glutathione metabolism of blood in patients with idiopathic pulmonary fibrosis. *Biochem Mol Med* 1995; 55:66–70.

180 Behr J, Maier K, Krombach F, Adelmann-Grill BC. Pathogenetic significance of reactive oxygen species in diffuse fibrosing alveolitis. *Am Rev Respir Dis* 1991; 144:146–150.

181 Gosset P, Wallaert B, Tonnel AB, Fourneau C. Thiol regulation of the production of TNF-alpha, IL-6 and IL-8 by human alveolar macrophages. *Eur Respir J* 1999; 14:98–105.

182 Cantin AM, Larivee P, Begin RO. Extracellular glutathione suppresses human lung fibroblast proliferation. *Am J Respir Cell Mol Biol* 1990; 3:79–85.

183 Junn E, Lee KN, Ju HR et al. Requirement of hydrogen peroxide generation in TGF-beta 1 signal transduction in human lung fibroblast cells: involvement of hydrogen peroxide and Ca2 + in TGF-beta 1-induced IL-6 expression. *J Immunol* 2000; 165:2190–2197.

184 Goldstein RH, Fine A. Potential therapeutic initiatives for fibrogenic lung diseases. *Chest* 1995; 108:848–855.

185 MacNee W, Rahman I. Oxidants/antioxidants in idiopathic pulmonary fibrosis. *Thorax* 1995; 50:S53-S58.

186 Borok Z, Buhl R, Grimes GJ et al. Effect of glutathione aerosol on oxidant-antioxidant imbalance in idiopathic pulmonary fibrosis. *Lancet* 1991; 338:215–216.

187 Hagiwara SI, Ishii Y, Kitamura S. Aerosolized administration of *N*-acetylcysteine attenuates lung fibrosis induced by bleomycin in mice. *Am J Respir Crit Care Med* 2000; 162:225–231.

188 Meyer A, Buhl R, Magnussen H. The effect of oral *N*-acetylcysteine on lung glutathione levels in idiopathic pulmonary fibrosis. *Eur Respir J* 1994; 7:431–436.

189 Meyer A, Buhl R, Kampf S, Magnussen H. Intravenous *N*-acetylcysteine and lung glutathione of patients with pulmonary fibrosis and normals. *Am J Respir Crit Care Med* 1995; 152:1055–1060.

190 Behr J, Maier K, Degenkolb B, Krombach F, Vogelmeier C. Antioxidative and clinical effects of high-dose *N*-acetylcysteine in fibrosing alveolitis. Adjunctive therapy to maintenance immunosuppression. *Am J Respir Crit Care Med* 1997; 156:1897–1901.

191 Teder P, Noble PW. A cytokine reborn? Endothelin-1 in pulmonary inflammation and fibrosis. *Am J Respir Cell Mol Biol* 2000; 23:7–10.

192 Yanagisawa M, Kurihara H, Kimura S et al. A novel potent vasoconstrictir peptide produced by vascular endothelial cells. *Nature* 1988; 332:411–415.

193 Mattoli S, Mezzetti M, Riva G, Allegra L, Fasoli A. Specific binding of endothelin on human bronchial smooth muscle cells in culture and secretion of endothelin-like material from bronchial epithelial cells. *Am J Respir Cell Mol Biol* 1990; 3:145–151.

194 Shahar I, Fireman E, Topilsky M et al. Effect of endothelin-1 on alpha-smooth muscle actin expression and on alveolar fibroblast proliferation in interstitial lung diseases. *Int J Immunopharmacol* 1999; 21:759–775.

195 Sessa WC, Kaw S, Hecker M, Vane JR. The biosynthesis of endothelin-1 by human polymorphonuclear leukocytes. *Biochem Biophys Res Commun* 1991; 174:613–618.

196 Gu J, Pinheiro JM, Yu CZ, D'Andrea M, Murlidharan S, Malik A. Detection of endothelin-like immunoreactivity in epithelium and fibroblasts of the human umbilical cord. *Tissue Cell* 1991; 23:437–444.

197 Halim A, Kanayama N, el Maradny E, Maehara K, Terao T. Activated neutrophil by endothelin-1 caused tissue damage in human umbilical cord. *Thromb Res* 1995; 77:321–227.

198 McMillen MA, Sumpio BE. Endothelins: polyfunctional cytokines. *J Am Coll Surg* 1995; 180:621–637.

199 Marini M, Carpi S, Bellini A, Patalano F, Mattoli S. Endothelin-1 induces increased fibronectin expression in human bronchial epithelial cells. *Biochem Biophys Res Commun* 1996; 220:896–899.

200 Peacock AJ, Dawes KE, Shock A, Gray AJ, Reeves JT, Laurent GJ. Endothelin-1 and endothelin-3 induce chemotaxis and replication of pulmonary artery fibroblasts. *Am J Respir Cell Mol Biol* 1992; 7:492–499.

201 Dawes KE, Cambrey AD, Campa JS et al. Changes in collagen metabolism in response to endothelin-1: evidence for fibroblast heterogeneity. *Int J Biochem Cell Biol* 1996; 28:229–238.

202 Giaid A, Michel RP, Stewart DJ, Sheppard M, Corrin B, Hamid Q. Expression of endothelin-1 in lungs of patients with cryptogenic fibrosing alveolitis. *Lancet* 1993; 341:1550–1554.

203 Uguccioni M, Pulsatelli L, Grigolo B et al. Endothelin-1 in idiopathic pulmonary fibrosis. *J Clin Pathol* 1995; 48:330–334.

204 Mutsaers SE, Foster ML, Chambers RC, Laurent GJ, McNulty RJ. Increased endothelin-1 and its localization during the development of bleomycin-induced pulmonary fibrosis in rats. *Am J Respir Cell Mol Biol* 1998; 18:611–619.

205 Park SH, Saleh D, Giaid A, Michel RP. Increased endothelin-1 in bleomycin-induced pulmonary fibrosis and the effect of an endothelin receptor antagonist. *Am J Respir Crit Care Med* 1997; 156:600–608.

206 Cambrey AD, Harrison NK, Dawes KE et al. Increased levels of endothelin-1 in bronchoalveolar lavage fluid from patients with scleroderma contribute to fibroblast mitogenic activity in vitro. *Am J Respir Cell Mol Biol* 1994; 11:439–445.

207 Rockey DC, Chung JJ. Endothelin antagonism in experimental hepatic fibrosis. Implications for endothelin in the pathogenesis of wound healing. *J Clin Invest* 1996; 98:1381–1388.

208 Mutsaers SE, Marshall RP, Goldsack NR, Laurent GJ, McAnulty RJ. Effect of endothelin receptor antagonists (BQ-485, Ro 47–0203) on collagen deposition during the development of bleomycin-induced pulmonary fibrosis in rats. *Pulm Pharmacol Ther* 1998; 11:221–225.

209 van Roon JA, Lafeber FP, Bijlsma JW. Synergistic activity of interleukin-4 and interleukin-10 in suppression of inflammation and joint destruction in rheumatoid arthritis. *Arthritis Rheum* 2001; 44:3–12.

210 Van Deventer SJ. Immunotherapy of Crohn's disease. *Scand J Immunol* 2000; 51:18–22.

211 Asadullah K, Docke WD, Sabat RV, Volk HD, Sterry W. The treatment of psoriasis with IL-10: rationale and review of the first clinical trials. *Expert Opin Investig Drugs* 2000; 9:95–102.

212 Moore KW, de Waal Malefyt R, Coffman RL, O'Garra A. Interleukin-10 and the interleukin-10 receptor. *Annu Rev Immunol* 2001; 19:683–765.

213 Akdis CA, Joss A, Akdis M, Blasser K. Mechanism of IL-10-induced T cell inactivation in allergic inflammation and normal response to allergens. *Int Arch Allergy Immunol* 2001; 124:180–182.

214 Kumar A, Creery WD. The therapeutic potential of interleukin 10 in infection and inflammation. *Arch Immunol Ther Exp* 2000; 48:529–538.

215 Reitamo S, Remitz A, Tamai K, Uitto J. Interleukin-10 modulates type I collagen and matrix metalloprotease gene expression in cultured human skin fibroblasts. *J Clin Invest* 1994; 94:2489–2492.

216 Wang SC, Ohata M, Schrum L, Rippe RA, Tsukamoto H. Expression of interleukin-10 by in vitro and in vivo activated hepatic stellate cells. *J Biol Chem* 1998; 273:302–308.

217 Martinez JA, King TE Jr, Brown K et al. Increased expression of the interleukin-10 gene by alveolar macrophages in interstitial lung disease. *Am J Physiol* 1997; 273:L676–683.

218 Arai T, Abe K, Matsuoka H et al. Introduction of the interleukin-10 gene into mice inhibited bleomycin-induced lung injury. *Am J Physiol Lung Cell Mol Physiol* 2000; 278:L914–922.

219 Hashimoto T, Nakamura M, Oshika Y et al. Interleukin-10 relieves the inhibitory effects of interferon-gamma on normal human lung fibroblasts. *Int J Mol Med* 2001; 7:149–154.

Infection

14

Current and future management of pneumonia

Mario Cazzola[1] and Maria Gabriella Matera[2]

[1] Department of Respiratory Medicine, Division of Pneumology and Allergology, A. Cardarelli Hospital, Naples, Italy, and
[2] Institute of Pharmacology and Toxicology, Medical School, Second Neapolitan University, Naples, Italy

Antimicrobial agents are the cornerstones of bacterial pneumonia therapy. In fact, there are convincing data to show that patients with pneumonia have a better chance of survival if given antibiotics[1]. Initial antibiotic choice should be based on expected etiological pathogens, while knowledge of local microbial epidemiology and susceptibility patterns is crucial. Characteristics of the antibiotic itself, such as microbiological activity (bactericidal or bacteriostatic mode of action) and the spectrum of activity of the compound are relevant to choice of treatment. The frequency of side-effects and the interference with immunological homeostasis, as well as the ability to pass from capillary bed to bronchial lumen across a series of membranes and diffusional paths (the so-called blood–bronchoalveolar barrier), also influence the choice of the antibiotic to be used[1].

Microbiological problems

Because antibiotic therapy is usually initiated before the results of bacteriological analysis are available, the physician must take into account the potential pathogens and their current susceptibilities to available antimicrobial agents.

Incidence

Epidemiological data, including geographic setting, seasonal timing and a history of occupational or unusual exposures, may be crucial in determining the aetiology of pneumonia. However, it is impor-

tant to differentiate between infections that are community acquired and those that are hospital-acquired (Table 14.1). The relative frequencies with which individual agents cause pneumonia are quite different in these two locations.

Community-acquired pneumonia (CAP) is a common illness associated with significant morbidity and mortality. It is an acute infection of the pulmonary parenchyma that is associated with at least some symptoms of acute infection and is accompanied by the presence of an acute infiltrate on chest radiograph or auscultatory findings consistent with pneumonia. CAP occurs in a patient who is not hospitalized or residing in a long-term care facility for ≥ 14 days before the onset of symptoms[2].

Nosocomial pneumonia is defined as an infection of lung parenchyma that was neither present nor incubating at the time of the patient's admission to the hospital[3].

Community-acquired pneumonia

Causal pathogens

Despite the best of exhaustive efforts, the etiology of CAP is not found in about 50–60% of all cases. Results from the Pneumonia Patient Outcomes Research Team (PORT) Cohort Study have recently demonstrated that only 29.7% of 944 outpatients had one or more microbiological tests performed, and only 5.7% had an assigned microbiological cause[4]. This is a true problem because information from the history, physical examination, laboratories, and chest radiograph is not very sensitive or specific

Table 14.1. Common etiological agents in pneumonia

Outpatient	Inpatient	Nursing home
Streptococcus pneumoniae	*Streptococcus pneumoniae*	*Streptococcus pneumoniae*
Mycoplasma pneumoniae	Atypicals	Gram-negative rods
Chlamydia pneumoniae	Gram-negative rods	*Haemophilus influenzae*
Haemophilus influenzae	*Haemophilus influenzae*	

for predicting etiology, or even for differentiating typical from atypical organisms or bacterial causes from viral ones. Besides, a thorough understanding of the microbiology of CAP is essential for appropriate diagnosis and management.

The best opportunity to make an etiological diagnosis is before antibiotics are administered. Identification of the microbial cause of pneumonia permits specific, narrow-spectrum antibiotic treatment that may be more effective, less toxic, and less expensive than empirical therapy. Unfortunately, determination of the etiological pathogens of CAP is still now problematic because of the lack of reliable rapid laboratory diagnostic tools as well as the controversy concerning diagnostic criteria[5]. In general, age and medical history, including travel and animal contacts, and the physical examination of the patient will offer important clues to the cause of the pneumonia.

Viral pneumonias account for at least 17% of cases of CAP in children and in adults[6], but up to 53% of outpatients with bacterial pneumonia have been found to have a concurrent viral infection. Viral pneumonias are predominant in the winter and spring[7]. Influenza virus types A and B account for over one half of viral pneumonias in adults[8], whereas respiratory syncytial virus (RSV) and parainfluenza viruses are the most frequent viral pathogens in infants and children. RSV is seasonal, with activity, which rises in the autumn, peaks in winter and returns to baseline in the spring. Peak attack rates for RSV occur in winter in children less than 6 months of age. People with pre-existing heart or lung diseases may be particularly susceptible to viral pneumonias, which may be further complicated by bacterial infections. Immunocompromised hosts are suscep-

tible to pneumonias caused by cytomegalovirus and other herpesviruses, as well as rubeola and adenovirus[9].

Before the 1930s, most cases of pneumonia were attributed to *Streptococcus pneumoniae*[10]. Improved techniques have helped to identify additional causative pathogens. *S. pneumoniae* is still the most common known cause of CAP, accounting for 20% to 60% of all cases[11]. It is the most common bacterial pathogen recovered in patients who develop CAP after an influenza virus infection. Up to 25% of cases of pneumococcal pneumonia may progress to bacteremia, which has a mortality rate of nearly 20%[12]. Pneumococcal infections occur predominantly in the winter and early spring. In developing countries, the attack rate of pneumococcal disease is high, particularly in children[13] and in crowded communities of adults in whom the attack rate may be as high as 100‰ population per year[14].

Haemophilus influenzae and *Moraxella catarrhalis* are increasingly being implicated in CAP, particularly in patients with chronic obstructive pulmonary disease (COPD). These organisms should always be considered in patients with recurrent pneumonia[15]. *M. catarrhalis* seems to be a rare cause of pneumonia in children[16]. On the contrary, non-typeable strains of *H. influenzae* are responsible for many cases of pediatric pneumonia. These strains rarely invade the bloodstream to cause widespread infections[17], whereas serotype b organisms cause life-threatening pneumonia in children[18]. *H. influenzae* should be a cause of pneumonia even in previously fit young adults[19].

Chlamydia pneumoniae and *Mycoplasma pneumoniae* are other common causes in younger persons. Together they may account for 25% of CAP cases[20]. Although pneumonia caused by either of these organisms tends to be mild, some cases have been life threatening. Until recently pneumonia due to atypical pathogens has been considered uncommon in old people. A review of 11 studies of pneumonia identified *Chlamydia* and *Coxiella* spp. as the cause in only 2% of patients aged over 65[21]. However, recent surveys have documented *C. pneumoniae* in up to 26% of cases, which suggest it is the second commonest cause of pneumonia in this age group[22]. There is evidence that *M. pneumoniae* also plays an important role in older adults; in fact, it has been implicated in 11–17% of pneumonias in patients older than 40 years[23]. *C. pneumoniae* is found both as a single etiological agent and as a mixed infection, most often with *S. pneumoniae*[24]. The synergistic effect may be due to the ciliostatic effect of *C. pneumoniae* rendering the host more susceptible to the second agent. Patients infected with both *S. pneumoniae* and *C. pneumoniae* have a more severe illness[25].

Legionella species have been reported in 2% to 6% of cases of CAP[26]. The frequency may be higher in some series because of local variation or laboratory (isolation) technique. Relative to other bacteria, *Legionella* accounts for a higher proportion of patients hospitalized with severe CAP. Both sporadic cases and epidemics of Legionnaire's disease have occurred. Low prevalence of *Legionella* spp. and *M. pneumoniae* infection is observed in older patients hospitalized for CAP[27].

Staphylococcus aureus and gram-negative bacilli are much less common causes of CAP. *S. aureus* predominantly affects the elderly and is mostly seen in association with influenza pandemics. It is more frequent in nursing home patients (25.7%) compared with community patients (14.3%)[28]. High alcohol intake is a risk factor for developing *S. aureus*-induced CAP in middle-aged people[29]. Also gram-negative bacilli are most likely to infect alcoholics and nursing home patients. However, while gram-negative bacilli account for an appreciable proportion of cases in CAP patients over the age of 65 years in the United States, they are absent in the elderly in the United Kingdom[30].

The frequency of anaerobe-induced CAP is unclear, mainly because of the difficulty in recovering these organisms[31], although CAP can be the result of infection by anaerobic bacteria. Dental plaque would seem to be a logical source of these bacteria, especially in patients with periodontal disease[32]. Anaerobes, mostly species of *Bacteroides*, *Fusobacterium*, *Peptococcus* and *Peptostreptococcus*, might be considered the causative pathogen in patients predisposed to aspiration (e.g. those with a history of altered consciousness or dysphagia)[33].

Pneumocystis carinii is the potential infectious agent in immunosuppressed patients and in those at high risk for HIV infection[34]. It can be isolated also in patients with severe CAP[35].

Although there are no good data on the local incidence of different CAP organisms, geography can be a strong predictor of causal organism. In New Zealand, a microbiological diagnosis was made in 181 cases (71%), *S. pneumoniae* (39%), *M. pneumoniae* (16%), *Legionella* spp. (11%), and *H. influenzae* (11%) being the most commonly identified organisms[36]. In Spain, *S. pneumoniae* was the most frequently isolated microorganism (43%), followed by *C. pneumoniae* (21%), *H. influenzae* (19%), and *M. pneumoniae* (11%)[37]. In Israel, the etiology of CAP was identified in 279 (80.6%) out 346 consecutive adult patients[38]. The distribution of causal agents was as follows: *S. pneumoniae* (42.8%), *M. pneumoniae* (29.2%); *C. pneumoniae* (17.9%); *Legionella* spp. (16.2%), respiratory viruses (10.1%); *C. burnetii* (5.8%); *H. influenzae* (5.5%), and other causes (6.0%). In Japan, causative pathogens were identified in 199 out of 336 episodes (61%)[39]. *S. pneumoniae* was the most common pathogen (23%), followed by *H. influenzae* (7.4%), *M. pneumoniae* (4.9%), and *Klebsiella pneumoniae* (4.3%). The *Streptococcus milleri* group and *C. pneumoniae* were detected in 3.7 and 3.4% of the episodes, respectively. Pneumonia due to *Legionella* spp. was recognized in only two patients.

Severity as a predictor of causal pathogen

Emphasis has always been placed on the assessment of the severity of disease. Patients with non-severe

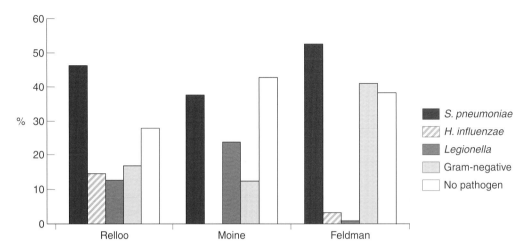

Fig. 14.1 Microbiological etiology of severe CAP. Data from three recent studies[42–44].

pneumonia have mortality rates less than 1%. Therefore, they could probably be treated as outpatients. Not only is severity a useful prognostic factor, but it may also give an indication of the likely causal pathogen.

Mild CAP

Although there is no uniform definition of mild pneumonia, clinicians usually define patients with mild pneumonia as those who are 'not too sick', have normal respiratory and mental status, and are able to maintain oral intake. By inference, mild pneumonia occurs in younger patients with less comorbidity and has a better outcome than pneumonia that is moderate to severe. Atypical pathogens such as *M. pneumoniae* and *C. pneumoniae*, and respiratory tract viruses are common causes of mild pneumonia[40].

Severe CAP

Severe CAP is emerging as an increasingly growing problem. Experimental evidence suggests that severe CAP is pathophysiologically distinct from other forms of CAP. In one report[41] examining cytokine levels in severe CAP, levels of IL-1 and TNF-α were highest in severe pneumonia patients, compared to patients without severe pneumonia. IL-6 levels did not discriminate between infected and

non-infected patients and appeared to reflect severity of stress whether of infectious or non-infectious origin. *S. pneumoniae* is the most common causative agent of severe CAP (Fig. 14.1). Other pathogens, such as *Legionella* and gram-negative enteric bacilli, especially *Pseudomonas aeruginosa*, are more common in patients with severe CAP than in milder forms of the disease. Patients with advanced age and serious comorbid illnesses, such as COPD, diabetes mellitus, carcinoma, bronchiectasis, renal failure and alcoholism, seem predisposed to infection with these pathogens[42–45]. A prospective study of 132 patients with severe CAP treated in the Intensive Care Unit (ICU) was carried out to determine the causative agents *S. pneumoniae* (45%), gram-negative bacilli (15%), and *H. influenzae* (15%) were the most frequent pathogens[46].

Nosocomial pneumonia

Causal pathogens

The spectrum of etiological agents for hospital-acquired pneumonia (HAP) differs from those likely to cause CAP. Factors that are associated with specific organisms include underlying risk factors, disease severity, and length of hospitalization before the onset of the pneumonia. As the most common route of pathogen entry is microaspiration of upper airway secretions[43,47,48], the Aetiology of HAP depends largely on pathogenic bacteria colonizing the oropharynx.

Most patients are colonized with a core group of organisms during their initial hospitalization (<5 days). These core organisms are the pathogens most commonly isolated with early-onset HAP and include *S. pneumoniae*, *H. influenzae*, methicillin-susceptible *S. aureus*, and the enteric gram-negative bacilli (*Escherichia coli*, *Enterobacter* spp., *Proteus* spp., *Klebsiella* spp., and *Serratia marcescens*)[49–52]. Among patients who have been hospitalized for longer periods of time (≥ 5 days) or have specific risk factors, the core organisms may still cause HAP. However, additional pathogens such as methicillin-resistant *S. aureus* (MRSA), *Pseudomonas* spp., *Enterobacter* spp., and *Acinetobacter* spp. need to be considered[53,54].

The reported distribution of etiological agents causing nosocomial pneumonia varies between hospitals because of differences in patient populations and diagnostic methods employed. In general, however, bacteria have been the most frequently isolated pathogens. In effect, nosocomial bacterial pneumonias are frequently polymicrobial[55,56] and gram-negative bacilli are the usual predominant organisms[56,57] although *S. aureus* (especially MRSA)[58] and other gram-positive cocci, including *S. pneumoniae*[59], have recently emerged as significant isolates.

Schaberg et al.[60] reported that in 1986–1989 aerobic bacteria comprised at least 73%, and fungi 4%, of isolates from sputum and tracheal aspirates of pneumonia patients at the University of Michigan Hospitals and hospitals participating in the National Nosocomial Infection Surveillance System (NNIS). Very few anaerobic bacteria and no viruses were reported, probably because anaerobic and viral cultures were not performed routinely in the reporting hospitals.

Legionnaires' disease
Since identification of the etiological agent, numerous outbreaks of nosocomial Legionnaires' disease have been reported[61]. The overall proportion of nosocomial pneumonias due to *Legionella* spp. has not been determined. One autopsy study estimated that 3.8% of all persons who died of nosocomial pneumonia at 40 hospitals participating in the NNIS system during the mid-1970s had Legionnaires' disease[62]. Data from a 1997 survey of hospitals participating in the NNIS system suggested that 29% of 196 hospitals have identified nosocomial transmission since 1990. In particular, 60% of hospitals in which transmission had been recognized have identified at least two cases[63]. Because diagnostic tests for *Legionella* spp. infection are not routinely performed on all patients with HAP in most hospitals, these ranges probably underestimate the incidence of Legionnaires' disease.

Persons with severe immunosuppression or chronic underlying illnesses, such as hematological malignancy or end-stage renal disease, are at markedly increased risk for legionellosis[64]. Persons in the later stages of acquired immunodeficiency syndrome are also probably at increased risk of legionellosis, but data are limited because of infrequent testing of patients. Persons with diabetes mellitus, chronic lung disease, or non-hematological malignancy, those who smoke cigarettes and the elderly are at moderately increased risk[65].

Ventilator-associated pneumonia
Ventilator-associated pneumonia (VAP) is a common infection in ICU patients that results in high mortality and morbidity and increased duration of hospital stay. VAP specifically refers to pneumonia developing in a mechanically ventilated patient more than 48 hours after intubation[66]. Aspiration of microorganisms colonizing the oropharynx is the main route of bacterial entry to lower airways in mechanically ventilated patients. Unfortunately, there are few data to suggest that individual patient characteristics predict the etiology of VAP. Early onset VAP that occurs within 72 hours of initiation of intubation is usually due to aspiration during that procedure. It is most often produced by antibiotic-sensitive organisms (*S. pneumoniae*, *S. aureus*, *H. influenzae*) except in

certain populations (e.g. COPD patients who may be colonized by *P. aeruginosa*)[67]. Late onset VAP is seen 72 hours post intubation, and is frequently due to antibiotic-resistant organisms, such as MRSA, *P. aeruginosa*, *Acinetobacter*, or *Enterobacter* spp.[67,68]. Fagon et al.[69] reported that gram-negative bacilli were present in 75% of protected-specimen brushings (PSB) quantitative cultures from patients who had received mechanically assisted ventilation and acquired nosocomial pneumonia; 40% of the cultures were polymicrobial. In the report by Torres et al.[70], 20% of pathogens recovered from cultures of PSB, blood, pleural fluid, or percutaneous lung aspirate were gram-negative bacilli in pure culture, and 17% were polymicrobial. However, 54% of specimens did not yield any microorganism, probably because of receipt of antibiotics by patients. Cultures of bronchoscopic specimens from mechanically ventilated patients with pneumonia have rarely yielded anaerobes.

Host factors, oropharyngeal and gastric colonization, cross-infection, and complications from the use of antibiotics and nasogastric and endotracheal tubes increases the risk of bacterial VAP[71].

Resistance patterns

Since the introduction of antibiotics into clinical use, bacteria have protected themselves by developing antibiotic resistance mechanisms. They may survive because of their ability to manipulate genetic information and to mutate rapidly, but more importantly to inherit, express, and disseminate exogenous genes[72]. The physical characteristics of the microbial community play a major role in gene exchange, but antimicrobial agents provide the selective pressure for the development of resistance and promote the transfer of resistance genes among bacteria. Resistant infections confront and thwart the treatment of some patients in the community as well as in the hospital[73]. Currently, there are increasing problems worldwide with multiresistant bacteria. These problems are especially evident within hospitals, where they frequently present as nosocomial epidemics. Risk groups include hospitalized

Table 14.2. Resistance to penicillin among *Streptococcus pneumoniae* isolates in New York City hospital laboratories

Number of isolates	Number (%)		
	1993	1994	1995
Screened with oxacillin disks[a]	3227	4133	4912
Zone size ≤19 mm[b]	273 (9)	549 (13)	995 (20)
Screened and confirmed with validated MICs[c]	1229	2491	3535
Zone size ≤19 mm	154 (13)	350 (14)	704 (20)
I[d]	70 (6)	209 (8)	310 (9)
R[d]	19 (2)	115 (5)	222 (6)

Notes:

[a] The number of operating laboratories in 1993, 1994, 1995 was 33, 40, and 51, respectively.

[b] Diffusion zone size of the oxacillin disk test.

[c] The number of operating laboratories in 1993, 1994, 1995 was 10, 22, and 35, respectively.

[d] I = intermediate sensibility to penicillin (MIC > 0.1 and < 1.0 μg/ml); R = penicillin-resistant (MIC > 2.0 μg/ml).

Adapted from Heffernan et al.[267].

and immunocompromised persons, children attending day-care and elderly patients in nursing homes.

S. pneumoniae

S. pneumoniae with reduced susceptibility to penicillin (defined as minimum inhibitory concentration (MIC) to penicillin > 0.1 μg/ml confirmed by an approved National Committee for Clinical Laboratory Standards (NCCLS) methodology) is becoming a healthcare concern, not only because of the high prevalence of infections caused by this pathogen but also because of the rate at which resistance has progressed[74] (Table 14.2). Recently, the

Centres for Disease Control and Prevention (CDC) reported data from the National Pneumococcal Sentinel Surveillance System during 1993–1994[75]. The penicillin non-susceptible *S. pneumoniae* (MIC = 0.1 μg/ml: intermediate) was shown to be 14.1%, with 3.2% penicillin-resistant (MIC = 2 μg/ml) strains. Pneumococcal strains become resistant by alterations in one or more of the penicillin binding proteins (PBP), which are responsible for growth and repair of the cell wall. The alteration in the PBP causes poor penicillin binding to PBP, so the drug cannot act. Although many penicillin-resistant isolates are sensitive to newer β-lactams such as cefotaxime, some strains have developed resistance to these drugs by producing simultaneous changes in more than one PBP. Recent use of β-lactam antibiotics, an age of 0–4 years, or day-care attendance by a member of the patient's household in the 3 months before the patient's illness, are predictive factors associated with invasive penicillin non-susceptible *S. pneumoniae* infections[76,77].

The penicillin non-susceptible *S. pneumoniae* may also be resistant to other antibiotic agents. For example, the National Pneumococcal Sentinel Surveillance System during 1993–1994 has shown that 64.4% of the penicillin non-susceptible *S. pneumoniae* isolates were also non-susceptible to one other class of antimicrobial drug[78]. Similar data were reported by other multicentre surveillance studies[79,80]. In particular, a prospective, Australia-wide, laboratory-based survey during 1994–1995 demonstrated that resistance rates were higher for most other antibiotics than for penicillin (penicillin, 6.7%; chloramphenicol, 6%; erythromycin, 11%; tetracycline, 15%; and co-trimoxazole, 42%)[81].

The overall prevalence of macrolide resistance in pneumococci varies by country. In Slovakia, almost all pneumococcal isolates are resistant[82], whereas in Portugal only 0.6% of isolates are resistant and the proportion appears to be declining[83]. In the United Kingdom, erythromycin resistance increased from 3.3% to 8.6% between 1989 and 1992[84]. In the United States, 10% of pneumococcal isolates appear to be erythromycin resistant[79]. The N^6-methylation of a specific adenine residue (A2058) in 23S rRNA with reduced affinity between the antibiotic and the ribosome[85], and the efflux of the antibiotic from the cell[86], are the mechanisms described for resistance to erythromycin in the pneumococcus. The reasons for the increasing resistance in *S. pneumoniae* worldwide are not completely understood, although antibiotic pressure appears to be a major factor[87]. While 90 serotypes exist, four serotypes (6B, 14, 19, 23F) account for most disease and drug-resistant *S. pneumoniae* strains.

S. aureus

At present, approximately 95% of staphylococci are penicillinase producers and, consequently, resistant to penicillin G and V, and to the amino-, carboxy- and acylureidopenicillins. Moreover, approximately 30% of *S. aureus* isolates obtained from patients hospitalized in the United States are resistant to methicillin[88]. The intrinsic resistance to β-lactam antibiotics in *S. aureus* is conferred by an additional PBP-2' (or PBP-2a, encoded by the *mecA* gene), which is absent in susceptible staphylococci. PBP-2' binds poorly with methicillin and most other β-lactams and can fulfill the functions of the other essential PBPs 1, 2 and 3. Thus, MRSA is resistant to all β-lactams, not just to methicillin and the isoxazoyl penicillins. The proportion of MRSA in the various European countries ranged from < 1% in Scandinavia to > 30% in Spain, France and Italy, in 1992–1993[89]. In Japan, analysis of approximately 7000 strains isolated from patients in various geographic areas during 1992–1993 indicated that 60% of *S. aureus* isolates were resistant to methicillin[90].

MRSA ventilator-associated pneumonia is a frequent complication in ICU, manifesting itself as late-onset pneumonia in patients who have been intubated for prolonged periods and/or have undergone previous bronchoscopy. Over the 5-year period from 1990 to 1994, of 2411 mechanically ventilated patients, 347 (14.4%) acquired MRSA, 220 (63.4%) had MRSA positive respiratory tract samples and 41 (18.6%) developed ventilator-associated MRSA pneumonia[91].

Vancomycin or other glycopeptide intermediately

resistant *S. aureus* (VISA/GISA; MIC = 8 μg/ml) also has emerged[92]. Evidence for cell-wall reorganization has been reported for GISA isolates. These changes in cell-wall structure may be responsible for the atypical phenotypic characteristics and decreased susceptibility to vancomycin[93].

The extensive use of quinolones has been associated with a rapid increase in resistance, particularly in MRSA, but also in methicillin-susceptible strains[94]. Ciprofloxacin resistance emerged rapidly in MRSA and developed particularly among strains resistant to co-trimoxazole. It was more common in patients with MRSA acquired nosocomially. In that group, no host or in-hospital factors were associated with ciprofloxacin resistance[95]. In the 1995 survey in individual hospitals in Melbourne, 16–24% of MRSA isolates were ciprofloxacin-resistant, compared with 80–100% in Sydney and 30–44% in Brisbane. There was great diversity of phage type patterns for ciprofloxacin-resistant strains, suggesting heterogeneous development of resistance[96].

H. influenzae

H. influenzae resistance has a geographical variation, reaching critical levels in some countries. β-Lactamase production is the primary mechanism for this resistance. Rates of resistance found among isolates of *H. influenzae* in 1996 were of around 20% or more in France, Belgium and Spain, and in excess of 10% in the UK and the Czech Republic[97]. In the same year in non-European centres, Mexico (25%), Saudi Arabia (27.9%), Hong Kong (37.1%) and the USA (30.4% of combined isolates) had a high prevalence of β-lactamase production. Isolates of β-lactamase-negative, ampicillin-resistant *H. influenzae* were generally very uncommon, with only Barcelona, Spain consistently associated with rates in excess of 1%. A national multicentre surveillance study of antibiotic resistance among clinical isolates of *H. influenzae* in the United States in 1994 and 1995 found 39 out of 1537 clinical isolates that were β-lactamase negative but ampicillin intermediate or resistant and, even more surprisingly, 17 β-

lactamase-positive isolates that were resistant to co-amoxiclav[98]. In any case, resistance rates of >5% with *H. influenzae* from patients with community-acquired respiratory tract infections were observed only with cefaclor (12.8%) and co-trimoxazole (16.2%) in the USA and Canada in 1997[99].

H. influenzae can also be resistant to other classes of antibiotics. For example, some strains of *H. influenzae* produce chloramphenicol acetyltransferase and are resistant to chloramphenicol[100]. Rare isolates of *H. influenzae* resistant to ofloxacin, ciprofloxacin and lomefloxacin in patients with recurrent respiratory infection have been noted in Europe, Asia and the USA[101].

The activity of macrolides is intrinsically low against *H. influenzae*. A survey of resistance was carried out in ten European countries, namely Slovakia, France, Germany, Great Britain, Hungary, the Republic of Ireland, Italy, The Netherlands, Portugal and Spain. Respiratory samples were collected from 4297 patients with lower respiratory tract infections and cultured for the presence of *S. pneumoniae*, *H. influenzae* and *M. catarrhalis*. Almost all of the strains of *H. influenzae* tested were resistant to erythromycin, (MIC$_{50}$ > or = 4 mg/l)[102].

M. catarrhalis

Many strains of *M. catarrhalis* produce β-lactamase and are resistant to several β-lactam antibiotics. In 1993, penicillin and amoxicillin resistance was more prevalent in the USA than in Europe[103]. All penicillin-resistant strains isolated in the USA exhibited β-lactamase activity, whilst 8% of β-lactamase-negative strains isolated in Europe were also penicillin resistant. In the same year, almost all strains were highly susceptible to erythromycin, clarithromycin, azithromycin, doxycycline and co-trimoxazole.

In 1995, the overall rate of β-lactamase production in the United States was 95.3%[104]. When the NCCLS MIC interpretative breakpoints for *H. influenzae* were applied, percentages of strains found to be susceptible to selected oral antimicrobial agents were as follows: azithromycin, clarithromycin, and erythromycin, 100%; tetracycline and chloramphenicol, 100%; co-amoxiclav, 100%; cefixime, 99.3%; cefpodoxime, 99.0%; cefaclor, 99.4%; loracarbef, 99.0%; cefuroxime, 98.5%; cefprozil, 94.3%; and co-trimoxazole, 93.5%.

The Alexander Project, a multicentre surveillance study of the antimicrobial susceptibility of community-acquired lower respiratory tract bacterial pathogens collected from geographically separate centres in countries of the European Union, various states in the USA, Mexico, Brazil, Saudi Arabia, South Africa, Hong Kong and other European countries, found β-lactamase production in over 90% of *M. catarrhalis* isolates tested in 1996[97].

Fluoroquinolone resistance in *M. catarrhalis* isolates has been quite rare. However, several documented cases of fluoroquinolone-resistant *M. catarrhalis* clinical isolates present a warning that resistances can emerge in at-risk patients[105].

The increase in numbers of β-lactamase-producing strains of *M. catarrhalis* has been associated with increased failure rates of penicillins in eradication of respiratory infections. The pathogenicity of these organisms is apparent through their ability not only to survive penicillin therapy but also to protect penicillin-susceptible pathogens, such as *S. pneumoniae*, from these drugs[106].

Enterobacteriaceae

In the last few years, the number of isolated clinical strains from the *Enterobacteriaceae* family, mainly *Enterobacter* and *Klebsiella* spp. resistant to third generation cephalosporins and other β-lactams, has rapidly increased. They are probably even more prevalent than is currently recognized because of difficulties in their detection by the clinical microbiology laboratory. In addition, several outbreaks associated with these multiresistant strains have been reported[107]. The production of β-lactamases is the most frequent manifestation of β-lactam resistance. The class A extended-spectrum β-lactamases hydrolyse extended-spectrum β-lactams and are inhibited by clavulanic acid. The plasmid-mediated

cephalosporinases hydrolyse extended-spectrum cephalosporins and cephamycins and are not inhibited by clavulanic acid. They have been reported in Europe and in the United States. The carbapenemases noted among *Enterobacteriaceae* are either the chromosomally located penicillinases found in rare *Enterobacter cloacae* or *Serratia marcescens* isolates or the plasmid-mediated metalloenzyme IMP-1 that is widespread in Japan[108].

Extended-spectrum β-lactamase-producing *Enterobacteriaceae* acquisition depends on length of stay in the ICU and the use of invasive procedures. In fact, risk for acquiring extended-spectrum β-lactamase-producing *Enterobacteriaceae* (*K. pneumoniae* in most cases) increases during the ICU stay, from 4.2% in the first week to 24% in the fourth week[109]. Urinary catheterization and arterial catheterization are independent risk factors for acquiring extended-spectrum β-lactamase-producing *Enterobacteriaceae* and probably reflect frequency of health care manipulations.

Non-fermentative gram-negative bacilli

Non-fermentative gram-negative bacilli [*P. aeruginosa*, *Acinetobacter baumannii* (previously *Acinetobacter calcoaceticus*), *Stenotrophomonas maltophilia* (previously *Pseudomonas* and *Xanthomonas maltophilia*), and *Burkholderia cepacia* (previously *Pseudomonas cepacia*)] are of substantial concern because of their similar high intrinsic resistances to antibiotics. The basis for the high intrinsic resistance of these organisms is the lower outer-membrane permeability of these species, coupled with secondary resistance mechanisms such as an inducible cephalosporinase or antibiotic efflux pumps. The latter mechanism confers co-resistance to quinolones, which take advantage of low outer-membrane permeability. Even a small change in antibiotic susceptibility of these organisms can result in an increase in the MIC of a drug to a level that is greater than the clinically achievable level[110]. Resistance to antimicrobial agents is common among *P. aeruginosa* in ICU[111].

Pharmacokinetics and pharmacodynamics of antibiotics

The potential therapeutic efficacy of an antibiotic depends not only on its spectrum of action, but also on the concentration that it reaches in the bloodstream and in the site where the infection is developing. In patients with bacterial pneumonia, the site of infection is in the alveolar spaces or in the pulmonary interstitium. With the improvements in the technique of bronchoalveolar lavage (BAL) it has been possible to obtain samples from the alveolar lining and alveolar macrophages. The alveolar lining is considered an important site of extracellular infection in pneumonia, whereas macrophages are an important site in intracellular infections. The concentrations reached by antibiotics in these two distal sites should be excellent predictors of their clinical efficacy in the treatment of pneumonia[112]. However, the presence of a correlation between antibiotic levels in the site of infection and their clinical efficacy in the lung has not been clearly demonstrated due to numerous methodological difficulties[113]. For example, the pulmonary disposition of vancomycin remains low for most mechanically ventilated patients with MRSA pneumonia 24 h after the onset of treatment compared with the MIC for most gram-positive organisms, although the drug is effective[114]. Moreover, high peak serum concentrations of tobramycin, which could be toxic, are necessary to obtain microbiologically active concentrations at the alveolar level[115], but this aminoglycoside is active in nearly all cases of pneumonia elicited by gram-negative bacteria

There is now growing consensus on the opinion that neither blood nor tissue levels are of primary importance, and that the tissue/blood ratio is equally scarcely important. More important, instead, is the correlation between blood or tissue concentrations of the drug and the MIC values for the infectious agent[116].

The use of the ratio of C_{max} to MIC_{90} is one way to predict possible clinical activity with pharmacokinetic and microbiological determinants. However, a simple comparison of MIC values with the drug

Table 14.3. Pharmacokinetic and pharmacodynamic parameters correlating with antibacterial efficacy in animal infection models

Parameter	Drugs
Time above the MIC	Penicillins, cephalosporins, carbapenems, aztreonam, macrolides, and clindamycin
24-hour AUC/MIC	Aminoglycosides, fluoroquinolones, azithromycin, tetracyclines, and vancomycin
Peak/MIC	Aminoglycosides and fluoroquinolones

concentrations available in the patients' serum is not sufficient to calculate the potential clinical effect of the drug[117]. In fact, the MIC does not represent the pharmacodynamic properties of an antibiotic, e.g. its killing ability in vivo. Pharmacodynamics of antibiotics deals with time course of drug activity and mechanisms of action of drugs on bacteria (Table 14.3). Probably, time above MIC (T > MIC) is the most crucial consideration. In fact, the bactericidal activity of β-lactams such as cephalosporins is dependent upon the time that serum concentrations remain above the MIC of a given organism[118]. A significant linear correlation exists between T > MIC and time to eradication of bacteria from respiratory secretions[119]. The goal of a dosing regimen for antibiotics of this type is to maximize the time during which the organism is exposed to the drug, since the bactericidal activity correlates more to duration than to magnitude of dose[117]. Consequently, we might expect that concentrations above the MIC for the entire dosing interval should achieve optimal clinical results. However, the pharmacodynamic effects of subinhibitory concentrations of different β-lactam antibiotics may also contribute to the performance against several pathogens[120].

Nevertheless, several studies from Craig's laboratory using a number of bacterial strains with different antibiotic susceptibility and more than 50 different dosing regimens in mice, have allowed the elaboration of an interesting new concept[121–125]. The

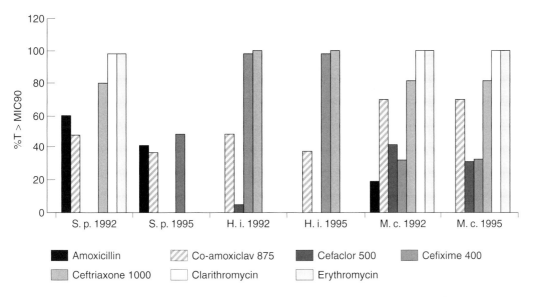

Fig. 14.2 The duration of time that serum concentrations of different antibiotics exceed MIC (%T > MIC$_{90}$) for *S. pneumoniae* (S.p.), *H. influenzae* (H.i.) and *M. catarrhalis* (M.c.): comparison between 1992 and 1995. Adapted from Drusano and Craig[126].

results of these studies showed that for β-lactam antibiotics, that have time-dependent killing and minimal-to-moderate post-antibiotic effect, an in vivo bacteriostatic effect was possible when levels were above the MIC for approximately 40% of the dosing interval, whereas maximum killing was approached when levels were above the MIC for 70% of the time. Therefore, the aim for a highly effective dosing regimen would be to provide levels above the MIC for at least 70% of the dosing interval[121]. This means that probably there are real differences amongst the β-lactam antibiotics in terms of how much coverage is needed to achieve static or fully bactericidal effect[126].

The duration of time that concentrations exceed MIC should be the pharmacodynamic parameter that best correlates with therapeutic efficacy of β-lactam antibiotics and, consequently, avoids resistance, although the abuse of drugs select resistant strains. This is an important remark because a rise in MIC values reduces the time above MIC when an antibiotic is used at the same dosing regimen (Fig. 14.2)[126,127].

The fluoroquinolones and aminoglycosides exhibit a concentration-dependent killing and prolonged post-antibiotic effect. The goal of a dose regimen for these classes of agents is to maximize the drug concentration. Thus, peak-MIC ratio and/or the area under the concentration-time curve (AUC) to MIC$_{90}$ (AUIC ratio) would be expected to be the major pharmacodynamic parameters correlating with efficacy for these drugs. In order to achieve optimal antibacterial efficacy, it has been documented that the AUIC ratio should be greater than 125 and peak-MIC ratio should be between 8 and 10[128].

We must stress that these are concepts and hard clinical evidence to substantiate them is not available. Consequently, the magnitude and duration by which concentrations must exceed the MIC remain controversial. In fact, papers that support the importance of the interrelationship between pharmacokinetics and pharmacodynamics in inducing a good clinical and bacteriological outcome are insufficient. Schentag et al.[120] reported a clear correlation between the length of time per day above the MIC and the time to eradicate the pathogen from the tracheal aspirate in intubated intensive care patients who were given cefmenoxime for nosocomial pneumonia. Correlations were also observed between the day of eradication and the length of time ciprofloxacin concentrations remained above the MIC[129]. Recently, Schentag et al.[128] have demonstrated that the achievement of minimally effective antibiotic action, consisting of an area under the inhibitory titre (AUIC) of at least 125, is associated with bacterial eradication in about 7 days for β-lactams and quinolones. Adding an aminoglycoside to β-lactams may produce a slight increase in their rate of bacterial killing in vivo, but because of their narrow therapeutic window, and the associated low doses in relation to MIC, there are situations in which the aminoglycosides may be unable to add sufficient additional AUIC.

Interaction between antibiotics and the host natural defences

The recovery from a bacterial infection requires the combined activity of host resistance and antimicrobial therapy. The ability of powerful antibiotics has improved the results of antimicrobial therapy, but host resistance is still the most important determinant of outcome.

A wide range of antibiotics administered in vivo or in vitro may modulate the host defence reaction elicited by pathogens: substantial data now exist on the direct or indirect effects of antibacterial agents on the immune system (Table 14.4). The synergistic interactions, which occur between the host immune system and antimicrobial agents, contribute to the successful outcome of antimicrobial chemotherapy[130]. Antibacterial agents can be classified into four groups: those that do not modify host defences (e.g. most β-lactams and chloramphenicol); those that depress immune functions in vitro and ex vivo (tetracyclines, aminoglycosides, sulphonamides, teicoplanin, and rifampicin); those that display synergy with the immune system (i.e. co-operate with the host antibacterial system, particularly as a result of intracellular penetration (macrolides and quinolones); and, finally, those that enhance

Table 14.4. Antibiotics and the host defence system

Antibiotic	Effect
Effects on human phagocyte motility	
Doxycycline	↓
Rifampicin	↓
Cotrimoxazole	↓
Effects on phagocyte oxidative burst	
Josamycin	↑
Rokitamycin	↓
Dirithromycin	↑
Effects on phagocytosis and bacterial killing by human phagocytes	
Tetracycline	↓
Sulfonamides	↓
Cefpimizole	↑
Cefotaxime	↑
Cefodizime	↑
Ceftriaxone	↑
Cefaclor	↑
Cefetamet	↑
Macrolides	↑
Effect on the specific immune system	
Cefotaxime	↑ IL-1
Cefodizime	↑ IL-1, IL-8, IFN-γ
	↓ IL-6, TNF-α
Cefaclor	↓ IL-6 and TNF-α
Cefetamet	↓ IL-6 and TNF-α
Ceftazidime	≈
Ceftriaxone	≈
Macrolides	↓ IL-2 and IL-5
Intracellular bioactivity	
Macrolides	↑

immune function in either healthy individuals or immunocompromised patients[131]. In vivo data seem to concur with the in vitro studies. Unfortunately, the contradictory nature of several in vitro observations and the small number of in vivo studies preclude any unequivocal conclusion regarding the role of antibiotics as potential immunomodulators in the treatment of inflammatory diseases.

By way of illustration, clinically relevant concentrations of most quinolones seem to have no direct

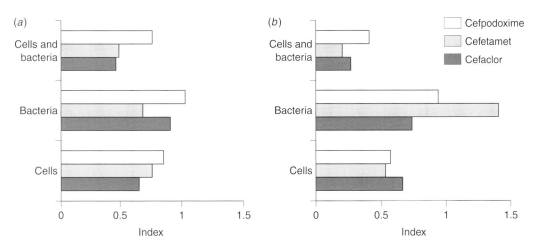

Fig. 14.3 Effects of preincubation with cefaclor, cefetamet and cefpodoxime on LTB$_4$ release from human granulocytes. (*a*); *E. coli* K12pANN5211. (*b*); *S. aureus* 121C. (Adapted from Scheffer and König[144].)

effect on isolated immune parameters such as phagocytic cell functions, lymphocyte proliferation, immunoglobulin production, IFN-γ secretion and bone marrow progenitor cell proliferation[132]. Nevertheless, synergistic phagocytosis and intracellular killing of *K. pneumoniae* is observed in the presence of macrophages and subinhibitory concentrations (one-half MIC) of pefloxacin. Pre-treatment of bacteria with pefloxacin leads to an increase in both bacterial uptake and microbicidal activity of phagocytes. Exposure of the macrophages to pefloxacin does not affect any phagocyte functions[133]. In contrast, the production of certain cytokines (IL-1, IL-2) and colony stimulating factors by stimulated lymphocytes and splenocytes is enhanced in the presence of clinically achievable concentrations of the drug[134], probably because they enhance IL-2 gene induction[135]. However, levofloxacin increases IL-2 production in a concentration-dependent manner with a significant increase at concentrations of 10 µg/ml or more and GM-CSG only at concentrations exceeding 50 µg/ml[136]. It is interesting to highlight that ciprofloxacin has a post-transcriptional differential effect on the production of IL-1α and IL-1β, reducing the total amount of IL-1β produced by LPS-stimulated human monocytes, while IL-1α is unaffected[137]. It also modulates IL-6 and IL-8 expression in a differentiated manner[138]. Moreover, it increases the concentrations of nuclear factor of activated T cells (NF-AT-1) and AP-1. Thus, ciprofloxacin interferes with regulative pathway common to several cytokines[139]

Among the β-lactam antibiotics, cephalosporins may modulate mediator release from various cells, e.g. basophils, mast cells, and polymorphonuclear neutrophils[139]. Whereas ceftriaxone and ceftazidime fail to show any modulatory effect on the release of inflammatory cytokines, cefodizime at the high concentrations of 200 µg/ml exerts a marked inhibitory activity on TNF-α release from human peripheral mononuclear cells[140]. At concentrations as low as 50–100 µg/ml, cefodizime inhibits the release of TNF-α and IL-6 and shows a significant stimulatory activity on IL-8 release[141]. Cefodizime also induces a significant dose-dependent increase in GM-CSF release from human bronchial epithelial cells[142]. Cefetamet and cefaclor decrease the secretion of IL-6 and TNF-α from human lymphocyte–monocyte–basophil suspension, but cefaclor does not alter the production of mRNA for IL-6 and TNF-α[143]. Moreover, cefetamet, cefpodoxime and cefaclor suppress the generation of LTB$_4$ from human neutrophil granulocytes (Fig. 14.3)[144]. LTB$_4$ is one of the most potent chemotactic factors for polymorpho-nuclear leukocytes.

Macrolides are a class of antibiotics taken up and concentrated by cells; consequently, they can reach intracellular concentrations far higher than those attained in the extracellular medium[145]. This property may alter the function of phagocytes, which are crucial for both antibacterial defence and inflammation. They are particularly attractive in the treatment of infectious asthma because they dose-dependently inhibit microvascular leakage and neutrophil recruitment induced by LPS[146]. A body of evidence highlights that macrolides may not only enhance the host defence system through increased cytokine synthesis by host cells, but also exhibit anti-inflammatory activity by including anti-inflammatory cytokines. Roche et al.[147] have shown that high concentrations (100 μg/ml) of erythromycin enhance extracellular IL-1 activity from human monocytes in vitro. Kita et al.[148] have shown that the administration of erythromycin to mice enhanced the production of IL-1 by macrophages and production of IL-2 and IL-4 by splenocytes. A 28-day treatment with roxithromycin induced an increased synthesis of IL-1 and TNF-α production by macrophages and the production of IL-2, IL-4 and IFN-γ by spenocytes[149], but a longer-term (for 42 days) administration inhibited both IL-1 and IL-2 production[150]. Erythromycin and clarithromycin have been reported to exert a suppressive effect on IL-6 expression in human bronchial epithelial cells[151]. This finding contrasts with the results of Bailly et al.[152] who showed that spiramycin and, to a lesser extent, erythromycin increased total IL-6 production without affecting IL-1 and IL-1β or TNF-α production, whereas roxithromycin had no effect. Moreover, erythromycin and clarithromycin, both 14-member macrolides, but not 16-member macrolide josamycin, have inhibitory effects on IL-8 expression in and suppress the release of IL-8 from normal and inflamed human bronchial epithelial cells[153]. Considering that IL-8 induces the migration of neutrophils to inflammatory sites, the impaired production and/or secretion of this cytokine may reduce neutrophil accumulation. Both 14-member and 16-member macrolides suppress the proliferative response of peripheral blood mononuclear cells stimulated by polyclonal T-cell mitogens and the IL-2 production by T-cells but not the expression of IL-2 receptor (CD25)[154]. An interesting study has shown that the incubation of the human bronchial epithelial cell cultures in the presence of 0.1–10 μg/ml erythromycin significantly blocked the H. influenzae endotoxin-induced release of IL-6, IL-8 and soluble intercellular adhesion molecule (sICAM)-1[155]. Moreover, pre-incubation with erythromycin prevented the endotoxin-induced expression of c-fos, c-jun, and NFkB, that are fundamental for the transcriptional regulation of TNF-α gene in monocytes[156].

It is unknown whether the efficacy of antimicrobial therapy can be improved by support of the impaired host resistance. The biological response-modifying activity of such drugs has not been proved to be of clinical significance except for the intracellular activity of those agents that have the ability to enter cells. The direct modification of immune responses is still a matter of debate; in fact, it remains difficult to relate the clinical situation to in vitro findings. However, it is likely that it is better to use antibiotics with immunomodulating activity for practical and timely treatment of patients with pneumonia, particularly those with diminished immune capacity or those who insidiously develop septic syndrome.

Treatment

Apart from antimicrobial therapy, management of pneumonias includes adequate hydration (oral or intravenous), maintenance of arterial blood gases with oxygen therapy or assisted ventilation. The antimicrobial treatment of pneumonia must always be early, prompt and, by necessity, empiric. Empiric therapy depends in part on the setting, epidemiological patterns in the hospital, and severity of illness. When choosing empirical treatments, clinicians should remember that clinical symptoms rarely predict the microbial etiology, antibiotic resis-

Table 14.5. Recommendations for initial empirical antibiotic treatment of CAP[158–161]

Country	Non-severely ill patient	Severely ill patient
France	Amoxicillin 1 g t.i.d or macrolide	Co-amoxiclav + (macrolide or fluoroquinolone) or third generation cephalosporin + (macrolide or fluoroquinolone)
Italy	β-lactam/β-lactamase inhibitor ± macrolide	Second/third generation cephalosporin ± macrolide
Spain	Procaine penicillin 1 200 000 U b.i.d or erythromycin (ethylsuccinate) 2–4 g/day	Third generation cephalosporin + erythromycin
Great Britain	Aminopenicillin (e.g. amoxicillin 500 mg t.i.d) or benzyl-penicillin (1.2 g q.i.d)	Erythromycin + second/third generation cephalosporin or ampicillin + flucloxacillin + erythromycin

tance is a worldwide problem and the route of administration may predict the response to therapy. Several other important points must be considered in designing treatment regimens. In fact, the initial antimicrobial regimen is important, the major pathogens include *S. pneumoniae*, *H. influenzae*, other aerobic gram-negative rods, and atypical pathogens, and copathogens may be present[157]. Assessment of therapy is essential after 2 or 3 days and the early and complete evaluation of all causes of failure is necessary, as failure of initial treatment is a factor for bad prognosis.

Guidelines or consensus statements for the administration of empirical antibiotic therapy have been developed by speciality society in many countries. They are available as a starting point for the selection of antimicrobial agents used for the treatment of CAP or HAP, although they have not been validated in randomized clinical trials. All statements stress that local epidemiological and susceptibility patterns should always be taken into account and that, ultimately, the physician is in the best position to determine the ideal antibiotic regimen for each patient.

Community-acquired pneumonia guidelines

Considering the guidelines on CAP of four European countries, Italy[158], France[159], Spain[160] and Great Britain[161], it is apparent that in all cases indications

are given for the management of two patient groups: severe and non-severe (Table 14.5). In particular, all the above guidelines suggest the use of a penicillin or a macrolide for non-severe patients. Although there is no universally accepted definition for severe CAP, some factors are certainly important. If one or more of the conditions listed in Table 14.6 are present, pneumonia is defined as severe. In this case, the guidelines differ in recommending a penicillin or an aminopenicillin, in suggesting single or combined use with a macrolide, and in the routine prescription of a β-lactamase inhibitor. Each document recommends the use of an association between a second or third generation cephalosporin and a macrolide in severe patients.

Although the scientific community has apparently accepted the above guidelines, there is widely differing antibiotic prescribing habits by general practitioners in Western Europe[162]. An analysis of the empirical prescribing behaviour of European clinicians in the treatment of CAP has shown that macrolides, aminopenicillins with or without clavulanic acid, and cephalosporins were the most commonly employed antibiotics, although the order with which they were prescribed varied greatly among different countries. Aminopenicillin was first or second choice in four out of seven nations. Cephalosporin use was very common in Germany and Southern Europe. In Italy, parenteral treatment with third generation cephalosporins or imipenem was the most

Table 14.6. Factors that allow the definition of CAP severity.

Respiratory rate >30 breaths min^{-1}

P$_a$O$_2$/FIO$_2$ ratio >250

Rapid radiographic worsening (≥50% increase in infiltrate size within 48 hours)

Bilateral or multilobar involvement

Shock

Need for vasopressors for more than 4 hours

Evidence of sepsis with organ dysfunction

Note:
Adapted from El-Ebiary[268]

common choice (almost 40% of cases). The differences in prescribing habits are certainly not attributable to guideline recommendations, nor can be explained by scientific reasoning, such as differences in aetiology, penicillin-resistant pneumococcus rate, pharmacokinetics, or safety, and are not linked with ecological or economical considerations. The differences are presumably multifactorial, and at least partly due to diversities in local health systems (for example, in the United Kingdom community-acquired patients are immediately admitted to hospital and not treated at home)[163] and the sources of information at the clinician's disposal. Local therapeutic traditions, marketing factors, and scientific rationale are probably equally important in the empirical choice of the treatment for CAP[164].

The North American guidelines for pneumonia are more articulate[165,166] including considerations on comorbidity, patient age, disease severity, need for hospitalization, and the selection of one or more appropriate antimicrobial agents (Fig. 14.4). Specifically, the Canadian guidelines[165] divide nonsevere patients into those aged <65 years without comorbidity, and those aged ≥ 65 years or with comorbidity. Among the former, macrolides are first choice antibiotics, followed by tetracyclines as second line treatment. In patients with comorbidity, second generation cephalosporins, a β-lactam/β-lactamase inhibitor combination, or cotrimoxazole

are recommended treatment choices. Macrolides may be added as an option to each of the above drugs. Severe patients require hospitalization and may be divided into those referred to a general ward or to an intensive care unit (Table 14.7). For the former, use of a second or third generation cephalosporin is suggested, with the addition of a macrolide as an option. For patients admitted to ICU, intravenous macrolide is recommended, with the possible addition of rifampicin and one or more anti-pseudomonas drugs, in view of the most commonly occurring pathogens in this setting. The American Thoracic Society (ATS)[166] recommendations are similar to the Canadian guidelines[165]. The major difference lies in taking 60 years as an age limit instead of 65, because American experts feel that patients over 60 years should not be treated outside the hospital since age becomes a co-morbidity factor in itself .

The North American guidelines[166] recommend erythromycin as first choice antibiotic in patients under 60 years of age treated at home, because of the vast experience accumulated in the use of this drug and its relatively low cost. However, approximately 40% of *H. influenzae* clinical isolates are resistant to erythromycin[167]. Moreover, gastrointestinal disturbances and pharmacological interactions following treatment with this drug are very common and there is a high risk of poor adherence to treatment due to significant side effects and need for frequent administrations (3–4 times daily).

In smokers and in patients needing wide-spectrum treatment, more recent macrolides, such as azithromycin and clarithromycin, should always be kept in mind, also considering the high probability of *H. influenzae* acting as causal pathogen[168]. In many patients, the clinical advantages and a reduced incidence of side effects counterbalance the greater cost of these macrolides. Both azithromycin and clarithromycin possess better pharmacokinetic profiles and more convenient administration schemes[169].

Even the very recent guidelines by the Infectious Diseases Society of America (Table 14.8)[170] suggest the empiric use of macrolides (erythromycin, cla-

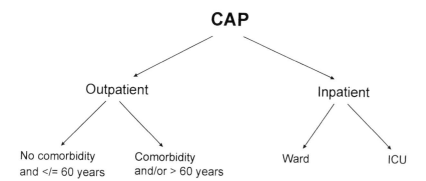

CAP

Outpatient

No comorbidity
and </= 60 years

Comorbidity
and/or > 60 years

Inpatient

Ward

ICU

Fig. 14.4 ATS patient categories for CAP. Appropriate placement of patient in specific division of outpatient or inpatient treatment should guide antimicrobial selection. (Adapted from Niederman et al. [166].)

rithromycin, and azithromycin), fluoroquinolones with high anti-*S. pneumoniae* activity (grepafloxacin, levofloxacin and trovafloxacin), or doxycillin in patients that do not require hospitalization (Table 14.9). Specifically, azithromycin and clarithromycin are to be preferred when *H. influenzae* infection is suspected. In hospitalized patients, macrolides must be associated with β-lactams, except when bronchiectasis is present, in which case it is preferable to add an anti-pseudomonas drug.

Currently available guidelines for the treatment of CAP are certainly useful, but their use has brought out new problems that must be evaluated with the utmost care. For example, the use of cephalosporins has increased considerably. This entails the risk of a selection of cephalosporin-resistant strains within hospital environments, such as vancomycin-resistant enterococci[171]. The British Thoracic Society[161] recommends the use of cefotaxime and cefuroxime in view of concerns regarding *S. pneumoniae* penicillin-resistant strains. However, the current resistance rate (MIC for penicillin > 0.1 mg/l) in England and Wales is as low as 3.8%[172] although regional variations are reported. Moreover, there is no solid proof that these levels of resistance are clinically relevant in pneumococcal pneumonia when adequate doses of penicillin are administered[173]. For this reason, Wort and Rogers[174] feel that

there is no need for cephalosporin use as first choice treatment in CAP, although local epidemiological considerations on penicillin resistance must be kept in mind. For many British clinicians, amoxicillin and ampicillin are still first choice oral treatment[175], with co-amoxiclav as an alternative for its greater activity towards *H. influenzae*. Intravenous penicillin is restricted to severe cases. Only if local resistance trends preclude such a line of treatment should parenteral cephalosporins be used. Because of the efficacy of β-lactam antibiotics in treating pneumococcal infections, there is no indication at this time that adding vancomycin to the therapeutic regimen would offer any further benefit for most patients.

The British approach, although scientifically correct, is not the most effective in clinical practice. It is likely that the 'Italian empirical model' according to which parenteral cephalosporins are first choice treatment in CAP is the best approach considering that the mortality rate for CAP in Italy is among the lowest in Europe[176]. In any case, the emerging trend in the United States is that parenteral treatment with a cephalosporin (primarily ceftriaxone, or, alternatively, ceftazidime or cefotaxime) outside the hospital setting is a valid, safe, and low cost alternative[177–179].

Antibiotics active towards intermediate resistance pneumococcus (MIC = 0.1–1 μg/ml) include high dose penicillin (12 million units daily), cefotaxime, and ceftriaxone[180]. Vancomycin is recommended for highly resistant strains (MIC > 2 μg/ml) Table 14.9). The above recommendations are supported by a recent study reporting that current rates of

Table 14.7. Treatment of severe CAP[a,b]

Macrolide + anti-Pseudomonas antibiotic

Third generation anti-Pseudomonas cephalosporin, imipenem, ciprofloxacin, aztreonam, anti-pseudomonas penicillin

Notes:
[a] If *Legionella* is identified, rifampin must be added.
[b] Due to the high mortality associated with *P. aeruginosa* pneumonia, an aminoglycoside should be added so as to obtain double coverage towards *Pseudomonas* (at least during the first few days of treatment) when using a third generation cephalosporin, imipenem or ciprofloxacin
Adapted from Mandel et al.[165]

S. pneumoniae intermediate resistance to penicillin and cephalosporins are not associated with an increase in mortality rate[181].

Certainly, considering the role of *C. pneumoniae* and its resistance to β-lactams, the addition of a macrolide must be kept in mind, unless laboratory data rapidly rules out involvement of this microorganism. Evidence is accumulating that new macrolides, such as clarithromycin, are superior to erythromycin, in terms of both antibiotic spectrum, and greater activity towards *C. pneumoniae*[182]. Several new fluoroquinolones possess a similar range of activity. Among these, grepafloxacin, levofloxacin, and sparfloxacin are the most promising. Specifically, levofloxacin has been shown particularly useful in infections caused by pneumococcus strains highly resistant to penicillin[183]. Should ongoing clinical trials and clinical practice demonstrate that these drugs are a valid monotherapy in CAP, it is likely that future guidelines will have to keep this class of drugs in due consideration[184].

A recent US study on elderly patients showed that the routine use of macrolides is not to be encouraged because only 7.5% of patients presented an organism needing macrolide treatment, and no mortality was present among these patients[185]. A true definition of the current frequency with which *C. pneumoniae* causes CAP is lacking. For this reason, Woodhead[186] has suggested that a random-

Table 14.8. Empirical antibiotic selection for patients with CAP according to the Infectious Diseases Society of America guidelines[170]

Non-hospitalized patients
  Generally preferred: macrolides[a], fluoroquinolones[b] or doxicycline
  Modifying factors:
    Suspected penicillin-resistant *Streptococcus pneumoniae*: fluorquinolones[b]
    Suspected aspiration: co-amoxiclav
    Young adult (>17–40 years): doxicycline

Hospitalized patients
  General Medicine Ward
    Generally preferred: β-lactams with or without macrolides[a], or fluorquinolones[b] (alone)
    Alternatives: cefuroxime with or without macrolides[a], or azithromycin (alone)

  Admitted to ICU for severe pneumonia
    Generally preferred: erythromycin, azithromycin or a fluorquinolone + cefotaxime, ceftriaxone or β-lactam/β-lactamase inhibitor[c]

  Modifying factors
    Structural lung disease: anti-pseudomonas penicillin, a carbapenemic, or cefepime + a macrolide[a] or a fluorquinolone[b] + an aminoglycoside
    Allergy to penicillin: a fluorquinolone with and without clindamycin
    Suspected aspiration: a fluorquinolone + clindamycin or metronidazole or β-lactam/β-lactamase inhibitor[c] (alone)

Notes:
[a] Azithromycin, clarithromycin or erythromycin.
[b] Levofloxacin, sparfloxacin, grepafloxacin, trovafloxacin, or other fluorquinolone highly active towards *S. pneumoniae*.
[c] Ampicillin/sulbactam, or ticarcillin/clavulanate or piperacillin/tazobactam (for structural lung disease, ticarcillin/clavulanate or piperacillin).

ized, comparative controlled study should be carried out to compare β-lactam alone with a β-lactam and a macrolide before recommending use of a macrolide in elderly patients with CAP.

During clinical trials, the presence of co-pathogens is a common occurrence. This suggests that *C.*

Table 14.9. Treatment of penicillin-resistant *Streptococcus pneumoniae*

MIC for penicillin	MIC for cephalosporins	Antibiotic
<2.0 μg/ml	—	Penicillin G
>2.0 μg/ml	<2.0 μg/ml	Ceftriaxone Cefotaxime
>2.0 μg/ml	>2.0 μg/ml	Vancomycin Imipenem

Notes:
MIC = Minimal inhibitory concentration.
Adapted from Anonymous[180].

pneumoniae may simply initiate pathological events, but a different pathogen is the true cause of pneumonia. Therefore, it is hardly surprising that treatment with an antibiotic ineffective towards *C. pneumoniae* is equally capable of obtaining clinical remission in approximately the same time span required following administration of an antibiotic presenting activity towards this atypical pathogen[187].

However, it may be supposed that co-infection with *C. pneumoniae* and other pathogens does have some effect on the course of pneumonia. In a recent study by Kauppinen et al.[188], three groups of patients with pneumonia were examined: those with *C. pneumoniae* infection, those with *S. pneumoniae* infection, and those with mixed infection. The authors report that, in the presence of *C. pneumoniae* infection alone, the clinical course was mostly mild, with a mean hospital stay of 8.4 days, although only 36% had received adequate antibiotic treatment for this infection. In the presence of *S. pneumoniae* infection, all patients had received adequate antibiotic treatment, and mean hospital stay was 10.5 days. However, when both pathogens were present and subjects were treated only for pneumococcus, the mean hospitalization reached 21.9 days. These data suggest a possible role for co-infection in determining increased pneumonia severity. Nevertheless, further confirmation is required before implementing routine treatment of atypical infections during pneumonia. Until these data are

available, macrolides should probably be used initially in severe patients only, particularly when infection with *Legionella* is suspected.

Unfortunately, therapeutic recommendations contained in guidelines often clash with factors affecting the total costs of treatment of pneumonia such as the need for hospitalization, attempts to reach an etiological diagnosis, the selection of empiric antibiotic therapy, time span needed for switching from parenteral therapy to oral treatment, and length of hospital stay. Moreover, the management habits of single clinicians, often reflecting local practices, must not be ignored and may equally substantially affect the total cost of treatment. For example, an interesting American study[189] has demonstrated that the use of medical procedures and consultations was more common for patients discharged from University Hospitals than from General Hospitals, causing an 11% increase in costs in the former hospitals. Similarly, costs were 15% greater in urban compared to rural hospitals. Internal medicine and lung disease clinicians made more use of diagnostic procedures, and were associated with greater expenses, than general practitioners. Notwithstanding the variability in procedure use and treatment expenses concerning CAP, there were no differences in mortality and in readmission rates.

One of the first and probably most important decisions concerning cost of treatment is not the choice of antibiotic, but rather the need for hospital admission. In fact, pneumonia is an important cause of hospital admission, but frequency varies greatly. This finding suggests the need for efficient and widely accepted predictive indexes for negative outcome. A large study involving over 50 000 patients identified valid criteria for predicting the outcome of CAP[190]. The predictive rule allots scores based on age and the presence of co-morbidity, abnormal physical examination (respiratory rate ≥ 30 or body temperature ≥ 40 °C), and laboratory findings (pH < 7.35, serum urea ≥ 30 mg/dl, or serum sodium < 130 mmol/l) on admission. Home treatment for class I patients (no risk factors), brief observation as inpatient for class II patients (score between 71 and 90), and hospital admission for class

IV (score between 91 and 130) and class V patients (score > 130) may significantly reduce the number of hospital admissions by approximately one third. However, the above scoring system seems to be too complex for use in routine clinical practice.

In hospitalized patients, the length of stay is a primary determinant of the management costs of pneumonia. Data from the National Healthcare Cost and Utilisation Project, of the National Ambulatory Medical Care Survey and the National Hospital Ambulatory Medical Care Survey were employed to determine the cost of treatment in patients aged 65 or over[191]. Figures soared to a total cost of 4.8 billion dollars for the treatment of patients aged over 65, and over 3.6 billion dollars for the treatment of patients aged under 65 years. The mean length of hospital stay was 7.8 days with a mean cost of $7166 for patients over 65, and 5.8 days with a mean cost of $6042 for younger patients.

Obviously, given the high cost of CAP requiring hospitalization, every treatment that allows home management may result in substantial savings, particularly among patients under 65 years of age.

One of the key elements determining length of hospital stay is the duration of parenteral treatment. Ehrenkranz et al.[192] reported a reduction in mean hospital stay by 2.4 days and an $884 reduction per patient/therapy when parenteral treatment was switched to oral treatment and the patient was discharged on the third day of hospitalization. In that study the disease severity indexes and the outcome following discharge were similar for those inpatients who had continued parenteral treatment and prolonged hospital stay. Generally, by cautiously applying specific criteria for the identification of candidates for switch therapy, most patients may be treated orally within three days from initiation of therapy (Table 14.10).

By altering the prescribing habits of hospital-based clinicians in CAP, it may be possible to lower costs with no significant increase in the risk of negative outcome. This finds proof in the study by Omidvari et al.[193]. The authors treated a group of patients with cefamandol 1 g intravenously every 6 hours for 7 days, and a second group with cefaman-

Table 14.10. Criteria used to identify candidates to switch from parenteral to oral treatment.

Improvement in cough

Improvement in respiratory distress

Absence of fever for > 24 hours

Absence of high risk for resistant pathogens, for example *S. aureus*

Absence of concomitant unstable medical disease

Absence of complications, for example congestive heart failure

Intact gastrointestinal absorbance

Improvement in leukocytosis

Note:
Adapted from Ramirez et al.[269], Fine et al.[270], and Ramirez[271].

dol (1 g intravenously every 6 hours for 2 days) followed by oral treatment with cefaclor (500 mg every 8 hours for 5 days). Between the two groups there was no difference in clinical course, remission rate, survival rate, and clearing of radiographic abnormalities. Average length of treatment (6.88 days for the conventional group compared to 7.30 days for the group with switch therapy), and the rate of overall symptom improvement (97% vs. 95%, respectively) was similar in both groups. Patients receiving early oral treatment required a shorter hospital stay (7.3 vs. 9.7 days), and overall expenses were lower ($2,953 vs. $5,002).

Nosocomial pneumonia guidelines

The aetiology of HAP is substantially different from that of CAP, and this explains the need for different guidelines. Gram-negative bacilli, including *P. aeruginosa*, *Klebsiella*, *Acinetobacter* species, *Enterobacter*, and gram-positive cocci such as *S. aureus* are common causes of nosocomial pneumonia[194,195]. Disease caused by these virulent pathogens is often severe and commonly complicated by pulmonary necrosis, multilobar involvement, micro-abscesses or empyema.

Guidelines on HAP are relatively scarce. Excepting US and Canadian guidelines, the only other national

Table 14.11. Organisms associated with nosocomial pneumonia and antibiotics recommended by the American Thoracic Society guidelines[197]

Group 1: Mild to moderate nosocomial pneumonia, no unusual risk factors, onset in any moment, or early onset severe nosocomial pneumonia

Key organisms	Key antibiotics
[a] Enteric gram-negative bacteria (non-Pseudomonas such as: *Enterobacter, Escherichia coli, Proteus, Klebsiella, Serratia marcescens, Haemophilus influenzae*	Cephalosporin (second or third generation, non-anti-Pseudomonas) or
	β-lactam/β-lactamase inhibitor or
[a] Methicillin susceptible *Staphylococcus aureus*	if allergic to penicillin, a fluorquinolone[b] or clindamycin +
[a] *Streptococcus pneumoniae*	aztreonam

Group 2: Mild to moderate nosocomial pneumonia with risk factors associated with specific additional organisms, onset in any moment

Risk factors	Key organisms + specific risk organisms	Key antibiotics + specific additional coverage
Abdominal surgery, aspiration	[a] Anaerobes	Clindamycin, or β-lactam/β-lactamase inhibitor
Coma, cranial trauma, diabetes, renal failure	[a] *S. aureus*	± vancomycin (until MRSA is not excluded)
High dose steroids	[a] *Legionella*	Erythromycin ± rifampin
Prolonged stay in Intensive Care, steroids, antibiotics, pulmonary disease	[a] *Pseudomonas aeruginosa*	Treat as severe nosocomial pneumonia (Group 3)

Group 3: Severe nosocomial pneumonia with risk factors, early onset, or severe nosocomial pneumonia, late onset

Key organisms	Antibiotics
[a] *Pseudomonas aeruginosa*	Aminoglycoside or ciprofloxacin, +
[a] *Acinetobacter* species	One of the following:
	anti-Pseudomonas penicillin,
	β-lactam/β-lactamase inhibitor
[a] Consider MRSA	and
	± vancomycin (if MRSA is a problem)

Notes:

[a] Recommended treatment does not include immunocompromised patients.

[b] If *S. pneumoniae* is not a problem.

MRSA = methicillin-resistant *S. aureus*.

recommendations have appeared in Australia, Sweden, and France[196]. However, due to the lack of useful data for the drawing up of guidelines based on clinical evidence, it is probably more appropriate to refer to these documents as consensus among experts rather than true guidelines.

Specifically, the ATS[197] recommends that antibiotic choice should take into account disease severity, length of hospital stay, and the presence of specific risk factors (Table 14.11). When pneumonia arises within 5 days from hospitalization, a β-lactam/β-lactamase inhibitor association or a second or third generation cephalosporin is recommended. When pneumonia arises later during hospital stay, it is imperative that antibiotics active against *P. aeruginosa* be used, such as the association between an aminoglycoside or a fluoroquinolone with a wide spectrum β-lactam. When anaerobic infection is present, clindamycin or a β-lactam/β-lactamase inhibitor association are suggested, whereas vancomycin is recommended when MRSA is suspected. Conversely, when *Legionella* infection is assumed, a macrolide should be used[198].

Clearly, the management of MRSA infection is limited by the small number of antibiotics with activity against these resistant strains. Vancomycin and teicoplanin are the only agents available with reliable activity against serious MRSA infections. Other agents, including doxycycline, fluoroquinolones, gentamicin, novobiocin, rifampin, and co-trimoxazole have been used to treat patients with MRSA in an ongoing effort to expand treatment options. However, physicians have less clinical experience with these agents, the efficacy of these agents is not always optimal, and resistance to these agents has developed[199].

Unfortunately, currently available guidelines do not suggest reliable alternatives, but rather consider risk factors and the severity of the disease, with little attention being brought to previously mentioned aspects.

It must be remembered that when using empirical antibiotic treatment in a hospital ward, unresponsive patients must be quickly identified and alternative treatment schemes must be available. Treatment may require modifications based on patient culture results and/or clinical response. The latter may be difficult to assess due to the variable course of nosocomial pneumonia, and is associated with host and bacterial factors, and the co-existence of other pathological processes.

Several studies demonstrate that all treatment approaches suggested by the different guidelines are ineffective in up to 30–40% of cases[200,201]. The presence of unresponsive pathogens is the main cause of treatment failures. These may be common pathogens that develop in unexpected environments or with unusual resistance patterns. The treatment failure is commonly observed in patients with prior antimicrobial therapy (with systemic administration of antibiotics), the late diagnosis of HAP resulting in the late onset of appropriate antibiotic therapy and/or the incorrect choice of antibiotic. In patients without satisfactory clinical outcome, the empiric therapeutic regimen rarely includes newer broad spectrum antimicrobial agents. In any case, many authors feel that two-drug regimens are insufficient to reduce the incidence of bacteria not covered by antibiotic therapy[202]. Presumably, only three-antibiotic regimens attain a high degree of efficacy, though carrying a higher cost and a heavier burden of side effects.

Future therapeutic options

The activity of antibiotics is diminishing by the increasing number of resistant strains and by the increase of infections with naturally resistant microorganisms. However, the rational use of antibiotics can slow this trend and perhaps reverse it. To reach this aim it is necessary to increase research activities in the field of pharmacodynamics in order to allow a more rational dosing.

Better technology documentation and statistics in microbiological diagnostics could improve calculated chemotherapy. Furthermore, we need more information about the epidemiology of resistant bacteria. The knowledge about receptors, mechanism of action and mechanism of resistance should help to elude these obstacles in antimicrobial chemotherapy. Therefore, future efforts to curtail antibiotic resistance will require a concerted effort in multiple areas, particularly enhanced epidemiological surveillance to better detect resistance trends, judicious use of antibiotics, and new drug development.

Unfortunately, it is probable that in the future we will have only a few new drugs due to the current demands for extensive preclinical and clinical documentation and the excessive costs involved in the development of a new chemical entity. While there is a need for continued development of new antibiotics, the growth of managed healthcare in the Western world is likely to have a significant impact on research and development activities. This is especially the case for compounds showing slight improvement over existing therapies.

In any case, with modern techniques of sequencing of the complete bacterial genus in order to find new targets, with combinatory chemistry and with the high throughput screening, some new drugs should be developed in the future. The research focusing on novel targets and on alternative approaches is most likely to yield breakthroughs against problem organisms in the future.

New antimicrobial agents

Screening of isolated biochemical targets and intact bacteria using high-throughput technologies, modifying existing compound classes to create more powerful compounds overcoming pathogen resistance, and introduction of completely new classes of antibiotics represent three areas that have been partially exploited in the past and continue to represent fertile fields for further investigation. In addition, a number of investigators are working to develop inhibitors of new bacterial targets and to develop inhibitors of genes relating to virulence or pathogenesis (Table 14.12)[203].

Development of novel 'classic' antimicrobial agents

New information on the binding of classical protein synthesis inhibitors to ribosomal RNA provides a rational explanation for their selective action against bacteria. It also explains why chromosomal point mutations conferring resistance by structural changes at the target site are relatively rare in the majority of bacteria.

The streptogramins are a class of antibiotics remarkable for their antibacterial activity and their unique mechanism of action[204,205]. These antibiotics are produced naturally, but the therapeutic use of

Table 14.12. Major areas of current research of novel antimicrobial agents.

Development of novel 'classic' antimicrobial agents	Streptogramins, ketolides, oxazolidinones, evernonomycins, cyclic thiazolyl peptide antibiotics
Chemical modification of currently known agents	Cephalosporins and carbacephalosporins bearing various thiazolylthio moieties at C-3, carbapenems bearing various thiazolylthio moieties at C-2, glycylcyclines, N-substituted derivatives of vancomycin, novel fluoroquinolones
Potentiators of known antimicrobials	Metallo-β-lactamases inhibitors, bacterial efflux pump inhibitors
Inhibitors of new targets	Inhibitors of aminoacyl-tRNA synthetases, inactivators of *FemA* or *FemX*, inhibitors of lipid A biosynthesis, natural toxins inhibiting bacterial topoisomerases, inhibitors of the protease or transpeptidase function
Antisense nucleotides	

Note:
Adapted from Moellering[203].

the natural compounds is limited because they do not dissolve in water. New semisynthetic derivatives, in particular the injectable streptogramin quinupristin/dalfopristin, offer promise for treating the rising number of infections that are caused by multiply resistant bacteria. The streptogramins consist of two structurally unrelated compounds, group A (dalfopristin) and group B (quinupristin). They inhibit bacterial growth by disrupting the translation of mRNA into protein. The natural streptogramins are produced as mixtures of the group A and B compounds, the combination of which is a more potent antibacterial agent than either type of compound alone. Whereas the type A or type B compound alone has, in vitro and in animal models of infection, a moderate bacteriostatic activity, the combination of the two has strong bacteriostatic activity and often bactericidal activity. MICs of quinupristin/dalfopristin range from 0.20 to 1 μg/ml for *S. pneumoniae*, from 0.25 to 2 μg/ml for *S. aureus* and from 0.50 to 4 μg/ml for *Enterococcus faecium*, the principal target organisms of this drug. Quinupristin/dalfopristin also has activity against mycoplasmas, *H. influenzae*, *Legionella* spp. and *M. catarrhalis*. It is the first antibiotic since vancomycin to offer potentially promising activity against MRSA.

Ketolides are derivatives of the 14-membered ring macrolides, in which a keto group at position 3 of the ring system replaces the L-cladinose moiety, which appears necessary for the induction of MLS_B resistance phenotype. Further modifications of the macrolactone backbone allowed us to obtain three different series of 9-oxime, 11,12-carbamate, and 11, 12-hydrazonocarbamate ketolides. These compounds are very active against penicillin/erythromycin-resistant pneumococci and non-inducers of MLS_B resistance. The 11,12-substituted ketolide 61 (HMR 3004) demonstrates a potent activity against multiresistant pneumococci associated with a well-balanced activity against all bacteria involved in respiratory infections including *H. influenzae*, *M. catarrhalis*, group A streptococci, and atypical bacteria. In addition, HMR 3004 displayed high therapeutic activity in animals infected by all major strains, irrespective of their resistance phenotype[206]. HMR 3647 is another ketolide. It is more active than HMR 3004 against *S. pneumoniae*[207]. ABT-773 is a novel ketolide derived from erythromycin. It is more potent in vitro than erythromycin and ciprofloxacin against *M. pneumoniae* and susceptible and multidrug resistant *S. pneumoniae*-208.

The oxazolidinones, such as eperezolid (formerly U-100592) and linezolid (formerly U-100766), are a new chemical class of synthetic antibacterial agents unrelated to any agent presently marketed that are active orally or intravenously against multidrug-resistant gram-positive bacteria. They possess a unique mechanism of bacterial protein synthesis inhibition. In fact, they inhibit the formation of the initiation complex in bacterial translation systems by preventing formation of the N-formylmethionyl-tRNA-ribosome-mRNA ternary complex[209]. There is a uniform susceptibility in sensitive bacteria independent of resistance to other antibiotics. The oxazolidinones have bacteriostatic activity against a number of important gram-positive pathogens including MRSA, penicillin-resistant *S. pneumoniae*, and vancomycin-resistant enterococci. They appear to be efficacious and well tolerated, both orally and parenterally, at doses which produce plasma concentrations in excess of the levels predicted to be necessary for efficacy[210].

Evernonomycins are chemically complicated oligosaccharides with molecular weights in the order of vancomycin. They are active against gram-positive bacteria, with slightly increased activity as compared to vancomycin. Ziracin (SCH27899) is an injectable everninomycin derivative with strong activity against glycopeptide-resistant enterococci, oxacillin-resistant staphylococci, and penicillin-resistant streptococci[211]. It is as effective as ceftriaxone in penicillin-resistant *S. pneumoniae* pneumonia[212].

Strain MJ347–81F4 has been found to produce two new cyclic thiazolyl peptide antibiotics, components A and B[213]. Taxonomic studies including morphological and physiological characteristics and chemical analysis of whole cells of the producing strain revealed this microorganism to belong to genus Amycolatopsis, and so the authors designated the strain *Amycolatopsis* spp. MJ347–81F4. After 10 to 12 days of fermentation, most of the antibacterial activity was present mainly in the mycelial cake and reached its maximum level. In comparison with reference compounds, A as the major component showed excellent in vitro activity against gram-positive bacteria including highly MRSA with MICs in the range of concentration of 0.006 to approximately 0.1 μg/ml. The results on the antimicrobial activity against thiazolyl peptide-resistant mutants of *Bacillus subtilis* NRRL B-558 indicated that the possible molecular target of MJ347–81F4 component A might be the 50S subunits of the ribosome, the inactivation of which would inhibit protein synthesis. Antibacterial agent, diperamycin has been produced in the culture broth of *Streptomyces griseoaurantiacus* MK393-AF2[214]. Various spectroscopic analyses of diperamycin suggest that it belongs to a member of cyclic hexadepsipeptide antibiotic. Diperamycin has potent inhibitory activity against various gram-positive bacteria including MRSA.

Chemical modification of currently known agents

Cephalosporins and carbacephalosporins bearing various thiazolylthio moieties at C-3 have been synthesized which show both in vitro antibacterial activity against MRSA and high affinity for PBP-2'[215]. RO-639141 and CP-6679 are promising agents. RO-639141, a pyrrolidinone-3-ylidenemethyl cephalosporin, induces a potent inhibition of PBP-2' through a high rate of acylation, a high affinity, and lower rate of deacylation, thus reversing all the factors that normally render this protein resistant to β-lactams[216]. CP-6679, a 3'-quaternary ammonium cephem with a fluoromethyl residue on the oxime group and an imidazothiazolium moiety at C-3 on the cephem nucleus, shows broad-spectrum activity that includes strains of MRSA and *P. aeruginosa*[217].

Carbapenems bearing various thiazolylthio moieties at C-2 also show potent in vitro and in vivo anti-MRSA activity and good affinity for PBP-2', demonstrating that the thiazolylthio moiety has an important role in improving the affinity for PBPO-2' and consequently the anti-MRSA activity of these drugs[215]. J-111225, J-114870, and J-114871 are novel carbapenems active against MRSA (Table 14.13) as well as gram-positive and gram-negative organisms including *P. aeruginosa*[218]. Studies on pharmacokinetic profile showed better plasma levels in rhesus monkeys and a greater stability to human DHP-1 compared to imipenem, indicating the potential of these compounds for use as a single agent in the treatment of bacterial infections in man [219]. The 1 β-

Table 14.13. In vitro anti-MRSA activities of J-111225, J-114870, and J-114871 in comparison to imipenem and vancomycin

Antibacterial agent	MIC$_{90}$ (µg/ml)
J-111225	4
J-114870	4
J-114871	4
imipenem	128
vancomycin	1

Note:
Adapted from Di Medugno and Felici[215].

methyl carbapenem antibiotics, BO-2727 and S-4661 are extremely active against *P. aeruginosa*. BO-2727 is a new injectable carbapenem antibiotic with broad-spectrum, potent antibacterial activity. It is four- to eight-fold more active in vitro than meropenem, imipenem and biapenem against MRSA. BO-2727 also shows superior activity against *P. aeruginosa*, and is two- to fourfold more active than imipenem against imipenem-resistant strains[220]. S-4661 is another promising new carbapenem for the treatment of infections caused by gram-positive and -negative bacteria, including penicillin-resistant *S. pneumoniae* and drug-resistant *P. aeruginosa*[221].

A new class of tetracyclines, named glycylcyclines, has been the subject of numerous reports[222]. The glycylcyclines are currently the only derivatives that exhibit antibacterial activity comparable to that of the early tetracyclines when they were first introduced. These compounds show potent activity against a broad spectrum of gram-positive and gram-negative bacteria, including strains that carry the two major tetracycline-resistance determinants, efflux and ribosomal protection. The spectrum of activity of the *N,N*-dimethylglycylamido derivative of minocycline and 6-demethyl-6-deoxytetracycline, two of the glycylcycline derivatives, includes organisms with resistance to antibiotics other than tetracyclines, e.g. methicillin-resistant *S. aureus*, penicillin-resistant *S. pneumoniae*, and vancomycin-resistant enterococci. The 9-*t*-butylglycylamido derivative of minocycline exhibited similar activity against MRSA, penicillin-resistant streptococci, and vancomycin-resistant enterococci, and activity against a wide diversity of gram-negative aerobic and anaerobic bacteria, most of which were less susceptible to tetracycline and minocycline[223].

The most rational approach to the chemical transformation of glycopeptides involves the modification of the internal 'binding pocket' and the peripheral regions of the molecule that participate in the stabilization of the antibiotic-target complex. Novel semisynthetic drugs of this group with enhanced antibacterial activities are now available. These new derivatives are particularly interesting because they do not appear to bind to the usual vancomycin target. Thus, they may have a unique mechanism of action. The enhanced antibacterial activities of N-substituted derivatives of vancomycin derive from the nature of the hydrophobic side chain, which can have a marked effect on dimerization and membrane binding[224]. A new glycopeptide antibiotic, LY333328, a semisynthetic N-alkyl derivative of LY264826, a naturally occurring structural analog of vancomycin, has improved in vitro activity over vancomycin and teicoplanin against a range of gram-positive organisms, including MRSA[225]. It is not only active against vancomycin resistant enterococci, but, in contrast to vancomycin, is also highly bactericidal. However, it is not yet clear whether VISA strains are also hit effectively or better by this new derivative, as compared to vancomycin.

Fluoroquinolones are antibacterial agents that attack DNA gyrase and topoisomerase IV on chromosomal DNA. The existence of two fluoroquinolone targets and stepwise accumulation of resistance suggested that new quinolones could be found that would require cells to obtain two topoisomerase mutations to display resistance. Compounds containing a C8-methoxyl group are particularly lethal, and incubation of wild-type cultures on agar containing C8-methoxyl fluoroquinolones produces no resistant mutant, whereas thousands arise during comparable treatment with control compounds lacking the C8 substituent[226].

Moxifloxacin, gatifloxacin, and clinafloxacin are three new quinolones that are currently undergoing clinical trials. Moxifloxacin is a new 8-methoxy-fluoroquinolone with broad-spectrum gram-positive and gram-negative activity. It is active against most *S. aureus* isolates tested ($MIC_{90} = 1$ µg/ml for ciprofloxacin-resistant isolates) and is little influenced by known mutations in the *grl* and *gyr* loci[227]. The new compound demonstrates bactericidal activity at concentrations 2, 4, 8 times the MIC against species commonly implicated in respiratory tract infections as well as viridans group streptococci. At a concentration of eight times the MIC[228], the frequency of spontaneous resistance ranged from 2.5×10^{-7} to $< 4 \times 10^{-8}$. Gatifloxacin, a novel 6-fluoro-8-methoxy quinolone, and clinafloxacin, another novel C8-substituted fluoroquinolone, have been shown active against multiresistant gram-positive species[229]. It has been suggested that moxifloxacin, gatifloxacin, and clinafloxacin are more active than ciprofloxacin against gram-positive cocci, probably because they carry an azabicyclo (moxifloxacin), 3-amino-pyrrolidinyl (clinafloxacin) or 3-methyl-piperazinyl (gatifloxacin) moiety at position C7[230]. Gemifloxacin and sitafloxacin are two other novel fluoroquinolones under development. Gemifloxacin is highly potent against *Streptococcus* spp. and retains high activity against strains of *S. pneumoniae* resistant to ciprofloxacin[231]. Moreover, gemifloxacin shows greatly improved potency against *Chlamydia* spp. compared to ciprofloxacin and either ofloxacin or levofloxacin[232]. The activity of sitafloxacin compares favourably with that of levofloxacin, trovafloxacin, clinafloxacin, gatifloxacin, and moxifloxacin against clinically important gram-negative pathogens[233] and is superior to that of the other quinolones against gram-positive cocci[234]. All these new quinolones have similar pharmacokinetic features to many earlier fluoroquinolones, including excellent oral bioavailability, moderate clearance and elimination half-lives, and volumes of distribution above 1.5 l/kg (Table 14.14)[235].

Table 14.14. Comparative pharmacokinetics and in vitro activity of novel fluoroquinolones against *S. pneumoniae*

Agent	Oral dose (mg)	AUC0–24 (mg/l h)	C_{max} (mg/l)	*S. pneumoniae* MIC_{90} (mg/l)
Clinafloxacin	200 bd	45	2.8	0.06
Moxifloxacin	400 od	34	3.2	0.12
Gatifloxacin	400 od	30	3.4	0.5
Gemifloxacin	600 od	24.4	3.8	0.03

Potentiators of known antimicrobials

Attempts are currently under way to find inhibitors of class I chromosomal β-lactamases, to discover specific inhibitors of tetracycline efflux systems, and to develop compounds that thwart the function of efflux pumps that lead to multiple resistance in organisms such as *P. aeruginosa* and other bacteria. Effective inhibition of AmpC cephalosporinases are to be found among the penems and monobactams, but none of these has yet proved suitable for pharmaceutical development[236]. BRL 42715, novel penem inhibitor, enhances the activity of the β-lactams for strains that constitutively expressed class I β-lactamase[237]. The penicillanic acid sulfone Ro 48–1220 inhibits class I chromosomal β-lactamases at lower concentrations than tazobactam[238]. Several inhibitors of carbapenem-idrolysing metallo-β-lactamases such as LL-10G568α, J-111225, some trifluoromethyl alcohol and ketone derivatives of L- and D-alanine, biphenyltetrazoles, and mercaptoacetic acid thiol esters, are in preclinical study[215]. However, none of these inhibitors has broad-spectrum activity against all known metallo-β-lactamases. Ro 07–3149 inhibits the tetracycline efflux pump without affecting the energy state, and exhibits very low antibacterial activity but shows weak synergy with tetracycline[239]. The development of compounds that thwart the function of efflux pumps and lead to multiple resistance in *P. aeruginosa* is very difficult because a tripartite efflux pump is necessary for the efflux of all substrate antibiotics[240].

Moreover, the intrinsic resistance of *P. aeruginosa* to most of the β-lactams is due to the interplay of both chromosomal β-lactamase and the MexAB-OprM efflux system[241]. Bacterial efflux pump inhibitors have been discovered, but their properties as revealed to date are not sufficiently attractive to warrant development[242].

Inhibitors of new targets

An alternative approach to the problem of emerging resistance to current antibiotics is to seek structural novel antibiotics that inhibit new molecular targets involved in bacterial growth or in bacterial infection[243].

Apart from isoleucyl-tRNA synthetase, bacteria contain additional aminoacyl-tRNA synthetases required for ligation of other amino acids to tRNAs. Therefore, these essential enzymes are attractive targets for new antibacterial agents[244]. A series of novel thiazoles, that has been prepared and evaluated for their inhibitory activity against aminoacyl-tRNA synthetases, displayed potent and selective enzyme activity against both gram-positive and gram-negative bacteria[245].

The formation of the *S. aureus* peptidoglycan pentaglycine interpeptide chain needs *FemX*, *FemA* and *FemB* for the incorporation of glycines Gly2–Gly3, and Gly4–Gly5, respectively. The complete pentaglycine interpeptide bridge is important for the sensitivity against β-lactam antibiotics and for the undisturbed activity of the staphylococcal cell wall synthesizing and hydrolysing enzymes. The drastic loss of β-lactam resistance after inactivation of *FemA* or partial impairment of *FemX* even beyond the level of the sensitive wild-type strains renders these proteins attractive anti-staphylococcal targets[246].

One obstacle to developing new drugs against gram-negative bacteria is their outer membrane, which acts as a very efficient permeability barrier. The outer leaflet of the outer membrane of gram-negative bacteria is composed mainly of lipopolysaccharides (LPS). Lipid A is the active component of LPS endotoxins responsible for the stimulation of immune cells[247]. Accordingly, inhibitors of lipid A biosynthesis should be bactericidal against most types of gram-negative bacteria, should increase the sensitivity of these bacteria to other antibiotics, and decrease the inflammatory response associated with sepsis by decreasing lipid A production. These features make lipid A a remarkable target for the discovery of new antibiotics. By enhancing outer membrane permeability to small molecules, anti-lipid A antibiotics should act synergistically with other available antibiotics, including some that are currently not used to treat gram-negative infections. Another advantage of anti-lipid A antibiotics is that their activity will be limited to certain major classes of gram-negative bacteria. This feature should preserve colonization resistance and reduce the selective pressure that often results in emergence of multidrug-resistant microorganisms such as vancomycin-resistant *Enterococcus*[248].

Promising candidates for development into clinically useful antibiotics also include natural toxins targeting bacterial topoisomerases, such as CcdB, microcin B17 and clerocidin[249,250]. They inhibit DNA replication, as do the currently available fluoroquinolones. These natural toxins target different domains of the *GyrA* and *GyrB* proteins compared with the quinolones, and no cross-resistance with quinolones has been observed.

There are several opportunities to target infection processes. For example, adherence is a potential multi-site target for antibiotic therapeutic development. The strategy behind the development of this new class of antibiotics is not intended to kill the pathogen but remove it from the host by allowing physical mechanisms and innate immunity to clear the organisms. One virulence factor of a pathogen is the ability to express adherence proteins/factors on the cell surface. Gram-negative bacteria assemble a variety of adhesive organelles on their surface, including the thread-like structures known as pili[251]. Pilus biogenesis is essential for bacterial pathogenesis, as in many cases the initial interaction between the pathogen and host occurs via the pilus. Two highly conserved proteins are essential for the production of pili: the periplasmic chaperone and the molecular usher. Molecular chaperones are currently defined as proteins that assist the non-covalent assembly/disassembly of protein-containing structures but are not normal components of these structures[252]. The usher forms a pore in the outer membrane through which the pilins are believed to pass as the pilus grows[253]. Small-molecule inhibitors of the periplasmic chaperone that block any of the functions along the biogenesis pathway would result in the production of 'bald' bacteria that would be unable to adhere to host tissues. Inhibitors of molecular usher function would be expected to block the polymerization of pilin subunits into functional pili. The chaperone–subunit complexes would remain trapped in the periplasm with no way across the outer membrane to the cell surface. Again, this is not expected to be lethal[254].

It is also possible to interfere with gram-positive surface protein expression pathway. Surface proteins of gram-positive organisms generally fulfil one of two roles in pathogenesis: either modifying the host immune response or directing adherence to host tissues[255]. It has been demonstrated in many laboratories that blocking such activities allows the host to repel the invading organisms. Inhibitors of the pathway, protease or transpeptidase function, will result in release of proteins from the cell and prevent adherence to host tissues. Moreover, the inability to anchor essential proteins to the cell wall will leave pathogenic microorganisms 'exposed' to the immune system and subject to mechanical forces that dislodge particulate matter from mucosal surfaces[252].

Antisense nucleotides

Antisense antinucleotides are an attractive concept because these small oligonucleotides could bind to and inactivate critical segments of DNA or RNA and this inactivation could severely cripple or kill bacterial cells. Unfortunately, attempts to produce antisense antinucleotides for use as antimicrobial agents has proven difficult because of problems such as non-specific binding and chemical and metabolic instability, and major problems in delivering intact oligonucleotides to intracellular targets[203]. In the past few years, the genome sequences of seven pathogenic bacterial species have been published and, in the near future, the complete sequence information of the genomes of a further 30 bacterial pathogens is likely to become available. The availability of whole bacterial genome sequences will provide a basis for new approaches to therapy of infectious diseases[256].

Endotoxin antagonists

The lipid As from the non-pathogenic bacteria *Rhodobacter capsulatus*, and *Rhodobacter sphaeroides*, have greatly attenuated toxicity and can block the activity of more agonistic endotoxins. The lipid A analogs E5531 and E5564, that elicit effects on phospholipid membranes that are different from those of lipid A[257], can antagonize the action of LPS in vitro and suppress the pathological effects of LPS in vivo in mice[258]. The bactericidal/permeability-increasing protein (BPI) of neutrophils, a superior lipid A-binding agent[259], is another endotoxin antagonist. It is currently undergoing clinical trials. It has both endotoxin-neutralizing activity and the ability to kill a variety of gram-negative bacilli. Several other basic peptides and lipid A-binding proteins are also being investigated as endotoxin-blocking agents, but they are at earlier stages of development[260,261].

Cytokines as immunoadjuvants in the treatment of pneumonia

The emergence of organisms with high-level antibiotic resistance patterns, in conjunction with a greater number of immunosuppressed patients at risk for infection, has made the treatment of pneumonia harder. Of more concern is the fact that poor outcomes often occur in the treatment of patients infected with organisms that are sensitive to the antibiotics used. Our understanding of the role of cytokines in lung host defence has greatly expanded over the past decade, with the obvious goal being identification of specific cytokines that can be targeted for immunotherapy (either by selective augmentation or depletion). However, the exact clinical setting and mechanism by which to administer or inhibit cytokines has not yet been fully realized. Most previous approaches to immunotherapy have involved the systemic augmentation or neutralization of specific cytokines and/or cytokine receptors. Unfortunately, significant dose-limiting toxicity or specific immune effects that are undesirable often complicate this form of immunotherapy when they occur systemically. This is especially true for the systemic administration of cytokines such as TNF-α, IL-2, and IL-12[262]. Therefore, in instances where the disease process is focal, local, and compartmentalized, delivery of specific immunotherapy is the most rational approach to treatment.

In order to avoid the complications of toxicity which are associated with the intravenous administration of cytokines such as TNF, IL-2 and IL-12, researchers are investigating the local, compartmentalized delivery of specific cytokines as a rational approach to the treatment of focal diseases such as pneumonia. This approach has been demonstrated to be of therapeutic utility in animal models of bacterial pulmonary infections. Greenberger et al.[263] have demonstrated that intratracheal delivery of an adenoviral vector expressing the pro-inflammatory cytokine IL-12 enhanced both bacterial clearance and survival in mice challenged with *K. pneumoniae*. Lei et al.[264] have investigated the treatment of pneumonia by adenovirus-mediated delivery of murine IFN-γ, a critical cytokine in pulmonary host defences against both intracellular and extracellular pathogens. After intratracheal inoculation in rats, prolonged expression of functional IFN-γ in vivo was demonstrated by enhanced host defences against *P. aeruginosa* and *K. pneumoniae*. Transfer of the IFN-γ gene has also been employed by this group in an attempt to enhance cell-mediated immunity against tuberculosis. In this setting, adenovirus-mediated delivery of the murine IFN gene resulted in a significant inhibition in the growth of *M. tuberculosis* in mice given a low-dose aerosol challenge with the organism.

Human trials are now underway to examine the effect of r-met HuG-CSF (filgrastim) as an adjuvant in the treatment of severe bacterial pneumonia and sepsis. Filgrastim is a human G-CSF produced by recombinant DNA technology by *E. coli* transformed with the human G-CSF gene. Although filgrastim has an amino acid sequence identical to the sequence predicted from analysis of the human gene, there is an N-terminal methionine [met] required for expression in *E. coli*. An open-label Phase I trial involving 30 patients with severe community-acquired pneumonia indicates that the subcutaneous administration of r-met HuG-CSF 75–600μg/day for 10 days, in combination with antibiotics, is well-tolerated, despite induction of significant peripheral neutrophilia[265]. However, no apparent dose-response effect of filgrastim on several pneumonia clinical variables, such as days of fever, duration of antibiotics, hospitalization days, or gas exchange was observed. In another study[266], filgrastim (300 μg/day up to 10 days) as an adjunct to antibiotics for hospitalized patients with CAP increased blood neutrophils threefold, but time to resolution of morbidity, mortality, and length of hospitalization were not affected. Treatment, however, accelerated radiological improvement and appeared to reduce serious complications, e.g. empyema, adult respiratory distress syndrome, and disseminated intravascular coagulation. Filgrastim administration was safe and well tolerated in these patients.

REFERENCES

1 Morbidity & Mortality Weekly Report. Pneumonia and influenza death rates – United States. *MMWR* 1995; 44:535–537.

2 Bartlett JG, Breiman RF, Mandell LA, File TM. Community-acquired pneumonia in adults: guidelines for management. *Clin Infect Dis* 1998; 26:811–838.

3 Mandell LA, Marrie TJ, Niederman MS, and the Canadian Hospital-Acquired Pneumonia Consensus Conference Group. Initial antimicrobial treatment of hospital-acquired pneumonia in adults: a conference report. *Can J Infect Dis* 1993; 4: 317–321.

4 Fine MJ, Stone RA, Singer DE et al. Processes and outcomes of care for patients with community-acquired pneumonia results from the pneumonia patient outcomes research team (PORT). *Cohort Study Arch Intern Med* 1999;159:970–980.

5 File TM Jr., Tan JS. Incidence, etiologic pathogens, and diagnostic testing of community-acquired pneumonia. *Curr Opin Pulm Med* 1997; 3:89–97.

6 Ruben FL. Viral pneumonias. The increasing importance of a high index of suspicion. *Postgrad Med* 1993; 93:57–60.

7 Lieberman D, Lieberman D, Porath A. Seasonal variation in community-acquired pneumonia. *Eur Respir J* 1996; 9:2630–2634.

8 Krech T, Wegmann T, Martin H, Hatz C, Sonnabend W. Die Atiologie atypischer Pneumonien. Eine serologische Studie an 1494 Patienten. *Schweiz Med Wochenschr* 1986; 116:2–7.

9 Greenberg SB. Viral pneumonia. *Infect Dis Clin North Am* 1991; 5:603–621.

10 Marrie TJ. Community-acquired pneumonia. *Clin Infect Dis* 1994; 18:501–513.

11 Bartlett JG, Mundy LM. Community-acquired pneumonia. *N Engl J Med* 1995; 333:1618–1624.

12 Mandell LA. Community-acquired pneumonia. Etiology, epidemiology and treatment. *Chest* 1995; 108:35S–42S.

13 Forgie IM, Campbell H, Lloyd-Evans N et al. Etiology of acute lower respiratory tract infections in children in a rural community in The Gambia. *Pediatr Infect Dis J* 1992;11:466–473.

14 Nathan EA. A report on pneumonia at the Premier Diamond Mine. *Transvaal Med J* 1907; 2:154–159.

15 Hedlund J, Kalin M, Ortqvist A. Recurrence of pneumonia in middle-aged and elderly adults after hospital-treated pneumonia: aetiology and predisposing conditions. *Scand J Infect Dis* 1997; 29:387–392.

16 Klein JO. Role of nontypeable *Haemophilus influenzae* in pediatric respiratory tract infections. *Pediatr Infect Dis J* 1997; 16 (2 Suppl):S5–S8.

17 Moxon ER, Wilson R. The role of *Haemophilus influenzae* in the pathogenesis of pneumonia. *Rev Infect Dis* 1991; 13 (Suppl 6):S518–S527.

18 Claesson BA, Leinonen M. *Moraxella catarrhalis* – an uncommon cause of community-acquired pneumonia in Swedish children. *Scand J Infect Dis* 1994; 26:399–402.

19 Woodhead MA, Macfarlane JT. *Haemophilus influenzae* pneumonia in previously fit adults. *Eur J Respir Dis* 1987; 70:218–220.

20 Heiskanen-Kosma T, Korppi M, Jokinen C et al. Etiology of

childhood pneumonia: serologic results of a prospective, population-based study. *Pediatr Infect Dis J* 1998; 17:986–991.

21 Woodhead MA. Pneumonia in the elderly. *J Antimicrob Chemother* 1994; 34 (Suppl A):85–92.

22 Lieberman D, Schlaeffer F, Porath A. Community-acquired pneumonia in old age. *Age Ageing* 1997; 26:69–75.

23 Murray HW, Masur H, Senterfit LB, Roberts RB. The protean manifestations of *Mycoplasma pneumoniae* infection in adults. *Am J Med* 1975; 58:229–242.

24 Kauppinen MT, Herva E, Kujala P, Leinonen M, Saikku P, Syrjala H. The etiology of community-acquired pneumonia among hospitalized patients during a *Chlamydia pneumoniae* epidemic in Finland. *J Infect Dis* 1995; 172:1330–1335.

25 Kauppinen MT, Saikku P, Kujala P, Herva E, Syrjala H. Clinical picture of community-acquired *Chlamydia pneumoniae* pneumonia requiring hospital treatment: a comparison between chlamydial and pneumococcal pneumonia. *Thorax* 1996; 51:185–189.

26 Bozzoni M, Radice L, Frosi A, Vezzoli S, Cuboni A, Vezzoli F. Prevalence of pneumonia due to Legionella pneumophila and *Mycoplasma pneumoniae* in a population admitted to a department of internal medicine. *Respiration* 1995; 62:331–235.

27 Janssens JP, Gauthey L, Herrmann F, Tkatch L, Michel JP. Community-acquired pneumonia in older patients. *J Am Geriatr Soc* 1996; 44:539–544.

28 Garb JL, Brown RB, Garb JR, Tuthill RW. Differences in etiology of pneumonias in nursing home and community patients. *JAMA* 1978; 240:2169–2172.

29 Fernandez-Sola J, Junque A, Estruch R, Monforte R, Torres A, Urbano-Marquez A. High alcohol intake as a risk and prognostic factor for community-acquired pneumonia. *Arch Intern Med* 1995; 155:1649–1654.

30 Venkatesan P, Gladman J, Macfarlane JT et al. A hospital study of community acquired pneumonia in the elderly. *Thorax* 1990; 45:254–258.

31 Bartlett JG. Anaerobic bacterial infections of the lung and pleural space. *Clin Infect Dis* 1993; 16 (Suppl 4):S248-S255.

32 Scannapieco FA, Mylotte JM. Relationships between periodontal disease and bacterial pneumonia. *J Periodontol* 1996; 67 (10 Suppl):1114–1122.

33 Lode H. Microbiological and clinical aspects of aspiration pneumonia. *J Antimicrob Chemother* 1988; 21 (Suppl C):83–90.

34 Mundy LM, Auwaerter PG, Oldach D et al. Community-acquired pneumonia: impact of immune status. *Am J Respir Crit Care Med* 1995; 152:1309–1315.

35 Leeper KV Jr. Severe community-acquired pneumonia. *Semin Respir Infect* 1996; 11:96–108.

36 Neill AM, Martin IR, Weir R et al. Community acquired pneumonia: aetiology and usefulness of severity criteria on admission. *Thorax* 1996; 51:1010–1016.

37 Gomez J, Banos V, Ruiz Gomez J et al. Prospective study of epidemiology and prognostic factors in community-acquired pneumonia. *Eur J Clin Microbiol Infect Dis* 1996;15:556–560.

38 Lieberman D, Schlaeffer F, Boldur I et al. Multiple pathogens in adult patients admitted with community-acquired pneumonia: a one year prospective study of 346 consecutive patients. *Thorax* 1996; 51:179–184.

39 Ishida T, Hashimoto T, Arita M, Ito I, Osawa M. Etiology of community-acquired pneumonia in hospitalized patients: a 3-year prospective study in Japan. *Chest* 1998; 114:1588–1593.

40 Marrie TJ. Epidemiology of mild pneumonia. *Semin Respir Infect* 1998; 13:3–7.

41 Puren AJ, Feldman C, Savage N, Becker PJ, Smith C. Patterns of cytokine expression in community-acquired pneumonia. *Chest* 1995; 107:1342–1349.

42 Feldman C, Ross S, Mahomed AG, Omar J, Smith C. The aetiology of severe community-acquired pneumonia and its impact on initial, empiric, antimicrobial chemotherapy. *Respir Med* 1995; 86:187–192.

43 Moine P, Vercken JB, Chevret S, Chastang C, Gajdos P. Severe community-acquired pneumonia etiology, epidemiology, and prognostic factors. French Study Group for Community-Acquired Pneumonia in the Intensive Care Unit. *Chest* 1994; 105:1487–1495.

44 Rello J, Quintana E, Ausina V, Net A, Prats G. A Three year study of severe community-acquired pneumonia with emphasis on outcome. *Chest* 1993; 103:232-235.

45 Marston BJ, Lipman HB, Breiman RF. Surveillance for Legionnaires' disease. *Arch Intern Med* 1994; 154:2417–2424.

46 Johanson WG Jr, Pierce AK, Sanford JP, Thomas GD. Nosocomial respiratory infections with gram-negative bacilli. The significance of colonization of the respiratory tract. *Ann Intern Med* 1972 77:701–706.

47 Craven DE, Driks MR. Pneumonia in the intubated patient. *Semin Respir Infect* 1987; 2:20–33.

48 Craven DE, Steger KA, Barber TW. Preventing nosocomial pneumonia: state of the art and perspectives for the 1990s. *Am J Med* 1991; 91 (Suppl 3B):44S-53S.

49 Torres A, Puig de la Bellacasa J, Xaubet A et al. Diagnostic value of quantitative cultures of bronchoalveolar lavage and telescoping plugged catheters in mechanically ventilated patients with bacterial pneumonia. *Am Rev Respir Dis* 1989; 140:306–310.

50 Rouby JJ, Martin De Lassale E, Poete P et al. Nosocomial bronchopneumonia in the critically ill: Histologic and bacteriologic aspects. *Am Rev Respir Dis* 1992; 146:1059–1066.

51 Schleupner CJ, Cobb DK. A study of the etiologies and treatment of nosocomial pneumonia in a community-based teaching hospital. *Infect Control Hosp Epidemiol* 1992; 13:515–525.

52 Prod'hom G, Leuenberger P, Koerfer J et al. Nosocomial pneumonia in mechanically ventilated patients receiving antacid, ranitidine, or sucralfate as prophylaxis for stress ulcer: A randomized controlled trial. *Ann Intern Med* 1994; 120:653–662.

53 Niederman MS. Gram-negative colonization of the respiratory tract:Pathogenesis and clinical consequences. *Semin Respir Infect* 1990; 5:173–181.

54 Rello J, Ausina V, Ricart M, Castella J, Prats G. Impact of previous antimicrobial therapy on the etiology and outcome of ventilator associated pneumonia. *Chest* 1993; 104:1230–1235.

55 Rodriguez de Castro F, Sole Violan J, Lafarga Capuz B et al. Reliability of the bronchoscopic protected catheter brush in the diagnosis of pneumonia in mechanically ventilated patients. *Crit Care Med* 1991; 19:171–175.

56 Pugin J, Auckenthaler R, Mili N, Janssens JP, Lew PD, Suter PM. Diagnosis of ventilator-associated pneumonia by bacteriologic analysis of bronchoscopic and nonbronchoscopic 'blind' bronchoalveolar lavage fluid. *Am Rev Respir Dis* 1991; 143:1121–1129.

57 Jimenez P, Torres A, Rodriguez-Roisin R et al. Incidence and etiology of pneumonia acquired during mechanical ventilation. *Crit Care Med* 1989; 17:882–885.

58 Inglis TJ, Sproat LJ, Hawkey PM, Gibson JS. Staphylococcal pneumonia in ventilated patients: a twelve-month review of cases in an intensive care unit. *J Hosp Infect* 1993; 25:207–210.

59 Chastre J, Fagon JY, Soler P et al. Diagnosis of nosocomial bacterial pneumonia in intubated patients undergoing ventilation: comparison of the usefulness of bronchoalveolar lavage and the protected specimen brush. *Am J Med* 1988; 85:499–506.

60 Schaberg DR, Culver DH, Gaynes RP. Major trends in the microbial etiology of nosocomial infection. *Am J Med* 1991; 91 (Suppl 3B):72S-75S.

61 Centers for Disease Control and Prevention. Guideline for prevention of nosocomial pneumonia. *MMWR* 1997; 46:28–79.

62 Cohen ML, Broome CV, Paris AL, Martin WT, Allen JR. Fatal nosocomial Legionnaires' disease: Clinical and epidemiologic characteristics. *Ann Intern Med* 1979; 90:611–613.

63 Fiore AE, Butler JC, Emori TG, Gaynes RP Jr. A survey of methods to detect and control nosocomial Legionnaires' disease among hospitals participating in the National Nosocomial Infections Surveillance System. 35th Annual Meeting of the Infectious Diseases Society of America, San Francisco, 1997. Abstract No. 332..

64 Carratala J, Gudiol F, Pallares R, Dorca J, Verdaguer R, Ariza J, Manresa F. Risk factors for nosocomial *Legionella pneumophila* pneumonia. *Am J Respir Crit Care Med* 1994; 149:625–629.

65 Marston BJ, Lipman HB, Breiman RF. Surveillance for Legionnaires' disease. Risk factors for morbidity and mortality. *Arch Intern Med* 1994; 154:2417–2422.

66 Meduri GU, Johanson WG Jr. International Consensus Conference: Clinical investigation of ventilator-associated pneumonia: Introduction. *Chest* 1992; 102 (Suppl 1):S551-S552.

67 Rello J, Torres A. Microbial causes of ventilator-associated pneumonia. *Semin Respir Infect* 1996; 11:24–31.

68 Ewig S, Torres A, El-Ebiary M et al. Bacterial colonization patterns in mechanically ventilated patients with traumatic and medical head injury. Incidence, risk factors, and association with ventilator-associated pneumonia. *Am J Respir Crit Care Med* 1999; 159:188–198.

69 Fagon JY, Chastre J, Domart Y et al. Nosocomial pneumonia in patients receiving continuous mechanical ventilation. Prospective analysis of 52 episodes with use of a protected specimen brush and quantitative culture techniques. *Am Rev Respir Dis* 1989; 139:877–884.

70 Torres A, Aznar R, Gatell JM et al. Incidence, risk, and prognosis factors of nosocomial pneumonia in mechanically ventilated patients. *Am Rev Respir Dis* 1990; 142:523–528.

71 Craven DE, Steger KA. Nosocomial pneumonia in mechanically ventilated adult patients: epidemiology and prevention in 1996. *Semin Respir Infect* 1996; 11:32–53.

72 Davies J. Origins and evolution of antibiotic resistance. *Microbiologia SEM* 1996; 12:9–16.

73 Cohen MT. Epidemiology of drug resistance: for a post-antimicrobial era. *Science* 1992; 257:1050–1055.

74 Goldstein FW, Garau J. 30 years of penicillin-resistant *S. pneumoniae*: myth or reality? *Lancet* 1997; 350:223–224.

75 CDC. Surveillance for penicillin-non-susceptible

Streptococcus pneumoniae – New York City. 1995. *JAMA* 1997; 277:1585–1586.

76   Kronenberger CB, Hoffman RE, Lezotte DC, Marine WM. Invasive penicillin-resistant pneumococcal infections: a prevalence and historical cohort study. *Emerg Infect Dis* 1996; 2:121–124.

77   Nava JM, Bella F, Garau J et al. Predictive factors for invasive disease due to penicillin-resistant *Streptococcus pneumoniae*: a population-based study. *Clin Infect Dis* 1994; 19:884–890.

78   Butler JC, Hofmann J, Cetron MS, Elliott JA, Facklam RR, Breiman RF. The continued emergence of drug-resistant *Streptococcus pneumoniae* in the United States: an update from the Centers for Disease Control and Prevention's Pneumococcal Sentinel Surveillance System. *J Infect Dis* 1996; 174:986–993.

79   Doern GV, Brueggemann A, Holley HP Jr, Rauch AM. Antimicrobial resistance of *Streptococcus pneumoniae* recovered from outpatients in the United States during the winter months of 1994 to 1995: results of a 30-center national surveillance study. *Antimicrob Agents Chemother* 1996; 40:1208–1213.

80   Simor AE, Louie M. The Canadian Bacterial Surveillance Network, Low DE. Canadian national survey of prevalence of antimicrobial resistance among clinical isolates of *Streptococcus pneumoniae*. *Antimicrob Agents Chemother* 1996; 40:2190–2193.

81   Collignon PJ, Bell JM. Drug-resistant *Streptococcus pneumoniae*: the beginning of the end for many antibiotics? Australian Group on Antimicrobial Resistance. *Med J Aust* 1996; 164:64–67.

82   Reichler MR, Rakovsky J, Sobotová A et al. Multiple antimicrobial resistance of pneumococci in children with otitis media, bacteremia, and meningitis in Slovakia. *J Infect Dis* 1995; 171:1491–1496.

83   Vaz Pato MV, Belo de Carvalho C, Tomasz A, the Multicenter Study Group. Antibiotic susceptibility of *Streptococcus pneumoniae* isolates in Portugal. A multicenter study between 1989 and 1993. *Microb Drug Resist* 1995; 1:59–69.

84   Aszkenasy OM, George RC, Begg NT. Pneumococcal bacteraemia and meningitis in England and Wales 1982 to 1992. *Commun Dis Rep CDR Rev* 1995; 5:R45-R50.

85   Weisblum B. Erythromycin resistance by ribosome modification. *Antimicrob Agents Chemother* 1995; 39:577–585.

86   Sutcliffe J, Tait-Kamradt A, Wondrack L. *Streptococcus pneumoniae* and *Streptococcus pyogenes* resistant to macrolides but sensitive to clindamycin: a common resis-

tance pattern mediated by an efflux system. *Antimicrob Agents Chemother* 1996; 40:1817–1824.

87   Lister PD. Multiply-resistant pneumococcus: therapeutic problems in the management of serious infection. *Eur J Clin Microbiol Infect Dis* 1995; 14 (Supp 1):18–25.

88   Panlilio AL, Culver DH, Gaynes RP et al. Methicillin-resistant *Staphylococcus aureus* in U.S. hospitals, 1975–1991. *Infect Control Hosp Epidemiol* 1992; 13:582–586.

89   Voss A, Milatovic D, Wallrauch-Schwarz C, Rosdahl VT, Braveny I. Methicillin-resistant *Staphylococcus aureus* in Europe. *Eur J Clin Microbiol Infect Dis* 1994 Jan;13(1):50–55.

90   Hashimoto H, Inoue M, Hayashi I. A survey of *Staphylococcus aureus* for typing and drug-resistance in various areas of Japan during 1992 and 1993 [Japanese]. *Jap J Antibiotics* 1994;47:618–26.

91   Pujol M, Corbella X, Pena C, Pallares R, Dorca J, Verdaguer R, Diaz-Prieto A, Ariza J, Gudiol F. Clinical and epidemiological findings in mechanically-ventilated patients with methicillin-resistant *Staphylococcus aureus* pneumonia. *Eur J Clin Microbiol Infect Dis* 1998; 17:622–628.

92   CDC. *Staphylococcus aureus* with reduced susceptibility to vancomycin – United States, 1997. *MMWR* 1997; 46:765–766.

93   Daum RS, Gupta S, Sabbagh R, Milewski WM. Characterization of *Staphylococcus aureus* isolates with decreased susceptibility to vancomycin and teicoplanin: isolation and purification of a constitutively produced protein associated with decreased susceptibility. *J Infect Dis* 1992; 166:1066–1072.

94   Hillery SJ, Reiss-Levy EA. Increasing ciprofloxacin resistance in MRSA. *Med J Aust* 1993; 158:861–863.

95   Hershow RC, Khayr WF, Schreckenberger PC. Ciprofloxacin resistance in methicillin-resistant *Staphylococcus aureus*: associated factors and resistance to other antibiotics. *Am J Ther* 1998; 5:213–220.

96   Gottlieb T, Mitchell D. The independent evolution of resistance to ciprofloxacin, rifampicin, and fusidic acid in methicillin-resistant *Staphylococcus aureus* in Australian teaching hospitals (1990–1995). Australian Group for Antimicrobial Resistance (AGAR). *J Antimicrob Chemother* 1998; 42:67–73.

97   Felmingham D, Washington J. Trends in the antimicrobial susceptibility of bacterial respiratory tract pathogens – findings of the Alexander Project 1992–1996. *J Chemother* 1999; 11 (Suppl 1):5–21.

98   Doern GV, Brueggemann AB, Pierce G, Holley HP Jr, Rauch A. Antibiotic resistance among clinical isolates of

Haemophilus influenzae in the United States in 1994 and 1995 and detection of beta-lactamase-positive strains resistant to amoxicillin-clavulanate: results of a national multicenter surveillance study. *Antimicrob Agents Chemother* 1997; 41:292–297.

99 Doern GV, Jones RN, Pfaller MA, Kugler K. *Haemophilus influenzae* and *Moraxella catarrhalis* from patients with community-acquired respiratory tract infections: antimicrobial susceptibility patterns from the SENTRY antimicrobial Surveillance Program (United States and Canada, 1997). *Antimicrob Agents Chemother* 1999; 43:385–389.

100 Powell M, Livermore DM. Mechanisms of chloramphenicol resistance in *Haemophilus influenzae* in the United Kingdom. *J Med Microbiol* 1988 Oct;27(2):89–93.

101 Vila J, Ruiz J, Sanchez F, Navarro F, Mirelis B, de Anta MT, Prats G. Increase in quinolone resistance in a *Haemophilus influenzae* strain isolated from a patient with recurrent respiratory infections treated with ofloxacin. *Antimicrob Agents Chemother* 1999; 43:161–162.

102 Richard MP, Aguado AG, Mattina R, Marre R Sensitivity to sparfloxacin and other antibiotics, of *Streptococcus pneumoniae*, *Haemophilus influenzae* and *Moraxella catarrhalis* strains isolated from adult patients with community-acquired lower respiratory tract infections: a European multicentre study. SPAR Study Group. Surveillance Programme of Antibiotic Resistance. *J Antimicrob Chemother* 1998; 41:207–214.

103 Berk SL, Kalbfleisch JH. Antibiotic susceptibility patterns of community-acquired respiratory isolates of *Moraxella catarrhalis* in western Europe and in the USA. The Alexander Project Collaborative Group. *J Antimicrob Chemother* 1996; 38 (Suppl A):85–96.

104 Doern GV, Brueggemann AB, Pierce G, Hogan T, Holley HP Jr; Rauch A. Prevalence of antimicrobial resistance among 723 outpatient clinical isolates of *Moraxella catarrhalis* in the United States in 1994 and 1995: results of a 30-center national surveillance study. *Antimicrob Agents Chemother* 1996; 40:2884–2886.

105 Di Persio JR, Jones RN, Barrett T, Doern GV, Pfaller MA. Fluoroquinolone-resistant *Moraxella catarrhalis* in a patient with pneumonia: report from the SENTRY Antimicrobial Surveillance Program (1998). *Diagn Microbiol Infect Dis* 1998; 32:131–135.

106 Hol C, Van Dijke EE, Verduin CM, Verhoef J, van Dijk H. Experimental evidence for *Moraxella*-induced penicillin neutralization in pneumococcal pneumonia. *J Infect Dis* 1994; 170:1613–1616.

107 Sader HS, Pfaller MA, Jones RN. Prevalence of important pathogens and the antimicrobial activity of parenteral drugs at numerous medical centers in the United States. II. Study of the intra- and interlaboratory dissemination of extended-spectrum beta-lactamase-producing *Enterobacteriaceae*. *Diagn Microbiol Infect Dis* 1994; 20:203–208.

108 Nordmann P. Trends in β-lactam resistance among *Enterobacteriaceae*. *Clin Infect Dis* 1998; 27 (Suppl 1):S100–S106.

109 Lucet JC, Chevret S, Decre D et al. Outbreak of multiply resistant *Enterobacteriaceae* in an intensive care unit: epidemiology and risk factors for acquisition. *Clin Infect Dis* 1996; 22:430–436.

110 Hancock RE. Resistance mechanisms in *Pseudomonas aeruginosa* and other nonfermentative gram-negative bacteria. *Clin Infect Dis* 1998; 27 (Suppl 1):S93-S99.

111 Spencer RC. Predominant pathogens found in the European Prevalence of Infection in Intensive Care Study. *Eur J Clin Microbiol Infect Dis* 1996; 15:281–285.

112 Cazzola M. Problems and perspectives in the antibiotic treatment of lower respiratory tract infections. *Pulm Pharmacol* 1994; 7:139–152.

113 Cazzola M, Diamare F, Vinciguerra A, Salzillo A, Calderaro F. La penetrazione polmonare degli antibiotici e il suo impatto clinico. *Rass Pat App Respir* 1996; 11:134–147.

114 Georges H, Leroy O, Alfandari S et al. Pulmonary disposition of vancomycin in critically ill patients. *Eur J Clin Microbiol Infect Dis* 1997; 16:385–388.

115 Carcas AJ, Garcia-Satue JL, Zapater P, Frias-Iniesta J. Tobramycin penetration into epithelial lining fluid of patients with pneumonia. *Clin Pharmacol Ther* 1999; 65:245–250.

116 Bergogne-Bérézin E, Vallée E. Pharmacokinetics of antibiotics in respiratory tissues and fluids. In: Pennington JE, Ed. *Respiratory Infections: Diagnosis and Management*. 3rd edn. New York, Raven Press, 1994; 715–740.

117 Cazzola M, Matera MG. Interrelationship between pharmacokinetics and pharmacodynamics in the design of dosage regimens for treating acute exacerbations of chronic bronchitis. *Respir Med* 1998; 92:895–901.

118 Cars O. Efficacy of β-lactam antibiotics: integration of pharmacokinetics and pharmacodynamics. *Diagn Microbiol Infect Dis* 1997; 27:29–34.

119 Odenholt-Tornqvist I, Lowdin E, Car O. Pharmacodynamic effects of subinhibitory concentrations of β-lactam antibiotics in vitro. *Antimicrob Agents Chemother* 1991; 35:1834–1839.

120 Schentag JJ, Smith H, Swanson DJ et al. Role of dual individualization with cefmenoxime. *Am J Med* 1984; 77 (Suppl 6A):43–50.

121 Craig WA. Interrelationship between pharmacokinetics and pharmacodynamics in determining dosage regimens for broad-spectrum cephalosporins. *Diagn Microbiol Infect Dis* 1995; 25:89–96.

122 Craig WA, Leggett J, Toutsuka K. Key pharmacokinetic parameters of antibiotic efficacy in experimental animal infections. *J Drug Dev* 1988; 1 (Suppl 3):7–15.

123 Craig WA, Ebert S, Watanabe Y. Differences in time above MIC required for efficacy of beta-lactams in aminal infection models. Abstract 86. In *Proceedings and Abstracts of the 35th Interscience Conference on Antimicrobial Agents and Chemotherapy* 1993; 135.

124 Andes D, Urban A, Craig WA. *In vitro* activity of amoxicillin and amoxicillin-clavulanate against penicillin-resistant pneumococci. Abstract A82. In *Proceedings and Abstracts of the 35th Interscience Conference on Antimicrobial Agents and Chemotherapy* 1995; 16.

125 Urban A, Andes D, Craig WA. *In vivo* activity of cefpodoxime against penicillin-resistant pneumococci. Abstract 2229. *Final Program and Abstracts of the 19th International Congress of Chemotherapy* 1995; 381C.

126 Drusano GL, Craig WA. Relevance of pharmacokinetics and pharmacodynamics in the selection of antibiotics for respiratory tract infections. *J Chemother* 1997; 9 (Suppl 3):38–44.

127 Cazzola M, Matera MG. Parenteral antibiotic therapy: strategies to minimize the development of antibiotic resistance. *J Antimicrob Chemother* (submitted).

128 Schentag JJ, Birmingham MC, Paladino JA et al. In nosocomial pneumonia, optimizing antibiotics other than aminoglycosides is a more important determinant of successful clinical outcome, and a better means of avoiding resistance. *Semin Respir Infect* 1997; 12:278–293.

129 Nix DE, Sands MF, Peloquin CA et al. Dual individualization of intravenous ciprofloxacin in patients with nosocomial lower respiratory tract infections. *Am J Med* 1987; 82 (4A):352–356.

130 Fernandes AC, Anderson R, Theron AJ, Joone C, van Rensburg CEJ. Enhancement of human polymorphonuclear leukocyte motility by erythromycin in vitro and in vivo. *S Afr Med J* 1984; 66:173–177.

131 Labro M-T. Cefodizime as a biological response modifier: a review of its in vivo, ex vivo and in vitro immunomodulatory properties. *J Antimicrob Chemother* 1990; 26 (Suppl C):37–47.

132 Shalit I. Immunological aspects of new quinolones. *Eur J Clin Microbiol Infect Dis* 1991; 10:262-266.

133 Cuffini AM, Tullio V, Fazari S, Allocco A, Carlone NA. Pefloxacin and immunity: cellular uptake, potentiation of macrophage phagocytosis and intracellular bioactivity for *Klebsiella pneumoniae*. *Int J Tissue React* 1992; 14:131–139.

134 Petit JC, Daguet GL, Richard G, Burghoffer B. Influence of ciprofloxacin and piperacillin on interleukin-1 production by murine macrophages. *J Antimicrob Chemother* 1987; 20:615–617.

135 Riesbeck K, Sigvardsson M, Leanderson T, Forsgren A. Superinduction of cytokine gene transcription by ciprofloxacin. *J Immunol* 1994; 153:343–352.

136 Yoshimura T, Kurita C, Usami E, Nakao T, Weatanabe S, Kobayashi J, Yamazaki F, Nagai H. Immunomodulatory action of levofloxacin on cytokine production by human peripheral blood mononuclear cells. *Chemotherapy* 1996; 42:459–464.

137 Bailly S, Mahe Y, Ferrua B et al. Quinolone-induced differential modification of IL-1α and IL-1β production by LPS-stimulated human monocytes. *Cell Immunol* 1990; 128:277–288.

138 Galley HF, Nelson SJ, Dubbels AM, Webster NR. Effect of ciprofloxacin on the accumulation of interleukin-6, interleukin-8, and nitrite from a human endothelial cell model of sepsis. *Crit Care Med* 1997; 25:1392–1395.

139 Tufano MA, Cipollaro de l'Ero G, Ianniello R, Baroni A, Galdiero F. Antimicrobial agents induce monocytes to release IL-1 alpha, IL-6, and TNF, and induce lymphocytes to release IL-4 and TNF tau. *Immunopharmacol Immunotoxicol* 1992; 14:769–782.

140 Ritts RE. Antibiotics as biological response modifiers. *J Antimicrob Chemother* 1990; 26 (Suppl C):37–48.

141 Meloni F, Ballabio P, Bianchi L, Grassi FA, Gialdroni Grassi G. Cefodizime modulates in vitro tumor necrosis factor-α, interleukin-6 and interleukin-7 release from human peripheral monocytes. *Chemotherapy* 1995; 41:289–295.

142 Pacheco Y, Hosni R, Dagrosa EE et al. Antibiotics and production of granulocyte-macrophage colony-stimulating factor by human bronchial epithelial cells in vitro. *Arzneimittelforschung* 1994; 44:559–563.

143 Scheffer J, Knöller J, Cullmann W, König W. Effects of cefetamet and cefaclor on inflammatory responses of human granulocytes, basophils and rat mast cells. *Méd Mal Infect* 1992; 22:548–555.

144 Scheffer J, König W. Cephalosporins and inflammatory host reactions. *Respiration* 1993; 60 (Suppl 1):25–31.

145 Labro MT. Penetration intracellulaire des macrolides. *Presse Med* 1997; 26 (Suppl 2):11–15.

146 Tamaoki J, Sakai N, Tagaya E, Konno K. Macrolide antibiotics protect against endotoxin-induced vascular leakage and neutrophil accumulation in rat trachea. *Antimicrob Agents Chemother* 1994; 38:1641–1643.

147 Roche Y, Fay M, Gougerot-Pocidalo MA. Interleukin-1 production by antibiotic-treated human monocytes. *J Antimicrob Chemother* 1988; 21:597–607.

148 Kita E, Sawaki M, Nishikawa F et al. Enhanced interleukin production after long-term administration of erythromycin stearate. *Pharmacology* 1990; 41:177–183.

149 Kita E, Sawaki M, Mikasa K et al. Alteration of host response by a long-term treatment of roxithromycin. *J Antimicrob Chemother* 1993; 32:285–294.

150 Konno S, Addachi M; Asano K, Kawazoe T, Okamoto K, Takahashi T. Influence of roxithromycin on cell-mediated immune response. *Life Sci* 1992; 51:PL107-PL112.

151 Takizawa H, Desaki M, Ohtoshi T, Kikutani T, Okazaki H, Sato M, Akiyama N, Shoji S, Hiramatsu K, Ito K. Erythromycin suppresses interleukin-6 expression by human bronchial epithelial cells: a potential mechanism of its anti-inflammatory action. *Biochem Biophys Res Commun* 1995; 210:781–786.

152 Bailly S, Pocidalo J-J, Fay M, Gougerot-Pocidalo M-A. Differential modulation of cytokine production by macrolides: interleukin-6 production is increased by spiramycin and erythromycin. *Antimicrob Agents Chemother* 1991; 35:2016–2019.

153 Takizawa H, Desaki M, Ohtoshi T et al. Erythromycin modulates IL-8 expression in normal and inflamed human bronchial epithelial cells. *Am J Respir Crit Care Med* 1997; 156:266–271.

154 Morikawa K, Oseko F, Morikawa S, Iwamoto K. Immunomodulatory effects of three macrolides, midecamycin acetate, josamycin, and clarithromycin, on human T-lymphocyte function in vitro. *Antimicrob Agents Chemother* 1994; 38:2643–2647.

155 Khair OA, Devalia JL, Abdelaziz MM, Sapsford RJ, Davies RJ. Effect of erythromycin on *Haemophilus influenzae* endotoxin-induced release of IL-6, IL-8 and soluble intercellular adhesion molecule (sICAM)-1 by cultured human bronchial epithelial cells. *Eur Respir J* 1995; 8:1451–1457.

156 Mandell LA. New treatment options for pneumonias. *Infect Med* 1998; 15 (Suppl E):34–45.

157 Sung SJ, Walters JA, Hudson J, Gimble JM. Tumor necrosis factor-α mRNA accumulation in human myelonocytic cell lines: role of transcriptional regulation by DNA sequence motifs and mRNA stabilization. *J Immunol* 1991; 147:2047–2054.

158 Gialdroni Grassi G, Bianchi L. Guidelines for the management of community-acquired pneumonia in adults. Italian Society of Pneumology. Italian Society of Respiratory Medicine. Italian Society of Chemotherapy. *Monaldi Arch Chest Dis* 1995; 50:21–27.

159 SPILF, Societe de Pathologie Infectieuse de Langue Francaise. Infections des voies respiratoires: conference de concensus en therapeutique anti-infectieuse. *Rev Med Infect* 1991; 21:1s-8s.

160 SEPAR. Spanish Thoracic Society. National recommendations for diagnosis and treatment of community acquired pneumonia. Barcelona, Spain: Ediciones Doyma, 1992.

161 British Thoracic Society. Guidelines for the management of community-acquired pneumonia in adults admitted to hospital. *Br J Hosp Med* 1993; 49:346–350.

162 Huchon GJ, Gialdroni-Grassi G, Leophonte P, Manresa F, Schaberg T, Woodhead M. Initial antibiotic therapy for lower respiratory tract infection in the community: a European survey. *Eur Respir J* 1996; 9:1590–1595.

163 Schaberg T, Gialdroni-Grassi G, Huchon G, Leophonte P, Manresa F, Woodhead M. An analysis of decisions by European general practitioners to admit to hospital patients with lower respiratory tract infections. The European Study Group of Community Acquired Pneumonia (ESOCAP) of the European Respiratory Society. *Thorax* 1996; 51:1017–1022.

164 Ortqvist A. Antibiotic treatment of community-acquired pneumonia in clinical practice: a European perspective. *J Antimicrob Chemother* 1995; 35:205–212.

165 Mandel LA, Niederman M. The Canadian Community Acquired Pneumonia Consensus Conference Group. Antimicrobial treatment of community-acquired pneumonia in adults: a conference report. *Can J Infect Dis* 1993; 4:25–28.

166 Niederman MS, Bass JB Jr, Campbell GD et al. Guidelines for the initial management of adults with community-acquired pneumonia: diagnosis, assessment of severity, and initial antimicrobial therapy. American Thoracic Society. Medical Section of the American Lung. *Am Rev Respir Dis* 1993; 148:1418–1426.

167 Thornsberry C, Ogilvie P, Kahn J, Mauriz Y. Surveillance of antimicrobial resistance in Streptococcus pneumoniae, Haemophilus influenzae, and Moraxella catarrhalis in the United States in 1996–1997 respiratory season. The Laboratory Investigator Group. *Diagn Microbiol Infect Dis* 1997; 29:249–257.

168 Cazzola M, Ariano R, Gioia V et al. Bacterial isolates and cigarette smoking in patients with chronic bronchitis: results from an Italian multicenter survey. *Clin Ther* 1990; 12:105–117.

169 Conte JE Jr, Golden J, Duncan S, McKenna E, Lin E, Zurlinden E. Single-dose intrapulmonary pharmacokinetics of azithromycin, clarithromycin, ciprofloxacin, and

cefuroxime in volunteer subjects. *Antimicrob Agents Chemother* 1996; 40:1617–1622.

170 Bartlett JG, Breiman RF, Mandell LA, File TM Jr. Guidelines from the Infectious Diseases Society of America. Community-acquired pneumonia in adults: guidelines for management. *Clin Infect Dis* 1998; 26:811–838.

171 French GL. Enterococci and vancomycin resistance. *Clin Infect Dis* 1998; 27(Suppl 1):S75–83.

172 Johnson AP, Speller D, George RC, Warner M, Domingue G, Efstratiou A. Prevalence of antibiotic resistance and sero-types in pneumococci in England and Wales: results of observational surveys in 1990 and 1995. *BMJ* 1996; 312:1454–1456.

173 Klugman KP. The clinical relevance of in-vitro resistance to penicillin, ampicillin, amoxycillin and alternative agents, for the treatment of community-acquired pneu-monia caused by *Streptococcus pneumoniae, Haemophilus influenzae* and *Moraxella catarrhalis. J Antimicrob Chemother* 1996; 38 (Suppl A):133–140.

174 Wort SJ, Rogers TR. Community-acquired pneumonia in elderly people. *BMJ* 1998; 316:1690.

175 Chan R, Hemeryck L, O'Regan M, Clancy L, Feely J. Oral versus intravenous antibiotics for community acquired lower respiratory tract infection in a general hospital: open, randomised controlled trial. *BMJ* 1995; 310:1360–1362.

176 Huchon G, Woodhead M. Management of adult commu-nity-acquired lower respiratory tract infections. *Eur Respir Rev* 1998; 8:391–426.

177 Trowbridge JF. Outpatient parenteral antibiotic therapy. Management of serious infections. Part II: Amenable infec-tions and models for delivery. Pneumonia and chronic lung disease. *Hosp Pract (Off Ed)* 1993; 28 (Suppl 2):20–24.

178 Tice AD. Experience with a physician-directed, clinic-based program for outpatient parenteral antibiotic therapy in the USA. *Eur J Clin Microbiol Infect Dis* 1995; 14:655–661.

179 Tice AD, Poretz D, Cook F, Zinner D, Strauss MJ. Medicare coverage of outpatient ambulatory intravenous antibiotic therapy: a program that pays for itself. *Clin Infect Dis* 1998; 27:1415–1421.

180 Anonymous. The choice of antibacterial drugs. *Med Lett Drugs Ther* 1996; 38:25–34.

181 Pallares R, Linares J, Vadillo M et al. Resistance to penicil-lin and cephalosporins and mortality from severe pneu-mococcal pneumonia in Barcelona, Spain. *N Engl J Med* 1995; 333:474–480.

182 Williams JD, Sefton AM. Comparison of macrolide anti-biotics. *J Antimicrob Chemother* 1993; 31 (Suppl C):11–26.

183 North DS, Fish DN, Redington JJ. Levofloxacin, a second-

generation fluoroquinolone. *Pharmacotherapy* 1998; 18:915–935.

184 Grossman RF. The role of fluoroquinolones in respiratory tract infections. *J Antimicrob Chemother* 1997; 40 (Suppl A):59–62.

185 Mundy LM, Oldach D, Auwaerter PG et al. Implications for macrolide treatment in community-acquired pneumonia. Hopkins CAP Team. *Chest* 1998; 113:1201–1206.

186 Woodhead M. Community acquired pneumonia in elderly people. Addition of erythromycin is not currently justified. *BMJ* 1998; 317:1524.

187 Kauppinen MT, Saikku P, Kujala P, Herva E, Syrjala H. Clinical picture of community-acquired Chlamydia pneu-moniae pneumonia requiring hospital treatment: a com-parison between chlamydial and pneumococcal pneumonia. *Thorax* 1996; 51:185–189.

188 Kauppinen MT, Saikku P, Kujala P, Herva E, Syrjala H. Clinical picture of Chlamydia pneumoniae requiring hos-pital treatment: a comparison between chlamydial and pneumococcal pneumonia. *Thorax* 1996;51:185–189.

189 Whittle J, Lin CJ, Lave JR et al. Relationship of provider characteristics to outcomes, process, and costs of care for community-acquired pneumonia. *Med Care* 1998; 36:977–987.

190 Fine MJ, Auble TE, Yealy DM et al. A prediction rule to identify low-risk patients with community-acquired pneu-monia. *N Engl J Med* 1997; 336:243–250.

191 Niederman MS, McCombs JS, Unger AN, Kumar A, Popovian R. The cost of treating community-acquired pneumonia. *Clin Ther* 1998; 20:820–837.

192 Ehrenkranz NJ, Nerenberg DE, Shultz JM, Slater KC. Intervention to discontinue parenteral antimicrobial therapy in patients hospitalized with pulmonary infec-tions: effect on shortening patient stay. *Infect Control Hosp Epidemiol* 1992; 13:21–22.

193 Omidvari K, de Boisblanc BP, Karam G, Nelson S, Haponik E, Summer W. Early transition to oral antibiotic therapy for community-acquired pneumonia: duration of therapy, clinical outcomes, and cost analysis. *Respir Med* 1998; 92:1032–1039.

194 Hessen MT, Kaye D. Nosocomial pneumonia. *Crit Care Clin* 1988; 4:245–257.

195 Scheld WM, Mandell GL. Nosocomial pneumonia: Pathogenesis and recent advances in diagnosis and therapy. *Rev Infect Dis* 1991; 13 (Suppl 9):S743-S751.

196 Mandell LA, Campbell GD Jr. Nosocomial pneumonia guidelines: an international perspective. *Chest* 1998; 113:188S-193S.

197 American Thoracic Society. Hospital-acquired pneumonia

in adults: diagnosis, assessment of severity, initial anti-microbial therapy, and preventive strategies. A consensus statement. *Am J Respir Crit Care Med* 1996; 153:1711–1725.

198 Hart CA, Makin T. *Legionella* in hospitals: a review. *J Hosp Infect* 1991; 18 (Suppl A):481–489.

199 Bradley SF. Methicillin-resistant *Staphylococcus aureus*: long-term care concerns. *Am J Med* 1999; 106 (Suppl 5A):2S–10S.

200 Sieger B, Berman SJ, Geckler RW, Farkas SA. Empiric treatment of hospital-acquired lower respiratory tract infections with meropenem or ceftazidime with tobramycin: a randomized study. Meropenem Lower Respiratory Infection Group. *Crit Care Med* 1997; 25:1663–1670.

201 Wolff M. Comparison of strategies using cefpirome and ceftazidime for empiric treatment of pneumonia in intensive care patients. The Cefpirome Pneumonia Study Group. *Antimicrob Agents Chemother* 1998;42:28–36.

202 Niederman MS. An approach to empiric therapy of nosocomial pneumonia. *Med Clin North Am* 1994; 78:1123–1141.

203 Moellering RC Jr. Antibiotic resistance: lessons for the future. *Clin Infect Dis* 1998; 27 (Suppl 1):S135–40.

204 Barriere JC, Berthaud N, Beyer D, Dutka-Malen S, Paris JM, Desnottes JF. Recent developments in streptogramin research. *Curr Pharm Des* 1998; 4:155–180.

205 Rubinstein E, Keller N. Future prospects and therapeutic potential of streptogramins. *Drugs* 1996; 51 (Suppl 1):38–42.

206 Agouridas C, Denis A, Auger JM et al. Synthesis and antibacterial activity of ketolides (6-O-methyl-3-oxoerythromycin derivatives): a new class of antibacterials highly potent against macrolide-resistant and -susceptible respiratory pathogens. *J Med Chem* 1998; 41:4080–4100.

207 Reinert RR, Bryskier A, Lutticken R. *In vitro* activities of the new ketolide antibiotics HMR 3004 and HMR 3647 against *Streptococcus pneumoniae* in Germany. *Antimicrob Agents Chemother* 1998; 42:1509–1511.

208 Nilius AM, Bui M, Almer L, Hensey D, Ma Z,Or YS, Glamm RK. Comparison of the in vitro activity of ABT-773, a novel antibacterial ketolide, with erythromycin and ciprofloxacin against respiratory pathogens. *J Antimicrob Chemother* 1999; 44 (Suppl A):76.

209 Swaney SM, Aoki H, Ganoza MC, Shinabarger DL. The oxazolidinone linezolid inhibits initiation of protein synthesis in bacteria. *Antimicrob Agents Chemother* 1998; 42:3251–2255.

210 Dresser LD; Rybak MJ. The pharmacologic and bacteriologic properties of oxazolidinones, a new class of synthetic antimicrobials. *Pharmacotherapy* 1998; 18:456–462.

211 Cormican MG, Marshall SA, Jones RN. Preliminary inter-pretive criteria for disk diffusion susceptibility testing of SCH 27899, a compound in the everninomicin class of antimicrobial agents. *Diagn Microbiol Infect Dis* 1995; 23:157–160.

212 Hill J, Barry A, Tsitsi J et al. Efficacy of Ziracin (SCH27899) vs ceftriaxone in patients with acute bacterial pneumonia due to penicillin resistant *Streptococcus pneumoniae*. *J Antimicrob Chemother* 1999; 44 (Suppl A):99–100.

213 Sasaki T, Otani T, Matsumoto H et al. MJ347–81F4 A & B, novel antibiotics from Amycolatopsis sp.: taxonomic characteristics, fermentation, and antimicrobial activity. *J Antibiot (Tokyo)* 1998; 51:715–721.

214 Matsumoto N, Momose I, Umekita M et al. Diperamycin, a new antimicrobial antibiotic produced by Streptomyces griseoaurantiacus MK393-AF2. I. Taxonomy, fermentation, isolation, physico-chemical properties and biological activities. *J Antibiot (Tokyo)* 1998; 51:1087–1092.

215 Di Modugno E, Felici A. The renewed challenge of β-lactams to overcome bacterial resistance. *Curr Opin Anti-infect Investig Drugs* 1999; 1:26–39.

216 Page M, Bur D, Hebeisen P et al. Inhibition of the penicillin-binding proteins of methicillin-resistant Staphylococci by pyrrolidinone-3-ylidenemethyl cephems. *ICAAC* 1998; 38:F-22.

217 Ida T, Kurazono M, Yoshida T et al. ME1209 (CP6679), a new parenteral cephalosporin. I. In vitro activity against MRSA. *ICAAC* 1998; 38:F-12.

218 Adachi Y, Nagano R, Shibata K, Kato Y, Hashizume T, Morishima H. *In vitro* activities if J-111,225, J-114,870, J-114,871, novel carbapenems having potent activities against MRSA and *Pseudomonas aeruginosa*. *ICAAC* 1998; 38:F-54.

219 Shibata K, Nagano R, Nagami K et al. Studies on pharmacokinetics and basic toxicity of novel trans-3,5-disubstituted pyrrolidinylthio-1β-methylcarbapenem. *ICAAC* 1998; 38:F-53.

220 Kato Y, Otsuki M, Nishino T. Antibacterial properties of BO-2727, a new carbapenem antibiotic. *J Antimicrob Chemother* 1997; 40:195–203.

221 Tsuji M, Ishii Y, Ohno A, Miyazaki S, Yamaguchi K. In vitro and in vivo antibacterial activities of S-4661, a new carbapenem. *Antimicrob Agents Chemother* 1998; 42:94–99.

222 Sum PE, Sum FW, Projan SJ. Recent developments in tetracycline antibiotics. *Curr Pharm Des* 1998; 4:119–132.

223 Petersen PJ, Jacobus NV, Weiss WJ, Sum PE, Testa RT. In vitro and in vivo antibacterial activities of a novel glycylcycline, the 9-t-butylglycylamido derivative of minocycline (GAR-936). *Antimicrob Agents Chemother* 1999; 43:738–744.

224 Allen NE, LeTourneau DL, Hobbs JN Jr. The role of hydro-

phobic side chains as determinants of antibacterial activity of semisynthetic glycopeptide antibiotics. *J Antibiot (Tokyo)* 1997; 50:677–684.

225 Harland S, Tebbs SE, Elliott TS. Evaluation of the in-vitro activity of the glycopeptide antibiotic LY333328 in comparison with vancomycin and teicoplanin. *J Antimicrob Chemother* 1998; 41:273–276.

226 Zhao X, Xu C, Domagala J, Drlica K. DNA topoisomerase targets of the fluoroquinolones: a strategy for avoiding bacterial resistance. *Proc Natl Acad Sci USA* 1997; 94:13991–13996.

227 Schmitz FJ, Hofmann B, Hansen B et al. Relationship between ciprofloxacin, ofloxacin, levofloxacin, sparfloxacin and moxifloxacin (BAY 12–8039) MICs and mutations in grlA, grlB, gyrA and gyrB in 116 unrelated clinical isolates of *Staphylococcus aureus. J Antimicrob Chemother* 1998; 41:481–484.

228 Souli M, Wennersten CB, Eliopoulos GM. In vitro activity of BAY 12–8039, a new fluoroquinolone, against species representative of respiratory tract pathogens. *Int J Antimicrob Agents* 1998; 10:23–30.

229 Blondeau JM. Expanded activity and utility of the new fluoroquinolones: a review. *Clin Ther* 1999; 21:3–40.

230 Bauernfeind A. Comparison of the antibacterial activities of the quinolones Bay 12–8039, gatifloxacin (AM 1155), trovafloxacin, clinafloxacin, levofloxacin and ciprofloxacin. *J Antimicrob Chemother* 1997; 40:639–651.

231 Jevons GM, Andrews JM, Wise R. The tentative BSAC breakpoint of gemifloxacin, a novel fluoroquinolone. *J Antimicrob Chemother* 1999; 44 (Suppl A):141.

232 Felmingham D, Robbins MJ, Dencer C, Salman H, Mathias I, Rudgway GL. *In vitro* activity of gemifloxacin against *S. pneumoniae, H. influenzae, M. catarrhalis, L. pneumophila* and *Chlamydia* spp. *J Anticrob Chemother* 1999; 44 (Suppl A):131.

233 Milatovic D, Fluit A, Schmitz F-J, Verhoef J. *In vitro* activity of sitafloxacin (DU-6859A) and six other fluoroquinolones. Part I: Gram-negative aerobic bacteria. *J Antimicrob Chemother* 1999; 44 (Suppl A):171.

234 Milatovic D, Fluit A, Schmitz F-J, Verhoef J. *In vitro* activity of sitafloxacin (DU-6859A) and six other fluoroquinolones. Part II: Gram-positive cocci. *J Antimicrob Chemother* 1999; 44 (Suppl A):171.

235 Turnidge J. Pharmacokinetic and pharmacodynamic profiles of the new quinolones. *J Antimicrob Chemother* 1999; 44 (Suppl A):27.

236 Maiti SN, Phillips OA, Micetich RG, Livermore DM. β-Lactamase inhibitors: agents to overcome bacterial resistance. *Curr Med Chem* 1998; 5:441–456.

237 Qadri SM, Ueno Y, Cunha BA. Susceptibility of clinical isolates to expanded-spectrum beta-lactams alone and in the presence of beta-lactamase inhibitors. *Chemotherapy* 1996; 42:334–342.

238 Tzouvelekis LS, Gazouli M, Prinarakis EE, Tzelepi E, Legakis NJ. Comparative evaluation of the inhibitory activities of the novel penicillanic acid sulfone Ro 48–1220 against beta-lactamases that belong to groups 1, 2b, and 2be. *Antimicrob Agents Chemother* 1997; 41:475–477.

239 Hirata T, Wakatabe R, Nielsen J, Satoh T, Nihira S, Yamaguchi A. Screening of an inhibitor of the tetracycline efflux pump in a tetracycline-resistant clinical-isolate of *Staphylococcus aureus* 743. *Biol Pharm Bull* 1998; 21:678–681.

240 Srikumar R, Kon T, Gotoh N, Poole K. Expression of *Pseudomonas aeruginosa* multidrug efflux pumps MexA-MexB-OprM and MexC-MexD-OprJ in a multidrug-sensitive *Escherichia coli* strain. *Antimicrob Agents Chemother* 1998; 42:65–71.

241 Masuda N, Gotoh N, Ishii C, Sakagawa E, Ohya S, Nishino T. Interplay between chromosomal beta-lactamase and the MexAB-OprM efflux system in intrinsic resistance to beta-lactams in *Pseudomonas aeruginosa. Antimicrob Agents Chemother* 1999; 43:400–402.

242 Coleman K, Athalye M, Clancey A, Davison M, Payne DJ, Perry CR, Chopra I. Bacterial resistance mechanisms as therapeutic targets. *J Antimicrob Chemother* 1994; 33:1091–1116.

243 Chopra I, Hodgson J, Metcalf B, Poste G. The search for antimicrobial agents effective against bacteria resistant to multiple antibiotics. *Antimicrob Agents Chemother* 1997; 41:497–503.

244 Schimmel P, Tao J, Hill J. Aminoacyl tRNA synthetases as targets for new anti-infectives. *FASEB J* 1998; 12:1599–1609.

245 Yu XY, Hill JM, Yu G et al. Synthesis and structure-activity relationships of a series of novel thiazoles as inhibitors of aminoacyl-tRNA synthetases. *Bioorg Med Chem Lett* 1999; 9:375–380.

246 Kopp U, Roos M, Wecke J, Labischinski H. Staphylococcal peptidoglycan interpeptide bridge biosynthesis: a novel antistaphylococcal target? *Microb Drug Resist* 1996; 2:29–41.

247 Rietschel ET, Kirikae T, Schade FU et al. Bacterial endotoxin: molecular relationships of structure to activity and function. *FASEB J* 1994; 8:217–225.

248 Wyckoff TJ, Raetz CR, Jackman JE. Antibacterial and anti-inflammatory agents that target endotoxin. *Trends Microbiol* 1998, 6:154–159.

249 Liu J. Microcin B17: posttranslational modifications and

their biological implications. *Proc Natl Acad Sci USA* 1994; 91:4618–4620.

250 Maxwell A. DNA gyrase as a drug target. *Trends Microbiol* 1997; 5:102–109.

251 Hultgren SJ, Abraham S, Caparon M, Falk P, St Geme JW 3d, Normark S. Pilus and nonpilus bacterial adhesins: assembly and function in cell recognition. *Cell* 1993; 73:887–901.

252 Jones CH, Danese PN, Pinkner JS, Silhavy TJ, Hultgren SJ. The chaperone-assisted membrane release and folding pathway is sensed by two signal transduction systems. *EMBO* J 1997; 16:6394–406.

253 Thanassi DG, Saulino ET, Hultgren SJ. The chaperone/usher pathway: a major terminal branch of the general secretory pathway. *Curr Opin Microbiol* 1998; 1:223–231.

254 Jones CH, Hruby DE. New targets for antibiotic development:biogenesis of surface adherence structures. *Drug Discovery Today* 1998, 3:495–504.

255 Jadoun J, Burstein E, Hanski E, Sela S. Proteins M6 and F1 are required for efficient invasion of group A streptococciinto cultured epithelial cells. *Adv Exp. Med Biol* 1997; 418:511–515.

256 Frosch M, Reidl J, Vogel U. Genomics in infectious diseases: approaching the pathogens. *Trends Microbiol* 1998, 6:346–349.

257 Asai Y, Iwamoto K, Watanabe S. The effect of the lipid A analog E5531 on phospholipid membrane properties. *FEBS Lett* 1998; 438:15–20.

258 Kobayashi S, Kawata T, Kimura A e t al. Suppression of murine endotoxin response by E5531, a novel synthetic lipid A antagonist. *Antimicrob Agents Chemother* 1998;42:2824–2829.

259 Weiss J, Elsbach P, Shu C et al. Human bactericidal/permeability-increasing protein and a recombinant NH2-terminal fragment cause killing of serum-resistant gram-negative bacteria in whole blood and inhibit tumor necrosis factor release induced by the bacteria. *J Clin Invest* 1992; 90:1122–1130.

260 Ried C, Wahl C, Miethke T et al. High affinity endotoxin-binding and neutralizing peptides based on the crystal structure of recombinant Limulus anti-lipopolysaccharide factor. *J Biol Chem* 1996; 271:28120–28127.

261 Pajkrt D, Doran JE, Koster F et al. Antiinflammatory effects of reconstituted high-density lipoprotein during human endotoxemia. *J Exp Med* 1996; 184:1601–1608.

262 Edwards MJ, Abney DL, Heniford BT, Miller FN. Passive immunization against tumor necrosis factor inhibits interleukin-2-induced microvascular alterations and reduces toxicity. *Surgery* 1992; 112:480–6.

263 Greenberger MJ, Kunkel SL, Strieter RM et al. IL-12 gene therapy protects mice in lethal Klebsiella pneumonia. *J Immunol* 1996; 157:3006–3012.

264 Lei DH, Lancaster JR, Joshi MS et al. Activation of alveolar macrophages and lung host defenses using transfer of the interferon-gamma gene. *Am J Physiol – Lung Cellular & Mol Physiol* 1997; 16:L852-L859.

265 deBoisblanc BP, Mason CM, Andresen J et al. Phase 1 safety trial of Filgrastim (r-metHuG-CSF) in non-neutropenic patients with severe community-acquired pneumonia. *Respir Med* 1997; 91:387–394.

266 Nelson S, Belknap SM, Carlson RW et al. A randomized controlled trial of filgrastim as an adjunct to antibiotics for treatment of hospitalized patients with community-acquired pneumonia. CAP Study Group. *J Infect Dis* 1998; 178:1075–1080.

267 Heffernan R, Henning K, Labowitz A, Hjelte A, Layton M. Laboratory survey of drug-resistant *Streptococcus pneumoniae* in New York City, 1993–1995. *Emerg Infect Dis* 1998; 4:113–116.

268 El-Ebiary M. Community-acquired pneumonia: assessment of therapy. *Eur Respir Rev* 1998; 8:295–298.

269 Ramirez JA, Srinath L, Ahkee S, Huang A, Raff MJ. Early switch from intravenous to oral cephalosporins in the treatment of hospitalized patients with community-acquired pneumonia. *Arch Intern Med* 1995; 155:1273–1276.

270 Fine MJ, Medsger AR, Stone RA et al. The hospital discharge decision for patients with community-acquired pneumonia. Results from the Pneumonia Patient Outcomes Research Team Cohort Study. *Arch Intern Med* 1997; 157:47–56.

271 Ramirez JA. Switch therapy in community-acquired pneumonia. *Diagn Microbiol Infect Dis* 1995; 22:219–223.

15

Current treatment of chronic bronchial suppuration

Robert Wilson

Royal Brompton Hospital, Sydney Street, London SW3 6N, UK.

Introduction

'Chronic bronchial sepsis' has been used as a term to describe chronic bronchial infection leading to daily production of purulent sputum. However, the term sepsis implies that bacteremia is part of the syndrome, but this is rare in these patients because an exuberant immune response confines the infection to the lung. 'Chronic bronchial suppuration' is therefore a better term to use. Chronic expectoration of mucopurulent or purulent sputum should lead to suspicion of the presence of bronchiectasis. Bronchiectasis is defined as abnormal chronic dilation of one or more bronchi. This structural abnormality results in poor mucus clearance from affected areas, predisposing the patient to recurrent or chronic bacterial infections.

There are a number of different types of bronchiectasis that are characterized by the form of airway dilation. Saccular or cystic bronchiectasis occurs when there is severe loss of structural elements in the bronchial wall leading to large balloon-like dilations. This type of bronchiectasis usually follows severe lung infections and is characterized by the production of large volumes of sputum and finger clubbing[1]. It is now infrequently seen in developed countries. In varicose bronchiectasis there are local constrictions superimposed on cylindrical changes. Traction bronchiectasis occurs in fibrotic lung conditions such as fibrosing alveolitis in which the airway walls are pulled apart by the fibrotic process. Much more frequently seen nowadays is a cylindrical form of bronchiectasis in which the damage to the bronchial wall is less severe than cystic bronchiectasis. This has been termed 'modern' bronchiectasis[2]. There is a copious lymphocytic infiltrate in the bronchial wall of these cases which strongly resembles the follicular type of bronchiectasis described by Whitwell in his classic study[3]. This type of bronchiectasis is usually bilateral and may be diffuse, although the lower lobes are usually worst affected.

There are a number of known causes of bronchiectasis (Table 15.1), and several other conditions that are associated with bronchiectasis (Table 15.2). However, we remain ignorant of many of the underlying causes of bronchiectasis, and over half of cases are still considered idiopathic[2]. Recognition of the presence of bronchiectasis should lead to investigation of possible causes (Table 15.3), some of which are treatable, and the construction of a management plan to alleviate symptoms and avoid progression of the disease. Since progression may be insidious, or occur in a stepwise rather than gradual manner, regular follow-up and re-assessment is required, in most cases for life.

The current prevalence of bronchiectasis is unknown. On the one hand, the prevalence of severe forms of bronchiectasis has decreased because of the introduction of vaccination against childhood infections, improved socio-economic conditions and the availability of antibiotics[1,4,5]. However, in parts of the world where social conditions are poor and health care less available bronchiectasis remains a more common cause of morbidity and mortality. On the other hand, chest radiographs are

Table 15.1. Causes of bronchiectasis

Congenital
e.g. defective bronchial wall, pulmonary sequestration

Postinfective
e.g. tuberculosis, whooping cough, non-tuberculous
    mycobacteria

Mechanical obstruction
intrinsic (e.g. tumour or foreign body) or extrinsic (e.g. lymph
    node) obstruction of airway lumen

Deficient immune response
e.g. panhypogammaglobulinemia, selective immunoglobulin
    deficiency, HIV

Excessive immune response
e.g. allergic bronchopulmonary aspergillosis, lung transplant
    rejection, chronic graft vs. host disease

Abnormal mucus clearance
e.g. primary ciliary dyskinesia, cystic fibrosis, Young's
    syndrome

Fibrosis
e.g. cryptogenic fibrosing alveolitis, sarcoidosis

Inflammatory pneumonitis
e.g. aspiration of gastric contents, inhalation of toxic gases

Table 15.2. Conditions associated with
bronchiectasis

Infertility
e.g. primary ciliary dyskinesia, cystic fibrosis, Young's
    syndrome

Inflammatory bowel disease
e.g. ulcerative colitis, Crohn's disease, celiac disease

Connective tissue disorders
e.g. rheumatoid arthritis, systemic lupus erythematosus

Malignancy
e.g. acute or chronic lymphatic leukemia

Diffuse panbronchiolitis
predominantly seen in Japanese

Yellow nail syndrome
Discoloured (usually yellow) nails, lymphedema and pleural
    effusions

α_1- antiproteinase deficiency
more commonly causes emphysema

Mercury poisoning
Pink's disease may cause Young's syndrome (obstructive
    azoospermia, sinusitis and bronchiectasis)

a very insensitive means of detecting bronchiectasis, and the advent of high resolution, thin section computed tomography (CT) scans has led to increased recognition of bronchiectasis in patients whose condition might otherwise not have been diagnosed or they would have been described as suffering from chronic bronchitis[6]. If a patient is currently smoking when seeking help for a chronic productive cough, it is likely that advice will be given about smoking cessation rather than a referral being made for investigation. This could be one reason that most patients with 'modern bronchiectasis' referred to our clinic are non-smokers. Some smoking-related chronic bronchitis patients produce purulent sputum each day and have persistent bronchial infection while in an otherwise stable condition[7]. At the present time the incidence of bronchiectasis in this group is unknown, but our own experience is that bronchiectasis defined by CT scan criteria is often present. CT scans are much less unpleasant for the patient than bronchograms, so they are performed more frequently and detect a milder disease condition than we have understood by the term bronchiectasis in the past. This must be kept in mind when comparing new to older studies. The true prevalence of bronchiectasis will only be determined if in the future we can develop an inexpensive imaging technique that can be applied to population surveys.

Pathophysiology

Chronic bronchial infection usually occurs because the lung defences are impaired in some way. The bacterial species that cause chronic infection adopt various strategies to avoid clearance by the lung defences, but they are not as virulent in terms of causing invasive disease. Patients carry the same bacterial strain for many months, and acquisition of a new strain is not necessarily associated with an exacerbation of symptoms[8,9]. The stable state repre-

Table 15.3. Investigation of bronchiectasis

All patients
Chest radiograph (PA and lateral)
Sinus radiographs
Respiratory function tests
Blood investigations[a]
Sputum microscopy including staining for eosinophils
Sputum culture
Sputum smear and culture for acid fast bacilli
Skin tests (atopy, aspergillus)
High-resolution thin-section CT scan
Sweat test (nasal potential difference, genotyping)
Nasal mucociliary clearance (cilia studies if abnormal)

Selected patients
Fibreoptic bronchoscopy
Barium swallow (video fluoroscopy)
Respiratory muscle function
Semen analysis
Tests for associated conditions
Antibody responses to vaccination
Blood tests for rarer immune deficiencies

Note:

[a] To include: differential white cell count; total
immunoglobulin (Ig) levels of IgG, IgM, IgA, IgE, and IgG
subclasses; *Aspergillus* RAST and precipitins; rheumatoid
factor and antinuclear antibodies; α_1-antiproteinase.

sents a 'stand-off' between bacteria and the host defences. Bacteria are confined to the airways and their numbers are contained by the host defences, but they are not eradicated. Bacterial numbers increase at the time of an exacerbation, in most cases because the host defences are further reduced, e.g. by a viral infection, or sometimes because the bacteria escape the host defences, either due to a change in the colonizing strain, e.g. in its antigenic structure, or on some occasions following infection with a new strain. The chronic host inflammatory response increases during an exacerbation and this, together with products of the bacteria themselves, causes lung damage. The relationship between bacteria and the host in chronic infection is very different from an acute infection such as pneumonia, when virulent bacteria may overcome intact host

defences, or capitalize on a weakened host, leading to a brief interchange during which either the host defences triumph (perhaps supported by antibiotics) and bacteria are eradicated, or the bacteria overwhelm the host defences and invade the body causing the host to succumb.

Large numbers of neutrophils are attracted from the bloodstream into the bronchial lumen during chronic infection by chemotactic factors derived from bacteria and by host factors (eg IL-8, C5a, LTB-4). The failure of this inflammatory response to eradicate the infection is partly due to the pathogenic mechanisms of the bacteria and partly due to the impairment in the host defences[9]. Neutrophils spill proteolytic enzymes such as elastase and reactive oxygen species during migration from the bloodstream and during phagocytosis that stimulate mucus secretion and damage the epithelium and structural proteins of the lung. Tissue damage in the affected area may spread to involve areas of normal bystander lung. Immune complexes are formed between antibodies that are produced locally, and those arriving via transudation, and bacterial antigens[10]. These complexes stimulate further inflammatory processes. The lung defences are weakened by the damage caused by bacterial products and inflammation, and this in turn promotes continued infection which stimulates more inflammation. This has been termed a 'vicious circle' of events (Fig. 15.1).

The walls of bronchi and bronchioles contain lymphoid follicles and nodes. As well as B-lymphocytes and plasma cells in the follicles there is a well-developed cell-mediated immune response present, with increased numbers of activated T-lymphocytes, mainly of the suppressor/cytotoxic CD8 – positive phenotype, antigen processing cells and mature macrophages[11]. Epithelial cells, lymphocytes and macrophages release cytokines and other factors which orchestrate and perpetuate the inflammatory processes.

The 'vicious circle' outlined above will damage the airway causing bronchiectasis and chronic bronchial suppuration, but the starting point of the circle is often poorly understood. Lung injury may have

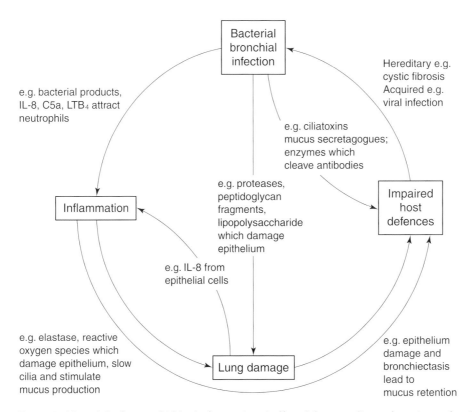

Fig. 15.1 A vicious circle of events which begins because impaired host defences predispose the patient to chronic bacterial bronchial infection. Bacteria utilize various mechanisms to persist in the airway. Persistent infection provokes chronic inflammation which damages lung tissue and further impairs host defences promoting continued infection.

occurred earlier during an acute event, e.g. inhalation of a toxic gas, or have been caused by a serious infection, e.g. tuberculosis or whooping cough. This event could have created local conditions which permitted bacteria to get a foothold and once they persisted in the lung and attracted chronic inflammation, the 'vicious circle' commenced and the extent of lung damage slowly spread. In some cases there may be a more generalized host defence problem, e.g. primary ciliary dyskinesia or hypogammaglobulinemia. However, most often when the patient presents there is already established bronchiectasis and chronic infection. Investigation of the patient at this time may not discover a known cause of bronchiectasis and the circumstances leading to the initial permissive conditions are either lost in the patient's history or unknown. The significance of an episode of whooping cough or measles in childhood, which was followed by a long period of good health prior to the onset of chronic bronchial suppuration is uncertain. Patients with 'modern bronchiectasis' in whom a cause is not found will often give a history of wheezy bronchitis in childhood, followed by a period of reasonably good health before the onset of chronic cough and sputum production in adult life. Patients may also describe the start of their problems as a severe 'viral illness' which went down onto their chest and did not resolve.

The end result of chronic inflammation is that subsegmental airways are permanently dilated, tortuous, and partially or totally obstructed by copious amounts of secretions. Side branches are frequently obliterated. Structural proteins are lost from the bronchial wall and there is a variable amount of fibrosis. The process often involves bronchioles, and long-standing obstruction may result in complete fibrosis of small airways. Characteristically, the elastin layer which supports the bronchial wall is deficient or absent, and the muscle and cartilage also shows signs of destruction. These changes weaken the wall and facilitate subsequent distortion of the normal architecture. The airway epithelium is usually damaged and ciliated cells are lost. There may be peribronchial pneumonic changes with evidence of parenchymal damage. The pulmonary arteries may thrombose and can recanalize. With long-standing disease there is hypertrophy of the bronchial arteries with anastomosis and sometimes considerable shunting to the pulmonary arteries[12].

Bacteriology

Infections are usually caused by bacterial species that form part of the nasopharyngeal commensal flora: non-typable *Haemophilus influenzae*, *Haemophilus parainfluenzae*, *Streptococcus pneumoniae* and *Moraxella catarrhalis* are the most common species; or are opportunistic pathogens, e.g. *Pseudomonas aeruginosa* and *Stenotrophomonas maltophilia*. Isolation of gram-negative bacilli such as *Escherichia coli* and *Proteus* sp. may reflect previous antibiotic treatment. Mixed infections are common. *Staphylococcus aureus* is quite an unusual pathogen in bronchiectasis, and when it is isolated repeatedly it should prompt investigations to determine whether the patient is a cystic fibrosis variant or has allergic bronchopulmonary aspergillosis. These are two conditions in which bronchiectasis is predominantly in the upper lobes and *S. aureus* is a more common pathogen[13].

We have found that our bronchiectasis patients infected with *H. influenzae* while in a stable condition have the same quality of life as those with sterile sputum[14]. This provocative finding suggests that chronic infection might not necessarily be harmful,

at least in the medium term, and the deciding factor may be the amount of inflammation that the bacterial infection induces, which in turn may depend upon not only the number of bacteria present, but also the particular strain involved[15].

The initial infection by *P. aeruginosa* is usually with a non-mucoid strain which becomes mucoid when the infection is chronic. *P. aeruginosa* is thought to be directly involved in the deterioration of pulmonary function and respiratory failure that ultimately leads to almost all deaths in cystic fibrosis. In bronchiectasis, it has also been shown that *P. aeruginosa* is associated with extensive lung disease and severe airflow obstruction[16], and that decline in lung function is faster in those colonized by *P. aeruginosa* than those colonized by other organisms[17]. Not surprisingly, we found that patients infected with *P. aeruginosa* had worse quality of life than patients infected with other species[14]. However, not all authors have found *P. aeruginosa* infection to be associated with clinical deterioration[18], and more studies are needed to confirm a direct cause and effect relationship between acquisition of *P. aeruginosa* and deterioration in health. For example, it could be that *P. aeruginosa* infection occurs in those patients whose lung function is already deteriorating, and thus it is a marker of deterioration occurring for some other reason rather than the cause[17].

Burkholderia (formerly *Pseudomonas*) *cepacia* infects patients with cystic fibrosis, but is a very rare pathogen in non-cystic fibrosis bronchiectasis. Tuberculosis is a rare complication of bronchiectasis, but non-tuberculous mycobacteria can infect bronchiectatic airways and in some, but not all cases lead to worsening of the condition. A sputum sample should be sent for smear and culture of acid fast bacilli if a patient fails to respond to appropriate antibiotic therapy, particularly if a new infiltrate appears on the chest radiograph. CT scan appearances of diffuse cylindrical bronchiectasis, small airways disease and peripheral nodules, which may be cavitating, suggest the diagnosis (Fig. 15.2). Some species of non-tuberculous mycobacteria, particularly *Mycobacterium avium-intracellulare*, can infect patients without pre-existing lung disease

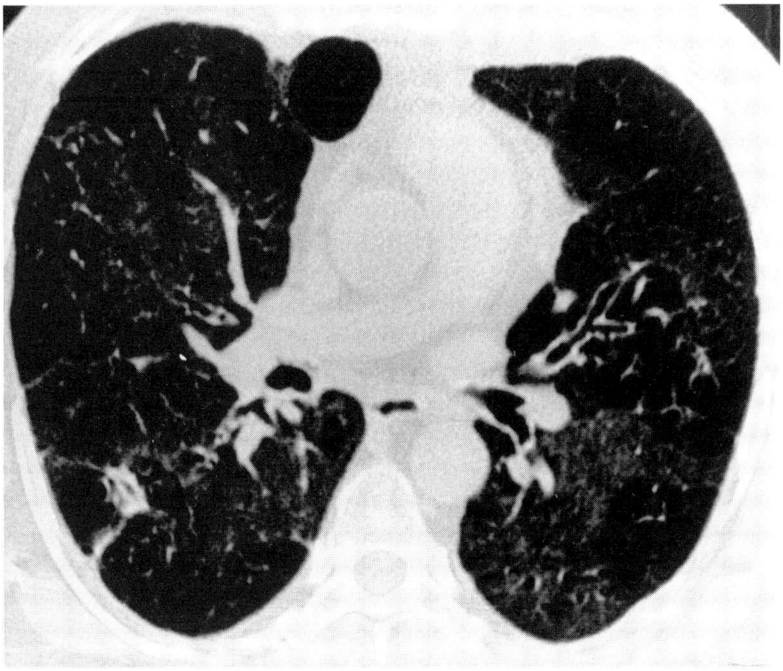

Fig. 15.2 CT scan of a patient with *Mycobacterium avium-intracellulare* infection. In the left lung a central bronchiectatic airway is seen. In the right lung a peripheral nodule is present which has a cavity. The combination of bronchiectatic airways and peripheral nodules which may be cavitating is suggestive of non-tuberculous mycobacterial infection.

or demonstrable immune deficiency. *M.avium-intracellulare* infection leads to small airways disease and bronchiectasis, and after several years of infection it can be difficult to determine whether the infection by non-tuberculous mycobacteria is primary or secondary [19].

Clinical features

The most common symptoms are chronic cough and sputum production. Patients suffer from recurrent infective exacerbations which are signalled by an increase in the purulence of the sputum. Although most often an exacerbation is associated with increased sputum production, sometimes the volume of sputum decreases because it becomes more sticky and difficult to clear. There is a high prevalence of chronic rhinosinusitis, which suggests that there might be an underlying abnormality

affecting the mucosa of the upper and lower respiratory tracts, or the association may be due to cross-infection between the two sites. Expiratory airflow obstruction is usually present, and there is a positive correlation between the severity of airflow obstruction and the severity of bronchiectasis[20]. There may be some reversibility indicating an asthmatic component, although in many patients airflow obstruction is relatively fixed[21,22]. Over half of patients had airway hyperresponsiveness to metacholine in one study[23]. Chest pains or discomfort are quite common, and arthralgia may occur[24]. Haemoptysis when present is usually small and complicates an exacerbation. Serious haemoptysis requiring selective arteriography and embolization or surgery to control it is a rare complication nowadays. Symptoms of poor concentration and undue tiredness are present in most patients, particularly during exacerbations.

There may be coarse crackles heard over the site of bronchiectasis, but sometimes there are no crackles in the lungs to suggest the diagnosis. Airflow obstruction can cause a hyperinflated chest and wheezes, and there may be late inspiratory squeaks suggesting small airways disease. Clubbing is quite unusual. Weight should be recorded since it may fall during ill health. A 24-hour sputum collection can be very informative, as patients tend to be inaccurate in their description of what they produce. A patient who describes continuous sputum production may present a collection that is largely saliva, whereas at the other extreme some patients produce several hundred millilitres of purulent sputum. Mucus plugs occur typically in allergic bronchopulmonary aspergillosis and can be sent for microscopy and culture.

In 1940 it was reported that 70% of 400 patients with bronchiectasis were dead before 40 years of age[25]. Nowadays the natural history of bronchiectasis has changed and the prognosis is much improved. However, in a recent study bronchiectasis was still the primary cause of death in 13% of patients with the condition[26]. The disease may progress slowly over many years and quality of life is usually impaired[27,28]. We have found that reduced exercise tolerance, frequent infective exacerbations and infection by *P. aeruginosa* are associated with poor quality of life[27]. Occasional patients deteriorate more rapidly and progress to respiratory failure at a relatively young age. The reason for this may not be clear.

Investigations

An unexpected diagnosis, such as atypical cystic fibrosis or primary ciliary dyskinesia, may be made by following the complete protocol outlined in Table 15.3. This may not be practical in all cases, but younger patients, those with associated conditions, e.g. infertility, and those in whom respiratory function is deteriorating and/or infective exacerbations becoming more frequent or prolonged should be referred to a respiratory physician with a special interest in bronchiectasis. Many of the investigations are widely available and should be performed in all patients.

Lung function tests are non-specific, but provide a measure of the amount of functional impairment that can be repeated to provide an assessment of change with time. Airflow obstruction is usually present and the degree of reversibility should be assessed. Gas transfer values that have been adjusted for alveolar volume are usually well preserved. The shuttle walking test is easy to perform and gives a reproducible measure of exercise capacity[27].

Sputum should be sent for microscopy, since eosinophils may cause purulence, and their presence in large numbers indicates asthma and/or allergic bronchopulmonary aspergillosis rather than infection; and for routine culture, as well as smear and culture for acid fast bacilli. Rapid growth by species such as *P. aeruginosa* can mask other important pathogens. A short transit time to the laboratory and judicious laboratory techniques such as sputum homogenization, dilution and quantitative counts, will ensure that useful information is obtained. Selective techniques which alter the culture conditions to suppress the growth of some species while encouraging growth of others can be used. Sputum samples should be sent routinely at each outpatient clinic visit to monitor the current bacteriology and antibiotic sensitivity, and a sample sent for acid fast bacilli once a year, or if patients are not responding to usual antibiotic treatment.

Bronchiectasis patients usually have high levels of the major immunoglobulin classes reflecting frequent or chronic infection. In the series reported by Cole[2], 83% of patients had one or more immunoglobulin classes G, A or M raised by more than 2 standard deviations above the mean. Blood tests should always include total serum immunoglobulins and immunoglobulin G subclasses, since immunoglobulin deficiency is a relatively common cause of bronchiectasis which requires particular treatment[29]. Antibody responses to vaccination should be measured as part of an immunological assessment in suspected cases, a twofold or greater response to pneumococcal and *Haemophilus influenzae* type b vaccine is normal. All cases of immune deficiency may be secondary to malignancy, particularly of the lymphoreticular system, so a high index of suspicion must be maintained. Peripheral blood eosinophilia and a positive RAST test (specific IgE) to aspergillus characterizes allergic bronchopulmonary aspergillosis. Aspergillus precipitins (IgG) are positive in about half of these cases, but multiple precipitin lines may indicate the presence of an aspergilloma.

Some investigations, such as ciliary function and ultrastructure, can only be performed in specialist centres. However, the saccharin test can be used as a simple screening test to determine whether there is a mucociliary problem[30], and more detailed ciliary studies need only be performed if this is abnormal. We also use exhaled nasal nitric oxide as a screening test, because levels of this gas are low in patients with primary ciliary dyskinesia for reasons that are not understood[31]. Other investigations will only be carried out in selected patients: bronchoscopy (presence of an obstructing lesion), semen analysis (primary ciliary dyskinesia patients may have immotile sperm, cystic fibrosis and Young's syndrome patients have azoospermia), barium swallow and video fluoroscopy together with oesophageal pH monitoring (aspiration of gastric contents), barium studies (inflammatory bowel disease), blood tests for rarer immune deficiencies (bronchiectasis can occur in patients infected with the human immunodeficiency virus, or more serious generalized infections beginning during childhood may indicate the need for tests such as neutrophil phagocytosis, chemiluminescence and chemotaxis).

A chest radiograph is a relatively insensitive test for bronchiectasis, in one study detecting less than 50% of patients who subsequently had positive bronchography[32]. Peribronchial fibrosis thickens the bronchial walls so that they are seen as tramlines, and when the bronchi run perpendicular to the X-ray beam they appear as small rings, often with thickened walls. Severe disease results in crowding of blood vessels and displacement of fissures due to volume loss in the affected lobes. Cystic bronchiectasis gives ring shadows varying in size

from 1 to 3 cm, usually with thin walls, and if these overlap it produces a honeycomb appearance. High resolution thin-section (1–2 mm) CT scans, performed with a fast scan time (1 second or less) to reduce artefacts from respiratory motion and cardiac pulsation, have replaced bronchography to establish the diagnosis and assess the extent of bronchiectasis, although they do not help in establishing the cause of the disease. The whole of both lungs should be examined with 10 mm intersection spacing. There is high sensitivity and specificity compared to bronchography[20]. The CT findings of bronchiectasis were established by Naidich and colleagues[33]. They are related to the presence of dilated air-filled bronchi, dilated fluid-filled bronchi, and loss of volume resulting from parenchymal loss which leads to crowding of bronchi. The appearance depends on the orientation of the bronchi to the scanning plane. When they lie in the same plane they appear as tramlines which do not decrease in diameter in the usual manner as they progress to the outside of the lung. The easiest method to tell whether a bronchus is dilated is to compare it to the adjacent pulmonary artery. Dilated bronchi that are perpendicular to the scanning plane have a circular appearance, and then the smaller pulmonary artery gives it a signet ring appearance (Fig. 15.3). Mucus filled bronchi appear as branching tubes or nodules. End expiratory scans identify increased trans-radiance in areas where air-trapping has occurred due to small airways disease.

Having established the presence and extent of bronchiectasis, the degree of functional impairment, and the presence or absence of a known cause, it is important to be in a position to monitor the progress of the patient. Lung function tests and chest radiographs are easy investigations to perform repeatedly, but are relatively insensitive. CT scans can monitor progression of disease, but only after damage has occurred, and radiation exposure may be of concern if many repeated scans are taken. We have found that blood markers of inflammation (neutrophil count, ESR, C-reactive protein) correlate with extent of bronchiectasis on CT scan and impairment of lung function, but the level of inflammation

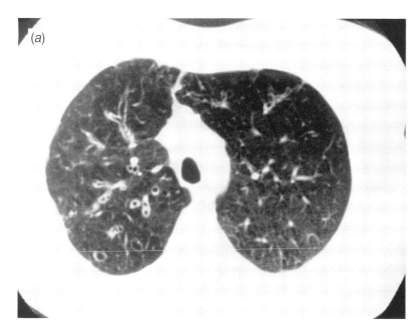

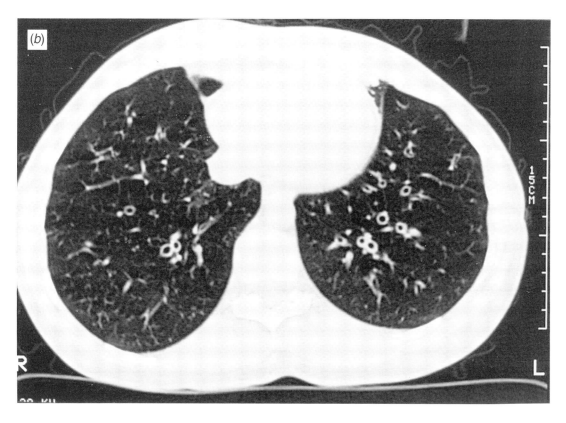

Fig. 15.3 CT scans of two patients with bronchiectasis. (*a*) A bronchiectatic airway in the right upper lobe which does not taper in the usual way is seen in the upper part of the film. Below this are several airways showing the signet ring appearance. Upper lobe bronchiectasis and chronic *Staphylococcus aureus* infection led to investigation of possible cystic fibrosis which was confirmed. (*b*) Several bronchiectatic airways in the left lung demonstrate the signet ring appearance. This appearance is caused by a dilated airway with its adjacent pulmonary artery.

in the lung may be a better index of disease activity[34]. Neutrophil elastase or myeloperoxidase might be useful measures in sputum, and hydrogen peroxide levels in exhaled air provide a measure of airway inflammation and oxidative stress[35]. Indium-III-labelled granulocyte scans measure not only inflammatory cell recruitment to the lung, but also show the sites in the bronchial tree that are affected[2].

Quality of life questionnaires provide a robust summary of the patients' symptoms and the impact of the disease on activities and lifestyle. They have proved useful measures of the benefit of therapeutic intervention in asthma and COPD. We have recently validated the St George's Respiratory Questionnaire in bronchiectasis and demonstrated that it was sensitive to change in the patients condition[27].

Non-antibiotic treatment of chronic bronchial suppuration

Physiotherapy

Poor clearance of mucus from bronchiectatic airways is probably the fundamental reason that patients become infected, and mucus contains bacterial products and inflammatory mediators which have the potential to both cause tissue damage and attract more inflammation. Therefore, physiotherapy is an important aspect of management, and it also allows the patient to expectorate sputum at chosen times during the day, rather than at inconvenient or socially embarrassing times. Patients are advised to perform postural drainage at least once daily, and increase the frequency to twice or three times if they suffer an exacerbation. Patients should be taught by a trained physiotherapist to adopt the correct position to drain affected areas, and clear mucus by controlled breathing techniques, sometimes aided by chest clapping by the patient or partner. Understandably compliance is poor, because of the nature of the process and the amount of time required, although the patient may not admit to this. Some patients, most commonly females, suppress their cough because of a dislike of sputum, and as a consequence their condition deteriorates. Physical exercise should be encouraged because it aids mucus clearance and since it is enjoyable compared to physiotherapy it may be more popular with the patient.

Nebulized saline may be given in an attempt to promote cough clearance and liquefy secretions, but other mucolytic agents have no role to play. Human recombinant DNase gives some benefit to patients with cystic fibrosis, but this approach was ineffective or may even have increased the frequency of exacerbations in bronchiectasis[36]. Asthmatic patients should take their short-acting bronchodilators before physiotherapy. Long-acting beta-agonists, inhaled corticosteroids and nebulized antibiotics should be taken after physiotherapy when the airways contain less secretions.

Treatment of airway inflammation

Any asthmatic component of bronchiectasis and chronic rhinosinusitis should be treated in the usual way. Infections may provoke an exacerbation of the asthmatic component, and this may be avoided by increasing the dosage of inhaled corticosteroids at the onset of the exacerbation. Exposure of the nasal and paranasal sinus mucosa to topical corticosteroids may be increased by using drops taken in the head down and forwards position[37]. Acid reflux may aggravate airway inflammation and should be enquired about and treated if present. Treatment of allergic bronchopulmonary aspergillosis with long-term oral or high-dose inhaled corticosteroids may prevent exacerbations. Systemic corticosteroids have unacceptable side effects when used long-term to reduce airway inflammation, although they may be used for short periods during severe exacerbations[38]. In severe cases long-term use may be unavoidable, in which case bone densitometry should be monitored and consideration given to protection by hormone replacement therapy (post-menopausal females) or biphosphonates.

Several treatments, other than antibiotics and systemic corticosteroids, have been investigated to see whether they reduce airway inflammation. These include high-dose inhaled corticosteroids[39], non-steroidal anti-inflammatory agents[40] and protease inhibitors[41]. Although, as yet there is little evidence of clinical benefit from these approaches, it may be that it is in this area that major advances are made in the future management of chronic bronchial suppuration. Annual influenza vaccination should be encouraged, and pneumococcal vaccination is probably worthwhile.

Treatment of hypogammaglobulinemia

Panhypogammaglobulinaemia and some selective immunoglobulin deficiencies respond well to regular replacement therapy with intravenous immunoglobulin. The interval between replacement can be varied depending on the clinical response, but 3 weeks is commonly chosen. The immunoglobulin **G** levels are measured prior to the next infusion and dosage adjusted to keep them within the normal range. In patients with selective immunoglobulin deficiency care should be taken to document whether benefit is obtained from replacement. This may involve a prolonged period of assessment since infective exacerbations and/or episodes of pneumonia may occur intermittently. Diary cards of symptoms should be kept before and after the introduction of (or a change in) treatment.

Respiratory failure

Patients with severe chronic respiratory failure and bronchiectasis require long-term oxygen treatment. Carbon dioxide retention is a problem that is sometimes encountered. Nasal intermittent positive pressure ventilation may provide some stabilization of their respiratory status and reduce the number of days spent in hospital. It is often surprisingly well tolerated despite a history of sinusitis[42]. This approach can also be used acutely during exacerbations **in order to** try to avoid the need for intubation and full ventilatory support.

Surgical treatment

The only curative treatment of bronchiectasis is surgical resection, although we have been surprised on occasions by the resolution of dilated bronchi on CT scan with medical treatment. The results of many apparently successful surgical series have been reported, but the indications for surgery are seldom made clear, and the causes of bronchiectasis are not defined to allow a comparison of like groups[2]. Very careful consideration should be given before proceeding with surgery. We have many middle-aged patients with generalized bronchiectasis who had lobectomies at an earlier age. The affected areas removed by surgery should be localized, and there should not be an underlying condition which predisposes to generalized bronchiectasis, e.g. primary ciliary dyskinesia. Indium-III-granulocyte scans have been used to confirm that inflammation is confined to the area of structural abnormality identified by the CT scan. More generalized inflammation would suggest that the patient will continue to have problems following surgery and may develop bronchiectasis elsewhere after several years[2]. 'Modern' cylindrical bronchiectasis tends to be bilateral and surgery is carried out infrequently for this reason. It is impossible to apply results from old surgical series, performed when case severity was very different from today, to 'modern' bronchiectasis. The best results are obtained when the cause is localized obstruction of an airway[43]. In such cases there is dramatic relief from disabling fever, malaise and pleuritic pain which can transform a patient's life.

Palliative surgical resection may be considered if a localized area of severe bronchiectasis defies medical management and acts as a sump for infection of other areas, even if less severe bronchiectasis is present elsewhere. Emergency surgical resection may be necessary for life threatening hemoptysis, but embolization of the appropriate bronchial artery is usually attempted first. The relevant anastomosing pulmonary artery may also require obstruction, e.g. by a balloon catheter[44].

Lung transplantation (single lung, two lungs or heart–lung transplantation) has been used to treat respiratory failure due to bronchiectasis, and can be considered if deterioration in the patient's condition occurs despite optimal medical treatment. Single lung transplantation is not usually considered because of fears of cross-infection from areas of bronchiectasis in the remaining lung, and the risk of disseminated infection in the presence of immunosuppression required to avoid rejection of the transplanted lung. However, this understandable dogma may need to be reconsidered because of the low number of donor organs available. There have also been some encouraging results in cystic fibrosis patients who have received live donor single lobe transplantation.

Antibiotics used in the treatment of chronic bronchial suppuration

Beta lactams

All beta-lactam antibiotics (penicillins, cephalosporins, carbapenems and monobactams) interfere with the biosynthesis of the peptidoglycan structure of the cell wall of actively dividing bacteria which causes lysis. They bind to transpeptidase and carboxypeptidase enzymes called penicillin binding proteins (PBPs), located beneath the cell wall outside the cytoplasmic membrane, and interfere with their function. Penicillins generally have a short half-life. They are divided into groups depending on their structure that have different spectra of activity and pharmacological properties[45,46].

Bacterial resistance to penicillins and other beta-lactam antibiotics arises either due to release of enzymes that break down the antibiotic, or due to changes in the PBPs, or due to failure of the antibiotic to penetrate through the outer wall porin channels. Pneumococcal penicillin resistance occurs due to alteration in PBPs. The most common group of beta-lactamases produced by clinical isolates is the plasmid-mediated TEM enzymes that exist in many Enterobacteriaceae, *H. influenzae* and *Neisseria* species. Development of new beta-lactam antimicrobial agents during the past decades has resulted in a number of drugs with increased, albeit not total, resistance to beta-lactamases. Another pharmacological approach has been the development of beta-lactamase inhibitors that can be used in combination with a beta-lactam drug to overcome the beta-lactamase-mediated resistance[47]. Clavulanic acid is currently combined with amoxycillin as Augmentin and ticarcillin as Timentin. Although it has a low level of antibacterial action itself, clavulanate inhibits beta-lactamases of numerous pathogenic gram-positive and gram-negative bacteria by forming a stable inactive complex, but does not inhibit the chromosomally mediated enzymes produced by some Enterobacteriaceae and *P. aeruginosa*. Sulbactam and tazobactam are other beta-lactamase inhibitors used in combination with ampicillin and piperacillin, respectively.

Allergic reactions to penicillin and its synthetic analogues are quite common (3–5% of general population), but true IgE-dependent anaphylaxis is rare. Most anaphylactic responses follow the drug being given parenterally, and there is no association with atopy. Some patients who are allergic to penicillin can tolerate the drug when given it again so sensitization may only be temporary. Confirmation of IgE-related sensitization may be obtained by standard skin prick testing. Almost all beta-lactam antibiotics show some cross-sensitization, although it happens infrequently with cephalosporins and quite rarely with the new beta-lactam antibiotics such as aztreonam and imipenem. Patients who have a strong history of penicillin anaphylaxis and need penicillin for a serious infection can be desensitized, but in practice an alternative antibiotic can usually be chosen[48].

Cephalosporins are classified as first- (e.g. cephradine, cephalexin), second- (e.g. cefaclor, cefuroxime), third- (e.g. cefotaxime, ceftriaxone, ceftazidime) or fourth-generation (e.g. cefepime) antibiotics. The second-generation cephalosporins extended the antibacterial spectrum of the first generation, not only against Enterobacteriaceae, but also *H. influenzae*. The third and fourth generation are represented by a very diverse group of potent antibiotics with a broader spectrum and with much more stability against beta-lactamase enzymes. Cephalosporins are a remarkably safe class of antibiotic. Anaphylactic reactions are very rare in spite of their structural similarity to penicillin. Some cephalosporins are potent inducers of chromosomally mediated beta-lactamases and can cause resistance to many agents by this mechanism. Linked to this inducibility is the ability of the bacteria to undergo mutation to high-level constitutive beta-lactamase production[46].

Thienamycin was the first available antibiotic of the new carbapenem class; it is co-administered with cilastatin, a specific inhibitor of the enzyme dehydropeptidase-1 (DHP-1), which prevents rapid renal metabolism of thienamycin. The combination, thienamycin plus cilastatin, is called imipenem and has very good activity against all categories of pathogenic bacteria. Meropenem is a broad spectrum carbapenem that is stable in the presence of DHP-1 and does not, therefore, require co-administration with an inhibitor. Meropenem is preferred to imipenem because it is generally more active against Enterobacteriaceae, it is given by an 8 hourly dosage schedule rather than 6 hourly that is usual for imipenem, and it has less central nervous system side effects. Several oral carbapenems are in development.

Aztreonam is the first synthetic monobactam and has a narrow spectrum of action. It has a high affinity for PBP-3 of susceptible gram-negative bacteria (including *P. aeruginosa*), but does not bind to the essential PBPs of gram-positive and anaerobic bacteria. Because aztreonam lacks the bicyclic nucleus of the penicillins and cephalosporins, cross-reactivity is rare. Superinfections by gram-positive organisms, especially enterococci and staphylococci, have occurred in patients treated with aztreonam alone.

Macrolides

Macrolides are so called because they possess a macrocyclic lactone nucleus. They inhibit protein synthesis of susceptible organisms by reversible binding to the 50S ribosomal subunit. A number of 14-, 15-, and 16-membered macrolides have been synthesized in recent years with the goal of overcoming some of the problems of the older erythromycin agents, such as variable activity against *H. influenzae*, gastrointestinal side effects, and the need to administer the drug four times a day. Erythromycin inhibits most hemolytic streptococci and *M. catarrhalis*. It also inhibits the atypical bacterial species *Mycoplasma pneumoniae, Legionella pneumophila*, and chlamydia species including *Chlamydia pneumoniae*, that are resistant to beta lactams. Activity against anaerobic species is extremely variable[49]. Macrolides have anti-inflammatory properties

which are independent of their antibiotic action. This has led to investigation of their wider use in bronchiectasis (see later).

Resistance to macrolides can be either chromosomal or plasmid mediated, and can be inducible or constitutively expressed. The biochemical basis is by methylation of adenine residues, which prevents binding of erythromycin to the binding site. Resistance of *S. pneumoniae* had remained low in most countries until recent years, but the multiply resistant (including penicillin) strains first described in South Africa are becoming much more common in some countries, particularly in Spain and the USA[50]. Resistance of *M. pneumoniae* and *L. pneumoniae* has not been noted. Bacterial strains resistant to erythromycin are usually resistant to the newer macrolides. Clarithromycin is a derivative of erythromycin with an alkylated hydroxyl group at C6. It has improved activity against legionella and chlamydia, but similar activity to erythromycin for *H. influenzae*. However, its 14-OH metabolite is also active against *H. influenzae*, and since the effects of the parent antibiotic and the metabolite are additive the overall action is superior. Clarithromycin is rapidly absorbed from the gastrointestinal tract and prolonged half-lives of the parent compound and the 14-OH metabolite allows twice daily dosing[51].

Azithromycin is the prototype of the semisynthetic macrolides called the azalides. This antibiotic has remarkable pharmacokinetics in that it rapidly penetrates into tissues and the highest concentrations are found in the intracellular environment. This might be an advantage when treating intracellular pathogens such as *Legionella* and *Chlamydia*, but clinical evidence is lacking. High tissue concentrations persist for up to 5 days after a single oral dose. Azithromycin need only be administered once daily and because of the long tissue half-life it has been recommended to be given for only 3 days to treat infective bronchitis[52]. Ketolides are semisynthetic derivatives of the 14-membered ring macrolides. They are active against multiresistant penicillin/macrolide resistant pneumococci, and have good activity against other bacterial species causing lower respiratory tract infections including atypical species. They may also retain the anti-inflammatory properties described with macrolide antibiotics.

Because they are more potent and have improved pharmacokinetics the newer macrolides can be taken less frequently at lower dosage and, therefore, have a much improved gastrointestinal side effect profile. Macrolides may result in alteration of hepatic enzyme systems and may therefore interact with many drugs including theophylline. The new macrolides are important antibiotics in the treatment of non-tuberculous mycobacteria infections. The interaction with rifabutin, an antibiotic commonly used to treat mycobacterial infections, is important to be aware of because of the increased risk of uveitis.

Quinolones

Uniquely among antimicrobials in clinical use, the primary bacterial targets of fluoroquinolones are enzymes involved in the replication of DNA[53,54]. They interfere with DNA replication, segregation of bacterial chromosomes, transcription, and other cellular processes. In general, second generation quinolones, e.g. ciprofloxacin and levofloxacin have good activity against most Enterobacteriaceae, fastidious gram-negative bacilli including *H. influenzae*, and gram-negative cocci such as *M. catarrhalis*. Ciprofloxacin is the most active against *P. aeruginosa* and provides the only oral option for treatment of infection by this bacterium. Second generation quinolones have good activity against *S. aureus*, but are less active against streptococci and enterococci, and have minimal activity against anaerobes. They are active in vitro against *Chlamydia*, *Mycoplasma*, and *Legionella* species, and have some activity against mycobacterial species[53]. Absorption is reduced by administration with antacids containing divalent cations and iron-containing preparations. Side effects include cytochrome P450 interactions, e.g. delayed theophylline clearance, phototoxicity and central nervous system problems including convulsions. Two mechanisms of quinolone resistance have been identified: alteration in the target DNA

enzymes and an efflux pump. Only chromosomal-mediated quinolone resistance has been found so far, and single-step mutation to high-level resistance is very rare, but high-level resistance can be selected by serial exposure of bacteria to increasing drug concentrations. In certain clinical settings, the emergence of resistance has been problematic, and *P. aeruginosa* and *S. aureus* have been particularly troublesome[54].

Temafloxacin was a new third-generation quinolone antibiotic with improved activity against *S. pneumoniae*. However, this antibiotic had to be withdrawn soon after launch as a result of serious adverse reactions which included severe hypoglycaemia, hepatic dysfunction, haemolytic anaemia and renal dysfunction, requiring dialysis in some instances, anaphylaxis and death. Subsequently, several other third-generation quinolones with improved gram-positive activity have been withdrawn or their use severely restricted because of side effects, e.g. trovafloxacin (eosinophilic hepatitis), grepafloxacin (cardiac arrhythmias) and sparfloxacin (photosensitivity). However, other third generation quinolones, e.g. moxifloxacin and gatifloxacin have been released and have not had these problems. They all have the advantage of improved gram-positive activity, and are active against penicillin-resistant pneumococcal strains. They will be much better suited than ciprofloxacin to the treatment of community-acquired respiratory infections, but concern has been expressed that widespread use may lead to an increase in levels of resistance particularly in the pneumococcus[54].

Tetracyclines

Tetracyclines are broad-spectrum oral antibiotics that work by binding to the bacterial 30S ribosomal subunit and inhibiting protein synthesis. Their use has been limited by emergence of resistance in respiratory pathogens, but since their popularity declined, levels of resistance have fallen. The semi-synthetic newer tetracyclines such as doxycycline and minocycline have advantages in that they have a much longer half-life in serum which allows once daily dosage. Plasmids impart resistance by coding for proteins that interfere with active transport through the cytoplasmic membrane. Tetracyclines pose a special danger to pregnant women because fatal reactions due to hepatotoxicity have occurred. With the exception of doxycycline, which is excreted in the faeces largely as an inactive conjugate and minocycline, they increase uremia in patients with chronic renal failure. They cause brown discolouration of the teeth and may retard growth of bone in the human foetus and in children[49].

Chloramphenicol

Chloramphenicol inhibits bacterial protein synthesis by binding to the 50S ribosomal subunit. The antibiotic is well absorbed, penetrates into tissues, and has good activity against common respiratory pathogens such as *H. influenzae* and *S. pneumoniae* and many anaerobic bacteria. However, its use is severely curtailed by its potential to cause bone marrow toxicity. This occurs in two forms, first dose-related bone marrow suppression, which usually begins 5 to 7 days after initiation of treatment and is reversible, and second, idiosyncratic aplastic anemia, which is very rare and unrelated to dose. Resistance to chloramphenicol occurs via plasmid-mediated acetylation, which prevents binding to the ribosome[49]. Chloramphenicol is sometimes used empirically to treat chronic bronchial suppuration when other oral agents have failed. The reason for the response that is sometimes seen is unclear, but may be due to its activity against *H.influenzae* or anaerobes.

Trimethoprim-sulfamethoxazole

This antibiotic combination acts synergistically by inhibiting sequential steps in the bacterial pathway generating folate cofactors that function as one carbon donors in the synthesis of nucleic acids. The commonest mechanism of trimethoprim resistance is plasmid mediated and involves dihydrofolate reductase with reduced affinity for trimethoprim. It is not recommended for infants under 2 months of age because of the risk of kernicterus, or for pregnant or lactating women. Use has declined because of bacterial resistance and also serious side effects. Although these are not common, the sulfonamide component can lead to hypersensitivity reactions such as rash, vasculitis, erythema nodosum, erythema multiforme, and Stevens–Johnson syndrome[55].

Aminoglycosides

The spectrum of activity is broad, and aminoglycosides are particularly active against aerobic gram-negative rods. They are usually used in combination with a beta-lactam to treat chronic bronchial suppuration or nosocomial infections. Aminoglycosides act at the ribosomal level to inhibit bacterial protein synthesis, and as they are not absorbed from the intestines can only be given parenterally. Their bactericidal effect is very much concentration dependent, and peak concentrations in serum correlate with clinical and bacteriological response, while low concentrations have little efficacy, but still accumulate and therefore increase the risk of toxicity. For this reason, aminoglycosides may be given as a once daily infusion over 30 minutes, clearance being checked by a single trough level just before the next dose. Otherwise they are given 8 hourly and the dosage and frequency of administration adjusted individually from peak and trough serum measurements.

Resistance to aminoglycosides can result from alterations in cellular permeability or the ribosomal target, but most commonly is due to enzymes that modify aminoglycoside structure (e.g. acetylation, adenylation or phosphorylation), which may be carried on plasmids, transposons or the chromosome. The toxicity of aminoglycosides is based on accumulation and the major side effects involve the kidney and ear. Reduced glomerular filtration and proteinuria both usually show gradual recovery after discontinuation of therapy. Cochlear ototoxicity is caused by permanent degeneration of hair cells in the organ of Corti, starting in the high-pitch region of the basilar membrane. Vestibular damage also occurs, but because the patient can compensate for this disturbance it is usually less serious[56].

Oxazolidones and streptogramins

These are new antibiotics which inhibit protein synthesis. They are active against multiresistant gram-positive cocci including methicillin-resistant *S. aureus*.

Antibiotic treatment of chronic bronchial suppuration

General principles

The outcome of antibiotic therapy depends mainly on the severity of the bronchiectasis. When bronchiectasis is mild to moderate, antibiotics can eradicate the infection and the lung defences may keep the airways sterile or bacterial numbers low for a prolonged period. An external event, such as a viral infection, may then precipitate an exacerbation which is associated with an increase in bacterial numbers. When lung damage is more severe, the bronchial tree is usually chronically infected and the patient's symptoms may gradually return over several weeks, or sometimes more quickly, after stopping an antibiotic. In these different circumstances antibiotics may be needed only during infective exacerbations associated with a change in sputum production, breathlessness and malaise, or continuously if relapse is rapid. Chronic inflammation may lead to disease progression, and antibiotic therapy can theoretically prevent this by decreasing the bacterial load and so reducing the level of inflammation[57,58]. However, long term studies to determine whether antibiotics are successful in preventing deterioration in lung function or increase in the extent of bronchiectasis have not been performed, except in cystic fibrosis patients where disease progression is more rapid[59]. Unfortunately, there have been very few antibiotic trials carried out in patients with chronic bronchial suppuration. In a recent review of the non-cystic fibrosis literature few published studies were identified[60–65]. These studies of small groups of patients have not provided any clear guidance about choice of antibiotic. Therefore, one has to rely on general principles to provide a logical approach to antibiotic treatment.

The choice of antibiotic is influenced by the high frequency of β-lactamase production by strains of *M. catarrhalis* and *H. influenzae*, the presence or absence of *P. aeruginosa* which is usually resistant to all oral antibiotics except ciprofloxacin, and by pharmacokinetic characteristics of antibiotics. The efficacy of an antibiotic is probably related to the concentration of antibiotic at the site of infection in the lung and the sensitivity of the bacterium. The site of infection in chronic bronchial suppuration is the airway lumen where bacteria are present in large numbers, often 10^9/ml of sputum or higher, and they are adherent to the respiratory mucosa and associated with secretions. The concentration of antibiotic in the lung may be markedly different from that observed in serum as there are significant barriers to the penetration of the antibiotic[66,67]. In the presence of inflammation, the partitioning of antibiotics in tissue compartments may be altered due to increased membrane permeability. Thus for drugs such as beta-lactams that do not cross membranes easily, penetration increases in the presence of inflammation. Conversely, during resolution antibiotic concentrations at the site of infection may fall, which at least theoretically could allow bacterial persistence and predispose to relapse. However, the situation is complicated because infection, particularly if it is chronic, may change tissue anatomy and physiology in various ways. For example, blood flow to the site of infection may be increased due to vasodilatation, or conversely may be reduced by poor blood supply to damaged and scarred airways. It has also been reasoned that antibiotics which penetrate well into cells, such as the quinolones, might be carried into the lumen within neutrophils. The secretions themselves also provide a barrier, as may the alginate substance which is secreted by mucoid pseudomonas strains and forms a gel layer around colonies, because most antibiotics do not pass into these sites easily.

Two important pharmacokinetic parameters have been defined. First, the peak concentration of the antibiotic at the site of infection compared to the sensitivity of the bacterium for the antibiotic. Second, the time after an antibiotic is administered

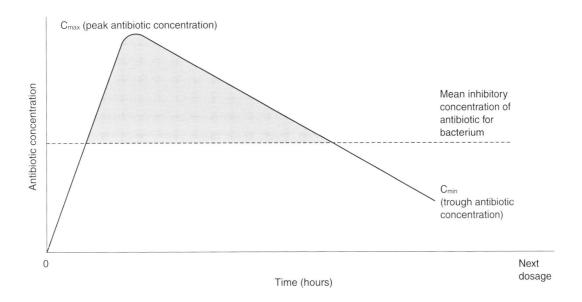

Fig. 15.4 Pharmacokinetic properties of antibiotics which may influence their clinical efficacy. The shaded part is the area under the curve which exceeds the antibiotic's inhibitory concentration for the bacterium.

that the concentration of the antibiotic at the site of infection exceeds the concentration required to inhibit the bacterium. The two parameters are combined by plotting a curve of antibiotic concentration against time and calculating the area under the curve which exceeds the inhibitory concentration for the bacterium. The larger the value the more effective the antibiotic is likely to be (Fig. 15.4). Although the concentrations of antibiotic at the site of infection are most relevant, they are difficult to obtain from the lung, and despite the reservations explained above serum concentrations are often used. Antibiotics vary in their ability to penetrate into the bronchial mucosa as well as in their activity against different species. In general beta lactams and aminoglycosides penetrate less well into the respiratory mucosa than macrolides, azalides and quinolones which gives the latter antibiotic classes an advantage in the treatment of chronic bronchial suppuration[68–71].

Damaged airways, high bacterial numbers and plentiful secretions in bronchiectasis makes it difficult to achieve a high concentration of antibiotic at the site of infection. The length of the course of antibiotics may need to be longer, and the dosage given higher, than is usual for bronchial infections in chronic bronchitis or community acquired pneumonia where the host defences are more intact and bacterial numbers are less. A patient's general well-being and the volume and colour of their sputum can be used to empirically judge the length of the course of treatment. Lung function may also improve, but this is not always the case[60]. If patients are severely unwell at presentation, or do not respond to oral antibiotics, then intravenous antibiotics are required. These achieve much higher concentrations in serum which is reflected at the site of infection, and particularly for treatment of *P. aeruginosa* most preparations only have an intravenous formulation. They should be commenced in hospital where supportive treatment (e.g. physiotherapy) can also be given. Increasingly, patients are being taught to administer their own intravenous antibiotics, so that once they are improving their stay in hospital can be shortened by completing the course of treatment at home. The fall in the level of the blood inflammatory markers (neutrophil count,

C-reactive protein and ESR) can also be used to judge response to intravenous treatment[34].

Oral antibiotic treatment

The following clinical parameters can be used to decide whether a patient is well enough to receive oral antibiotics as an outpatient: general well-being; lack of significant pyrexia (>38 °C might indicate that pneumonia is present); spirometry (compared to values obtained when the patient is well); oxygen saturations; lack of consolidation on the chest radiograph; level of home support. The presence of chest pain which would limit coughing and physiotherapy is an important reason to admit to hospital, because this can lead to a rapid deterioration in the patient's condition.

The choice of antibiotic may be guided by previous sputum bacteriology and antibiotic sensitivity, particularly the presence or absence of P. aeruginosa. The lack of clinical trial data means that choice is influenced by personal experience. In the absence of P. aeruginosa high dose amoxycillin (1 gram three times daily up to a dose of three grams twice daily for 7 to 14 days), amoxycillin/clavulanate (625 mg three times daily for 7 to 14 days), azithromycin (500 mg once daily for 3 to 6 days), doxycycline (100 mg or 200 mg once daily for 7 to 14 days) and ciprofloxacin (750 mg twice daily for 7 to 14 days) are our antibiotics of choice. We do not tend to use oral cephalosporins because of poor activity against H.influenzae (e.g. cephalexin and cefaclor) or poor absorption after oral administration (e.g. cefuroxime axetil and cefixime). We do not use clarithromycin because of data from chronic bronchitis trials showing persistence of H.influenzae after treatment[72].

The commonest mistakes are to underdose or to stop antibiotic treatment too quickly. Underdosing leads to subinhibitory concentrations of antibiotic at the site of infection which in turn leads to persistence of the infection and promotes development of antibiotic resistance; and stopping antibiotic treatment before the exacerbation has fully resolved leads to persistent inflammation and can result in a rapid relapse. In chronic bronchitis a short course of antibiotics is usually successful because the host defences are relatively intact and can facilitate clearance of the infection, but this is not the case in bronchiectasis.

In the presence of P. aeruginosa only quinolone antibiotics are active and ciprofloxacin is the antibiotic of choice. Unfortunately repeated courses of ciprofloxacin lead to stepwise development of resistance if they are given too frequently. Patients with P. aeruginosa infection may respond to oral antibiotics that have no activity against P. aeruginosa. We have had success using azithromycin 500 mg once daily for 6 days. This unexpected outcome may be due to spontaneous recovery, the benefit of adjunct treatment, e.g. physiotherapy or corticosteroids, successful treatment of coinfection with a sensitive species, or due to the anti-inflammatory properties of the macrolide antibiotic.

Intravenous antibiotic treatment

In the absence of P. aeruginosa we usually use a second- (e.g. cefuroxime 750 mg or 1.5 g three times daily) or third- (e.g. ceftriaxone 1 g or 2 g once daily) generation cephalosporin. Ceftriaxone is preferred to cefotaxime because it is given once instead of three times daily, which reduces the nursing time and is important if the patient is to complete the course of treatment at home. Amoxycillin/clavulanate would be an acceptable alternative, but may be less well tolerated.

In the presence of P. aeruginosa the antibiotic options are shown in Table 15.4. The choice may be made on the basis of the most recent sensitivity results. There seems to be a poor correlation between in vitro antibiotic susceptibility testing and in vivo antibiotic efficacy. This may be partly explained by bacterial population dynamics where resistant strains are a small subpopulation of the total bacterial load. Another explanation is that some antibiotics can inhibit bacterial production of virulence factors despite in vitro resistance[73]. A semi-synthetic penicillin (e.g. piperacillin) or third-generation cephalosporin with pseudomonas activity (e.g. ceftazidime) is usually used, most often in combination with an aminoglycoside antibiotic. There are several reports showing synergism

Table 15.4. Intravenous antibiotics used in the treatment of *Pseudomonas aeruginosa*

Antibiotic	Usual adult dosage	Comment
Azlocillin	5 g 8 hourly	Ureidopenicillin[a]. Withdrawn by manufacturers
Piperacillin	4 g 8 hourly	Ureidopenicillin[a]. Not used in cystic fibrosis due to incidence of allergic reactions. Also available with the beta lactamase inhibitor tazobactam as Tazocin given 4.5 g 8 hourly
Ticarcillin	5 g 6 or 8 hourly	Caboxypenicillin[a]. Not available in all countries, but is available with the beta lactamase inhibitor clavulanic acid as Timentin given 3.2 g 6 or 8 hourly
Ceftazidime	2 g 8 hourly	Third-generation cephalosporin
Aztreonam	2 g 8 hourly	Monobactam. No gram-positive activity therefore should be given in combination
Meropenem	1 g 8 hourly	Carbapenem. Simpler formulation, better pharmacokinetics and fewer side effects than imipenem with cilastatin
Gentamicin	2 to 5 mg/kg daily in divided doses 8 hourly[b]	Aminoglycoside. Given in combination with one of above antibiotics. Side effects of oto- and nephro-toxicity are dose related. Excretion via kidney so dosage and frequency require adjustment in renal failure. Other aminoglycosides are available, e.g. tobramycin
Amikacin	15 mg/kg daily in divided doses 8 or 12 hourly[b]	Aminoglycoside. Stable to many of bacterial enzymes that inactivate other aminoglycosides.

Notes:

[a] Sodium content of these antibiotics may cause hypernatraemia/fluid overload.

[b] Monitor peak (1 hour after injection) and trough (just before dose) levels after third dose, and subsequently after dosage adjustment if this result is abnormal or there are concerns about accumulation. Aminoglycosides can also be given once daily as a single infusion over 30 minutes which has several advantages including efficacy since this is related to peak serum level, reduced risk of toxicity, and that it is only necessary to monitor a single trough level taken just before the next dose. Expert advice should be sought on dosage.

between beta-lactams and aminoglycosides against *P. aeruginosa*, but these results have been produced in animal models or in clinical studies of pneumonia, e.g. in neutropenic patients when there is a likelihood of bacteremia[74]. Therefore, the benefit of using an aminoglycoside for chronic bronchial suppuration involving *P. aeruginosa* has to be balanced against the side effects of this class of antibiotic. Monobactams, e.g. aztreonam, carbapenems, e.g. meropenem and antibiotic combinations with a beta lactamase inhibitor, e.g. piperacillin/tazobactam have increased the antibiotic options available to treat *P. aeruginosa* infection. However, infection by multi-resistant strains still occurs, particularly in patients with severe bronchiectasis who have required multiple courses of intravenous antibiotics. In these circumstances *P. aeruginosa* usually retains

sensitivity to colistin sulphomethate, which has to be used intravenously with caution because of nephrotoxicity and neurotoxicity[75].

The course of intravenous antibiotics should be continued for 7 to 14 days. The aim of treatment is to reduce the bacterial load in the bronchial tree to low numbers, leading to a reduction in the level of inflammation and recovery of host defences such as mucus clearance which are impaired during the exacerbation by increased mucus viscosity, bronchospasm and epithelial damage. An early switch to oral therapy as the patient improves, which would be appropriate in an acute community acquired pneumonia, should not be made in chronic bronchial suppuration, particularly when using beta lactam antibiotics, because their pharmacokinetics will mean that reduced concentrations of antibiotic reach the site of infection, and this may result in incomplete resolution of the infection and early relapse.

Prophylactic antibiotics

Patients who quickly relapse following intravenous treatment may be considered for long-term prophylactic antibiotics. This decision should only be taken after careful consideration and when other aspects of management have been optimized. There is justifiable concern that this approach promotes antibiotic resistance, or infection by more resistant species, e.g. *P. aeruginosa*, or that there may be side effects from the treatment. Three different approaches have been used: oral antibiotics[63,76], inhaled antibiotics given as an isotonic solution via a nebulizer[61,65,77,78], and regular pulsed courses of intravenous antibiotics[79].

Because the concentration of antibiotics at the site of infection in the airway is important, the idea of delivering high concentrations of antibiotic directly onto the mucosa by inhalation is appealing. A number of regimens are used, including beta-lactams, aminoglycosides and colistin sulphomethate, either singly or in combination. At the moment only colistin sulphomethate has a licence for this route of administration, and a formulation of tobramycin is being investigated in clinical trials. Most experience of nebulized antibiotics has been gained in cystic fibrosis where they have been used to treat *P. aeruginosa*. Benefit has been demonstrated in terms of improved well-being and lung function, and reduced frequency of exacerbations and hospital admissions[77]. Nebulized gentamicin reduced airway inflammation and mucus secretion in bronchiectasis, and there was some improvement in lung function and exercise tolerance[78]. Nebulized antibiotics are best given in a prophylactic manner to delay relapse following a course of intravenous treatment, and they are less effective during acute exacerbations, probably because they are deposited in the central airways due to obstruction of smaller airways by secretions and bronchospasm[80]. The antibiotic should be delivered by a suitable air compressor and nebulizer device to allow effective dispersal through the bronchial tree, with a one way valve system and an outlet so that exhaled antibiotics can be discharged via a window, preventing exposure of family or other patients to the antibiotic. Nebulized antibiotics are most commonly used in patients with chronic *P. aeruginosa* infection and we usually prefer colistin sulphomethate because resistance is rare and it is not an antibiotic we commonly use via other routes of administration. Some patients experience bronchospasm which can be severe enough to exclude this approach, and treatment should be commenced in hospital. Another antibiotic can be tried empirically if bronchospasm occurs. Peak flows and spirometry should be recorded before and after the first dose and for several days as in some cases the onset of bronchospasm is delayed.

Similar benefits to nebulized antibiotics have been demonstrated with regular oral antibiotics[63,76]. This approach is limited by the patient's tolerance of the antibiotic (particularly gastrointestinal side effects) or development of resistance. Sometimes a number of different antibiotics are rotated to try to avoid these problems. Regular pulsed courses of intravenous antibiotics have been advocated in cystic fibrosis and clinical benefits have been claimed[79]. The course of intravenous antibiotics is given before full relapse has occurred, so maintaining suppression of the bacterial load in the lung, and thus keeping the level of inflammation under control. We have used a similar protocol in severe bronchiectasis. The length of time between the courses of antibiotics can be tailored to the particular patient's history, but 4 to 8 weeks is commonly chosen. This period can be increased as the patient's condition improves, and in some cases we have been able to revert to a conventional 'on demand' antibiotic policy. We have found improvement in patients' quality of life using this approach, but in a recent prospective randomized study of cystic fibrosis patients carried out by the British Thoracic Society, regular elective treatment was compared to symptomatic treatment; patients in the symptomatic group receive a mean of 3 antibiotic treatments each year and the elective group 4, and there were no significant differences in changes in lung function and survival over 3 years [81].

Macrolide antibiotics

Diffuse panbronchiolitis is a condition of unknown aetiology described in Japanese patients[82]. There is chronic inflammation which is initially located predominantly in the respiratory bronchioles, but in advanced cases bronchiectasis develops. Continuous erythromycin is commonly used to treat these patients, even when there is chronic bronchial infection involving *P. aeruginosa*[83]. Several recent experimental observations might explain the unexpected benefits that have been reported, and justify further clinical studies in a wider bronchiectasis population. Erythromycin reduces exotoxin production by *P. aeruginosa* at concentrations which do not affect bacterial growth[73]. Macrolides suppress biofilm mode of bacterial growth, which otherwise gives bacteria some protection against neutrophil phagocytosis[84]. Macrolides also have anti-inflammatory actions such as inhibition of neutrophil chemotaxis[85] and generation of reactive oxygen species[86], and are also inhibitors of mucus secretion in vitro[87]. Roxithromycin, a new semisynthetic macrolide, decreased airway hyperresponsiveness to methacholine challenge in a group of children with bronchiectasis[88].

We have used prolonged courses of erythromycin, clarithromycin or azithromycin in patients with chronic bronchial suppuration including those chronically infected with *P. aeruginosa*. Benefits in some patients have included decreased sputum production, improved lung function and reduced frequency of infective exacerbations. Azithromycin has the advantage of once daily dosage, and its peculiar pharmacokinetics of persisting in lung tissue has enabled us to use an intermittent dosage regimen, e.g. alternate days following a 6-day 'loading' course of treatment, which reduces the incidence of gastrointestinal and other side effects. Some patients have complained of tinnitus and/or reduced hearing after several months' treatment and patients should be warned to stop the antibiotic if this occurs. Liver function tests should also be monitored. The number of patients that we have treated in this way is small, and the long-term use of macrolide antibiotics has not been the subject of a controlled trial.

Benefits of an antibiotic policy designed to minimize chronic bronchial suppuration

In the 'vicious circle' illustrated in Fig. 15.1 persistent bacterial infection causes lung damage by stimulating chronic inflammation, and this leads to progression of the bronchiectasis and deterioration in lung function. Furthermore, we have shown that the frequency of infective exacerbations and chronic inflammation are both associated with a poor quality of life[27,34]. Antibiotics suppress inflammation by decreasing the bacterial load, and it could be argued that they should be given in whatever volume and frequency is required to achieve this aim. However, there may be several drawbacks to such an approach both in terms of side effects involving the patients themselves, e.g. antibiotic-induced colitis, and with respect to antibiotic resistance in the patient and the species overall. Superinfections may also occur during long-term antibiotic treatment, and the resident chronic infection may be driven towards a more antibiotic-resistant species, e.g. *P. aeruginosa*.

The level of inflammation generated by bacterial infection may not just be related to bacterial load. Different bacterial species[34], and even the strain involved[15], attract variable inflammatory responses. There may also be genetic differences on the host side in the response to infection. The marked difference in the rates of disease progression between cystic fibrosis and bronchiectasis suggests that the 'vicious circle' described above is accelerated in cystic fibrosis. This has been ascribed to abnormal ion transport causing impaired mucociliary clearance resulting in a greater bacterial load, but recent experimental results have suggested a different explanation. The cystic fibrosis mouse is a powerful model to investigate basic mechanisms. Experimental mice homozygous for the cystic fibrosis gene, that have been raised in pathogen-free conditions, have greater numbers of lymphocytes in the airway submucosa compared with wild-type litter-mates[89]. This suggests that possibly there is an exaggerated immune response in cystic fibrosis. In a second study cystic fibrosis mice had a higher mortality than their normal littermates in a *P. aeruginosa* bronchopneumonia model which used bacteria embedded in agar beads to set up a chronic infection. The agar beads prevent the mucociliary system clearing bacteria in both groups of mice, so should exclude this aspect of the cystic fibrosis condition contributing to the result. Bacterial counts in the lungs were the same in the two groups and the excess mortality in the cystic fibrosis mice was associated with increased levels of inflammatory mediators in the lungs[90]. These results suggest that the basic defect in cystic fibrosis may in some way cause an exaggerated inflammatory response which increases tissue damage. The possibility that some cases of idiopathic bronchiectasis who progress rapidly might be explained in a similar way deserves further investigation.

Future developments

The pharmaceutical industry will continue to produce new antibiotics with increased potency against resistant strains, but bacteria with their rapid generation time are always likely to stay one step ahead. Several studies are investigating whether vaccines might benefit susceptible patients, but the number of species that are involved in chronic bronchial suppuration may limit this approach, and once established infection persists in chronic bronchial suppuration despite an exuberant antibody response which suggests that this strategy would only be successful as a preventative measure[10]. Indeed, one might expect that vaccination might lead to a deterioration in the presence of chronic infection by enhancing inflammation.

Improvements in our management of chronic bronchial suppuration are most likely to arise from a better understanding of the basic mechanisms involved in idiopathic 'modern' bronchiectasis. We need to understand the host defence abnormalities that permit infection to become established, and the factors which govern the level of the inflammatory response. Presently the discovery of better ways of reducing lung damage by controlling the chronic inflammatory response and drugs that are effective in enhancing mucus clearance seem to be the two most fruitful areas for new drug development.

REFERENCES

1 Field CE. Bronchiectasis. Third report on a follow-up study of medical and surgical cases from childhood. *Arch Dis Child* 1969; 44:551–561.

2 Cole PJ. Bronchiectasis, in Brewis RAL, Corrin B, Geddes DM, Gibson GJ ed: *Respiratory Medicine*, 2nd edn., London, WB Saunders Company Ltd, 1995:1286–1317.

3 Whitwell F. A study of the pathology and pathogenesis of bronchiectasis. *Thorax* 1952; 7:213–239.

4 Konietzko NFJ, Carton RW, Leroy EP. Causes of death in patients with bronchiectasis. *Am Rev Respir Dis* 1969; 100:852–858.

5 Sanderson JM, Kennedy MCS, Johnson MF, Manley DCE. Bronchiectasis: results of surgical and conservative management. *Thorax* 1974; 29:407–416.

6 Munro NC, Cooke J, Currie DC, Strickland B, Cole PJ. Comparison of thin-section computed tomography with bronchography in the identification of bronchiectatic segments in patients with chronic sputum production. *Thorax* 1990; 45:135–139.

7 Wilson R. Bacterial infection and chronic obstructive pulmonary disease. *Eur Respir J* 1999; 13:233–235.

8 Klingman KL, Pye A, Murphy TF, Hill SL. Dynamics of respiratory tract colonization by *Branhamella catarrhalis* in bronchiectasis. *Am J Respir Crit Care Med* 1995; 152:1072–1078.

9 Wilson R, Dowling RB, Jackson AD. The biology of bacterial colonization and invasion of the respiratory mucosa. *Eur Respir J* 1996; 9:1523–1530.

10 Hill SL, Mitchell JL, Burnett D, Stockley RA. IgG subclasses in the serum and sputum from patients with bronchiectasis. *Thorax* 1998; 53:463–468.

11 Lapa e Silva JR, Jones JAH, Cole PJ, Poulter LW. The immunological component of the cellular inflammatory infiltrate in bronchiectasis. *Thorax* 1989; 44:668–673.

12 Liebow AA, Hales MR, Lindsberg GE. Enlargement of the bronchial arteries and their anastomoses with pulmonary arteries in bronchiectasis. *Am J Pathol* 1949; 25:211–231.

13 Shah PL, Mawdsley S, Nash K, Cullinan P, Cole PJ, Wilson R. Determinants of chronic infection with *Staphylococcus aureus* in patients with bronchiectasis. *Eur Respir J* 1999; 14:1340–1344.

14 Wilson CB, Jones PW, O'Leary CJ, Hansell DM, Cole PJ, Wilson R. Effect of sputum bacteriology on the quality of life of patients with bronchiectasis. *Eur Respir J* 1997; 10:1754–1760.

15 Bresser P, van Alphen L, Habets FJM. Persisting *Haemophilus influenzae* strains induce lower levels of interleukin-6 and interleukin-8 in H292 lung epithelial cells than non-persisting strains. *Eur Respir J* 1997; 10:2319–2326.

16 Miszkiel KA, Wells AU, Rubens MB, Cole PJ, Hansell DM. Effects of airway infection by *Pseudomonas aeruginosa*: a computed tomographic study. *Thorax* 1997; 52:260–264.

17 Evans SA, Turner SM, Bosch BJ, Hardy CC, Woodhead MA. Lung function in bronchiectasis: the influence of *Pseudomonas aeruginosa. Eur Respir J* 1996; 9:1601–1604.

18 Kerem E, Corey M, Gold R, Levinson H. Pulmonary function and clinical course in patients with cystic fibrosis after pulmonary colonization with *Pseudomonas aeruginosa. J Pediatr* 1990; 116:714–719.

19 Wilson R, Abdallah S. Pulmonary disease in immunocompetent patients caused by non-tuberculous mycobacteria. In: *Tuberculosis.* Ed. Wilson R. *Eur Respir Monograph* 1997; 12:247–272.

20 Hansell DM. Imaging of obstructive pulmonary disease. Bronchiectasis. *Radiol Clin N Am* 1998; 36:107–128.

21 Murphy MB, Reen DJ, Fitzgerald M. Atopy, immunological changes and respiratory function in bronchiectasis. *Thorax* 1984; 39:179–184.

22 Nogrady SG, Evans WV, Davies BH. Reversibility of airways obstruction in bronchiectasis. *Thorax* 1978; 33:635–637.

23 Bahous J, Cortier A, Pineua L et al. Pulmonary function tests and airway responsiveness to metacholine in chronic bronchiectasis of the adult. *Bull Eur Physiopathol Respir* 1984; 20:375–380.

24 Steinfort CL, Smith MJ, Harrison NK, Prince C, Cole PJ. Reactive arthritis in bronchiectasis. *Am Rev Respir Dis* 1987; 135:A42.

25 Perry KMA, King DS. Bronchiectasis: a study of prognosis based on a follow-up of 400 patients. *Am Rev Tuberc* 1940; 41:531–548.

26 Keistinen T, Saynajakangas O, Tuuponen T, Kivela SL. Bronchiectasis: an orphan disease with a poorly-understood prognosis. *Eur Respir J* 1997; 10:2784–2787.

27 Wilson CB, Jones PW, O'Leary CJ, Cole PJ, Wilson R. Health status assessment in bronchiectasis using the St. George's Respiratory Questionnaire. *Am J Respir Crit Care Med* 1997; 156:536–541.

28 Ellis DA, Thornley PE, Wightman AJ, Walker M, Chalmers J, Crofton JW. Present outlook in bronchiectasis: clinical and social study and review of factors influencing prognosis. *Thorax* 1981; 36:659–664

29 De Gracia J, Rodrigo MK, Morell F et al. IgG subclass deficiencies associated with bronchiectasis. *Am J Respir Crit Care Med* 1996; 153:650–655.

30 Stanley P, MacWilliam L, Greenstone M, Mackay IS, Cole PJ. Efficacy of a saccharin test for screening to detect abnormal mucociliary clearance. *Br J Dis Chest* 1984; 78:62–65.

31 Lundberg JON, Weitzberg E, Nordvall ST, Kuylenstierna R, Lundberg JM, Alving K. Primary nasal origin of exhaled nitric oxide and absence of Kartenger's syndrome. *Eur Respir J* 1994; 7:1501–1504.

32 Currie DC, Cooke JC, Morgan AD et al. Interpretation of bronchograms and chest radiographs in patients with chronic sputum production. *Thorax* 1987; 42:278–284.

33 Naidich DP, McCauley DI, Khouri NF et al. Computed tomography of bronchiectasis. *J Comput Assist Tomogr* 1982; 6:437–444.

34 Wilson CB, Jones PW, O'Leary CJ et al. Systemic markers of inflammation in stable bronchiectasis. *Eur Respir J* 1998; 12:820–824.

35 Loukides S, Horvath I, Wodehouse T, Cole PJ, Barnes PJ. Elevated levels of expired breath hydrogen peroxide in bronchiectasis. *Am J Respir Crit Care Med* 1998; 158:991–994.

36 O'Donnell AE, Barker AF, Howite JS, Fick RB. Treatment of idiopathic bronchiectasis with recombinant human DNase 1. *Chest* 1998; 113:1329–1334.

37 Charlton R, Mackay IS, Wilson R, Cole PJ. A double blind, placebo controlled trial of betamethasone nasal drops in the treatment of nasal polyposis. *Br Med J* 1985; 291–788.

38 Rosenstein BJ, Eigen H. Risks of alternate-day prednisolone in patients with cystic fibrosis. *Pediatrics* 1991; 87:245–246.

39 Tsang KWT, Ho PL, Lam WK et al. Inhaled fluticasone reduces sputum inflammatory indices in severe bronchiectasis. *Am J Respir Crit Care Med* 1998; 158:723–727.

40 Konstan MW, Byard PJ, Hoppel CL, Davis PB. Effect of high-dose ibuprofen in patients with cystic fibrosis. *N Engl J Med* 1995; 332:848–854.

41 McElvaney NG, Nakamura H, Birrer P et al. Modulation of airway inflammation in cystic fibrosis. *In vivo* suppression of interleukin-8 levels on the respiratory epithelial surface by aerosolization of recombinant secretory leukoprotease inhibitor. *J Clin Invest* 1992; 90:1296–1301.

42 Gacouin A, Desrues B, Lena H, Quinquenel ML, Dassonville J, Delaval PH. Long-term nasal intermittent positive pressure ventilation (NIPPV) in sixteen consecutive patients with bronchiectasis: a retrospective study. *Eur Respir J* 1996; 9:1246–1250.

43 Agasthian T, Deschamps C, Trastek VF, Allen MS, Pairotero PC. Surgical management of bronchiectasis. *Ann Thorac Surg* 1996; 62:976–980.

44 Bredin CP, Richardson PR, King TKC, Sniderman KW, Sos TA,

Smith JP. Treatment of massive haemoptyses by combined occlusion of pulmonary and bronchial arteries. *Am Rev Respir Dis* 1978; 117:969–973.

45 Wright AJ, Wilkowske CJ. The penicillins. *Mayo Clinic Proc* 1987; 62:806–820.

46 Thompson RL. Cephalosporin, carbapenem, and mono-bactam antibiotics. *Mayo Clin Proc* 1987; 62:821–834.

47 Parker RH, Eggleston M. Beta lactamase inhibitors: another approach to overcoming antimicrobial resistance. *Infect Control* 1987; 8:36–40.

48 Holgate ST. Penicillin allergy: how to diagnose and when to treat. *Br Med J* 1988; 296:1213–1214.

49 Wilson WR, Cockerill FR. Tetracyclines, chloramphenicol, erythromycin, and clindamycin. *Mayo Clin Proc* 1987; 62:906–915.

50 Bacquero F, Martinez-Beltran J, Loza E. A review of antibiotic resistance patterns in Europe. *J Antimicrob Chemother* 1991; 28 (Suppl C):31–28.

51 Hardy DJ, Swanson RN, Rode RA, Marsh K, Shipkowitz NL, Clement JJ. Enhancement of the in vitro and in vivo activities of clarithromycin against *Haemophilus influenzae* by 14 hydroxy clarithromycin, its major metabolite in humans. *Antimicrob Agents Chemother* 1990; 34:1407–1413.

52 Baldwin DR, Wise R, Andrews JM, Ashby JP, Honeybourne D. Azithromycin concentrations at the sites of pulmonary infection. *Eur Respir J* 1990; 3:886–90.

53 Hooper DC, Wolfson JS. Fluoroquinolone antimicrobial agents. *N Engl J Med* 1991; 324:384–394.

54 Drlica K, Zhao X. DNA gyrase, topoisomerase IV, and the 4-quinolones. *Microb Molec Biol Rev* 1997; 61:377–392.

55 Foltzer MA, Reese RE. Trimethoprim – sulfamethoxazole and other sulfonamides. *Med Clin N Am* 1987; 71:1177–1193.

56 Laskin OL, Longstreth JA, Smith CR, Lietman PS. Netilmicin and gentamicin multidose kinetics in normal subjects. *Clin Pharmacol Ther* 1983; 34:644–650.

57 Stockley RA, Hill SL, Morrison HM. Effect of antibiotic treatment on sputum elastase in bronchiectatic outpatients in a stable clinical state. *Thorax* 1984; 39:414–419.

58 Currie DC, Higgs E, Metcalfe S, Roberts DE, Cole PJ. Simple method of monitoring microbial load in chronic bronchial sepsis: pilot comparison of reduction in colonising microbial load with antibiotics given intermittently and continuously. *J Clin Pathol* 1987; 40:830–836.

59 Suter S. New perspectives in understanding and management of the respiratory disease in cystic fibrosis. *Eur J Pediatr* 1994; 153:144–150.

60 Hill SL, Stockley RA. Effect of short and long-term antibiotic response on lung function in bronchiectasis. *Thorax* 1986; 41:798–800.

61 Hill SL, Morrison HM, Burnett D, Stockley RA. Short-term response of patients with bronchiectasis to treatment with amoxycillin given in standard or high doses orally or by inhalation. *Thorax* 1986; 41:559–565.

62 Lam WK, Chau PY, So SY et al. Ofloxacin compared with amoxycillin in treating infective exacerbations in bronchiectasis. *Resp Med* 1989; 83:299–303.

63 Currie DC, Garbett ND, Chan KL et al. Double-blind randomized study of prolonged higher-dose amoxycillin in purulent bronchiectasis. *Q J Med* 1990; 76:799–816.

64 Chan TH, Ho SS, Lai CK et al. Comparison of oral ciprofloxacin and amoxycillin in treating infective exacerbations of bronchiectasis in Hong Kong. *Chemotherapy* 1996; 42:150–156.

65 Lin H-C, Cheng H-F, Wang C-H, Liu C-Y, Yu C-T, Kuo H-P. Inhaled gentamicin reduces airway neutrophil activity and mucus secretion in bronchiectasis. *Am J Respir Crit Care Med* 1997; 155:2024–2029.

66 Valcke Y, Pauwels R, Van Der Straeten M. Pharmacokinetics of antibiotics in lungs. *Eur Respir J* 1990; 3:715–722.

67 Baltimore RS, Christie CD, Smith GJ. Immunohisto-pathological localisation of *Pseudomonas aeruginosa* in lungs from patients with cystic fibrosis. Implications for the pathogenesis of progressive lung deterioration. *Am Rev Respir Dis* 1989; 140:1650–1661.

68 Wilson R, Tsang KWT. Antibiotics and the lung. In: Page CP, Metzger WJ, eds. *Drugs and the Lung*. New York: Raven Press; 1994:347–381.

69 Bergogne-Berezin E. Pharmacokinetics of antibiotics in respiratory secretions. In: Penington JE, ed. *Respiratory Infections: Diagnosis and Management*, 2nd edn. New York: Raven Press, 1989:608–631.

70 Firsov AA, Vostrov SN, Shevenko AA, Cornaglia G. Parameters of bacterial killing and antimicrobial effect examined in terms of area under the concentration-time curve relationships: action of ciprofloxacin against *Escherichia coli* in an in-vitro dynamic model. *Antimicrob Agents Chemother* 1997; 41:1281–1287.

71 Thomas JK, Forrest A, Bhavnavi SM et al. Pharmacodynamic evaluation of factors associated with the development of bacterial resistance in acutely ill patients during therapy. *Antimicrob Agents Chemother* 1998; 42:521–527.

72 Wilson R, Kubin R, Ballin I et al. Five day moxifloxacin therapy compared with seven day clarithromycin therapy for the treatment of acute exacerbations of chronic bronchitis. *J Antimicrob Chemother* 1999; 44:501–513.

73 Tanaka E, Kanthakumar K, Cundell DR et al. The effect of erythromycin on *Pseudomonas aeruginosa* and neutrophil mediated epithelial damage. *J Antimicrob Chemother* 1994; 33:765–775.

74 Pennington JE. Hospital-acquired pneumonia. In: Pennington JE, ed, *Respiratory Infections: Diagnosis and Management*, 3rd edn. New York: Raven Press; 1994:207–227.

75 Conway SP, Pond MN, Watson A, Etherington C, Robey HL, Goldman MH. Intravenous colistin sulphomethate in acute respiratory exacerbations in adult patients with cystic fibrosis. *Thorax* 1997; 52:987–993.

76 Rayner CFJ, Tillotson G, Cole PJ, Wilson R. Efficacy and safety of long term ciprofloxacin in the management of severe bronchiectasis. *J Antimicrob Chemother* 1994; 34:149–156.

77 Mukhopadhyay S, Singh M, Cater JI, Ogston S, Franklin M, Olver RE. Nebulised antipseudomonal antibiotic therapy in cystic fibrosis: a meta-analysis of benefits and risks. *Thorax* 1996; 51:364–368.

78 Hodson ME, Penketh ARL, Batten JC. Aerosol carbenicillin and gentamicin treatment of *Pseudomonas aeruginosa* infection in patients with cystic fibrosis. *Lancet* 1981; ii:1137–1139.

79 Szaff M, Hoiby N, Flensborg EW. Frequent antibiotic therapy improves survival of cystic fibrosis patients with chronic *Pseudomonas aeruginosa* infection. *Acta Paediatr Scand* 1983; 72:651–657.

80 Mukhopadhyay S, Staddon GE, Eastman C, Palmer M, Davies ER, Carswell F. The quantitative distribution of nebulised antibiotic in the lung in cystic fibrosis. *Respir Med* 1994; 88:203–211.

81 Elborn JS. Precott RJ, Stack BHR et al. Elective versus symptomatic antibiotic treatment in cystic fibrosis patients with chronic *Pseudomonas aeruginosa* infection of the lungs. *Thorax* 2000; 55:355–358.

82 Homma H, Yamanaka A, Tanimoto S et al. Diffuse panbronchiolitis. A disease of the transitional zone of the lung. *Chest* 1983; 83:63–69.

83 Kudoh S, Uetake T, Hagiwara K et al. Clinical effects of low dose long-term erythromycin chemotherapy on diffuse panbronchiolitis. *Jap J Thorac Dis* 1987; 25:632–642.

84 Ichimiya T, Yamasaki T, Nasu M. *In vitro* effects of antimicrobial agents on *Pseudomonas aeruginosa* biofilm formation. *J Antimicrob Chemother* 1994; 34:331–241.

85 Eyraud A, Desnotes J, Lombard JY et al. Effects of erythromycin, josamycin and spiramycin on rat polymorphonuclear leukocyte chemotaxis. *Chemotherapy* 1986; 32:379–382.

86 Anderson R. Erythromycin and roxithromycin potentiate human neutrophil locomotion in vitro by inhibition of leukoattractant-activated superoxide generation and auto-oxidation. *J Infect Dis* 1989; 159:966–973.

87 Goswami SK, Kivity S, Marom Z. Erythromycin inhibits respiratory glycoconjungate secretion from human airways in vitro. *Am Rev Respir Dis* 1990; 141:72–78.

88 Koh YY, Lee MH, Sun YH, Sung KW, Chae JH. Effect of roxithromycin on airway responsiveness in children with bronchiectasis: a double-blind placebo controlled study. *Eur Respir J* 1997; 10:994–999.

89 Zahm JM, Gaillard D, Dupuit F et al. Early alterations in airway mucociliary clearance and inflammation of the lamina propria in cystic fibrosis mice. *Am J Physiol* 1997; 272:C853–859.

90 van Heeckeren A, Walenga R, Konstan MW, Bonfield T, Davies PB, Fenkol T. Excessive inflammatory response of cystic fibrosis mice to bronchopulmonary infection with *Pseudomonas aeruginosa*. *J Clin Invest* 1997; 100:2810–2815.

16

Current and future treatment of cystic fibrosis

R.G. Gary Ruiz, Hilary H. Wyatt and John F. Price

Department of Child Health, King's College Hospital, Denmark Hill, London, UK

Introduction

Respiratory failure remains the most common cause of death in people with cystic fibrosis (CF). The median survival has increased, however, from 14 years in 1969, to 28 years in 1990[1]. This dramatic improvement in health has arisen primarily through effective treatment of the characteristic respiratory infections, but also through greatly improved management of nutrition. Even in the absence of any innovative treatment for the lungs it is predicted that the median survival for babies born in the early 1990s will be 40 years. The advent of therapies aimed at the basic defect in CF will have the greatest benefit for those with the least pre-existing lung damage but such therapies remain in investigative stages. Aggressive management of respiratory infections will remain the mainstay of treatment for minimising CF lung disease for the foreseeable future. The pulmonary damage in CF seems to arise from a two-stage process. First, there is a predisposition to respiratory tract infection with certain bacteria coupled with the inability to eradicate this infection, and secondly an escalating inflammatory response. It is thought that this intense inflammation causes ultimately more of the progressive lung damage than the inciting organisms.

Cystic fibrosis was identified as an autosomal recessive condition in 1952. The gene was traced to the long arm of chromosome 7 in 1985, and 4 years later the full sequence of its 250 Kbp structure was determined[2–4]. The product of this gene is a transmembrane protein of the adenosine triphosphate (ATP)-binding cassette family, and is present at the luminal surface of epithelial cells, and in other sites such as intracellular organelles. In health this gene product, or cystic fibrosis transmembrane conductance regulator (CFTR), is thought to have a number of functions that primarily influence ion and water movement, and thence ultimately the composition of secretions in the lumina of the various tissues affected. Following identification of the CF gene CFTR was shown to be a chloride channel regulated by cyclic adenosine monophosphate (AMP) mediated protein kinase A phosphorylation[5,6]. Impaired outward ion movement through the mutated CFTR chloride channel is associated with an inability to secrete liquid into the lumen. CFTR also appears to have a regulatory function on other ion transport systems, and in CF there is excessive (amiloride sensitive) reabsorption of salt and water. Over 900 mutations in the CF gene have been identified so far, although many of them are extremely rare (http://genet.sickkids.on.ca/cftr/). Debate continues about the exact composition of the altered secretions, and the mechanism by which the CF airway is predisposed to infection with certain micro-organisms is also not fully elucidated. The CF lung appears structurally normal at birth, but is peculiarly susceptible to infection with a number of pathogens, many of which do not usually colonize healthy lungs. No specific abnormality of the humoral immune system has been identified and this is supported by the lack of infections that develop in non-pulmonary CF tissues. The secretions are thought to be rendered more viscous by inadequate hydration, which has direct adverse effects on mucociliary clearance. It has also been postulated that abnormal CFTR function results in a high salt concentration in ESL, which in turn inactivates local antibacterial substances such as beta defensin 1[7]. This theory, however, is controversial[8]. Defective acidification within intracellular organelles results in decreased sialylation of glycoproteins[9]. Increased expression of asialoGM1 residues on the surface of respiratory epithelial cells in CF has been shown to be associated with increased binding of *Pseudomonas aeruginosa* pili and *Staphylococcus aureus* to those cells[10,11]. Other work has suggested that normal CFTR itself acts as a cellular receptor for the binding, endocytosis, and clearance of *Pseudomonas aeruginosa* from the airway, and that the increase in *Pseudomonas aeruginosa* adherence in CF is therefore a direct result of the presence of defective CFTR[12]. *Staphylococcus aureus* is one of the first bacteria that infect the CF lung. Once this organism has entered the airways, stripping of fibronectin is thought to expose additional bacterial receptor sites. Initial infection with *Pseudomonas aeruginosa* is usually silent. Subsequent transformation of this organism to a mucoid phenotype is almost invariable and associated with more rapid deterioration in lung function[13].

An intense inflammatory response is stimulated within the lungs but, even with appropriate antibiotic therapy, is usually unable to eradicate the infection. A massive infiltration of neutrophils into the lungs follows the release of chemoattractants such as IL-8, tumour necrosis factor-α (TNFα) and leukotrienes[14,15]. The granulocytes release proteases and oxidants that directly contribute to structural damage of the airways. In particular, neutrophil elastase destroys opsonins such as IgG and C3bi in the airway lumen and opsonin receptors such as CR1 on phagocytes. It also further stimulates the release of neutrophil chemoattractants, promotes hypertrophy and hyperplasia of mucus glands and causes structural damage to the airways[16]. Decaying neutrophils also release large quantities of DNA that contribute to airway obstruction by increasing the viscoelasticity of CF airway secretions[17]. Continuing infection and inflammation develop into a vicious cycle that causes extensive tissue damage. Without treatment, progressive pulmonary destruction ensues with widespread cystic and bronchiectatic change and ultimately insufficient functioning respiratory units to maintain adequate gaseous exchange. Without lung transplantation the patient dies from type II respiratory failure. There are difficulties conducting clinical research in CF due to the relative rarity of the condition, great variability in phenotype and many confounding variables that can influence outcome. Also, the current improved management has led to a slow rate of progression of lung disease such that clinical studies need to be conducted over many years to detect any change. Many studies involve relatively small numbers of patients and results must be interpreted with some caution.

There is, however, good evidence to suggest that the uncontrolled inflammatory response to infection within the lung begins early in the course of lung disease. A number of studies have demonstrated the presence of pathogens in bronchoalveolar lavage (BAL) samples taken from the lower respiratory tract of infants and older children with no clinical evidence of infection[18,19]. The detection of large numbers of neutrophils, and high levels of interleukin-8 and neutrophil elastase in the BAL fluid from the same patients indicate that this is not a benign colonization, rather an active, pathological process. These same studies also demonstrated inflammation within the respiratory lumina of some patients, in the absence of any positive bacterial or viral culture. It was suggested that inflammation may precede initial colonization, and it was speculated that the basic defect somehow directly contributes to the exaggerated inflammatory response[19,20]. More recently, however, there has been evidence that has led to the conclusion that inflammation occurs primarily in response to infection and that the inflammatory response can be successful initially in eradicating infection[21,22]. Until stategies for correcting the basic defect become the norm early in life, anti-inflammatory and anti-infective drugs will remain the mainstays of treatment.

Anti-inflammatory drugs

Corticosteroids

It has long been hypothesized that therapies aimed at diminishing the inflammatory response might have a beneficial impact on the course of the disease. Daily corticosteroids for 3 weeks in patients with stable but severe airway obstruction, however, showed no significant improvement in lung function[23]. The effects of long-term, alternate day, oral corticosteroids were first investigated in the early 1980s[24]. A further, 4 year, study 10 years later compared 2 mg/kg, and 1 mg/kg, of alternate day prednisolone with placebo and both demonstrated beneficial effects on pulmonary function and nutrition. A high incidence of growth retardation, glucose intolerance and cataracts required the premature termination of the higher dose arm in the latter study. Even the use of lower dose corticosteroids was associated with significant side effects, particularly when the drug was given for more than 24 months. Two weeks of daily prednisolone, followed by 10 weeks of alternate day steroids was associated, however, with an improvement in lung function and a decline in serum cytokine and immunoglobulin levels[25]. The use of corticosteroids for an intermediate duration, for instance in association with infective exacerbations, may prove the most effective course. The use of inhaled corticosteroids has been under investigation, as the side effects would potentially be minimized. Two studies have failed to demonstrate any benefit on pulmonary function or inflammatory markers in sputum[26,27], but other work has shown a beneficial effect[28]. It is suggested that, as the penetration of inhaled steroid into viscous, purulent secretions is poor, the dose of steroid required to inhibit neutrophil migration can only be achieved systemically or by using very high doses via the inhaled route. A beneficial effect of inhaled steroids may only be achieved if they are commenced soon after diagnosis through newborn screening when inflammation is likely to be at its least.

Non-steroidal anti-inflammatory drugs (NSAIDs)

High dose ibuprofen has been shown to inhibit neutrophil migration, adherence, swelling, aggregation and release of lysosomal contents[29]. A 4-year randomized, double blind, placebo-controlled study of high dose ibuprofen (20–30 mg/kg twice daily) has been shown to slow the progression of CF lung disease, particularly in children with mild lung disease[30]. No significant side effects were reported, but concern about side effects remains and this treatment is not in widespread use in this country (it seems more popular in the US). Plasma monitoring of ibuprofen levels is recommended to ensure that a therapeutic concentration of 50–100 µg/ml is achieved. There is no strong evidence to support its use in adults with moderate to severe lung disease ($FEV_1 < 60\%$ predicted), particularly in view of the increased risk of haemoptysis and other complications. Piroxicam, another NSAID, decreased in a dose-related fashion pulmonary polymorphonuclear leukocyte recruitment, and subsequent perivascular and peribronchial infiltration. A double-blind, placebo-controlled trial over a 12–19-month period demonstrated fewer hospitalizations and less deterioration in lung function in the group treated with piroxicam[31].

Antiproteases

The effects of proteases from bacteria and neutrophil elastase (NE), are normally balanced by naturally occurring antiproteases such as secretory leukoprotease inhibitor (SLPI) and α_1-antitrypsin. In CF the release of a large amount of NE into the lung overwhelms these antiproteases, enhances mucus secretion and directly injures airway tissue. NE also acts as a chemoattractant for other neutrophils by up-regulating production of Il-8, and interferes with opsonization by degrading immunoglobulins and other associated proteins. A recombinant form of SLPI has been developed and early work has shown it has potential for minimizing the effects of inflammation by two mechanisms. First it suppressed respiratory epithelial neutrophil elastase and Il-8 levels in CF patients[32]. In vitro and animal work has also shown that it increases levels of reduced glutathione (GSH), a naturally occurring antioxidant[33,34]. There are indications that SLPI also has local antimicrobial activity, with effects on viruses, bacteria and fungi[35]. This apparent multiple action makes it an attractive therapeutic option. Alpha 1-antitrypsin derived from pooled human serum (Prolastin) has been available since 1988 and has been administered by inhalation. Animal studies of chronic *Pseudomonas aeruginosa* lung infection have found that aerosolized Prolastin significantly decreased elastase activity, lung neutrophil counts and bacterial colony counts[36]. An early study in 12 CF patients given aerosolized alpha 1 anti-trypsin showed that neutrophil elastase in respiratory epithelial lining fluid (ELF) was suppressed, and also that the inhibitory effect of cystic fibrosis ELF on *Pseudomonas* killing by neutrophils was reversed[37]. The risks of blood-borne infections from Prolastin will be abolished with the advent of alpha 1 anti-trypsin produced from either transgenic sheep or as a recombinant human protein. It has been suggested that the combination of SLPI with alpha 1 antitrypsin could have complementary effects[38].

Antioxidants

Oxidative stress arises within the lung when the production of reactive oxygen species (ROS), or free radicals, exceeds the neutralizing capacity of available antioxidant defences. The lung has a range of antioxidant defences that help to maintain a balanced redox status. These antioxidants are present in the intracellular, vascular and extracellular respiratory tract lining fluid (RTLF) compartments. Free radicals are normally transformed into less reactive species by local antioxidants such as scavenging molecules, and enzyme systems such as superoxide dismutase (SOD) and the glutathione redox cycle. Non-enzymatic antioxidants include vitamins A, E and C, and reduced glutathione (GSH). GSH is an efficient intracellular and extracellular scavenger of oxygen

radicals and is the major local antioxidant in the lung, being present at high concentration in normal epithelial lining fluid[39]. Also, oxidants can inactivate antiproteases and proteases can inactivate antioxidants, which further perpetuates the inflammatory process. A number of studies have shown plasma antioxidant depletion and increased free radical production by inflammatory cells in CF. In particular, low levels of GSH have been found in RTLF and plasma in CF and attributed to the high levels of free radicals[40]. Recently, however, it has been suggested that low glutathione in RTLF is a direct result of impaired transport of this molecule through CFTR[41]. Whatever the mechanism of depletion, there is potential for improving local antioxidant status with the use of aerosolized GSH[41]. Oral supplementation of fat-soluble vitamins is routine in most CF clinics and supranormal levels of vitamin E are often encouraged. Vitamin A is used more cautiously in view of its potential hepatotoxicity. It is not usual to give additional vitamin C. One uncontrolled study has suggested there may be attenuation of pulmonary inflammation when the diet is supplemented with the vitamin A precursor beta-carotene[42].

Interleukin-10

Interleukin (IL)-10 is an important regulator of the inflammatory response, in part through inhibition of production of TNF-alpha, IL-1beta, IL-6 and IL-8. A preliminary study detected significantly less soluble IL-10 in the epithelial lining fluid of CF patients compared to controls[43]. They also concluded that there was down-regulation of IL-10 production from bronchial epithelial cells in CF and that this deficiency may be as important as the increase in proinflammatory cytokines in the excessive inflammatory response. Later work from the same group showed increased lung inflammation and more systemic morbidity in IL-10 knockout mice with chronic endobronchial *Pseudomonas aeruginosa* infection[44]. These changes were to some extent reversed when the mice were treated with IL-10.

Heparin

Heparin is a naturally occurring proteoglycan released from pulmonary mast cells and has a wide range of biological properties. It has an inhibitory effect on the heparinase enzyme secreted by T cells that, in turn, contributes to inhibition of neutrophil influx and T-cell trafficking across vascular endothelium[45]. A preliminary, uncontrolled study in six CF patients chronically infected with *Burkholderia cepacia* demonstrated a significant reduction in sputum and serum IL-6 and IL-8 after 1 week of nebulized heparin[46]. There was also a subjective improvement in ease of sputum expectoration and a trend towards thinner sputum. It was postulated that the latter effects were due to changes in the electrostatic properties of mucin molecules consequent on the negative charge of heparin.

Macrolides

The anti-inflammatory effects of macrolide antibiotics in respiratory diseases have received increasing attention over the last few years. Diffuse panbronchiolitis (DPB) is a disease seen predominantly in Japan and, like CF, is characterized by persistent pulmonary infection with mucoid *Pseudomonas aeruginosa* and neutrophil infiltration[47]. A dramatic improvement in survival in DPB was demonstrated with the long term use of low dose erythromycin[48]. Isolated reports of the clinical benefit of macrolides in CF followed[49,50]. The benefit occurs below the minimum inhibitory concentration of the drug for *Pseudomonas aeruginosa*. The mechanism of action is unclear but may involve the influence of macrolides on a number of inflammatory pathways. The inhibition of neutrophil chemotaxis and chemotactic activity, suppression of neutrophil oxidant burst, accelerated neutrophil apoptosis, reduced *Pseudomonas aeruginosa* adherence, a decrease in mucus hypersecretion by airway cells and interference with *Pseudomonas aeruginosa* biofilm formation have all been suggested[51]. It has also been suggested that macrolides exert their anti-inflammatory effect in CF through the up-regulation of a P-

glycoprotein called multidrug-resistant-associated protein that transports various compounds out of cells[52]. Multidrug-resistant-associated protein is homologous to CFTR and the two proteins can complement each other. Several double-blind, placebo-controlled trials are in progress.

Pentoxifylline

Pentoxifylline, a xanthine derivative, suppresses TNF-alpha production and is probably one of the mechanisms by which it modulates neutrophil activity. It also has antioxidant activity through scavenging of hydroxyl radicals. A double-blind placebo-controlled trial of pentoxifylline given for 6 months in CF patients showed some beneficial effects on sputum elastase concentrations, forced vital capacity and frequency of respiratory infective exacerbations in the treatment group compared to placebo[53].

Fatty acid supplementation

Many studies since the 1960s have demonstrated an abnormal fatty acid profile in CF plasma, consistent with a relative deficiency of essential fatty acids. The deficiencies were most marked in pancreatic insufficient patients and were thought to contribute to the predisposition of CF patients to infection. The fatty acid composition of plasma in CF does not completely resemble that of a dietary deficiency and it is considered to be a primary defect, rather than the result of fat malabsorption[54,55]. Increased eicosatrienoic acid (ETA), and decreased linoleic acid and docosahexaenoic acid (DHA) levels are seen in plasma of patients with CF[55]. Arachidonic acid, and its inflammatory mediators, normally increases in response to infection. A deficiency of DHA leads to abnormal membrane fluidity and membrane trafficking as well as a compensatory increased production of arachidonic acid via the n-6 pathway. This, in turn, increases the balance towards inflammation. A number of studies have shown that fatty acid supplements improve, but do not normalize, the abnormal biochemical profile. Fish oil preparations containing the omega-3 fatty acids eicosapentaenoic acid (EPA) and DHA appear to have anti-inflammatory properties. They inhibit leukotriene B_4 release from neutrophils and reduce IL-1 and TNFalpha production. Studies are under way to investigate the benefit on membrane fluidity and arachidonic acid metabolism by supplementation with high dose DHA alone because it appears to compete with EPA in these pathways[56].

Deoxyribonuclease (DNase)

Improved clearance of thick secretions from the airways may have an indirect but beneficial effect on inflammation. The 1950s saw the first attempts at reducing the tenacity of viscous infected sputum by using bovine DNase to break up long strands of DNA released from dead neutrophils. The studies were halted because of adverse reactions, in particular anaphylaxis and marked bronchospasm. The advent of a recombinant human DNase led to a number of trials, culminating in a large phase III randomized, double-blind study that compared placebo with once or twice daily nebulized rhDNase[57]. The study demonstrated improvement in lung function in the groups treated with rhDNase of an approximately 6% increase in FEV_1 from baseline, and around 30% reduction in age-adjusted risk of pulmonary exacerbations in both treated groups, compared to placebo. The differences in the once and twice daily treated groups were small, so a once daily regime is recommended. The study population consisted largely of older, sicker patients and a longer open study period has shown that treated patients still experience a decline in lung function. A recent study has looked at the effects of early intervention with DNase in children aged 6–10 years with mild lung disease (forced vital capacity greater than 85% of that predicted). A preliminary report indicated that, over a 2-year period, those treated with DNase had a 3% predicted treatment benefit in FEV_1 and a 34% reduction in the risk of an infective exacerbation, compared to placebo[58]. The high cost of this treatment (around £8000 per year) has led to variable usage worldwide. In the UK, guidelines have been introduced in many areas for the use of DNase, with

improvement in FEV_1 and other clinical indicators being used to determine whether it should be continued in the long term. Those patients with declining lung function, an increasing need for parenteral antibiotics and sticky sputum that is difficult to clear are most likely to benefit. Clinical experience has shown that there is a wide range of response from individual patients. There is some evidence that alternate day dosing is as effective as daily use in the long term, which will significantly reduce costs[59]. In practice, most patients do not want to spend unnecessary time in their already busy day administering a treatment that they perceive has little benefit. There has been some concern that treatment with rhDNase increases proteolytic activity within the bronchial lumen as a result of the release of neutrophil elastase and cathepsin G from complexes with antiproteases or DNA. Study results, however, have been conflicting[60,61]. Whatever the mechanism, the high levels of elastase in the lungs in all studies has led to the conclusion that combination therapy with an inhaled antiprotease may be more effective in reducing the inflammatory load[62].

Nebulized hypertonic saline enhances mucociliary clearance, improves hydration and reduces viscosity of mucus[63]. Hypertonic saline improves lung function in some studies, although comparative studies indicate a greater benefit from DNase[64]. As with DNase, the response to treatment is very variable between patients and individual assessment is recommended.

Leukotriene receptor antagonists

Leukotrienes (LTs) are potent proinflammatory mediators and are products of the 5-lipoxygenase metabolic pathway from arachidonic acid. LTB_4 is a potent neutrophil chemotactic and chemokinetic agent, and the cysteinyl leukotrienes (LTC_4, LTD_4 and LTE_4) cause increased mucus production, leukocyte chemotaxis, bronchoconstriction and increased vascular permeability. Elevated levels of LTs, capable of exerting significant biological effects, have been previously found in CF sputum[65]. A number of approaches to antileukotriene therapy are possible. Agents that block their production by inhibition of the action of 5-lipoxygenase enzyme, or antagonize receptors for the molecules have been developed, originally for use in asthma. They may have greatest effect in atopic CF patients who have been shown to produce higher levels of leukotrienes[66]. Also, a short-term study of dietary supplementation of omega-3 fatty acids was associated with increased levels of eicosapentaenoic acid and docosahexaenoic acid, with concomitant reduction in serum levels of LTB_4[67]. There has been little work reported so far of attempts to modulate the effects of excessive leukotriene production in CF.

Treatment of infection

Pulmonary infection is the major cause of morbidity as well as mortality in CF. Ultimately infection results from defective mucociliary clearance of inhaled bacteria. There is a relatively small range of common bacterial pathogens. The four most important organisms are *Staphylococcus aureus*, *Haemophilus influenzae*, *Pseudomonas aeruginosa* and *Burkholderia cepacia*. *S. aureus* and *H. influenzae* are usually the first pathogens to be encountered in childhood. *P. aeruginosa* may be cultured intermittently at first but eventually mutates to a mucoid form, which is impossible to eradicate so that chronic infection ensues. *B. cepacia* is highly transmissible and also produces chronic infection. Other organisms now recognized as CF pathogens such as *Stenotrophomonas maltophilia* and non-tuberculous mycobacteria are cultured less frequently at present, but may become increasingly important in the future. Although more than one pathogen may be cultured from the same sputum the regular isolation of a particular organism has prognostic implications. On the US CF Foundation database, the median survival for patients with chronic infection with *P. aeruginosa* was 28 years and with *B. cepacia* was 16 years, but for those with neither infection it was 39 years[68].

Clearly different organisms demand treatment with different antibiotics, which can be delivered in different ways. Antibiotics may be given orally, intra-

Table 16.1. Commonly used antibiotics in CF

Target pathogen	Oral agents	Intravenous agents
S. aureus	Flucloxacillin	Flucloxacillin
	Co-amoxiclav	Gentamicin
	Erythromycin, clarithromycin	Cefuroxime
	Clindamycin	
	Fucidin	
	Rifampicin	
	Doxycycline	
	Cefuroxime, cephalexin	
H. influenzae	Amoxycillin, co-amoxiclav	Cefuroxime
	Cefaclor, cefuroxime	Co-amoxiclav, amoxycillin
	Erythromycin, clarithromycin	
	Doxycycline	
P. aeruginosa	Ciprofloxacin	Ceftazidime
	Azithromycin	Tobramycin, gentamicin, amikacin
		Meropenem, imipenem/cilastin
		Aztreonam
		Ticarcillin/clavulanic acid

venously or nebulized. Table 16.1 lists some of the antibiotics in common usage. The choice of antibiotic should be guided by sputum culture and sensitivities. A number of general principles distinguish antibiotic therapy in CF from treatment elsewhere. They will be described briefly before discussing a number of specific issues in the drug treatment for infection in CF.

General principles

Better and more aggressive use of antibiotics are among the major factors associated with the improved median survival of CF patients in recent years[69]. The main indications for antibiotics in CF are:

- prophylaxis against specific infection
- positive routine sputum culture without symptoms
- increased respiratory symptoms which may be associated with initial viral respiratory infection
- acute respiratory infective exacerbations
- suppression of chronic infection

In general, antibiotics are given in higher doses for longer periods in CF patients than non-CF individuals. Reasons cited for the inadequacy of ordinary treatment regimes in CF have included altered pharmacokinetics, poor sputum penetration, inactivation of antibiotics by CF sputum, idiosyncratic bacterial behaviour (such as the development of mucoidity by *P. aeruginosa*) and the need to target mixed bacterial populations[70]. Altered pharmacokinetics in CF have been explained by increased renal clearance of antibiotics and a relatively greater volume of distribution[71]. This has been shown for aminoglycosides[72] and β-lactams[73] but not for fluoroquinolones[74]. One study showed much greater enhancement of non-renal than renal clearance of cloxacillin in CF patients[75]. However, more recently it has been argued that many older studies would have contained relatively malnourished patients with increased lean body mass, into which aminoglycosides and β-lactam are primarily distributed. If volume of distribution is corrected for lean body mass instead of total weight values, CF and non-CF are similar[76]. However, regardless of the explanation most antibiotics still need to be given in higher dosage to achieve a therapeutic effect in CF patients[71].

Antistaphylococcal prophylaxis

S. aureus was cultured from bronchoalveolar lavage in 40% of CF infants during the first 3 months of life in an Australian prospective cross-sectional study[18]. Importantly more than a third were symptom free. Many centres give continuous antistaphylococcal prophylaxis for at least the first 2–3 years of life, some give lifelong prophylaxis, and others give treatment when clinically indicated[77]. The clinical effectiveness of the latter policy would clearly be affected by the regularity of bacterial surveillance.

A systematic review of 13 trials of antistaphylococcal therapy concluded that treatment frequently cleared the sputum of *S. aureus* and that young children are likely to benefit from prophylaxis[78]. The latter conclusion was largely based on the only published randomized placebo-controlled trial of continuous flucloxacillin, which was given for 2 years after diagnosis on a neonatal screening programme[79]. Infants on prophylaxis had less cough, fewer *S. aureus* isolates, fewer hospital admissions that were of shorter duration, and less need for additional antibiotic courses. Their lung function after 1 year, however, was no different to control infants[80]. The most recent Cochrane Review of prophylactic antibiotics for CF[81] considered trials of at least 1 year of continuous treatment. Data from only two unpublished studies in addition to the Weaver et al. study were eligible for the analysis giving a total of 177 patients aged 0–7 years. Prophylaxis from early infancy up to three years was thought to be of benefit, but no conclusions could be drawn for older children and adults, or for extending treatment beyond 3 years. Nor could any rigorous assessment of adverse effect of antistaphylococcal prophylaxis be made.

Generation of resistant organisms by prophylactic use of antibiotics is always a concern. Although there is a lack of data from randomized trials, resistance seems less likely with flucloxacillin than with cephalosporins or macrolides[82] and widespread methicillin resistance has not been the experience of centres using flucloxacillin prophylactically[83]. Nevertheless the overall prevalence of methicillin-resistant *S. aureus* is increasing in some centres [84].

Perhaps of greater concern is whether antistaphylococcal prophylaxis predisposes to acquisition of *P. aeruginosa* infection. Although not published in a peer reviewed journal, a large US CF Foundation multicentre controlled trial of giving prophylactic cephalexin or placebo for 5–7 years to newly diagnosed CF infants showed no advantage of prophylaxis over placebo apart from reduced cultures of *S.*

aureus. However, 25% of the cephalexin group compared to 13% of the placebo group cultured *P. aeruginosa*[85]. However, the majority of centres using antistaphylococcal prophylaxis would choose a penicillinase-resistant penicillin rather than a cephalosporin. On the European Registry for CF, German patients on continuous antistaphylococcal therapy were noted to have higher rates of *P. aeruginosa* acquisition than patients on intermittent or 'no' therapy[86]. It is difficult to draw firm conclusions from such observations and a randomized trial would be needed.

In summary so far, antistaphylococcal prophylaxis has only been shown to be of clinical benefit in CF during the first 2–3 years of life. Concerns about resistance generation and predisposing to *P. aeruginosa* acquisition have yet to be substantiated with the commonly used antibiotics such as flucloxacillin.

Antibiotics for *H. influenzae* infection

H. influenzae is cultured more frequently in CF children than age-matched asthmatic controls[87]. In this study the isolation rate was significantly higher during chest exacerbations suggesting that it was a pathogen. The true prevalence of *H. influenzae* infections in CF is probably underestimated because of the difficulty in culturing the organism in the presence of *P. aeruginosa*[88]. However, 30% of sputa from 55 consecutive patients attending an adult CF clinic cultured non-typeable *H. influenzae* in a study designed specifically to look for this organism[89]. Under-recognition of *H. influenzae* infection in CF may help to explain why patients who only appear to culture *P. aeruginosa* can sometimes respond to a β-lactam without activity against the latter[90]. *H. influenzae* cultured from CF sputa is usually ampicillin-sensitive[91]. Suitable alternatives are given in Table 16.1.

Kaiser et al.[92] assessed the efficacy of coamoxiclav in 300 non-CF patients with common colds (aged 16–64 years) and found a significant benefit in 61 patients who cultured *H. influenzae*, *Moraxella catarrhalis* or *Streptococcus pneumoniae* from nasopharyngeal aspirates. Upper respiratory tract infections are not commoner in CF patients than healthy controls but do cause significant respiratory deterioration and predispose to secondary bacterial infection[93]. Many would recommend CF patients to start an anti-*H. influenzae* antibiotic, such as amoxycillin, at the onset of a cold pending the result of sputum culture unless they are chronically infected with *P. aeruginosa*[83].

Oral treatment for *P. aeruginosa* infection

The quinolones are the only specifically antipseudomonal agents that can be given orally. (The recently recognized role of macrolides in chronic *P. aeruginosa* infection in CF is discussed in the section of this chapter dealing with anti-inflammatory therapies.) Ciprofloxacin is the quinolone that has most widespread use in CF[94], although ofloxacin appears to be equally efficacious[95]. The important place of ciprofloxacin therapy in conjunction with nebulized colistin for preventing or delaying chronic infection with *P. aeruginosa* is discussed in the ensuing section on nebulized antibiotics.

The advantages of oral over intravenous therapy with regard to convenience and reduced cost are obvious. Ten days' treatment with oral ciprofloxacin in adult CF patients with acute infective exacerbations was found to be as good as intravenous azlocillin and gentamicin in one small, randomized trial[96]. However, the Danish clinic compared their conventional 3-monthly intravenous antibiotic regime (using an aminoglycoside and β-lactam) in CF patients colonized with *P. aeruginosa* with 2 weeks of ciprofloxacin for two consecutive 3-monthly cycles. They found that conventional treatment was significantly better than quinolone treatment especially in the most seriously ill patients[97]. Indeed, a 1-year randomized placebo-controlled trial of 3-monthly oral ciprofloxacin for 10 days in adult CF patients did not show any significant improvement in FEV_1 or in the need for intravenous antibiotics in the treatment group. More ominously, a rise in the median MIC to ciprofloxacin was seen in *P. aeruginosa* cultured from the treatment group[98].

The rapid development of resistance to ciprofloxacin is a concern. In one study with 29 adult CF patients who all had sensitive strains of *P. aeruginosa* initially, 45% had resistant isolates after 14 days' treatment with ciprofloxacin in spite of clinical improvement[99]. Furthermore, ciprofloxacin has been shown to select imipenem-resistant variants of *P. aeruginosa* in vitro[100], suggesting a potential risk of resistance to agents in addition to quinolones from indiscriminate use.

Quinolones are very safe antibiotics with rare gastrointestinal and central nervous system side effects. The adverse effect most likely to be encountered is photosensitivity to sunlight[101], which can be countered using sun block. Reports of quinolone-associated arthropathy and damage to growing cartilage in beagle puppies have delayed official recommendation for the use of ciprofloxacin in children. However, ciprofloxacin has been used in children with CF on a compassionate basis for years with a similar safety profile to adults[102]. A review of the cumulated published findings of quinolone use in over 7000 children and adults concluded that concerns over chondrotoxicity were unfounded[103]. There is, however, still little published data on use in children below the age of 5 years[94].

Inhaled antipseudomonal antibiotics

Less than 20% of the serum concentration of β-lactam agents[104] and 12% of the serum level of aminoglycosides may be found in the sputum[105]. Delivering antibiotics directly to the site of infection in cystic fibrosis by inhalation is therefore an attractive option. It theoretically enables much higher sputum concentrations than could be achieved by maximal non-toxic doses given by the intravenous route. Obstructed CF airways may, however, result in uneven distribution of antibiotic through the lungs. Mainly antipseudomonal antibiotics have been given by inhalation and this has generally been by nebulization. The efficiency of drug delivery by nebulization is notoriously variable and many factors including the device, the drug and the patient will affect the small proportion of the original dose that

is ultimately deposited in the airways[106]. There have been three main areas where nebulized antibiotics have been employed in CF:

- chronic suppressive therapy in stable patients with chronic *P. aeruginosa* infection
- prevention or delay of chronic infection with *P. aeruginosa*
- adjunct therapy for pulmonary infective exacerbations

Chronic suppressive therapy

The first randomized double-blind trial of inhaled antibiotics in CF was performed in 1981[107]. A cross-over design was used to compare nebulized gentamicin and carbenicillin with placebo over a year in 20 adult patients with chronic *P. aeruginosa* colonization. Mean FEV_1 and FVC and subjective symptom scores were significantly better during active treatment than when taking placebo.

There followed a number of studies using different nebulized antibiotics, including colistin, gentamicin, tobramycin and ceftazidime most of which reported some clinical benefit[108]. The trials were relatively small and it is difficult to draw any general conclusions from them because differing antibiotics, doses, durations of treatment, nebulizer devices, measures of response, etc. were used. Nevertheless, a 1996 meta-analysis of five randomized trials concluded that continuous nebulized antipseudomonal antibiotics reduced pulmonary exacerbations and respiratory pseudomonal load and improved lung function[109]. There was a trend towards increased resistance of cultured *P. aeruginosa*. A subsequent Cochrane review of nebulized antibiotics in CF[110] included 758 patients from ten randomized trials and concluded that lung function was better in the treated groups. Three of the trials (581 patients) enabled an analysis of hospital admissions, which were reduced in treated groups. Only two trials (591 patients) could be analysed for additional antibiotic requirement, which was also reduced by continuous nebulized antibiotics. Again, nebulized antibiotics were associated with increased bacterial resistance but not with renal or auditory toxicity. This meta-analysis was heavily influenced by a single trial that contributed 68% of the patients.

This was a multicentre double-blind placebo-controlled trial of intermittent nebulized tobramycin with a treatment period of 24 weeks. Over 500 CF patients were recruited with a mean age of 21 years[111]. Patients were monitored over three consecutive 8-week cycles comprising nebulized tobramycin or placebo for 4 weeks followed by 4 weeks off nebulized treatment. This was a phase III study that followed a much smaller earlier study with a higher dose of tobramycin, which demonstrated efficacy and safety[112]. In the 24-week study, the dose of tobramycin was reduced to 300 mg twice daily and it was given in 5 ml instead of 30 ml. The monthly on/off design was chosen as animal studies had shown histological resolution of any toxic changes after a month, there was some evidence that therapeutic effect persisted after stopping the nebulized drug, it was likely to encourage compliance, and it attempted to lessen the emergence of resistant strains of *P. aeruginosa*. Patients on nebulized tobramycin showed a significant improvement in lung function within 2 weeks of starting which was maintained. At 20 weeks the mean FEV_1 was still 10% above baseline while patients on placebo had fallen to 2% below baseline at the equivalent time. The density of *P. aeruginosa* in the sputum was dramatically decreased in the tobramycin group, although this effect decreased with each successive treatment cycle. Patients on tobramycin were less likely to require hospitalization or intravenous antibiotics than those on placebo. Ototoxicity, nephrotoxicity and accumulation of drug in the serum were not seen.

Patients who elected to receive tobramycin in an open-label extension to the study maintained FEV_1 above baseline, but the effect diminished with time to 4.7% above baseline at 92 weeks[113]. A subanalysis of teenagers (aged 13–17 years) in the study revealed that the mean weight gain at the end of the 24-week randomized trial was 2.3 kg for those on tobramycin but only 1.0 kg for those on placebo[114]. Placebo patients who elected to go on to intermittent nebulized tobramycin in the open-label study subsequently showed an impressive catch-up in weight.

In summary, long-term treatment with nebulized antipseudomonal antibiotics appears to prevent clinical deterioration in CF patients with chronic *P. aeruginosa* infection and is generally safe. Increasing bacterial resistance associated with regular tobramycin use, but not with colistin[115], may be a concern but does not appear to affect clinical efficacy.

Prevention or delay of chronic infection with *P. aeruginosa*

End-stage lung disease in CF is, most often, primarily related to chronic infection with *P. aeruginosa* (at least three positive cultures over a minimum of 6 months, with at least a month between cultures and signs of infection[94]). A period of intermittent colonization[94], which averaged 12 months in one series[116], usually precedes chronic infection. The prophylactic use of antipseudomonal antibiotics to prevent initial colonization with *P. aeruginosa* has not been studied, although other prophylactic strategies have future potential. However, once initial colonization is recognized, there may be a window of opportunity for eradicating the organism before mucoid change and increased sputum volume make it impossible.

In an open 27-month trial, 26 consecutive Danish CF children who had cultured *P. aeruginosa* but never received antipseudomonal therapy previously, were randomized to receive nebulized colistin and oral ciprofloxacin for 3 weeks whenever they cultured *P. aeruginosa* on routine monthly sputum cultures[117]. During the trial 7 (58%) of the untreated but only 2 (14%) of the treated children developed chronic *P. aeruginosa* infection. A placebo-controlled double-blind randomized study of continuous nebulized tobramycin for a year after first isolation of *P. aeruginosa* suggested that this too could prevent or delay chronic infection[118].

The Danish clinic subsequently adopted a three-step protocol for first isolation of *P. aeruginosa* in 1989. Initially nebulized colistin (1 megaunit twice daily) and oral ciprofloxacin was given for 3 weeks. If *P. aeruginosa* were cultured again a higher dose of nebulized colistin (2 megaunits thrice daily) would be given with ciprofloxacin for 3 weeks. If cultured a third time within 6 months the higher dose colistin and ciprofloxacin would be given for 3 months. They compared 48 patients treated with this aggressive protocol with 43 historic controls. Chronic infection after 3 years occurred in only 16% of the treated patients compared to 72% of controls. They concluded that 3 months' was more effective than 3 weeks' treatment[119]. The use of historic controls is always open to criticism, but they argued that there were no other significant treatment policy differences between the comparative periods. The magnitude of the differences would certainly complicate ethical considerations for a randomized-controlled trial. Furthermore, aggressive treatment of initial *P. aeruginosa* colonization is cited as one of the primary reasons that the Danish clinic were unique in actually managing to *decrease* the incidence of chronic *P. aeruginosa* infection from 16% to 2%[120].

Adjunct therapy for acute exacerbations

A number of small studies have been performed to assess the benefit of giving a drug by nebulizer in addition to the intravenous route to treat acute respiratory exacerbations. The drugs have included carbenicillin[121], tobramycin in conjunction with IV ticarcillin and tobramycin[122] and amikacin in conjunction with IV ceftazidime and amikacin[123]. None showed any additional benefit. This may have been due to inadequate power of the studies to show a difference. However, the practice cannot be recommended on the current evidence.

Intravenous antipseudomonal antibiotics

Although intravenous (IV) antibiotics may be necessary to treat infection with any of the CF pathogens they are most commonly given for *P. aeruginosa* infection. IV antibiotics are used:

- for acute respiratory exacerbations
- after failure of oral treatment (e.g. to improve chest symptoms or eradicate *P. aeruginosa* after first isolation)
- for routine 3-monthly maintenance therapy

Acute respiratory exacerbations may be associated with symptoms such as increased cough, sputum and breathlessness and reduced exercise tolerance and appetite, and signs such as increase in respiratory distress and added sounds, reduction in lung function and weight, fever and new chest X-ray infiltrates[124]. They are normally treated with IV antibiotics for at least two weeks[94] as objective measures of improvement usually only start to occur towards the end of the first week.

Monotherapy vs. combination therapy

A number of small studies have suggested that monotherapy with ceftazidime may be effective treatment[125,126]. The recent Cochrane review of single vs. combination IV antibiotics was inconclusive[127]. However, most centres would use a combination of two antibiotics[77] to reduce the risk of resistant *P. aeruginosa* strains emerging. Indeed, a recent report of an outbreak of a ceftazidime-resistant epidemic strain of *P. aeruginosa* in a clinic where ceftazidime monotherapy used to be practised cautions against antipseudomonal monotherapy[128].

There is also good evidence of synergy between antibiotics used in combination against *P. aeruginosa* in vitro that may occur even when there is resistance to one of the combination[129]. This occurs particularly when combining an aminoglycoside with a β-lactam (which have different modes of action) and this is the recommended clinical combination[94]. Some of the commonly used antibiotics are listed in Table 16.1. No one combination will be universally superior to another and the choice is made primarily according to susceptibility testing on sputum culture but also to history of allergic responses, ease of administration, cost, etc.

Optimal aminoglycoside dosing

The relatively increased dose requirement by weight in CF is readily demonstrated with the aminoglycosides[130]. Repeated high dose courses clearly pose the risk of aminoglycoside (vestibular-auditory and renal) toxicity. Renal toxicity can be manifested by hypomagnesemia in the absence of a rise in creatinine due to renal magnesium wasting[131]. The concentration-dependent killing demonstrated by aminoglycosides and the fact that toxicity is related to trough serum levels, have led to the use of once daily aminoglycoside dosing.

A meta-analysis of 21 randomized trials in non-CF patients concluded that once daily dosing was as effective as multiple dosing, had a lower risk of toxcity and no greater risk of ototoxicity[132]. However, the data in CF is limited. Giving 12-hourly tobramycin to CF adults may be less toxic but as effective as 8-hourly dosing[133]. One randomized trial of 22 CF children and adolescents concluded that, in combination with ceftazidime, once daily was as effective and safe as thrice daily tobramycin[134] but this and other data may simply have inadequate power[135]. Although large multicentred trials are in progress in the UK and USA to determine the optimal aminoglycoside dosing, many centres already use once daily dosing particularly with home IV therapy where the increased convenience to the patient is considerable.

Allergic reactions

Most allergic reactions to IV antibiotics in CF patients involve the β-lactams. Piperacillin has been particularly associated with adverse reactions in CF[136] and is not recommended for routine use. Anaphylaxis can occur and patients on home IV treatment should always receive at least the first dose in hospital as a precaution[83]. However, serum sickness-like drug fever and rash are the commonest allergic manifestations. A retrospective analysis of reactions in a large US centre gave a mean time to onset of drug-induced fever or rash of 9.1 days[137]. In addition to piperacillin the highest frequency of allergic reactions occurred with another acylaminopenicillin, mezlocillin and imipenem/cilastin. In patients who have developed reactions to ceftazidime, successful desensitization using a continuous infusion regimen starting at very low dose and gradually increasing has been described[138]. There have also been case reports of desensitization of patients with tobramycin hypersensitivity[139].

Elective vs. symptomatic therapy

There are two approaches to the use of IV antibiotics in CF patients with chronic *P. aeruginosa* infection.

One is to give courses of IV antibiotics only when there is evidence of clinical deterioration. The other is to give regular courses usually every 3 months in an attempt to prevent clinical deterioration and lung damage[69]. The former was the policy in the Copenhagen clinic before 1976 but thereafter the latter approach was adopted. The annual mortality in these patients was 10–20% before and fell to 1–2% after the change in policy[140]. The 5-year survival increased from 54% to 82%[69]. However, this was a retrospective comparison and this may not have been the only significant intervention associated with the improvement.

The only randomized trial comparing elective IV antibiotics to IV therapy when symptomatic in 60 adult CF patients did not show any advantages of either policy[141]. However, this may have been because the average number of IV courses in the symptomatic group (3) was not far off that for the elective group (4). Thus although a recent Cochrane review[142] highlighted the need for an adequately powered multicentre trial, the two policies may approximate to the same thing as the threshold for elective IV antibiotics continues to diminish.

Intravenous colistin

Colistin-resistant *P. aeruginosa* is extremely unusual even after years of continuous nebulized colistin treatment[115]. Concerns over potential nephrotoxicity and neurotoxicity have limited intravenous colistin usage. However, IV colistin by slow infusion has been used in adult CF centres in the UK for several years with success[143,144]. More recently, bolus IV colistin administration has been found to be safe[145].

Treatment for other infections

Burkholderia cepacia complex

Chronic infection with *Burkholderia cepacia* in CF has been a recognized problem since the early 1980s[146]. The consequences vary from no additional symptoms, to decline in lung function and respiratory exacerbations similar to those with *P. aeruginosa*, to fatal rapidly progressive 'cepacia syndrome'.

There are no randomized trials of antibiotic treatment regimes. Respiratory exacerbations are treated according to in vitro sensitivities where possible. *B. cepacia* is typically resistant to colistin and amino-glycosides[147]. However, aminoglycosides may still act synergistically in combination with other anti-biotics. In one in vitro study of 119 *B. cepacia* iso-lates, triple antibiotic combinations were more likely to be bactericidal than double combinations or single antibiotics[148]. Triple combinations of tobramycin, meropenem and another antibiotic such as ceftazidime were most effective in this series. Orally, combinations of ciprofloxacin, rifam-picin, chloramphenicol and minocycline have been used[149]. First isolates of *B. cepacia* are usually treated aggressively as with *P. aeruginosa*. Nebulized anti-biotics (e.g. ceftazidime or ticarcillin) are also com-monly given to treat chronic infection, although currently, there is no evidence from clinical trials to support this practice.

Methicillin-resistant *Staphylococcus aureus* (MRSA)

The increasing prevalence of MRSA in the general population has been reflected in CF patients[84]. Methicillin resistance restricts the choice of antibio-tic for treating respiratory infections, necessitates increased social isolation and may contraindicate lung transplantation, but does not appear otherwise to increase respiratory morbidity or mortality in adult CF patients[84]. In CF children, acquisition of MRSA may have a negative impact on growth but not on respiratory function[150].

Distinguishing between colonization of the nose and throat, and true lung infection with MRSA can sometimes be difficult. Identification of MRSA from the nose, throat or skin should be followed by topical eradication measures using standard regimens[151]. For acute respiratory exacerbations a glycopeptide such as teicoplanin or vancomycin should be included in the intravenous antibiotic regime[83], although some strains of MRSA are also sensitive to aminoglycosides. Oral agents such as fusidic acid, rifampicin, trimethoprim and sometimes quino-lones and tetracycline can be useful for less severe infections, but are better used in combination than

as single agents to reduce emergence of resis-tance[151]. Aerosolized aminoglycosides and even vancomycin have been used in chronic MRSA infec-tion in CF[152].

Stenotrophomonas maltophilia

S. maltophilia is another organism that has been cultured with increasing frequency from CF sputa[153]. It is still not clear whether to regard it as a CF patho-gen. One US study found that CF patients colonized with *S. maltophilia* had poorer growth and lung function than age matched controls and that treat-ment with long-term antibiotics and days of i.v. anti-biotic therapy were significant risk factors for acquisition of the organism[154]. This does not, of course, answer whether *S. maltophilia* is a cause or simply a marker of poorer clinical outcome. While new data is awaited, most would reserve treatment against this organism for clinical deterioration without any other obvious cause[83].

S. maltophilia is a highly resistant organism[155] and most antipseudomonal antibiotics including colis-tin are ineffective. The organism is often sensitive to co-trimoxazole and sometimes to monocycline, co-amoxiclav, ticarcillin/clavulanate or astreonam[83].

Non-tuberculous mycobacteria

A number of reasons have been cited for the increas-ing frequency with which non-tuberculous myco-bacteria (NTB) are being cultured from CF sputum. These include more active searching, better culture techniques, increasing prevalence in the general population and greater likelihood of exposure due to increasing survival[156]. Meeting the ATS criteria for NTM infection[157] in CF is usually difficult because 'other reasonable causes of the disease' cannot often be excluded unequivocally. Although most CF patients who regularly culture NTM may be colo-nized with little clinical impact[158], some patients undoubtedly have true infection requiring treat-ment[159].

Treatment of NTM infection in CF patients may be complicated by the need to use higher drug doses than in non-CF patients[160]. There may also be unusual resistance patterns due to previous multiple antibiotic use, and difficulty in assessing a true therapeutic effect because of susceptibility of other pathogens to the same drugs[156]. A variety of NTM have been isolated from CF sputum[158]. Unfortunately, the one that is most likely to be associated with progressive lung disease is *M. abscessus* (formerly *M. chelonae* subspecies abscessus)[157] which is notoriously difficult to treat. *M. abscessus* is often only sensitive to the newer macrolides (clarithromycin and azithromycin) and the parenteral antibiotics amikacin, cefoxitin and imipenem[157]. Continuous intravenous therapy for 6 months may produce clinical improvement but fail to eradicate the organism and prevent relapses[159] and treatment is often continued for one year or longer.

Some future anti-infective strategies

Vaccines against *Pseudomonas aeruginosa*
Immunization against *P. aeruginosa* is an obvious strategy to prevent chronic colonization and infection. Boosting an antibody response to *P. aeruginosa* may prevent bacterial attachment, neutralize toxic bacterial products and enhance bacterial killing through opsonization and the activation of complement. However, an enhanced inflammatory response to *P. aeruginosa* that is ineffective is also potentially detrimental[161]. Indeed, naturally acquired hypergammaglobulinemia is a poor prognostic indicator in CF[162].

There has only been one pseudorandomized trial of a *P. aeruginosa* vaccine that has been published to date. This used a polyvalent pseudomonas vaccine (a freeze-dried blended extract of 16 serotypes) and concluded that immunization did not reduce *P. aeruginosa* colonization or confer a clinical advantage[163]. However, there were only 34 children in the study.

Phase I studies of a flagella vaccine IMMUNO in healthy subjects showed that it was well tolerated and gave rise to persistently high antibody levels not only in the blood but in the secretory immune system of the airways[164]. A Phase III multicentre randomized placebo-controlled study involving 400 CF patients who were not colonized with *P. aeruginosa* was begun in 1998.

Naturally produced antilipopolysaccharide (LPS) antibodies to *P. aeruginosa* in CF patients have low affinity and are non-opsonic. However, those produced following immunization with an O-polysaccharide toxin A conjugate vaccine had high affinity and promoted opsonophagocytic killing of *P. aeruginosa*[165]. There also appeared to be a lower rate of *P. aeruginosa* infection amongst a small number of immunized CF subjects compared to matched retrospective controls[165]. A large (330 patients) multicentre Phase III randomized placebo-controlled trial is also in progress with this vaccine.

There may also be a place for passive immunization to prevent *P. aeruginosa* infection[166]. There have been promising reports of the effectiveness of nightly gargling with an extract containing chicken derived antibodies (IgY) to *P. aeruginosa* and Phase II and III studies have been planned[167].

New antimicrobials
The prevention and treatment of lung infection will remain a mainstay of CF treatment in patients even with the advent of gene therapy. Gene therapy attempts to avoid the vicious cycle of infection, inflammation and lung damage. It is therefore likely to be most effective in patients prior to the onset of widespread irreversible lung damage. The patient with CF alive today is unlikely to come into such a category without aggressive anti-infective therapy. Developing new antimicrobials with activity particularly against resistant *P. aeruginosa* and the emerging pathogens, more effective antibiotic treatment protocols, better methods of delivery, etc. all have high priority in CF drug research.

A catechol-containing monobactam called PA-1806 (formerly BMS-180680) has excellent in vitro activity against gram-negative bacteria including *P. aeruginosa*, *B. cepacia* and *S. maltophilia*[168]. It enters the bacteria through iron transport mechanisms and inhibits cell wall synthesis. Phase I trials delivering the drug by nebulizer to CF patients are underway.

Taurolidine, which is used as an antiseptic peritoneal lavage solution, has good activity against *B. cepacia*. A small double-blind placebo-controlled crossover trial in CF patients colonized with *B. cepacia* gave disappointing results[169]. However, the authors have subsequently suggested that reformulation of taurolidine and its derivatives would increase the concentration that could be delivered and may improve efficacy[170].

Agents that prevent adherence of *P. aeruginosa* to respiratory tract epithelial cells would have potential for use in CF. Dextran and other neutral polysaccharides have been shown to have this effect in vitro[171]. Pneumonia after intranasal innoculation of *P. aeruginosa* in mice was significantly reduced by prior administration of aerosolized dextran[172]. Dextran also has the additional benefit of reducing viscoelasticity of CF sputum in vitro[173]. One mechanism that may enhance *P. aeruginosa* adherence to CF respiratory epithelium is increased numbers of asialoglycolipid receptors. Adherence of *P. aeruginosa* to CF nasal epithelial cells in vitro can be significantly reduced in the presence of polyclonal antiasialoGM1 antibody, which may have potential in vivo application[174].

Manipulation of airway surface liquid (ASL) may provide another antimicrobial strategy in CF. Xylitol can decrease ASL salt concentration which may enhance natural antimicrobial factors such as human β-defensins, lactoferrin, and lysozyme. Intranasal xylitol spray has been shown to reduce the number of nasal coagulase-negative *Staphylococcus* compared to saline control in healthy volunteers in a double-blind randomized crossover study[175].

REFERENCES

1 FitzSimmons SC. The changing epidemiology of cystic fibrosis. *J Pediatr* 1993; 122(1):1–9.

2 Kerem B, Zielenski J Markiewicz D et al. Identification of the cystic fibrosis gene: genetic analysis. *Science* 1989; 245:1073–1080.

3 Riordan JR, Rommens JM, Kerem B et al. Identification of the cystic fibrosis gene: cloning and characterization of complementary DNA. *Science* 1989; 245:1066–1073.

4 Rommens JM, Iannuzzi MC, Kerem B et al. Identification of the cystic fibrosis gene: chromosome walking and jumping. *Science* 1989; 245:1059–1065.

5 Bear CE, Li CH, Kartner N et al. Purification and functional reconstitution of the cystic fibrosis transmembrane conductance regulator (CFTR). *Cell* 1992; 68(4):809–818.

6 Tilly BC, Winter MC, Ostedgaard LS, et al. Cyclic AMP-dependent protein kinase activation of cystic fibrosis transmembrane conductance regulator chloride channels in planar lipid bilayers. *J Biol Chem* 1992; 267(14):9470–9473.

7 Goldman MJ, Anderson GM, Stolzenberg ED et al. Human beta-defensin-1 is a salt-sensitive antibiotic in lung that is inactivated in cystic fibrosis. *Cell* 1997; 88(4):553–560.

8 Knowles MR, Robinson JM, Wood RE et al. Ion composition of airway surface liquid of patients with cystic fibrosis as compared with normal and disease-control subjects. *J Clin Invest* 1997; 100(10):2588–2595.

9 Barasch J, Kiss B, Prince A, Saiman L, Gruenert D and Al-Awqati Q. Defective acidification of intracellular organelles in cystic fibrosis. *Nature* 1991; 352(6330):70–73.

10 Saiman L, Prince A. *Pseudomonas aeruginosa* pili bind to asialoGM1 which is increased on the surface of cystic fibrosis epithelial cells. *J Clin Invest* 1993; 92(4):1875–1880.

11 Imundo L, Barasch J, Prince A, Al-Awaqati Q. Cystic fibrosis epithelial cells have a receptor for pathogenic bacteria on their apical surface. *Proc Natl Acad Sci USA* 1995; 92:3019–3023.

12 Pier GB, Grout M, Zaidi TS. Cystic fibrosis transmembrane conductance regulator is an epithelial cell receptor for clearance of *Pseudomonas aeruginosa* from the lung. *Proc Natl Acad Sci* 1997; 94(22):12088–12093.

13 Henry RL, Mellis CM, Petrovic L. Mucoid *Pseudomonas aeruginosa* is a marker of poor survival in cystic fibrosis. *Pediatr Pulmonol* 1992; 12:158–161.

14 Richman-Eisenstat JB, Jorens PG, Hebert CA, Ueki I, Nadel JA. Interleukin-8: an important chemoattractant in sputum of patients with chronic inflammatory airway diseases. *Am J Physiol* 1993; 264:L413-L418.

15 Greally P, Hussein MJ, Cook AJ, Sampson AP, Piper PJ, Price JF. Sputum tumour necrosis factor-α and leukotriene concentrations in cystic fibrosis. *Arch Dis Child* 1993; 68:389–392.

16 Bruce MC, Poncz L, Klinger JD, Stern RC, Tomashefski JF, Jr, Dearborn DG. Biochemical and pathologic evidence for proteolytic destruction of lung connective tissue in cystic fibrosis. *Am Rev Respir Dis* 1985; 132:529–535.

17 Chernick WS, Barbero GJ. Composition of tracheobronchial secretions in cystic fibrosis of the pancreas and bronchiectasis. *Pediatrics* 1959; 24:739–745.

18 Armstrong DS, Grimwood K, Carzino R, Carlin JB, Olinsky A, Phelan PD. Lower respiratory infection and inflammation in infants with newly diagnosed cystic fibrosis. *BMJ* 1995; 310:1571–1572.

19 Khan TZ, Wagener JS, Bost T, Martinez J, Accurso FJ, Riches DW. Early pulmonary inflammation in infants with cystic fibrosis. *Am J Respir Crit Care Med* 1995; 151:1075–1082.

20 Balough K, McCubbin M, Weinberger M et al. The relationship between infection and inflammation in the early stages of lung disease from cystic fibrosis. *Pediatr Pulmonol* 1995; 20(2):63–70.

21 Armstrong DS, Grimwood K, Carlin JB, Carzino R, et al. Lower airway inflammation in infants and young children with cystic fibrosis. *Am J Respir Crit Care Med* 1997; 156:1197–1204.

22 Scheid P, Kempster L, Griesenbach U et al. Inflammation in cystic fibrosis airways: relationship to increased bacterial adherence. *Eur Respir J* 2001; 17:27–35.

23 Pantin CF, Stead RJ, Hodson ME, Batten JC. Prednisolone in the treatment of airflow obstruction in adults with cystic fibrosis. *Thorax* 1986; 41:34–38.

24 Auerbach HS, Williams M, Kirkpatrick JA et al. Alternate day prednisolone reduces morbidity and improves pulmonary function in cystic fibrosis. *Lancet* 1985; 2:686–688.

25 Greally P, Hussein MJ, Vergani D, Price JF. Interleukin-1α, soluble interleukin-2 receptor and IgG concentrations in cystic fibrosis treated with prednisolone. *Arch Dis Child* 1994; 71:35–39.

26 Schiotz PO, Jorgensen M, Flensborg EW et al. Chronic Pseudomonas aeruginosa lung infection in cystic fibrosis. A longitudinal study of immune complex activity and inflammatory response in sputum sol-phase of cystic fibrosis patients with chronic *Pseudomonas aeruginosa* lung infections: influence of local steroid treatment. *Acta Paed Scand* 1983; 72(2):283.

27 Balfour-Lynn IM, Klein NJ, Dinwiddie R. Randomised controlled trial of inhaled corticosteroids (fluticasone propionate) in cystic fibrosis. *Arch Dis Child* 1997; 77(2):124–30.

28 Bisgaard H, Pedersen SS, Nielsen KG et al. Controlled trial of inhaled budesonide in patients with cystic fibrosis and chronic bronchopulmonary *Pseudomonas aeruginosa* infection. *Am J Resp Crit Care Med* 1997; 156(4 Pt 1):1190–6.

29 Konstan MW, Vargo KM, Davis PB. Ibuprofen attenuates the inflammatory response to *Pseudomonas aeruginosa* in a rat model of chronic pulmonary infection. Implications for antiinflammatory therapy in cystic fibrosis. *Am Rev Respir Dis* 1990; 141:186–192.

30 Konstan MW, Byard PJ, Hoppel CL et al. Effect of high-dose Ibuprofen in patients with cystic fibrosis. *N Engl J Med* 1995; 332:848–854.

31 Sordelli DO, Macri CN, Maillie AJ, Cerquetti MC. A preliminary study on the effect of anti-inflammatory treatment in cystic fibrosis patients with *Pseudomonas aeruginosa* lung infection. *Int J Immunopathol Pharmacol* 1994; 7:109.

32 McElvaney NG, Nakamura H, Birrer P et al. Modulation of airway inflammation in cystic fibrosis. *In vivo* suppression of interleukin-8 levels on the respiratory epithelial surface by aerosolization of recombinant secretory leukoprotease inhibitor. *J Clin Invest* 1992; 90(4):1296–1301.

33 Vogelmeier C, Gillissen A, Buhl R. Use of secretory leukoprotease inhibitor to augment lung antineutrophil elastase activity. *Chest* 1996; 110(6 Suppl):261S-266S.

34 Gillissen A, Birrer P, McElvaney NG et al. Recombinant secretory leukoprotease inhibitor augments glutathione levels in lung epithelial lining fluid. *J Appl Physiol* 1993; 75(2):825–832.

35 Tomee JFC, Koëter GH, Hiemestra PS, Kauffman HF. Secretory leukoprotease inhibitor: a native antimicrobial protein presenting a new therapeutic option? *Thorax* 1998; 53:114–116.

36 Cantin AM, Woods DE. Aerosolized prolastin suppresses bacterial proliferation in a model of chronic *Pseudomonas aeruginosa* lung infection. *Am J Resp Crit Care Med* 1999; 160(4):1130–1135.

37 McElvaney NG, Hubbard RC, Birrer P, Chernick MS et al. Aerosol alpha 1-antitrypsin treatment for cystic fibrosis. *Lancet* 1991; 337(8738):392–394.

38 Bingle L, Tetley TD. Secretory leukoprotease inhibitor: partnering α₁-proteinase inhibitor to combat pulmonary inflammation. *Thorax* 1996; 51:1273–1274.

39 Kelly FJ. Gluthathione: in defence of the lung. *Food Chem Toxicol* 1999; 37(9–10):963–966.

40 Roum JH, Buhl R, McElvaney NG, Borok Z, Crystal RG. Systemic deficiency of glutathione in cystic fibrosis. *J Appl Physiol* 1993; 75(6):2419–2424.

41 Hudson VM. Rethinking cystic fibrosis pathology: the critical role of abnormal reduced glutathione (GSH) transport caused by CFTR mutation. *Free Rad Biol Med* 2001; 30(12):1440–61.

42 Winkelhofer-Roob BM, Schlegel-Hauter SE, Khoschsorur G, van't Hof MA, Suter S, Shmerling DH. Neutrophil elastase/alpha 1-proteinase inhibitor complex levels decrease in plasma of cystic fibrosis patients during long-term oral beta-carotene supplementation. *Ped Res* 1996; 40(1):130–134.

43 Bonfield TL, Konstan MW, Burfeind P, Panuska JR, Hilliard JB, Berger M. Normal bronchial epithelial cells constitu-

tively produce the anti-inflammatory cytokine interleukin-10, which is downregulated in cystic fibrosis. *Am J Respir Cell Mol Biol* 1995; 13(3):257–261

44 Chmiel JF, Konstan MW, Knesebeck JE et al. IL-10 attenuates excessive inflammation in chronic *Pseudomonas* infection in mice. *Am J Respir Crit Care Med* 1999; 160:2040–2047.

45 Page CP. Proteoglycans: the 'Teflon' of the airways? *Thorax* 1997; 52:924–925.

46 Ledson M, Gallagher M, Hart CA, Walshaw M. Nebulized heparin in *Burkholderia cepacia* colonized adult cystic fibrosis patients. *Eur Respir J* 2001; 17:36–38.

47 Koyama H, Geddes DM. Erythromycin and diffuse panbronchiolitis. *Thorax* 1997; 52:915–918.

48 Høiby N. Diffuse panbronchiolitis and cystic fibrosis: East meets West. *Thorax* 1994; 49:531–532.

49 Jaffé A, Francis J, Rosenthal M, Bush A. Long-term azithromycin may improve lung function in children with cystic fibrosis. *Lancet* 1998; 351:420.

50 Pirzada OM, Taylor CJ. Long-term macrolide antibiotics improve pulmonary function in cystic fibrosis. *Paediatr Pulmonol* 1999; 19(Suppl.):263.

51 Jaffé A and Bush A. Anti-inflammatory effects of macrolides in lung disease. *Ped Pulmonol* 2001; 31:464–473,

52 Altschuler EL. Azithromycin, the multidrug-resistant-protein, and cystic fibrosis. *Lancet* 1998; 351:1286.

53 Aronoff SC, Quinn FJ Jr, Carpenter LS, Novick WJ Jr. Effects of pentoxifylline on sputum neutrophil elastase and pulmonary function in patients with cystic fibrosis: preliminary observations. *J Pediatr* 1994; 125(6 Pt 1):992–997.

54 Henderson WR Jr, Astley SJ, McCready MM et al. Oral absorption of omega-3 fatty acids in patients with cystic fibrosis who have pancreatic insufficiency and in healthy control subjects. *J Pediatrics* 1994; 124(3):400–408.

55 Roulet M, Frascarolo P, Rappaz I, Pilet M. Essential fatty acid deficiency in well nourished young cystic fibrosis patients. *Eur J Pediatr* 1997; 156(12):952–956.

56 Freedman SD, Shea JC, Blanco PG, Alvarez JG. Fatty acids in cystic fibrosis. *Curr Opin Pulm Med* 2000; 6(6):530–532.

57 Fuchs HJ, Borowitz DS, Christiansen DH et al. Effect of aerosolized recombinant human DNase on exacerbations of respiratory symptoms and on pulmonary function in cystic fibrosis. The Pulmozyme Study Group. *N Engl J Med* 1994; 331:637–642.

58 Konstan MW, Tiddens HA, Quan JM, McKenzie S, Wohl ME et al. A randomised, placebo-controlled trial of two years treatment with dornase alfa (Pulmozyme) in cystic fibrosis patients aged 6–10 years with early lung disease (abstract). *Pediatr Pulmonol* 2000; 20(Suppl.):299.

59 Suri R, Metcalfe C, Lees B et al. A randomised comparative trial of hypertonic saline, alternate day and daily rhDNase in children with cystic fibrosis. *Thorax* 2000; 55(Suppl. 3):A75.

60 Rochat T, Dayer Pastore F, Schlegel-Haueter SE et al. Aerosolized rhDNase in cystic fibrosis: effect on leucocyte proteases in sputum. *Eur Respir J* 1996; 9:2200–2206.

61 Shah PL, Scott SF, Knight RA, Hodson ME. The effects of recombinant human DNase on neutrophil elastase activity and interleukin-8 levels in the sputum of patients with cystic fibrosis. *Eur Respir J* 1996; 9:531–534.

62 Vogelmeier C, Doring G. Neutrophil proteinases and rhDNase therapy in cystic fibrosis. *Eur Respir J* 1996; 9:2193–2195.

63 Wallis C. Mucolytic therapy in cystic fibrosis. *J R Soc Med* 2001; 94(suppl40):17–24.

64 Suri R, Wallis C, Bush A. *In vivo* use of hypertonic saline in CF. *Ped Pulmonol* 2000; Suppl 20; 125–126.

65 Sampson AP, Spencer DA, Green CP, Piper PJ, Price JF. Leukotrienes in the sputum and urine of cystic fibrosis children. *Br J Clin Pharmac* 1990; 30:861–869.

66 Greally P, Cook AJ, Sampson AP et al. Atopic children with cystic fibrosis have increased urinary leukotriene E4 concentrations and more severe pulmonary disease. *J Allergy Clinl Immunol* 1994; 93(1 Pt 1):100–107

67 Kurlandsky LE, Bennink MR, Webb PM, Ulrich PJ, Baer LJ. The absorption and effect of dietary supplementation with omega-3 fatty acids on serum leukotriene B4 in patients with cystic fibrosis. *Ped Pulmonol* 1994; 18(4):211–217.

68 FitzSimmons S. The Cystic Fibrosis Foundation Patient Registry Report, 1996. Pediatr Pulmonol 1996; 21:267–275.

69 Szaff M, Høiby N, Flensborg EW. Frequent antibiotic therapy improves survival of cystic fibrosis patients with chronic *Pseudomonas aeruginosa* infection. *Acta Paediatr Scand* 1983; 72:651–657.

70 Mouton JW, Kerrebijn KF. Antibacterial therapy in cystic fibrosis. *Med Clin N. Am* 1990; 74:837–850.

71 Strandvik B. Antibiotic therapy of pulmonary infections in cystic fibrosis. Dosage schedules and duration of treatment. *Chest* 1988; 94:146S-149S.

72 Horrevorts AM, Driessen OMJ, Michel MF, Kerribijn KF. Pharmacokinetics of antimicrobial drugs in cystic fibrosis. Aminoglycoside antibiotics. *Chest* 1988; 94:120S-125S.

73 Lietman PS. Pharmocokinetics of antimicrobial drugs in cystic fibrosis. β-lactam antibiotics. *Chest* 1988; 94:115S-119S.

74 Reed MD, Stern RC, Myers CM, Yamashita TS, Blumer JL. Lack of unique ciprofloxacin pharmacokinetics in cystic fibrosis. *J Clin Pharmacol* 1988; 28:691–699.

75 Spino M, Chai RP, Isles AF et al. Cloxacillin absorption and disposition in cystic fibrosis. *J Pediatr* 1984; 105:829–835.

76 Touw DJ, Vinks AA, Mouton JW, Horrevorts AM. Pharmacokinetic optimisation of antibacterial treatment in patients with cystic fibrosis. Current practice and suggestions for future directions. *Clin Pharmacokinet* 1998; 35:437–459.

77 Taylor RF, Hodson ME. Cystic fibrosis: antibiotic prescribing practices in the United Kingdom and Eire. *Respir Med* 1993; 87:535–539.

78 McCaffery K, Olver RE, Franklin M, Mukhopadhyay S. Systematic review of antistaphylococcal antibiotic therapy in cystic fibrosis. *Thorax* 1999; 54:380–383.

79 Weaver LT, Green MR, Nicholson K et al. Prognosis in cystic fibrosis treated with continuous flucloxacillin from the neonatal period. *Arch Dis Child* 1994; 70:84–89.

80 Beardsmore CS, Thompson JR, Williams A et al. Pulmonary function in infants with cystic fibrosis: the effect of antibiotic treatment. *Arch Dis Child* 1994; 71:133–137.

81 Smyth A, Walters S. Prophylactic antibiotics for cystic fibrosis (Cochrane Review). In: *The Cochrane Library*, Issue 4, 2001. Oxford: Update Software.

82 Elborn JS. Treatment of *Staphylococcus aureus* in cystic fibrosis, Thorax 1999; 54:377–379.

83 Littlewood J et al. Antibiotic treatment for cystic fibrosis. Report of the UK Cystic Fibrosis Trust's antibiotic group. April 2000.

84 Thomas SR, Gyi KM, Gaya H, Hodson ME. Methicillin-resistant *Staphylococcus aureus*: impact at a national cystic fibrosis centre. *J Hosp Infect* 1998; 40:203–209.

85 Stutman HR, Marks MI. Antibiotic prophylaxis study group. Cephalexin prophylaxis in newly diagnosed infants with cystic fibrosis. Sixth Annual North American Cystic Fibrosis Conference, Orlando, 1994.

86 Ratjen F, Comes G, Paul K, Posselt HG, Wagner TO, Harms K. Effect of continuous antistaphylococcal therapy on the rate of *P. aeruginosa* acquisition in patients with cystic fibrosis. *Pediatr Pulmonol* 2001; 31:13–16.

87 Rayner RJ, Hiller EJ, Ispahani P, Baker M. *Haemophilus* infection in cystic fibrosis. *Arch Dis Child* 1990; 65:255–258.

88 Roberts DE, Cole P. Use of selective media in bacteriological investigation of patients with chronic suppurative respiratory infection. *Lancet* 1980; 1:796–797.

89 Bilton D, Pye A, Johnson MM et al. The isolation and characterization of non-typable *Haemophilus influenzae* from the sputum of adult cystic fibrosis patients. *Eur Resp J* 1995; 8:948–953.

90 Geddes DM. Antimicrobial therapy against *Staphyloccus aureus*, *Pseudomonas aeruginosa* and *Pseudomonas cepacia*. *Chest* 1988; 94:1405–1445.

91 Pressler T, Szaff M, Høiby N. Antibiotic treatment of *Haemophilus influenzae* and *Haemophilus parainfluenzae* infections in patients with cystic fibrosis. *Acta Paediatr Scand* 1984; 541–547.

92 Kaiser L, Lew D, Hirschel B et al. Effects of antibiotic treatment in the subset of common-cold patients who have bacteria in nasopharyngeal secretions. *Lancet* 1996; 347:1507–1510.

93 Collinson J, Nicholson KG, Cancio E et al. Effects of upper respiratory tract infections in patients with cystic fibrosis. *Thorax* 1996; 51:1115–1122.

94 Döring G, Conway SP, Heijerman HGM et al. Antibiotic therapy against *Pseudomonas aeruginosa* in cystic fibrosis: a European consensus. *Eur Respir J* 2000; 16:749–767.

95 Jensen T, Pedersen SS, Nielsen CH, Høiby N, Koch C. The efficacy and safety of ciprofloxacin and ofloxacin in chronic *Pseudomonas aeruginosa* infection in cystic fibrosis. *J Antimicrob Chem* 1987; 20:585–594.

96 Hodson ME, Roberts CM, Butland RJ, Smith MJ, Batten JC. Oral ciprofloxacin compared with conventional intravenous treatment for *Pseudomonas aeruginosa* infection in adults with cystic fibrosis. *Lancet* 1987; 1:235–237.

97 Jensen T, Pedersen SS, Høiby N, Koch C. Efficacy of oral fluoroquinolones versus intravenous antipseudomonal chemotherapy in treatment of cystic fibrosis. *Eur J Clin Microbiol* 1987; 6:618–622.

98 Sheldom CD, Assoufi BK, Hodson ME. Regular three monthly oral ciprofloxacin in adult cystic fibrosis patients infected with *Pseudomonas aeruginosa*. *Respir Med* 1993; 87:587–593.

99 Shalit I, Stutman HR, Marks MI, Chartrand SA, Hilman BC. Randomized study of two dosage regimens of ciprofloxacin for treating chronic bronchopulmonary infection with cystic fibrosis. *Am J Med* 1987; 82:189–195.

100 Radberg G, Nilsson LE, Svensson S. Development of quinolone-imipenem cross resistance in *Pseudomonas aeruginosa* during exposure to ciprofloxacin. *Antimicrob Agents Chemother* 1990; 34:2142-2147.

101 Norrby SR. Side-effects of quinolones: comparison between quinolones and other antibiotics. *Eur J Clin Micro Infect Dis* 1991; 10:378–383.

102 Chysky V, Kapila K, Hullman R, Arcieri G, Schacht P, Echols R. Safety of ciprofloxacin in children: worldwide clinical experience based on compassionate use. Emphasis on joint evaluation. *Infection* 1991; 19:289–296.

103 Burkhardt JE, Walterspiel JN, Schaad UB. Quinolone arthropathy in animals versus children. *Clin Infect Dis* 1997; 25:1196–1204.

104 Lietman PS. Pharmacokinetics of antimicrobial drugs in cystic fibrosis. Beta-lactam antibiotics. *Chest* 1988; 94; 115S-120S.

105 Mendelman PM, Smith AL, Levy J, Weber A, Ramsey B, David RL. Aminoglycoside penetration, inactivation and efficacy in cystic fibrosis sputum. *Am Rev Resp Dis* 1985; 32:761–765.

106 Laube BL. In vivo measurements of aerosol dose and distribution clinical relevance. *J Aerosol Med* 1996; 9:S77-S91.

107 Hodson ME, Penketh ARL, Batten JC. Aerosol carbenicillin and gentamicin treatment of *Pseudomonas aeruginosa* infection in patients with cystic fibrosis. *Lancet* 1981; 2:1137–1139.

108 Campbell PW, Saiman L. Use of aerosolized antibiotics in patients with cystic fibrosis. *Chest* 1999; 116:775–788.

109 Mukhopadhyay S, Singh M, Cater JI, Ogston S, Franklin M, Olver RE. Nebulised antipseudomonal antibiotic therapy in cystic fibrosis: a meta-analysis of benefits and risks. *Thorax* 1996; 51:364–368.

110 Ryan G, Mukhopadhyay S, Singh M. Nebulised antipseudomonal antibiotics for cystic fibrosis (Cochrane Review). In: *The Cochrane Library*, Issue 3, 2001. Oxford: Update Software.

111 Ramsey B, Pepe M, Quan JM et al. Intermittent administration of inhaled tobramycin in patients with cystic fibrosis. *N Engl J Med* 1999; 340:23–30.

112 Ramsey BW, Dorkin HL, Eisenberg JD et al. Efficacy of aerosolized tobramycin in patients with cystic fibrosis. *N Engl J Med* 1993; 328:1740–1746.

113 Nickerson B, Montgomery AB, Kylstra JW et al. Safety and effectiveness of 2 years of treatment with intermittent inhaled tobramycin in cystic fibrosis patients. *Paediatr Pulmonol* 1999 Suppl 19: 243, abstr 280.

114 Moss R, Kylstra JW, Montgomery AB, Gibson R. Who benefits more? An analysis of FEV1 and weight in adolescent (age 13 to<18) cystic fibrosis patients using inhaled tobramycin. *Paediatr Pulmonol* 1999 Suppl 19: 243, abstr 279.

115 Littlewood JM, Koch C, Lambert PA et al. A ten year review of Colomycin. *Respir Med* 2000; 94:632–640.

116 Johansen HK, Høiby N. Seasonal onset of initial colonisation and chronic infection with *Pseudomonas aeruginosa* in patients with cystic fibrosis in Denmark. *Thorax* 1992; 47:109–111.

117 Valerius NH, Koch C, Høiby N. Prevention of chronic *Pseudomonas aeruginosa* colonisation in cystic fibrosis by early treatment. *Lancet* 1991; 338:725–726.

118 Wieseman HG, Steinkamp G, Ratjen F et al. Placebo-controlled, double-blind, randomized study of aerosolized tobramycin for early treatment of *Pseudomonas aeruginosa* colonization in cystic fibrosis. *Pediatr Pulmonol* 1998; 25:88–92.

119 Frederiksen B, Koch C, Høiby N. Antibiotic treatment of initial colonization with *Pseudomonas aeruginosa* postpones chronic infection and prevents deterioration of pulmonary function in cystic fibrosis. *Pediatr Pulmonol* 1997; 23:330–335.

120 Frederiksen B, Koch C, Høiby N. Changing epidemiology of *Pseudomonas aeruginosa* infection in Danish cystic fibrosis patients (1974–1995). *Pediatr Pulmonol* 1999; 28:159–166.

121 Huang NN, Hiller EJ, Macri CM, Capitanio M, Cundy KR. Carbenicillin in patients with cystic fibrosis: clinical pharmacology and therapeutic evaluation. *J Pediatr* 1971; 78:338–345.

122 Stephens D, Garey N, Isles A, Levison H, Gold R. Efficacy of inhaled tobramycin in the treatment of pulmonary exacerbations in children with cystic fibrosis. *Pediatr Infect Dis* 1983; 3:209–211.

123 Schaad UB, Wedgewood-Krucko J, Suter S, Kramer R. Efficacy of inhaled amikacin as adjunct to intravenous combination therapy (ceftazidime and amikacin) in cystic fibrosis. *J Pediatr* 1987; 111:599–605.

124 Ramsey BW. Management of pulmonary disease in patients with cystic fibrosis. *N Engl J Med* 1996; 335:179–188.

125 Permin H, Koch C, Høiby N, Christensen HO, Moller AF, Moller S. Ceftazidime treatment of chronic *Pseudomonas aeruginosa* respiratory tract infection in cystic fibrosis. *J Antimicrob Chemo* 1983; 12:313–323.

126 Gold R, Overmeyer A, Knie B, Fleming PC, Levison H. Controlled trial of ceftazidime vs. ticarcillin and tobramycin in the treatment of acute respiratory exacerbations in patients with cystic fibrosis. *Pediatr Infect Dis* 1985; 4:172–177.

127 Elphick HE, Tan A. Single versus combination intravenous antibiotic therapy for people with cystic fibrosis (Cochrane Review). In: *The Cochrane Library*, Issue 4, 2001. Oxford: Update Software.

128 Cheng K, Smyth RL, Govan JR et al. Spread of beta-lactam-resistant *Pseudomonas aeruginosa* in a cystic fibrosis clinic. *Lancet* 1996; 348:639–642.

129 Weiss K, Lapointe JR. Routine susceptibility testing of four

antibiotic combinations for improvement of laboratory guide to therapy of cystic fibrosis infections caused by *Pseudomonas aeruginosa*. *Antimicrob Agents Chemo* 1995; 39:2411–2414.

130 Mann HJ, Canafax DM, Cipolle RJ, Daniels CE, Zaske DE, Warwick WJ. Increased dosage requirements of tobramycin and gentamicin for treating *Pseudomonas pneumonia* in patients with cystic fibrosis. *Pediatr Pulmonol* 1985; 1:238–243.

131 Von Vigier RO, Truttmann AC, Zindler-Schmocker K et al. Aminoglycosides and renal magnesium homeostasis in humans. *Nephrol Dial Transpl* 2000; 15:822–826.

132 Barza M, Ioannidis JP, Cappelleri JC, Lau J. Single or multiple daily doses of aminoglycosides: a meta-analysis. *BMJ* 1996; 312:338–345.

133 Wood PJ, Ioannides-Demos LL, Li SC et al. Minimisation of aminoglycoside toxicity in patients with cystic fibrosis. *Thorax* 1996; 51:369–373.

134 Vic P, Ategbo S, Turck D et al. Efficacy, tolerance and pharmacokinetics of once daily tobramycin for pseudomonas exacerbations in cystic fibrosis. *Arch Dis Child* 1998; 78:536–539.

135 Tan K, Bunn H. Once daily versus multiple daily dosing with intravenous aminoglycosides for cystic fibrosis (Cochrane Review). In: *The Cochrane Library*, Issue 4, 2000. Oxford: Update Software.

136 Wills R, Henry RL, Francic JL. Antibiotic hypersensitivity reactions in cystic fibrosis. *J Paediatr Child Health* 1998; 34:325–329.

137 Pleasants RA, Walker TR, Samuelson WM. Allergic reactions to parenteral beta-lactam antibiotics in patients with cystic fibrosis. *Chest* 1994; 106:1124–1128.

138 Battersby NC, Patel L, David TJ. Increasing dose regimen in children with reactions to ceftazidime. *Clin Exp Allergy* 1995; 25:1211–1217.

139 Earl HS, Sullivan TJ. Acute desensitization of a patient with cystic fibrosis allergic to both beta-lactam and aminoglycoside antibiotics. *J Allergy Clin Immunol* 1987; 79:477–483.

140 Pedersen SS, Jensen T, Høiby N, Koch C, Flensborg EW. Management of *Pseudomonas aeruginosa* lung infection in Danish cystic fibrosis patients. *Acta Paediatr Scand* 1987; 76:955–961.

141 Elborn JS, Prescott RJ, Stack BHR et al. Elective versus symptomatic antibiotic treatment in cystic fibrosis patients with chronic *Pseudomonas* infection of the lungs. *Thorax* 2000; 55:355–358.

142 Breen L, Aswani N. Elective versus symptomatic intravenous antibiotic therapy for cystic fibrosis (Cochrane Review). In: *The Cochrane Library*, Issue 4, 2001. Oxford: Update Software.

143 Conway SP, Pond MN, Watson A, Etherington C, Robey HL, Goldman MH. Intravenous colistin sulphomethate in acute respiratory exacerbations in adult patients with cystic fibrosis. *Thorax* 1997; 52:987–993.

144 Ledson MJ, Gallagher MJ, Cowperthwaite C, Convery RP, Walshaw MJ. Four years' experience of intravenous colomycin in an adult cystic fibrosis unit. *Eur Respir J* 1998; 12:592–594.

145 Conway SP, Etherington C, Munday J, Goldman MH, Strong JJ, Wootton M. Safety and tolerability of bolus intravenous colistin in acute respiratory exacerbations in adults with cystic fibrosis. *Ann Pharmacother* 2000; 34:1238–1242.

146 Isles A, Maclusky I, Corey M et al. *Pseudomonas cepacia* infection in cystic fibrosis: an emerging problem. *J Pediatr* 1984; 104:206–210.

147 Pitt TL, Kaufman ME, Patel PS, Benge LC, Gaskin S, Livermore DM. Type characterisation and antibiotic susceptibility of *Burkholderia* (*Pseudomonas*) cepacia isolates from patients with cystic fibrosis in the United Kingdom and the Republic of Ireland. *J Med Microbiol* 1996; 44:203–210.

148 Aaron SD, Ferris W, Henry DA, Speert DP, MacDonald NE. Multiple combination bactericidal antibiotic testing for patients with cystic fibrosis infected with Burkholderia cepacia. Am J Resp *Crit Care Med* 2000; 161:1206–1212.

149 Jones AM, Dodd ME, Webb AK. Burkholderia cepacia: current clinical issues, environmental controversies and ethical dilemmas. *Eur Respir J* 2001; 17:295–301.

150 Miall LS, McGinley NT, Brownlee KG, Conway SP. Methicillin resistant *Staphylococcus aureus* (MRSA) infection in cystic fibrosis. *Arch Dis Child* 2001; 84:160–162.

151 Fraise AP. Guidelines for the control of methicillin-resistant *Staphylococcus aureus*. *J Antimicrob Chemother* 1998; 42:287–289.

152 Maiz L, Canton R, Mir N, Baquero F, Escobar H. Aerosolized vancomycin for the treatment of methicillin-resistant *Staphylococcus aureus* infection in cystic fibrosis. *Pediatr Pulmonol* 1998; 26:287–289.

153 Demko CA, Stern RC, Doershuk CF. *Stenotrophomonas maltophilia* in cystic fibrosis: incidence and prevalence. *Pediatr Pulmonol* 1998; 25:304–308.

154 Talmaciu I, Varlotta L, Mortensen J, Schidlow DV. Risk factors for emergence of *Stenotrophomonas maltophilia* in cystic fibrosis. *Pediatr Pulmonol* 2000; 30:10–15.

155 Denton M, Kerr KG. Microbiological and clinical aspects of infection associated with *Stenotrophomonas maltophilia*. *Clin Microbiol Rev* 1998; 11:57–80.

156 Olivier KN, Yankaskas JR, Knowles MR. Nontuberculous mycobacterial pulmonary disease in cystic fibrosis. *Semin Respir Infect* 1996; 11:272-284.

157 American Thoracic Society. Diagnosis and treatment of disease caused by nontuberculous mycobacteria. *Am J Respir Crit Care Med* 1997; 156:S1-S25.

158 Torrens JK, Dawkins P, Conway SP, Moya E. Non-tuberculous mycobacteria in cystic fibrosis. *Thorax* 1998; 53:182–185.

159 Cullen AR, Cannon CL, Mark EJ, Colin AA. *Mycobacterium abscessus* infection in cystic fibrosis. Colonization or infection? *Am J Respir Crit Care Med* 2000; 161:641–645.

160 Gilljam M, Berning SE, Peloquin CA, Strandvik B, Larsson LO. Therapeutic drug monitoring in patients with cystic fibrosis and mycobacterial disease. *Eur Respir J* 1999; 14:347–351.

161 Keogan MT, Johansen HK. Vaccines for preventing infection with Pseudomonas aeruginosa in people with cystic fibrosis (Cochrane Review). In: *The Cochrane Library*, Issue 4, 2001. Oxford: Update Software.

162 Wheeler WB, Williams M, Matthews WJ, Colten HR. Progression of cystic fibrosis lung disease as a function of serum immunoglobulin G levels: a 5-year longitudinal study. *J Pediatr* 1984; 104:695–699

163 Langford DT, Hiller J. Prospective, controlled study of a polyvalent pseudomonas vaccine in cystic fibrosis – three year results. *Arch Dis Child* 1984; 59:1131–1134.

164 Döring G, Dorner F. A multicenter vaccine trial using the *Pseudomonas aeruginosa* flagella vaccine IMMUNO in patients with cystic fibrosis. *Behring Institute Mitteilungen* 1997; 98:338–344.

165 Cryz SJ Jr, Lang A, Rudeberg A et al. Immunization of cystic fibrosis patients with *Pseudomonas aeruginosa* O-polysaccharide-toxin A conjugate vaccine. *Behring Institute Mitteilungen* 1997; 98:345–349.

166 Pier GB. Rationale for development of immunotherapies that target mucoid *Pseudomonas aeruginosa* infection in cystic fibrosis patients. *Behring Institute Mitteilungen* 1997; 98:350–360.

167 Kollberg H, Johannesson M, Schuster A, Carlander D, Larsson A. IgY to prevent infection with *Pseudomonas aeruginosa*. Results from phase I study and how to go on with phase II-III studies. In: Proceedings of XIIIth International Cystic Fibrosis Congress, Stockholm, 2000.

168 Fung-Tomc J, Bush K, Minassian B et al. Antibacterial activity of BMS-180680, a new catechol-containing monobactam. *Antimicrob Agents Chemother* 1997; 41:1010–1016.

169 Ledson MJ, Gallagher MJ, Robinson M et al. A randomised double blind placebo controlled crossover trial of nebulised taurolidine in adult cystic fibrosis patients colonised with *Burkholderia cepacia*. Proceedings of the 22nd *European Cystic Fibrosis Conference*, Berlin, 1998.

170 Ledson MJ, Cowperthwaite C, Walshaw MJ, Gallagher MJ, Williets T, Hart CA. Nebulised taurolidine and *B. cepacia* bronchiectasis. *Thorax* 2000; 55:91.

171 Barghouti S, Guerdoud LM, Speert DP. Inhibition by dextran of *Pseudomonas aeruginosa* adherence to epithelial cells. *Am J Respir Crit Care Med* 1996; 154:1788–1793.

172 Bryan R, Feldman M, Jawetz SC et al. The effects of aerosolized dextran in a mouse model of *Pseudomonas aeruginosa* pulmonary infection. *J Infect Dis* 1999; 179:1449–1458.

173 Feng W, Garrett H, Speert DP, King M. Improved clearability of cystic fibrosis sputum with dextran treatment in vitro. *Am J Resp Crit Care Med* 1998; 157:710–714.

174 Davies J, Dewar A, Bush A et al. Reduction in the adherence of *Pseudomonas aeruginosa* to native cystic fibrosis epithelium with anti-asialoGM1 antibody and neuraminidase inhibition. *Eur Respir J* 1999; 13:565–570.

175 Zabner J, Seiler MP, Launspach JL et al. The osmolyte xylitol reduces the salt concentration of airway surface liquid and may enhance bacterial killing. *Proc Natl Acad Sci USA* 2000; 97:11614–11619.

Part IV

Pulmonary vascular diseases

17

Pathophysiology of pulmonary vascular disease

Sanjay Mehta and David G. McCormack

A. C. Burton Vascular Research Laboratory, Division of Respirology, London Health Sciences Centre, Departments of Medicine, Pharmacology and Toxicology, University of Western Ontario, London, Ontario, Canada

Introduction

Primary disorders of the pulmonary vasculature are decidedly uncommon. However, secondary involvement of pulmonary blood vessels is very common, being a feature or a complication of many cardiac, pulmonary and other medical conditions. Although we understand more about diseases of the pulmonary blood vessels than just a few decades ago, there is still much less known about the pulmonary vessels than about the systemic blood vessels. However, the presence of similar types of cells in both systemic and pulmonary vessels and a limited range of pathological responses to injury permit students of both to learn from each other.

In this chapter, we will review our understanding of the pathogenesis and pathophysiology of pulmonary vascular disease (PVD). PVD may be primary (idiopathic) or secondary to an underlying medical disorder, especially of the heart and lungs. We will focus on one particular entity, primary pulmonary hypertension (PPH) as a prototypical human example of PVD. Although there is much overlap between proposed mechanisms of pulmonary vascular injury in PPH and in secondary PVD, significant clinical and biological heterogeneity exists. Thus, wherever possible, hypothesized mechanisms will be presented with representative, supporting data from studies of patients with PPH. When no such data exist, we will present data from other clinical disorders of PVD, e.g. congenital heart disease (CHD)-associated pulmonary arterial hypertension

(PAH), as well as from studies using various animal models of PVD.

General mechanisms of pulmonary arterial hypertension

A prerequisite to understanding the pathogenesis of PAH, and having a logical approach to the clinical problem is a knowledge of the various mechanisms that can raise pulmonary artery pressure (P_{PA}) and/or pulmonary vascular resistance (PVR). These mechanisms include: (i) vasoconstriction, (ii) intravascular thrombosis, (iii) proliferation (or thickening) of the media or intima, (iv) loss of cross sectional surface area of the pulmonary vascular bed, and (v) increase in pulmonary blood flow. The latter two mechanisms are important in the pathogenesis of secondary PAH (SPH) such as occurs in severe emphysema (with destruction of lung parenchyma) or CHD with left to right shunts and increased pulmonary blood flow. To a greater or lesser degree, the first three mechanisms may play a role in the pathogenesis of PPH. An early hypothesis was that PPH progressed from a vasoconstrictive component to a fixed obstruction of the pulmonary vascular bed. It is now widely held that vasoconstriction is less important, and chronic pulmonary vascular thrombosis, remodelling and inflammation are more important in the pathogenesis of PVD. Thus, the following discussion will reflect this evolving thinking by focusing on the latter mechanisms.

It is important to note that a variety of seemingly diverse stimuli (such as portal hypertension, shear stress, viral infection and drugs) all lead to the same plexogenic pulmonary arteriolar lesions. Most investigators agree that some genetic predisposition is needed for the development of severe, progressive PAH following exposure to an inciting stimulus. The progressive vascular remodelling leads to increased endothelial shear stress which, in turn, leads to more remodelling. It remains unclear precisely what (if any) link exists between endothelial cell proliferation and pulmonary vasoconstriction.

Although many cells and soluble components in the vessel wall probably contribute to the pathogenesis of PVD, a critical, central role of the endothelium is incontrovertible. Alterations and dysfunction of endothelial cells are common, unifying features of different PVD, and of the various pathogenetic mechanisms that contribute to such disease. Thus, endothelial dysfunction will serve as a common thread through our discussion of the pathogenesis of PVD.

Pulmonary vasoconstriction

For many years investigators subscribed to the concept that active vasoconstriction was the key mechanism in the pathogenesis of PPH[1]. This concept was supported by early observations that administration of vasodilators resulted in a lowering of P_{PA} in this disease[2,3]. Further, the observation that resistance vessels in the lungs of these patients had medial hypertrophy was interpreted as evidence supporting vasoconstriction[4].

Despite the fact that pulmonary vascular smooth muscle constriction contributes to the pathogenesis of PPH, most investigators now feel that, while active pulmonary vasoconstriction is present in some patients with PPH, it is unlikely to be the initiating mechanism. Although there is no truly representative model of PPH, the monocrotaline rat model has been extensively used to examine the pathogenesis of the disease. Four weeks following injection into the animal, there is pulmonary hypertension and

medial hypertrophy of the pulmonary vessels. Importantly, preceding this hypertrophy, there is proliferation and increased metabolic activity of the endothelial cell (EC) layer[5]. Results such as these have shifted current thinking to the concept that medial hypertrophy is a consequence of endothelial dysfunction and that there may be abnormal control of the endothelium over pulmonary vascular smooth muscle. Nevertheless, pulmonary vasoconstriction is contributory to the increase in pulmonary vascular resistance (PVR) characteristic of PPH. Vascular tone (pulmonary or systemic) in vivo is likely a consequence of a complex balance between competing vasoconstrictor and vasodilator mediators.

A variety of mediators have been implicated in the alteration of pulmonary vascular tone in PPH. Examples are the vasoactive metabolites of arachidonic acid, prostacyclin (PGI_2) and thromboxane A2 (TxA_2). PGI_2 is synthesized by endothelial cells via PGI2 synthase and is both a potent inhibitor of platelet aggregation and a vasodilator. TxA2, synthesized predominantly by platelets and macrophages is a potent vasoconstrictor which has a very short circulating half-life (30 s). There is abundant evidence that there is endothelial dysfunction and altered eicosanoid synthesis in patients with PAH. Rich et al.[6] reported decreased serum levels of 6-keto-$PGF_{1\alpha}$ (the stable metabolite of prostacyclin) in patients with PPH. Subsequently Badesch and coworkers[7] demonstrated decreased PGI2 production by pulmonary vascular endothelial cells obtained from animals with PAH secondary to hypobaric hypoxic exposure. This work has been elaborated on by Christman and colleagues[8] who evaluated patients with both PPH and SPH and found increased urinary excretion of TxA_2 metabolites in all patients with pulmonary hypertension, regardless of whether it was primary or secondary disease. Further, there was also a decreased urinary excretion of PGI_2 metabolites, in patients with all forms of PAH. These data suggest that, in PAH, there is an imbalance in vasodilator and vasoconstrictor eicosanoids derived from either circulating platelets or pulmonary vascular cells. Supporting this hypothesis, Rabinovitch et al. have demonstrated that increasing endothelial prostacyclin release prevents hypoxic PAH[9] and Geraci et al. have reported that pulmonary prostacyclin synthase overexpression in mice prevents the development of hypoxic PAH[10].

Another circulating vasoactive mediator that may be important in the pathogenesis of PAH is serotonin. Serotonin is known to be a pulmonary vasoconstrictor, perhaps to an even greater degree than hypoxia[11]. Further, plasma serotonin levels are increased in patients with PPH (see below)[12]. It is at least partly through inhibition of serotonin uptake that the appetite suppressants fenfluramine and dexfenfluramine may lead to PPH in susceptible individuals.

Two other important vasoactive mediators produced by the pulmonary vascular endothelium are the vasodilator nitric oxide (NO) and the vasoconstrictor endothelin-1 (ET-1). ET-1 receptors include ETA receptors located predominantly on smooth muscle cells (which mediate vasoconstriction) and ETB receptors which are mainly on endothelial cells (and mediate vasodilation). An increase in ET-1 has been demonstrated in experimental PAH[13]. In patients with PPH, increased plasma levels of ET-1 and increased pulmonary vascular ET-1 immunoreactivity have been reported[14,15]. Further, blockade of ETA receptors, or the use of ETB receptor agonists improves P_{PA} in animal models of PAH secondary to increased pulmonary flow or increased left atrial pressure[16,17].

The role of NO in the pathogenesis of PAH has been the subject of many investigations. It is generally thought that release of the endogenous vasodilator NO contributes to the normal low resting tone of the pulmonary circulation. This is supported by the observation that inhibition of nitric oxide synthase (NOS) in humans (with L-NMMA) causes both an increase in P_{PA} and PVR[18]. Further, mice that have the eNOS gene deleted have PAH[19]. Whether eNOS expression is increased or decreased in many different models of SPH is controversial[20–22]. Similarly, in patients with PPH there is conflicting data on pulmonary vascular ecNOS expression, with evidence both for decreased expression and increased expression[23–25]. Nevertheless, the collected evidence supports the concept that an imbalance between vasoconstrictor and vasodilator mediators may play a fundamental role in the vasoconstrictive component of PAH.

In addition to an imbalance in the production of vasodilator and vasoconstrictor mediators leading to PAH, it is possible that there is inherent abnormal vasoreactivity of the pulmonary circulation in some patients. For example, consistent with an underlying endothelial dysfunction in patients with PPH, there is loss of endothelium-dependent relaxation to acetylcholine and substance-P in vivo[26–28]. Abnormal vasoreactivity may be a consequence of a perinatal insult[29]. Alternatively, there may be genetic susceptibility to the development of PAH (and increased vasoreactivity) as suggested by the observation that 5–10% of cases of PPH have a familial predisposition (see below).

In addition to endothelial dysfunction contributing to abnormal pulmonary vascular reactivity, there may be defects in the pulmonary vascular smooth muscle itself. A potential mechanism that may contribute to vasoconstriction in patients with PPH is down-regulation or absence of voltage-gated potassium (Kv) channels. Thus, inhibition of Kv channels in pulmonary artery smooth muscle cells, for example by hypoxia[30], or dexfenfluramine[31] causes pulmonary vasconstriction. Consistent with Kv channels being important in the pathophysiology of the disease, it has been reported that isolated smooth muscle cells (SMC) from pulmonary arteries of patients with PPH are relatively depolarized (less negative resting membrane potential, EM) and have an attenuated response to 4-aminopyridine, a blocker of Kv channels[32]. Moreover, the more depolarized EM results in a higher resting intracytoplasmic calcium concentration, which may promote vasoconstriction. This group has gone on to describe decreased SMC mRNA levels of the pore-forming Kv α 1.5 subunit, suggesting that a genetic defect in SMC Kv expression contributes to PPH in some patients[33].

In summary, several abnormalities in endothelial function, SMC function, and in the balance of circulating vasoconstrictor and vasodilator mediators clearly contribute to enhanced pulmonary vasoconstriction in PPH. Although this vasoconstriction is no longer believed to be the major factor in the pathogenesis of PAH, it clearly contributes to the elevation of P_{PA} and PVR in most patients with PAH.

Pulmonary vascular thrombosis and thrombotic arteriopathy

Introduction

Among its critical roles in the regulation of many vascular homeostatic processes, the endothelium regulates the interaction of the vascular wall with both cellular components, e.g. platelets, and soluble components, e.g. coagulation proteins, of the blood. Thus, in the presence of endothelial dysfunction, pulmonary vascular thrombosis may contribute to the pathogenesis of PVD, and especially PPH. This could be a result of either pulmonary emboli from distant sources, or active *in situ* pulmonary vascular thrombosis. Furthermore, this concept has advanced our understanding of the pathogenesis of PAH in recognizing that other factors could contribute to the increase in PVR besides just pulmonary vasoconstriction. As discussed below, collected evidence from pathological specimens, studies of blood coagulation parameters, and clinical observations on the results of systemic anticoagulation therapy in PPH strongly support a role for pulmonary vascular thrombosis in the pathogenesis and pathophysiology of PVD.

Pathological evidence

Pulmonary vascular thrombosis and thrombotic arteriopathy are among the most common pathological findings in PVD, and especially PPH[34–36]. Thrombotic lesions are most commonly recognized as non-laminar, eccentric intimal fibrotic lesions, suggesting chronic organization of a previous thrombotic event. Occasionally, complete vascular obliteration by pulmonary vascular thrombosis may be seen, with evidence of organization as well as re-

Table 17.1. Prevalence of isolated and combined thrombotic and plexogenic arteriopathy in 48 patients with PPH

	Thrombotic arteriopathy n (%)	Plexogenic arteriopathy n (%)
Only 1 type of pathological lesion present	19 (40)	20 (42)
Both types of pathological lesion present	9 (19)	
Overall prevalence	28 (58)	29 (60)

Notes:
Adapted from data[40].
Abbreviations: PPH, Primary pulmonary hypertension.

canalization of the organized thrombus. When such thrombotic lesions predominate in the pulmonary vasculature, the term thrombotic arteriopathy may be applied. Although such thrombotic lesions may be seen in the pulmonary vasculature of individuals without underlying cardiac or pulmonary disease, these lesions are much more frequent in the presence of PAH, both PPH and SPH related to CHD or chronic hypoxia[37].

In two large case series describing the pulmonary vascular pathology in patients with PPH, the prevalence of isolated thrombotic arteriopathy was between 60 and 70%, although evidence for pulmonary vascular thrombosis was also present in many patients with the more classic plexogenic pulmonary arteriopathy[38,39]. Similarly, a more recent description of pulmonary vascular histopathology in 48 patients from a PPH registry (Table 17.1) showed isolated thrombotic arteriopathy in 40%, and thrombotic lesions in other patients with plexogenic arteriopathy, yielding an overall prevalence of thrombotic lesions of 58%[40]. In this study, the presence of chronic thrombotic arteriopathy did not identify patients with regard to specific symptomatology, age, presentation, functional class or family history of PPH. However, these authors found a significant difference in the severity of PAH, which was

Table 17.2. Effect of underlying pathology of pulmonary arteriopathy on severity of pulmonary arterial hypertension and survival in patients with PPH

	Thrombotic arteriopathy ($n = 10$)	Plexogenic arteriopathy ($n = 20$)
PVR (mmHg / l / min)	29 ± 13[a]	44 ± 22
Mean Ppa (mm Hg)	61 ± 11	76 ± 22
Median survival (days)	1070[a]	297

Notes:

Adapted from data[40].

Data represents mean ± SEM.

Abbreviations: PPH, Primary pulmonary hypertension; PVR, pulmonary vascular resistance; Ppa, pulmonary artery pressure.

Significance: [a], $P < 0.05$ for thrombotic vs. plexogenic arteriopathy.

less severe in patients with thrombotic vs. plexogenic arteriopathy (Table 17.2). Moreover, these differences in severity of PAH were reflected in better survival in patients with thrombotic arteriopathy[40].

Chronic thrombotic lesions have also been described in PVD associated with exogenous toxins (e.g. aminorex) and in the setting of PAH associated with portal hypertension[41]. Given that organized thrombotic lesions are not specific for PPH, they are not thought to be an essential feature of this disease, but rather a complication related to the severity and duration of the pulmonary hypertensive vascular state. In this regard, such thrombotic lesions are quite unusual in children, but quite common in adults with PAH; in fact a significant linear correlation has been found between the prevalence of these lesions and age ($r = 0.5$, $P < 0.001$)[37]. There was also a significant correlation with the duration of clinical disease in patients; multiple linear regression analysis identified a relationship between the presence of thrombotic lesions and both age ($P = 0.002$) and duration of illness ($P = 0.007$)[37]. In grouping patients according to the decade of their death (1940s to 1980s), there were no significant differences in the prevalence of thrombotic lesions or in the apparent contribution of the thrombotic arteriopathy to the pathogenesis of PPH.

Thus, in summary, it is clear that chronic pulmonary vascular thrombosis is present in many forms of PAH including PPH.

Abnormalities of blood coagulation and fibrinolysis

Blood coagulation is a complex process characterized by an interaction of the endothelial cell with both soluble and cellular components of blood. The latter consist predominantly of soluble plasma coagulation proteins and both the intracellular components and integral membrane components of platelets. In the healthy state, a fine balance exists between the tendency to thrombosis and prevention of significant blood coagulation by both antithrombotic and fibrinolytic mechanisms. Disruption of this balance, as for example with congenital deficiencies of a single antithrombotic factor, e.g. antithrombin-3 [AT-3], may be associated with premature, recurrent and widespread vascular thrombotic events.

The critical role of the vascular endothelium in the regulation of this thrombotic–antithrombotic balance has been recognized[42]. The endothelium participates actively in the process of coagulation, as it sustains the activation of factor X, facilitates new formation of the prothrombinase complex ($X_A V_A$), releases tissue factor which is critical in the activation of the extrinsic pathway of coagulation, and produces and liberates Von Willebrand Factor (vWF), which functions as an adhesive protein in the interaction of platelets with the vessel wall, as well as a carrier for factor VIII[42,43].

Endothelial cells not only facilitate the thrombotic process, but also actively inhibit thrombosis and promote fibrinolysis. The production and release of NO and PGI_2, two potent platelet aggregation inhibitors, is an important mechanism in the prevention of thrombosis[44]. As well, the expression of thrombomodulin, a high affinity receptor for thrombin, on the surface of endothelial cells prevents the conversion of fibrinogen to fibrin[45]. Endothelial cells are a source of tissue plasminogen activator (t-PA), a key activator of plasminogen (factor XIII) in the fibrinolytic cascade[46]. Of note, endothelial cells also synthesize and release plasminogen activator inhibitor-1 (PAI-1), an inhibitor of t-PA, highlighting the role of the endothelium in regulating the balance of prothrombotic and antithrombotic mediators and cascades[47].

The recognition of the critical role of the endothelium in this balance between prothrombotic and antithrombotic tendencies suggested that endothelial dysfunction in the setting of PAH may contribute to the pathogenesis of the pulmonary hypertensive vascular disease state through abnormalities of the blood coagulation and fibrinolytic systems. Thus, active intravascular thrombosis may be present in PPH. Plasma levels of fibrinopeptide A (FP-A), a by-product and thus a marker of fibrin generation, were elevated in all 31 PPH patients in one study, and markedly so in 19/31 patients (61%)[48]. In another report of a single patient with PPH, an actual gradient of FP-A was found across the lung suggestive of pulmonary vascular-specific fibrin formation rather than a generalized vascular prothrombotic state[49]. Furthermore, in a family of patients with PPH and an abnormal hemoglobin variant, elevated fibrinopeptide levels were also found[50]. These blood abnormalities were associated with evidence of thrombotic pulmonary arteriopathy on lung histology[51].

Abnormalities of fibrinogen plasma levels and metabolism have also been described in patients with PPH. For example, a decreased half-life of plasma fibrinogen was found in patients with PPH[52]. However, fibrinogen levels were found to be higher ($P<0.01$) in patients with PPH ($n=25$) or SPH secondary to recurrent pulmonary thromboembolism ($n=11$) in contrast to both control patients ($n=28$) and patients with SPH due to CHD ($n=12$)[53]. Furthermore, basal plasma levels of t-PA antigen, t-PA activity and PAI-1 activity did not differ between control and PAH patients. However, upper extremity venous occlusion for 15 minutes, known to activate

Table 17.3. Fibrinolysis is impaired in patients with PPH and SPH as evidenced by a lack of increase in t-PA postvenous occlusion

	n	Increased t-PA postvenous occlusion n (%)
PPH	25	11 (44)[a]
Thromboembolism-related SPH	11	5 (45)[a]
Healthy controls	28	24 (86)

Notes:
Adapted from data[53].
Abbreviations: PPH, Primary pulmonary hypertension; SPH, secondary pulmonary hypertension; t-PA, tissue plasminogen activator.
Significance: [a], $P<0.05$ vs. healthy controls.

the fibrinolytic system, was associated with a blunted increase in the t-PA activity levels in patients with PPH or SPH due to thromboembolism when compared to control patients ($P<0.03$; Table 17.3). In summary, an impaired fibrinolytic response to stimulation, as well as a possible prothrombotic state due to increased fibrinogen levels was demonstrated in patients with PPH and SPH due to recurrent pulmonary thromboembolism. Similarly, abnormalities of the fibrinolytic system, e.g. increased PAI-1 levels, have been reported in the basal state in patients with PPH compared to control[48,54–56]. In one of these studies, the increased PAI-1 levels in 12 patients with PPH were associated with decreased plasma soluble thrombomodulin and a prolonged euglobulin lysis time, a global in vitro measure of fibrinolytic activity[56]. Lower fibrinolytic activity correlated with higher mean P_{PA} ($r=0.41$, $P=0.003$). In another study of 16 patients with PPH, not only was plasma PAI-1 activity elevated, but there was also a trans-pulmonary gradient with higher arterial than mixed venous levels, suggesting locally impaired fibrinolysis in the pulmonary vascular bed[55]. Finally, 10% of patients with PPH in one

Table 17.4. Abnormalities in activity and composition of vWF in patients with PPH and SPH

	n	vWF activity (%)	Proportion of low-MW vWF multimers (%)
PPH	11	231 ± 89[b,c]	60 ± 13[b]
SPH	19	122 ± 48[a]	52 ± 11[b]
Healthy control normal range		87 ± 23	35 ± 12

Notes:

Adapted from data[58].

Data represents mean ± SD.

Abbreviations: vWF, von Willebrand factor; MW, molecular weight; PPH, Primary pulmonary hypertension; SPH, secondary pulmonary hypertension.

Significance: [a], $P < 0.05$ and [b], $P < 0.001$ vs. healthy controls; [c], $P < 0.001$, PPH vs. SPH.

study had antibodies to fibrin-bound t-PA, suggesting another possible mechanism for an impaired fibrinolytic state[73].

vWF is a protein synthesized and stored in endothelial cells, megakaryocytes and platelets that is essential in the interaction of platelets with endothelial cells. Abnormalities have been described in vWF levels and activity in patients with PPH[55,57,58]. For example, measurement of vWF activity by an in vitro ristocetin cofactor activity assay revealed an elevated vWF activity relative to immunologically measured vWF antigen levels in 6/6 patients with PPH, and only mildly increased vWF activity in 2/17 patients with SPH due to CHD and 1/13 patients with CHD without PAH[57]. In another study, baseline levels of vWF activity were also found to be significantly greater in both PPH and SPH patients than in controls (Table 17.4)[58]. Moreover, PPH patients had greater levels of vWF activity than SPH patients ($P < 0.001$). Enhanced endothelial secretion of vWF can be stimulated by thrombin, fibrin, various cytokines, complement, and increased shear stress in the setting of PVD. vWF abnormalities in PPH are likely a marker of endothelial injury or dysfunction rather than platelet defects since the ristocetin cofactor activity assay is done with normal platelets from healthy blood donors.

Besides changes in activity, abnormalities in the composition of vWF have also been noted (Table 17.4). vWF normally exists as a population of multimers of a basic subunit, with an apparent molecular weight of 1×10^6–20×10^6 D. Increased proteolytic degradation of the main vWF subunit in PAH produces an abnormal vWF multimeric pattern, characterized by an increased proportion of smaller vWF multimers[57–59]. Furthermore, vWF activity levels and the proportion of smaller vWF multimers were significantly higher in PPH and SPH patients who died during the first year of follow-up than in survivors. In multivariate regression analysis, both a proportion of smaller vWF multimers ≥68% and vWF activity ≥220% were significantly associated with 1 year mortality; each had an overall predictive value of 80% and were 95% specific, although only 67% and 44% sensitive, respectively. All four patients with greater than 70% low molecular weight multimeric forms died during the first year, and all four PPH patients with vWF activity greater than 250% died during the first year. It is of note that neither vWF activity nor the proportion of low molecular weight vWF multimers correlated with P_{PA}, and neither P_{PA} or right atrial pressure were associated with survival in these patients, most of whom received Coumadin but not vasodilators[58].

Inherited thrombophilic states

Deficiencies of several classic inhibitors of coagulation, e.g. AT-3, and the presence of abnormal procoagulant factors, e.g. factor V Leiden, are well recognized risk factors for pulmonary thromboembolic disease. Overall, there is no evidence to suggest an increased tendency to PAH in these thrombophilic states, or an increased prevalence of these inherited disorders in patients with PPH[60]. For example, a study of 42 Caucasian patients with PPH found that only one patient (2.4%) was heterozygous for the single point mutation associated with factor V Leiden, similar to the normal population prevalence of 3–4%[61].

The presence of antibodies to the phospholipid component of cell membranes is thought to be a common cause of thrombophilia. This antiphospholipid antibody (aPLa) syndrome may be either primary (idiopathic), or more commonly seen in the setting of connective tissue disorders such as systemic lupus erythematosus (SLE) and is associated with an increased tendency to both arterial and venous thrombosis. PAH related to chronic, recurrent pulmonary vascular thromboembolic disease has been well described in the aPLa syndrome. However, the association between the aPLa syndrome and PAH appears uncommon. For example, 18 patients had pulmonary thromboembolic disease in a cohort of 70 patients with aPLa syndrome; only 2 patients had developed PAH, in one of whom PAH was idiopathic and resembled PPH[62]. Furthermore, these same investigators described 24 patients with PAH in a SLE Clinic, 1 of whom had idiopathic PAH associated with the aPLa syndrome[63]. Thus, in summary, although there appears to be weak association, idiopathic PAH resembling PPH is quite uncommon in the aPLa syndrome, and PAH in this setting is usually related to pulmonary thromboembolic disease.

Abnormalities of platelet function

Platelets are capable of releasing many vasoactive substances that promote smooth muscle contraction and vasoconstriction (e.g. TxA_2, serotonin), as well as mitogenic factors stimulating proliferation of smooth muscle cells, endothelial cells and fibroblasts, e.g. serotonin, PDGF, TGF-β. Thus, platelets may contribute very significantly to the remodelling of the pulmonary vasculature in PVD. In addition, increased platelet aggregation would be expected from the altered balance of vasoactive mediators in PPH, i.e. the increase in TxA_2 (pro-aggregatory) and the decrease in PGI_2 (anti-aggregatory)[8].

Experimental models have implicated platelet abnormalities in the thrombotic tendency of PAH. For example, in the commonly used monocrotaline model of PVD, vascular thrombi are often found in the pulmonary vasculature[64]; moreover, the development of monocrotaline-induced PAH in rats is attenuated by experimentally induced thrombocytopenia[65]. There are only a few clinical studies of platelet function and activation in patients with PPH. For example, as mentioned above, a case report described thrombocytosis in a single patient with PPH and evidence for increased pulmonary vascular-specific fibrin generation and platelet activation[49]. Moreover, since TxA_2 production is predominantly from platelets, the above-described increase in the urinary metabolites of TxA_2 in PPH vs. SPH and control subjects is consistent with significant platelet activation in PPH[8]. A study of patients with moderately severe SPH (mean P_{PA} 39–84 mmHg) due to various etiologies demonstrated circulating platelet aggregates by scanning electron microscopy in 7/12 patients vs. 1/6 controls[66]. In addition, platelet activation was indicated by increased plasma β-thromboglobulin levels in SPH patients vs controls ($P<0.025$).

One of the key mechanisms for platelet involvement in the pathogenesis of PVD may be the production and release of serotonin, a vasoactive substance with important effects on cell growth and proliferation. A family with a documented platelet serotonin storage disorder, resulting in high plasma serotonin levels, has been described in which one family member developed PPH more than 20 years after the identification of the platelet defect[67]. A similar inherited platelet defect associated with increased plasma serotonin levels in the Fawn-hooded rat is associated with a genetically determined, idiopathic form of PAH[68,69]. In 16 patients with PPH, marked elevations of plasma serotonin were found in contrast to normal age and sex-matched control patients (Table 17.5)[12]. Given that virtually all blood serotonin is stored in platelets, these authors then studied platelet serotonin levels, finding lower levels in PPH patients vs. controls (Table 17.5). Moreover, in vitro platelet stimulation studies demonstrated greater serotonin release by platelets from PPH

Table 17.5. Abnormalities in plasma and platelet serotonin levels in patients with PPH

	n	Plasma serotonin (nM)	Platelet serotonin $(10^{-18}\,mol\,/\,platelet)$
PPH	16	30.1 ± 9.2^{b}	1.8 ± 0.6^{a}
Healthy control normal range		0.6 ± 0.1	3.2 ± 0.2

Notes:

Adapted from data[12].

Data represents mean $\pm$ SEM.

Abbreviations: PPH, Primary pulmonary hypertension.

Significance: [a], $P<0.01$ and [b], $P<0.001$ vs. healthy controls.

patients than from control patients in response to epinephrine, ADP, and collagen ($P<0.05$ for each). Finally, 6 of 16 subjects underwent heart-lung transplantation; in these patients studied before and 350 ± 30 days after transplantation, the abnormal platelet and plasma serotonin concentrations were not significantly affected by transplantation. In summary, a platelet defect characterized by increased serotonin release, associated with low platelet serotonin levels and markedly increased plasma levels, is a consistent finding in PPH that persisted despite improved pulmonary vascular hemodynamics following heart–lung transplantation. This suggests a primary platelet defect rather than a secondary abnormality related to the abnormal pulmonary vascular hemodynamics in PPH.

Supportive evidence for coagulation factor and platelet function abnormalities in PPH also comes from studies looking at the long term response to epoprostenol. Although this agent is a potent pulmonary vasodilator, long-term benefit in severe PPH has been shown even in patients without an acute vasodilator response to epoprostenol[70,71]. For example, plasma factor VIII levels and vWF antigen levels were abnormally high in 24/26 (92%) and 18/25 (72%) adult patients with PPH, respectively[72]. Both abnormalities were significantly less frequent (29% and 16%, respectively) in 38 children with PPH. Similarly, vWF activity was abnormally high (greater

than 120% normal) in 13/25 adult patients (52%), but only 6/37 children (16%). Furthermore, ex vivo platelet aggregation studies demonstrated depressed responses in 87% of adults and 79% of children. One year of continuous intravenous epoprostenol therapy was associated with significant decreases in factor VIII levels, vWF antigens levels, and vWF activity in both adults and children. Platelet aggregation abnormalities had fully normalized in 83% of adults and 80% of children following long-term epoprostenol. Furthermore, hemodynamic improvement was associated with improved platelet function, as there were significant correlations between the decrease in P_{PA} and both the improvement in platelet aggregation ($P<0.005$) and the vWF activity: vWF antigen level ratio ($P<0.01$).

In summary, platelet abnormalities are not only associated with PVD, but may contribute to the pathogenesis of PPH. Chronic epoprostenol therapy may be associated with improvements in platelet function and severity of PVD. Whether the improvement is dependent on vasodilation remains uncertain, as there is no data available following chronic vasodilator therapy, e.g. with calcium-channel blockers (CCB).

Antibodies to fibrin-bound t-PA

In a study assessing the immunogenetic response to fibrin-bound t-PA, 9% of adults (4/45) and 10% of children (4/41) with PPH had antibodies to fibrin-bound t-PA, compared to only 2.5% (1/40) children with PAH due to congenital cardiac lesions[73]. In this small minority of patients with antibodies to fibrin-bound t-PA, there was a very high frequency (6/7, 86%, OR = 14.4, $P=0.05$) of HLA-DQ7 compared to 29% in healthy control subjects. Furthermore, PPH patients with antibodies to fibrin-bound t-PA commonly had a HLA amino acid epitope profile associated with the aPLa syndrome. In summary, HLA-DQ7 and antibodies to fibrin-bound t-PA appear to define a small subset of both children and adults with PPH with a possible pathogenetic similarity to the aPLa syndrome.

Clinical studies of anticoagulation in PPH

Two clinical studies support the hypothesis that ongoing pulmonary vascular thrombosis contributes to the pathogenesis and the progression of PVD in PPH. The first is a retrospective review of 120 patients with PPH followed for an average of 14 years between 1955 and 1977 at the Mayo Clinic[38]. In these patients, many with severe PAH (mean P_{PA} 64 mmHg), 57% had evidence for chronic organized pulmonary vascular thromboses at autopsy. Overall survival was quite poor with only 21% surviving 5 years, and in a multiple linear regression analysis, one of the strongest, positive prognostic factors was the use of systemic anticoagulation therapy ($P=0.01$). The long-term effect of anticoagulation has also been looked at in a prospective study, although a non-randomized one in which systemic anticoagulation was selectively prescribed for 35 of 64 patients with PPH in whom the perfusion lung scan revealed non-uniform pulmonary blood flow[74]. Survival was better in those treated with anticoagulation than those not receiving anticoagulants ($P=0.025$). The improvement in survival was especially apparent in patients not receiving CCB therapy over the 5-year follow-up period because of a lack of an acute CCB vasodilator response; 91, 62, and 47% survival at 1, 3, and 5 years, respectively, with anticoagulation vs. 52, 31, and 31%, respectively, without anticoagulation. Although both clinical studies of systemic anticoagulation in PPH are methodologically flawed, the apparent survival benefit has led to widespread recommendation and clinical use of anticoagulants in PPH.

In summary, several lines of evidence from many studies suggest that abnormalities of blood coagulation factors, antithrombotic factors and the fibrinolytic system contribute to a prothrombotic state in patients with PPH. Nevertheless, there is some controversy about the above described alterations of the coagulation and fibrinolytic systems given some evidence to the contrary. For example, in a methodologically well-done small study that tried to eliminate all sources of artifactual activation of platelets and coagulation proteins, no significant differences in markers of platelet activation (platelet factor 4 and β-thromboglobulin), fibrin formation (fibrinopeptide A), and fibrin dissolution (fibrinopeptide BB1–42) were found in 10 patients with PPH and 9 patients with SPH due to CHD[75]. It is clear that the evidence in favour of alterations in the coagulation and fibrinolytic systems in PPH is derived from many small, often poorly controlled, non-definitive studies. However, the weight of evidence supports an important prevalence, pathogenetic significance and biological relevance of ongoing pulmonary vascular thrombosis in PPH.

A primary underlying disorder favouring thrombosis does not appear to be present in the majority of patients with PPH. Rather, a thrombotic tendency appears to be more a consequence of PVD both in the setting of PPH as well as SPH. Whereas a thrombotic tendency may be a marker of less severe disease with a better prognosis, interruption of ongoing thrombosis with effective anticoagulant therapy appears to predict a better prognosis, especially for patients with more advanced or severe disease not responsive to vasodilators.

Pulmonary vascular remodelling

Introduction

The lack of vasodilator response in many patients with PPH suggests the presence of pulmonary vascular abnormalities other than simply increased vasomotor tone. Pathological studies have demonstrated chronic alterations in the structure and composition of the walls of the pulmonary arteries (PAs), commonly referred to as remodelling. These complex changes of SMC, EC and fibroblast phenotype and function, as well as ultrastructural and functional matrix changes determine the functional changes in pulmonary vascular tone, resistance and reactivity that characterize chronic PAH. The degree to which vasoconstriction and vascular remodelling contribute to the increase in PVR varies between disease states associated with PAH, e.g. PPH vs. SPH due to chronic hypoxia, and between individuals with the same disease state, for example, PPH.

Vessel wall structural changes

Detailed observations of pathological specimens from patients with PPH have been instrumental in demonstrating vascular wall remodelling, and in furthering our thinking of the pathogenesis of PPH. Abnormalities at all levels of the pulmonary circulation have been described, involving all layers of the blood vessel wall, and essentially all vascular cell types. These alterations include SMC hyperplasia and hypertrophy, neomuscularization of smaller PAs, concentric intimal and subintimal fibrosis and cellular proliferation, ultrastructural and functional endothelial changes, matrix and adventitial changes, as well as plexiform vascular lesions. All of these changes significantly contribute to pulmonary vascular luminal narrowing, decreased total pulmonary vascular cross-sectional surface area, and increased PVR. For example, in 19 PPH patients, the vessel wall accounted for $63.5 \pm 11.8\%$ of the cross-sectional area of resistance vessels, compared to values of 15% or less in normal subjects[76]. There are also physiological implications of these vascular wall changes, including decreased pulmonary vascular compliance and altered pulmonary vascular reactivity.

Among the local changes in the pulmonary vascular wall in patients with PPH, the important presence of inflammatory cells and cytokines has recently been recognized[77-79]. For example, moderate-to-intense perivascular mononuclear (lymphocyte and macrophage) cell infiltration was seen in 7/10 cases of PPH characterized by plexogenic lesions, with most inflammatory cells clustered around dilatatory and plexiform lesions in muscular PAs, infiltrating the adventitia and outer media[77]. Moreover, intense expression of 5-lipoxygenase (5-LO; role in production of proinflammatory leukotrienes) and 5-LO associated protein (FLAP; role in control of gene expression and cell growth) have also been described in EC of remodelled PAs and in perivascular macrophages[80]. Based on animal models of PAH, other cytokines that may play a role in pulmo-

nary vascular remodelling in human PVD include IL-1, PAF, bFGF, as well as the vasoactive mediators TxA_2, angiotensin-II (AII), endothelin, and serotonin. Indeed, elevated serum levels of the pro-inflammatory cytokines IL-1β and IL-6 have been reported in 29 patients with severe PPH[79].

Proliferation and phenotypic alterations of EC and SMC are controlled by a plethora of growth factors. There is strong evidence to suggest that increased expression and activity of several of these growth factors contribute to the vascular remodelling in PVD. For example, in the remodelled PAs of patients with PPH, there is increased protein expression of transforming growth factor (TGF)-β in medial SMCs[81], and PDGF-A (role in stimulating proliferation of fibroblasts and SMC) in perivascular macrophages[82]. Similarly, markedly increased immunoreactivity for endothelin and angiotensin converting enzyme (ACE) have been noted in the PAs of patients with PPH undergoing transplant vs healthy donor lungs; these observations are consistent with a role for both endothelin and AII in vascular remodelling of PAs[15,83]. Among the growth factors, the possible role of VEGF deserves special consideration. VEGF is highly expressed in SMC and in EC lining plexiform lesions in patients with PPH. Given its important roles in angiogenesis, enhanced endothelial permeability and monocyte adhesion to EC, VEGF may contribute to pathophysiological vascular remodelling[78]. However, there is also intriguing animal data to suggest the opposite: VEGF-induced angiogenesis and EC proliferation may actually be compensatory in PAH. For example, antibody neutralization of VEGF's effects exacerbates PAH in animal models of hypoxic and monocrotaline-induced PVD, whereas exogenous recombinant VEGF attenuates PAH[84]. Thus, EC proliferation and plexiform lesions may actually be adaptive mechanisms in response to PAH and pulmonary vascular obliteration, rather than manifestations of the PVD process[77].

Abnormalities in EC structure and function are likely central not only to initiation of PVD in some patients, e.g. PPH, but to progression of disease in the majority of patients with PAH, regardless of the

Table 17.6. Abnormalities in BAL nitrite/nitrate levels and exhaled NO in patients with PPH

	n	BAL NOx- (μM)	Exhaled NO (ppb)
PPH	8	0.7 ± 0.2^a	2.8 ± 0.9^a
Healthy controls	8	3.3 ± 1.1	8 ± 1

Notes:
Adapted from data[87].
Data represents mean $\pm$ SEM.
Abbreviations: NO, nitric oxide; BAL, bronchoalveolar lavage; PPH, Primary pulmonary hypertension; NOx-, nitrites/nitrates.
Significance: [a], $P < 0.05$ vs. healthy controls.

Table 17.7. Blunted increase in exhaled NO excretion on exercise in patients with PPH

	n	Exhaled NO excretion (nl/min)	
		Rest	Exercise
PPH	9	142 ± 84	155 ± 81^a
Healthy controls	20	117 ± 45	268 ± 85

Notes:
Adapted from data[88].
Data represents mean $\pm$ SEM.
Abbreviations: NO, nitric oxide; PPH, Primary pulmonary hypertension.
Significance: [a], $P < 0.001$ vs. healthy controls.

underlying disease state, e.g. PPH or SPH. The normal role of the endothelium in maintaining a low resistance pulmonary circulation and an antithrombotic state has been discussed above. However, possibly even more important are the endothelium's anti-mitogenic effects on vascular wall SMCs and fibroblasts, normally inhibiting excessive growth, differentiation and metabolic activity of these cells. As such, endothelial dysfunction is likely necessary for the pulmonary vascular wall remodelling that contributes to the pathogenesis of PVD. The endothelium contributes to pulmonary vascular homeostasis through several mechanisms. One of the most important is the release of NO. As reviewed above, NO has many roles in vascular homeostasis, including pulmonary vasodilatation, and inhibition of platelet aggregation and thrombosis. NO also has a potent antimitotic effect on SMC and fibroblasts in vitro[85].

A deficiency of endogenous NO has been proposed to contribute to the pathophysiology of PAH[86]. Although this is an attractive hypothesis, given the many pulmonary vascular homeostatic effects of NO described above, it remains controversial. Several lines of evidence support a deficiency of NO. For example, decreased exhaled NO levels and BAL levels of the oxidative metabolites of NO ($NO_x^- = NO_2^- + NO_3^-$) were found at bronchoscopy in PPH patients vs controls (Table 17.6)[87]. Moreover, BAL

NOx- levels were inversely correlated with mean PAP ($r = -0.776$, $P = 0.047$). In another study, 9 patients with PPH had a blunted exercise-induced increase in exhaled NO excretion, despite similar levels at rest as 20 control subjects (Table 17.7)[88]. Similarly, stimulated NO release was attenuated in isolated perfused lungs from PPH patients in contrast to unused normal transplant donor lungs[89].

As reviewed above, an intriguing study has suggested decreased endothelial expression of eNOS in the elastic and muscular PAs of PPH patients[23]. Furthermore, these authors found an inverse correlation between histological grade and immunohistochemical staining intensity ($r = -0.787$, $P < 0.001$). However, this has been challenged, as increased eNOS expression has also been reported in PA lesions in patients with PPH[24,25]. Unfortunately, equally conflicting data on NOS expression has been reported in animal models of PAH; whether cNOS expression is increased, decreased or unchanged depends on the model, e.g. hypoxia vs. monocrotaline, the animal species studied, and the time point at which NOS expression is assessed after injury[90–93]. Finally, recent work with eNOS genetic knockout (-/-) mice showed pulmonary vascular hyperresponsiveness to mild hypoxia, suggesting a compensatory role for eNOS in at least chronic hypoxic PAH, and a contributory role of NO deficiency in this model[94]. It is our opinion that there is strong evidence for an inadequate biological activity of endothelial-derived NO, in the setting of a pulmonary vascular hypertensive state, regardless of possible changes in actual endothelial NOS expression.

In summary, it is possible that vascular wall inflammation, cellular necrosis, and locally produced cytokines and growth factors contribute to the above-described structural changes, although it remains uncertain whether vessel wall inflammation is a cause, or simply a result of PVD. It is intriguing that anti-inflammatory therapy may have a role in PVD. In this regard, a single case report describes a young woman with pathological PPH and a 5-year history of constitutional features and non-specific laboratory evidence of an inflammatory process, e.g. elevated ESR, fibrinogen, and AT-3 as well as hyper-gammaglobulinemia; although she did not have an acute vasodilator response, significant hemodynamic improvement was seen after treatment with low-dose methotrexate and prednisone for 1 year, without anticoagulants or vasodilators[95].

Smooth muscle changes

As discussed above, abnormal pulmonary vascular SMC function may contribute to the enhanced vasoconstrictor state typical of PAH. Furthermore, chronic histological and functional changes in these SMCs are an important part of pulmonary vascular remodelling in PAH[96]. Abnormalities in SMC growth include hyperplasia and hypertrophy in large PAs, as well as neomuscularization of normally poorly or non-muscularized pulmonary blood vessels. Pulmonary vascular SMC hyperplasia and hypertrophy are the most common histological findings in patients with PAH[97]. SMC hyperplasia/hypertrophy is the only pathological finding in many patients dying with PPH, especially in children and younger adults[36]. Neomuscularization is characterized by the differentiation of SMC precursors into mature SMC, and their migration into normally poorly muscularized small PAs and non-muscular alveolar and pre-capillary vessels[97].

SMC growth and proliferation are controlled by a complex network of many physical, chemical and immune factors, both stimulatory and inhibitory. SMC proliferation, hypertrophy and increased matrix protein synthesis in the setting of PVD likely occur in response to local and systemic mitogens, local hypoxia, and mechanical stress. The various stimuli likely act through a variety of intracellular signalling pathways, including tyrosine kinases, calcium fluxes and protein kinases. Increased SMC responsiveness to such stimuli and such signalling mechanisms is likely in the presence of extracellular matrix degradation and disturbed homeostatic anti-proliferative mechanisms such as endothelial-derived NO and prostacyclin. Finally, SMC responses likely depend upon regional phenotypic heterogeneity as well as intrinsic, e.g. genetic or acquired, SMC differences in the capacity to respond[96].

Histological changes occur in isolated SMC in vitro, and thus presumably in pulmonary vascular SMC in vivo, in response to various cell mitogens, e.g. PDGF-A and -B. Intensive research is identifying a role for an increasing number of such substances, including ET-1, TxA_2, and serotonin. For example, increased levels of polyamines, known to have a major regulatory role in cell growth and differentiation, have been found in chronically hypoxic lungs[98]. It has also been suggested that this enhanced growth, proliferation, and maturation of SMC may be related, in part, to chronic, active SMC contraction and resulting vasoconstriction. For example, in chronic hypoxic models of PAH, SMC hyperplasia/hypertrophy can be significantly attenuated by prolonged vasodilator therapy with CCB. However, it is clear that increased intracellular calcium may also directly stimulate SMC growth and maturation, independent of SMC contraction[96].

A decline in the presence of anti-proliferative factors is at least as important as an increased presence of the above mitogenic substances. Thus, endothelial dysfunction with decreased elaboration of NO and PGI_2, two well-recognized, potent, endogenous antimitotic factors, likely contributes to a local environment favouring SMC and fibroblast growth, proliferation and differentiation, leading to vascular wall remodelling[8]. In summary, SMC alterations contribute importantly to the pathogenesis of PVD, both through chronic changes in the composition and function of the vascular wall, as well as alterations in pulmonary vascular physiology.

Endothelial cell alterations

As is apparent from our discussion, the EC plays a critical, central role in normal pulmonary vascular function, and an equally important role in the physiological and structural alterations that contribute to the pathophysiology of PVD. This hypothesis is strongly supported by observations of altered levels and expression of mediators derived from the endothelium, as well as pathological descriptions of EC changes, both with regard to ultrastructural appearance and metabolic function[8].

As described above in the relevant sections, normal endothelial function is essential to the maintenance of a low-resistance, vasodilated pulmonary circulation, to an anti-thrombotic nature of the interaction of blood components with the vessel wall, and to an anti-proliferative state of the cellular components of the vessel wall. Disturbances in EC function have been hypothesized based on observed abnormalities in each of these systems in the pulmonary vascular bed in the setting of PVD, e.g. a vasoconstricted, prothrombotic state with evidence for disturbed SMC and fibroblast growth and maturation.

There exists great controversy surrounding the nature of the endothelial defect in PVD. EC dysfunction occurs in response to physical factors, e.g. stretch, biochemical factors, e.g. drugs such as anorectic agents), and immune factors, e.g. infection with the human immunodeficiency virus (HIV)[96]. Moreover, regardless of the underlying etiology of PVD, ongoing EC damage is a result of the disturbed pulmonary vascular hemodynamics, e.g. increased P_{PA}, enhanced EC-platelet interaction, and local, in situ thrombus formation. In this 'vicious cycle' of PVD, EC damage then itself contributes to progression of the individual mechanistic features of PVD, including abnormal pulmonary vasoconstriction, thrombosis and vascular wall remodelling.

Alternatively, an intriguing hypothesis proposes that EC dysfunction is a primary, basic abnormality in at least some types of PVD, for example, PPH. Thus, a congenital (inherited or prenatal) defect of EC function may be a latent predisposition to PVD, manifesting clinically either spontaneously as PPH or as SPH following a postnatal insult. For example, although an increased risk of PAH is well accepted after exposure of humans to anorexigenic medication (e.g. dexfenfluramine), the overall risk is at most 1 in 10000 exposed individuals, suggesting some underlying predisposition that is unmasked by the exposure[99,100]. The nature of this putative basic EC defect remains undefined, although active investigation is pursuing a genetic etiology (see below).

An alternative hypothesis comes from a developing understanding of the pathogenesis of a classic pathological pulmonary vascular lesion in patients with PPH, the plexiform lesion. Plexiform lesions are aneurysmal dilatations in the walls of predominantly muscular PAs, often at branch points, that histologically consist of loose connective tissue and a network of multiple, irregular, small, thin-walled blood vessels formed by EC proliferation[77]. Although initially described in PPH, they are recognized in many other settings, including SPH associated with connective tissue disorders, HIV infection, and cyanotic CHD. Exciting recent work into the genetic character of the ECs lining the multiple channels of a plexiform lesion has indicated a monoclonal, e.g. tumour-like, single cell origin, proliferation of EC[101]. A similar monoclonality has been reported in plexiform lesions in patients with anorexigen-associated PAH[78]. Thus, a somatic genetic defect in a growth-regulatory gene element may underlie EC proliferation and dysfunction in a subset of patients with PVD.

In summary, although basic, primary defects in EC function remain under intense investigation, it is clear that EC dysfunction, regardless of etiology, contributes to the pathophysiology of PVD.

Matrix and adventitial changes

Although pulmonary vascular remodelling is largely characterized by cellular changes, alterations in the composition of the extracellular matrix of the pulmonary vascular wall have also been proposed[102,103]. For example, histological studies reveal eccentric intimal fibrotic lesions, as well as a lamellar pattern of reduplication of elastic laminae and medial fibrosis[40,97]. Thus, pulmonary vascular wall fibrosis and changes in elastin and collagen content appear to contribute to the pathophysiology of PVD, including disturbed pulmonary vascular hemodynamics[104]. Furthermore, activation of matrix degrading enzymes, e.g. elastase, matrix metalloproteinases, can release mitogenically active growth factors, which can then influence SMC and EC proliferation.

Many factors appear to contribute to vascular wall extracellular matrix changes. Based on much work in animal models of PAH, these factors include physical, biochemical, immunological and inflammatory influences. With regard to physical factors, it is widely held that the presence of abnormal pulmonary vascular hemodynamics in PAH itself contributes to ongoing vascular remodelling and to the propagation of PAH[105]. Both static transmural mechanical stress related to increased P_{PA}, as well as dynamic shear stress related to disturbed pulmonary vascular flow profiles probably contribute importantly to matrix changes and vascular wall remodelling. For example, it has been demonstrated that acute cyclic stretch of PAs produced increased collagen and elastin synthesis[106]. Furthermore, in monocrotaline-exposed rats, pulmonary vascular neointimal remodelling and PAH is limited unless blood flow is also increased, either with contralateral pneumonectomy or with subclavian-PA anastomosis[28,105]. The vascular SMC and EC likely play central roles in responding to, and modulating, these various influences on the local matrix composition and function[102,106].

Although there is a paucity of human data on the direct hemodynamic effects of extracellular matrix changes, there is evidence of an important func-

tional correlate of this remodelling in animal models of PAH. For example, treatment with the antifibrotic agent, β-aminopropionitrile, is associated with less structural changes, lower vascular wall matrix collagen and elastin content, and attenuated pulmonary vascular hemodynamic abnormalities following chronic hypoxia in rats[107]. Similar results have been reported with cis-hydroxyproline, an inhibitor of collagen synthesis[108].

In summary, pulmonary abnormalities other than simply increased vasomotor tone contribute significantly to pulmonary hypertension. Chronic remodelling of both cellular and matrix components of the intima, media, and adventitia contribute to pulmonary vascular luminal narrowing and also determine the functional changes in pulmonary vascular tone and reactivity. The pathogenesis of these changes include roles for inflammatory cells and cytokines, matrix breakdown, growth factors such as VEGF, endothelial dysfunction and monoclonal proliferation, as well as smooth muscle cell growth and proliferation.

Genetic contributions to pulmonary vascular disease

Introduction

Based on active research over the past 20 years, it is likely that there is a significant genetic component to the pathogenesis of PAH in general, and specifically to PPH. Initial support for an underlying genetic predisposition came from the earliest clinical observations of PPH: (i) the absence of any inciting event or toxic exposure in the majority of patients, (ii) the not infrequent onset of disease in childhood and young adulthood, and (iii) the identification of an increased familial risk of PPH, although this was true only in a minority of patients.

Given the heterogeneity of clinical disease in patients with PAH and PPH, it is unlikely that a single genetic abnormality is the basis of disease in the majority of patients. Hence, such disorders are probably polygenic. Several basic pathophysiological defects have been identified in PPH, providing clues to candidate genes and genetic defects. These include abnormal platelet function, e.g. a disorder of excessive serotonin release, abnormalities of SMC K_V channel function, and immunogenetic abnormalities related to aPLa, as described above.

Familial tendency of PPH

Although PPH is most frequently a sporadic, non-familial disease, an increased risk in the twin siblings of patients with PPH, as well as in other family members, has been recognized for over 30 years[109,110]. Although only 5 to 10% of all cases of PPH are thought to be familial, an intriguing report has suggested that this might be an underestimate because of an overlooked possibility of coancestry. The family histories of 13 patients with apparently sporadic PPH were extensively reviewed, leading to the identification of coancestry in the families of two of these patients ($P = 0.004$)[111].

It has been suggested that the clinical features and mortality of familial PPH do not differ from sporadic cases of PPH[112,113]. A wide range of survival in familial cases has been observed, from sudden death at presentation to death 27 years after presentation. However, the overall distribution of survival after symptom onset was found to be virtually identical to that previously reported for non-familial disease[112].

The genetics of familial PPH remain controversial, although features have been established. Although some investigators have previously suggested X-linked genetic transmission, two well reported instances exclude this possibility; these include a case of father-to-son transmission, as well as transmission from a grandfather to a granddaughter through an unaffected father[112]. As well, the involvement of most or all members of a sibship in several reported families has suggested that the gene may be autosomally dominant. However, there is highly variable penetrance in different families, explaining in part one of the features of familial PPH, that is the infrequent expression of the gene in some families[112,113]. For example, in some families there are large numbers of healthy relatives in each generation of affected siblings, and there are families in which the gene appears to have been asymptomatically transmitted over at least two generations before being re-expressed as disease.

One of the most striking genetic aspects of PPH appears to be a gender bias. The female to male predominance of disease has been reported between 2:1 and 10:1 in non-familial disease, and from 2:1 to 2.7:1 in familial disease[112,113]. There is a very significant, skewed gender ratio at birth in the offspring of individuals known to have the gene; 160/282 children were female (57%, $P < 0.01$) and 122 (43%) were male[113]. Furthermore, out of 124 patients with the gene for PPH, 72 of 84 females (86%) developed PPH, whereas only 27 of 40 males (68%) developed PPH. Through an intriguing set of calculations, these authors suggested that the female-predominant gender distribution of PPH may be due to selective loss in utero of male embryos affected by PPH.

The observation has been repeatedly made that PPH appears to manifest itself at an earlier age and more severely in subsequent generations. This is the phenomenon of genetic anticipation. For example, in a thorough characterization of the genetic and familial aspects of PPH in 124 individuals from 24 families, genetic anticipation was confirmed as the age of death significantly decreased through three successive generations from 46 ± 15 to 36 ± 13 to 24 ± 11 years of age[113]. The phenomenon of genetic anticipation supports a genetic contribution to familial PPH, and further, suggests a possible molecular basis for the genetic mutation. Genetic anticipation in the neurological conditions of the fragile X syndrome and myotonic dystrophy is thought to be due to the presence of increased numbers of short tandem repeat (STR) sequences of 3 nucleotides. STRs are associated with misaligned hybridization during meiosis, leading to STR expansion in subsequent generations. A greater number of STR sequences in sequential generations is associated with a greater risk of impaired gene expression or unstable transcripts or peptide products. It remains unconfirmed whether STRs are the genetic basis of familial PPH.

Disease associations of PPH

Besides an increased risk of PPH in the family members of affected individuals, associations between PPH in families and various abnormal hemoglobin variants have been described. For example, PAH and a low oxygen affinity β-chain variant hemoglobin, Hb Warsaw, appeared to cosegregate in a family[50]. Furthermore, two asymptomatic family members with Hb Warsaw had evidence for early PVD including slightly raised P_{PA} in 1 individual, and an abnormal ventilation–perfusion scan in another individual. A second family study described a new, low oxygen affinity β-chain variant hemoglobin, Hb Washtenaw. In this family, the index case had severe PPH and the abnormal hemoglobin, and two siblings with the abnormal hemoglobin were found to have elevated P_{PA} on exercise echocardiography suggestive of early PPH[114]. Both of these reports have suggested that one of the putative genes for familial PPH may be located near the β-globin gene on chromosome 11.

One of the most striking clinical observations in patients with PPH has been an association with autoimmune diseases such as the connective tissue diseases, e.g. progressive systemic sclerosis, antiphospholipid antibody syndrome, and autoimmune thyroiditis[115–117]. Even in the absence of an associated autoimmune disease, patients with PPH often express autoantibodies typical of the connective tissue disorders, including antinuclear antibodies (ANA), and rheumatoid factor (RF)[115]. Furthermore, an association between PPH and specific immunogenetic markers on leukocytes, the human leukocyte antigens (HLA) has been reported. For example, in a detailed immunogenetic study of 3 families with familial PPH, 8/15 members carrying the PPH gene expressed HLA-DRw52 and 7/15 expressed HLA-DR3,DRw52,DQw2[118]. Although immunoglobulin isotype deficiencies were seen including IgA deficiency and mild IgD deficiency, they were unusual, being present in only one member of each family who was DR3 positive. A fourth family was distinguished by the presence of both PPH and PAH associated with CHD, as well as the presence of varying autoantibodies and different HLA associations as compared to the first three families. Thus, two clinical subsets of familial PPH can be distinguished by the presence or absence of autoantibodies, the association with autoimmune disorders, and different HLA markers. As above, this suggests that a single genetic defect is not the basis for familial PPH. It is possible that at least one gene underlying familial PPH may be found near the HLA locus on chromosome 6.

Genetic studies

The above clues have suggested a genetic basis for the disease in at least some patients with PPH. Two recent studies have used the powerful genetic tool of linkage analysis to statistically identify the region of the chromosome where the familial PPH gene locus (*PPH1*) likely resides[119,120]. One of these studies used microsatellite markers in a large family with PPH to identify a candidate region, and confirmed the identified chromosome region in a second, ethnically distinct family[121]. In calculating a lod (logarithm of the odds ratio of likelihood of a gene being in a particular region of the chromosome) score, these authors were able to exclude the hemoglobin β-chain region on chromosome 11 as well as the HLA region on chromosome 6 as potential sites of *PPH1*. The final analysis with more closely spaced markers localized *PPH1* to a 27-cM region on chromosome 2q31–q32, with a maximal lod score of 3.87, indicating $>$1000 to 1 odds in favour of linkage in this region. The other study of 6 ethnically homogeneous families confirmed linkage of familial PPH to 2q with a maximum lod score of 7.86[120]. Furthermore, these authors suggested that a single, major gene might account for all cases of familial PPH in Caucasian patients of Western European or North American descent.

Very recently, the gene that is associated with familial PPH at this locus on chromosome 2 has been identified as coding for the bone morphogenetic protein receptor II (BMPR2)[122]. This is a member of the family of TGF-β type II receptors, many of which have important roles in inhibiting cell proliferation and differentiation[81]. The five missense and termination mutations in BMPR2 result in EC proliferating uncontrollably following injury. This exciting work holds promise for relating the genetic defect to the actual pathogenesis and pathophysiology of PVD.

In summary, the above described important clinical observations and investigations, the familial tendency of PPH and association of PPH with abnormal hemoglobin variants and autoimmune phenomena have all suggested a possible genetic basis to PPH in at least some patients. Extensive studies of multiple families have confirmed an autosomally dominant genetic disease with variable, but often high penetrance in various families, with a striking female predilection based on what may be a greater loss of affected males in utero.

Detailed linkage analysis of the entire chromosome, and subsequent molecular cloning have now identified a single gene defect in *BMPR2* that is associated with familial PPH. Whether this tremendous advance will help us in understanding the pathophysiology of PVD, and more importantly either preventing disease expression or perhaps treating PVD more effectively and at an earlier stage remains to be seen.

Conclusion

PVD has evolved from a clinical–physiological syndrome into a condition characterized by newly-identified genetic mutations, multiple disease associations, and a complex pathogenesis including pulmonary vascular constriction, thrombosis, remodelling and inflammation. Ongoing exciting research and our developing understanding of this complex pathogenesis and pathophysiology of PVD hold great promise not only for better understanding the biology of the pulmonary circulation, but also for intervening to lessen the morbidity and mortality of such conditions as PPH.

REFERENCES

1   Reeves JT, Groves BM, Turkevich D. The case for treatment of selected patients with primary pulmonary hypertension. *Am Rev Resp Dis* 1986; 134(2):342–346.

2   Dresdale DT, Schultz M, Michton RJ. Primary pulmonary hypertension. *Am J Med* 1951; 11:686–705.

3   Wood P. Pulmonary hypertension with special reference to the vasoconstrictive factor. *Br Heart J* 1958; 20: 557–570.

4   Wagenvoort CA. The pathology of primary pulmonary hypertension. *J Pathol* 1970; 101(4):i.

5   Rosenberg HC, Rabinovitch M. Endothelial injury and vascular reactivity in monocrotaline pulmonary hypertension. *Am J Physiol* 1988; 255(6 Pt 2):H1484–H1491.

6   Rich S, Dantzker DR, Ayres SM et al. Primary pulmonary hypertension: a national prospective study. *Ann Intern Med* 1987; 107:216–223.

7   Badesch DB, Orton EC, Zapp LM et al. Decreased arterial wall prostaglandin production in neonatal calves with severe chronic pulmonary hypertension. *Am J Respir Cell Mol Biol* 1989; 1(6):489–498.

8   Christman BW, McPherson CD, Newman JH et al. An imbalance between the excretion of thromboxane and prostacyclin metabolites in pulmonary hypertension. *N Engl J Med* 1992; 327:70–75.

9   Rabinovitch M, Mullen M, Rosenberg HC, Maruyama K, O'Brodovich H, Olley PM. Angiotensin II prevents hypoxic pulmonary hypertension and vascular changes in rat. *Am J Physiol* 1988; 254(3 Pt 2):H500–H508.

10 Geraci MW, Gao BF, Shepherd DC et al. Pulmonary prostacyclin synthase overexpression in transgenic mice protects against development of hypoxic pulmonary hypertension. *J Clin Invest* 1999; 103(11):1509–1515.

11 al-Tinawi A, Krenz GS, Rickaby DA, Linehan JH, Dawson CA. Influence of hypoxia and serotonin on small pulmonary vessels. *J Appl Physiol* 1994; 76(1):56–64.

12 Herve P, Launay JM, Scrobohaci ML et al. Increased plasma serotonin in primary pulmonary hypertension. *Am J Med* 1995; 99(3):249–254.

13 Miyauchi T, Yorikane R, Sakai S. et al. Contribution of endogenous endothelin-1 to the progression of cardiopulmonary alterations in rats with monocrotaline-induced pulmonary hypertension. *Circ Res* 1993; 73(5):887–897.

14 Stewart DJ, Levy RD, Cernacek P, Langleben D. Increased plasma endothelin-1 in pulmonary hypertension: marker or mediator of disease? *Ann Intern Med* 1991; 114:464–469.

15 Giaid A, Yanagisawa M, Langleben D et al. Expression of endothelin-1 in the lungs of patients with pulmonary hypertension. *N Engl J Med* 1993; 328:1732–1739.

16 Wong J, Reddy VM, Hendricks-Munoz K, Liddicoat JR, Gerrets R, Fineman JR. Endothelin-1 vasoactive responses in lambs with pulmonary hypertension and increased pulmonary blood flow. *Am J Physiol* 1995; 269(6 Pt 2):H1965-H1972.

17 Sakai S, Miyauchi T, Sakurai T et al. Pulmonary hypertension caused by congestive heart failure is ameliorated by long-term application of an endothelin receptor antagonist. Increased expression of endothelin-1 messenger ribonucleic acid and endothelin-1-like immunoreactivity in the lung in congestive heart failure in rats. *J Am Coll Cardiol* 1996; 28(6):1580–1588.

18 Blitzer ML, Loh E, Roddy MA, Stamler JS, Creager MA. Endothelium-derived nitric oxide regulates systemic and pulmonary vascular resistance during acute hypoxia in humans. *J Am Coll Cardiol* 1996; 28:591–596.

19 Steudel W, Ichinose F, Huang PL et al. Pulmonary vasoconstriction and hypertension in mice with targeted disruption of the endothelial nitric oxide synthase (nos 3) gene. *Circ Res* 1997; 81(1):34–41.

20 Black SM, Fineman JR, Steinhorn RH, Bristow J, Soifer SJ. Increased endothelial NOS in lambs with increased pulmonary blood flow and pulmonary hypertension. *Am J Physiol* 1998; 275(5 Pt 2):H1643–H1651.

21 Le Cras TD, Xue C, Rengasamy A, and Johns RA. Chronic hypoxia upregulates endothelial and inducible NO synthase gene and protein expression in rat lung. *Am J Physiol* 1996; 270(1 Pt 1): L164-L170.

22 Villamor E, Le Cras TD, Horan MP, Halbower AC, Tuder RM, Abman SH. Chronic intrauterine pulmonary hypertension impairs endothelial nitric oxide synthase in the ovine fetus. *Am J Physiol* 1997; 272(5 Pt 1):L1013–L1020.

23 Giaid A, Saleh D. Reduced expression of endothelial nitric oxide synthase in the lungs of patients with pulmonary hypertension. *N Engl J Med* 1995; 333:214–221.

24 Xue C, Johns RA. Endothelial nitric oxide synthase in the lungs of patients with pulmonary hypertension. *N Engl J Med* 1995; 333:1642–44.

25 Mason NA, Springall DR, Burke M et al. High expression of endothelial nitric oxide synthase in plexiform lesions of pulmonary hypertension. *J Pathol* 1998; 185(3):313–318.

26 Conraads VM, Bosmans JM, Claeys MJ et al. Paradoxic pulmonary vasoconstriction in response to acetylcholine in patients with primary pulmonary hypertension. *Chest* 1994; 106(2):385–390.

27 Brett SJ, Gibbs JSR, Pepper JR, Evans TW. Impairment of endothelium-dependent pulmonary vasodilation in patients with primary pulmonary hypertension. *Thorax* 1996; 51:89–91.

28 Okada K, Tanaka Y, Bernstein M, Zhang W, Patterson GA, Botney MD. Pulmonary hemodynamics modify the rat pulmonary artery response to injury – a neointimal model of pulmonary hypertension. *Am J Pathol* 1997; 151(4):1019–1025.

29 Sartori C, Allemann Y, Trueb L, Delabays A, Nicod P, Scherrer U. Augmented vasoreactivity in adult life associated with perinatal vascular insult. *Lancet* 1999; 353(9171):2205–2207.

30 Weir EK, Archer SL: The mechanism of acute hypoxic pulmonary vasoconstriction: the tale of two channels. *FASEB J* 1995; 9(2):183–189.

31 Weir EK, Reeve HL, Huang JM et al. Anorexic agents aminorex, fenfluramine, and dexfenfluramine inhibit potassium current in rat pulmonary vascular smooth muscle and cause pulmonary vasoconstriction. *Circulation* 1996; 94(9):2216–2220.

32 Yuan JX, Aldinger AM, Juhaszova M et al. Dysfunctional voltage-gated K^+ channels in pulmonary artery smooth muscle cells of patients with primary pulmonary hypertension. *Circulation* 1998; 98(14):1400–1406.

33 Yuan XJ, Wang J, Juhaszova M, Gaine SP, Rubin LJ. Attenuated $K+$ channel gene transcription in primary pulmonary hypertension. *Lancet* 1998; 351(9104):726–727.

34 Wagenvoort CA. Lung biopsy specimens in the evaluation of pulmonary vascular disease. *Chest* 1980; 77(5):614–625.

35 Harris P, Heath D. *The Human Pulmonary Circulation*. 1986.

36 Wagenvoort CA, Wagenvoort N. Primary pulmonary hypertension: a pathologic study of the lung vessels in 156 clinically diagnosed cases. *Circulation* 1970; 72:1163–84.

37 Wagenvoort CA, Mulder PG. Thrombotic lesions in primary plexogenic arteriopathy. Similar pathogenesis or complication? *Chest* 1993; 103(3):844–849.

38 Fuster V, Steele PM, Edwards WD, Gersh BJ, McGoon MD, Frye RL. Primary pulmonary hypertension: natural history and the importance of thrombosis. *Circulation* 1984; 70(4):580–587.

39 Bjornsson J, Edwards WD. Primary pulmonary hypertension: A histopathologic study of 80 cases. *Mayo Clin Proc* 1985; 60:16–25.

40 Pietra GG, Edwards WD, Kay JM et al. Histopathology of primary pulmonary hypertension. A qualitative and quantitative study of pulmonary blood vessels from 58 patients in the National Heart, Lung, and Blood Institute, Primary Pulmonary Hypertension Registry. *Circulation* 1989; 80(5):1198–1206.

41 Edwards BS, Weir EK, Edwards WD, Ludwig J, Dykoski RK, Edwards JE. Coexistent pulmonary and portal hyperten-

sion: morphologic and clinical features. *J Am Coll Cardiol* 1987; 10(6):1233–1238.

42 Rodgers GM, Greenberg CS, Shuman MA. Characterization of the effects of cultured vascular cells on the activation of blood coagulation. *Blood* 1983; 61:1155–1162.

43 Stern DM, Nawroth PP, Kisiel W, Vehar G, Esmon CT. The binding of factor IXa to cultured bovine aortic endothelial cells: induction of a specific site in the presence of factors VIII and X. *J Biol Chem* 1985; 260: 6717–6722.

44 Moncada S, Palmer RM, Higgs EA. Nitric oxide: physiology, pathophysiology, and pharmacology. *Pharmacol Rev* 1991; 43:109–142.

45 Esmon CT. The regulation of natural anticoagulant pathways. *Science* 1987; 235:1348–1352.

46 Loskutoff DJ, Edgington TE. Synthesis of a fibrinolytic activator and inhibitor by endothelial cells. *Proc Natl Acad Sci USA* 1977; 74(9):3903–3907.

47 Sakata Y, Okado M, Noro A, Matsuda M. Interaction of tissue-type plasminogen activator and plasminogen activator inhibitor-1 on the surface of endothelial cells. *J Biol Chem* 1988; 263:1960–1969.

48 Eisenberg PR, Lucore C, Kaufman L, Sobel BE, Jaffe AS, Rich S. Fibrinopeptide A levels indicative of pulmonary vascular thrombosis in patients with primary pulmonary hypertension. *Circulation* 1990; 82(3):841–847.

49 Rostagno C, Prisco D, Abbate R, Poggesi L. Pulmonary hypertension associated with long-standing thrombocytosis. *Chest* 1991; 99(5):1303–1305.

50 Rich S., Hart K. Familial pulmonary hypertension in association with an abnormal hemoglobin: insights into the pathogenesis of primary pulmonary hypertension. *Chest* 1991; 99:1208–1210.

51 Rich S, Pietra GG, Kieras K, Hart K, Brundage BH. Primary pulmonary hypertension: radiographic and scintigraphic patterns of histologic subtypes. *Ann Intern Med* 1986; 105:499–502.

52 Langleben D, Moroz LA, McGregor M, Lisbona R. Decreased half-life of fibrinogen in primary pulmonary hypertension. *Thrombos Res* 1985; 40(4):577–580.

53 Huber K, Beckmann R, Frank H, Kneussl M, Mlczoch J, Binder BR. Fibrinogen, t-PA, and PAI-1 plasma levels in patients with pulmonary hypertension. *Am J Resp Crit Care Med* 1994; 150(4):929–933.

54 Boyer-Neumann C, Brenot F, Wolf M et al. Continuous infusion of prostacyclin decreases plasma levels of t-PA and PAI-1 in primary pulmonary hypertension. *Thrombos Haemosta* 1995; 73(4):735–736.

55 Hoeper MM, Sosada M, Fabel H. Plasma coagulation profiles in patients with severe primary pulmonary hypertension. *Eur Resp J* 1998; 12:1446–1449.

56 Welsh CH, Hassell KL, Badesch DB, Kressin DC, Marlar RA. Coagulation and fibrinolytic profiles in patients with severe pulmonary hypertension. *Chest* 1996; 110(3):710–717.

57 Geggel RL, Carvalho AC, Hoyer LW, Reid LM. von Willebrand factor abnormalities in primary pulmonary hypertension. *Am Rev Resp Dis* 1987; 135(2):294–299.

58 Lopes AA, Maeda NY, Bydlowski SP. Abnormalities in circulating von Willebrand factor and survival in pulmonary hypertension. *Am J Med* 1998; 105(1):21–26.

59 Lopes AA, Maeda NY. Abnormal degradation of von Willebrand factor main subunit in pulmonary hypertension. *Eur Resp J* 1995; 8(4):530–536.

60 Chaouat A, Weitzenblum E, Higenbortam TW. The role of thrombosis in severe pulmonary hypertension. *Eur Resp J* 1996; 9:356–63.

61 Elliott CG, Leppert MF, Alexander GJ, Ward K, Nelson L, Pietra GG. Factor V Leiden is not common in patients diagnosed with primary pulmonary hypertension. *Eur Resp J* 1998; 12(5):1177–1180.

62 Asherson RA, Khamashta MA, Ordi-Ros J et al. The 'primary' antiphospholipid syndrome: major clinical and serological features. *Medicine* 1989; 68:366–74.

63 Asherson RA, Higenbottam TW, Dinh-Xuan AT, Khamashta MA, Hughes GR. Pulmonary hypertension in a lupus clinic: experience with twenty-four patients. *J Rheumatol* 1990; 17:1292–8.

64 Merkow L, Kleinerman J. An electron microscopic study of pulmonary vasculitis induced by monocrotaline. *Laboratory Investigation* 1966; 15:547–564.

65 Kanai Y, Hori S, Tanaka T et al. Role of 5-hydroxytriptamine in the progression of monocrotaline-induced pulmonary hypertension in rats. *Cardiovasc Res* 1993; 27:1619–1623.

66 Lopes AA, Maeda NY, Almeida A, Jaeger R, Ebaid M, Chamone DF. Abnormalities in circulating von Willebrand factor and survival in pulmonary hypertension. *Angiology* 1993;701–706.

67 Herve P, Drouet L, Dosquet C et al. Primary pulmonary hypertension in a patient with a familial platelet storage pool disease: role of serotonin. *Am J Med* 1990; 89:117–120.

68 Kentera D, Susic D, Veljkovic V, Tucakovic G, Koko V. Pulmonary artery pressure in rats with hereditary platelet function defect. *Respiration* 1988; 54(2):110–114.

69 Sato K, Webb S, Tucker A et al. Factors influencing the idiopathic development of pulmonary hypertension in the fawn hooded rat. *Am Rev Resp Dis* 1992; 145(4 Pt 1):793–797.

70 Barst RJ, Rubin LJ, McGoon MD, Caldwell EJ, Long WA, Levy PS. Survival in primary pulmonary hypertension with long-term continuous intravenous prostacyclin. *Ann Intern Med* 1994; 121(6):409–415.

71 Barst RJ, Rubin LJ, Long WA et al. A comparison of continuous intravenous epoprostenol (prostacyclin) with conventional therapy for primary pulmonary hypertension. The Primary Pulmonary Hypertension Study Group. *N Engl J Med* 1996; 334(5):296–302.

72 Friedman R, Mears JG, Barst RJ. Continuous infusion of prostacyclin normalizes plasma markers of endothelial cell injury and platelet aggregation in primary pulmonary hypertension. *Circulation* 1997; 96(9): 2782–2784.

73 Morse JH, Barst RJ, Fotino M et al. Primary pulmonary hypertension, tissue plasminogen activator antibodies, and HLA-DQ7. *Am J Resp Critical Care Med* 1997; 155(1):274–278.

74 Rich S, Kaufmann E, Levy PS: The effect of high doses of calcium-channel blockers on survival in primary pulmonary hypertension. *N Engl J Med* 1992; 327:76–81.

75 Schulman LL, Grossman BA, Owen J. Platelet activation and fibrinopeptide formation in pulmonary hypertension. *Chest* 1993; 104(6):1690–1693.

76 Palevsky HI, Schloo BL, Pietra GG et al. Primary pulmonary hypertension. Vascular structure, morphometry, and responsiveness to vasodilator agents. *Circulation* 1989; 80(5):1207–1221.

77 Tuder RM, Groves B, Badesch DB, Voelkel NF. Exuberant endothelial cell growth and elements of inflammation are present in plexiform lesions of pulmonary hypertension. *American J Pathol* 1994; 144(2):275–285.

78 Tuder RM, Voelkel NF. Pulmonary hypertension and inflammation. *J Laborat Clin Med* 1998; 132(1):16–24.

79 Humbert M, Monti G, Brenot F et al. Increased interleukin-1 and interleukin-6 serum concentrations in severe primary pulmonary hypertension. *Am J Resp Crit Care Med* 1995; 151:1628–1631.

80 Wright L, Tuder RM, Wang J, Cool CD, Lepley RA, Voelkel NF. 5-lipoxygenase and 5-lipoxygenase activating protein (FLAP) immunoreactivity in lungs from patients with primary pulmonary hypertension. *Am J Resp Crit Care Med* 1998; 157:219–229.

81 Botney MD, Bahadori L, and Gold LI. Vascular remodeling in primary pulmonary hypertension. Potential role for transforming growth factor-B. *Am J Pathol* 1994; 114:286–295.

82 Humbert M, Maitre S, Capron F, Rain B, Musset D, Simonneau G. Pulmonary edema complicating continuous intravenous prostacyclin in pulmonary capillary hemangiomatosis. *Am J Resp Crit Care Med* 1998; 157(5):1681–1685.

83 Schuster DP, Crouch EC, Parks WC, Johnson T, Botney MD. Angiotensin converting enzyme expression in primary pulmonary hypertension. *Am J Resp Crit Care Med* 1996; 154(4 Pt 1):1087–1091.

84 Tuder RM, Allard I, Voelkel NF. Role of vascular endothelial growth factor in hypoxia and monocrotaline induced pulmonary hypertension. *Circulation* 1996; 94:I647.

85 Garg UC, Hassid A. Nitric oxide-generating vasodilators and 8-bromo-cyclic guanosine monophosphate inhibit mitogenesis and proliferation of cultured rat vascular smooth muscle cells. *J Clin Invest* 1989; 83:1774–1777.

86 Sperling RT, Creager MA. Nitric oxide and pulmonary hypertension. *Coron Artery Dis* 1999; 10(5):287–294.

87 Kancko FT, Arroliga AC, Dweik RA et al. Biochemical reaction products of nitric oxide as quantitative markers of primary pulmonary hypertension. *Am J Resp Crit Care Med* 1998; 158:917–23.

88 Riley MS, Porszasz J, Miranda J, Engelen MPKJ, Brundage BH, Wasserman K. Exhaled nitric oxide during exercise in primary pulmonary hypertension and pulmonary fibrosis. *Chest* 1997; 111:44–50.

89 Cremona G, Higenbottam TW, Bower EA, Wood AM, Stewart S. Hemodynamic effects of basal and stimulated release of endogenous nitric oxide in isolated human lungs. *Circulation* 1999; 100(12):1316–1321.

90 Resta TC, Gonzales RJ, Dail WG, Sanders TC, Walker BR. Selective upregulation of arterial endothelial nitric oxide synthase in pulmonary hypertension. *Am J Physiol* 1997; 272:H806–H813.

91 Everett AD, Lecras TD, Xue C, Johns RA. eNOS expression is not altered in pulmonary vascular remodeling due to increased pulmonary blood flow. *Am J Physiol* 1998; 18(6):L1058–L1065.

92 Xue C, Rengasamy A, Le Cras TD, Koberna PA, Dailey GC, Johns RA. Distribution of NOS in normoxic vs hypoxic rat lung: upregulation of NOS by chronic hypoxia. *Am J Physiol* 1994; 267:L667–L678.

93 Tyler RC, Muramatsu M, Abman SH et al. Variable expression of endothelial NO synthase in three forms of rat pulmonary hypertension. *Am J Physiol – Lung Cell Molec Physiol* 1999; 20(2):L297–L303.

94 Fagan KA, Fouty BW, Tyler RC et al. The pulmonary circulation of homozygous or heterozygous eNOS-null mice is hyperresponsive to mild hypoxia. *J Clin Invest* 1999; 103:291–299.

95 Bellotto F, Chiavacci P, Laveder F, Angelini A, Thiene G, Marcolongo R. Effective immunosuppressive therapy in a

patient with primary pulmonary hypertension. *Thorax* 1999; 54(4):372–374.

96 Stenmark KR, Mecham RP. Cellular and molecular mechanisms of pulmonary vascular remodeling. *Ann Rev Physiol* 1997; 59:89–144.

97 Heath D, Wood E, Dushane J, Edwards JE. The structure of the pulmonary trunk at different ages and in cases of pulmonary hypertension and pulmonary stenosis. *J Pathol Bacteriol* 1959; 77:443–450.

98 Hoet PHM, Nemery B. Polyamines in the lung: polyamine uptake and polyamine-linked pathological or toxicological conditions. *Am J Physiol – Lung Cell Molec Physiol* 2000; 278(3):L417–L433.

99 Brenot F, Herve P, Petitpretz P, Parent F, Duroux P, Simonneau GR. Primary pulmonary hypertension and fenfluramine use. *Br Heart J* 1993; 70:537–541.

100 Abenhaim L, Moride Y, Brenot F et al. Appetite-suppressant drugs and the risk of primary pulmonary hypertension. *N Engl J Med* 1996; 335:609–616.

101 Lee KM, Tsai KY, Wang N, Ingber DE. Extracellular matrix and pulmonary hypertension – control of vascular smooth muscle cell contractility. *Am J Physiol: Heart and Circ Physiol* 1998; 43(1):H76–H82.

102 Botney MD, Kaiser LR, Cooper JD et al. Extracellular matrix protein gene expression in atherosclerotic pulmonary arteries. *Am J Pathol* 1992; 140:357–364.

103 Rabinovitch M: Pulmonary hypertension – updating a mysterious disease. *Cardiovasc Res* 1997; 34(2):268–272.

104 Botney MD, Liptay MJ, Kaiser LR, Cooper JD, Parks WC, Mecham RP. Active collagen synthesis by pulmonary arteries in human primary pulmonary hypertension. *Am J Pathol* 1993; 143:121–129.

105 Tanaka Y, Schuster DP, Davis EC, Patterson GA, Botney MD. The role of vascular injury and hemodynamics in rat pulmonary artery remodeling. *J Clin Invest* 1996; 98:434–442.

106 Tozzi CA, Poiani J, Harangozo AM, Boyd CD, Riley DJ. Pressure-induced connective tissue synthesis in pulmonary artery segments is dependent on intact endothelium. *J Clin Invest* 1989; 84:1005–1012.

107 Kerr JS, Riley DJ, Frank MM, Trelstad RL, Frankel HM. Reduction of chronic hypoxic pulmonary hypertension in the rat by beta-aminopropionitrile. *J Appl Physiol* 1984; 57(6):1760–1766.

108 Poiani GJ, Tozzi CA, Choe JK, Yohn SE, Riley DJ. An anti-fibrotic agent reduces blood pressure in established pulmonary hypertension in the rat. *J Appl Physiol* 1990; 68(4):1542–1547.

109 Melmon KL, Braunwald E. Familial pulmonary hypertension. *N Engl J Med* 1963; 269:770–775.

110 Rogge JD, Mishkin ME, Genovese PD. The familial occurrence of primary pulmonary hypertension. *Ann Intern Med* 1966; 65:672–684.

111 Elliott G, Alexander G, Leppert M, Yeates S, Kerber R. Coancestry in apparently sporadic primary pulmonary hypertension. *Chest* 1995; 108(4):973–977.

112 Loyd JE, Primm RK, Newman JH. Familial primary pulmonary hypertension: clinical patterns. *Am Rev Resp Dis* 1984; 129(1):194–197.

113 Loyd JE, Butler MG, Foroud TM, Conneally PM, Phillips JA3, Newman JH. Genetic anticipation and abnormal gender ratio at birth in familial primary pulmonary hypertension. *Am J Resp Crit Care Med* 1995; 152(1):93–97.

114 Wille RT, Krishnan K, Cooney KA, Bach DS, Martinez F. Familial association of primary pulmonary hypertension and a new low-oxygen affinity beta-chain hemoglobinopathy, Hb Washtenaw. *Chest* 1996; 109(3):848–850.

115 Rich S, Kieras K, Hart K, Groves BM, Stobo JD, Brundage BH. Antinuclear antibodies in primary pulmonary hypertension. *J Am Col Cardiol* 1986; 8:1307–1311.

116 Badesch DB, Wynne KM, Bonvallet S, Voelkel NF, Ridgway C, Groves BM. Hypothyroidism and primary pulmonary hypertension: an autoimmune pathogenetic link? *Ann Intern Med* 1993; 119(1):44–46.

117 Curnock AL, Dweik RA, Higgins BH, Saadi HF, Arroliga AC. High prevalence of hypothyroidism in patients with primary pulmonary hypertension. *Am J Med Sci* 1999; 318(5):289–292.

118 Morse JH, Barst RJ, Fotino M. Familial pulmonary hypertension: immunogenetic findings in four Caucasian kindreds. *Am Rev Resp Dis* 1992; 145(4 Pt 1):787–792.

119 Morse JH, Jones AC, Barst RJ, Hodge SE, Wilhelmsen KC, Nygaard TG. Mapping of familial primary pulmonary hypertension locus (pph1) to chromosome 2q31-q32. *Circulation* 1997; 95(12):2603–2606.

120 Nichols WC, Koller DL, Slovis B. Localization of the gene for familial primary pulmonary hypertension to chromosome 2q3 1–22. *Nat Genet* 1997; 15:277–820.

121 Morse JH, Barst RJ. Detection of familial primary pulmonary hypertension by genetic testing. *N Engl J Med* 1997; 337(3):202-203.

122 Deng Z, Morse JH, Slager SL et al. Familial primary pulmonary hypertension (gene PPH1) is caused by mutations in the bone morphogenetic protein receptor-II gene. *Am J Hum Genet* 2000; 67(3):737–744.

18

Current treatment of pulmonary vascular diseases

Tarek Saba and Andrew Peacock

Scottish Pulmonary Vascular Unit, Western Infirmary, Glasgow, UK

Introduction

The normal pulmonary circulation is an adaptable compliant system, allowing for large variations in blood flow with relatively small changes in resistance and pulmonary artery pressure. This flexibility is gradually lost in the face of progressive vascular damage due to an intrinsic disease process or a recurrent acute insult, and results in pulmonary hypertension.

The pathological changes were first described by Romberg in 1891[1] in a patient with unexplained pulmonary arteriosclerosis. In 1951, Dresdale et al. coined the term primary pulmonary hypertension[2] and widespread awareness of the disease came with the epidemic of pulmonary hypertension, blamed on the use of the appetite suppressant aminorex fumarate, that swept Europe in 1967. It took almost 90 years for the first effective medical and surgical treatment to become available, but in the past 10 years there have been dramatic improvements in both quality of life and survival with the use of calcium channel blockers and prostacyclin. This has led to increasing recognition of the important role that pulmonary vascular disease plays in many disease processes, and renewed interest in early diagnosis and intervention.

Definition and classification

Pulmonary hypertension is defined as a mean pulmonary artery pressure of over 25 mmHg at rest or 30 mmHg during exercise[3]. It has traditionally been classified as either primary or secondary after clinical assessment (Table 18.1), but the realization that the underlying pathological abnormalities in some types of secondary disease were very similar to those seen in primary pulmonary hypertension prompted a new classification based on histology (Table 18.2). This was proposed at the second World Health Organization symposium held in Evian, France in 1998[4]. However, the traditional classification will be used throughout this chapter to avoid confusion, since this has been used almost exclusively in the recent literature.

Epidemiology

Primary pulmonary hypertension (PPH) is rare, with an estimated incidence of one to two cases per million people per year. It is commoner in women (ratio 1.7:1), perhaps due to a lower survival rate of male foetuses with the disease[5], and the mean age at the time of diagnosis is in the mid-30s. Untreated, the prognosis is bleak with a 3-year survival of 48% in one large series (NIH). The familial form of the disease probably accounts for 6%[6] and is indistinguishable clinically from the sporadic form[7]. It is inherited in an autosomal dominant fashion, and displays genetic anticipation[5].

The overall incidence of secondary pulmonary hypertension (SPH) is unknown, but has been estimated at 0.5% to 53% depending upon the underlying disorder (Table 18.3)[8–10]. Little is known about

Table 18.1. Classical classification of pulmonary hypertension

Primary pulmonary hypertension
(including Familial disease)

Secondary pulmonary hypertension

Connective tissue disease
Scleroderma/CREST syndrome
Mixed connective tissue disease
Overlap syndrome
Systemic lupus erythematosus

Chronic hypoxic lung disease
Chronic obstructive pulmonary disease
Sleep disordered breathing
Interstitial lung disease

Thromboembolic disease
Pulmonary thromboembolism
In situ thrombosis
Sickle cell disease

Congenital heart disease
Ventricular septal defect
Atrial septal defect

Left-sided heart disease
Valvular disease
Left ventricular failure

Drugs
Appetite suppressants
Amphetamines
L-tryptophan
Cocaine

Portal hypertension

HIV

Other
Chronic high altitude
Neonatal lung disease
Pulmonary veno-occlusive disease
Sarcoidosis
Schistosomiasis

Table 18.2. New WHO classification of pulmonary hypertension[4] 1998

1. **Pulmonary arterial hypertension**
   1.1 Primary pulmonary hypertension
       (a) Sporadic
       (b) Familial
   1.2 Related to:
       (a) Collagen vascular disease
       (b) Congenital systemic to pulmonary shunts
       (c) Portal hypertension
       (d) HIV infection
       (e) Drugs/toxins
           (1) Anorexigens
           (2) Other
       (f) Persistent pulmonary hypertension of the newborn
       (g) Other

2. **Pulmonary venous hypertension**
   2.1 Left-sided atrial or ventricular heart disease
   2.2 Left-sided valvular heart disease
   2.3 Extrinsic compression of central pulmonary veins
       (a) Fibrosing mediastinitis
       (b) Adenopathy/tumours
   2.4 Pulmonary veno-occlusive disease
   2.5 Other

3. **Pulmonary hypertension associated with disorders of the respiratory system and/or hypoxaemia**
   3.1 Chronic obstructive pulmonary disease
   3.2 Interstitial lung disease
   3.3 Sleep disordered breathing
   3.4 Alveolar hypoventilation disorders
   3.5 Chronic exposure to high altitude
   3.6 Neonatal lung disease
   3.7 Alveolar-capillary dysplasia
   3.8 Other

4. **Pulmonary hypertension due to chronic thrombotic and/or embolic disease**
   4.1 Thromboembolic obstruction of proximal pulmonary arteries
   4.2 Obstruction of distal pulmonary arteries
       (a) Pulmonary embolism (thrombus, tumour, OVA and/or parasites, foreign material)
       (b) *In situ* thrombosis
       (c) Sickle cell disease

Table 18.2 (*cont.*)

5. **Pulmonary hypertension due to disorders directly affecting the pulmonary vasculature**
    5.1 Inflammatory
        (a) Schistosomiasis
        (b) Sarcoidosis
        (c) Other
    5.2 Pulmonary capillary hemangiomatosis

Functional assessment[a]

A. **Class I** – Patients with pulmonary hypertension but without resulting limitation of physical activity. Ordinary physical activity does not cause undue dyspnea or fatigue, chest pain or near syncope.
B. **Class II** – Patients with pulmonary hypertension resulting in slight limitation of physical activity. They are comfortable at rest. Ordinary physical activity causes undue dyspnea or fatigue, chest pain or near syncope.
C. **Class III** – Patients with pulmonary hypertension resulting in marked limitation of physical activity. They are comfortable at rest. Less than ordinary activity causes undue dyspnea or fatigue, chest pain or near syncope.
D. **Class IV** – Patients with pulmonary hypertension with inablility to carry out any physical acitivity without symptoms. These patients manifest signs of right heart failure. Dyspnea and/or fatigue may even be present at rest. Discomfort is increased by any physical activity.

[a] Modified after the New York Heart Association Functional Classification.

prognosis in different types of SPH, although the outlook for connective tissue disease seems poor[8].

Clinical assessment

History

Symptoms are not very helpful in the diagnosis of pulmonary hypertension (Table 18.4). The commonest symptom is exercise intolerance due to shortness of breath and tiredness, but the disorder may have been present for years before medical

Table 18.3. Estimated prevalence of secondary pulmonary hypertension (SPH) in some disorders

Disease/condition	SPH (%)
Connective tissue diseases overall	10
CREST syndrome	<50
Mixed connective tissue disease	23–53
Scleroderma	2.3–35%
Systemic lupus erythematosus	0.5–14%
Rheumatoid arthritis/ Sjögren's syndrome/ dermatomyositis	Rare
Chronic obstructive pulmonary disease	Unknown
Fibrosing lung disease	Unknown
Portal hypertension	? 0.5–2
HIV infection	? 0.5–2
Use of anorectic agents	? 25 – 50 per million per year

advice is sought. In retrospect, symptoms often predated presentation, but were explained away as trivial or caused by concurrent disease.

Other symptoms occur later as pulmonary artery pressures rise. Chest pain, when it occurs, is atypical for cardiac disease. It is sharp, stabbing, can be retrosternal or left sided, and often has no relationship to exertion. It can be associated with palpitations or a sensation of a pounding heartbeat. When syncope occurs, it is a bad prognostic sign. It can be due to postural hypotension, arrhythmias, or be exercise induced. As the disease progresses right heart failure develops with edema, worsening shortness of breath and tiredness, and eventually orthopnea. Another symptom frequently described by patients with advanced disease is intractable dry cough, the cause of which remains unclear.

When taking a history, attention should be paid to symptoms of diseases known to predispose to pulmonary hypertension. Ocular discomfort, a dry mouth, dysphagia and arthritis suggest underlying connective tissue disease, although Raynaud's

Table 18.4. Symptoms/signs of primary pulmonary hypertension

Symptoms	Signs
Exercise intolerance	Cyanosis
Shortness of breath	Right ventricular heave
Tiredness	Third/fourth heart sound
Atypical chest pain	Wide splitting of second heart sound
Palpitations	Postural hypotension
Dizziness	Edema
Syncope	Raised jugular venous pressure
Dry cough	
Orthopnea	

phenomenon, which also occurs in PPH, is often the only symptom at presentation. A personal or family history of thromboembolic disease may be relevant. Direct questions should be asked about risk factors for pulmonary hypertension such as the use of anorectic agents, recreational drug use or the possibility of HIV infection. A history of exercise intolerance in childhood may indicate congenital heart disease. Chronic hypoxic lung disease is common, and a small proportion will develop clinically significant pulmonary hypertension.

Examination

There are no pathognomonic signs of pulmonary hypertension, but there are a number of useful clinical findings. There may be a right ventricular heave, a third and/or a fourth heart sound, and widened splitting of the second heart sound. Postural hypotension is often present and the signs of right heart failure develop as the disease progresses. Cyanosis is common and may be the result of pulmonary vascular disease or related to the cause.

In addition to the above, there are also signs indicating an underlying cause. Patients with connective tissue disease may have cutaneous changes such as telangiectasia, calcinosis and sclerodactyly. Finger clubbing and end-inspiratory crackles suggest pul-

monary fibrosis. A fixed and widely split second heart sound is heard in left to right shunt, and there may be a mid-diastolic murmur in pulmonary hypertension due to mitral stenosis. Signs of liver disease raise the possibility of portopulmonary hypertension and obesity may be causing chronic ventilatory failure and/or obstructive sleep apnoea, although the latter is probably not an independent risk factor for pulmonary hypertension.

Investigation

There is a need for a reliable non-invasive method for the diagnosis and assessment of pulmonary hypertension. The advent of echocardiography made the screening of small numbers of 'at risk' patients possible, but it is not suitable for larger-scale screening since it is time consuming and insensitive in certain patient groups, such as those with chronic obstructive pulmonary disease or the overweight.

Simple first line tests can be useful but are frequently normal in 'pulmonary arterial hypertension' (WHO classification)[4]:

Chest radiography   May show cardiomegaly and prominent pulmonary arteries with peripheral pruning. Right atrial enlargement may also be seen.

Electrocardiography   May show right heart strain and right ventricular hypertrophy.

Pulmonary function tests   Normal dynamic and static lung volumes with disproportionately reduced gas transfer factor reflecting reduced pulmonary capillary blood volume.

Transthoracic echocardiography   Can give an estimate of systolic pulmonary artery pressure and cardiac output, as well as right heart chamber size.

Ventilation/perfusion scan   Normal ventilation component with patchy loss of perfusion.

Arterial blood gases   Hypoxemia (and hypocapnia).

Table 18.5. Specific investigations to detect underlying disease associated with pulmonary hypertension

Connective tissue disease	High resolution computed tomographic scanning (HRCT)
	Autoimmune studies
	Inflammatory markers
Pulmonary thromboembolic disease	Magnetic resonance angiography (MRA)
	Computerized axial tomography angiography (CTA)
	Thrombophilia screen
Portal hypertension	Hepatitis serology
	Autoimmune studies
	Abdominal ultrasonography
	Endoscopy
Chronic hypoxic lung disease	Sleep studies
Congenital heart disease	Transesophageal echocardiography
Other	Human immunodeficiency viral serology (HIV)
	Genetic studies

Other useful investigations include:

Six-minute walk test   Decrease in distance covered with rapid rise in heart rate and fall in oxygen saturation.

Cardiopulmonary exercise testing   Characteristic pattern of abnormalities including reduced work capacity, maximum oxygen uptake (VO_2) and oxygen pulse (VO_2/heart rate), and raised ventilatory equivalents for oxygen and carbon dioxide.

Magnetic resonance imaging (MRI)   Useful for non-invasive assessment of right ventricular morphology and function. Can also study blood flow patterns in pulmonary circulation.

Specific investigations to exclude underlying disorders associated with pulmonary hypertension are listed in Table 18.5.

Right heart catheterization

This is the definitive investigation for pulmonary hypertension. Measurements are taken of right atrial pressure, right ventricular systolic and end-diastolic pressures, pulmonary artery pressure and pulmonary artery occlusion pressure (wedge). Cardiac output is usually measured by thermodilution as the mean of three readings. If pulmonary artery pressure is raised then an acute vasodilator assessment should be done (see below).

If underlying congenital heart disease is suspected, then an oxygen saturation run should be performed. Blood samples are taken from superior vena cava, high right atrium, mid right atrium, low right atrium, inferior vena cava, right ventricle and pulmonary artery, and oxygen saturation analysed. A step-up in readings would indicate a left to right shunt. A ventricular septal defect is usually diagnosed at echocardiography.

If the pulmonary artery pressure is normal, the patient should be asked to perform exercise sufficient to raise the heart rate, in order to investigate the presence of exercise-induced pulmonary hypertension. Three minutes of straight leg raising is usually adequate. Further useful information can also be obtained by ambulatory pulmonary artery pressure monitoring with a micromanometer-tipped catheter[11], but this is not widely available.

The effect of oxygen on pulmonary artery pressure and cardiac output should also be assessed, in particular where hypoxia is present and thought to be a contributing factor. Oxygen is also a vasodilator in this situation, reversing hypoxic pulmonary vasoconstriction.

If ventilation/perfusion scanning suggested the possibility of pulmonary thromboembolism, or if there is high clinical suspicion, pulmonary angiography should be performed. This can usually be performed safely in these patients, but should not be undertaken lightly since it carries an increased risk due to sudden rises in pressure in hypertensive non-compliant vessels[12]. In our laboratory angiography is performed by selective cannulation.

Table 18.6. Vasodilators for acute vasodilator assessment

	Mode of delivery	Half-life	Adverse effects	Cost
Prostacyclin	Intravenous	3 minutes	Hypotension, nausea, jaw pain, abdominal pain, headache, flushing	Very expensive
Nitric oxide	Inhaled	1–2 minutes	None reported, but metabolites are toxic.	Cheap, but needs delivery system
Adenosine	Intravenous	10 seconds	Hypotension, bradycardia, heart block, bronchospasm, chest pain, flushing, paresthesia, headache	Expensive
Calcium channel blockers	Oral	2–4 hours	Hypotension, bradycardia or tachycardia, heart block, negatively inotropic, headaches, nausea and vomiting, dizziness, agitation	Cheap

Acute vasodilator studies

If pulmonary artery pressures are raised, then an acute vasodilator assessment should be performed. A positive response is thought to be an accurate predictor of long-term vasodilator response, at least in primary pulmonary hypertension[13,14]. Vasodilator assessments should only be carried out in pulmonary vascular units since they can be dangerous in inexperienced hands. They are done in the cardiac catheterization laboratory or in an intensive care facility with continuous hemodynamic monitoring, including pulmonary artery pressure, heart rate, oxygen saturation, and invasive or frequent non-invasive blood pressure measurement.

Which patients should be tested?

An acute vasodilator assessment should be done in all patients with pulmonary hypertension who are being considered for long-term vasodilator treatment. In particular, those in whom exercise capacity is preserved are more likely to have a positive response[15]. However, there is an increased risk of adverse events during testing in patients with right heart failure especially if right atrial pressure exceeds 20 mmHg or cardiac output is less than 2 l/min[16,17]. In the *Experience from the NIH Registry* published in 1989, eight patients out of 163 developed hypotension requiring treatment during acute

testing, and two patients died[18]. They were found to have higher right atrial pressures than the other patients (15 ± 2 mmHg vs. 9 ± 1 mmHg and $P < 0.05$).

The proportion of patients with primary pulmonary hypertension who respond to vasodilators is less than 30%[9,19], and the figure may be even lower for some types of secondary pulmonary hypertension[8].

Which vasodilator to use for an acute assessment?

A number of vasodilators have been used for this purpose including nitric oxide gas[20,21], adenosine[22,23], prostacyclin[21,24], and calcium channel blockers[16]. The choice of drug depends upon local experience, availability of delivery systems, and rapidity of effect required (see Table 18.6).

Prostacyclin

Prostacyclin was the first acute vasodilator to be tested in primary pulmonary hypertension[24] and it is now used as a long term treatment by continuous intravenous infusion. It is a naturally occurring prostaglandin with a potent effect on vascular endothelium. Its half-life of approximately 3 minutes means that an acute assessment can be completed during diagnostic catheterization, and any side effects should resolve quickly after stopping the infusion. There is a close correlation between prostacyclin responsiveness and efficacy of treatment with calcium channel blockers[14,17].

The main disadvantages of prostacyclin as an acute vasodilator are cost and availability. It also has a relatively long half-life when compared to adenosine and nitric oxide. Initial small studies found a high proportion of patients reporting intolerable side effects[24] but this has not been confirmed by larger studies.

Administration (acute)

Infusion should be started at 1 ng/kg/min and increased by 1–2 ng/kg/min every 5–15 minutes until a positive response is obtained or adverse effects intervene, with a maximum dose in adults of 12 ng/kg/min[14]. Expected adverse effects are systemic hypotension, nausea, headache, flushing, abdominal pain and jaw pain, and should rapidly resolve with a reduction in the infusion rate.

There is evidence that prostanoids can be given in aerosolized form with a similar effect to nitric oxide[25].

Nitric oxide

In 1980 Furchgott and Zawadzki reported that an intact endothelium was required for certain vasodilators to be effective[26]. Endothelium-derived relaxing factor was isolated and later shown to be nitric oxide[27,28]. It is produced in endothelial cells by the enzyme nitric oxide synthase (NOS). It then leaves the endothelium and binds to soluble guanylate cyclase, stimulating production of cyclic 3,5-monophosphate (cGMP) which triggers smooth muscle relaxation.

Nitric oxide (NO) is an odourless, colourless gas. It is an unstable radical and has a short half-life in the presence of oxygen. It has been shown to be a potent vasodilator in patients with pulmonary hypertension[20,29,30] and was the first agent capable of selectively reducing pulmonary artery pressure without causing systemic hypotension because it is rapidly taken up by hemoglobin[31–33]. It has similar effects to calcium channel blockers and prostacyclin in primary pulmonary hypertension[20,29] and there is evidence of a synergistic effect when tested in combination with oxygen[34]. It has the advantages of rapid onset and offset, with no significant acute adverse effects, and it is cheap to produce. Its therapeutic use has been limited by the requirement for a metered gas delivery system. This problem is compounded by the fact that several of its metabolites are toxic including nitrogen dioxide (NO_2), necessitating careful environmental monitoring.

Administration (acute)

NO is commercially available in cylinders either pure or as a mixture with nitrogen. An example of a delivery system is shown in Fig. 18.1. The gas is entrained into the circuit proximally by a continuous preset fresh gas flow of air. It is allowed to mix before being sampled continuously by an NO concentration sensor downstream and then being delivered to the patient via a facemask or mouthpiece. The one-way pressure-release valve allows expired air to leave the system. The adequacy of total gas flow can be assessed by movement of the reservoir bag during breathing. There is as yet no agreed testing protocol, but Sitbon et al. found a maximal effect was obtained at concentrations of 10 ppm given for 6–10 minutes[29]. There are no guidelines on monitoring, but inspired NO, NO_2 and oxygen should be measured, as well as environmental NO_2. Scavenging of expired gas is probably unnecessary for acute testing, on current evidence.

Adenosine

Adenosine has been shown to be a potent vasodilator[22], and acts by increasing intracellular cyclic AMP in vascular smooth muscle. It also causes coronary vasodilatation and reduces systemic vascular resistance[35]. It has a very short half-life of approximately 10 seconds, which makes it a convenient and rapidly

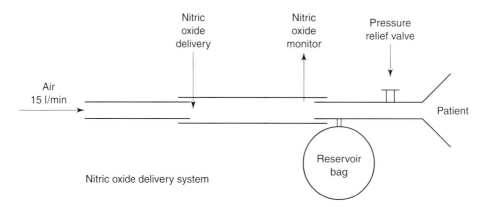

Fig. 18.1 Nitric oxide (NO) is entrained into the circuit proximally by a continuous flow of air at 15 litres/minute. It is allowed to mix before being sampled by an NO concentration monitor downstream and then being delivered to the patient via a facemask or mouthpiece. The one-way pressure relief valve allows expired air to leave the system and minimizes rebreathing. Inspired NO, NO_2 and oxygen should be measured, as well as environmental NO_2. Scavenging of expired gas is probably unnecessary during acute testing.

reversible agent for acute vasodilator testing. It is also cheaper than prostacyclin, readily available, and appears to have similar effects on pulmonary hemodynamics in primary pulmonary hypertension[36]. In one study, some patients with no response to nifedipine did respond to adenosine[37], and it may cause further vasodilatation in those already taking high dose calcium channel blockers[38].

Administration

Adenosine has been successfully infused both centrally[22] and peripherally[36]. The infusion should be started at 50–100 µg/kg/min and increases at 2 minute intervals until a positive response is obtained or side effects develop, up to a limit of 500 µg/kg/min[37].

Adenosine is contraindicated in asthma and should be used with caution in patients with significant reversible airflow obstruction, since it may cause wheezing and chest tightness. It is also a potent blocker of conduction in the atrioventricular node and should be avoided in those with second or third degree heart block. Side effects include flushing, chest pain, breathlessness, headache, tingling or numbness of the extremities, hypotension and bradycardia. All rapidly resolve when the infusion is discontinued.

Calcium channel blockers

Calcium channel blockers cause vasodilatation by reducing the influx of extracellular calcium into muscle cells. They are a heterogeneous group of compounds with varying half-lives and side effect profiles, but the most commonly used drugs are nifedipine and diltiazem. They are cheap and widely available, and have been shown to be effective at identifying patients who will respond to long term vasodilator treatment[16,39,40].

Unfortunately there are a number of disadvantages to their use. Their relatively long half-lives mean that assessments can take up to 12 hours to complete, and high doses are often required[39,40]. They are not selective for the pulmonary vasculature, and can cause hypotension by systemic vasodilatation. In addition, they are negatively inotropic, especially verapamil which should be avoided[41]. They have been known to delay conduction in the atrioventricular node resulting in variable heart block, and nifedipine may cause tachycardia.

Administration (acute)

In 1987, Rich and Kaufman described a method of acutely assessing vasodilator response using incremental doses of nifedipine and diltiazem[16]. After diagnostic right heart catheterization and baseline measurements, patients should be given hourly doses of nifedipine 20 mg or diltiazem 60 mg until either a positive response occurs or intolerable side effects develop. Careful observation is needed, preferably in a coronary care setting, with invasive systemic and pulmonary hemodynamic monitoring. If a positive response is achieved, the total cumulative dose given should be halved and administered three to four times per day.

As well as the problems already discussed, other side effects include nausea, vomiting, dizziness and agitation.

What is a positive vasodilator response?

There is still no agreement on the definition of a positive vasodilator response. Some investigators have relied simply upon a reduction in calculated pulmonary vascular resistance of between 20% and 50%[4]. The main criticism of relying only upon resistance is that marked changes can occur without there being significant alterations in pulmonary artery pressure and cardiac output, both of which have been shown to be prognostic indicators[4]. Other investigators have therefore required both a significant fall in pulmonary artery pressure and a rise in cardiac output. The situation is further complicated by the observation that prostacyclin and adenosine appear to have a predominant effect on cardiac output[36], whereas calcium channel blockers have relatively more effect on pulmonary artery pressure[4,39]. There is also evidence of a negative effect on systemic oxygen delivery in some patients during acute vasodilator treatment with an increase in ventilation-perfusion mismatching, due to an effect on hypoxic pulmonary vasoconstriction.

While the question was not answered at the recent World Convention on Advances in the Management of Primary Pulmonary Hypertension in France in 1998[4], a working definition of a 20% fall in pulmonary artery pressure and a 20% rise in cardiac output was used in designing a management algorithm.

Most of the reported experience with acute vasodilator testing has been in patients with primary pulmonary hypertension, and it is difficult to make recommendations for secondary pulmonary hypertension. It seems likely that the principles of assessment and interpretation will be similar, although more studies are needed to clarify the issue.

Long-term treatment: general principles

The aims of treatment in pulmonary hypertension are twofold: to improve exercise tolerance and thereby quality of life, and to prolong survival. Although there has been some recent evidence that the pathophysiological process can be reversed, the disease is relentlessly progressive in the majority of patients with no realistic prospect of a cure.

As will be seen, most of the studies of treatment efficacy have looked at patients with primary pulmonary hypertension, and there is relatively little published information to guide therapy in secondary forms of the disease. The recent reclassification of some forms of secondary pulmonary hypertension into the same category as primary pulmonary hypertension (see Table 18.2) raises the possibility that these conditions will respond similarly to treatment. This remains to be seen, but evidence is mounting of important differences in outcome with intravenous prostacyclin, particularly with regard to adverse effects, in patients with connective tissue disease and portopulmonary hypertension[42,43]. Until firmer evidence is available, it seems reasonable to apply the same management principles in most forms of the disease (Fig. 18.2).

Vasodilators

The hypothesis that vasoconstriction plays a part in the pathogenesis of pulmonary hypertension

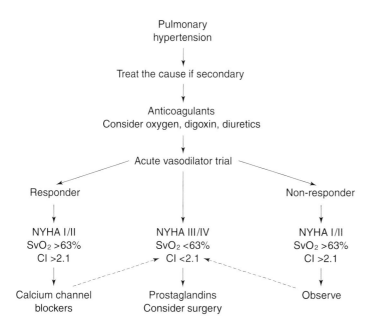

Fig. 18.2 A suggested management algorithm for pulmonary arterial hypertension (WHO classification). NYHA = New York Heart Association classification, SvO_2 = mixed venous oxygen saturation, CI = cardiac index.

naturally led to the use of vasodilators in the treatment of pulmonary hypertension, and there have been a number of studies with different vasodilators over the past 20 years. The aim of treatment is to reduce pulmonary artery pressure and increase cardiac output, thereby reducing pulmonary vascular resistance and right ventricular afterload. In 1980 Rubin and Peter[44] reported a 52% reduction in pulmonary vascular resistance following hydralazine in 4 patients with primary pulmonary hypertension. Since then a wide range of vasodilators have been tried but there are still no prospective randomized controlled trials of oral therapy, although a number of uncontrolled studies[39,40,45] have shown marked improvements in pulmonary hemodynamics, exercise tolerance and survival in carefully selected patients.

The evidence for a role for vasodilators in secon-

dary pulmonary hypertension is weaker, although vasoconstriction is thought to be involved in the pathogenesis (see previous chapter). Many studies of the effect of vasodilators on patients with pulmonary hypertension due to hypoxic lung disease have been performed, and the only drug that is consistently beneficial is oxygen. The current consensus is that there may be a role for a selective pulmonary vasodilator in these patients[46] and there is some evidence that the newer calcium channel blockers may be useful (see later). However, there is still controversy about the advisability or necessity of treating raised pulmonary artery pressures in this context[18,47,48] with some authors casting doubt over the contribution of the pulmonary circulatory changes to the pathophysiological process[49,50]. The rise in pulmonary artery pressure in these patients is mild, even in severe disease, and the annual change seems to be less than 1 mmHg on average[51,52]. However, several investigators have shown a correlation between survival and pulmonary hemodynamics[53,54] and there is evidence that acute rises in pressure take place during exercise, sleep and episodes of acute respiratory failure (see previous chapter). In pulmonary vascular disease related to connective tissue disease, evidence is accumulating of sustained benefit from both prostacyclin and calcium channel blockers, but there is still no consensus.

Choice of vasodilator for chronic therapy

All vasodilators have significant side effects that limit their use, and can be life threatening in some situations. Since there is no way of differentiating responders from non-responders without formal vasodilator testing, a vasodilator assessment should always be carried out under controlled conditions (as above). There is evidence that the acute response to vasodilator challenge accurately identifies patients who will benefit from long term treatment[13,14]. In primary pulmonary hypertension, treatment with calcium channel blockers is recommended if there is a positive response. If there is no response to an acute assessment then continuous intravenous prostacyclin should be considered. There is less consensus on treatment in secondary pulmonary hypertension, but it seems reasonable to apply the same criteria.

Calcium channel blockers

Background

These are the most widely used class of vasodilators in pulmonary hypertension. They consist of a number of different compounds, and were classified by Opie in 1987[55]. The dihydropyridines are the group most widely studied and prescribed. They are thought to act by binding to the slow membrane channels of cardiac and vascular smooth muscle cells thereby inhibiting the influx of extracellular calcium and reducing muscle contraction.

Diltazem and nifedipine are the most commonly used oral vasodilators for long term therapy although newer drugs such as nicardipine and amlodipine are now also being used[9]. Verapamil is not recommended due to its significant negative inotropic properties[41].

Primary pulmonary hypertension

Calcium channel blockers were initially used in the same doses as those used to treat systemic hypertension and angina but only had a small effect on pulmonary artery pressure[56,57]. Since then a series of important studies have shown a dramatic effect in carefully selected patients treated with significantly higher doses[39,40,45].

In 1985 Rich et al.[45] studied 23 patients with relatively severe primary pulmonary hypertension. Although vasodilator responders did have better long-term survival overall, the results were disappointing, with no relationship between drug treatment and clinical outcome. This may have been due to treatment with low drug doses or selection bias, in that the mean survival for the study patients was significantly shorter than the two to three year mean survival of untreated patients reported at the time. In addition, the definition of a favourable vasodilator response used in this study did not require a drop in pulmonary artery pressure, which may explain the high proportion of responders found.

In 1987 Rich and Brundage reported on a series of 13 patients whom they assessed in a novel way[40]. Thirteen consecutive patients with primary pulmonary hypertension referred to the University of Illinois were given consecutive hourly doses of either diltiazem 60 mg or nifedipine 20 mg with serial invasive measurements of hemodynamic variables. Doses continued until a positive response was obtained or side effects intervened, with a positive response defined as both a reduction in pulmonary vascular resistance of 50% and a fall in mean pulmonary artery pressure of 33% (unlike the 1985 study). When a positive response was achieved, the cumulative effective dose was then given every 6 to 8 hours over a 24-hour period to ensure that the effect was sustained. Patients were then discharged on the total daily dose received in divided doses, and all were given digoxin to counter possible negative inotropic effects.

Eight individuals responded to acute challenge and all reported improvement in NYHA functional class. Five patients were studied after 1 year of treatment and all were found to have an improvement in their echocardiographic appearances and in the electrocardiac manifestations of right ventricular hypertrophy and in four patients there was sustained hemodynamic improvement.

Rich et al. continued to assess all new referrals with primary pulmonary hypertension with some modifications of their protocol, including redefining a favourable vasodilator response as a 20% decrease in both pulmonary artery pressure and pulmonary vascular resistance. In 1992, they published the results of 64 patients assessed between 1/7/85 and 31/3/91[39], and compared their survival with that of patients enrolled in the National Institutes of Health Registry (NIH) of primary pulmonary hypertension[58]. Thirteen 'responders' were treated with a mean nifedipine dose of 172 mg (± 41 mg) and four with a mean diltiazem dose of 720 mg (± 208 mg) for up to 5 years.

The results were remarkable. They found a 5-year survival of 94% (16 out of 17) in those treated with calcium channel blockers as compared to 1-, 3-, and 5-year survival rates of 68%, 47% and 38%, respectively, in the NIH registry cohort (Fig. 18.3). This difference remained after accounting for concurrent administration of diuretics and digoxin. Warfarin treatment was associated with significantly better survival, especially in the group of non-responders.

This was a landmark study, which was the first to show that treatment could significantly improve prognosis in carefully selected patients with pulmonary hypertension. However, they noticed that the overall survival of their cohort was no better than that of the NIH patients, which raised the possibility that those individuals who responded to acute treatment were a subgroup with a better prognosis. In addition, the proportion of responders was only 26%, lower than the 62% (8 out of 13) reported in the 1987 study.

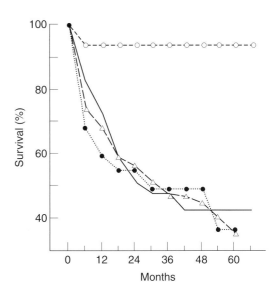

Fig. 18.3 Kaplan–Meier estimates of survival among patients who responded to treatment (open circles), those who did not respond (solid line), patients enrolled in the NIH registry who were treated at the University of Illinois (solid circles), and the NIH registry cohort (triangles). The percentages were calculated every 6 months for 5.5 years. The rate of survival was significantly better in patients who responded ($P = 0.003$) than in the other groups.

Secondary pulmonary hypertension

There have been a number of case reports and small studies but no large series looking at the effects of calcium channel blockers in secondary pulmonary hypertension. There is evidence, mainly through case reports, of acute and long term improvement in pulmonary hemodynamics in pulmonary vascular disease associated with connective tissue disease[8]. In 1991 Alpert et al.[59] studied ten patients with a mean pulmonary artery pressure of 42 mmHg, six of whom had CREST syndrome, three mixed connective tissue disease and one systemic sclerosis. They were given 10 mg of nifedipine orally at 90-minute intervals until pulmonary vascular resistance fell to normal levels, up to a maximum of 30 mg.

There was a significant fall in pulmonary artery pressure and pulmonary vascular resistance in nine out of ten patients, which was sustained in all six patients in whom hemodynamic measurements were repeated, with subjective improvement in dyspnea. There were no reported adverse reactions. The authors hypothesized that the high response rate may have been due the presence of only mild or moderate pulmonary hypertension in the majority of patients, perhaps reflecting less advanced disease with reversible vasoconstriction, although three out of four patients with severe pulmonary hypertension also improved. The long-term effects and benefits of treating this group of patients with high doses of calcium channel blockers remain unknown.

The majority of studies looking at the effect of calcium channel blockers in pulmonary hypertension due to hypoxic lung disease have been acute assessments, mainly on patients with relatively severe irreversible chronic airflow obstruction, hypoxemia and mild or moderate pulmonary hypertension[46]. The results have been conflicting, with some investigators showing an improvement in pulmonary hemodynamics and evidence of reduced progression[60], and others demonstrating worsening gas exchange[61,62], the development of tolerance[60,63] and an unacceptable incidence of side effects. The most recent study was by Sajkov et al.[64] who compared the effects of amlodipine and felodipine on ten patients with moderately severe irreversible airflow obstruction and an average mean pulmonary artery pressure of 41 mmHg in an open blind crossover study. Patients received increasing doses of one of the drugs (2.5, 5, 10 mg) with weekly increments for 3 weeks, followed by a 1-week washout period before receiving the other drug in similar fashion. Pulmonary hemodynamics were measured by Doppler echocardiography after 1 week on each treatment dose. They found a significant fall in pulmonary artery pressure with both drugs at the 2.5 mg dose with no added benefit from higher doses and no adverse effects on arterial oxygen tension or calculated oxygen delivery. Unlike felodipine, amlodipine was well tolerated, with significantly fewer side effects. The effects on symptoms and exercise tolerance were not reported.

Administration/adverse effects

Calcium channel blockers have potentially serious side effects in this group of patients and should only be prescribed to patients with a favourable acute vasodilator study. The assessment process described above for primary pulmonary hypertension is clearly expensive and time consuming, and involves considerable morbidity for the patient. Current practice is usually for patients to start treatment on a low dosage regime, such as 60 mg diltiazem twice daily, under close non-invasive observation in hospital. The dose can then be increased steadily on an outpatient basis until adequate symptom relief is obtained or adverse effects supervene.

These drugs are negatively inotropic and should be avoided in patients with overt right ventricular dysfunction[18]. They can also cause peripheral oedema due to salt and water retention, which may mask the development of right heart failure. They are not selective vasodilators, and systemic hypotension may occur, which can be refractory to treatment. More usually they will cause dizziness due to postural hypotension which can be troublesome. Diltiazem may cause bradycardia or heart block by inhibiting conduction through the atrioventricular node. Nifedipine may cause tachycardia, and has been reported to precipitate pulmonary edema[65].

Prostacyclin

Background

Prostacyclin was discovered in 1976 [66] and synthesized as a sodium salt in 1977[67]. It is a naturally occurring prostaglandin produced by the arachidonic acid cascade, and primarily secreted by vascular endothelium[68]. It is involved in local homeostasis and the regulation of vascular tone and is not a circulating hormone[69]. It has a number of properties which make it potentially useful. It is a potent pulmonary and systemic vasodilator with a short half-life. It inhibits platelet aggregation and adherence to damaged vascular endothelium and has a similar effect on white cells. It also has mild fibrinolytic activity and a cytoprotective effect has been demonstrated in ischaemic organs. It acts by increasing intracellular levels of cyclic adenosine monophosphate and inhibiting smooth muscle contraction[70].

It was first marketed for clinical use in 1983 and renamed epoprostenol (Flolan), but currently is only licensed for use in the United Kingdom as an antiplatelet aggregator in renal dialysis, although it is licensed for use in primary pulmonary hypertension in France, Spain and the United States. Its usefulness has been limited by expense, a short half-life and the need for it to be given intravenously.

Primary pulmonary hypertension

There is now strong evidence of a beneficial effect of continuous intravenous prostacyclin with or without a favourable acute vasodilator response[71–8]. In 1982 Rubin et al demonstrated the vasodilator properties of prostacyclin on the pulmonary circulation in seven patients with primary pulmonary hypertension[24]. Total pulmonary resistance fell by more than 20% and there was a small but statistically significant fall in mean pulmonary artery pressure; however, four patients developed intolerable side effects. The effects were rapid and dose dependent.

In 1984 Higenbottam et al. successfully used a continuous intravenous infusion of prostacyclin to restore a 27-year-old woman to independence after being almost bedbound with severe progressive pulmonary hypertension[71]. This case report led to a study of ten patients referred for consideration for heart–lung transplantation, all of whom had clinical and hemodynamic evidence of worsening primary pulmonary hypertension despite oral vasodilators[72]. After obtaining baseline measurements, prostacyclin was infused peripherally in a dose of 2 ng/kg/min and increased by 1 ng/kg/min every 15 minutes until a 20% fall in pulmonary vascular resistance or systemic arterial pressure was observed, or side effects intervened. Long-term treatment was then commenced at the maximal tolerated dose via a tunnelled sterile cannula in the subclavian vein, and patients were taught to manage the infusions at home. All patients showed an initial improvement in exercise performance during treatment, and all but one noticed rapid subjective improvement. Side effects were mild and transient, but there were three episodes of septicaemia and three patients developed unexplained ascites. Patients coped reasonably well overall showing the feasibility of this mode of treatment.

Rubin et al. published similar results in the first prospective randomized trial of continuous intravenous prostacyclin vs. conventional oral vasodilator treatment (primarily calcium channel blockers)[73]. Twenty-four patients with primary pulmonary hypertension, who had been referred because they were either unresponsive to or intolerant of vasodilators, were studied. All underwent right heart catheterization, and an incremental prostacyclin infusion until systemic blood pressure fell by 40%, heart rate rose by 40% or side effects intervened. Eleven were randomized to receive prostacyclin, and were given the hemodynamically optimal dose determined during the incremental study. Twelve were assigned to maximal conventional treatment including oral vasodilators, if thought beneficial. Right heart catheterization was repeated after 2 months of treatment.

After two months, the patients treated with prostacyclin showed significant haemodynamic changes from baseline, unlike the conventional therapy group. The benefits of prostacyclin therapy were sustained for up to 18 months, although they found that the mean dose had to be doubled every 6 to 12 months. Adverse effects did not increase, suggesting that this was partially due to tachyphylaxis and not simply disease progression. The eighteen surviving patients were then enrolled in a study of the long term effects of prostacyclin and followed up for up to 6 years in some cases[74]. Despite a number of serious complications, clinical and hemodynamic improvements were maintained, and there was evidence of improved survival when compared to historical controls. This was in spite of the fact that several of these patients has not displayed a positive response to the initial acute testing.

The clearest evidence for the therapeutic effect of prostacyclin in primary pulmonary hypertension came in the first prospective, randomized, multicentre open trial comparing the effects of continuous intravenous prostacyclin plus conventional therapy with conventional therapy alone[75]. Eighty-one patients underwent an acute prostacyclin assessment using the same protocol as Rubin et al.[73], before being randomized into two treatment groups. Right heart catheterization was repeated after 12 weeks.

There was a marked improvement in exercise capacity in the 41 patients on prostacyclin and conventional treatment as opposed to a reduction in the 40 patients on conventional treatment alone, with improved quality of life indices. Mean pulmonary artery pressure fell by 8% on average in the prostacyclin group, and pulmonary vascular resistance dropped by 21%. There were eight deaths during the study, all from the conventional treatment only group. Once again, no attempt was made to limit treatment with prostacyclin to those patients with a positive acute vasodilator response. This suggests that the benefits of prostacyclin are not simply due to vasodilation, although it is possible that a subgroup of patients with a good acute response were responsible for the overall improvement. There were frequent minor side effects and four episodes of catheter-related sepsis, as well as 26 episodes of malfunction of the drug delivery system.

Interestingly, a later study[76] has reported that the mean reduction in pulmonary artery pressure over the course of the period studied was greater than that expected from an acute vasodilator study with adenosine. In a group of 27 patients, all but one had a greater long-term benefit from prostacyclin than that predicted by adenosine, including seven patients with no significant acute vasodilator response. There is also evidence of right ventricular and pulmonary vascular remodelling, and less endothelial injury and platelet aggregation in these patients[77,78]. These studies suggest an additional effect of long-term prostacyclin, perhaps a reversal of the histological disease process.

Secondary pulmonary hypertension

There have only been three sizeable series looking at the long-term effects of continuous intravenous prostacyclin in secondary pulmonary hypertension[42,43,79]. None of the studies had a control group,

and in one of them[42] there were several major complications, including severe sepsis and pulmonary edema. In the first study, McLaughlin et al.[79] reported on 33 patients with a mean pulmonary artery pressure of 60 mmHg, all of whom were classified as New York Heart Association (NYHA) 3 or 4. The causes of pulmonary hypertension were connective tissue disease (14 patients), congenital heart disease (7 patients), portopulmonary hypertension (7 patients), thromboembolic disease (3 patients) and sarcoidosis (2 patients). Patients with a favourable acute vasodilator response to adenosine were excluded. All patients reported improved symptoms, with a significant improvement in NYHA classification and exercise time. At repeat right heart catheterization after three to 28 months, mean pulmonary artery pressure fell by 23%, pulmonary vascular resistance fell by 50% and cardiac output rose by 62%. There were no significant differences when the three largest subgroups were analysed separately, suggesting that the severity of pulmonary hypertension may be more important than the underlying cause. Minor side effects were common and there were several episodes of local infection and sepsis.

Humbert et al. treated 17 patients with underlying connective tissue disease with prostacyclin for 6 weeks[42]. All had severe pulmonary hypertension unresponsive to oral vasodilators, with a mean pulmonary artery pressure of 52 mmHg and none responded favourably to acute vasodilator challenge with nitric oxide. There was a significant improvement in mean pulmonary artery pressure, cardiac index, pulmonary vascular resistance and mixed venous oxygen saturation at both 6 weeks and long-term follow-up. However, seven patients died while on treatment as a result of sepsis and disease progression.

The third series was by Krowka et al., who studied the acute and long-term effects of continuous intravenous prostacyclin in portopulmonary hypertension[43]. They studied fifteen patients with advanced liver disease and mean pulmonary artery pressure over 35 mmHg. They confirmed the observation by Kuo et al.[80] that cardiac output is significantly higher in this condition than other forms of pulmonary hypertension, and found an acute improvement in pulmonary hemodynamics of similar magnitude to that previously reported in studies of primary pulmonary hypertension using equivalent doses of prostacyclin. They went on to study the long term effects of prostacyclin in ten patients over a mean of 8.7 months, and reported sustained improvement in all of them with evidence of further benefit when compared to the acute changes. Six of the ten patients died during the course of the study, leading the authors to postulate that intravenous prostacyclin may exacerbate the consequences of advanced liver disease, perhaps as a result of increasing splenic blood flow and portal venous congestion following a rise in cardiac output. It remains unclear whether prostacyclin confers an overall benefit in this group of patients.

A number of other studies have shown significant improvement in hemodynamics in subjects with secondary pulmonary hypertension, in response to a short-term infusion of prostacyclin. These include hypoxic lung disease[81], congestive heart failure[82], congenital heart disease[83], thromboembolic disease[81], and pulmonary fibrosis[81]. The long-term effects of treatment are unknown.

Administration/adverse effects

Prostacyclin is manufactured as a powder in vials of 0.5 mg and 1.5 mg, and is reconstituted with a solution of pH 10.5. Patients need to be taught how to manage their own infusion because the drug must be stored at 2–8 °C and used within 24 hours of reconstitution. Additionally, its half life of about 3 minutes[66] means that pumps need reloading quickly with minimal interruption. The infusion site should be kept sterile and medical advice sought as soon as symptoms and signs of infection appear.

The drug should be delivered by continuous intravenous infusion into a large vein via a single lumen indwelling central catheter, which should preferably be tunnelled to minimize the risk of infection. Where treatment cannot be deferred pending catheter placement, the infusion can initially be started

Table 18.7. Side effects of prostacyclin

Flushing
Sweating
Jaw pain
Nausea
Vomiting
Postural hypotension
Palpitations
Headaches
Skin rashes

peripherally. There is no general agreement on the correct therapeutic dose. Usual practice is to start at two nanograms per kilogram per minute and increase in increments of two nanograms per kilogram per minute until limited by side effects, which include flushing, sweating, jaw pain, postural hypotension, palpitations, nausea and diarrhea, headaches and skin rashes (Table 18.7)[84]. Almost all patients will develop some adverse effects but they often fade with time and the dose can be increased further. The aim is to improve symptoms and objective measures of exercise tolerance. Prostacyclin is contraindicated in pulmonary veno-occlusive disease[73] and pulmonary capillary hemangiomatosis[85] due to reports of acute pulmonary edema. There have also been reports of ascites[72] that were not confirmed by later studies.

All the studies of outpatient continuous intravenous prostacyclin have reported complications due to drug delivery systems, either through failure or contamination, and a number of deaths have been reported. Clearly, this treatment is suitable for selected patients only after appropriate training, and is best managed by specialist centres.

Alternative delivery methods and prostacyclin analogues

There has been interest recently in alternative methods of delivering prostacyclin and its analogues.

Beraprost, an orally active prostacyclin analogue with a half-life of between 3 and 6 hours has given promising results in seven patients with primary and secondary pulmonary hypertension[86]. Mikhail et al. compared the effects of nebulized prostacyclin with intravenous prostacyclin and nitric oxide in an acute vasodilator study of 12 patients with primary and secondary pulmonary hypertension. They found that nebulized prostacyclin gave the greatest improvement in hemodynamics[25].

Randomized placebo-controlled studies are currently in progress using nebulized iloprost and subcutaneous prostacyclin analogue.

Oxygen

Background

Oxygen is a selective pulmonary vasodilator by virtue of its effect on hypoxic pulmonary vasoconstriction. Although Euler and Liljestrand first described this reflex in 1946[87], the precise mechanism has still not been elucidated. It is thought to be involved in the development of pulmonary hypertension in chronic hypoxic lung disease (see previous chapter).

Clinical studies

Oxygen treatment should be considered in all patients with pulmonary hypertension who are hypoxic at rest or desaturate with exercise. This is most important in those with raised pulmonary artery pressure as a result of chronic obstructive pulmonary disease, in whom two large multicentre controlled studies have shown a marked improvement in disease progression and mortality with long term oxygen therapy (15 to 17 hours/day). However, the improvement in survival was not clearly linked to an improvement in pulmonary haemodynamics. In the NOTT trial[88] there was a small decrease in pulmonary vascular resistance in the continuous oxygen therapy group compared to an increase in those receiving only nocturnal oxygen, but improved survival was only seen in those with an initially low pulmonary vascular resistance. In the British MRC study[89], mean pulmonary artery pressure increased by approximately 3 mmHg annually in the control group, whereas there was no change in the group treated with oxygen for 15 hours per day, but there was no direct link between pulmonary hemodynamics and survival. Later studies have demonstrated a fall in pulmonary artery pressure with oxygen therapy[90] and an association with improved survival[91]; however, some authors have considered the reduction in pulmonary artery pressure too small to account for the reduced mortality.

There is no evidence for anything other than a palliative role for oxygen in patients with primary pulmonary hypertension and other causes of secondary pulmonary hypertension. However, there is good reason to believe that similar benefits may occur in any chronic hypoxaemia state where hypoxic pulmonary vasoconstriction may be contributing to pulmonary artery pressure and right ventricular afterload. Therefore many clinicians would advocate prescribing long-term oxygen therapy in pulmonary hypertension where there is persistent hypoxia at rest. Those who become hypoxic with exercise should have oxygen available for short-term use.

Administration/adverse effects

The need for long-term oxygen therapy should be assessed in the usual way in line with national guidelines, bearing in mind the risk where there are smokers in the household. An oxygen concentrator is usually more cost effective, and the dose required should be reassessed at regular intervals.

Other vasodilators

A number of other oral vasodilators have been tried in the past and found wanting (see Table 18.8). There was particular interest in angiotensin-converting

Table 18.8. Other vasodilators

Angiotensin-converting enzyme inhibitors
Hydralazine
Diazoxide
Isoproterenol
Intravenous nitroglycerin

enzyme inhibitors initially but results were disappointing.

Anticoagulation

Most authors agree that, in the absence of any contraindications, all patients with significant pulmonary hypertension should be given anticoagulants to achieve an INR of 2[9,19].

In primary pulmonary hypertension, post mortem studies have shown the presence of thrombotic lesions with evidence of recanalization[92], and fresh intrapulmonary thrombus is frequently found in patients after sudden death. In a retrospective study, Fuster et al.[93] reported evidence of improved survival in those treated with anticoagulants. Rich et al.[39] demonstrated improved survival with warfarin treatment after subgroup analysis of a prospective study, in particular in those who did not respond to treatment with calcium channel blockers.

In secondary pulmonary hypertension the story is less clear, although many of these patients are at high risk of thromboembolism due to dilated right heart chambers and a low cardiac output state, venous insufficiency, secondary polycythemia, and relative. In connective tissue disease, where there may be antiphospholipid antibodies, there is some evidence from pathological studies of similar thrombotic lesions to those seen in primary pulmonary hypertension[8], but there are no studies of the effects of anticoagulant treatment upon outcome. Patients with pulmonary vascular disease due to proven or suspected recurrent thromboembolism should clearly be given anticoagulants. Where this is contra- indicated, insertion of a caval filter should be considered.

Inotropic agents

Cardiac glycosides

Cardiac glycosides have been widely prescribed by physicians treating pulmonary hypertension for many years. Their benefit in left ventricular dysfunction has been demonstrated[94], but there has been no clear evidence of a long term effect in right ventricular dysfunction. Some authors have advised against their use in cor pulmonale[95], while others have recommended their use to counter the negative inotropic effects of high dose calcium channel blockers in primary pulmonary hypertension[40].

Several small controlled trials have failed to show an improvement in haemodynamics and right ventricular function with conventional doses of digoxin. Brown et al. found no significant change in exercise tolerance or right ventricular ejection fraction at rest or during exercise in 12 patients with stable chronic airflow obstruction[96]. Another study looking at 15 patients with severe chronic airflow obstruction found an improvement in right ventricular ejection fraction after 8 weeks of digoxin treatment, but only in those individuals with a coexisting reduction in left ventricular ejection fraction[97]. Aubier et al. studied the effects of an intravenous infusion of digoxin on eight artificially ventilated patients with acute respiratory failure and chronic airflow obstruction[98]. They had a mean pulmonary artery pressure of 39 mmHg and normal cardiac output measurements at baseline. There was a significant improvement in diaphragmatic strength during supramaximal electrical stimulation, but no change in hemodynamics.

More recently, Rich et al. studied the effects of a 1 mg intravenous infusion on seventeen patients with severe primary pulmonary hypertension and normal left ventricular function[99]. Subjects had a mean pulmonary artery pressure of 61 mmHg and a mean cardiac output of 3.49 litres/minute and served as their own controls. They found a 10% rise in cardiac output with a similar rise in mean pulmonary artery pressure and no change in pulmonary vascular resistance. There was a reduction in circulating norepinephrine and an unexpected rise in atrial natriuretic peptide levels. There were no adverse effects. There have been no studies to date for the long term effects of digoxin in pulmonary hypertension.

Beta agonists

Isoproterenol, a beta 2-adrenoceptor agonist, has been shown to increase cardiac output in patients with primary pulmonary hypertension with no effect on pulmonary artery pressure, and therefore a reduction in calculated pulmonary vascular resistance[100]. It was initially thought to act as a vasodilator, but its effects are probably more easily explained by a direct inotropic effect. There is a theoretical risk of inducing right ventricular ischaemia with beta agonists by a chronotropic effect that has been implicated in patients with congestive heart failure[101], although small uncontrolled studies have shown sustained symptomatic benefit with sublingual isoproterenol[102].

Dopamine and dobutamine may be useful in the event of acute deterioration of right ventricular function, but insufficient evidence is available in pulmonary hypertension to make any recommendations.

Diuretics

Diuretics are useful in right heart failure due to pulmonary hypertension, to reduce excessive right ventricular preload and control edema. Their role is probably purely palliative, with no evidence of a beneficial effect on survival. However, they should be administered with caution for a number of reasons. First, patients with pulmonary hypertension depend upon a high filling pressure to maintain right ventricular cardiac output, and it is safer to err

on the side of fluid overload than hypovolemia and risk exacerbating postural hypotension.

Secondly, the presence and degree of edema is a useful clinical sign of disease progression or response to treatment. It is better to see edema resolve following more intensive vasodilator therapy than with the addition of a diuretic.

Thirdly, a diuresis may raise the haematocrit and increase the risk of intravascular thrombosis in patients already at increased risk of thromboembolism.

If diuretics are prescribed or the dose modified, patients should be carefully monitored and encouraged to weigh themselves at frequent intervals.

Antiarrhythmics

There have been no studies looking for a beneficial effect on survival with the use of prophylactic antiarrhythmics in patients with pulmonary hypertension. There is no evidence that calcium channel blockers (see above) reduce the risk of life-threatening rhythm disturbances, and no other antiarrhythmic drugs have been widely prescribed.

Venesection

Venesection has been shown to improve exercise tolerance in polycythemic patients with chronic obstructive pulmonary disease[103]. It has also been shown to lower pulmonary artery pressure and pulmonary vascular resistance and increase right ventricular ejection fraction in this group of patients[104]. It seems reasonable to expect similar benefits in all those with polycythemia secondary to chronic hypoxia.

Secondary pulmonary hypertension: specific points and treatment summary

It is important that the underlying disease process is treated at the same time, and this will often require joint management with other specialist services. Good communication is essential, especially before instituting prostacyclin therapy.

In the absence of contraindications, all patients should probably be started on anticoagulant therapy, although there is no evidence of benefit except in pulmonary thromboembolic disease. It seems likely that, where there is evidence of endothelial damage, there will be increased risk of *in situ* thrombosis, however the benefits of treating mild pulmonary hypertension have yet to be established.

Long-term oxygen therapy should be given to all those who are hypoxic at rest, and a cylinder of oxygen to those who desaturate with exercise.

Venesection should be considered in those with polycythaemia due to chronic hypoxia.

Connective tissue diseases

There is sufficient evidence of benefit from vasodilators for prostacyclin[42,79] and calcium channel blockers[8,59] to be considered in all patients. Those on immunosuppressive treatment may be at relatively high risk of infection while on intravenous prostacyclin although no link was found in the study by Humbert et al.[42]. Some of these patients have disabilities that may make management of a continuous infusion difficult.

Pulmonary thromboembolic disease

The effects of calcium channel blockers are unknown, but there is some evidence of a benefit from prostacyclin, especially in distal thromboembolism[79]. The possibility of thromboendarterectomy should always be considered (see later). If there is evidence of proximal pulmonary arterial thrombosis at perfusion scanning or angiography, a specialist surgical opinion should be sought. CT and MR angiography are also useful for excluding resectable thrombus. A search should be made for the source of thrombosis.

Chronic hypoxic lung disease

In spite of a number of studies, it remains unclear whether calcium channel blockers have a beneficial role to play in this group of patients[46,60–64]. Nifedipine appears to be the most effective overall, but a large prospective placebo-controlled trial will be required to resolve the issue. There have been no studies of the effects of prostacyclin. This is the only group of patients with pulmonary hypertension where oxygen has been shown to reduce disease progression and prolong survival[88–91].

Congenital heart disease

There is a theoretical risk of inducing right to left shunting and thereby worsening hypoxaemia with prostacyclin in patients with established Eisenmenger's syndrome, by preferential dilatation of the systemic vasculature. There have been few studies in this group of patients, but no adverse effects have been reported, and there is evidence of benefit with acute[83] and long-term therapy[79]. The effects of calcium channel blockers are unknown.

Pulmonary venous hypertension

A complete discussion on the management of pulmonary hypertension due to heart failure and valve disease is beyond the scope of this chapter. Calcium channel blockers are negatively inotropic which limits their usefulness. Although there is evidence of an improvement in hemodynamics acutely with prostacyclin in congestive heart failure[82], one recent study of long-term therapy was halted early due to an increased mortality in the treatment arm, and therefore this treatment cannot be recommended at the present time. Short-term infusion of prostacyclin has been reported to cause pulmonary edema in pulmonary veno-occlusive disease because of increased pulmonary perfusion in the presence of downstream vascular obstruction[73].

Portopulmonary hypertension

Two recent studies have suggested a beneficial long-term effect of prostacyclin on pulmonary haemodynamics in these patients, although this may have been at the expense of worsening liver disease[43,80]. More studies are needed before recommendations can be made. The effects of calcium channel blockers are unknown.

Human immunodeficiency virus infection (HIV)

There is increasing awareness that HIV infection predisposes towards the development of pulmonary hypertension, perhaps due to a direct effect of the virus on the pulmonary vasculature[105,106]. It is one of the commonest causes of the disease in France but at the time of writing there was only one case identified in the UK. All patients with unexplained pulmonary hypertension should be screened for HIV infection after appropriate counselling.

The long-term effects of calcium channel blockers are unknown, and the infection risk from an indwelling catheter for continuous intravenous prostacyclin would be unacceptable.

Surgical options

There are three surgical options currently available at a number of specialist centres for patients with pulmonary hypertension. The most recent development has been the success of pulmonary thromboendarterectomy in carefully selected patients

Transplant

The first heart–lung transplantation was performed in a patient with primary pulmonary hypertension[107], and this was the standard treatment for severe pulmonary hypertension until the advent of effective medical therapy in the past 15 years.

Nowadays, it is very much a treatment of last resort and should always be preceded by a trial of medical therapy. Survival rates are better than those of medical therapy for patients unresponsive to vasodilators, but slightly worse than medical therapy for those with a positive vasodilator response, with 1 year and 3 year survival rates of 70% and 47%, respectively[108]. There is little difference between single, double and heart/lung transplantation[19]. Early complications include acute graft rejection and infection, and the main late complication is chronic rejection (bronchiolitis obliterans syndrome) which occurs in between 35% and 50% of recipients. The timing of referral to a transplant centre is a difficult issue, and the shortage of organ donors is the principal rate-limiting step.

Atrial septostomy

Atrial septostomy appears to have a useful role in the management of patients with severe progressive pulmonary vascular disease after the failure of medical therapy, and in whom the atrial septum is intact. The natural history of pulmonary hypertension is rising pulmonary artery pressure, falling cardiac output and progressive right heart failure. Right atrial pressure correlates better than other hemodynamic indices with survival and there is evidence that primary pulmonary hypertension patients with a patent foramen ovale have better survival rates than those without[109]. The rationale for atrial septostomy is to artificially create a right to left shunt thereby increasing cardiac output and systemic oxygen delivery, and reducing right atrial pressure.

Rich and Lam first used this approach in 1983, and since then several investigators have reported a beneficial effect on pulmonary hemodynamics[110–113]. In 1998, the World Symposium on Primary Pulmonary Hypertension published guidelines after reviewing the evidence, and a suggested therapeutic algorithm is shown (Fig. 18.4)[4]. Relative contraindications are a mean right atrial pressure of more than 20 mmHg, a

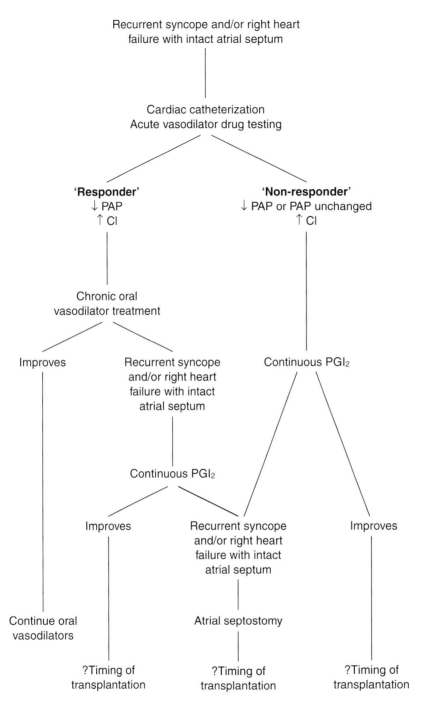

Fig. 18.4 Indications for performing palliative artrial septostomy in selected patients with advanced pulmonary vascular disease. PAP = pulmonary artery pressure; CI = cardiac index; PGI2 = prostacyclin I2.

pulmonary vascular resistance index of greater than 55 units/m^2, a predicted 1 year survival of less than 40%, and a systemic arterial oxygen saturation on room air of less than 90%. Unresolved issues include mechanism of action, optimal timing of intervention, choice of technique (blade balloon or graded balloon dilation), and long-term effects[114].

Thromboendarterectomy

In carefully selected patients with proximal thromboembolic disease demonstrated at angiography, the outcome of pulmonary endarterectomy is good. There is an increase in pulmonary blood flow and cardiac output, extended survival, and improved quality of life[115]. There is also evidence of resolution of peripheral thromboembolic disease postoperatively.

Monitoring

There are two aspects to monitoring these patients: pulmonary hemodynamics and exercise tolerance. Cardiac catheterization is invasive and carries a significant risk and an accurate and reproducible noninvasive method of measuring hemodynamics is needed. The best method currently available is echocardiography, but there are considerable difficulties in some groups of patients, in particular those with airways obstruction and the overweight. Exercise hemodynamics are difficult to assess with echocardiography, and cardiopulmonary exercise testing is useful, either with a simple 6-minute walk test or by means of formal cycle ergometry and analysis of expired gases. This approach not only gives a measure of exercise tolerance, but also provides variables that can be correlated with pulmonary artery pressure. Changes in chest radiograph appearance, electrocardiography and oxygen saturation may also be helpful, in addition to clinical assessment. Magnetic resonance imaging is also being increasingly used in some centres to assess pulmonary

Table 18.9. Negative prognostic factors in pulmonary hypertension

Negative acute vasodilator assessment
Worsening haemodynamics
Deteriorating exercise tolerance
Syncope
Pericardial effusion
SvO2 < 63%
Onset of right heart failure

blood flow characteristics, and right ventricular morphology and function[116,117]. Where there is evidence of significant disease progression, repeat cardiac catheterization may be necessary.

Prognosis

The overall prognosis for these patients remains poor, but recent advances are cause for optimism. Median survival after diagnosis was only 2.5 years in one series, but the use of anticoagulants, calcium channel blockers and prostacyclin has made an appreciable difference. A suggested management algorithm for pulmonary arterial hypertension (WHO classification) is shown in Fig. 18.2. Poor prognostic factors include worsening pulmonary hemodynamics and exercise tolerance, a negative acute vasodilator assessment, signs of right heart failure, arrhythmias, a pericardial effusion and a mixed venous oxygen saturation below 63%[4,39,58,75] (Table 18.9). Death is most often due to progressive right heart failure and arrhythmias.

Pulmonary hypertension in children

Introduction

There are important differences in the causes and management of pulmonary hypertension between children and adults. What follows serves as an introduction to the drug treatment of the disorder, and the reader requiring detailed information is referred to the following reviews[118–121].

The commonest causes of childhood pulmonary hypertension are persistent pulmonary hypertension of the newborn and congenital heart defects: however, all of the known causes of adult disease have been recognized in children (see Table 18.1). Primary pulmonary hypertension (PPH) is a much less common diagnosis in children than in adults.

Persistent pulmonary hypertension of the newborn

This is a syndrome of persistently raised pulmonary vascular resistance and diminished pulmonary vasoreactivity shortly after birth, causing right to left shunting of blood through the foramen ovale and patent ductus arteriosus, and often resulting in severe hypoxemia. There may be a clearly defined precipitant such as meconium aspiration or sepsis, or it may be idiopathic.

Treatment has until recently been supportive concentrating on oxygen delivery and maintenance of systemic blood pressure. Vasodilator drug therapy has been hampered by the lack of a selective pulmonary vasodilator, but the discovery of nitric oxide has raised the prospect of lowering pulmonary vascular resistance without causing systemic vasodilation. Inhaled nitric oxide has been shown to improve gas exchange in term or near term infants, and reduce the need for extracorporeal membrane oxygenation (ECMO)[119,122]. However, a beneficial effect on survival has not been shown.

Congenital heart defects

Any cardiac abnormalities with potential for left to right shunting may cause pulmonary hypertension, and an estimated 30% of individuals with a congenital lesion will go on to develop clinically significant pulmonary vascular disease[123]. The age at which this happens depends mainly upon the type of defect, but also upon the presence of concomitant chronic lung disease such as cystic fibrosis. Symptoms may not occur until adult life, or may be evident before the end of the first year.

Clearly, the most effective treatment is early surgical repair of the defect; however, medical therapy is still needed when there is established or progressive pulmonary vascular disease, or where an Eisenmenger's complex has developed.

Treatment should be with anticoagulation, correction of hypoxia and venesection. No vasodilator has yet been studied in a placebo-controlled trial, but there is evidence of a role for inhaled nitric oxide as a diagnostic and therapeutic agent[120]. There have also been reports of a synergistic effect on pulmonary vasodilation of nitric oxide and oral beraprost, a prostacyclin analogue[124].

Primary pulmonary hypertension

The pathophysiology of primary pulmonary hypertension in children is similar to that of the disorder in adults, and the same investigations should be performed, including an acute vasodilator assessment (see above). Unlike adults, where less than 30% respond with a fall in mean pulmonary artery pressure and pulmonary vascular resistance[9,19], over 40% of children have a positive response and should be treated with oral calcium channel blockers. The remainder, including all those responders who fail to improve on oral therapy, should be offered continuous intravenous prostacyclin.

The use of vasodilators has revolutionized the prognosis of children with pulmonary hypertension. Using this approach, Barst et al. reported 3-year survival rates of 97%, 94% and 92%, respectively, for responders on oral therapy, responders on oral and intravenous therapy and non-responders on intravenous therapy alone[125]. This compares with a median survival of only ten months for children in the NIH Registry[58]. All patients should also be treated with warfarin, digoxin, diuretics and oxygen if required.

REFERENCES

1 Romberg E. Uber sklerose der Lungen arterie. *Dtsch Archiv Klin Med* 1891; 48:197–206.

2 Dresdale DT, Schultz M, Michtom RJ. Primary pulmonary hypertension: clinical and haemodynamic study. *Am J Med* 1951; 11:686–705.

3 Rubin L. ACCP consensus statement: primary pulmonary hypertension. *Chest* 1987; 104:236–250.

4 Rich S, ed. *Primary Pulmonary Hypertension: Executive Summary from the World Symposium–Primary Pulmonary Hypertension 1998.* Available from the World Health Organisation via the Internet (*http://www.who.int/ncd/cvd/pph.html*).

5 Loyd JE, Butler MG, Foroud TM, Conneally PM, Phillips JA III, Newman JH. Genetic anticipation and abnormal gender ratio at birth in familial primary pulmonary hypertension. *Am J Respir Crit Care Med* 1995; 152:93–97.

6 Rich S, Dantzker DR, Ayres SM et al. Primary pulmonary hypertension: a national prospective study. *Ann Intern Med* 1987; 107:216–223.

7 Loyd JE, Atkinson JB, Pietra GG, Virmani R, Newman JH. Heterogeneity of pathologic lesions in familial primary pulmonary hypertension. *Am Rev Respir Dis* 1988; 138:952–957.

8 Sanchez O, Humbert M, Sitbon O, Simonneau G. Treatment of pulmonary hypertension secondary to connective tissue diseases. *Thorax* 1999; 54:273–277.

9 Gaine SP. Rubin LJ. Primary pulmonary hypertension. *Lancet* 1998; 352:719–725.

10 Rubin LJ. Primary pulmonary hypertension. *N Engl J Med* 1997; 336:111–117.

11 Raeside DA, Chalmers G, Clelland J, Madhok R, Peacock AJ. Pulmonary artery pressure variation in patients with connective tissue disease: 24 hour ambulatory pulmonary artery pressure monitoring. *Thorax* 1998; 53:857–862.

12 Nicod P, Peterson K, Levine M et al. Pulmonary angiography in severe chronic pulmonary hypertension. *Ann Intern Med* 1987; 107:565–568.

13 Barst RJ. Pharmacologically induced pulmonary vasodilation in children and young adults with primary pulmonary hypertension. Chest 1986; 89:497–503.

14 Groves BM, Badesh DB, Turkevitch D et al. Correlation of acute prostacyclin response in primary (unexplained) pulmonary hypertension with efficacy of treatment with calcium channel blockers and survival. In: Hume JR, Reeves JT, Weir EK, eds. *Ion Flux in Pulmonary Vascular Control.* New York: Plenum Press; 1993:317–330.

15 Rhodes J, Barst R, Garofano RP, Thoele DG, Gersony WM. Haemodynamic correlates of exercise function in patients with primary pulmonary hypertension. *J Am Coll Cardiol* 1991; 18:1738–1744.

16 Rich S, Kaufman E. High dose titration of calcium channel blockers for primary pulmonary hypertension: guidelines for short-term drug testing. *J Am Coll Cardiol* 1991; 18:1323–1328.

17 Rozkovec A, Stradling J, Shepherd G, MacDermot J, Oakley CM, Dollery CT. Prediction of favourable responses to long term vasodilator treatment of pulmonary hypertension by short term administration of epoprostenol (prostacyclin) or nifedipine. *Br Heart J* 1988; 59:696–705.

18 Weir EK, Rubin LJ, Ayres SM et al. The acute administration of vasodilators in primary pulmonary hypertension. Experience from the National Institutes of Health Registry on Primary Pulmonary Hypertension. *Am Rev Respir Dis* 1989; 140:1623–1630.

19 Peacock AJ. Primary pulmonary hypertension. *Thorax* 1999; 54:0–12.

20 Sitbon O, Umbert M, Jagot JL et al. Inhaled nitric oxide as a screening agent for safely identifying responders to calcium channel blockers in primary pulmonary hypertension. *Eur Respir J* 1998; 12:265–270.

21 Jolliet P, Bulpa P, Thorens JB, Ritz M, Chevrolet JC. Nitric oxide and prostacyclin as test agents of vasoreactivity in severe precapillary pulmonary hypertension: predictive ability and consequences on haemodynamics and gas exchange. *Thorax* 1997; 52:369–372.

22 Morgan JM, McCormack DG, Griffiths MJD, Morgan CJ, Barnes PJ, Evans TW. Adenosine as a vasodilator in primary pulmonary hypertension. *Circulation* 1991; 84:1145–1149.

23 Baer S, Schrader BJ, Kaufman E. Effects of adenosine in combination with calcium channel blockers in patients with primary pulmonary hypertension. *J Am Coll Cardiol* 1993; 21:413–418.

24 Rubin LJ, Groves BM, Reeves JT, Frosolono M, Handel F, Cato AE. Prostacyclin-induced acute pulmonary vasodilation in primary pulmonary hypertension. *Circulation* 1982; 66:334–338.

25 Mikhail G, Gibbs SR, Richardson M et al. An evaluation of nebulised prostacyclin in patients with primary or secondary pulmonary hypertension. *Eur Heart J* 1997; 18:1499–1504.

26 Furchgott R, Zawadzki J. The obligatory role of endothelial cells in the relaxation of arterial smooth muscle by acetylcholine. *Nature* 1980; 288:373–376.

27 Palmer RMJ, Ferrige AG, Moncada S. Nitric oxide release

accounts for the biological activity of endothelium-derived relaxing factor. *Nature* 1987; 327:524–526.

28 Ignarro LJ, Buga GM, Wood KS et al. Endothelium-derived relaxing factor produced and released from artery and vein is nitric oxide. *Proc Natl Acad Sci USA* 1987; 84:9265–9269.

29 Sitbon O, Brenot F, Denjean A et al. Inhaled nitric oxide as a screening vasodilator agent in primary pulmonary hypertension: a dose-response study and comparison with prostacyclin. *Am J Respir Crit Care Med* 1995; 151:384–389.

30 Williamson DJ, Hayward C, Rogers P et al. Acute hemodynamic responses to inhaled nitric oxide in patients with limited scleroderma and isolated pulmonary hypertension. *Circulation* 1996; 94:477–482.

31 Pepke-Zaba J, Higenbottam TW, Dinh-Xuan AT, Stone D, Wallwork J. Inhaled nitric oxide as a cause of selective pulmonary vasodilation in pulmonary hypertension. *Lancet* 1991; 338:1173–1174.

32 Frostell CG, Blomqvist H, Hedenstierna G, Lundberg J, Zapol WM. Inhaled nitric oxide selectively reverses human hypoxic pulmonary vasoconstriction without causing systemic vasodilation. *Anaesthesiology* 1993; 78:427–435.

33 Adnot S, Kouyoumdjian C, Defouilloy C et al. Hemodynamic and gas exchange responses to infusion of acetylcholine and inhalation of nitric oxide in patients with chronic obstructive lung disease and pulmonary hypertension. *Am Rev Respir Dis* 1993; 148:310–316.

34 Atz MA, Adatia I, Lock JE, Wessel DL. Combined effects of nitric oxide and oxygen during acute pulmonary vasodilator testing. *J Am Coll Cardiol* 1999; 33:813–819.

35 Kneussl MP, Lang IM, Brenot FP. Medical management of primary pulmonary hypertension. *Eur Respir J* 1996; 9:2401–2409.

36 Nootens M, Schrader B, Kaufmann E, Vestal R, Long W, Rich S. Comparative acute effects of adenosine and prostacyclin in primary pulmonary hypertension. *Chest* 1995; 107:54–57.

37 Schrader B, Inbar S, Kaufmann L, Vestal RE, Rich S. Comparison of the effects of adenosine and nifedipine in pulmonary hypertension. *J Am Coll Cardiol* 1992; 19:1060–1064.

38 Inbar S, Schrader BJ, Kaufmann E, Vestal R, Rich S. The effects of adenosine in combination with calcium channel blockers in patients with primary pulmonary hypertension. *J Am Coll Cardiol* 1993; 21:413–418.

39 Rich S, Kaufman E, Levy PS. The effect of high doses of calcium channel blockers on survival in primary pulmonary hypertension. *N Engl J Med* 1992; 327:76–81.

40 Rich S, Brundage BH. High-dose calcium channel-block-ing therapy for primary pulmonary hypertension: evidence for long-term reduction in pulmonary arterial pressure and regression of right ventricular hypertrophy. *Circulation* 1987; 76:135–141.

41 Packer M, Medina N, Yushak M. Adverse haemodynamic and clinical effects of calcium channel blockade in pulmonary hypertension secondary to obliterative pulmonary vascular disease. *J Am Coll Cardiol* 1984; 4:890–901.

42 Humbert M, Sanchez O, Fartoukh M et al. Short-term and long-term epoprostenol (prostacyclin) therapy in pulmonary hypertension secondary to connective tissue diseases: results of a pilot study. *Eur Respir J* 1999; 13:1351–1356.

43 Krowka MJ, Frantz RP, McGoon MD, Severson C, Plevak DJ, Wiesner RH. Improvement in pulmonary haemodynamics during intravenous epoprostenol (prostacyclin): a study of 15 patients with moderate to severe portopulmonary hypertension. *Hepatology* 1999; 30:641–648.

44 Rubin LJ, Peter RH. Oral hydralazine therapy for primary pulmonary hypertension. *N Engl J Med* 1980; 302:69.

45 Rich S, Brundage BH, Levy PS. The effect of vasodilator therapy on the clinical outcome of patients with primary pulmonary hypertension. *Circulation* 1985; 71:1191–1196.

46 Peacock AJ. The role of vasodilators in treating pulmonary hypertension secondary to hypoxic lung disease. In: Peacock AJ 1996 *Pulmonary Circulation*. Chapman and Hall 16; 195–209.

47 Weitzenblum E, Kessler R, Oswald M. Medical treatment of pulmonary hypertension in chronic lung disease. *Eur Respir J* 1994; 7:148–152.

48 Salvaterra CG, Rubin LJ. Investigation and management of pulmonary hypertension in chronic obstructive pulmonary disease. *Am Rev Respir Dis* 1993; 148:1414–1417.

49 Macnee W, Wathen C, Flenley DC, Muir AD. The effects of controlled oxygen therapy on ventricular function in patients with stable and decompensated cor pulmonale. *Am Rev Respir Dis* 1988; 137:1289–1295.

50 Macnee W. Pathophysiology of cor pulmonale in chronic obstructive pulmonary disease (part two). *Am J Respir Crit Care Med* 1994; 150:1158–1168.

51 Weitzenblum E, Loiseau A, Hirth C, Mirhom R, Rasaholinjanahary J. Course of pulmonary haemodynamics in patients with chronic obstructive pulmonary disease. *Chest* 1979; 75:656–662.

52 Weitzenblum E, Sautegeau A, Ehrhart M, Mammosser M, Pelletier A. Long term course of pulmonary pressure in chronic obstructive pulmonary disease. *Am Rev Respir Dis* 1984; 130:993–998.

53 Traver G, Cline MG, Burrow S. Predictors of mortality in chronic obstructive pulmonary disease. *Am Rev Respir Dis* 1979; 119:895–902.

54 Cooper R, Ghali J, Simmons BE, Castaner A. Elevated pulmonary artery pressure: an independant predictor of mortality. *Chest* 1991; 99:112–120.

55 Opie LH. International Society and Federation of Cardiology: Working group on classification of calcium antagonists for cardiovascular disease. *Am J Cardiol* 1987; 80:630–632.

56 Rubin LJ, Nicod P, Hillis LD, Firth BG. Treatment of primary pulmonary hypertension with nifedipine. *Ann Intern Med* 1983; 99:433–438.

57 Olivari M, Levine T, Weir E, Cohn J. Haemodynamic effects of nifedipine at rest and during exercise in primary pulmonary hypertension. *Chest* 1984; 86:14–19.

58 D'Alonzo GE, Barst RJ, Ayres SM et al. Survival in patients with primary pulmonary hypertension: results from a National Prospective Registry. *Ann Intern Med* 1991; 115:343–349.

59 Alpert MA, Pressly TA, Mukerji V et al. Acute and long term effects of nifedipine on pulmonary and systemic haemodynamics in patients with pulmonary hypertension associated with diffuse systemic sclerosis, the CREST syndrome and mixed connective tissue disease. *Am J Cardiol* 1991; 68:1687–1691.

60 Agustoni P, Doria E, Galli C, Tamborini G, Guazzi MD. Nifedipine reduces pulmonary pressue and vasodilator tone during short but not long term treatment of pulmonary hypertension in patients with chronic obstructive pulmonary disease. *Am Rev Respir Dis* 1989; 139:120–125.

61 Karla L, Bone MF. Effect of nifedipine on physiological shunting and oxygenation in chronic obstructive pulmonary disease. *Am J Med* 1993; 94:419–423.

62 Melot C, Hallemans R, Naeije R, Mols P, Lejeune P. Deleterious effect of nifedipine on pulmonary gas exchange in chronic obstructive pulmonary disease. *Am Rev Respir Dis* 1984; 130:612–616.

63 Mookherjee S, Ashutosh K, Dunsky M et al. Nifedipine in chronic cor pulmonale: acute and relatively long term effects. *Clin Pharmacol Ther* 1988; 44:289–296.

64 Sajkov D, Wang T, Frith PA, Bune AJ, Alpers JA, McEvoy RD. A comparison of two long acting vasoselective calcium antagonists in pulmonary hypertension secondary to COPD. *Chest* 1997; 111(6):1622–1630.

65 Batra AK, Segall PH, Ahmed T. Pulmonary edema with nifedipine in primary pulmonary hypertension. *Respiration* 1985; 47:161–163.

66 Moncada S, Gryglewski R, Bunting S, Vane JR. An enzyme isolated from arteries transforms prostaglandin endoperoxides to an unstable substance that inhibits platelet aggregation. *Nature* 1976; 263:663–665.

67 Johnson RA, Lincoln FH, Thompson JL, Nidy EG, Mizak SA, Axen U. Synthesis and stereochemistry of prostacyclin and synthesis of 6-keto-prostaglandin F1-alpha. *J Am Chem Soc* 1977; 99:4182–4184.

68 Moncada S, Herman AG, Higgs EA, Vane JR. Differential formation of prostacyclin (PGX or PGI2) by layers of the arterial wall. An explanation for the anti-thrombotic of vascular endothelium. *Thromb Res* 1977; 11:323–344.

69 Blair IA, Barrow SE, Wadell KA, Lewis PJ, Dollery CT. Prostacyclin is not a circulating hormone in man. *Prostaglandins* 1982; 23:579–589.

70 Jones K. Prostacyclin. In Peacock AJ 1996 *Pulmonary Circulation.* Chapman and Hall 9; 115–122.

71 Higenbottam T, Wheeldon D, Wells F, Wallwork J. Long-term treatment of primary pulmonary hypertension with continuous intravenous epoprostenol (prostacyclin). *Lancet* 1984; 1046–1047.

72 Jones DK, Higenbottam TW, Wallwork J. Treatment of primary pulmonary hypertension with intravenous epoprostenol (prostacyclin). *Br Heart J* 1987; 57:270–278.

73 Rubin LJ, Mendoza J, Hood M et al. Treatment of primary pulmonary hypertension with continuous intravenous prostacyclin (epoprostenol): results of a randomised trial. *Ann Intern Med* 1990; 112:485–491.

74 Barst RJ, Rubin LJ, McGoon MD, Caldwell EJ, Long WA, Levy PS. Survival in primary pulmonary hypertension with long term continuous intravenous prostacyclin. *Ann Intern Med* 1994; 121:409–415.

75 Barst RJ, Rubin LJ, Long WA et al. A comparison of continuous intravenous epoprostenol (prostacyclin) with conventional therapy for primary pulmonary hypertension. *N Engl J Med* 1996; 334:296–301.

76 McLaughlin VV, Genthner DE, Panella MM, Rich S. Reduction in pulmonary vascular resistance with long-term epoprostenol (prostacyclin) therapy in primary pumonary hypertension. *N Engl J Med* 1998; 338:273–277.

77 Friedman R, Mears G, Barst RJ. Continuous infusion of prostacyclin normalizes plasma markers of endothelial cell injury and platelet aggregation in primary pulmonary hypertension. *Circulation* 1997; 96:2782–2784.

78 Hinderliter AL, Willis PW 4th, Barst RJ et al. Effects of long term infusion of prostacyclin (epoprostenol) on echocardiographic measures of right ventricular structure and function in primary pulmonary hypertension. Primary

Pulmonary Hypertension Study Group. *Circulation* 1997; 95(6):1479–1486.

79 McLaughlin VV, Genthner DE, Panella MM, Hess DM, Rich S. Compassionate use of continuous prostacyclin in the management of secondary pulmonary hypertension: a case series. *Ann Intern Med.* 1999; 130:740–743.

80 Kuo PC, Plotkin JS, Rubin LJ. Distinctive clinical features of portopulmonary hypertension. *Chest* 1997; 112:980–986.

81 Jones K, Higenbottam T, Wallwork J. Pulmonary vasodilation with prostacyclin in primary and secondary pulmonary hypertension. *Chest* 1989; 96:784–789.

82 Yui Y, Nakajima H, Kawai C, Murakami T. Prostacyclin therapy in patients with congestive heart failure. *Am J Cardiol* 1982; 50:320–324.

83 Bush A, Busst C, Knight WB, Shinebourne EA. Modification of pulmonary hypertension secondary to congenital heart disease by prostacyclin therapy. *Am Rev Respir Dis* 1987; 136:767–769.

84 Pickles H, O'Grady J. Side effects occurring during administration of epoprostenol (prostacyclin, PGI2) in man. *Br J Clin Pharmacol* 1982; 14:177–185.

85 Humbert M, Maitre S, Capron F, Rain B, Musset D, Simonneau G. Pulmonary edema complicating continuous intravenous prostacyclin in pulmonary capillary hemangiomatosis. *Am J Respir Crit Care Med* 1998; 157:1681–1685.

86 Saji T, Ozawa Y, Ishikita T, Matsuura H, Matsuo N. Short-term haemodynamic effect of a new oral PGI2 analogue, Beraprost, in primary and secondary pulmonary hypertension. *Am J Cardiol* 1996; 78:244–247.

87 Euler U.S Von and Liljestrand G. Observations on the pulmonary arterial blood pressure in the cat. *Acta Physiol Scand* 1946; 12:301–320.

88 Nocturnal Oxygen Therapy Trial Group. Continuous or nocturnal oxygen therapy in hypoxemic chronic obstructive lung disease. *Ann Intern Med* 1980; 93:391–398.

89 Report of the Medical Research Council Working Party. Long-term domiciliary oxygen therapy in chronic hypoxic cor pulmonale complicating chronic bronchitis and emphysema. *Lancet* 1981; 1:681–685.

90 Weitzenblum E, Sautegeau A, Ehrhart M, Mamosser M, Pelletier A. Long-term oxygen therapy can reverse the progression of pulmonary hypertension in patients with chronic obstructive pulmonary disease. *Am Rev Respir Dis* 1985; 131:493–498.

91 Timms R, Khaja F, Williams G and The Nocturnal Oxygen Therapy Trial Group. Hemodynamic response to oxygen therapy in chronic obstructive pulmonary disease. *Ann Intern Med* 1985; 102:29–36.

92 Bjornsson J, Edwards WD. Primary pulmonary hypertension: a histopathologic study of 80 cases. *Mayo Clin Proc* 1985; 60:16–25.

93 Fuster V, Steele PM, Edwards WD, Gersh BJ, McGoon MD, Frye RL. Primary pulmonary hypertension: natural history and the importance of thrombosis. *Circulation* 1984; 70:580–587

94 Packer M, Gheorghiade M, Young JB et al. Withdrawal of digoxin from patients with chronic heart failure treated with angiotensin converting enzyme inhibitors. *N Engl J Med* 1993; 329:1–7.

95 Green LH, Smith TW. The use of digitalis in patients with pulmonary disease. *Ann Intern Med* 1977; 87:459.

96 Brown SE, Pakron FJ, Milne N et al. Effects of digoxin on exercise capacity and right ventricular function during exercise in chronic airflow obstruction. *Chest* 1984; 85:187–191.

97 Mathur PN, Powles P, Pugsley SO, McEwan MP, Campbell MEJ. Effect of digoxin on right ventricular function in severe chronic airflow obstruction: a controlled clinical trial. *Ann Intern Med* 1981; 95:283–288.

98 Aubier M, Murciano D, Viires N et al. Effects of digoxin on diaphragmatic strength generation in patients with chronic obstructive pulmonary disease during acute respiratory failure. *Am Rev Respir Dis* 1987; 135:544–548.

99 Rich S, Seidlitz M, Dodin E et al. The short-term effects of digoxin in patients with right ventricular dysfunction from pulmonary hypertension. *Chest* 1998; 114:787–792.

100 Shettigar UR, Hultgren HN, Specter M, Martin R, Davier DH. Primary pulmonary hypertension: favourable effects of isoproterenol. *N Engl J Med* 1976:1414–1415.

101 Curlman G. Inotropic therapy for heart failure. An unfulfilled promise. *N Engl J Med* 1991; 325:1509–1510.

102 Di Pietro DA, La Bresh KA, Shulman RM, Foland ED, Parisi AF, Sashara AA. Sustained improvement in primary pulmonary hypertension during six years of treatment with sublingual isoproterenol. *N Engl J Med* 1984; 310:1032–1034.

103 Wedzicha JA, Rudd RM, Apps, MC, Cotter FE, Newland AC, Empey DW. Erythrapheresis in patients with polycythaemia secondary to hypoxic lung disease. *Br Med J* 1983; 286:511–514.

104 Weisse AB, Moschos CB, Frank MJ, Levinson GE, Cannilla JE, Regan TJ. Haemodynamic effects of staged haematocrit reduction in patients with stable cor pulmonale and severely elevated haematocrit levels. *Am J Med* 1975; 58:92–98.

105 Mitchell DM. New developments in the pulmonary diseases affecting HIV infected individuals. *Thorax* 1995; 50:294–302.

106 Petitpret ZP, Brenot F, Azarian R. Pulmonary hypertension

patients with human immunodeficiency virus infection: comparison with primary pulmonary hypertension. *Circulation* 1994; 89:2722–2727.

107 Reitz BA, Wallwork JL, Hunt SA et al. Heart–lung transplantation. Successful therapy for those with pulmonary vascular disease. *N Engl J Med* 1982; 306:557–564.

108 Nootens M, Freels S, Kaufman E, Levy PS, Rich S. Timing of single lung transplantation for primary pulmonary hypertension. *J Heart Lung Transpl* 1994; 13:276–281.

109 Rozkovec A, Montanes P, Oakley CM. Factors that influence the outcome of primary pulmonary hypertension. *Br Heart J* 1986; 55:449–458.

110 Kerstein D, Levy PS, Hsu DT, Hordof AJ, Gersony WM, Barst RJ. Blade balloon atrial septostomy in patients with severe primary pulmonary hypertension. *Circulation* 1995; 91:2028–2035.

111 Rich S, Dodin E, McLaughlin VV. Usefulness of atrial septostomy as a treatment for primary pulmonary hypertension and guidelines for its application. *Am J Cardiol* 1997; 80:369–371.

112 Sandoval J, Gaspar J, Pulido T et al. Graded balloon atrial septostomy in severe primary pulmonary hypertension. *Intervent Cardiol* 1998; 32:297–304.

113 Rothman A, Sklansky MS, Lucas VW et al. Atrial septostomy as a bridge to lung transplantation in patients with severe pulmonary hypertension. *Am J Cardiol* 1999; 84:682–686.

114 Barst RJ. Role of atrial septostomy in the treatment of pulmonary vascular disease. *Thorax* 2000; 55:95–96.

115 Mayer E, Dahm M, Hake U et al. Mid-term results of pulmonary thromboendarterectomy for chronic thromboembolic pulmonary hypertension. *Ann Thorac Surg* 1996; 61:1788–1792.

116 Tardivon AA, Mousseaux E, Brenot F et al. Quantification of haemodynamics in primary pulmonary hypertension with magnetic resonance imaging. *Am J Respir Crit Care Med* 1994; 150:1075–1080.

117 Boxt LM. MR imaging of pulmonary hypertension and right ventricular dysfunction. *MRI Clin N Am* 1996 4, 2:307–325.

118 Abman SH. An overview of pulmonary hypertension in pediatrics. In: Peacock AJ 1996 *Pulmonary Circulation.* Chapman and Hall 32; 425–436.

119 Finer NN, Barrington KJ. Nitric oxide for respiratory failure in infants born at or near term. *The Cochrane Database of Systematic Reviews* 2000; Volume 1.

120 Atz AM, Wessel DL. Inhaled nitric oxide in the neonate with cardiac disease. *Sem Perinatol* 1997; 21(5):441–455.

121 Barst RJ. Recent advances in the treatment of pediatric pulmonary artery hypertension. *Pediat Clin of N Am* 1999 46(2):331–345.

122 Clark RH, Kuesser TJ, Walker MW, et al. Low-dose nitric oxide therapy for persistent pulmonary hypertension of the newborn. Clinical Inhaled Nitric Oxide Research Group. *N Engl J Med* 2000; 342(7):469–474.

123 Friedman WF. Proceedings of National Heart, Lung, and Blood Institute Pediatric Cardiology Workshop: pulmonary hypertension. *Pediatr Res* 1986; 20(9): 811–822.

124 Ichida F, Uese K, Hashimoto I et al. Acute effect of oral prostacyclin and inhaled nitric oxide on pulmonary hypertension in children. *J Cardiol* 1997; 29(4):217–224.

125 Barst RJ, Maislin G, Fishman AP. Vasodilator therapy for primary pulmonary hypertension in children. *Circulation* 1999; 99:1197–1208.

19

Future treatment of pulmonary vascular diseases

Norbert F. Voelkel, Mark W. Geraci and Steven Abman

Division of Pulmonary Sciences and Critical Care Medicine, University of Colorado Health Sciences Center, Denver, CO, USA

Introduction

Different parts of the pulmonary vasculature can be affected or involved during the course of a variety of lung diseases, for example, small pulmonary arteries show frequently *in situ* thrombosis and the capillary endothelium is leaky in the lungs of patients with the adult respiratory distress syndrome (ARDS)[1]. The pulmonary vasculature is certainly involved and structurally altered in COPD and emphysema[2,3]. There is pulmonary vascular involvement in eosinophilic granulomatosis[4], and it is often overlooked that there is significant vascular involvement in many forms of interstitial fibrosis, as well as in collagen vascular disorders[5,6]. Table 19.1 gives a list of lung diseases with pulmonary vascular involvement.

Pulmonary vascular remodelling is also a prominent feature of mitral valve stenosis, chronic left ventricular dysfunction, kyphoscoliosis and sleep apnea syndromes[7–9].

The recommendation for treatment of the pulmonary vascular disease component in these conditions has been and continues to be to treat the underlying primary lung disease. Unfortunately, some of the disorders that are associated with pulmonary hypertension or pulmonary vascular abnormalities are difficult to treat, for example interstitial lung diseases (ILD) or ARDS. On the other hand, treatment of patients with COPD with supplemental continuous oxygen has been shown to improve pulmonary hypertension (PH) and patient survival[10] yet it is not at all clear whether the patient survival is

Table 19.1. Pulmonary vascular involvement in lung diseases

Adult respiratory distress syndrome	small arteries, capillaries
Respiratory bronchiolitis	small precapillary arteries
COPD, emphysema	loss of capillaries, muscular arteries
Eosinophilic granuloma	precapillary arteries
ILD, including sarcoid	muscularization of arteries
Collagen vascular diseases	muscularization of arteries, plexiform lesions

causally related to a reduced pulmonary arterial pressure.

Against this backdrop it becomes clear that it is the group of pulmonary vascular diseases that more or less originate within the pulmonary vessels which require specific and new treatments. Pathogenetically, investigators in previous years have mainly considered pulmonary precapillary vasoconstriction, vascular injury and inflammation[11–13] as important factors that cause PH. Although treatment strategies can be built on these mechanisms no specific pulmonary vascular treatment regimens have been developed. A recent proposal for a new categorization of severe PH[14] makes a distinction between disease associated with angiogenic/endothelial cell proliferative diseases and stress-adaptive diseases (Fig. 19.1), i.e. a group of diseases where endovascular endothelial cell proliferation[15] is prominent and a group of disorders where vascular

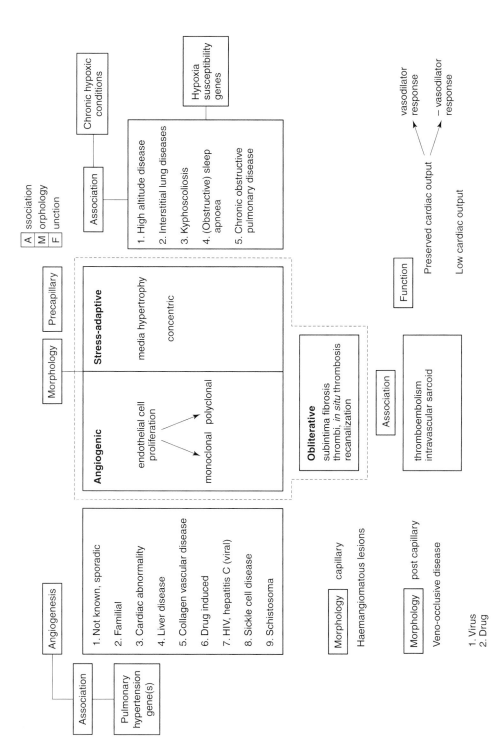

Fig. 19.1 Classification of severe pulmonary hypertension. Histology can separate an angiogenic form from a stress-adaptive form. The angiogenic manifestations include the so-called primary (sporadic) pulmonary hypertension and familial primary pulmonary hypertension. Angiogenic and stress-adaptive forms of pulmonary hypertension require different treatments. Patients with a preserved cardiac output have a better prognosis than those with a reduced cardiac output.

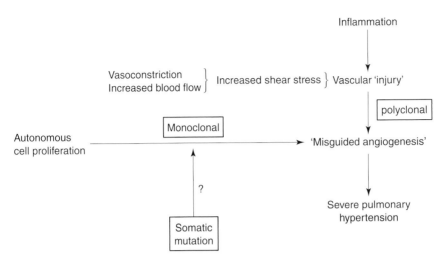

Fig. 19.2 Conceptually either increased shear stress or autonomous cell growth can explain mechanistically how obliterating lesions form in the small precapillary resistance vessels. Endothelial cell proliferation in 'primary' pulmonary hypertension is monoclonal but polyclonal in secondary forms of severe pulmonary hypertension.

media thickening is characteristic. Conceptually, these two groups probably require different treatments. If we consider the endothelium and the vascular smooth muscle a functional syncytium, then endothelial cell dysfunction or damage is likely to influence the behaviour of the VSMC, i.e. their role in vascular remodelling.

As a consequence of this syncytium concept treatment strategies should target the remodelled vessel as a whole. Fig. 19.2 organizes current concepts of the pathobiology of severe PH. The critical issue underlying our incomplete knowledge of the pathobiology of pulmonary hypertensive diseases is our lack of understanding of their natural history and the lack of animal models which display pulmonary plexogenic arteriopathy (Fig. 19.3, see colour plate section). The complete understanding of the pathobiology of severe PH requires the understanding of the initiating cellular and molecular events, the nature and role of progression factors and the final outcome. The final outcome clinically is right heart failure and we now appreciate that different patients – for identical degrees of PH – may have more or less efficient mechanisms of adaptation or compensation for the pressure overload[16].

Returning to pulmonary vascular remodelling and the pathobiology of severe PH (Fig. 19.4) we now know that plexiform pulmonary artery lesions occur as monoclonal endothelial cell proliferation in primary – spontaneous and familial – pulmonary hypertension (PPH), but in secondary PH the endothelial cell proliferation is polyclonal[17,18]. This strongly indicates that somatic endothelial cell mutations are a cause of endothelial cell proliferation in PPH. Hypothetically, proliferation of mutated endothelial cells could explain the vascular remodelling in PPH[19] – and one must not necessarily evoke vasoconstriction as a mechanism. A point mutation in the gene coding for the TGF-β II receptor has been identified in the endothelial cells microdissected from PPH patients' plexiform lesions[19]. In this context it is important to mention that only 25% of all patients with severe PH (at the time of their first heart catheter study) show a vasoreactive component. The traditional explanation for this fact is that the diagnosis of severe PH is always late, since there are no early symptoms. Although it is true that symptoms of dyspnea and fatigue are associated with severe hemodynamic compromise, an alternative hypothesis for the lack of a vascular reactive

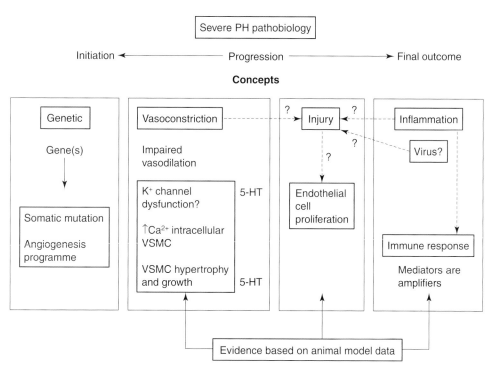

Fig. 19.4 This diagram attempts to synthesize the pathobiologically relevant elements of severe pulmonary hypertension. Genetic determinants are likely to play an important role. The pathogenetic concepts of vasoconstriction, endothelial cell injury and inflammation are based on animal model data only. The natural history of severe human pulmonary hypertension and therefore the factors responsible for initiation and progression of this disease are largely unknown.

component in many patients might be that vasoconstriction may not be important in these patients.

Treatment of the remodelled lung circulation

One treatment goal for severely pulmonary hypertensive states is to 'deremodel' the lung circulation. This probably implies the reversal of altered vascular cell phenotypes (Table 19.2).

This, in turn, may occur as the originally altered phenotype dies out or by reversing the selection pressure that has caused the emergence of the altered phenotype in the first place. As stated above, we still know too little about the process of vascular remodelling and the nature of the altered vascular

cell phenotype to recommend highly specific strategic targets. But if endothelial cells in the pulmonary hypertensive circulation break with the dogma of monolayer formation and resort to a phenotype that proliferates, forms clusters and finally pseudolumen very similar to an angiogenic process then antiangiogenesis treatment could be an option.

Angiogenesis factors

Angiogenesis is a complex process where a large number of factors are activated at the site and interact towards endothelial cell growth, smooth muscle cell migration and recruitment of pericytes. Although angiogenesis associated with inflammatory processes or associated with wound healing may differ from PH angiogenesis, activated macrophages

Table 19.2. Endothelial cell pulmonary hypertensive (proliferative?) phenotype

VEGF	+	Prostacyclin	−
KDR	+	synthase	
Angiopoetin	+	Prostacyclin	−
5-LO	+	receptor	
FLAP	+	p27	−
HIF-1α	+	PPARγ	−
ARNT	+		
Endothelin	+		

Note:

Present or increased gene expression: +.

absent or reduced gene expression: −.

and the action of growth factors are common to all these forms of angiogenesis[20–25]. Table 19.3 lists some of the angiogenesis factors.

Of these factors VEGF, its receptor KDR and angiopoetin II and its receptor Tie/Tek have been localized to the plexiform lesions[26]. There is also overexpression of eNOS in these lesions[27]. Whether any other factor listed above is expressed in the vascular lesions is presently unknown. Antibodies directed against VEGF have been shown to enhance hypoxic pulmonary hypertension in rats[28] and short-term adenovirus-VEGF-gene expression conversely has reduced chronic hypoxic pulmonary hypertension[29]. However, these experiments do not reflect on angiogenesis since angiogenesis is not a feature of hypoxic pulmonary hypertension in rodents; rather VEGF likely reduces pulmonary hypertension via NO production[30]. In contrast, anti-VEGF treatment inhibits granulomatous blood vessel growth in vivo. Conceptually blockers of the VEGF receptor KDR, which block the receptor's kinase activity[31], could be used to inhibit VEGF driven pulmonary vascular angiogenesis. However, experiments using a KDR blocker in rats show that chronic KDR blockade causes pulmonary arterial VSMC growth and increases pulmonary arterial pressures[32]. Drugs with this activity profile are currently in cancer treatment trials. Angiostatin is an endogenous angiogenesis inhibitor[33] that also might have future therapeutic potential, matrix metalloprotease inhibitors potentially would also be useful as angiogenesis inhibitors[34].

Inhibitors of metalloproteinases

The breakdown of extracellular matrix by metalloproteinases is important for initiation and progression of angiogenesis[34]. It has been shown that a number of matrix metalloproteinase inhibitors block angiogenesis induced by carcinoma cells implanted in the cornea[35]. In addition, VEGF can upregulate the expression of matrix metalloproteinases in vascular smooth muscle cells[21]. The group of Rabinovitch has shown inhibition of pulmonary vascular remodelling in rats made pulmonary hypertensive with the alkaloid monocrotaline treating the animals with a selective serine elastase inhibitor[36–40].

Inhibitors of inflammation

Presently treatment of inflammation is not a consideration in the clinical management of severe PH – although calcium entry blockers, especially in higher doses, may have anti-inflammatory actions. The evidence for the presence of inflammation in severe PH comes from the examination of lung tissue and plasma samples. Inflammatory cells are clearly present in the complex vascular lesions and clusters of macrophages surround small, remodelled arteries[15–41] (Table 19.4).

What remains unclear is whether the accumulation of inflammatory cells in the vascular lesions – and for that matter the increased levels of cytokines (in particular IL-1 and IL-6[43]) – are cause or consequence of the vascular remodelling. The presence of lymphocytes may be consistent with a local immune response. If so, then what are the antigens? The presence of inflammatory cells may be part of the angiogenic process and activated macrophages may amplify angiogenic activity. In addition, the expression of 5- and 15-lipoxygenase by endothelial cells in lungs from patients with severe PH[44,45] may indicate that the altered endothelial cell has assumed a role

Table 19.3. Angiogenic growth factors

Growth factor	Cell source	Target cells and major action
Basic fibroblast growth factor – bFGF	Macrophages Endothelial cells	Angiogenesis Fibroblast proliferation
Acidic fibroblast growth factor – aFGF	Macrophages Endothelial cells	Angiogenesis Fibroblast Proliferation
Vascular endothelial growth factor – VEGF	Epithelial cells Macrophages Neutrophils Platelets	Endothelial cell growth Increased vascular permeability Increased expression of 　metalloproteinases
Leptin	Adipose tissue cells	Endothelial cell growth
Platelet activating factor – PAF	Inflammatory cells	Increased VEGF expression Angiogenesis
Tumour necrosis factor – TNF	Inflammatory cells	Increased PAF expression Angiogenesis
Nitric oxide synthase – NOS	Endothelial cells	Angiogenesis
Insulin-like growth factor I – IGF-1	Fibroblast	Endothelial cell growth
Angiopoetin I – Ang 1		Maturation of vessel
Angiopoetin II – Ang 2	Vascular smooth muscle cells	Antagonist of Ang-1
Ephrin B2	Endothelial cells	Fusion of smaller vessels
Tryptase	Mast cells	Vessel tube formation

in inflammation[45] or, alternatively that these inflammatory proteins contribute to a cell growth programme.

It is of interest that, experimentally, inhibitors of platelet activating factor (PAF) drastically reduce the development of PH both in chronically hypoxic and in monocrotaline treated rats[46,47]. PAF affects production of leukotrienes in the lungs[48] and has been associated with angiogenesis[49] and mice deficient in 5-lipoxygenase (5-LO knock-out) are protected against PH[50], yet neither leukotriene antagonists nor 5-LO inhibitors or PAF receptor blockers have been used clinically in PH patients.

Suppression of vascular smooth muscle cell growth and hypertrophy

The thickening of the media in the precapillary pulmonary arteries is clearly an important part of the pulmonary vascular remodelling. Perhaps pulmonary VSMC hypertrophy is more prominent than VSMC proliferation. The hypertensive VSMC is less contractile, the phenotype likely has switched to a 'secretory' cell type[51].

The proto-oncogene c-myb regulates cell growth and is involved in mitogen-induced VSMC growth; heparin blocks VSMC cell cycle progression and blocks the induction of c-myb expression. In the model of chronic hypoxia-induced pulmonary hypertension in neonatal calves it has been shown that chronic treatment with heparin reduces the amount of vascular remodelling, i.e. the development of media thickening[52].

Agents that increase intracellular cGMP are postulated to inhibit pulmonary vascular remodelling since cGMP inhibits the mitogenesis and proliferation of VSMC. Endogenous factors like atrial natriuretic peptide (ANP) for which guanylate cyclase is

Table 19.4. Inflammatory cells in severe pulmonary hypertension and potential mediators involved in remodelling

Mast cells	Heath et al.[42]	histamine, serotonin, leukotrienes, tryptase
Macrophages	Tuder et al.[15]	TNF-α, IL-1, IL-6, bFGF, leukotriene, TGF-β
T-lymphocytes	Tuder et al.[15]	
B-lymphocytes	Tuder et al.[15]	

the receptor, and nitric oxide itself, inhibit vascular wall thickening in the lungs of experimental animals. Again, whether chronic treatment with nitric oxide via inhalation or whether nitric oxide donors have such an effect in patients with severe pulmonary hypertension is presently unknown. A future treatment based on the above developed principle would be the inhibition of the ANP clearance receptor. Conceptually, agents blocking the ANP clearance receptor would increase the circulating endogenous ANP, potentially leading to activation of the guanylate cyclase.

With the recent increase in anorexigen-related severe pulmonary hypertension[53–55] investigators have again focused their attention on serotonin since most of the appetite suppressant drugs either release serotonin or inhibit serotonin uptake. Serotonin is a VSMC mitogen and a pulmonary vasoconstrictor[56], and finally circulating serotonin levels may be elevated in patients with PPH[57]. Taken together these findings may justify the exploration of the usefulness of specific serotonin blockers.

Gene therapy for the remodelled lung circulation

Initially, information concerning the modification of vascular diseases via gene therapy came from studies of the systemic circulation. First attempts were directed towards modification of smooth muscle cell proliferation and hypertrophy in the setting of restenosis following angioplasty therapy; some of these studies made use of rodent models of

carotid artery injury obtained after rubbing a balloon catheter within the vessel lumen. Anti-sense strategies have been used aimed at the oncogene c-myb since this oncogene is expressed by proliferating smooth muscle cells. Morishita and coworkers delivered anti-sense oligonucleotides directed against CDK2 kinase or the transcription factor decoy of E2F binding sites. CDK2 kinase forms a complex with cyclin A and E2F; this approach reduced significantly, but not completely, the smooth muscle cell proliferation subsequent to the arterial injury[58]. Presently, only short-term transfection studies have been successful targeting the lungs of experimental animals. Both endothelial nitric oxide synthase (eNOS) and VEGF have been delivered via adenovirus vectors to the lungs of rats and the overexpression of either eNOS or VEGF have produced inhibition of acute pulmonary vasoconstriction.

Another candidate to consider for gene therapy is the prostacyclin synthase. Given the success of the presently recommended continuous IV infusion of prostacyclin in many forms of severe pulmonary hypertension[59,60] and the fact that the prostacyclin synthase gene is reduced in its expression in pulmonary hypertensive lungs[61] it would make sense to attempt strategies to reexpress prostacyclin synthase, a gene coding for a critical enzyme in the production of the very important vasodilator prostacyclin. Adenovirus vectors are likely to have, even under best conditions, a relatively short survival time, retroviral vectors may be available for permanent transfection either via the vascular or the airway route. As has been shown with eNOS and VEGF transfections short-term expression in rat lungs has been accomplished with an adenovirus vector transfection of the PGI2 synthase. Recently, Geraci and coworkers demonstrated overexpression of the prostacyclin synthase and continuously elevated levels of prostacyclin in the lungs of mice where the transgene was selectively overexpressed in surfactant producing alveolar cells. These animals lack an acute hypoxic pressor response and do not develop pulmonary hypertension when exposed to chronic hypoxia illustrating how chronic overproduction of prostacyclin in the lung can alter both vascular reactivity and prevent chronic hypoxia-induced pulmonary vascular remodelling[62]. These experiments should be seen as proof of principle and encourage investigators to continue to work on projects dedicated to overcome the defect in prostacyclin synthesis in the pulmonary hypertensive lung. Furthermore, these experiments indicate that strategies which increase epithelial cell production of endogenous vasodilators may hold promise for the treatment of pulmonary hypertension.

Treatment of the pressure overloaded right ventricle

It is the clinical experience of many investigators that in adult severe pulmonary hypertension the survival of the patient is less related to the magnitude of the pulmonary artery pressure but rather to the cardiac output and the right atrial pressure, i.e. to the absence or presence or the degree of right ventricular failure[63]. For unclear reasons, there are patients that present to their physicians at the time of diagnosis with manifest right ventricular failure, whereas other patients suffer mostly from dyspnea and fatigue and appear to develop right ventricular failure signs later in the course of their disease. Conceptually, it is necessary to consider the problem of severe pulmonary hypertension as a combined issue of progressive pulmonary vascular remodelling and the problem of the right ventricular reserve. As stated, why some patients with severe pulmonary hypertension fail early and other patients late is not at all clear; however, one might postulate that the 'quality' of the right ventricular myocardium might be different from patient to patient and therefore the ability to withstand the chronic pressure overload. The mechanism leading to 'appropriate' adaptation to the high pressure and the development of concentric right ventricular hypertrophy may code for the state of a compensated RV failure and longer survival. If one accepts this concept as developed then one may ask further questions.

First, is there a myocardial failure programme that is potentially reversible when the afterload has been removed? Second, are there individual and genetic determinants of right ventricular reserve? Stated differently, does the right ventricle have genetically based choices, for example, to activate a failure programme or to activate a pressure-adaptation programme? Further questions are whether the pressure-overloaded right ventricle is exposed to a different degree of wall stress based on the concentric or excentric hypertrophy of the chamber and whether concentric or excentric hypertrophy predispose the myocardium to a greater or lesser degree of RV ischemia? Availability of such specific information regarding the performance and contractile reserve of the right ventricular muscle may lead toward new treatments.

Combination therapy

Future treatment regimens for patients with severe pulmonary hypertension may not only include anti-inflammatory agents, but agents which target vascular remodelling. Patients in the future may receive a combination of drugs; for example, a patient with moderately severe pulmonary hypertension may receive an oral prostacyclin analogue, an endothelin receptor blocker, an anticoagulant plus a phosphodiesterase inhibitor. Other patients displaying a pattern of progressive angiogenic remodelling may receive a short course treatment with agents which induce apoptosis or inhibit matrix metalloproteinases.

Therapeutic approach to neonatal pulmonary hypertension

Pulmonary hypertension during the early postnatal period presents challenges and opportunities for therapeutic intervention that are unique from pulmonary hypertension in the adult. At birth, the pulmonary circulation undergoes a striking vasodilation, leading to an 8–10-fold increase in pulmonary blood flow due to marked vasodilation. This fall in pulmonary vascular resistance (PVR) is critical for normal cardiopulmonary adaptation at birth, and allows for gas exchange to occur during postnatal life. Some newborns fail to achieve this normal fall in PVR at birth, and develop severe hypoxemic cardio-respiratory failure. Persistent pulmonary hypertension of the newborn (PPHN) is a clinical syndrome that is characterized by failure of the pulmonary circulation to achieve and sustain the normal vasodilation at birth[64,65]. As a clinical syndrome, PPHN is associated with diverse neonatal heart and lung disorders, including asphyxia, meconium aspiration syndrome, respiratory distress syndrome, congenital diaphragmatic hernia, sepsis and pneumonia, or can be idiopathic (the so-called 'persistent fetal circulation'). These disorders are included within the syndrome of PPHN because they share physiological features, including high pulmonary artery pressure, leading to right-to-left extra-pulmonary shunting of blood flow across the foramen ovale or ductus arteriosus, and causing marked hypoxemia. High PVR in PPHN is also associated with abnormal vasoreactivity, as demonstrated by an inability to dilate to normal birth related stimuli (e.g. oxygen, ventilation and shear stress) and marked vasoconstriction to mild hypoxia or stress. In addition, newborns who die with PPHN have marked hypertensive remodelling of small pulmonary arteries, suggesting that structural pulmonary vascular disease can also contribute to high PVR in PPHN.

Mechanisms that cause PPHN are incompletely understood. Familial cases of PPHN have been reported, but most cases lack a positive family history of past cardiovascular or pulmonary disease. Although chronic hypoxia has long been considered as a likely etiology of PPHN, animal models of maternal hypoxia in rats and guinea pigs have not supported this hypothesis. Although newborns have low birth weight after exposure to chronic hypoxia in utero, there were no differences in pulmonary artery pressure or pulmonary artery wall thickness in comparison with control animals[66]. In contrast, intrauterine hypertension may be sufficient to cause PPHN. An animal model of partial compression of the ductus arteriosus (DA) in fetal lambs has demon-

strated marked changes in pulmonary vascular structure and sustained elevation of PVR after delivery[67]. These studies suggest that mechanisms that elevate pulmonary arterial pressure in utero, such as systemic hypertension or closure of the DA, can alter pulmonary vascular structure and reactivity, leading to functional and structural changes that characterize PPHN.

Physiologically, high PVR may be due to impaired release of vasodilators, enhanced production of vasoconstrictors, altered smooth muscle cell responsiveness, excessive production of an abnormal extracellular matrix production, and altered growth of smooth muscle cells. Experimental studies suggest that PPHN may be associated with decreased production and responsiveness to nitric oxide (NO). Impaired production of NO may lead to decreased vasodilation at birth[68–70], increased myogenic tone[71], and increased smooth muscle cell growth, that characterize PPHN. Similarly, decreased soluble guanylate cyclase and increased cGMP-specific phosphodiesterase (PDE5) activities may further impair NO-mediated vasodilation in PPHN by lowering smooth muscle cell cGMP content and limiting vasodilation[72,73]. Alternate mechanisms that have been suggested by this model include increased production of the potent vasoconstrictor and smooth muscle mitogen, endothelin-1 (ET-1), and altered expression of ET receptors[74]. Whether these mechanisms are operative in clinical PPHN are uncertain; however, clinical studies have demonstrated marked elevation of circulating ET levels in newborns with PPHN[75].

In the recent past, therapy of PPHN was limited to the use of hyperventilation, metabolic alkalosis, cardiotonic drugs and non-selective pharmacologic vasodilators[65]. Failure to respond to these agents often lead to treatment with extracorporeal membrane oxygenation (ECMO), which is expensive, labour intensive and associated with significant neurological and cardiopulmonary sequelae. More recently, several clinical studies have demonstrated that inhaled NO improves oxygenation and lowers PVR in newborns with PPHN, reducing the need for ECMO utilization[76–78]. Clinical responses to inhaled

NO have been achieved at relatively low doses (2–20 ppm), and are not associated with potential problems of NO-related toxicities, such as increased methemoglobinemia or exposure to high nitrogen dioxide levels. In addition, long-term follow-up studies of children who received NO during the immediate newborn period have demonstrated normal lung function and good developmental outcomes.

Although inhaled NO has been proven to be an effective pulmonary vasodilator in PPHN, not all newborns respond to this therapy. Several mechanisms may contribute to partial or poor responsiveness to inhaled NO. These include poor lung inflation, leading to an inability to deliver NO to the pulmonary circulation and increasing intrapulmonary shunting due to low lung volumes. Clinical studies have demonstrated that improved lung recruitment during high frequency oscillatory ventilation, enhances the vasodilator response to inhaled NO in many patients who demonstrated poor responsiveness during conventional ventilation[79].

In addition, PPHN may be characterized by decreased responsiveness to NO due to altered smooth muscle cell responsiveness to NO because of decreased soluble guanylate cyclase and increased PDE5 activities. Clinical reports have suggested that dypyridamole, a PDE5 inhibitor, may augment pulmonary vasodilation to inhaled NO in some patients with PPHN[80,81]. Further studies are underway to determine whether the combination of inhaled NO and PDE5 inhibitors will improve clinical outcome in PPHN.

Potential future therapies include the use of aerosolized prostacyclin, endothelin antagonists or perhaps K+ channel openers. These have not been studied in newborns with severe pulmonary hypertension, but may contribute to additional improvement in the responses of infants with severe PPHN. Some newborns who die with PPHN have extensive structural remodelling of small pulmonary arteries, that are predominantly characterized by excessive growth of vascular smooth muscle. In addition, extensive increases in extracellular matrix production consisting of altered collagen content, is also commonly present, and likely increases PVR by decreasing vascular compliance. In some cases, intimal hyperplasia is also present, causing intraluminal obstruction, even in newborns dying in the first weeks of life. These striking structural features of fatal PPHN suggest that new interventions that specifically target cell proliferation and synthetic function, independent of vasodilator properties, will provide an important therapeutic strategy in newborns who fail to respond to standard therapy, including inhaled NO. Finally, the subgroup of patients with severe PPHN with poor responsiveness to current therapy include those with lung hypoplasia, e.g. congenital diaphragmatic hernia or primary lung hypoplasia. These diseases continue to be a difficult subgroup to treat and survivors have significant long-term sequelae, including late pulmonary hypertension. In this group, novel strategies of enhancing vascular growth may be necessary to improve outcome. Recent studies in the developing rat lung suggest that disruption of normal lung vascular growth, induced by pharmacological inhibition of angiogenesis during the first 2 weeks of postnatal life, causes lung hypoplasia due to a marked reduction in septation and alveolarization[81]. In particular, treatment of the developing rat with SU5416, a novel inhibitor of the VEGF-KDR/flk-1 receptor, reduces alveolarization and arterial density, and causes striking pulmonary hypertension[81]. These findings suggest that disruption of VEGF-KDR/flk-1 signalling may be a critical mechanism underlying the development of PPHN, especially in the setting of lung hypoplasia. This hypothesis needs to be tested in the clinical setting, but may suggest that therapies directed toward enhancing VEGF signalling and lung vascular growth may provide a new approach to severe PPHN.

REFERENCES

1 Zapol WM, Snider MT. Pulmonary hypertension in severe acute respiratory failure. *N Engl J Med* 1977; 296:476–480.

2 Shaw, DB, Grover RF, Reeves JT, Blount G. Pulmonary circulation in chronic bronchitis and emphysema. *Br Heart J* 1965; 27:674–683.

3 Liebow AA, Gough J. Pulmonary emphysema with special reference to vascular changes. *Am Rev Resp Dis* 1959; 80:67–93.

4 Crausman R, Jennings CA, Tuder RM, Ackerson LM, Irvin GG, King TE. Pulmonary histiocytosis X: pulmonary function and exercise pathophysiology. *Am J Respir Crit Care Med* 1996; 153:426–435.

5 Tuder RM, Cool CD, Jennings C, Voelkel NF. Pulmonary vascular involvement in interstitial lung disease. In Schwarz MS, King TEJ, eds. *Interstitial Lung Disease*. Hamilton, Ontario, Canada: BC Decker; 1998:. 251–263.

6 Perez HD, Kramer N. Pulmonary hypertension in systemic lupus erythematosus: report of four cases and review of the literature. *Semin Arthritis Rheum* 1981; 11:177–181.

7 Harris P, Segal N, Bishop JM. The relation between pressure and flow in the pulmonary circulation in normal subjects and in patients with chronic bronchitis and mitral stenosis. *Cardiovasc Res* 1968; 2:73–83.

8 Bergosfsky EH, Turino GM, Fishman AP. Cardiorespiratory failure in kyphoscoliosis. *Medicine* 1959; 38:263–317.

9 Weil JV. Pulmonary hypertension and cor pulmonale in hypoventilating patients. In Weir EK, Reeves JT, eds, *Pulmonary Hypertension*, Future Publishing Co, Mount Cisco, New York; 1984: 321–339.

10 Weitzenblum E, Sautegeau A, Ehrhart M, Mammosser M, Pelletier A. Long-term oxygen therapy can reverse the progression of pulmonary hypertension in patients with chronic obstructive pulmonary disease. *Am Rev Respir Dis* 1985; 131:493–498.

11 Voelkel NF, Tuder RM. Cellular and molecular mechanisms in the pathogenesis of severe pulmonary hypertension. *Eur Respir J* 1995; 8:2129–2138.

12 Voelkel NF, Cool C, Lee SD, Wright L, Geraci MW, Tuder RM. Primary pulmonary hypertension between inflammation and cancer. *Chest* 1998; 114:225S-230S.

13 Voelkel NF, Tuder RM, Weir EK. Pathophysiology of primary pulmonary hypertension: from physiology to molecular mechanism. *Lung Biol Health Dis* 1997; 99:83–129.

14 Voelkel NF, Tuder RM. Severe pulmonary hypertension diseases – a perspective. *Eur Respir J* 1999, 14:1246–1250.

15 Tuder RM, Groves GM, Badesch DB, Voelkel NF. Exuberant endothelial cell growth and elements of inflammation and present in plexiform lesions of pulmonary hypertension. *Am J Pathol* 1994; 114:275–285.

16 Lowes BD, Minobe W, Abraham WT et al. Changes in gene expression in the intact human heart: downregulation of α-myosin heavy chain in hypertrophied, failing ventricular myocardium. *J Clin Invest* 1997; 100:2315–2324.

17 Lee SD, Shroyer KR, Markham NE, Cool CD, Voelkel NF, Tuder RM. Monoclonal endothelial cell proliferation is present in primary but not secondary pulmonary hypertension. *J Clin Invest* 1998; 101:927–934.

18 Tuder RM, Radisvljevic Z, Shroyer KR, Polak JM, Voelkel NF. Monoclonal endothelial cells in appetite suppressant-associated pulmonary hypertension. *Am J Respir Crit Care Med* 1998; 158:1999–2001.

19 Yeager M, Halley GR, Voelkel NF, Tuder RM. Microsatellite instability of endothelial cell growth and apoptosis genes within plexiform lesions in primary pulmonary hypertension. *Circ Res* 2001; 88:E2–E11.

20 Maisonpierre PC, Suri C, Jones PF et al. Angiopoietin-2, a natural antagonist for Tie2 that disrupts in vivo angiogenesis. *Science* 1997; 277:55–60.

21 Wang H, Keiser JA. Vascular endothelial growth factor upregulates the expression of matrix metalloproteinases in vascular smooth muscle cells: role of flt-1. *Circ Res* 1998; 83:832–840.

22 Jackson JR, Seed MP, Kircher CH, Willoughby DA, Winkler JD. The codependence of angiogenesis and chronic inflammation. *Faseb J* 1997; 11:457–465.

23 Sunderkotter C, Steinbrink K, Goebeler M, Bhardwaj R, Clemens S. Macrophages and angiogenesis. *J Leukoc Biol* 1994; 55:410–422.

24 Yancopoulos GD, Klagsbrun, Folkman J. Vasculogenesis, angiogenesis, and growth factors: ephrins enter the fray at the border. *Cell* 1998; 93:661–664.

25 Adams RH, Wilkinson GA, Weiss C et al. Roles of ephrinB ligands and EphB receptors in cardiovascular development: demarcation of arterial/venous domains, vascular morphogenesis, and sprouting angiogenesis. *Genes Dev* 1999; 13:295–306.

26 Tuder RM, Chacon M, Alger L et al. Expression of angiogenesis-related molecules in plexiform lesions in severe pulmonary hypertension: evidence for a process of disordered angiogenesis. *J Pathol* 2001; 195:367–374.

27 Mason NA, Springall DR, Burke M et al. High expression of endothelial nitric oxide synthase in plexiform lesions of pulmonary hypertension. *J Pathol* 1998; 185:313–318.

28 Tuder RM, Allard J, Voelkel NF. Role of vascular endothelial growth factor in hypoxia and monocrotaline induced pulmonary hypertension. *Circulation* 1996; 94:164.

29 Partovian C, Adnot S, Raffestin B, Levame M, Lemarchand P, Eddahibi S. Adenoviral mediated VEGF overexpression reduces chronic hypoxic pulmonary hypertension in rats. *Am J Resp Crit Care Med* 1999; 159:A217.

30 Shen BQ, Lee DY, Zioncheck TF. Vascular endothelial growth

factor governs endothelial nitric-oxide synthase expression via a KDR-Flk-1 receptor and a protein kinase C signaling pathway. *J Biol Chem* 1999; 274:33051–33063

31 Appleton L, Brown NJ, Willis D, Colville-Nash PR, Alam C, Brown JR, Willoughby DA. The role of vascular endothelial growth factor in a murine chronic granulomatous tissue air pouch model of angiogenesis. *J Pathol* 1996; 180:90–94.

33 Oreilly MS, Holmgren L, Folkman J. Endogenous angiogenesis inhibitors. *Mol Biol Cell* 1995; 6:672.

34 Galardy RE, Grobelny D, Foellmer HG, Fernandez LA. Inhibition of angiogenesis by the matrix metalloprotease inhibitor N-[2R-2-(hydroxamidocarbonymethyl)-4-methylpentanoyl)]-L-tryptophan methylamide. *Cancer Res* 1994; 54:4715–4718.

36 Ye C, Rabinovitch M. Inhibition of elastolysis by SC-37698 reduces development and progression of monocrotaline pulmonary hypertension. *Am J Physiol* 1991; 261:H1255–H1267.

37 Zhu L, Hinek A, Wigle D, et al. The vascular elastase which governs the development and progression of pulmonary hypertension is related to adipsin. *Mol Biol Cell* 1993; 4:410a.

38 Jones PL, Cowan KN, Rabinovitch M. Induction of tenasein and fibronectin are features associated with increased smooth muscle cell proliferation during the development of progressive pulmonary hypertension in children. *Am J Pathol* 1997; 150:1349–1360.

39 Rabinovitch M. Pulmonary hypertension: updating a mysterious disease. *Cardiovasc Res* 1997; 34:268–372.

40 Rabinovitch M. Elastase and the pathobiology of unexplained pulmonary hypertension. *Chest* 1998; 114:213S–224S.

41 Tuder RM, Voelkel NF. Pulmonary hypertension and inflammation. *J Lab Clin* 1998; 132:16–24.

42 Heath D, Yacoub M, Lung mast cells in plexogenic pulmonary arteriopathy. *J Clin Pathol* 1991; 44:1003–1006.

43 Humbert M, Monti G, Brenot F et al. Increased interleukin-1 and interleukin-6 serum concentrations in severe primary pulmonary hypertension. *Am J Respir Crit Care Med* 1995; 151:1628–1631.

44 Wright L, Tuder RM, Wang J, Cool CD, Lepley RA, Voelkel NF. 5-lipoxygenase and 5-lipoxygeanse activating protein (FLAP) immunoreactivity in lungs from patients with primary pulmonary hypertension. *Am J Respir Crit Care Med* 1998; 157:219–229.

45 Kasahara Y, Tuder RM, Cool CD, Lynch DA, Flores SC, Voelkel NF. Endothelial cell death and decreased expression of vascular endothelial growth factor and its receptor KDR/Flk-1 in emphysema. *Am J Resp Crit Care Med* 2001; 163:737–744.

46 Ono S, Westcott JY, Voelkel NF. PAF-antagonists inhibit pulmonary vascular remodeling induced by hypobaric hypoxia in rats. *J Appl Physiol* 1992; 73:1084–1092.

47 Ono S, Voelkel NF. PAF antagonists inhibit monocrotaline-induced lung injury and pulmonary hypertension. *J Appl Physiol* 1991; 71:2483–2492.

48 Voelkel NF, Worthen S, Reeves JT, Henson PM, Murphy RC. Nonimmunological production of leukotrienes induced by platelet-activating factor. *Science* 1982; 218:286–288.

49 Ahmed A, Dearn S, Shams N et al. Localization, quantification, and activation of platelet activating factor receptor in human endometrium during

50 Voelkel NF, Tuder RM, Wade K et al. Inhibition of 5-lipoxygenase-activating protein (FLAP) reduces pulmonary vascular reactivity and pulmonary hypertension in rats. *J Clin Invest* 1996; 97:2491–2498.

51 Voelkel NF, Tuder RM. Cellular and molecular biology of vascular smooth muscle cells in pulmonary hypertension. *Pulm Pharm Therap* 1997; 10:1–11.

52 Dempsey EC, Fasules J, Orton EC, Mecham RP, Das M, Stenmark K. Heparin attenuates severe pulmonary vascular remodeling in hypoxia-exposed neonatal calves: in vivo and in vitro effects. *Am Rev Respir Dis* 1995; 151:A733.

53 Abenhaim L, Moride Y, Brenot F, et al. Appetite-suppressant drugs and the risk of primary pulmonary hypertension. *N Engl J Med* 1996; 335:609–616.

54 Mark EJ, Patalas ED, Change HT, Evans RJ, Kessler SC. Fatal pulmonary hypertension associated with short-term use of fenfluramine and phentermine. *N Engl J Med* 1997; 337:602–605.

55 Voelkel NF. Appetite suppressants and pulmonary hypertension. *Thorax* 1997; 3:S63–S67.

56 Fanburg B, Lee SL. A role for the serotonin transporter in hypoxia-induced pulmonary hypertension. *J Clin Invest* 2000; 105:1521–1523.

57 Herve P, et al. Increased plasma serotonin in primary pulmonary hypertension. *Am J Med* 1995; 99:249–254.

58 Morishita R, Gibbons GH, Ellison KE et al. Intimal hyperplasia after vascular injury in inhibited by antisens cdk 2 kinase oligonucleotides. *J Clin Invest* 1994; 93:1458–1464,

59 Barst RJ, Rubin LJ, Long WA et al. A comparison of continuous intravenous epoprostenol (prostacyclin) with conventional therapy for primary pulmonary hypertension. *N Engl J Med* 1996; 334:296–301.

60 Mclaughlin VV, Genthner DE, Panella MM, Rich S. Reduction in pulmonary vascular resistance with long-term epoprostenol (prostacyclin) therapy in primary pulmonary hypertension. *N Engl J Med* 1998; 338:273–277.

61 Tuder R, Geraci MW, Wang J et al. Prostacyclin synthase expression is decreased in lungs from patients with severe pulmonary hypertension. *Am J Resp Crit Care Med* 1999; 159:1925–1932,

62 Geraci MW, Gao B, Shepherd DC et al. Pulmonary prostacyclin synthase overexpression in transgenic mice protects against development of hypoxic pulmonary hypertension. *J Clin Invest* 1999; 103:1509–1515.

63 Abraham WT, Raynolds, MV Gottschall B et al. Importance of angiotensin-converting enzyme in pulmonary hypertension. *Cardiology* 1995; 86:9–15.

64 Levin DL, Heymann MA, Kitterman JA, Gregory GA, Phibbs RH, Rudolph AM. Persistent pulmonary hypertension of the newborn. *J Pediatr* 1976; 89:1894–1898.

65 Kinsella JP, Abman SH. Recent developments in the pathophysiology and treatment of persistent pulmonary hypertension of the newborn. *J Pediatr* 1995; 126:853–864.

66 Geggel RL, Reid LM. The structural basis of PPHN. *Clin Perinatol* 1984; 3:525–549.

67 Abman SH, Shanley PF, Accurso FJ. Failure of postnatal adaptation of the pulmonary circulation after chronic intrauterine pulmonary hypertension in fetal lambs. *J Clin Invest* 1989; 83:1849–58.

68 Abman SH, Chatfield BA, Hall SL, McMurtry IF. Role of endothelium-derived relaxing factor during the transition of the pulmonary circulation at birth. *Am J Physiol* 1990; 259:H1921–1927.

69 Villamor E, Le Cras TD, Horan M, Halbower AC, Tuder R, Abman SH. Chronic intrauterine pulmonary hypertension impairs endothelial nitric oxide synthase in the ovine fetus. *Am J Physiol* 1997; 272:L1013–1020.

70 McQueston JA, Kinsella JP, Ivy DD, McMurtry IF, Abman SH. Chronic pulmonary hypertension in utero impairs endothelium-dependent vasodilation. *Am J Physiol* 1995; 268:H288–294.

71 Storme L, Rairigh RL, Parker TA, Kinsella JP, Abman SH. In vivo evidence for a myogenic response in the fetal pulmonary circulation. *Pediatr Res.* 1999; 45:425–431.

72 Steinhorn RH, Russell JA, Morin FC. Pulmonary arteries from newborn lambs with PPHN have decreased sensitivity to NO (abstract). *Pediatr Res* 1994; 35: 354A.

73 Hanson KA, Ziegler JW, Rybalkin SD, Miller J, Abman SH, Clarke WR. Chronic pulmonary hypertension increases lung cGMP phosphodiesterase activity by post-translational modification in the ovine fetus. *Am J Physiol* 1998; 275: L931–41.

74 Ivy DD, Abman SH. Role of endothelin in perinatal pulmonary vasoregulation. In: Weir EK, Archer SL, Reeves JT. eds. *Fetal and Neonatal Pulmonary Circulations*, NY: Futura, 1999:279–302.

75 Rosenberg AA, Kennaugh J, Koppenhafer SL, Loomis M, Chatfield BA, Abman SH. Increased immunoreactive endothelin-1 levels in persistent pulmonary hypertension of the newborn. *J Pediatr* 1993; 123:109–114.

76 Roberts JD, Polaner DM, Lang P, Zapol WM. Inhaled NO in PPHN. *Lancet* 1992; 340:818–819.

77 NINOS. Inhaled NO in full-term and nearly full-term infants with hypoxic respiratory failure. *N Engl J Med* 1997; 336:597–604.

78 Kinsella JP, Neish SR, Shaffer E, Abman SH. Effect of low dose inhalational nitric oxide in pulmonary hypertension of the newborn. *Lancet* 1992; 340:819–820.

79 Kinsella JP, Troug W, Walsh W et al. Randomized multicenter trial of inhaled nitric oxide and high frequency oscillatory ventilation in severe PPHN. *J Pediatr* 1997; 131:55–62.

80 Ziegler JW, Ivy DD, Fox JJ, Kinsella JP, Clarke WR, Abman SH. Dipyridamole, a cGMP phosphodiesterase inhibitor, causes pulmonary vasodilation in the ovine fetus. *Am J Physiol* 1995; 269:H473–9.

81 Kinsella JP, Toriella F, Ziegler JW, Ivy DD, Abman SH. Dipyridamole augmentation of the response to inhaled NO. *Lancet* 1995; 346:647–8.

82 Jakkula M, Le Cras TD, Gebb S et al. Inhibition of angiogenesis decreases alveolarization in the developing rat lung. *Am J Physiol Lung Cell Mol Physiol* 2000; 279:L600–L607.

Part V

Lung cancer

20

Molecular pathology of lung cancer

Ignacio I. Wistuba[1] and Adi F. Gazdar[2]

[1] Department of Pathology, Pontificia Universidad Catolica de Chile, Santiago, Chile
[2] Hamon Center for Therapeutic Oncology Research and Department of Pathology,
University of Texas Southwestern Medical Center, Dallas, USA

Lung cancer is classified into two major clinico-pathological groups, namely small cell lung carcinoma (SCLC) and non-small cell lung carcinoma (NSCLC)[1]. Squamous cell carcinoma, adenocarcinoma and large cell carcinoma are the major histological types of NSCLC[1]. Large cell carcinoma probably represents poorly differentiated variants of the other NSCLC types[1]. As with other epithelial malignancies, lung cancers are believed to arise after a series of progressive pathological changes (preneoplastic lesions) in the bronchial epithelium[2]. However, this sequence has been well established only for squamous cell carcinoma[2]. Many mutations, especially involving recessive oncogenes, have been described in clinically evident lung cancer[3]. While some of these are common to all lung cancer types, some are more frequent in specific tumour types[3]. For risk assessment and very early lung cancer detection it would be helpful to know about molecular events in the respiratory epithelial molecule preceding the development of lung carcinoma.

Preneoplasia and the development of lung cancer

Lung cancers are believed to arise after a series of progressive pathological changes (preneoplastic or precursor lesions) in the respiratory mucosa[4]. While the sequential preneoplastic changes have been defined for centrally arising squamous carcinoma (Fig. 20.1)[4], they have been poorly documented for the other cell types[1].

Epithelial changes in the large airways that may precede or accompany invasive squamous cell carcinoma include hyperplasia (basal cell hyperplasia and goblet cell hyperplasia), squamous metaplasia, squamous dysplasia and carcinoma *in situ* (CIS)[4]. The early abnormal epithelial changes such as hyperplasia and squamous metaplasia (without dysplasia) are probably reactive, regress after smoking cessation and are probably not true preneoplastic changes. The sequential preneoplastic changes associated with squamous carcinoma may also be present in adenocarcinomas and SCLCs. Hyperplasia of the bronchial epithelium and squamous metaplasia are extremely common findings, especially as a response to cigarette smoking[5,6]. Both changes have generally considered reversible and not premalignant. Dysplasia and CIS with squamous differentiation are the changes most frequently associated with the development of squamous cell lung carcinoma[7]. In some instances, a direct continuity can be shown between the invasive carcinoma and increasing degrees of dysplasia and CIS in the adjacent mucosa. Because dysplasia and CIS are usually not visible to the naked eye, their reported frequencies are relatively low and their natural history has not been elucidated. Recently, the use of the fluorescence bronchoscope has increased the recognition of dysplastic lesions of the large airways[8,9]. Since dysplastic lesions tend to show less autofluorescence than normal mucosa, they may be visualized by fluorescence bronchoscopy although not visible by conventional white light bronchoscopy.

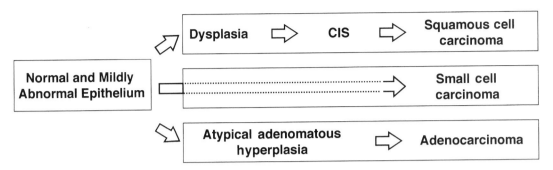

Fig. 20.1 Histopathological and genetic pathways of the three major histological types of lung cancer. While squamous cell carcinoma and adenocarcinoma appear to develop after a sequence of histopathological and genetic steps, small cell carcinoma (SCLC) seems to arise directly either from normal or mildly abnormal bronchial epithelium, without passing through the entire histological sequence.

Adenocarcinomas may be accompanied by hyperplastic and dysplastic changes including atypical adenomatous hyperplasia (AAH)[10] in peripheral airway cells, although the malignant potential of these lesions has not been demonstrated. However, lesions with AAH features are frequently detected accompanying adenocarcinomas, especially when a bronchioloalveolar carcinomatous pattern at the edge of less differentiated adenocarcinomas is seen[10,11]. The concept of the adenoma–carcinoma sequence as it applies to AAH and adenocarcinoma of the lung suggests there is a continuum from AAH to bronchioalveolar carcinoma.

Bronchiolar neuroendocrine cell hyperplasia represents a proliferation of neuroendocrine cells in and around small airway[12]. Because of their association with peripheral carcinoid tumours, they have been suggested as precursors to the carcinoid tumour[12]. While no specific preneoplastic changes have been described for SCLC, smoking related changes including squamous dysplasia and CIS may lie adjacent to SCLC tumours[13].

Information currently available suggests that lung preneoplastic lesions frequently are multifocal and widely dispersed, indicating a field effect ('field cancerization') by which much of the respiratory epithelium has been mutagenized, presumably from exposure to carcinogens[14]. Thus, lung carcinoma may occur anywhere in the vast and anatomically complicated respiratory tree including the peripheral lung, and second tumours are relatively frequent after one upper aerodigestive tract carcinoma[15].

Molecular abnormalities in invasive lung cancer

Several allelotyping and comparative genomic hybridization (CGH) studies have revealed that multiple genetic changes (estimated to be between 10 and 20) are found in clinically evident lung cancer involving known and putative recessive oncogenes and several dominant oncogenes[3].

Dominant oncogenes

Examples of abnormal dominant oncogenes in lung cancer are the *RAS* family members (*K-RAS*, *H-RAS* and *N-RAS*), the *MYC* family members (*C-MYC*, *N-MYC*, and *L-MYC*) and the *HER-2/NEU* gene. *RAS* mutations occur in approximately 20% of NSCLC, mainly in adenocarcinomas (90% involving *K-RAS* gene at codon 12), while *RAS* mutations have not been detected in any small cell lung cancer tumour or cell line[3,16]. Another example of a dominant oncogene in lung cancer is overexpression of the *MYC* family of genes, which occurs in nearly all SCLC and in many NSCLC[17–19]. Amplification of *MYC* family genes has been reported in SCLC, especially after administration of cytotoxic therapy[20]. Recent CGH studies have shown that lung cancer demonstrates increased copy number consistent with amplification of underlying dominant oncogenes at several chromosomal regions, including 1p, 1q, 2p, 3q, 5q, 11q, 16p, 17q, 19q, and Xq[21–24]. Some of these regions, like 1p32 (*L-MYC*), 2p25 (*N-MYC*), and 8q24 (*C-MYC*), contain known dominant oncogenes, while in others, the genes remain unidentified.

Recessive oncogenes

The list of recessive oncogenes that are involved in lung cancer is likely to include as many 10 to 15 known and putative genes[3]. These include changes in *TP53* (17p13), *RB* (13q14), *CDKN2* (9p21), and as yet unidentified candidate recessive oncogenes located in the short arms of chromosome 3 (3p) at 3p12 (*DUTT1* gene)[25], 3p14.2 (*FHIT* gene)[26,27], 3p21 (*BAP-1* gene) and 3p25 regions[3]. Recessive oncogenes are inactivated via a two-step process involving both alleles. Knudson has proposed that the first 'hit' frequently is a point mutation, while the second allele is subsequently inactivated via a chromosomal deletion, translocation, or other event such as hypermethylation[28]. Two key examples in lung cancer are the *TP53* and the *RB* genes. Mutations of *TP53* gene are very common in lung cancer, occurring in over 90% of SCLC and approximately 50% of NSCLC[3]. There is evidence that *TP53* gene mutations occur in association with specific carcinogen exposure and those carcinogens predispose to specific mutations. Of interest, similar mutational hot-spots at the *TP53* gene have been found in invasive lung carcinomas and adducts formed by benzo[α]pyrene metabolites derived from cigarette smoke[29]. The *RB* tumour suppressor gene has been extensively studied in lung cancer. In more than 80% of SCLC and some 20% to 30% of NSCLC the protein has been mutated, so it cannot fulfil its normal cell cycle regulatory function[30–32]. Another well documented genetic change that occurs frequently in lung cancer is inactivation of the *CDKN2* gene[3,33], and abnormalities have been found frequently in NSCLC, but rarely in SCLC. A variety of mechanisms inactivating *CDKN2* have been reported and each one seems to represent a substantial percentage of the *CDKN2* inactivation mechanism in NSCLC[34]. Those mechanisms include point mutations, heterozygous and homozygous deletions, and epigenetic changes as the promoter region hypermethylation[34–36]. Both *RB* and *CDKN2* gene inactivation targets the cell cycle, and removes checkpoints at G1/M. The major mechanism by which this occurs thus varies between lung cancer types: in SCLC it is *RB* inactivation, while in NSCLC it is *CDKN2* inactivation.

Many recessive oncogenes remain to be identified, although in most instances their chromosomal locations are known from cytogenetic and molecular analysis. Loss of heterozygosity analysis (LOH) using polymorphic microsatellite markers are frequently used to identify allelic losses at specific chromosomal regions, suggesting the involvement of other tumour suppressor genes in lung cancer pathogenesis[37]. The chromosomal regions include 1q, 2q, 4p, 4q, 5q, 6p, 6q, 8p, 8q, 9q, 10q, 11p, 11q, 14q, 17q, 18q, 21q and 22q[37–50]. Although several of these chromosomal arms contain known or candidate tumour suppressor genes (such as *MCC* and *APC* at 5q21, *TSCI* at 9q34, *WT1* at 11q13, *DCC* at 18q221, *NF2* at 22q12), these genes are not known to be mutated in lung cancer. Recently, three new candidate tumour suppressor genes called *PTEN/MMAC1*[51], *DMBT1*[52] and *PPP2R1B*[53] located on 10q23.3, 10q25.3–26.1 and 11q22–24, respectively, have demonstrated somatic alterations in lung cancer at varying frequencies[53–55].

Tumour type specific genetic changes in lung cancer

Studies of a large number of lung cancers have demonstrated different patterns of genetic changes between the two major groups of lung carcinoma (SCLC and NSCLC)[37]. Similar differences have been detected between the three major histological types of lung carcinoma (SCLC, squamous cell carcinoma and adenocarcinoma)[40,41,43,56,57], especially in the frequency of *K-RAS* mutations[58]. Thus, genetic abnormalities in lung cancer can be classified into two groups, those that are common to all lung cancers and those that segregate to some histological types of lung cancers. In general, *RB* mutations are usually limited to SCLC, *CDKN2* mutations to NSCLC, and *RAS* mutations to adenocarcinomas. Our published[37,41,43] and unpublished allelotyping studies of lung cancer cell lines and microdissected invasive primary tumours indicate that SCLC demonstrate more frequent losses at 4p, 4q, 5q21 (*APC–MCC* region), 10q and 13q14 (*RB*), while losses at 9p21 and 8p21–23 are more frequent in NSCLCs. Of interest, we have found different patterns of allelic loss involving the two major types of NSCLC (squamous cell and adenocarcinoma), with higher incidences of deletion at 17p13 (*TP53*), 13q14 (*RB*), 9p21 (*CDKN2*), 8p21–23 and several 3p regions in squamous cell carcinomas[122]. These results suggest that more genetic changes accumulate during tumorigenesis in squamous cell carcinomas than in adenocarcinomas. These differences may be related to differences in pathogenesis, such as etiological factors, e.g. smoking exposure, operating via separate pathways. In fact, different patterns of allelic losses[40] and *TP53* gene mutations have been reported in lung carcinomas arising in non-smokers vs. smokers[59,60].

Genetic abnormalities in the multistage development of lung cancer

Although our knowledge of the molecular events in invasive lung cancer is relatively extensive, until recently we knew little about the sequence of events which occur in preneoplastic lesions. Some studies have provided evidence that molecular lesions can be identified at the earliest stages of the pathogenesis of lung cancer[61–68]. *MYC* and *RAS* up-regulation, cyclin D1 expression, p53 immunostaining, and DNA aneuploidy have been detected in the dysplastic epithelium adjacent to invasive lung carcinomas[67,69–75]. *K-RAS* mutations and 3p allelic losses have also been detected in atypical adenomatous hyperplasia[76], which may be a potential precursor lesion of adenocarcinoma. Although *TP53* mutations have been demonstrated in non-malignant epithelium of lung specimens resected for lung cancer[65,67], and widely dispersed in bronchial epithelium in a smoker without lung cancer[77], little information is available on the chronology of *TP53* mutation in preneoplastic epithelium. Whether or when *RB* genetic abnormalities occur prior to the occurrence of invasive tumour is not known.

To further understand the sequential molecular changes involved in lung cancer pathogenesis, we have developed a four-step scheme to systematically search for mutations by examining: (i) lung cancer cell lines[37,41,43]; (ii) microdissected primary lung tumours of the three major histological types[41,43]; (iii) normal and abnormal respiratory epithelium accompanying lung cancer specimens[43,78]; and (iv) bronchoscopy biopsies from smokers without lung cancer[43,79]. Recently, we demonstrated that most lung cancer cell lines retain the properties of their parental tumours for lengthy culture periods[80]. Thus, lung cancer cell lines appear very representative of the lung tumours from which they were derived and provide suitable material for screening of genetic abnormalities in this neoplasm. Those genetic changes were then examined in the different tumour histological type archival specimens[43], and their accompanying normal and abnormal respiratory epithelia[43,78]. The most frequent and earliest genetic abnormalities present during the multistage development of lung cancer were investigated in the bronchial epithelium of smoker subjects[43,79]. Using a precise microdissection technique (micromanipulator or laser capture microdissection) under direct microscopic observation a variable number of cells from invasive primary tumour, stromal lymphocytes (as a source of normal constitutional DNA) and epithelial foci were obtained. Using PCR-based techniques, these different specimens were examined for point mutations and allelic losses at chromosomal regions fre-

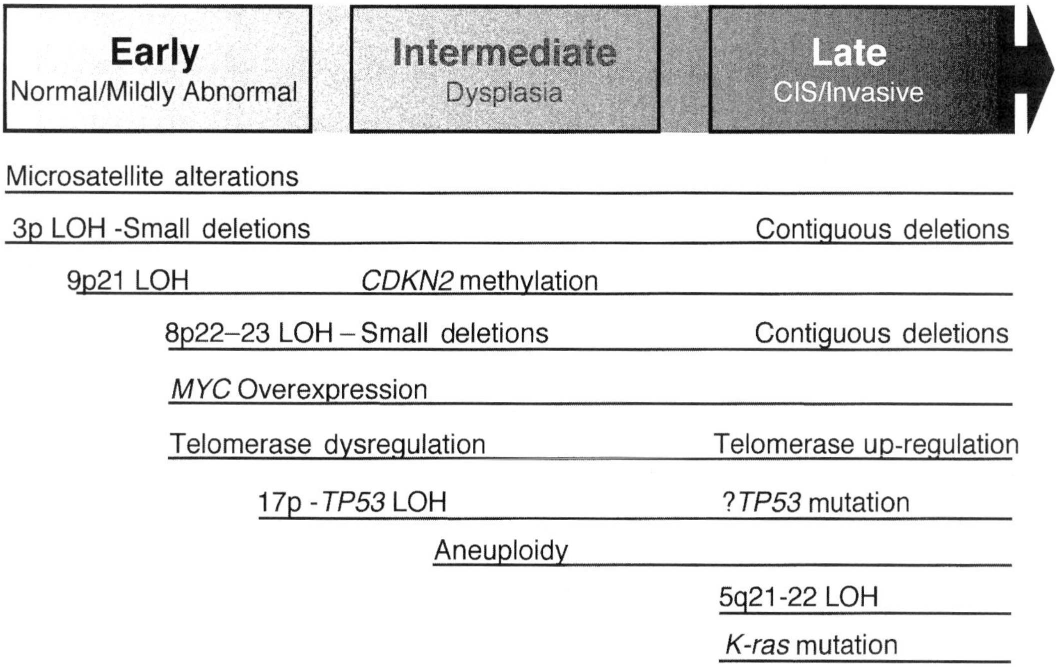

Early Normal/Mildly Abnormal	Intermediate Dysplasia	Late CIS/Invasive	

Microsatellite alterations		
3p LOH -Small deletions		Contiguous deletions
9p21 LOH	CDKN2 methylation	
8p22–23 LOH – Small deletions		Contiguous deletions
MYC Overexpression		
Telomerase dysregulation		Telomerase up-regulation
17p -TP53 LOH		?TP53 mutation
Aneuploidy		
		5q21-22 LOH
		K-ras mutation

Fig. 20.2 Sequential genetic changes during the multistage pathogenesis of lung cancer. Molecular changes occurring during lung cancer pathogenesis may commence early at normal or mildly abnormal (hyperplasia/metaplasia) epithelium, at an intermediate (dysplasia) stage, or relatively late (carcinoma *in situ*, CIS, or invasive carcinoma).

quently mutated or deleted in clinically evident lung carcinoma specimens.

Sequential genetic changes in the pathogenesis of lung cancers

Our data have demonstrated that in lung cancer the developmental sequence of molecular changes is not random (Fig. 20.2). Allelic loss at one or more 3p regions (especially telomeric regions 3p21, 3p22-24 and 3p25) and 9p21, and to a lesser extent at 8p21–23, 13q14 (*RB*) and 17p13 (*TP53*), being detected frequently very early in pathogenesis, commencing in histologically normal epithelium[43,78]. In contrast, LOH at 5q21 (*APC–MCC* region) and *K-RAS* mutations were only detected at the CIS stage, and *TP53* mutations appear at variable times. By exam-

ining all our material for the early losses at 3p, 9p and 8p, we suggest that the order of events is normally either 3p→9p→8p or 3p→8p→9p deletions followed by *TP53* deletion[43].

Recent attention has focused on the *FHIT* gene at 3p14.2, a candidate tumour suppressor gene for lung and other cancers, which spans FRA3B, the most common of the aphidocolin-inducible fragile sites[26,81,82]. While it is tempting to speculate that breaks at FRA3B destabilize the entire short arm of chromosome 3, leading to multiple deletions, our data indicated that allelic losses at other more telomeric 3p regions (3p21, 3p22-24 and 3p25) appeared at histologically earlier stages than losses within and around the *FHIT* gene[78]. This is in agreement with the published findings of frequent loss of the Fhit protein immunostaining from dysplasia stage in the multistage development of NSCLCs[83].

Table 20.1. Major genetic alterations in the three major histological types of lung cancer

Genetic alteration	Small cell (%)	Squamous cell (%)	Adenocarcinoma (%)
RAS mutation	<1	<1	20–30
MYC amplification	18–31	8–20	<1
BCL-2 expression	75–95	25–35	~10
TP53 gene			
Mutation	75–100	40	30
LOH (17p13)	90	82	44
Abnormal protein (IHC)	40–70	50–60	40
RB gene			
LOH (13q14)	67	29	33
Abnormal protein (IHC)	~90	12	11
CDKN2 gene			
Mutation	<1	30	30
Methylation	<1	30	30
LOH (9p21)	40	63	69
Abnormal protein (IHC)	0–10	45–80	39–46
FHIT gene			
Aberrant transcripts	79	50	80
LOH (3p14.2)	95	91	45
Abnormal protein (IHC)	90–100	87	57
Loss of heterozygosity			
3p12	85	95	35
3p 21.3	100	96	50
3p22–24	91	87	48
4p	100	~35	0
4q	100	~40	~33
5q21–22	70	27	0
6q	50	44	25
8p21–23	86	100	81
Microsatellite alterations	50	32	24
Telomerase activity	~100	~90	~90

The percentages are obtained from the literature cited in the text, and reflect consensus approximations.

Belinsky and coworkers[35] recently determined the timing of *CDKN2* methylation event in the multistage pathogenesis of lung squamous cell carcinoma. Of interest, *CDKN2* gene was coordinately methylated in 75% of CIS lesions adjacent to invasive squamous cell carcinomas harbouring this change. Moreover, the frequency of this event increased during disease progression from basal cell hyperplasia (17%) to squamous metaplasia (24%) to CIS (50%) lesions. This study shows that an epigenetic alteration, aberrant methylation of the *CDKN2* gene, can be an early event in the pathogenesis of lung cancer.

Our data also indicate that different patterns of sequential deletions are detected in the pathogenesis of the major histological types of lung cancers (Table 20.1). Overall, more cumulative and earlier allelic loss at several chromosomal regions frequently deleted in invasive tumours are found in bronchial epithelium accompanying centrally arising SCLC and squamous cell carcinomas than peripheral adenocarcinomas[123].

Accumulation of genetic changes in the development of lung cancer

The development of epithelial cancers requires multiple mutation[84], the stepwise accumulation of which may represent a mutator phenotype[85,86]. Thus, it is possible that those preneoplastic lesions that have accumulated multiple mutations are at higher risk for progression to invasive cancer. Using a panel of microsatellite markers targeting chromosomal regions frequently deleted in invasive lung carcinomas, we have detected similar incidences of LOH between histologically normal epithelium and slightly abnormal epithelial changes (hyperplasia and squamous metaplasia) accompanying the major types of lung tumours[78]. These findings indicate they may not be at higher risk of progression for those slightly abnormal epithelia. However, high grade dysplasia and CIS accompanying invasive squamous cell lung carcinomas demonstrated a significant increase of LOH[78], suggesting that the accumulation of mutations correlates with the morphological changes and may lead to development of these tumour types (sequential theory of lung cancer development, Fig. 20.1). In particular, the allelic loss patterns of CIS lesions were identical or nearly identical to those present in the corresponding invasive carcinoma[78]. As some specimens of histologically normal or mildly abnormal epithelia, especially those accompanying SCLCs, have demonstrated a very high incidence of allelic loss, equal to or greater than that present in some high grade dysplasia and CIS samples, we suggest that CIS and invasive carcinoma may arise directly from histologically normal or from mildly abnormal epithelium, without passing through the entire histological sequence (parallel theory of cancer development, Fig. 20.1).

Of great interest, our complete allelotyping analyses of chromosome arms 3p and 8p in the multistage development of squamous cell carcinomas have demonstrated that the extent of the deletions increase with progressive histological changes[43,78]. Thus, in all squamous cell invasive carcinomas and CIS lesions most of the 3p and 8p arms were deleted, and in all patients the extent of the losses in CIS and invasive carcinomas was greater than the 3p and 8p allelic losses found in the corresponding normal and preneoplastic foci.

Our recent analyses have indicated that four patterns of allelic loss could be determined (negative, early, intermediate, and advanced) in histologically normal and precursor lesions accompanying squamous cell lung carcinomas[78]. Histologically normal or mildly abnormal foci have a negative pattern (no allelic loss) or early pattern of loss while all foci of CIS and invasive tumour had an advanced pattern. However, dysplasias demonstrated the entire spectrum of allelic loss patterns, and they were the only histological category having the intermediate pattern. These findings suggest that dysplasias represent a heterogeneous group of lesions at a molecular level. As only a fraction (10% of moderate dysplasia, 40–80% of severe dysplasia) are believed to progress to cancer[87–89], molecular studies may aid in the identification of the subgroups of smokers with dysplasia who are at the greater risk of progression to lung cancer.

In summary, our findings demonstrate that, despite similar smoking exposures, different pathways and genotypic changes are involved in the pathogenesis of three major histological types of lung carcinoma, namely SCLC, squamous cell carcinoma and adenocarcinoma. It seems that more allele deletions accumulate during the tumorigenesis in centrally arising SCLC and squamous cell carcinomas than in peripherally located adenocarcinomas. The finding of different patterns of LOH between all the three major types of lung cancers is consistent with their different basis of histopathological and clinical characteristics.

Lung cancer precursor lesions represent outgrowth of multiple clones

Molecular analyses suggested that precursor lesions represented outgrowths of multiple clones, a finding compatible with the field effect theory[90]. Our analysis of 58 normal and non-invasive foci accompanying 12 invasive squamous cell carcinomas and having any molecular abnormality indicated that 30 (52%) probably arose as independent clonal events, while 28 (48%) were potentially of the same clonal origin as the corresponding tumour. If the potentially clonal lesions are truly clonal in origin, subclonal drift[91] must have occurred as an early and widespread event, as only 4 foci (6%) (from two subjects) of 62 lesions had identical patterns of mutations. However, we cannot exclude the possibility that some other earlier molecular event occurred in a single cell whose progeny were dispersed widely throughout the bronchial epithelium and subsequently gave rise to all of the foci we examined. If this event occurred, then subclonal drift[91] must have occurred as an early and widespread event. These findings suggest that histologically normal bronchial epithelium and lung cancer precursor lesions having smoking related genetic damage represent outgrowths of multiple small clones of genetically abnormal cells, a finding compatible with the field effect theory.

Similar genetic changes are detected in invasive lung cancers and their precursor lesions

We and others have noted that the specific parental allele lost in chromosomal deletions in preneoplastic lesions and their accompanying cancers are similar[43,61,62,67,78]. We have referred to this phenomenon as allele specific mutations (ASM). While others have noted ASM in advanced bronchial lesions (severe dysplasias)[67], which are believed to be the immediate precursors of invasive cancers and which were located adjacent to centrally arising squamous cell carcinomas, we have detected ASM in preneoplastic lesions located in all regions of the respiratory epithelium (bronchi, bronchioles, and alveoli) and encompassed a variety of differentiated cell types (mucous cells, metaplastic squamous cells, Clara cells, and type II alveolar pneumocytes)[43,61,62,78]. In addition, we have detected this phenomenon in a wider spectrum of preneoplastic lesions, including hyperplasia, squamous metaplasia, dysplasia and CIS[43,61,62,78]. Of great interest, we have detected ASM in smoking related damaged epithelium, even in biopsy samples obtained from different lungs[79].

What possible mechanism could account for allele specific mutations? We have proposed two possibilities for allele loss. First, the lesions could be clonal in origin, and a single cell or small clone of cells develops loss or point mutations at a specific allele at one or more loci, migrates widely throughout the respiratory epithelium of both lungs and eventually gives rise to a tumour. For the reasons stated above, this is highly unlikely. This possibility would require an unexpected fluidity of the bronchial epithelium, or at least of those cells in which the initial genetic change occurs. The second possibility is that, in individuals, one of any pair of alleles has a greater tendency to be lost, perhaps as a results of some form of genomic imprinting or the presence of fragile sites resulting in an inherited propensity to lose one of the two alleles.

However, not all the genetic analyses of physically distinct lesions have identified the same pattern of genetic damage. Multicentric development is supported by a study by Sozzi et al. of five patients with multiple lesions in their bronchial tree, detecting losses of different alleles on chromosome 3p regions and different mutations in the *TP53* and *K-RAS* genes between invasive lung tumours and accompanying preneoplastic lesions[64]. In addition, Franklin et al. studied the entire bronchial tree of a smoker dying without lung carcinoma[77]. A single, identical point mutation, G to T transversion in codon 245 was identified in the bronchial epithelium from seven of ten widely dispersed bilateral epithelial tissues. The morphology of the involved sites varied from normal to squamous metaplasia to moderate dysplasia. These findings support the alternative theory that a single clone of cells can be widely dispersed throughout the respiratory epithelium. However, our recent findings of ASM phenomenon in lung cancer precursor lesions that appeared to be of independent clonal origin suggests that ASM occurs via an alternative mechanism[78]. Whatever its mechanism, ASM is likely to be a phenomenon of major biological significance.

Genomic instability in the pathogenesis of lung cancer

In addition to the specific genetic changes discussed above, other evidence indicates that genomic instability occurs in lung cancer and its preneoplastic lesions. This evidence includes our finding of widespread aneuploidy throughout the respiratory epithelium of lung cancer patients[72]. Another molecular change frequently present in a wide variety of cancer types is microsatellite alterations (MAs) (also known as genomic alterations).

In hereditary non-poplyposis colon cancer (HNPCC), inherited defects in DNA mismatch repair enzymes result in large-scale genetic instability, with the formation of a ladder like pattern replacing the normal allele pattern[92]. Another form of microsatellite change, where only a single band of altered size is found, has been described in many forms of sporadic cancers, including lung cancer (range 0–45%)[93–96] referred to as microsatellite alterations[78,93,97–99]. The relationship of MAs to DNA repair mechanism has not been established, and they probably represent evidence of some form of genomic instability[86]. Because they arise in non-coding regions of the genome, they are not in the direct pathway of tumorigenesis MAs represent changes in the size of polymorphic microsatellite markers compared to the normal germline in individual persons. Nevertheless, MAs are attractive candidates for the early molecular detection of cancer[93,98]. Our data demonstrated the presence of MAs in a subset (50%) of lung carcinomas[78,99], as well as in their accompanying preneoplastic lesions and normal appearing epithelium[78]. Unlike allelic losses,

the frequency of MAs did not increase with more advanced histological changes. Of interest, MAs, when present in non-malignant foci, were always of a different size than those present in the corresponding invasive tumours. These findings indicate that either the preneoplastic lesions are not clonally related to the corresponding tumours or that the MAs arose during subclonal evolution. The finding of MAs in exfoliated cells present in sputum[98] from patients suggest that they may be markers for lung cancer or those at increased risk of developing lung cancer. While the MAs present in preneoplastic lesions were not present in the corresponding tumours, the presence of MAs may still predict for increased risk, as they probably represent a form of genomic instability[86]. Of interest, our recent findings indicated that a higher frequency of MAs are detected in bronchial epithelium accompanying SCLCs compared to the other lung cancer histological types[123], suggesting that more widespread and more extensive genetic damage is present in bronchial epithelium in patients with SCLC.

Telomerase dysregulation in the pathogenesis of lung cancer

Telomerase is currently recognized as a nearly ubiquitous tumour marker. Telomerase is a specialized ribonucleoprotein polymerase that adds TTAGGG repeats at the ends of vertebrate chromosomal DNA called telomeres[100]. Human telomeres undergo progressive shortening with cell division through replication of dependent sequence loss at DNA termini[101]. Telomerase is thought to compensate for the loss of telomeric repeats and is associated with the acquisition of the immortal phenotype. A variety of immortal cell lines, malignant tumours and germ cells have been found to specifically express telomerase activity[102–105], whereas most normal somatic cells do not express this activity[106]. In NSCLC, the telomerase positive percentage is 73% with weak to moderate activities whereas 100% of SCLC are positive and show strong signal activities[103].

Telomerase has been detected in preinvasive

lesions in a number of tumour systems, including lung[107]. In lung, low levels of telomerase activity have been detected in hyperplasia, dysplasia and CIS compared to invasive cancer. While weak telomerase RNA expression is detected in basal layers of normal and hyperplastic epithelium from lung cancer patients, dysregulation of telomerase expression increases with tumour progression with moderate to strong expression throughout the multilayers of the epithelium in metaplasia, dysplasia and CIS[107]. Of interest, foci of intense telomerase up-regulation are seen in CIS lesions in the vicinity of the invasive component of lung cancers. In addition, similar pattern of dysregulation in telomerase expression with increasing histological grade has also been noted in bronchoscopic biopsies of smoking damaged epithelium of current and former smokers, suggesting that telomerase could also be used as a potential marker for risk assessment (Rahti et al., unpublished data).

Molecular markers for early detection of lung cancer

Mutant *K-RAS* has been detected in the sputum up to several months prior to diagnosis of cancer[66] and *K-RAS* mutation has been detected in bronchoalveolar lavage fluid in a high proportion of patients with adenocarcinoma (56%), but not in patients with squamous cell carcinoma or with other diagnosis[108]. Recently, Ahrendt et al.[109] have reported that molecular assays could identify cancer cells in bronchoalveolar lavage fluid from patients with early-stage lung cancers. Using PCR-based assays for *K-RAS* and *TP53* gene mutations, CpG-islands methylation status of the *CDKN2* gene and for microsatellite instability, they were able to detect identical molecular abnormality in the bronchoalveolar fluid and corresponding tumours in 23 of 43 (53%) of the cases. These findings suggest that molecular strategies may detect the presence of neoplastic cells in the proximal airway of patients with early-stage lung carcinomas.

Smoking damaged bronchial epithelium

It has been established that advanced lung preneoplastic changes occur far more frequently in smokers than in non-smokers and increase in frequency with amount of smoking, adjusted by age[5,7]. Although morphological recovery occurs after smoking cessation[7,110], elevated lung cancer risk persists[111]. Changes in bronchial epithelium, including metaplasia and dysplasia, have been utilized as surrogate end points for chemoprevention studies[112,113]. Risk factors that identify normal and premalignant bronchial tissue at risk for malignant progression need to be better defined. However, most of the molecular studies of lung preneoplastic lesions have been performed in material from small number of subjects with concurrent lung cancer, and only scant information is available about molecular changes in the respiratory epithelium of smokers without cancer[43,67,68,79,114].

Two independent studies describing genetic changes in bronchial biopsy specimens from current and former smokers have been reported[79,114]. Mao et al.[114] described their analyses of the LOH and histological abnormalities present in biopsies from 54 current and former smokers and nine non-smokers. In each of the current and former smokers, bronchoscopy biopsies from six preselected sites demonstrated histological changes, including squamous metaplasia and dysplasia. In addition, LOH using three microsatellite markers at chromosomal region 3p14, 9p21 and 17p13 (*TP53*) were used as surrogate markers of tumour suppressor gene inactivation in the tissues. Although some differences were seen when the specimens of current smokers were compared with those of former smokers, allelic losses were surprisingly common in the non-malignant lung epithelial tissue of both groups. Whereas 76% of the smoker subjects demonstrated allelic loss at one or more of the three chromosomal regions analysed, deletions were detected in 75%, 57% and 18% of the subjects at 3p14, 9p21 and 17p13 (*TP53*), respectively.

Our results[79], which are in agreement with the above findings, also indicate that genetic changes similar to those found in lung cancers can be detected in non-malignant bronchial epithelium from current and former smokers and may persist for many years after smoking cessation. In our study, multiple biopsy specimens were obtained from 18 current smokers, 24 former smokers, and 21 non-smokers. PCR-based assays for 15 polymorphic microsatellite DNA markers were used to examine eight chromosomal regions (3p14.2 at *FHIT* gene, 3p14–21, 3p21, 3p22–24, 5q21 at *APC–MCC* region, 9p21, 13q14 at *RB*, and 17p13 at *TP53*) for genetic changes (LOH and MAs). High frequencies of LOH and MAs were observed in biopsies from current and former smokers, and no significant differences were observed between the two groups. Of great interest, no molecular changes were detected in non-smoker subjects. Among individuals who smoked, 86% demonstrated LOH in one or more biopsies and 24% showed LOH in all biopsies. Somewhat surprisingly, about half of the histologically normal epithelium showed LOH; however, the frequency of LOH and the severity of histological changes did not correspond until the CIS stage. A subset of the biopsies from smokers with either normal or preneoplastic histology showed LOH at multiple chromosomal sites, a phenomenon frequently observed in CIS and invasive cancer. Our findings suggest that CIS and other histologically normal and abnormal foci having multiple regions of allelic loss are at increased risk for progressing to invasive cancer. As it has been observed in epithelial foci accompanying invasive lung carcinoma[78], allelic losses on chromosome 3p and 9p were more frequent than deletions in chromosomes 5q21, 17p13 (*TP53* gene) and 13q14 (*RB* gene). Recently, we have also demonstrated frequent chromosome 8p21–23 allelic losses in bronchial samples from former and current smokers, confirming the findings that 8p deletions commence early during the pathogenesis of lung cancer[43]. All these findings suggest the hypothesis that identifying biopsies with extensive or certain patterns of allelic loss may provide new methods for assessing the risk in smokers of developing invasive lung cancer and for monitoring response to chemoprevention. As with all diagnostic tests, this concept will need to be validated in clinical trials.

Size of the patches with genetic changes in the pathogenesis of lung cancer

Although all or almost all of the current chemoprevention studies in the USA utilize serial bronchoscopic biopsies to evaluate response, there is no information available on the efficacy of this approach. While histopathological evaluation is the 'gold standard', many studies utilize molecular or other biological endpoints. For these reasons, we undertook an evaluation of the size and frequency of the molecularly altered (allelic loss and microsatellite alterations) clonal patches in smoking damaged bronchial epithelium. Our findings indicated that multiple small clonal and subclonal patches of molecular abnormalities (not much larger in size than the average bronchial biopsy obtained by fluorescence bronchoscopy) can be detected in the normal and slightly abnormal bronchial epithelium of patients with lung cancer[115]. The clonal patches of bronchial epithelium having molecular changes were usually small, and they were estimated to be approximately 40000 to 360000 cells. Based on the size of the average biopsy obtained by fluorescence bronchoscopy, we estimated the average surface area of the clonally altered patches to be between 4 and 80 sq. mm[115]. Thus, we estimate that there may be 8 or more independent molecularly altered clonal patches per sq. cm. These findings are consistent with the findings of Hittelman and coworkers who found evidence for the presence of numerous small monosomic and trisomic clonal and subclonal patches in smoking damaged upper aerodigestive epithelium as determined by FISH analyses[116,117]. All these findings suggest that the process of obtaining a biopsy may result in 'spontaneous' reversion of molecularly altered foci of bronchial epithelium to normal. Thus, our recent findings may help in the design of chemoprevention studies utilizing sequential bronchial biopsies for the monitoring of intermediate biomarkers as endpoints.

Molecular changes in the spectrum of lung neuroendocrine tumours

Recent classifications identify four categories of neuroendocrine tumours of the lung: low-grade typical carcinoid, intermediate grade atypical carcinoid, and high-grade large cell neuroendocrine carcinoma and SCLC[118]. While the pattern of genetic changes in SCLC has been well studied, relatively little is known regarding the genetic changes associated with the other histological types of lung neuroendocrine tumours. Recently, we studied molecular abnormalities (allele loss at 3p, 5q, 11q, 13q, and 17p chromosomal regions, and *TP53* and *RAS* gene mutations) present in a series of 59 neuroendocrine tumours of the lung representing the entire spectrum of histological types[119]. With the exception of *RAS* gene mutations, most of the studied changes were frequently present in neuroendocrine carcinomas and were present at lower frequencies in carcinoids. Allelic loss at one or more 3p regions was the most frequent change found in the carcinoids. A relatively high incidence LOH at the recently cloned *MEN1* (11q13) gene[120] was common in all neuroendocrine lung tumours, including carcinoids. This is in agreement with previous observations of relatively high incidence of MEN1 gene inactivation in lung carcinoids[121]. The patterns of *TP53* gene mutations were different between atypical carcinoid and high-grade neuroendocrine tumours. Of interest, 5q21–22 (*APC-MCC* region) allelic loss was correlated with poor survival in the carcinoid group. Although neuroendocrine lung tumours have varied etiologies, the results of our recently published study[119] support the clinico-pathological concept that they represent a spectrum ranging from low grade typical carcinoid and intermediate grade atypical carcinoid to the highly malignant large cell neuroendocrine carcinoma and SCLC.

Conclusions

In conclusion, our understanding of the molecular pathology of lung cancer is advancing rapidly with several specific genes and chromosomal regions being identified. Lung cancer appears to require many mutations in both dominant and recessive oncogenes before they become invasive. Several genetic changes are common to all lung cancer histological types, while others appear to be tumour type specific. The identification of those specific genes undergoing such mutations and the sequence of cumulative changes that lead the neoplastic changes for each lung tumour histological type remain to be fully elucidated. Recent findings in normal and preneoplastic bronchial epithelium from lung cancer patients and smoker subjects suggest that genetic changes may provide in this neoplasm new methods for early diagnosis, risk assessment and for monitoring response to chemoprevention.

Acknowledgements

Supported by contract N01-CN-45580-01 from the Early Detection Research Network, and Specialized Program of Research Excellence grant 1-P50-CA70907–01 from the National Cancer Institute, Bethesda, MD.

REFERENCES

1 Colby TV, Koss MN, Travis WD. *Tumors of the Lower Respiratory Tract*, 3rd. series, Fascicle 13, p. 1–554. Washington, D.C.: Armed Forces Institute of Pathology, 1995.

2 Colby TV, Wistuba II, Gazdar A. Precursors to pulmonary neoplasia. *Adv Anat Pathol* 1998; 5:205–215.

3 Sekido Y, Fong KM, Minna JD. Progress in understanding the molecular pathogenesis of human lung cancer. *Biochim Biophys Acta* 1998; 1378:F21–F59,

4 Saccomanno G, Archer VE, Auerbach O, Saunders RP, Brennan LM. Development of carcinoma of the lung as reflected in exfoliated cells. *Cancer* 1974; 33:256–270.

5 Auerbach O, Hammond EC, Garfinkel L. Changes in bronchial epithelium in relation to cigarette smoking, 1955–1960 vs. 1970–1977, *N Engl J Med*. 1979; 300:381–5.

6 Peters EJ, Morice R, Benner SE et al. Squamous metaplasia of the bronchial mucosa and its relationship to smoking. *Chest* 1993; 103:1429–3142.

7 Auerbach O, Stout AP, Hammond EC, Garfinkel L. Changes

in bronchial epithelium in relation to smoking and cancer of the lung. *New Engl J Med* 1961; 265:253–226.

8 Lam S, Kennedy T, Unger M et al. Localization of bronchial intraepithelial neoplastic lesions by fluorescence bronchoscopy. *Chest* 1998; 113:696–702.

9 Lam S, MacAulay C, LeRiche JC, Ikeda N, Palcic B. Early localization of bronchogenic carcinoma. *Diagnos Therapeut Endos* 1994; 1:75–78.

10 Shimosato Y, Noguchi M, Matsumo Y. Adenocarcinoma of the lung: Its development and malignant progression. *Lung Cancer* 1993; 9:99–108.

11 Mori M, Chiba R, Takahashi T. Atypical adenomatous hyperplasia of the lung and its differentiation from adenocarcinoma. Characterization of atypical cells by morphometry and multivariate cluster analysis. *Cancer* 1993; 72:2331–2340.

12 Miller RR., Muller NL. Neuroendocrine cell hyperplasia and obliterative bronchiolitis in patients with peripheral carcinoid tumors. *Am J Surg Pathol* 1995; 19:653–658.

13 Gazdar AF, Cohen MH, Ihde DC, Minna JD, Matthews MJ. Bronchial epithelial changes in association with small cell carcinoma of the lung. In: Muggia F, Rozencweig M, eds., *Proceedings of the Second National Cancer Institute Conference on Lung Cancer Treatment*, New York: Raven Press; 1979:167–174.

14 Slaughter DP, Southwick HW, Smejkal W. 'Field cancerization' in oral stratified squamous epithelium: clinical implications of multicentric origin. *Cancer* 1954; 6:963–968.

15 Johnson BE. Second lung cancers in patients after treatment for an initial lung cancer. *J Natl Cancer Inst* 1998; 90:1335–1345.

16 Mitsudomi T, Viallet J, Mulshine JL, Linnoila RI, Minna JD, Gazdar AF. Mutations of *ras* genes distinguish a subset of non-small-cell lung cancer cell lines from small-cell lung cancer cell lines. *Oncogene* 1991; 6:1353–1362.

17 Nau MM, Carney DN, Battey et al. Amplification, expression and rearrangement of c-*myc* and N-*myc* oncogenes in human lung cancer. *Curr Top Microbiol Immunol* 1984; 113:172–177.

18 Nau MM, Brooks BJ, Carney DN et al. Human small cell lung cancers show amplification and expression of the N-myc gene. *Proc Natl Acad Sci USA* 1986; 83:1092–1096.

19 Little CD, Nau MM, Carney DN, Gazdar AF, Minna JD. Amplification and expression of the c-myc oncogene in human lung cancer cell lines. *Nature* 1983; 306:194–196.

20 Johnson BE, Russell E, Simmons AM et al. MYC family DNA amplification in 126 tumor cell lines from patients with small cell lung cancer. *J Cell Biochem Suppl* 1996; 24:210–217.

21 Levin NA, Brzoska P, Gupta N, Minna JD, Gray JW,

Christman MF. Identification of frequent novel genetic alterations in small cell lung carcinoma. *Cancer Res* 1994; 54:5086–5091.

22 Levin NA, Brzoska PM, Warnock ML, Gray JW, Christman MF. Identification of novel regions of altered DNA copy number in small cell lung tumors. *Genes Chromosomes Cancer* 1995; 13:175–185.

23 Petersen I, Langreck H, Wolf G et al. Small-cell lung cancer is characterized by a high incidence of deletions on chromosomes 3p, 4q, 5q, 10q, 13q and 17p. *Br J Cancer* 1997; 75:79–86.

24 Schwendel A, Langreck H, Reichel M et al. Primary small-cell lung carcinomas and their metastases are characterized by a recurrent pattern of genetic alterations. *Int J Cancer* 1997; 74:86–93.

25 Sundaresan V, Chung G, Heppell-Parton A et al. Homozygous deletions at 3p12 in breast and lung cancer. *Oncogene* 1998; 1723–1729.

26 Ohta M, Inoue H, Cotticelli MG et al. The *FHIT* gene, spanning the chromosome 3p14.2 fragile site and renal carcinoma-associated t(3; 8) breakpoint, is abnormal in digestive tract cancers. *Cell* 1996; 84:587–597.

27 Sozzi G, Veronese ML, Negrini M et al. The FHIT gene at 3p14.2 is abnormal in lung cancer. *Cell* 1996; 85:17–26.

28 Knudson AG. Hereditary cancers: clues to mechanisms of carcinogenesis. *Br J Cancer* 1989; 59:661–666.

29 Denissenko MF, Pao A, Tang M-S, Pfeifer GP. Preferential formation of benz[a]pyrene adducts in lung cancer mutational hotspots in p53. *Science* 1996; 274:430–433.

30 Horowitz JM, Yandell DW, Park SH et al. Point mutational inactivation of the retinoblastoma antioncogene. *Science* 1989; 243:937–940.

31 Harbour JW, Sali SL, Whang-Peng J, Gazdar AF, Minna JD, Kaye FJ. Abnormalities in structure and expression of the human retinoblastoma gene in SCLC. *Science* 1988; 241:353–357.

32 Hensel CH, Hsieh CL, Gazdar AF et al. Altered structure and expression of the human retinoblastoma susceptibility gene in small cell lung cancer. *Cancer Res* 1990; 50:3067–3072.

33 Geradts J, Fong KM, Zimmerman PV, Maynard R, Minna JD. Correlation of abnormal RB, p16ink4a, and p53 expression with 3p loss of heterozygosity, other genetic abnormalities, and clinical features in 103 primary non-small cell lung cancers. *Clin Cancer Res* 1999; 5:791–800.

34 Shapiro GI, Park JE, Edwards CD et al. Multiple mechanisms of p16INK4A inactivation in non-small cell lung cancer cell lines. *Cancer Res* 1995; 55:6200–6209.

35 Belinsky SA, Nikula KJ, Palmisano WA et al. Aberrant methylation of p16(INK4a) is an early event in lung cancer and a

potential biomarker for early diagnosis. *Proc Natl Acad Sci USA* 1998; 95:11891–11896.

36 Vonlanthen S, Heighway J, Tschan MP et al. Expression of p16INK4a/p16alpha and p19ARF/p16beta is frequently altered in non-small cell lung cancer and correlates with p53 overexpression. *Oncogene* 1998; 17:2779–2785.

37 Virmani AK, Fong KM, Kodagoda D et al. Allelotyping demonstrates common and distinct patterns of chromosomal loss in human lung cancer types. *Genes Chromosomes Cancer* 1998; 21:308–319.

38 D'Amico D, Carbone DP, Johnson BE, Meltzer SJ, Minna JD. Polymorphic sites within the MCC and APC loci reveal very frequent loss of heterozygosity in human small cell lung cancer. *Cancer Res* 1992; 52:1996–1999.

39 Ohata H, Emi M, Fujiwara Y et al. Deletion mapping of the short arm of chromosome 8 in non-small cell lung carcinoma. *Genes Chromosomes Cancer* 1993; 7:85–88.

40 Sato S, Nakamura Y, Tsuchiya E. Difference of allelotype between squamous cell carcinoma and adenocarcinoma of the lung. *Cancer Res* 1994; 54:5652–5655.

41 Shivapurkar N, Virmani AK, Wistuba II et al. Deletions of chromosome 4 at multiple sites are frequent in malignant mesothelioma and small cell lung carcinoma. *Clin Cancer Res* 1999; 5:17–23.

42 Shiseki M, Kohno T, Nishikawa R, Sameshima Y, Mizoguchi H, Yokota J. Frequent allelic losses on chromosomes 2q, 18q, and 22q in advanced non-small cell lung carcinoma. *Cancer Res* 1994; 54:5643–5648.

43 Wistuba II, Behrens C, Virmani AK et al. Allelic losses at chromosome 8p21–23 are early and frequent events in the pathogenesis of lung cancer. *Cancer Res* 1999; 59:1973–1979.

44 Bepler G. and Garcia-Blanco M.A. Three tumor-suppressor regions on chromosome 11p identified by high-resolution deletion mapping in human non-small-cell lung cancer. *Proc Natl Acad Sci USA* 1994; 91:5513–5517.

45 Iizuka M, Sugiyama Y, Shiraishi M, Jones C Sekiya T. Allelic losses in human chromosome 11 in lung cancers. *Genes Chromosomes Cancer* 1995; 13:40–46.

46 Wang SS, Virmani A, Gazdar AF, Minna JD, Evans GA. Refined mapping of two regions of loss of heterozygosity on chromosome band 11q23 in lung cancer. *Genes Chromosomes Cancer* 1999; 25:154–159.

47 Ottaviano YL, Issa JP, Parl FF, Smith HS, Baylin SB, Davidson NE. Methylation of the estrogen receptor gene CpG island marks loss of estrogen receptor expression in human breast cancer cells. *Cancer Res* 1994; 54:2552–2555.

48 O'Briant, KC, Bepler G. Delineation of the centromeric and telomeric chromosome segment 11p15.5 lung cancer suppressor regions LOH11A and LOH11B. *Genes Chromosomes Cancer* 1997; 18:111–114.

49 Suzuki K, Ogura T, Yokose T et al. Loss of heterozygosity in the tuberous sclerosis gene associated regions in adenocarcinoma of the lung accompanied by multiple atypical adenomatous hyperplasia. *Int J Cancer* 1998; 79:384–389.

50 Kohno,T, Kawanishi M, Matsuda S et al. Homozygous deletion and frequent allelic loss of the 21q11.1-q21.1 region including the ANA gene in human lung carcinoma. *Genes Chromosomes Cancer* 1998; 21:236–243.

51 Li J, Yen C, Liaw D et al. PTEN, a putative protein tyrosine phosphatase gene mutated in human brain, breast and prostate cancer. *Science* 1997; 275:1943–1947.

52 Wu W, Kemp BL, Proctor ML et al. Expression of DMBT1, a candidate tumor suppressor gene, is frequently lost in lung cancer. *Cancer Res* 1999; 59:1846–1851.

53 Wang SS, Esplin ED, Li JL et al. Alterations of the PPP2R1B gene in human lung and colon cancer. *Science* 1998; 282:284–287.

54 Forgacs E, Biesterveld EJ, Sekido Y et al. Mutation analysis of the PTEN/MMAC1 gene in lung cancer. *Oncogene* 1998; 17:1557–1565.

55 Yokomizo A, Tindall DJ, Drabkin H et al. PTEN/MMAC1 mutations identified in small cell, but not in non-small cell lung cancers. *Oncogene* 1998; 17:475–479.

56 Yokoyama S, Yamakawa K, Tsuchiya E, Murata M, Sakiyama S, Nakamura Y. Deletion mapping on the short arm of chromosome 3 in squamous cell carcinoma and adenocarcinoma of the lung. *Cancer Res* 1992; 52:873–877.

57 Petersen I, Bujard M, Petersen S et al. Patterns of chromosomal imbalances in adenocarcinoma and squamous cell carcinoma of the lung. *Cancer Res* 1997; 57:2331–2335.

58 Suzuki Y, Orita M, Shiraishi M, Hayashi K, Sekiya T. Detection of ras gene mutations in human lung cancers by single-strand conformation polymorphism analysis of polymerase chain reaction products. *Oncogene* 1990; 5:1037–1043.

59 Gealy R, Zhang L, Siegfried JM, Luketich JD, Keohavong P. Comparison of mutations in the p53 and K-ras genes in lung carcinomas from smoking and nonsmoking women. *Cancer Epidemiol Biomarkers Prev* 1999; 8:297–302.

60 Takeshima Y, Seyama T, Bennett WP et al. p53 mutations in lung cancers from non-smoking atomic-bomb survivors. *Lancet* 1993; 342:1520–1521.

61 Hung J, Kishimoto Y, Sugio K et al. Allele-specific chromosome 3p deletions occur at an early stage in the pathogenesis of lung carcinoma. *JAMA* 1995; 273:558–563.

62 Kishimoto Y, Sugio K, Mitsudomi T et al. Allele specific loss of chromosome 9p in preneoplastic lesions accompanying non-small cell lung cancers. *J Natl Cancer Inst* 1995; 87:1224–1229.

63 Sozzi G, Miozzo M, Tagliabue E et al. Cytogenetic abnormalities and overexpression of receptors for growth factors in normal bronchial epithelium and tumor samples of lung cancer patients. *Cancer Res* 1991; 51:400–404.

64 Sozzi G, Miozzo M, Pastorino U et al. Genetic evidence for an independent origin of multiple preneoplastic and neoplastic lung lesions. *Cancer Res* 1995; 55:135–140.

65 Sozzi G, Miozzo M, Donghi R et al. Deletions of 17p and p53 mutations in preneoplastic lesions of the lung. *Cancer Res* 1992; 52:6079–6082.

66 Mao L, Hruban RH, Boyle JO, Tockman M, Sidransky D. Detection of oncogene mutations in sputum precedes diagnosis of lung cancer. *Cancer Res* 1994; 54:1634–1637.

67 Sundaresan V, Ganly P, Hasleton P et al. p53 and chromosome 3 abnormalities, characteristic of malignant lung tumours, are detectable in preinvasive lesions of the bronchus. *Oncogene* 1992; 7:1989–1997.

68 Thiberville L, Payne P, Vielkinds J et al. Evidence of cumulative gene losses with progression of premalignant epithelial lesions to carcinoma of the bronchus. *Cancer Res* 1995; 55:5133–5139.

69 Nuorva K, Soini Y, Kamel D et al. Concurrent p53 expression in bronchial dysplasias and squamous cell lung carcinomas. *Am J Pathol* 1993; 142:725–732.

70 Bennett WP, Colb, T., Travis WD et al. p53 protein accumulates frequently in early bronchial neoplasia. *Cancer Res* 1993; 53:4817–4822.

71 Hirano T, Franzen B, Kato H, Ebihara Y, Auer G. Genesis of squamous cell lung carcinoma. Sequential changes of proliferation, DNA ploidy, and p53 expression. *Am J Pathol* 1994; 144:296–302.

72 Smith AL, Hung J, Walker L et al. Extensive areas of aneuploidy are present in the respiratory epithelium of lung cancer patients. *Br J Cancer* 1996; 73:203–209.

73 Li ZH, Zheng J, Weiss LM, Shibat, D. c-k-ras and p53 mutations occur very early in adenocarcinoma of the lung. *Am J Pathol* 1994; 144:303–309.

74 Satoh Y, Ishikawa Y, Nakagawa K, Hirano T, Tsuchiya E. A follow-up study of progression from dysplasia to squamous cell carcinoma with immunohistochemical examination of p53 protein overexpression in the bronchi of ex-chromate workers. *Br J Cancer* 1997; 75:678–683.

75 Betticher DC, Heighway J, Thatcher N, Hasleton PS. Abnormal expression of CCND1 and RB1 in resection margin epithelia of lung cancer patients. *Br J Cancer* 1997; 75:1761–1768.

76 Westra WH, Baas IO, Hruban RH et al. K-ras oncogene activation in atypical alveolar hyperplasias of the human lung. *Cancer Res* 1996; 56:2224–2228.

77 Franklin WA, Gazdar AF, Haney J et al. Widely dispersed *p53*

mutation in respiratory epithelium. *J Clin Invest* 1997; 100:2133–2137.

78 Wistuba II, Behrens C, Milchgrub S et al. Sequential molecular abnormalities are involved in the multistage development of squamous cell lung carcinoma. *Oncogene* 1999; 18:643–650.

79 Wistuba II, Lam S, Behrens C et al. Molecular damage in the bronchial epithelium of current and former smokers. *J Natl Cancer Inst* 1997; 89:1366–1373.

80 Wistuba II, Bryant D, Behrens C et al. Comparison of features of human lung cancer cell lines and their corresponding tumors. *Clin Cancer Res* 1999; 5:991–1000.

81 Fong KM, Biesterveld EJ, Virmani A et al. *FHIT* and FRA3B allele loss are common in lung cancer and preneoplastic bronchial lesions and are associated with cancer-related *FHIT* cDNA splicing aberrations. *Cancer Res* 1997; 57:2256–2267.

82 Sozzi G, Veronese ML, Negrini M et al. The FHIT gene 3p14.2 is abnormal in lung cancer. *Cell* 1996; 85:17–26.

83 Sozzi G, Pastorino U, Moiraghi L et al. Loss of FHIT function in lung cancer and preinvasive bronchial lesions. *Cancer Res* 1998; 58:5032–5037.

84 Fisher JC. Multiple mutation theory of carcinogenesis. *Nature* 1958; 181:651–652.

85 Loeb LA. Mutator phenotype may be required for multistage carcinogenesis. *Cancer Res* 1991; 51:3075–3079.

86 Loeb LA. Microsatellite instability: marker of a mutator phenotype in cancer. *Cancer Res* 1994; 54:5059–5063.

87 Band PR, Feldstein M, Saccomanno G. Reversibility of bronchial marked atypia: implication for chemoprevention. *Cancer Detect Prevent* 1986; 9:157–160.

88 Frost JK, Ball WJ, Levin, ML et al. Sputum cytopathology: use and potential in monitoring the workplace environment by screening for biological effects of exposure. *J Occupat Med* 1986; 28:692–703.

89 Risse E, Vooijs G, van't Hof M. Diagnostic significance of 'severe dysplasia' in sputum cytology. *Acta Cytol* 1988; 32:629–634.

90 Strong MS, Incze J, Vaughan CW. Field cancerization in the aerodigestive tract – its etiology, manifestation, and significance. *J Otolaryng* 1984; 13:1–6.

91 Nowell PC. The clonal evolution of tumor cell populations. *Science* 1976; 194:23–28.

92 Liu B, Parsons R, Papadopoulos N et al. Analysis of mismatch repair genes in hereditary non-polyposis colorectal cancer patients. *Nat Med* 1996; 2:169–174.

93 Mao L, Lee DJ, Tockman MS, Erozan YS, Askin F, Sidransky D. Microsatellite alterations as clonal markers for the detection of human cancer. *Proc Natl Acad Sci USA* 1994; 91:9871–9875.

94 Fong KM, Zimmerman PV, Smith PJ. Microsatellite instability and other molecular abnormalities in non-small cell lung cancer. *Cancer Res* 1995; 55:28–30.

95 Adachi JI, Shiseki M, Okazaki T et al. Microsatellite instability in primary and metastatic lung carcinomas. *Genes Chromosom Cancer* 1995; 14:301–206.

96 Merlo A, Mabry M, Gabrielson E, Vollmer R, Baylin SB, Sidransky D. Frequent microsatellite instability in primary small cell lung cancer. *Cancer Res* 1994; 54:2098–2101.

97 Orlow I, Lianes P, Lacombe L, Dalbagni G, Reuter VE, Cordon-Cardo C. Chromosome 9 allelic losses and microsatellite alterations in human bladder tumors. *Cancer Res* 1994; 54:2848–2851.

98 Miozzo M, Sozzi G, Musso K et al. Microsatellite alterations in bronchial and sputum specimens of lung cancer patients. *Cancer Res* 1996; 56:2285–2288.

99 Wistuba II, Behrens C, Milchgrub S et al. Comparison of molecular changes in lung cancers in HIV-positive and HIV- indeterminate subjects. *JAMA* 1998; 279:1554–1559.

100 Morin GB. The human telomere terminal tranferase enzyme is a ribonucleoprotein that synthesizes TTAGGG repeats. *Cell* 1989; 59:521–529.

101 Hastie ND, Dempster M, Dunlop MG, Thompson AM, Green DK, Allshire RC. Telomere reduction in human colorectal carcinoma and with ageing. *Nature* 1990; 346:866–868.

102 Chadeneau C, Hay K, Hirte HW, Gallinger S, Bacchetti S. Telomerase activity associated with acquisition of malignancy in human colorectal cancer. *Cancer Res* 1995; 55:2533–2536.

103 Hiyama K, Hiyama E, Ishioka S et al. Telomerase activity in small-cell and non-small-cell lung cancer. *J Natl Cancer Inst* 1995; 87:895–902.

104 Hiyama E, Yokoyama T, Tatsumoto N et al. Telomerase activity in gastric cancer. *Cancer Res* 1995; 55:3258–3262.

105 Hiyama E, Gollahon L, Kataoka T et al. Telomerase activity in human breast tumors. *J Natl Cancer Inst* 1996; 88:116–122.

106 Counter CM. The roles of telomeres and telomerase in cell life span. *Mutat Res Rev Genet Toxicol* 1996; 366:45–63.

107 Yashima K, Litzky LA, Kaiser L et al. Telomerase expression in respiratory epithelium during the multistage pathogenesis of lung carcinomas. *Cancer Res* 1997; 57:2373–2377.

108 Mills NE, Fishman CL, Scholes J, Anderson SE, Rom WN, Jacobson DR. Detection of K-ras oncogene mutations in bronchoalveolar lavage fluid for lung cancer diagnosis. *J Natl Cancer Inst* 1995; 87:1056–1060.

109 Ahrendt SA, Chow JT et al. Molecular detection of tumor cells in bronchoalveolar lavage fluid from patients with early stage lung cancer. *J Natl Cancer Inst* 1999; 91:332–339.

110 Bertram JF, Rogers AW. Recovery of bronchial epithelium on stopping smoking. *Br Med J (Clin Res Ed)* 1981; 283:1567–1569,

111 Anon Office of Smoking and Health, U.S. Centers for Disease Control. *Morbid Mortal Weekly Rep* 1994; 43.

112 Schantz SP. Chemoprevention strategies: the relevance of premalignant and malignant lesions of the upper aerodigestive tract. *J Cell Biochem Suppl* 1993; 17F:18–26.

113 Boone CW, Kelloff GJ. Intraepithelial neoplasia, surrogate endpoint biomarkers, and cancer chemoprevention. *J Cell Biochem* Suppl 1993; 17F:37–48.

114 Mao L, Lee JS, Kurie JM et al. Clonal genetic alterations in the lungs of current and former smokers. *J Natl Cancer Inst* 1997; 89:857–862.

115 Park I-W, Wistuba II, Maitra A et al. Multiple clonal abnormalities in bronchial epithelium of lung cancer patients. *J Natl Cancer Inst* 1999; 91:1863–1868.

116 Hittelman WN. Genetic instability in the lung cancerization field. In: Brambilla C, Brambilla E, eds, *Lung Tumors: Fundamental Biology and Clinical Management*. New York: Marcel Dekker, Inc.; 1998:255–267.

117 Hittelman WN. Molecular cytogenetic evidence for multistep tumorigenesis: implications for risk assessment and early detection. In: S. Srivastava S, Gazdar AF, Henson DE, eds, *Molecular Pathology of Early Cancer*. Van Demanstratt, Netherlands: IOS Press; 1999:385–404.

118 Travis WD, Colby TV, Corrin B, Shimosato Y, Brambilla E, Countries CF. *World Health Organization Classification of Lung and Pleural Tumors*, 3rd edition. Berlin: Springer-Verlag, 1999.

119 Onuki N, Wistuba II, Travis WD et al. Genetic changes in the spectrum of neuroendocrine lung tumors. *Cancer* 1999; 85:600–607.

120 Chandrasekharappa SC, Guru SC, Manickam P et al. Positional cloning of the gene for multiple endocrine neoplasia-type 1. *Science* 1997; 276:404–407.

121 Debelenko LV, Brambilla E, Agarwal SK et al. Identification of MEN1 gene mutations in sporadic carcinoid tumors of the lung. 1997; 6:2285–2290.

122 Wistuba II, Behrens C, Virmani AK et al. High resolution chromosome 3p allelotyping of human lung cancer and preneoplastic/preinvasive bronchial epithelium reveals multiple discontinuous sites of 3p allele loss and three regions of frequent breakpoints. *Cancer Res* 2000; 60:1949–1960.

123 Wistuba II, Berry J, Behrens C et al. Molecular changes in the bronchial epithelium of patients with small cell lung cancer. *Clin Cancer Res* 2000; 6:2604–2610.

21

Small cell lung cancer

Desmond N. Carney

Department of Medical Oncology, Mater Hospital, Dublin, Ireland

Introduction

Small cell lung cancer (SCLC) accounts for 20–25% of all newly diagnosed patients with lung cancer[1–3]. Up to the early 1970s surgery and/or radiation therapy were the most frequent forms of treatment used. However, it was rapidly recognized that, even with such therapies, the majority of patients developed widespread disseminated disease in a short period with most patients dying within 3 months of diagnosis. More detailed staging procedures coupled with autopsy studies of patients who died within 28 days of 'curative surgical resection' for small cell lung cancer led to our current understanding of the biological behaviour of this tumour. With few exceptions all patients will have metastatic disease at diagnosis (clinically evident or not) and that treatment aimed solely at the primary tumour (radiotherapy or surgery) is purely palliative in nature for almost all patients and has little impact upon overall survival.

It soon became recognized that SCLC (unlike all other forms of lung cancer) demonstrates unique sensitivity to many different chemotherapeutic agents and radiation therapy. In subsequent trials carried out over the past two decades, the central role of combination chemotherapy in the treatment of all patients with small cell lung cancer, irrespective of their disease extent, has emerged. With combination chemotherapy and with the use in selective cases of chest radiotherapy and/or prophylactic cranial radiation therapy, responses to treatment will be observed in 80–90% of patients including complete remissions in 30–40%. Coupled with these significant response rates to cytotoxic therapy, the overall survival has increased 3–5-fold, compared with that observed in the prechemotherapy days. The median survival for all patients has improved from 2 to 3 months to 10 to 11 months; while up to 20–25% of patients with limited disease stage can achieve long-term disease-free survival (greater than 2 years)[1,2].

In the past decade considerable knowledge has been gained into understanding the important prognostic factors in this disease as they predict for responsiveness to chemotherapy and long-term survival. In addition, through large-scale randomized clinical trials the importance of chest radiation as part of the overall treatment strategy of patients with limited stage disease, and the benefit in selected patients with prophylactic cranial radiation, have been more clearly defined. While some answers have been obtained, many questions still remain regarding how best to integrate radiotherapy with chemotherapy; in addition to important radiation questions of dose, volume, and which chemotherapy agents are best combined with radiotherapy to gain maximal benefit with acceptable toxicity.

Perhaps in the past decade the greatest advance is the explosion in our knowledge of the biology of SCLC[4–6]. Our understanding of unique tumour cell associated antigens and the unique growth factors for this tumour has helped us consider alternative or different strategies for treating this disease, e.g. monoclonal antibodies. Moreover, as we increase our understanding of the role of dominant and tumour recessive oncogenes in the pathogenesis and biology of SCLC, the hope exists for the development of treatment approaches for both the early detection through screening techniques using molecular markers, and the chemo-prevention of this disease.

Although for many patients with SCLC cure is currently not achievable with our different regimens of treatment, for most a significant improvement both in median survival and quality of life can be obtained with treatment. The future remains optimistic, however, as with the hope of combining conventional therapies and biology therapies, combined with screening and early detection, we may finally achieve a greater overall survival and cure rate for patients with SCLC diagnosed in the next decade or so. As most cases of SCLC are due to cigarette smoking, elimination of tobacco from our society will continue to be the key factor in the elimination of this disease.

Staging of SCLC[7–14]

The mainstay of treatment of newly diagnosed patients with SCLC is combination chemotherapy. However, accurate and detailed staging procedures are required, both to more clearly define as much as possible, prognosis and the likelihood of achieving long-term survival. In addition, detailed staging procedures allows the identification of that subset of patients for whom combined modality therapy of chemotherapy with chest radiotherapy will be the treatment of choice and for whom optimism of long term disease free survival and cure may be achieved. Although the traditional TNM (tumour node metastases) staging system for other types of lung cancer (non-small cell lung cancer) has generally not been useful for the management of patients with SCLC, with some modifications a revised TNM system has been recently introduced and may be used in the future.

It is recognized that almost all patients with small cell lung cancer, have either locally advanced inoperable disease (Stage IIIB) or metastatic disease

Table 21.1. Staging of patients with SCLC

History and physical examination
Full blood count; biochemistry profile (LDH)
Chest radiograph
CT scan thorax and abdomen
Radionuclide bone scan
Bone-marrow aspirate and biopsy
Pathology review
Brain scan/MRI scan

(Stage IV). For these reasons, the classic veterans administration lung cancer study group (VALCSG) system of limited and extensive stage small cell lung cancer remains the most universally utilized staging system, and the one in which outcome of almost all clinical trials are defined[7].

Limited disease (LD) includes disease confined to one hemi-thorax and the regional lymph nodes including the ipsilateral mediastinal, ipsilateral supraclavicular and contralateral hilar and mediastinal lymph nodes. Thus LD may be defined as localized tumour that can be encompassed within a radiotherapy port. Patients with cytologically negative or positive ipsilateral pleural effusions are also designated as LD. Extensive disease (ED) includes all patients beyond the confines of LD.

In most studies at the time of initial presentation and after completion of standard staging procedures (Table 21.1) about 66% of patients will have extensive disease and the remaining one-third LD[8–13]. The variability in different series of the proportion of patients with ED or LD may be a consequence of both the number of staging procedures performed, and the sensitivity of these procedures in detecting metastatic disease. It must also be recognized that over the past decade with the introduction of more exhaustive and more sensitive staging techniques more patients with 'small volume' ED have been identified. This phenomenon of stage migration, i.e. the movement of patients with small volume metastatic disease from LD to ED will improve the survival of patients in both groups without any impact upon overall survival. This so-called 'Will Rogers phenomenon' may account for marginal improvements in treatment outcome when one compares more recently completed clinical trials with historical reported trials[13].

As treatment consideration will depend upon the stage of disease at diagnosis, most patients will undergo detailed staging procedures following the histological diagnosis of SCLC (Table 21.1). Staging procedures should include a complete history and physical examination, chest radiograph, a computed tomography scan of the thorax and upper abdomen (to include liver and adrenal glands), a radio-nucleide bone scan, and unilateral bone marrow aspirate and biopsy. Laboratory investigations should include routine FBC, biochemistry including hepatic, bone and renal profile, and serum lactate dehydroagenous levels (LDH). Measurement of serum tumour markers such as neuron specific enolase (NSE) or chromogrannina (neuroendocrine markers) are not routine[14]. Other detailed procedures including brain CT scan or MRI, lumbar puncture with CSF analysis etc. are not routinely performed unless there is a clinical suspicion of disease in these locations. The impact of other tests on outcome and treatment planning such as in vitro cell culture techniques, monoclonal staining of bone marrow cells etc. remain to be determined and are not part of routine staging procedures for this disease.

It might be argued that outside of the context of clinical trials exhaustive staging procedures as outlined are not essential once one site of extensive disease is identified, as results of further tests will have little bearing on treatment selection or outcome and may both delay the commencement of treatment and add to the overall cost of the care of the patient.

Serum tumour markers in SCLC[8,14]

Studies of SCLC in vivo and in vitro have confirmed the presence of neuroendocrine markers in these cells including L-DD, NSE, chromogranin A, etc. Many studies have reported on the utilization of serum levels of such markers as indicators of disease extent, response to treatment and early indicators of relapse in patients with SCLC. While results of these studies have shown a close correlation between levels of the tumour markers and the disease extent, etc., these markers in general are neither sensitive enough nor specific enough to consider their routine use in the care of patients with SCLC, nor that their initial levels have any impact on treatment selection. While rising serum tumour markers may antedate clinical or radiological evidence of disease progression by several months, these changes are not used to alter patient management and thus have little use in the routine care and follow-up of patients with SCLC.

Serum LDH levels, however, continue to be a useful marker of disease extent in patients with SCLC as indeed in patients with many other tumours. While non-specific and therefore non-diagnostic of an underlying tumour cell type, elevated levels in patients with SCLC frequently reflect extensive disease and may reflect the presence of bone marrow infiltration.

Prognostic factors in patients with SCLC[8-11] (Tables 21.2 and 21.3)

The most important prognostic factors in SCLC patients include the stage of disease at presentation and the performance status of the patients. These two factors above all others most accurately predict outcome in terms of response to therapy, medium and long-term survival. The median survival of approximately 18 months for patients with LD is significantly superior to that observed for patients with ED (7–9 months). In addition, while long-term survival (i.e. greater than 2 years) may be observed in 20–25% of patients with LD, some of whom will be cured of their disease, this is rarely if ever observed in patients with extensive disease.

The performance status (PS) of the patients has a major bearing on both outcome and survival with chemotherapy, and indeed on tolerance to chemotherapy. The survival of patients with ESOG PS 0, 1

Table 21.2. Prognostic factors in SCLC

Stage of disease
Performance status
Age
Serum biochemistry (LDH)
Sites of metastatic disease (liver/CNS)
Number of metastatic sites
Response to initial chemotherapy regimen

Table 21.3. Survival among patients with SCLC

Stage	Median survival time (weeks)
Limited	54
Extensive	35
Extensive (+1 site)	38
Extensive (≥2 sites)	31
Extensive: bone	49
Liver/bone marrow	36
Brain	22

Adapted from: Feld et al.[8]

and 2 is significantly better than that observed in patients with performance status 3 and 4. Indeed in many clinical trials patients with poor PS (PS 2–4) are frequently excluded because of their poor tolerance to chemotherapy and its associated side effects.

Considerable heterogeneity may exist among patients with ED SCLC. Patients included in this category may have one, two or more sites of metastatic disease, or may have disease in certain sites such as liver or CNS where responsiveness to chemotherapy is poor and thus median survival is reduced. Thus the outcome of patients with ED SCLC may vary considerably depending on the sites of metastatic disease identified and the number of sites positive for disease (Table 21.3).

It is clear that, while the current staging system of LD/ED SCLC remains in widespread use both in treatment planning and in predicting prognosis, it has become clear in recent years that within these two main groups many subsets of patients exist with very varied prognosis. Several investigators have proposed models to take into consideration such factors as LDH level, number and sites of metastatic disease, PS, etc. in addition to disease extent. While such models may more accurately reflect the prognosis of individual patients, they have yet to achieve widespread acceptance and application in clinical trials and standard practice. However, it remains important that a prognostic index incorporating all of the above factors be developed, so that we may better define patient prognosis and better select patients for clinical trials. Finally, it should also be recognized that, given the heterogeneity that exists amongst subsets of patients defined as having ED which may have a median survival ranging from 22 to 46 weeks, it is clear how patient selection may have such an important impact on the outcome of clinical trials and median survival.

Chemotherapy in small cell lung cancer[1-3,15-24]

The recognition in the 1960s and 1970s from both clinical and autopsy studies that from the time of diagnosis SCLC was a disseminated disease led to detailed studies of the efficacy of systemic chemotherapy with or without radiation treatment in the treatment of this tumour. Today, the mainstay of treatment of SCLC is the use of combination systemic chemotherapy with the aim of achieving the highest response rate and long-term disease free survival ('cure') with the lowest possible and acceptable morbidity. In selected cases thoracic radiation and/or prophylactic cranial irradiation would be part of the overall treatment strategy (see below). Prior to the use of chemotherapy for SCLC, when the treatment was usually of a palliative nature including chest radiotherapy and best supportive care, the median survival of patients with LD was 12–18 weeks and for those with ED approximately 6 weeks. Few patients if any ever achieved long-term survival. With current approaches of combination chemotherapy, clinical and radiological documented responses are seen in 80–90% of patients with

Table 21.4. Active chemotherapy agents in SCLC

'Old' agents	'New' agents
Cyclophosphamide	Paclitaxel
Ifosphamide	Docetaxel
Etoposide	Topotecan
Teniposide	Irinotecan (CPT-11)
Cisplatin	Vinorelbine
Carboplatin	Gemcitabine
Vincristine	
Doxorubicin	
Methotrexate	
Nitrosoureas	
Nitrogen mustard	

Table 21.5. Commonly used regimens in SCLC

EP	Etoposide
	Cisplatin
EC	Etoposide
	Carboplatin
CA	Cyclophosphamide
	Doxorubicin
	Vincristine
CDE	Cyclophosphamide
	Doxorubicin
	Etoposide

30–60% of patients achieving a complete remission. Complete remissions are most frequently seen in patients with LD. The median survival of all patients has improved significantly to approximately 11 months with 5–10% of patients achieving long term survival. As might be expected among patients with good performance status and limited stage disease, higher complete response rates and median (18–24 months) and long term (20–25% at 2 years) survival would be observed compared to a median survival of 7–9 months in patients with extensive disease.

Many agents demonstrate significant activity in the treatment of SCLC (Table 21.4). However, when used as single agents complete response rates are rare and responses are not often of a durable nature. For these reasons the majority of newly diagnosed patients are treated with combinations of two, three or four cytotoxic agents which have both different modes of action and different pattern of toxicities. The most commonly used regimens are listed in Table 21.5. While earlier studies suggest that 4-drug combination, or schedules of alternating regimens might yield superior results, such optimism has not been confirmed in randomized clinical trials. An analysis of recent trials suggest that Etoposide with either Cisplatin or Carboplatin is a regimen that is as effective as any other multidrug regimen in the treatment of SCLC and which have manageable and acceptable toxicity. The substitution of Cisplatin by

Carboplatin does not appear to lead to any loss of activity but does improve the toxicity profile and permits ease of administration of this regimen on an outpatient basis[23]. Moreover, this combination can be combined with concurrent chest radiotherapy with acceptable toxicity.

The choice of regimen may well be dictated by the general performance status of the patient, the presence of coexisting medical condition (e.g. congested cardiac failure or renal failure) in whom agents such as Doxorubicin or Cisplatin might be contra-indicated, or where chest radiotherapy is part of the planned treatment.

Side effects of chemotherapy include severe myelosuppression which occurs in 25–75% of patients with the greatest frequency observed in patients receiving combined modality therapy (chemotherapy and radiation). Other frequent toxicities include total alopecia, nausea, vomiting, peripheral neuropathy and late effects including cardiomyopathy and second cancers. Other toxicities may be noted in patients receiving chest radiotherapy (oesophagitis, pulmonary fibrosis) or patients receiving prophylactic cranial radiotherapy where a variety of neurotoxicities including mild dementia, ataxia, memory loss may occasionally be observed.

In general, chemotherapy is administered every 3 to 4 weeks for 4 to 6 months. Ideally, treatment is administered on an outpatient basis to minimize any disruption in the patient's lifestyle. The optimal duration of chemotherapy for newly diagnosed patients is not clearly defined. However, there are no convincing data to support the theory that maintenance chemotherapy is beneficial in SCLC patients: moreover prolongation of chemotherapy beyond four to six cycles, while not improving outcome may, however, lead to a deterioration in the quality of life due to the development and persistence of unacceptable toxicities[19,20].

Improving outcome in patients with SCLC with systemic chemotherapy[24-35]

SCLC remains a most frustrating disease to manage either by oncologists, chest physicians, radiotherapists or general physicians. For most patients, within a short time of their initial course of chemotherapy, clinical and radiological responses are observed in up to 90% of patients with an associated marked improvement in quality of life and decrease in disease-related symptoms. Unfortunately, most patients will relapse and in spite of further chemotherapy/radiotherapy, death from disease progression follows for almost all relapsing patients with a median survival from the time of relapse ranging from 3 to 6 months. Over the past two decades with few minor exceptions no significant improvements in outcome or long-term survival have been noted in patients with SCLC. Any minor gains observed may purely be a reflection of patient selection or stage migration.

Major efforts have been made to improve the outcome of patients receiving chemotherapy for SCLC. These attempts at dose intensification include:

1. The use of alternating non-cross resistant chemotherapy regimens.
2. Dose intensification including:
   (a) The use of high dose induction chemotherapy.
   (b) The use of weekly chemotherapy regimens.
   (c) The use of late intensification chemotherapy with autologous bone marrow transplantation or peripheral blood stem cell transplantation with growth factor cytokine support.

Table 21.6. Alternating non-cross resistant chemotherapy

	Chemotherapy	Patients	MS	P
Evans[26]	CAV	289	8.0	0.03
	CAV/PE			
Roth[25]	CAV	473	8.6	
	EP		8.3	0.425
	CAV/EP		8.1	

Alternating chemotherapy regimens

Drug resistance is a major problem for many tumours including SCLC. Although initially a very chemo-sensitive tumour, at the time of relapse drug resistance is the norm which is presumed to be due to the emergence of drug-resistant clones. It has long been postulated that the use of alternating non-cross-resistant regimens might reduce the emergence of drug-resistant clones thereby improving both the disease free survival and overall survival. However, as indicated (Table 21.6) a review of 13 randomized Phase III trials of alternating versus sequential combination chemotherapy regimens provides no convincing data suggesting an added benefit from alternating chemotherapy in this disease. In many of these trials the most frequently used regimens in either a sequential or alternating fashion were VAC or EP as both are highly active in newly diagnosed patients. However, these regimens may not be truly cross-resistant. Among patients who relapse after VAC, EP produces response rates of 40–60%. Conversely, however, among patients failing on EP, VAC therapy demonstrates much fewer responses in the region of 10–15%.

Dose intensification

Several approaches have been investigated for increasing the dose intensity of chemotherapy in SCLC. These include:

1. the use of modestly higher (usually 2–4-fold)

Table 21.7. High dose(a) vs. standard dose chemotherapy (b)

			Patients	RR	MS
Johnson[34]	CDV	SD	174	53%	34.7 wk
		HD	124	63%	29.3 wk
Ihde[33]	PE	SD	46	83%	10.7 mo
		HD	44	86%	11.4 mo
Arriagade[35]	PCDE	SD	50	56%	14 mo
		HD	55	67%	18 mo

Table 21.8. Weekly vs. 3-weekly chemotherapy

		Patients	RR	MS
Souhami[31]	Weekly	221	82%	10.8 mo
	3-weekly	217	81%	10.6 mo
Murray[30]	Weekly	110	87%	0.98 yr
	3-weekly	109	70%	0.91 yr

chemotherapy regimens without growth factor support,

2. the administration of chemotherapy at shorter intervals (i.e. weekly),

3. the use of high dose chemotherapy with either ABMT or PBSCT support with growth factor support.

In general, there are few data to show that, for most patients, the use of modestly higher doses of chemotherapy leads to any significant improvement in overall survival when compared to the use of chemotherapy administered in standard doses (Table 21.7) and on schedule. While higher doses of chemotherapy including high dose chemotherapy with growth factor support may be associated with higher initial response rates including complete response rates, this does not translate into improved long-term survival. It is clear, however, that such dose intensification is associated with increasing toxicity and cost.

Studies of high dose chemotherapy regimens with either ABMT or PBSCT rescue have also been carried out in many clinical trials using highly selected patients with excellent performance status. Again while improving overall response rates, the impact and long term survival is marginal when compared to standard chemotherapy and may be more a reflection of patient selection rather than impact on chemotherapy itself.

SCLC affects persons who are usually long-term cigarette smokers. Thus cormorbid medical problems including COAD and cardiac disease in addition to other cigarette related illnesses are quite common. In addition, the average age for persons who get lung cancer is 65 years. In the assessment of clinical trials of dose intensification most studies that yield a positive result usually include small numbers of patients with an excellent performance status with the majority of patients young with LD. Thus, the applicability of such dose intensification studies with increased toxicity to large national populations remains unanswered and to most patients is probably not applicable.

Weekly chemotherapy (Table 21.8)

Based on the data from the use of weekly chemotherapy in the treatment of aggressive non-Hodgkin's lymphoma and in other chemosensitive tumours, the use of weekly chemotherapy schedules has also been evaluated in patients with SCLC. Several randomized trials of weekly vs. 3-weekly chemotherapy regimens have been reported. Although initial response rates were somewhat higher in the weekly regimens, no differences in median or long-term survival have been noted. In general, as might be expected, hematological toxicity was greater in the weekly chemotherapy regimen often leading to delays in chemotherapy administration. While weekly chemotherapy has been tested predominantly in patients with extensive stage disease, the lack of benefit observed with these patients suggests that such an approach would be of questionable value in patients with LD.

Dose-intensive chemotherapy regimens including weekly chemotherapy, high dose chemotherapy, alternating chemotherapy etc., have all failed to demonstrate any significant improvement over standard chemotherapy regimens in the treatment of SCLC. Moreover, such approaches particularly in patients with ED are frequently associated with increasing toxicity, in particular myelosuppression. More data is required in young good performance status patients with limited disease to determine the exact role of dose intensification and high dose chemotherapy in the management of such patients.

Chemotherapy in relapsed patients[36–41]

In spite of the very high initial response rates observed with induction chemotherapy, the majority of patients will either progress while on initial chemotherapy or relapse sometime after completion of the planned schedule of chemotherapy. Relapses may be observed at a previous site of disease (e.g. thorax) or some distal site (e.g. CNS) or both. In general, while relapses may occasionally appear localized at the time of recurrence, rapid dissemination is usually the normal course of events. Treatment at the time of relapse will be dictated by the site of relapse, the prior treatment administered including chest radiotherapy and the timing of relapse in relation to the prior treatment.

For localized thoracic recurrence, in patients who have not yet received chest radiotherapy, thoracic radiation is a treatment of choice. All patients who have more distal relapses should, where possible, be considered for inclusion in clinical trials of new agents in this situation.

The use of chemotherapy in patients not suitable for inclusion in clinical trials will be dictated by (i) response observed to initial chemotherapy, (ii) the chemotherapy-free interval from initial treatment cessation to subsequent relapse, and (iii) the induction regimen used. In addition, the choice of treatment for a patient who has relapsed will also be dictated by their overall PS, the sites of relapse and the patient's wishes after receiving full information of the disease status. The patient who initially had either complete response or partial response to chemotherapy and a chemotherapy-free interval greater than 6 months is likely to respond again to the same or different chemotherapy regimens, with response rates observed of 25–75%. In general, response durations are short, in the region of 2–4 months. The choice of chemotherapy used will depend upon the prior chemotherapy regimen and may include CAV, EP, chronic oral Etoposide or some of the newer agents. As noted, for patients who progress on VAC, there is a greater likelihood of response to subsequent EP than for patients failing EP, treated with VAC. While there is no established salvage chemotherapy regimen, clearly EP is one choice for VAC failures with expected response rates of 40–50%. Chronic oral Etoposide induced responses in patients recurring after initial treatment. Other active agents include Topotecan and Ifosphamide (see below).

Treatment of elderly patients or patients with poor performance status[42–45]

With current treatment strategies only the minority of patients with SCLC are candidates for treatment with curative intent. Patients who are 65 years or less with good performance status (ECOG 01), LD and no significant cormorbid medical illnesses, have a potential for cure, including a very high response rate to initial chemotherapy, a 2-year disease-free survival of 20–40% and perhaps a long-term survival of 20% when treated with combined modality therapy. However, as lung cancer in general is a disease of the elderly with more than 50% of patients 65 years or over at diagnosis, and as most patients (two-thirds) will have extensive stage disease at diagnosis, this optimistic outcome is applicable only to the minority of newly diagnosed patients. The remainder of patients will be elderly (with LD/ED), LD patients with poor PS (ECOG 2–4), or patients with extensive stage disease. These patients who represent approximately 75% of all newly diagnosed patients are incurable with current treatment approaches. The treatment goal for these patients is to achieve maximum palliation of disease with improved quality of life and improved overall survival.

To obtain the maximum response to treatment and unless medically contra-indicated, all such patients if possible should be treated with combination chemotherapy. While studies of single agent Etoposide administered orally over 5 days or more, have revealed response rates of 50–80% and median survival of 7–9 months with acceptable toxicity, more recently reported randomized trials of combination chemotherapy versus single agent Etoposide have demonstrated superiority with the combination chemotherapy arm in terms of response rate, overall survival and quality of life. However, as such patients tolerate chemotherapy less well, dose modifications of standard chemotherapy regimens may be required although not desirable.

Chemotherapy for CNS metastases[46-48]

CNS metastases are frequently noted among patients with SCLC. Cerebral metastases are present in up to 10% of newly diagnosed patients. However, with long-term survival CNS metastases as a site of recurrent disease rises to as high as 40–50%. For patients with clinical or radiological apparent CNS metastases, cranial radiation is the treatment of choice leading to significant improvement in symptoms and improved quality of life.

Recent evidence suggests that, in previously untreated patients, chemotherapy alone can be associated with an intracranial response rate of up to 75% including complete resolution of disease. For such patients where intracranial metastases represent the sole site of metastatic disease at diagnosis, the median survival of these patients will approximate that of patients with otherwise limited stage disease. CNS metastases are a common site of relapse for patients following prior chemotherapy. In many, CNS metastases are often observed concurrently with relapsed disease at another site. With these patients radiotherapy remains the primary modality of treatment, as CNS responses to systemic chemotherapy are much lower at relapse than for newly diagnosed patients. Leptomeningeal metastases are also common in small cell lung cancer,

most notably detected in patients with progressive disease. Systemic treatment is of modest value and treatment with intrathecal chemotherapy with or without local field radiotherapy to symptomatic regions is the preferred treatment option. For patients with SCLC who develop spinal cord compression, a combination of high dose steroids with local field radiotherapy is the treatment of choice. Surgical intervention is rarely required owing to the sensitivity of this tumour to radiotherapy.

Thoracic ionizing radiation in limited stage small cell lung cancer[49-58]

In a retrospective analysis in the late 1980s of the use of thoracic radiation with systemic chemotherapy in limited stage small cell lung cancer it was shown that thoracic radiation was associated with an increased response rate and an improved median and long-term survival. However, several randomized trials at that time yielded conflicting data. In addition, combined modality therapy (CMT) was shown to be associated with increased toxicity including pneumonitis, cardiac toxicity, oesophagitis and pulmonary fibrosis. In the early 1990s two published meta-analyses of studies in excess of 2000 patients with limited stage small cell lung cancer disease demonstrated a survival advantage with the use of thoracic field radiation with chemotherapy. The 2- and 3-year survival were significantly improved with the addition of radiation therapy. Thus it is now generally accepted that patients with limited stage small cell lung cancer benefit from thoracic radiation and should receive combined modality therapy.

In the two meta-analyses which involved >1900 patients each, both showed an improvement in survival rates in those patients receiving thoracic radiation. At 3 years, about 9% of the chemotherapy only group remained alive and disease free compared to 14% of the combined modality group. This corresponded to a 14% reduction in mortality rate. In addition patients receiving combined modality therapy showed a marked reduction in local failure rate from 23% in the combined modality arm versus 48% in the chemotherapy alone arm. These benefits were associated with only a marginal increase in mortality rate increasing by approximately 1% in the combined modality therapy arm.

Several questions remain regarding the optimal way of integrating radiation and chemotherapy. The optimal total dose, volume dimensions and timing of thoracic radiation remain to be determined. While some difficulties were encountered in addressing this issue when Doxoribicin was part of the chemotherapy regimen, since the combination of Cisplatin or Carboplatin with Etoposide is the usual chemotherapy combination used and which can be more readily combined in full dose and schedule with radiation therapy, several investigators have addressed the importance of these radiotherapy issues. The results of the sequential therapeutic approach, i.e. radiation after completion of chemotherapy, have been disappointing, whereas studies of hyperfraction radiation therapy and the rapid alternation of combined modality therapy have yielded improved results. Moreover, it also appears that early rather than delayed radiation therapy also yields improved results.

Recent studies have addressed the use of hyperfractionation (twice daily) radiation therapy with once daily thoracic radiation in limited stage small cell lung cancer. Pilot studies of hyperfractionation radiation therapy appear to yield results superior to daily radiation. In the intergroup study of Turrisi et al. twice daily radiotherapy was initiated with a first cycle of chemotherapy (Etoposide and Cisplatin).[58] This showed a significantly improved survival as compared with concurrent once daily radiation therapy. At a median follow-up of 8 years the median survival for twice daily radiation was 23 months vs. 19 months for once daily radiation with a 2-year (47% vs. 41%) and a 5-year (26% vs. 16%) survival favouring twice daily radiation therapy. Of note, grade 3 esophagitis was significantly more frequent in the hyperfractionated group. These survival data are a considerable improvement over previous results in limited stage small cell lung cancer. The improved local control in this study did appear to lead to improved distal control and subsequent improved overall survival.

Further studies are needed to confirm the above and also to determine the optimum timing of chemotherapy and radiation. Most studies suggest that early as opposed to late or delayed radiation therapy yield better results and that concurrent chemotherapy and radiation therapy is superior to sequential therapy. The more widespread use of Etoposide and Cisplatin chemotherapy as initial chemotherapy for small cell lung cancer may greatly facilitate the integration of concurrent and/or hyperfraction radiation therapy in the management of limited stage small cell lung cancer with resultant acceptable toxicity.

Prophylactic cranial irradiation and small cell lung cancer[59-65]

Brain metastases remain a major cause of both morbidity and mortality among patients with SCLC. At the time of diagnosis up to 10% of patients will have intracranial metastases, most often associated with other sites of disseminated disease. However, in 1–2% of patients it is the sole site of extensive disease. Among patients who receive combination chemotherapy and thus achieve a significant prolongation of survival, brain metastases will become clinically apparent in 30–70% of these. Autopsy series show this figure to be even greater. The greater the survival, the greater the risk of developing brain metastases. Among patients who achieve a complete remission with chemotherapy, brain metastases may be the sole site of relapse in 10–15%, especially in patients diagnosed with limited disease. Thus, as combined modality therapy becomes more effective in the management of LD SCLC, the frequency of brain metastases later in the course of the disease may continue to rise.

For many years prophylactic cranial irradiation has been used in patients with SCLC in the belief that the treatment of microscopic subclinical metastases would prevent or delay the onset of symptomatic brain metastases. However, the efficacy of prophylactic cranial irradiation (PCI) has been questioned. Supporters of prophylactic cranial irradiation indicate that it is a safe way to reduce the overall incidence of brain metastases even if only a small number of patients benefit. Others who argue against the routine use point out that the brain is rarely the sole site of recurrence; radiation can be neurotoxic, and the data supporting the use of radiation therapy has not demonstrated it to have any major impact upon prolonged survival[64]. Recent data, however, would suggest that the use of PCI, particularly in patients who obtain a complete remission, will have a major impact upon prolonging survival. A meta-analysis of more than 900 patients, the majority of whom had limited stage disease and who took part in seven trials, evaluated the role of PCI. All of these patients had obtained a complete remission with systemic chemotherapy with or without thoracic radiation. Prophylactic cranial irradiation was associated with an absolute decrease of 25.3% in the cumulative incident of brain metastases at 3 years from 58.6% in the control group to 33.3% in the treatment group. More important, PCI was also associated with an absolute increase in overall survival of 5.4% at 3 years, from 15.3% in the control group to 20.7% in the treatment group. Of note, PCI was beneficial in patients with either limited or extensive disease. In the two largest trials included in this meta-analysis in which neuro-psychological tests were performed on most but not all patients, before, during and after treatment, no significant deterioration in neurocognitive function was found after PCI. Thus, this detailed meta-analysis confirms that there was a small absolute survival advantage for patients who receive PCI. Even though this advantage is small, it achieves a significance somewhat similar to the benefits of thoracic radiation therapy combined with chemotherapy in the treatment of patients with LD SCLC. Thus PCI should now be considered for most patients who achieve a complete remission with induction systemic treatment, chemotherapy or radiotherapy or both.

Several questions remain regarding the role and use of PCI in patients with SCLC. The optimal dose of radiation, volume of tissue to be irradiated and duration and timing of PCI have not yet been clearly defined. Also questions still remain regarding the safety and long term neuro-psychological consequences of PCI. On the current evidence, it is now reasonable to include PCI as part of the treatment of patients with LD SCLC who are in complete remission and of patients with extensive disease who have isolated metastases and who also achieve complete remission with systemic chemotherapy. It may be possible to minimize neurological damage by avoiding the concurrent administration of PCI with systemic chemotherapy and perhaps by minimizing its use in elderly patients.

New drugs in small cell lung cancer (Table 21.4)[3,66-69]

The relatively modest improvement in overall survival for patients with small cell lung cancer stresses the important need for the evaluation of new agents in the treatment of this disease (Table 21.4). Several phase I/II studies have identified agents with activity in SCLC[3]. These include the taxanes, the topoisomerase inhibitors, the antimetabolites and vinorelbines. In studies of previously untreated patients using these compounds as single agents response rates ranging from 5–39% have been observed, with lower response rates being observed in previously treated patients. The single agent activity of some of these compounds compare favourably with some of the 'established' active agents in small cell lung cancer. The evaluation of these agents in combination with established agents needs urgent assessment in phase II/phase III trials.

More recent studies have incorporated these 'newer' agents in the management of SCLC. In the study reported by Johnson et al. patients with ES SCLC received initial CT with Cisplatin/Etoposide[67]. At completion of this standard CT, responding patients were randomized to no further treatment (observation) or to 4 cycles of Topotecan 1.5 mg/m^2/d $\times$ 5 days every 21 days for four cycles. Of the initial 405 patients registered in this trial, 227 were randomized either to observation (112 patients) or Topotecan (115 patients). There was no difference observed between two study arms in either median survival (8.9 vs. 9.3 mo) or 1 year survival (27% vs. 25%). The disease-free survival was prolonged by 5 weeks in the Topotecan arm. However, toxicity was increased in the Topotecan arm. There have been several other reports of studies incorporating Topotecan with standard regimens in the treatment of SCLC. Thus far no significant benefits have been observed. However, and in particular in patients with poor PS, significant myelotoxicity has been noted. In no trial has the addition of Topotecan produced an overall survival greater than the standard of CE alone.

Irinotecan has also demonstrated considerable activity in SCLC patients including those who have failed previous CT and CE. In a most provocative study, Noda et al. reported on the randomized trial of Irinotecan (CPT-11) and Cisplatin versus Cisplatin/Etoposide in patients with ES SCLC[66]. One hundred and fifty four patients were randomized between the two study arms. The overall response rate between CPT-11/Cisplatin and Etoposide/Cisplatin was similar (83% vs. 67.5%). However, there was a significantly better median survival (12.8 vs. 9.8 mo) and 1- and 2-year survival advantage for the CPT-11/Cisplatin arm of the study. This observation at an interim analysis led to the closure of the study. This combination is one of the first examples of utilizing a newer agent to show a survival advantage over standard treatment and if confirmed may become a new standard of treatment in SCLC.

Surgery as the primary treatment of SCLC[70]

Approximately 5% or less of patients with SCLC will have very early stage disease (i.e. stage I and stage II) and will be candidates for surgical resection followed by systemic chemotherapy. Among these 'select' patients, a 5-year survival of 30–40% has been reported. However, a review of operable patients with small cell lung cancer demonstrated

no survival advantage of surgery prior to chemotherapy vs. chemotherapy alone. Currently, several investigators are evaluating surgery following initial neo-adjuvant chemotherapy in limited stage patients. While the resectability rate is as high as 85% the impact upon survival of this approach needs to be determined. Thus outside of clinical trials surgical resection of primary small cell lung cancers appear to be of limited value. The exception remains where the tumour remains undiagnosed (histologically) preoperatively. In these situations, usually where the tumour is peripheral, surgical resection is the initial treatment of choice. Once the diagnosis of SCLC is confirmed post-operative chemotherapy remains indicated.

Second primary cancers after surviving small cell lung cancer[71,72]

SCLC is that type of lung cancer most strongly linked to cigarette smoking with less than 3% of patients having no history of active exposure. While recent trials of CMT in particular in patients with LD have demonstrated improvements in MS, OS and long-term survival, this modest success is diminished in these patients by the high death rate due to second primary cancers, and other causes, often tobacco related.

In a recent review of patients treated for SCLC and who survived >2 years from diagnosis, the risk of developing a second lung cancer was 2–14% per patient per year and the risk increased 2–7-fold at 10 years from initial diagnosis. The majority of second cancers were squamous cell and few were resectable when diagnosed. As might be expected, the risk was greater among those who continued to smoke after their initial diagnosis of SCLC. Fewer than 20% survived >5 years from the diagnosis of the second cancer.

The recognition that such second cancers can develop in patients 'cured' of SCLC indicates the importance of intensive surveillance at the completion of treatment for SCLC, and the importance of smoking cessation at the time of diagnosis of SCLC. Such patients may also be candidates for chemo-prevention studies.

Summary and future directions of small cell lung cancer

1. Four to six months of initial chemotherapy is effective treatment for both limited and extensive stage small cell lung cancer. Maintenance chemotherapy beyond this time does not improved small cell lung cancer survival.
2. In patients with limited disease, combined modality therapy would appear to be the treatment of choice leading to improved response rates, local control and overall survival. The optimum use of radiation including its integration with chemotherapy, fractionation and total dose still remains to be determined. Studies do suggest that the early use of combined modality therapy appears to be associated with an improved outcome.
3. The use of Etoposide and Cisplatin or Carboplatin as initial chemotherapy appears to allow the integration of radiation therapy (in combined modality therapy) with acceptable toxicity as compared to Doxorubicin containing regimens.
4. There are no data to support the use of dose-intensive therapy requiring cytokine support, bone marrow support or peripheral blood stem cell support outside the realm of clinical trials.
5. The use of prophylactic cranial radiation should be reserved for patients (both limited and extensive) who achieve a complete remission with induction treatment. Delaying PCI until completion of chemotherapy may also decrease long-term neurological sequelae.
6. Late recurrences (i.e. >6 months after completion of initial chemotherapy) may be chemosensitive and such patients should be considered for further chemotherapy.
7. The development of second cancers in small cell lung cancer patients 2 years after initial diagnosis continues to be a problem. As a significant proportion of very late relapses may be non-small cell lung cancer, further biopsies of such patients for histological evaluation is indicated before the institution of further specific therapy.
8. The evaluation of new cytotoxic agents and their integration with currently proven active regimens offer some optimism for the future treatment of small cell lung cancer.

REFERENCES

1 Hansen HH. Management of small-cell cancer of the lung. *Lancet* 1992; 339:846–849.
2 Kristensen CA, Jensen PB, Poulsen HS et al. Small cell lung cancer: biological and therapeutic aspects. *Crit Rev Oncol Hematol* 1996; 22:27–60.
3 Edelman MJ, Gandara DR. Small cell lung cancer: current status of new chemotherapeutic agents. *Crit Rev Onc Hematol* 1998; 27:211–228.
4 Carney DN. Biology of small-cell lung cancer. *Lancet* 1992; 339:843–849.
5 Sozzi G, Carney DN. Molecular biology of lung cancer. *Curr Opin Pulm Med* 1998; 4:207–212.
6 Salgia R, Skarin AT. Molecular abnormalities in lung cancer. *J Clin Oncol* 1998; 16:1207–1217.
7 Mountain CF. Staging of lung cancer. The new international system. *Lung Cancer* 1987; 4–11.
8 Feld R, Sagman U, Le Blanc M. Staging and prognostic factors in small cell lung cancer. In: Pass HI, Mitchell JB, Johnson DH, Turrisi A, Minna JD, eds, *Lung Cancer*. Lippincott Williams and Wilkins; 2000:612–627
9 Cerny T, Blair V, Anderson A et al. Pretreatment prognostic factors and system in 407 small-cell lung cancer patients. *Int J Cancer* 1987; 39:146–149.
10 Lassen U, Osterlind K, Hansen M et al. Long-term survival in small-cell lung cancer: posttreatment characteristics in patients surviving 5 to 18+ years – an analysis of 1714 consecutive patients. *J Clin Oncol* 1995; 13:1215–1220.
11 Sagman U, Feld R, DeBoer G et al. Small cell carcinoma of the lung – derivation of a prognostic index. *Clin. Invest* 1986; 27:189–189.
12 Dearing MP, Steinberg SM, Phelps R et al. Outcome of patients with small-cell lung cancer: effect of changes in staging procedures and imaging technology on prognostic factors over 14 years. *J Clin Oncol* 1990; 8:1042–1049.

13 Feinstein AR, Sosin DM, Wells CK. The Will Rogers phenomenon. Stage migration and new diagnostic techniques as a source of misleading statistics for survival in cancer. *N Engl J Med* 1985; 312:1604–1608.

14 Carney DN, Marangos PJ, Ihde DC et al. Serum neuron specific enolase. A marker for disease extent and response to therapy in patients with small cell lung cancer. *Lancet* 1982; 1:583–585.

15 Grant SC, Gralla RJ, Kris MF, Orozem J, Kris EA. Single agent chemotherapy trials in small cell lung cancer. 1970–1990. The case for studies in previously treated patients. *J Clin Oncol* 1992; 10:482–498.

16 Kiasa RF, Murray N, Coldman AF. Dose-intensity meta-analysis of chemotherapy regimens in small-cell carcinoma of the lung. *J Clin Oncol* 1991; 9:499–508.

17 Chute JP, Chen T, Feigal E, Simon R, Johnson BE. Twenty years of phase III trials for patients with extensive stage small cell lung cancer: Perceptible progress. *J Clin Oncol* 1999; 17:1794–1801.

18 Elias A, Ibrahim J, Skarin AT et al. Dose-intensive therapy for limited stage small cell lung cancer. Long term outcome. *J Clin Oncol* 1999; 17:1175–1184.

19 Spriro SG, Souhami RL, Geddes DM et al. Duration of chemotherapy in small cell lung cancer: a Cancer Research Campaign trial. *Br J Cancer* 1989; 59:578–583.

20 Giaccone G, Dalesio O, Mcvie JG et al. Maintenance chemotherapy in small-cell lung cancer: long-term results of a randomized trial. *J Clin Oncol* 1993; 11:1230–1240.

21 Aisner J. Extensive disease small cell lung cancer. The thrill of victory; the agony of defeat. *J Clin Oncol* 1996; 14:658–665.

22 Lassen UN, Hirsch FR, Osterlind K et al. Outcome of combination chemotherapy in extensive stage small-cell lung cancer: any treatment related progress? *Lung Cancer* 1998; 20:151–160.

23 Kosmidis PA, Samantas E, Fountzilas G et al. Cisplatin/etoposide versus carboplatin/etoposide chemotherapy and irradiation in small cell lung cancer. A randomized phase III study. *Semin Oncol* 1994; 21:23–30.

24 DeVore III RF, Johnson DH. Chemotherapy for small cell lung cancer. In: Pass HI, Mitchell JB, Johnson DH, Turrisi A, Minna JD, eds, *Lung Cancer.* Lippincott Williams and Wilkins; 2000:923–939.

25 Roth BJ, Johnson DH, Einhorn et al. Randomized study of cyclophosphamide, doxorubicin, and vincristine versus etoposide and cisplatin versus alternation of these two regimens in extensive small-cell lung cancer: a Phase II trial of the Southeastern Cancer Study Group. *J Clin Oncol* 1992; 10:282-291.

26 Evans WK, Feld R, Murray N et al. Superiority of alternating non-cross-resistant chemotherapy in extensive small cell lung cancer. A multicenter, randomized clinical trial by the National Cancer Institute of Canada. *Ann Int Med* 1987; 107:451–458.

27 Ettinger DS, Finkelstein DM, Abeloff MD et al. A randomized comparison of standard chemotherapy versus alternating chemotherapy and maintenance versus no maintenance therapy for extensive-stage small-cell lung cancer: a phase III study of the Eastern Cooperative Oncology Group. *J Clin Oncol* 1990; 8:230–240.

28 Fukuoka M, Furuse K, Saijo N et al. Randomized trial of cyclophosphamide, doxorubicin and vincristine versus cisplatin and etoposide versus alternation of these regimens in small-cell lung cancer. *J Natl Cancer Inst* 1991; 83:855–861.

29 Fujol J-L, Douillard JY, Riviere A et al. Dose intensity of a four drug chemotherapy regimen with or without recombinant human granulocyte colony stimulating factor in small lung cancer. *J Clin Oncol* 1997; 15:2082–2089.

30 Murray N, Shepherd E, James K et al. A randomized study of CODE versus alternating CAV/EP for extensive stage small cell lung cancer. *J Clin Oncol* 1999; 17:2300–2307.

31 Souhami RL, Rudd R, Ruiz de Elvira M-L et al. Randomized trial of comparing weekly versus 3 weekly in small cell lung cancer. *J Clin Oncol* 1994; 12 1806–1812.

32 Feruse K, Fukuda M, Nishiwaki Y et al. Phase III study of intensive weekly chemotherapy with recombinant human granulocyte colony-stimulating factor versus standard chemotherapy in extensive-disease small-cell lung cancer. *J Clin Oncol* 1998; 16:2126–2132.

33 Ihde DC, Mulshine JL, Kramer BS et al. Prospective randomized comparison of high-dose and standard-dose etoposide and cisplatin chemotherapy in patients with extensive-stage small-cell lung cancer. *J Clin Oncol* 1994; 12:2022–2034.

34 Johnson DH, Einhorn LH, Birch R et al. A randomized comparison of high-dose versus conventional-dose cyclophosphamide, doxorubicin, and vincristine for extensive-stage small-cell lung cancer: a phase III trial of Southeastern Cancer Society. *J Clin Oncol* 1987; 5:1731–1738.

35 Arriagade R, Le Chevalier T, Pignon J. Initial chemotherapeutic doses and survival in patients with limited stage small cell lung cancer. *N Engl J Med* 1993; 329:1848–1856.

36 Chute JP, Kelley MJ, Venzon D et al. Retreatment of patients surviving cancer-free 2 or more years after initial treatment of small cell lung cancer. *Chest* 1996; 110:165–170.

37 Andersen M, Kristjansen PEG, Hansen HH. Second-line chemotherapy in small cell lung cancer. *Cancer Treat Rev* 1990; 17:427–436.

38 Schiller J, von Pawel J, Shepard FA et al. Topotecan versus cyclophosphamide, doxorubicin and vincristine for the treatment of patients with recurrent small cell lung cancer: a phase III study [Abstract]. *Proc Am Soc Clin Oncol* 1998; 17:456.

39 Ettinger DS, Finkelstein DM, Abeloff MD. Justification for evaluating new anticancer drugs in selected untreated patients with extensive-stage small-cell lung cancer: an Eastern Cooperative Oncology Group randomized study. *J Natl Cancer Inst* 1992; 84:1077–1084.

40 Ardizzoni A, Hansen HH, Dombernowsky P et al. Topotecan, a new active drug in the second-line treatment of small-cell lung cancer: a phase II trial in patients with refractory and sensitive disease. *J Clin Oncol* 1997; 15:2090–2096.

41 Huisman C, Postmus PE, Giaccone G et al. Second line chemotherapy and its evaluation in small cell lung cancer. *Cancer Treat Rev* 1999; 25:199–206.

42 Carney DN, Byrne A. Etoposide in the treatment of elderly/poor-prognosis patients with small-cell lung cancer. *Cancer Chemother Pharmacol* 1994; 34:S96–S100.

43 Johnson DH, Greco Fa, Strupp J et al. Prolonged administration of oral etoposide in patients with relapsed or refractory small-cell lung cancer: a phase II trial. *J Clin Oncol* 1990; 8:1613–1617.

44 Souhami RL, Spiro SG, Rudd M et al. Five-day oral etoposide treatment for advanced small-cell lung cancer: randomized comparison with intravenous chemotherapy. *J Natl Cancer Inst* 1997; 89:577–580.

45 Girling DJ, Thatcher N, Clark PI et al. Comparison of oral etoposide and standard multidrug intravenous chemotherapy for small cell lung cancer: a stopped multicentre randomized trial. *Lancet* 1996; 348:563–566.

46 Kristjansen PEG, Sorensen PS, Hansen MS et al. Prospective evaluation of the effect on initial brain metastases from small cell lung cancer of platinum-etoposide based induction chemotherapy followed by alternating multidrug regimen. *Ann Oncol* 1993; 4:579.583.

47 Kristensen CA, Kristjansen PEG, Hansen HH. Systemic chemotherapy of brain metastases from small-cell lung cancer: a review. *J Clin Oncol* 1992; 10:1498–1502.

48 Postmus PE, Sleijger DTh, Haaxma-Reiche H. Chemotherapy for central nervous system metastases from small cell lung cancer. A review. *Lung Cancer* 1989; 5:254–263.

49 Osterlind K, Hansen JJ, Hansen HS et al. Chemotherapy versus chemotherapy plus irradiation in limited small cell lung cancer. Results of a controlled trial with 5 years follow-up. *Br J Cancer* 1986; 54:7–17.

50 Souhami RL, Geddes DM, Spiro SG et al. Radiotherapy in small cell lung cancer of the lung treated with combination chemotherapy: a controlled trial. *Br Med J* 1984; 288:1643–1646.

51 Perry MC, Eaton WL, Propert KJ et al. Chemotherapy with or without radiation therapy in limited small-cell carcinoma of the lung. *N Engl J Med* 1987; 316:912–918.

52 Pignon J-P, Arriagada R, Ihde DC et al. A meta-analysis of thoracic radiotherapy for small cell lung cancer. *N Engl J Med* 1992; 327:1618–1824.

53 Warde P, Payne D. Does thoracic irradiation improve survival and local control in limited-stage small-cell carcinoma of the lung? A meta-analysis. *J Clin Oncol* 1992; 10:890–895.

54 Murray N, Coy P, Pater JL et al. Importance of timing for thoracic irradiation in the combined modality treatment of limited-stage small-cell lung cancer. *J Clin Oncol* 1993; 11:336–344.

55 Gregor A, Drings P, Burghouts J et al. Randomized trials of alternating versus sequential radiotherapy/chemotherapy in limited disease patients with small cell lung cancer: a EORTC study. *J Clin Oncol* 1997; 15:2840–2849.

56 Jeremic B, Shibamoto Y, Acimovic L et al. Initial versus late accelerated hyperfractionated radiotherapy and concurrent chemotherapy in limited small-cell lung cancer: a randomized study. *J Clin Oncol* 1997; 15:893–900.

57 Work E, Nielsen OS, Bentzen SM et al. Randomized study of initial versus late chest irradiation combined with chemotherapy in limited-stage small-cell lung cancer. *J Clin Oncol* 1997; 15:3030–3037.

58 Turrissi At, Kyungmann K, Glum R et al. Twice daily compared with once daily thoracic radiotherapy in limited small cell lung cancer treated concurrently with Cisplatin and Etoposide. *N Engl J Med* 1999; 340:265–271.

59 Nugent JL, Bunn PA Jr, Matthews MJ et al. CNS metastases in small cell bronchogenic carcinoma: increasing frequency and changing pattern with lengthening survival. *Cancer* 1979; 44:1885–1893.

60 Arriagada R, Le Chevalier T, Borie F et al. Prophylactic cranial irradiation for patients with small-cell lung cancer in complete remission. *J Natl Cancer Inst* 1995; 87:183–190.

61 Gregor A, Cull A, Stephens RJ et al. Prophylactic cranial irradiation is indicated following complete response to induction therapy in small cell lung cancer: results of a multicentre randomized trial. *Eur J Cancer* 1996; 33:1752–1758.

62 Johnson BE, Patronas N, Hayes W et al. Neurologic, computed cranial tomographic, and magnetic resonance imaging abnormalities in patients with small-cell lung cancer: further follow-up of 6- to 13-year survivors. *J Clin Oncol* 1990; 8:48–56.

63 Bunna PA Jr, Kelly K. Prophylactic cranial irradiation for patients with small-cell lung cancer. *J Natl Cancer Inst* 1995; 87:161–162.

64 Auperin A, Arriagada R, Pignon J-P et al. Prophylactic cranial irradiation for patients with small-cell lung cancer in complete remission. *N Engl J Med* 1999; 341:476–484.

65 Carney DN. Prophylactic cranial irradiation and small cell lung cancer. *N Engl J Med* 1999; 341:524–525.

66 Noda K, Nishiwaki Y, Kawahara M et al. Randomized phase III study of Irinotecan (CPT-11) and Cisplatin versus Etoposide and Cisplatin in extensive-disease small-cell lung cancer: Japan Clinical Oncology Group Study (JCOG9511). [Abstract 1887] 36th Annual Meeting of the American Society of Clinical Oncology, New Orleans, LA, 2000.

67 Johnson D, Adak S, Cella D et al. Topotecan (T) vs Observation (OB) following Cisplatin (P) plus Etoposide (E) in extensive stage small cell cancer (ES SCLC) (E77593): a phase III trial of Eastern Cooperative Oncology Group (ECOG). [Abstract 1886] 36th Annual Meeting of the American Society of Clinical Oncology, New Orleans, LA, 2000.

68 Lynch T, Herndon J, Lyss A et al. Paclitaxel (P) + Topotecan (T) + GCSF for previously untreated extensive small cell lung cancer (E-SCLC): Preliminary analysis of cancer and leukaemia group B (CALGB) 9430. [Abstract 1922] 36th Annual Meeting of the American Society of Clinical Oncology, New Orleans, LA, 2000.

69 Jett J, Hatfield A, Bauman M et al. Phase II trial of Topotecan and Paclitaxel (TP) with G-CSF support alternating with Etoposide and Cisplatin (EC) in previously untreated extensive stage small cell lung cancer (ED-SCLC). [Abstract 1921] 36th Annual Meeting of the American Society of Clinical Oncology, New Orleans, LA, 2000.

70 Shepherd FA. Surgical management of small cell lung cancer. In: Pass HI, Mitchell JB, Johnson DH, Turrissi A, Minna JD, eds, *Lung Cancer*. Lippincott Williams and Wilkins; 2000:967–980.

71 Tucker M.A., Murray N, Shaw EG et al. Second primary cancers related to smoking and treatment of small cell lung cancer. *J Natl Cancer Inst* 1997; 89:1782–1788.

72 Glisson BG, Hong WK. Survival after treatment of small cell lung cancer – an endless uphill battle. *J Natl Cancer Inst* 1997; 89:1745–1747.

Part VI

Cough

22

Mechanisms of cough

John J. Adcock

Pneumolabs (UK) Limited, Harrow, Middlesex, UK

Introduction

Cough is probably the most powerful and commonest normal physiological reflex. It is essential for the clearance of the respiratory tract, but in disease it may become pathological such that it impairs bodily functions and becomes an embarrassment for the patient. It is characterized by a violent expiration, which provides the high flow rates that are required to shear away mucus and remove foreign particles from the larynx, trachea and large bronchi. Its function to expel excess secretions and inhaled irritants from the airways is immediately obvious. However, the causes of cough are not necessarily associated with excessive bronchial secretions, as for example in chronic bronchitis, but are often related to lung diseases such as asthma and viral infection of the upper respiratory tract. Intensive and frequent cough may impair breathing and cardiac circulation, increase oxygen consumption and interfere with eating, sleep and rest.

Coughing is initiated when sensory receptors in the respiratory tract receive stimuli of sufficient intensity to evoke an increase in afferent nerve impulse activity[1,2]. Cough reflexes can be provoked easily by mechanical and chemical stimuli applied to the epithelium of either the larynx or tracheobronchial tree[3]. There are three main groups of airway sensory receptors which may be involved in the cough reflex initiated from these sites: the slowly adapting stretch receptors (SARs), the rapidly adapting stretch receptors (irritant, RARs) and the pulmonary and bronchial C-fibre receptors. Each is distributed throughout the tracheobronchial tree and the last group is also present in the alveolar wall. RARs and C-fibre receptors have also been identified in the larynx[4].

Action potential studies with the vagus nerve have demonstrated that agents that evoke coughing cause an enhanced activity in both myelinated Aδ-fibres from RARs and in non-myelinated fibres from C-fibre receptors[5]. It is well established that RARs are involved in the cough reflex, based on evidence from reflex and nerve recording experiments[4]. In contrast, most of the evidence that C-fibres are involved in coughing is derived from the fact that agents which are reputedly 'selective' stimulants of C-fibre receptors, such as capsaicin, evoke cough when administered by inhalation to animals and man[6,7]. Unfortunately, only a few studies have been undertaken to record action potentials in single fibres from the larynx and lower airways when these 'selective' agents are administered as aerosols. Until such experiments are carried out, the suggestion that stimulation of C-fibre receptors directly causes cough remains speculative. Evidence suggests that stimulation of pulmonary C-fibre receptors by capsaicin actually exerts an inhibitory influence on cough[8]. C-fibres, however, may be involved indirectly in the cough reflex by releasing tachykinins such as substance P that, in turn, may directly or indirectly evoke the cough reflex by stimulating RARs[9]. The other group of sensory receptors in the airways, the SARs, may facilitate coughing when stimulated[10,11].

Surprisingly little is known about the role of the

central nervous organization of the cough reflex. There is supposedly a 'cough centre' in the brainstem that is connected with the respiratory rhythm generator in the respiratory centre but this is unclear[12]. Motor output to respiratory and other muscles is, however, common to both centres. There is also a cortical input to cough and subjects can voluntarily induce and inhibit cough. The final act of the cough reflex is that transmitted by the motor pathways from the CNS which result in the powerful contractions of the abdominal muscles, collapse of the bronchi and opening of the glottis. Other motor responses associated with cough involve the autonomic nervous system producing reflex bronchoconstriction, secretion of mucus and airway vasodilatation[13,14], all of which increase the turbulence and shear forces in the bronchi.

Cough is a complex reflex pathway and this chapter examines in detail the peripheral and central mechanisms involved in the reflex. The potential sites and mechanisms of action of known antitussive drugs are also considered, since it is this area of research and the development of novel, more selective drugs which will eventually help to elucidate the exact role for each of the groups of peripheral sensory receptors in the cough reflex.

Sensory physiology of the cough reflex

Cough is due to activation of sensory receptors in the larynx and lower respiratory tract, sending impulses to the brainstem. Once in the brainstem the subsequent generation and central organization of the cough reflex is poorly understood. Mechanically, a cough generally starts with a deep inspiration due to increased contraction of the diaphragm and other inspiratory muscles acting in concert with muscles that enlarge the upper airways. The next compression phase is brief and is characterized by continuous tone in the diaphragm and concurrent activation of the rib cage/abdominal expiratory muscles and muscles that close the laryngeal folds. In the subsequent expulsive phase, the diaphragm ceases activity and the glottis is opened; the contin-

ued strong expiratory muscle activity results in high airflow velocities.

Cough usually occurs when sensory receptors in the respiratory tract receive stimuli of sufficient intensity to evoke an increase in sensory/afferent nerve impulse activity. Cough reflexes can be provoked easily by mechanical and chemical stimuli applied to either the larynx or tracheobronchial tree, for it is here that the greatest protection against the ingress of foreign materials is required. Sensory information from the respiratory tract which initiates the cough reflex is carried in the vagus nerves, since cough from stimulation of one side of the bronchial tree is abolished by ipsilateral vagotomy[15]. The three main groups of airway sensory receptors that may be involved in the cough reflex initiated from these sites are as follows.

Slowly adapting stretch receptors (SARs)

Slowly adapting stretch receptors with myelinated fibres in the Aδ–Aβ range are localized mainly to the airway smooth muscle of the trachea and larger bronchi and have the ultrastructural appearance of mechanoreceptors. They discharge during inflation and adapt slowly to maintained stretch of the airways. Collapse of the airways may either inhibit or stimulate them. In general, their role is to signal the degree of stretch of the lungs, but their activity may be affected by various mechanical and chemical factors, including contraction of airway smooth muscle[13,16].

Rapidly adapting stretch receptors (irritant, RARs)

RARs may be inactive during quiet breathing or may fire occasionally in respiratory cycles. They are identified by rapidly adapting bursts of impulse activity evoked by large inflations or deflations of the lungs, often with a prominent off response[1]. Lung RARs have their terminals in the airway epithelium and probably also deeper in the airway wall[13]. Although the vagal fibres are myelinated and in the Aδ range, the terminals are non-myelinated. The most superficial endings lie less than 1 μm from the airway lumen, where they are well sited for intraluminal irritation[17]. They occur throughout the trachea and larger bronchi, with concentration at the carina and the points of bronchial bifurcation[13,16]. They have also been identified physiologically in the larynx[18], but unlike in the tracheobronchial tree there seems to be a deficiency in our knowledge of laryngeal reflexes related to an analysis of nerve and receptor histology. RARs are stimulated by all the stimuli that can induce coughing, although most of them can also activate bronchial C-fibre receptors. However, the RARs compared with C-fibre receptors are particularly sensitive to mechanical stimuli. The evidence that RARs cause cough is extensive and has been reviewed by a number of groups[13,19,20].

It has been shown recently that RARs are activated by an increase in interstitial airway liquid volume caused by drug-induced plasma extravasation from mucosal post-capillary blood vessels[21]. This very important finding has strong implications because many inflammatory mediators and chemical agents that induce cough, such as histamine, bradykinin, capsaicin or substance P also cause plasma extravasation and, therefore, could evoke cough indirectly as well as directly. The relevance of this will be discussed later.

C-fibre endings

These are subdivided into pulmonary C-fibre endings and bronchial C-fibre endings, depending on the source of their blood supply[13]. They are distributed throughout the larynx, bronchial tree and the pulmonary C-fibre endings are also present in the alveolar wall. The non-myelinated C-fibres from these sensory receptors are sometimes silent or have irregular, sparse discharges under normal conditions. Moreover, their action potentials are usually small and inconspicuous compared to those of myelinated fibres. The receptors are activated by almost the same group of stimuli as those that affect RARs, although in general they are less sensitive to mechanical stimuli such as lung volume changes[13]. The reflex responses to stimulation of C-fibre recep-

tors include apnoea followed by rapid shallow breathing. C-fibre activation also causes reflex bronchoconstriction and tracheal mucus secretion[13]. The strongest evidence for C-fibre receptors as a pathway for cough is reviewed by Karlsson[22] and is based largely on the supposition that capsaicin is selective for C-fibres. In guinea pigs which had been given capsaicin at doses large enough to destroy their airway C-fibres, the cough response to capsaicin and citric acid was lost. However, capsaicin is not selective for C-fibres[23] and also activates RARs. In addition, capsaicin degeneration is not selective for non-myelinated fibres, but also affects small diameter myelinated fibres. Furthermore, since RARs have non-myelinated terminals, it is difficult to be precise about what sensory neurones are affected by capsaicin.

Relative roles of airway sensory receptors in the cough reflex

The functional role of sensory receptors in the respiratory tract is well established in relation to vagally mediated airway reflexes such as cough and bronchoconstriction, although the exact role for each group of receptors still remains to be elucidated. Their potential contribution to the cough reflex is summarized in Fig. 22.1. In animals, electrophysiological recordings from the vagus neurones have demonstrated that agents evoking cough cause an increased impulse activity in both myelinated Aδ-fibres originating from RARs and non-myelinated C-fibres originating from C-fibre receptors. There is considerable evidence that RARs are the main group or maybe even the only type of sensory receptor responsible for cough in the respiratory tract[19], including that caused by capsaicin. Indeed, capsaicin, which may be selective for C-fibres in vitro[24], stimulates both C-fibres and RARs in vivo[19,23]. Furthermore, cough, in cats and dogs, due to the so-called selective C-fibre stimulants, sulfur dioxide and capsaicin, is attenuated by cooling the vagus nerves to a temperature of 7–8°C, which blocks conduction in the Aδ-fibres originating from RARs but

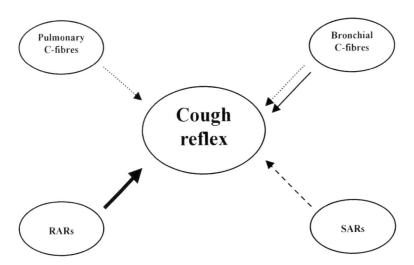

Fig. 22.1 Schematic representation of the potential role of airway sensory receptors in the cough reflex. Excitation of rapidly adapting stretch receptors (RARs) evokes the cough reflex. Stimulation of pulmonary C-fibre receptors inhibits the cough reflex, whereas activation of bronchial C-fibre receptors may either inhibit or evoke the reflex indirectly. Excitation of slowly adapting stretch receptors (SARs) may have a permissive role and thus facilitate the cough reflex.

leaves C-fibres intact. This technique may not completely differentiate afferent pathways, since it is still possible to evoke cough from sites other than the tracheobronchial tree when the nerves are at 7–8 °C and C-fibre reflexes other than cough can still be induced.

Stimulation of bronchial C-fibre receptors causes apnoea in animals and in humans[25]. A bronchoconstrictor reflex from bronchial C-fibres is also well established[22]. If stimulation of bronchial C-fibre receptors can also cause cough, one would have to postulate two or even three populations of C-fibre receptors for cough, apnoea and bronchoconstriction, presumably responding to different varieties or concentrations of stimulants, since one cannot have cough and apnea simultaneously. All of the stimuli used to excite C-fibre receptors can also activate RARs in vivo and the latter are an established and agreed pathway for cough. Therefore, it seems likely that the C-fibre receptors cause apnoea and bronchoconstriction, and not cough directly. Although pulmonary C-fibres were implicated in cough many years ago, most animal experiments point against

the idea[25]. A large number of studies using selective stimuli to these receptors have never established cough in any of the several species used. Activation of pulmonary C-fibre receptors inhibits cough induced mechanically in cats and dogs[8,26], which may also be true of the bronchial C-fibre receptors in dogs[27].

It seems reasonable to suggest that capsaicin and other 'selective' C-fibre stimulants may cause cough by activating RARs. Activation of C-fibres by these and many other agents probably leads to apnoea, rapid shallow breathing, bronchoconstriction and may cause reflex inhibition of cough through a central connection. This doesn't completely rule out a causative role for C-fibres in cough, since evidence now points to involvement of tachykinins in the cough reflex pathway. These substances, in particular substance P and neurokinin A, which are found in airway C-fibres, when administered exogenously by aerosol, can induce cough in animals and humans[28]. Furthermore, tachykinin antagonists inhibit capsaicin and citric acid-induced cough in conscious guinea pigs[29,30]. This important evidence suggests that agents which stimulate C-fibres, in addition to activating RARs, evoke the release of tachykinins probably from the C-fibres themselves and these tachykinins in turn stimulate the RARs to cause cough. Substance P has been shown to stimulate RARs and also sensitize RARs to other irritant agents in a number of species[19,31]. Alternatively, tachykinins such as substance P may act on postcapillary venules causing plasma extravasation and stimulation of adjacent RARs[25]. The increase in interstitial liquid volume might also affect the structure of the epithelium with stimulation of the branches of RARs there. This may explain why in vitro RARs were not stimulated by a number of agents known to cause cough in vivo, including histamine, bradykinin and substance P[24], since if these agents do stimulate RARs indirectly via plasma extravasation they would require an intact vascular circulation to exert their effects. Recent studies demonstrate how neutral endopeptidase inhibitors such as phosphoramidon, which prevent the breakdown of substance P, enhance the cough reflex due to substance P in guinea-pigs[19,28]. This is particularly interesting since it is well established that angiotensin converting enzyme (ACE) inhibitors cause cough in humans[32,33,34]. ACE inhibitors that inhibit the breakdown of substance P, also augment the cough response to capsaicin in guinea-pigs[35].

Thus, the activation of C-fibres could contribute indirectly to cough in animals and humans. It seems likely, therefore, that tussive agents such as citric acid and capsaicin may induce cough by two pathways: a direct activation of RARs and indirectly by facilitation of the cough reflex, mediated by the release of tachykinins from C-fibres (Fig. 22.2). The strength and pattern of the cough reflex will depend on the relative excitations of RARs and C-fibre receptors, the former reflexly exciting and the latter inhibiting cough, and the degree to which the local release of tachykinins causes plasma extravasation and excites RARs.

For completeness, SARs with myelinated $A\alpha$ and $A\beta$ afferent nerves have to be mentioned. These sensory receptors facilitate the cough reflex but are probably not directly involved since chemicals evoking cough do not alter their activity.

The anatomical site for initiation of the cough reflex

When assessed by single nerve fibre recording, the larynx has a far higher density of sensory receptors than do other sites in the respiratory tract and a far lower proportion of C-fibre receptors[36]. The importance of the larynx in cough induced by inhaled irritants such as citric acid and capsaicin has recently been reviewed[18]. Up until relatively recent times there seemed to be undisputed evidence on the involvement of the reflexogenic function of the larynx in relation to cough. However, several contradictory findings have been reported recently concerning the larynx as a source of respiratory reflexes. For instance denervation of the larynx in guinea pigs actually enhanced cough due to citric acid aerosol[37]. In addition, block of the superior laryngeal nerves in man caused no difference to cough also evoked by citric acid aerosol[38]. Furthermore, similar findings were reported for rats, rabbits and guinea pigs[39]. It remains possible in all of these studies that the area of deposition of the aerosols was not specific for the larynx and may also have included the tracheobronchial tree with regions endowed with RARs with a greater sensitivity to the stimuli being used. Had a stimulus more localized to the laryngeal mucosa been used a different effect of superior laryngeal nerve section may have been observed. Nevertheless, the evidence for the larynx as the primary site for initiating the cough reflex to inhaled irritants is not as convincing as that for the tracheobronchial tree as the primary site.

Central nervous mechanisms in cough

In addition to the obvious peripheral pathways in the cough reflex, constant stimulation of the sensory nerves by tachykinins or other inflammatory

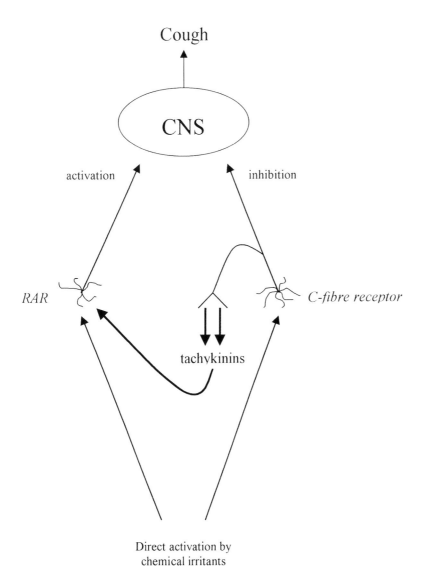

Cough

CNS

activation   inhibition

RAR

tachykinins

C-fibre receptor

Direct activation by
chemical irritants

Fig. 22.2 Diagrammatic representation of the possible role of airway sensory receptors in the cough reflex. Direct stimulation of RARs by chemical irritants evokes the cough reflex whereas direct activation of C-fibre receptors inhibits the cough reflex. Tachykinins may be released from C-fibre receptors and stimulate RARs either directly or indirectly via plasma extravasation. Tachykinins may also sensitize RARs and reduce the threshold to subsequent activation by chemical irritants.

mediators, which may be present in the inflamed airway in disease when the cough reflex is exaggerated, may lead to a phenomenon described as central sensitization. Central sensitization is a well-known mechanism in the processing of other sensory systems, such as pain[40]. The extent to which central sensitization contributes to the mechanism of cough is unknown. However, the sensitivity of the cough reflex in healthy volunteers can be increased by the exogenous application of a number of inflammatory mediators including prostaglandins $F_{2\alpha}$ and E_2[41,42].

Relatively little is known about the role of the central nervous organization of the cough reflex and the existence, anatomically, of a 'cough centre'. However, it is now clear that airway sensory afferents, irrespective of whether they are myelinated or non-myelinated, terminate within the brainstem in the nucleus tractus solitarus (NTS)[12]. Although functionally distinctive afferents terminate in discrete areas of the NTS, there is also a certain amount of overlap of their respective terminal fields that, along with the possibility of convergence onto polysynaptic neurones, could provide the neural substrate necessary to explain the apparent wide range of inputs evoking cough. Whilst the terminations of the airway afferents have been studied in some detail, much fewer data are available concerning the second and higher order neurones within the reflex pathways. $I\beta$ neurones, a subgroup of the inspiratory neurones in the dorsal respiratory group (DRG)[43], can be inactivated by lung inflation during expiration. Since the response adapts and needs relatively large inflations it has been suggested that this response may be mediated by RAR inputs. The pontine respiratory group is known to modulate activity in the DRG[44]. However, there is no information on the interaction of the two regions during cough. It has also been shown that the discharge pattern of some neurones in the midline raphe nuclei are altered during fictive cough in cats[44]. Neurones in the raphe nuclei are known to be influenced by respiratory reflexes via the NTS and can alter the pattern of breathing through actions on pontine, medullary and spinal respiratory neurones suggesting that the raphe neurones may modulate the cough reflex.

The processing of cough receptor inputs and coordination of brainstem neuronal networks to produce cough motor patterns in upper airway and thoracic-abdominal muscle is poorly understood. In order to elucidate the role of various populations of neurones in cough, it will be necessary to function-ally identify them. The sensitivity of the cough reflex and the strength and pattern of its response is, therefore, due to a complex interaction between C-fibre receptors and RARs, with peripheral and CNS interactions. How these mechanisms apply to clinical cough in patients is at present poorly understood, but is beginning to be clarified.

Cough mechanisms in humans

Inhalation cough challenge has been used for many years in the investigation of the cough reflex in humans[45] during which time a wide variety of methodological and practical problems have been overcome. The administration of inhaled irritants has been a useful pharmacological and epidemiological tool. Unfortunately because our knowledge of the physiology of the cough reflex is still at a basic level the precise nature and clinical relevance of each individual cough challenge in humans remains uncertain. However, despite this lack of knowledge it has become clear that agents such as citric acid, capsaicin and low chloride solutions have proved useful in studying cough in humans[46].

Citric acid was the first tussive agent to be used in man[45]. It is likely that the actual stimulus causing the firing of the sensory receptors, probably RARs, is a change in pH within the airway surface liquid rather than an effect of an individual ion[46] leading to the opening of a pH gated ion channel[47]. Capsaicin is another popular protussive agent in humans. At a cellular level, in sensitive neurones, capsaicin opens a relatively non-selective cation channel[48]. This allows sodium and calcium to enter and potassium ions to leave the cell resulting in depolarization and excitation of the neurone[48]. Once again the sensory receptor involved is probably the RAR (see above).

The production of cough by nebulized distilled water seems likely to be due to the absence of chloride from the solution[49]. Since ACE has an absolute requirement for the chloride ion as a cofactor, it has been suggested that the distilled water reduces the chloride content of the milieu surrounding the sensory receptor to a level below that required for ACE activity thus inhibiting the enzyme, which could ultimately lead to cough[46]. However, despite its possible physiological role the distilled water challenge has been rarely used in the investigation of antitussive drugs.

Cough in disease

Clinically, cough is one of the most frequent presenting symptoms of many diseases affecting the airways and lungs, and is often an early symptom of disease. The clinical spectrum of chronic cough has changed over the years. Tuberculosis which had been the leading cause of persistent cough has been replaced by chronic bronchitis. The commonest conditions that are associated with a chronic dry cough, excluding diseases such as carcinoma of the lung, include postnasal drip associated with chronic sinusitis/rhinitis, asthma, gastroesophageal reflux, upper respiratory tract virus infection, smoking, occupational exposures, air pollution and iatrogenic factors such as ACE inhibitor therapy[33,34].

The reason for the abnormal cough responses in humans is poorly understood. Cough frequently occurs in asthma and during upper respiratory tract infections that are accompanied by inflammation of the airways. There are many varied agents that can evoke cough in a number of different situations. These include citric acid, bradykinin, distilled water, SO_2, capsaicin, metabisulfite, cigarette smoke and ACE inhibitors. The sensitivity of the sensory nerve endings, probably the RARs, that mediate the cough reflex evoked by tussive agents is increased in asthmatics with cough, following upper respiratory tract infections in otherwise healthy individuals and in patients with ACE-inhibitor-evoked cough[32]. It is clear, therefore, that many different factors can influence the sensitivity of the cough reflex. In addition, the sensitivity of the cough reflex in healthy volunteers can be increased by the exogenous application of a number of inflammatory mediators including prostaglandins $F_{2\alpha}$ and E_2[33,34]. In many cases, treatment of the underlying cause of cough can reduce the increased sensitivity of the cough reflex. For instance, in individuals with an upper respiratory tract infection the sensitivity of the cough reflex is reduced to normal when the infection subsides. In addition, treatment of asthma can reduce the sensitivity of the cough reflex. Furthermore, in patients with ACE-inhibitor-induced cough, the cough subsides when the treatment is discontinued. Assuming that the central nervous system connections have not changed, it seems likely that the sensory information originating from the sensory receptors in the larynx and tracheobronchial tree is increased in these conditions to enhance the cough reflex. Thus, a similar phenomenon to that of hyperalgesia that occurs in inflamed tissues such as the skin may occur in the airways, where the airway sensory receptors are sensitized by inflammatory mediators, including the tachykinins, leading to an abnormal cough reflex[50]. This is particularly interesting in the light of ACE-inhibitor-evoked cough. ACE breaks down many peptides, notably the tachykinins substance P and neurokinin A. These tachykinins are released from sensory nerves and may evoke the cough reflex either directly by activating sensory nerve endings or indirectly by sensitising the sensory nerve endings to other irritants. Notwithstanding, elevation of these tachykinins by ACE-inhibitors could contribute to the cough observed in patients on this therapy.

Site and mechanisms of action of antitussive agents

It is not the purpose of this chapter to review current and future treatments of cough, since this is in a later chapter. However, it is important to examine the potential sites and mechanisms of action of some known antitussive drugs, because it is this area of research and the development of novel, more selective drugs which will eventually help to elucidate the exact role for each of the groups of peripheral sensory receptors in the cough reflex.

When cough is associated with excess production

of mucus within the lung, suppression of the cough reflex is generally undesirable, since mucus retention may occur which may present serious complications. When cough is non-productive and becomes a nuisance, preventing sleep and rest, suppression becomes desirable, although complete suppression can be dangerous as the lung is then deprived of an essential defence mechanism. An ideal drug would reduce the increased sensitivity of the cough reflex to normal, preferably by removing the disease process or by reducing the responsiveness of the airway sensory receptors. In the latter the most obvious airway sensory receptors to target would be the RARs. Drugs that affect cough can also do so indirectly. For example, drugs that cause bronchodilatation, such as the β-receptor agonists and cholinoceptor antagonists used in asthma, reduce the cough reflex without having any significant central effects.

Agents which inhibit cough may act at a variety of sites, both peripherally and centrally. Thus, antitussive agents may suppress peripheral airway sensory nerves, depress central neuronal function or suppress efferent nerves involved in the cough reflex. The number of potential sites of action of antitussive agents, therefore, includes all components of the cough reflex pathway from its initiation to its final synchronized motor response.

Drugs with antitussive activity are loosely classified into two groups based on their assumed site of action, peripheral or central. Centrally acting antitussive drugs act inside the central nervous system to depress one or more components of the central cough pathway. By definition, peripherally acting agents exert their mode of action outside the central nervous system, probably by inhibiting the activation of the airway sensory receptors responsible for initiating the cough reflex. The most frequently used cough suppressants are the opiates, local anesthetics, demulcents, expectorants, antihistamines and decongestants. Their proposed mechanisms of action have been extensively reviewed elsewhere[51] and apart from the opiates will not be considered here.

Until recently the antitussive effects of the classical opiates, such as codeine and morphine, were generally reported to be mediated centrally. With the identification of opioid receptors on the afferent/sensory neurones of the vagus nerves and with the unequivocal demonstration that agents with μ opioid-receptor-mediated antitussive actions can modulate impulse activity in airway sensory neurones originating from RARs and C-fibre receptors[52,53], this is clearly not the case. It seems reasonable to suggest, therefore, that the antitussive activity of drugs such as codeine is not restricted entirely to the central nervous system, but that some of its activity is also exerted peripherally. There is a vast array of numerous different types of drugs which have been shown to produce antitussive actions in a variety of animal and human models (Table 22.1), but the mechanism of antitussive action of most of these agents is far from clear. Since the sensory receptors, RARs and C-fibre endings, together with the vagal sensory neurones that carry their impulses are so obviously important in the cough reflex, it is somewhat surprising to find that there is such a paucity of data on the action of these agents at these peripheral sites. This may be due to the fact that it was always assumed that most of the antitussive drugs, apart from the local anaesthetics, acted exclusively via a central mechanism. Recently, increased interest has been directed towards drugs that act peripherally on the sensory receptors in the airways, since these might be expected to lack any secondary and undesirable central nervous actions. The sensory receptors for cough are known to have opioid receptors in their membranes and opioid agonists and the classical opiates may activate these receptors to inhibit cough (see above). Neurokinin antagonists are effective against cough in humans and experimental animals[31], via mechanisms described previously and this is a therapeutic approach that needs to be explored. Even capsaicin, a strong stimulant to cough, is included in some antitussive mixtures, and it can be shown in experimental animals to activate reflex pathways that inhibit cough[8].

The pharmacology of the central pathways for cough is increasingly being studied. The presence of

Table 22.1. Modulation of airway sensory receptors and cough

Agent	RARs	Pulmonary C	Bronchial C	Antitussive/inhibition of cough reflex
Morphine	?	(+)	?	✔
Codeine	− +	(+)	?	✔
Dextromethorphan	?	?	?	✔
443c81	−	+ → −	+ → −	✔
Cromoglycate	NE	−	−	✔
Nedocromil sodium	NE	NE	+	✔
Moguisteine	−	?	?	✔
Phenylbiguanide	+	+	+	✔
Capsaicin	+	+	+	✔
Lidocaine	−	−	−	✔
5-HT	+	+	+	✔
$GABA_B$- receptor agonists	?	?	?	✔
α_2-adrenoceptor agonists	?	?	?	✔
NMDA antagonists	?	?	?	✔
Ca^{2+} channel blockers	?	?	?	✔
Frusemide	−	NE	NE	✔
Theophylline	?	?	?	✔
β_2-adrenoceptor agonists	?	?	?	✔
anticholinergics	?	?	?	✔
Neurokinin antagonists	?	?	?	✔

Notes:

[1] +, activation of sensory nerve activity; -, inhibition of sensory nerve activity; (+), activation implied from evoked pulmonary reflex; + → −, initial activation, followed by inhibition; − +, inhibition low dose, activation high dose; NE, no effect; ?, effect unknown; ✔, inhibition.

opioid receptors at the synapses is well established, and is the likely central site of antitussive agents such as codeine[54]. Recent studies have demonstrated the presence of receptors in the central pathways for 5-HT, γ-aminobutyric acid (GABA), tachykinins, *N*-methyl-$_D$-aspartate and adenosine[54,55]. The way these receptors interact in the cough pathways has not been determined, but they point to possible important therapeutic advances in the future.

Conclusions

The involvement of airway sensory nerves in the cough reflex is beyond doubt. While there is much evidence that cough can be caused by stimulation of RARs in the tracheobronchial tree, the role of C-fibres is more uncertain. They can cause apnoea, bronchoconstriction and rapid shallow breathing, but a subpopulation that causes cough has not been established. When stimulated, C-fibres may release tachykinins, such as substance P, which could cause cough by direct stimulation of RARs or indirectly by promoting plasma extravasation which in turn may excite RARs and produce cough. Despite this knowledge, the information regarding the effects of known antitussives on these sensory nerves is far from complete. Although our understanding of the peripheral mechanisms of the cough reflex has improved in recent years, less is known about the central nervous pathways in cough and clearly much research is still required to clarify the interactions between the peripheral and central pathways. In addition, an increased understanding of the physiological and pharmacological events of the complete cough reflex from its initiation to the final motor act of coughing will lead to novel therapeutic approaches for its treatment.

REFERENCES

1 Widdicombe JG. Receptors in the trachea and bronchi of the cat. *J Physiol* 1954; 123:71–104.

2 Widdicombe JG. Respiratory reflexes from the trachea and bronchi of the cat. *J Physiol* 1954; 123:55–70.

3 Boushey HA, Richardson PS, Widdicombe JG, Wise JCM. The response of laryngeal afferent fibres to mechanical and chemical stimuli. *J Physiol* 1974; 240:153–175.

4 Widdicombe JG. Vagal reflexes in the airways. In *Lung Biology in Health and Disease*, vol 33; *The Airways: Neural Control in Health and Disease*, eds. MA Kaliner and PJ Barnes. Marcel Dekker, New York, Basel; 1988:187–202.

5 Coleridge JCG, Coleridge HM. Afferent vagal C-fibre innervation of the lungs and airways and its functional significance. *Rev Physiol Biochem Pharmacol* 1984; 99:1–110.

6 Collier JG, Fuller RW. Capsaicin inhalation in man and the effect of sodium cromoglycate. *Br J Pharmacol* 1984; 81:113–117.

7 Forsberg K, Karlsson J-A. Cough induced by stimulation of capsaicin-sensitive sensory neurons in conscious guinea-pigs. *Acta Physiol Scand* 1986; 128:319–320.

8 Tatar M, Webber SE, Widdicombe JG. Lung C-fibre receptor activation and defensive reflexes in anaesthetised cats. *J Physiol* 1988; 402:411–420.

9 Widdicombe JG. Neurophysiology of the cough reflex. *Eur Respir J* 1995; 8:1193–1202.

10 Sant'Ambrogio G, Sant'Ambrogio FB, Davies A. Airway receptors in cough. *Clin. Respir Physiol* 1984; 20:43–47.

11 Hanacek J, Davies A, Widdicombe JG. Influence of lung stretch receptors on the cough reflex in rabbits. *Respiration* 1984; 45:161–168.

12 Jordan D. Central nervous mechanism in cough. *Pulm Pharmacol* 1996; 9:389–392.

13 Coleridge HM, Coleridge JCG. Reflexes evoked from the tracheobronchial tree and lungs. In: Cherniak NS, Widdicombe JG, eds, *Handbook of Physiology*, III. *Respiratory System*, vol 2, Washington, DC: American Physiological Society; 1986:395–430.

14 Widdicombe JG. Nervous receptors in the tracheobronchial tree. *Prog Brain Res* 1989; 67:49–64.

15 Korpas J, Tomori Z. In *Cough and Other Respiratory Reflexes* 1979; Karger.

16 Sant'Ambrogio G. Information arising from the tracheobronchial tree of mammals. *Physiol Rev* 1982; 62:531–569.

17 Das RM, Jeffery PK, Widdicombe JG. The epithelial innervation of the lower respiratory tract of the cat. *J Anat* 1978; 126:123–131.

18 Sant'ambrogio G. Role of the larynx in cough. *Pulm Pharmacol* 1996; 9:379–382.

19 Widdicombe JG. Sensory mechanisms. *Pulm Pharmacol* 1996; 9:383–387

20 Karlsson J-A, Sant'Ambrogio G, Widdicombe JG. Afferent neural pathways in cough and reflex bronchoconstriction. *J Appl Physiol* 1988; 65:1007–1023.

21 Bonham AC, Kott KS, Ravi K, Kappagoda CT, Joad JP. Substance P contributes to rapidly adapting receptor responses to pulmonary venous congestion in rabbits. *J Physiol Lond* 1996; 493:229–238.

22 Karlsson J-A. The role of capsaicin-sensitive C-fibre afferent nerves in the cough reflex. *Pulm Pharmacol* 1996; 9:315–322.

23 Mohammed SP, Higenbottam TW, Adcock JJ. Effects of aerosol applied capsaicin, histamine and prostaglandin E_2 on airway sensory receptors of anaesthetised cats. *J Physiol* 1993; 469:51–66.

24 Fox AJ. Modulation of cough and airway sensory fibres. *Pulm Pharmacol* 1996; 9:335–342.

25 Widdicombe JG. Afferent receptors in the airways and cough. *Respiration Physiol* 1998; 114:5–15.

26 Tatar M, Sant'Ambrogio G, Sant'ambrogio FB. Laryngeal and tracheobronchial cough in anaesthetised dogs. *J Appl Physiol* 1994; 76:2672–2679.

27 Jackson DM, Norris AA, Eady RP. Nedocromil sodium and sensory nerves in the dog lung. *Pulm Pharmacol* 1989; 2:179–184.

28 Sekizawa K, Jia YX, Ebihara T, Hirose Y, Hirayama Y, Sasaki H. Role of substance P in cough. *Pulm Pharmacol* 1996; 9:323–328

29 Girard V, Naline E, Vilain P, Emonds-Alt X, Advenier C. Effect of two tachykinin antagonists, SR 48968 and SR 140333, on cough induced by citric acid in the unanaesthetised guinea-pig. *Eur Respir J* 1995; 8:1110–1114.

30 Yasumitsu R, Hirayama Y, Imai T, Miyayasu K, Hiroi J. Effect of specific tachykinin receptor antagonists on citric acid-induced cough and bronchoconstriction in unanaesthetised guinea-pigs. *Eur J Pharmacol* 1996; 300:215–219.

31 Advenier C, Emonds-Alt X. Tachykinin receptor antagonists and cough. *Pulm Pharmacol* 1996; 9:329–333

32 Spina D, Page CP. Airway sensory nerves in asthma: targets for therapy. *Pulm Pharmacol* 1996; 9:1–18

33 Chung KF, Lalloo UG. Diagnosis and management of chronic persistent dry cough. *Postgrad Med J* 1996; 72:594–598

34 Milgrom H. In Weiss ED, Stein M, eds, *Bronchial Asthma: Mechanisms and Therapeutics*, Little, Brown and Company 1993:644–649.

35 Ebihara T, Sekizawa K, Ohrui T, Nazakawa H, Sasaki H. Angiotensin-converting enzyme inhibitor and danazol increase sensitivity of cough reflex in female guinea pigs. *Am J Respir Crit Care Med.* 1996; 153:812–819.

36 Sant'Ambrogio G, Sant'Ambrogio FB. Role of the laryngeal afferents in cough. *Pulm Pharmacol* 1996; 9:309–314.

37 Forsberg K, Karlsson J-A, Lundberg JM, Zackrisson C. Effect of partial laryngeal denervation on irritant-induced cough and bronchoconstriction in conscious guinea pigs. *J Physiol Lond* 1990; 422:34P.

38 Stockwell M, Land S, Yip R, Zintel T, White C, Gallagher CG. Lack of importance of the superior laryngeal nerves in citric acid cough in humans. *J Appl Physiol* 1993; 75:613–617.

39 Tatar M, Karkolova D, Pecova R, Brozmanova M. The role of partial laryngeal denervation on the cough reflex in awake guinea pigs, rats and rabbits. *Pulm Pharmacol* 1996; 9:371–272.

40 McMahon SB, Lewin GR, Wall PD. Central hyperexcitability triggered by noxious inputs. *Curr Opin Neurobiol* 1993; 3:602–610.

41 Choudry NB, Fuller RW, Pride NB. Sensitivity of the human cough reflex: effects of inflammatory mediators, prostaglandin E_2, bradykinin and histamine. *Am Rev Respir Dis* 1989; 140:137–141

42 Nichol G, Nix A, Barnes PJ, Chung KF. Prostaglandin F_2 alpha enhancement of capsaicin-induced cough in man: modulation by beta$_2$ adrenergic and anticholinergic drugs. *Thorax* 1990; 45:694–698

43 Von Euler C. Brainstem mechanisms In: N.S. Cherniack and J.G. Widdicombe eds, *Handbook of Physiology, The Respiratory System*, II.Vol 2, *Control of Breathing*. Bethesda: American Physiological Society; 1986:1–67.

44 Shannon R, Baekey DM, Morris KF, Lindsey BG. Brainstem respiratory networks and cough. *Pulm Pharmacol* 1996; 9:343–347.

45 Bickerman HA, Barach AL, Itkin S, Drimmer F. Experimental production of cough in human subjects induced by citric acid aerosols. Preliminary studies on the evaluation of antitussive agents. *Am J Med Sci* 1954; 228:156–163.

46 Morice AH. Inhalation cough challenge in the investigation of the cough reflex and antitussives. *Pulm Pharmacol* 1996; 9:281–284.

47 Lowry RH, Wood AM, Higenbottam TW. Effects of pH and osmolality on aerosol-induced cough in normal volunteers. *Clin Sci* 1988; 74:373–378.

48 Beva, S, Docherty RJ. Cellular mechanisms of action of capsaicin. In: Wood J ed., *Neurosciences Perspective: Capsaicin in the Study of Pain*. New York: Academic Press; 1993:27–44.

49 Stone RA, Barnes PJ, Chung KF. Effect of frusemide on cough responses to chloride-deficient solution in normal and mild asthmatic subjects. *Eur Respir J* 1993; 6:862–867.

50 Adcock JJ, Garland LG. In: Page CP, Gardiner PJ, eds, *Airway Hyperresponsiveness: Is It Really Important for Asthma?* Blackwell Scientific; 1993:234–255.

51 Fuller RW, Jackson DM. Physiology and treatment of cough. *Thorax* 1990; 45:425–430.

52 Adcock JJ. Peripheral opioid receptors and the cough reflex. *Respir Med* 1991; 85:43–46.

53 Bolser DC, DeGennaro FC, O'Reilly S et al. Peripheral and central sites of action of GABA-B agonists to inhibit the cough reflex in the cat and guinea-pig. *Br J Pharmacol* 1994; 113:1344–1348.

54 Kamei J. Role of opioidergic and serotonergic mechanism in cough and antitussives. *Pulm Pharmacol* 1996; 9:349–356.

55 Bolser DC. Mechanisms of action of central and peripheral antitussive drugs. *Pulm Pharmacol* 1996; 9:357–364.

23

Current treatment of cough

Peter V. Dicpinigaitis

Department of Medicine, Albert Einstein College of Medicine, Bronx, New York, USA

Introduction

Cough is a protective reflex that serves to prevent the entry of foreign material into the respiratory tract, as well as to promote the expulsion of mucus from the airways. Often, however, persistent cough appears to serve no useful purpose, and results in significant morbidity, especially in terms of quality of life, among afflicted individuals[1]. Cough is the most common complaint for which outpatient medical attention is sought in the United States[2].

Acute cough, most commonly associated with an upper respiratory tract infection, is usually self limited. However, since the acute onset of cough may also indicate more serious underlying conditions such as pneumonia, malignancy, pulmonary embolism, congestive heart failure, or endobronchial foreign body, clinical judgment must dictate the extent of initial evaluation. Chronic cough, defined as cough present for greater than 3 weeks, is more likely to stimulate a patient to seek medical evaluation, and may present the clinician with a difficult diagnostic challenge. Fortunately, studies have confirmed that with the use of a systematic, diagnostic protocol, the etiology of cough can be established in the vast majority of patients[3-7].

Pharmacological therapy for cough can be most broadly categorized as antitussive or protussive. The goal of antitussive therapy is to eliminate bothersome, maladaptive cough, whereas protussive therapy is used to enhance the efficiency of cough in situations where mobilization of respiratory secretions is desired. Antitussive therapy may be further subdivided into specific therapy, which is aimed at an established or presumed specific etiology of cough, and non-specific therapy, whose goal is to suppress the cough reflex.

Chronic cough

Specific antitussive therapy

An organized, systematic approach to the evaluation of the patient with chronic cough is essential, since a definitive diagnosis will allow the initiation of specific antitussive therapy, which is highly effective. Recently, the American College of Chest Physicians published a consensus statement on the management of cough[8], which includes a diagnostic algorithm (Fig. 23.1). In the vast majority of patients who are non-smokers, not receiving angiotensin-converting enzyme (ACE) inhibitors, and who have normal or stable (with inconsequential chronic, postinflammatory changes) chest radiographs, chronic cough is due to postnasal drip syndrome (PNDS), asthma, or gastroesophageal reflux disease (GERD). These three etiologies, alone or in combination, have been demonstrated in prospective studies to account for chronic cough in 82–100% of such patients[4-7]. Multiple causes of chronic cough are often present simultaneously (23–29% of patients[4-7]), therefore, a partial response may indicate that only one of multiple etiologies of cough has been treated.

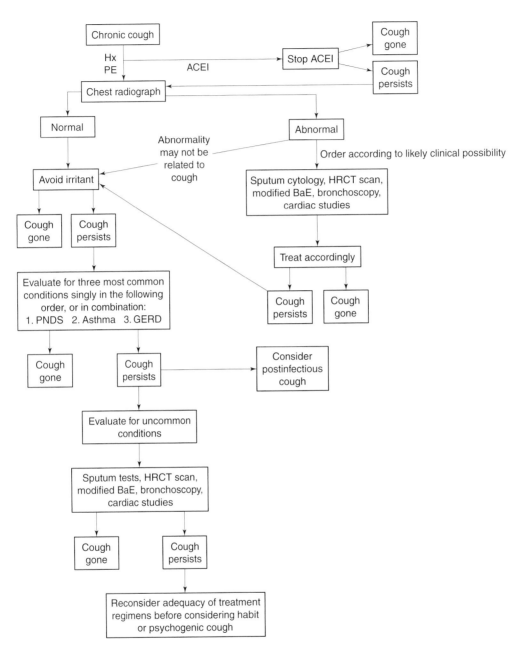

Fig. 23.1 Guidelines for evaluating chronic cough in immunocompetent adults. ACEI = angiotensin-converting enzyme inhibitor; BaE = barium esophagography; GERD = gastroesophageal reflux disease; HRCT = high-resolution computed tomography; HX = history; PE = physical examination; PNDS = postnasal drip syndrome. (Reprinted from [reference 8] Irwin RS, Boulet LP, Cloutier MM, et al. Managing cough as a defence mechanism and as a symptom: a consensus panel report of the American College of Chest Physicians. Chest 1998;114(suppl.):133S-181S, with permission from the American College of Chest Physicians.)

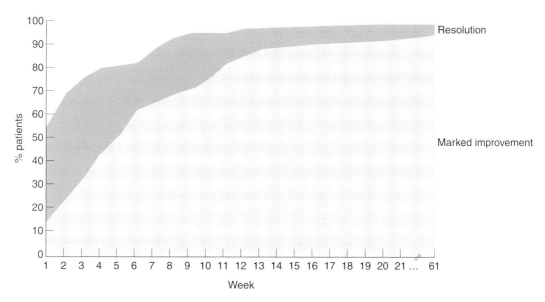

Fig. 23.2 Cough response to a stepwise diagnostic and therapeutic algorithm that emphasized initial treatment of all patients with an antihistamine-decongestant for postnasal drip, followed by further evaluation in nonresponders and partial responders. Marked improvement included patients with resolution. Note the gap between weeks 21 and 61. (Reprinted[5], with permission from the American College of Physicians–American Society of Internal Medicine.)

Evaluation of chronic cough in a cigarette smoker must begin with abstinence from tobacco, since cough due to smoking should significantly improve or resolve within four weeks of smoking cessation[9]. Cough due to ACE inhibitors usually resolves within 1–4 days after discontinuation of the drug, although some patients may have a slower response[10]. ACE inhibitor-induced cough is discussed in more detail below.

The clinician evaluating patients with chronic cough should bear in mind that complete resolution of cough, even with appropriate, specific antitussive therapy, may take weeks to months, especially in the case of cough due to GERD. However, initial improvement in symptoms, particularly with PNDS and cough-variant asthma, may occur within the first week (Fig. 23.2).

Postnasal drip syndrome (Table 23.1)

Multiple prospective studies have concluded that postnasal drip syndrome (PNDS) is the most common etiology of chronic cough[4–7,11]. PNDS itself may have numerous causes, the diagnosis of which will indicate specific therapeutic options (Table 23.1). In the minority of patients with PNDS who present with excessive sputum production, chronic bacterial sinusitis must be suspected, and four-view sinus radiography should be performed[12]. Unlike other etiologies of PNDS, the presence of chronic bacterial sinusitis mandates aggressive (minimum of 3 weeks) therapy with antibiotics effective against *S. pneumoniae, H. influenzae,* and oral anaerobic organisms.

The combination of a first-generation antihistamine and decongestant is considered to be the most consistently effective sole form of therapy for patients with PNDS-induced cough not due to sinusitis[8]. Whereas the older, potentially sedating, first generation antihistamine/decongestant combinations have been demonstrated to be effective in treating chronic cough due to PNDS[4,5,12,13], the newer-generation, relatively non-sedating antihistamines, such as terfenadine and loratadine/pseudoephedrine, have been shown, in randomized,

Table 23.1.

Etiologies of postnasal drip syndrome	Therapeutic options
chronic (bacterial) sinusitis	antibiotics; oral A/D[a]; nasal D[b]
seasonal allergic rhinitis	nasal CS; nasal cromolyn; oral A or A/D; avoidance of allergens
perennial allergic rhinitis	nasal CS; nasal cromolyn; oral A or A/D; avoidance of allergens
perennial non-allergic rhinitis	oral A/D; nasal CS; nasal IB
vasomotor rhinitis	avoidance of triggers; nasal IB; oral or nasal D; nasal CS
postinfectious 'postviral' rhinitis	oral A/D; nasal CS; nasal IB
rhinitis medicamentosa[c]	avoidance of irritant; nasal CS
rhinitis associated with pregnancy	therapy based on underlying etiology[d]

CS = corticosteroids; A = antihistamine; D = decongestant; A/D = antihistamine plus decongestant combination; IB = ipratropium bromide. [a] First-generation antihistamines preferred over newer-generation, non-sedating agents (see text); [b] topical decongestants should be used for no more than 5 days, since rebound congestion may develop; [c] can be induced by prescription therapy (i.e. inhaled nasal decongestants) or illicit drug use (i.e. inhaled cocaine); [d]rhinitis associated with pregnancy most often due to allergic rhinitis, sinusitis, rhinitis medicamentosa, and vasomotor rhinitis.

controlled trials, to be ineffective in treating acute cough due to the common cold[14–16]. Presumably, the first-generation antihistamines demonstrate greater antitussive efficacy because of greater anticholinergic potency and, perhaps, due to enhanced penetration into the central nervous system, thus explaining their sedating properties. It is interesting, therefore, that recent animal studies have shown that the antitussive actions of antihistamines are independent of their sedative effects[17]. The author initiates therapy of suspected PNDS-induced cough with a first-generation antihistamine/decongestant combination, azatadine maleate, 1 mg, plus sustained-release pseudoephedrine sulfate, 120 mg (Trinalin repetabs, Key Pharmaceuticals, Kenilworth, New Jersey, USA) twice daily. If daytime sedation occurs, a single, nightly dose is prescribed. If an unacceptable degree of sedation persists, therapy is changed to a newer-generation antihistamine/decongestant combination.

A subgroup of patients will present with cough as their sole symptom of PNDS, so-called 'silent PNDS'[5]. Therefore, since PNDS is the most common cause of chronic cough[4–7,11], and, since many patients with PNDS-induced cough will describe none of the typical symptoms of PNDS, it appears reasonable to initiate empiric therapy for PNDS in a patient with chronic cough in whom other etiologies are not evident. Such a strategy was prospectively evaluated by Pratter and colleagues[5], who found that first-generation antihistamine/decongestant therapy was beneficial in 87%, and the only treatment necessary in 36%, of 45 patients presenting with chronic cough of unknown etiology. Subjects unresponsive or only partially responsive to therapy were further evaluated according to a stepwise diagnostic algorithm[5].

Asthma

Asthma has been shown in several prospective studies to be the second most common cause of chronic cough in non-smoking adults[4–7]. In most patients with asthma, cough may accompany the more significant symptoms of dyspnea and wheezing. In a subgroup of asthmatics, however, cough is the predominant or sole symptom[18]. This condition is termed cough-variant asthma (CVA)[19].

Asthmatic cough is likely induced by inflammatory stimulation of sensory receptors, the rapidly adapting receptors (RARs) and C-fibre receptors, within the bronchial epithelium, whose afferent fibres stimulate a central cough centre[20]. It is important to note that cough and bronchoconstriction are separate entities, controlled by distinct afferent neural pathways[21].

Although demonstration of bronchial hyper-responsiveness by methacholine inhalation challenge (MIC) testing is commonly regarded as the diagnostic gold standard for CVA, the clinician must bear in mind that a positive MIC is merely consistent with CVA. A definitive diagnosis cannot be made until resolution of cough is achieved with appropriate specific therapy. A recent study of 15 patients with chronic cough and positive MIC demonstrated CVA to be present in only nine[22].

In general, the treatment of CVA is similar to that of typical asthma. Inhaled β_2-agonists or ipratropium bromide may offer acute, temporary relief of symptoms. For chronic, persistent cough, anti-inflammatory therapy is also indicated. Inhaled corticosteroids have been shown in prospective studies to be effective therapy for CVA[23]. It is important to note, however, that in some patients with CVA, cough may actually be exacerbated by inhaled steroid therapy, most likely due to a constituent of the aerosol. For example, cough occurs more commonly after inhalation of beclomethasone dipropionate than after triamcinolone acetonide, probably due to a component of the dispersant in the former[24]. Therefore, if corticosteroid aerosol-induced exacerbation of cough is suspected, or if cough on presentation is severe, oral corticosteroid therapy, alone or followed by inhaled therapy[25], is appropriate. The author begins with a 7-day course of oral prednisone, 40 mg daily, as an initial diagnostic therapeutic trial.

Although an initial improvement in cough is often achieved after 1 week of therapy with an inhaled β_2-agonist, complete resolution of cough due to asthma may require up to 8 weeks of treatment with inhaled corticosteroids[22].

Other agents shown prospectively to be effective in CVA include the inhaled anti-inflammatory agent nedocromil sodium[26] (double-blind, placebo-controlled trial), and the antiallergic compound, azelastine hydrochloride[27] (unblinded, uncontrolled study) which is thought to act through inhibition of substance P, a potent endogenous cough-inducing agent[20].

Recently, drugs that modulate the synthesis or activity of leukotrienes have become available for the treatment of asthma. Preliminary investigational data support previous anecdotal reports[28,29] suggesting that these agents may be particularly effective in CVA. In a randomized, double-blind, placebo-controlled, cross-over study, a 2-week course of zafirlukast, a cysteinyl leukotriene receptor antagonist, significantly improved subjective cough scores and inhibited capsaicin-induced cough in seven of eight subjects[30]. Of interest is the ability of zafirlukast to suppress cough which had been refractory to inhaled β_2-agonists in all subjects, and refractory to β_2-agonists plus inhaled corticosteroids in five of eight patients. Perhaps the leukotriene inhibitors more effectively modulate the hyperstimulated cough receptors within the bronchial epithelium of patients with CVA. An identical 14-day course of zafirlukast did not inhibit capsaicin-induced cough in healthy volunteers[31] or stable asthmatics without cough[32], suggesting that sensory afferent fibres inducing cough are hypersensitive only in the subgroup of asthmatics with CVA.

Gastroesophageal reflux disease

Gastroesophageal reflux disease (GERD) is among the most common causes of chronic, non-productive cough, exceeded in frequency only by PNDS and asthma[4–7]. Although gross aspiration and microaspiration from proximal esophageal reflux can cause cough, a significant percentage of patients with GERD-induced cough will have no evidence of such events after an extensive diagnostic evaluation. In most patients, chronic cough likely results from the presence of gastric acid in the distal esophagus stimulating a vagally mediated distal esophageal–tracheobronchial reflex[33,34]. Interestingly, patients with GERD but without respiratory symptoms have a reduced cough threshold, as measured by inhaled capsaicin[35]. This appears to be due to acid reflux irrespective of the presence of esophagitis, suggesting that the entry of gastric acid into the distal esophagus, rather than esophageal mucosal damage, is the major cause of GERD-induced cough[35].

It has been suggested that a self-perpetuating, positive feedback cycle exists between cough and

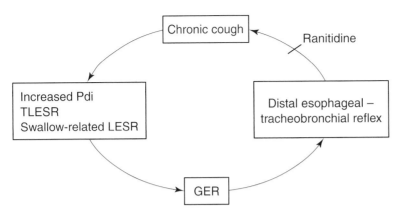

Fig. 23.3 The relationship between cough and gastroesophageal reflux (GER). See text for discussion. P_{di} = transdiaphragmatic pressure; TLESR = transient lower esophageal sphincter relaxation; LESR = lower esophageal sphincter relaxation. (Reprinted[36], with permission from Excerpta Medica, Inc.)

gastroesophageal reflux, in which cough from any cause may induce further reflux[36]. Although the mechanisms by which acid reflux is exacerbated by cough remain speculative, one model proposes that chronic, persistent cough, in addition to elevating transdiaphragmatic pressure (P_{di}), may promote swallow-related lower esophageal sphincter relaxation (LESR), or transient lower esophageal sphincter relaxation (TLESR), thereby enhancing reflux and further stimulating the distal esophageal–tracheobronchial reflex (Fig. 23.3). A goal of therapy, therefore, is to interrupt this vicious cycle.

Chronic cough due to GERD often presents a diagnostic dilemma for several reasons: most patients with GERD-induced cough do not experience typical reflux symptoms[34,37]; cough may be the sole manifestation of GERD[38]; reflux symptoms may occur subsequent to the development of chronic cough[39]; many patients recall the onset of cough to be temporally related to an upper respiratory tract infection[34,36]. Hence, the clinician must maintain a high index of suspicion.

In patients with unexplained cough without other symptoms, the initial test of choice to evaluate for the presence of GERD is 24-hour ambulatory esophageal pH monitoring[8]. However, since this modality is cumbersome and not universally available, empiric antireflux therapy may be indicated. As noted above, in the vast majority of nonsmoking patients who have normal chest radiographs and are not receiving ACE-inhibitor therapy, chronic cough is due to PNDS, asthma or GERD. Therefore, in such patients, after PNDS and asthma have been reasonably excluded, GERD is by far the most likely etiology of chronic cough, and hence empiric therapy is appropriate.

Initial empiric therapy for GERD-induced cough should include conservative measures such as high-protein, low-fat, antireflux diet, avoidance of coffee and tobacco, and elevation of the head of the bed[36]. This strategy, in combination with pharmacologic therapy using metaclopramide and/or H_2-antagonists, has been demonstrated to abolish cough in 70–100% of patients. However, the mean time to full resolution of cough was in the range of 5–6 months[4,38,40]. The clinician should be aware that resolution of GERD-induced cough is often a lengthy process; initial improvement in symptoms may not occur for 2–3 months with appropriate therapy.[8]

Although therapy with H_2-antagonists has been reported to have a success rate in GERD-induced cough of approximately 80%[4,41], a significant subgroup of patients may demonstrate refractory cough. In such cases, more aggressive acid suppression with proton-pump inhibitors, such as omeprazole and lansoprazole, may be indicated. Because

H_2-antagonist therapy alone may be ineffective[8], some clinicians initiate empiric antireflux therapy with proton-pump inhibitors. If successful, a transition to less expensive H_2-antagonists can be attempted if prolonged therapy with proton-pump inhibitors is deemed undesirable.

If prolonged therapy with a proton-pump inhibitor is unsuccessful, a formal diagnostic evaluation for GERD is indicated, since medical therapy may have been insufficient or ineffective. Some patients with GERD-induced cough will require high-dose proton-pump inhibitor therapy for symptomatic relief[8]. Furthermore, there appears to be a subgroup of patients in whom cough persists despite documentation, by 24-hour esophageal pH monitoring, of total or near-total suppression of esophageal acid, raising the possibility that GERD-induced cough may not be mediated solely by acid[42].

Antireflux surgery, including open or laparoscopic fundoplication, should be considered in patients with documented failure of intensive medical therapy, including high-dose proton-pump inhibitors[8]. Surgical intervention has been demonstrated to be successful in eliminating or improving GERD-induced cough, with sustained symptomatic improvement 6[43] and 12 months[44] postoperatively.

Postinfectious cough

Not uncommonly, patients without history of pulmonary disease or respiratory symptoms develop a non-productive cough temporally related to the occurrence of an acute respiratory tract infection. Although the cough is usually transient and self limited, a subgroup of patients will suffer persistent cough for weeks to months following resolution of other symptoms. The mechanism of postinfectious cough remains poorly understood, but is likely to involve airway inflammation[45–47] with resultant enhancement of the sensitivity of cough-inducing afferent nerves within the airway epithelium[48]. Cough may occur with[45,46] or without[3,48] simultaneous increase in bronchial hyperresponsiveness. Postinfectious cough is likely caused predominantly by viral infections, although infection with *M. pneumoniae*, *C. pneumoniae*, strain TWAR, and *B. pertus-*

sis have also been implicated in adults[8]. Interestingly, a recent study of patients with acute Mycoplasma pneumonia did not demonstrate enhanced cough sensitivity to inhaled capsaicin or tartaric acid[49].

Pharmacological intervention is necessary for persistent or debilitating symptoms. Postinfectious cough is often refractory to standard antitussive therapy, including codeine[50,51]. On the presumption that inflammatory mechanisms are involved in postinfectious cough, corticosteroid therapy seems appropriate, and has been used with success[3]. The author treats severe, presumed postinfectious cough with oral prednisone, 40 mg daily for one week, followed by tapering doses during the subsequent 1–2 weeks. Inhaled corticosteroids may be used following oral therapy for any residual symptoms, or may be attempted as initial therapy for less severe cough. No published data exist regarding the use of inhaled steroids to treat postinfectious cough.

Other agents that have been shown to be useful in prospective, randomized studies include inhaled ipratropium bromide[52] (double-blind, cross-over design) and the oral H_1-antagonist oxatomide[53] (open-label design, used in conjunction with dextromethorphan).

Cough due to angiotensin-converting enzyme (ACE) inhibitors

Approximately 10–20% of patients treated with ACE inhibitors develop a dry, persistent cough which is usually refractory to standard antitussive therapy[10,54]. The incidence of cough appears to be higher in women[10], patients treated with ACE inhibitors for congestive heart failure as opposed to hypertension[54], non-smokers[55], and Chinese persons[56]. The cough is a class effect of the ACE inhibitors, and is not dose related[10]. The onset of ACE inhibitor-induced cough is variable, occurring as soon as hours after the initial dose, or months later[8,10]. The cough usually resolves within four days of cessation of therapy[10], but may take up to four weeks[57].

The etiology of ACE inhibitor-induced cough remains unclear. Proposed mediators include bradykinin, a bronchial irritant metabolized by ACE[58];

prostaglandins, the increased production of which may be mediated by bradykinin[59]; and substance P, a tachykinin and potent bronchoconstrictor that is also degraded by ACE and is a presumed neurochemical mediator of the cough reflex[60,61].

The only definitive treatment of ACE inhibitor-induced cough is discontinuation of the offending drug. Agents that have demonstrated the ability to attenuate ACE inhibitor-induced cough in small, randomized, double-blind, placebo-controlled, cross-over studies include: inhaled sodium cromoglycate[62], theophylline[63], indomethacin[59], the calcium-channel antagonists amlodipine and nifedipine[59], and the thromboxane synthase inhibitor/thromboxane receptor antagonist, picotamide[64]. Drugs shown to suppress ACE inhibitor-induced cough in open-label, uncontrolled studies include the GABA-agonist baclofen[65], and the thromboxane synthetase inhibitor ozagrel[66].

A newer class of therapeutic agents, the angiotensin II (A-II) receptor antagonists, by not degrading ACE and thereby not producing elevated tissue levels of bradykinin and substance P, theoretically should not induce cough. Losartan, the first A-II receptor antagonist approved for clinical use, has been associated with a low incidence of cough, similar to that observed with the diuretic hydrochlorothiazide[57].

Chronic bronchitis and bronchiectasis

Unlike the predominantly dry cough caused by PNDS, asthma, GERD, viral infections and ACE inhibitors, cough due to chronic bronchitis and bronchiectasis is usually associated with significant sputum production[67,68]. A thorough history will assist in the diagnosis of these conditions.

Chronic bronchitis is predominantly a disease of smokers. Although persistent cough is a major component of chronic bronchitis, patients with this condition tend not to seek medical attention nearly as often as do patients with cough due to other etiologies[8]. Because cigarette smoke probably stimulates cough via induction of bronchial inflammation, mucus hypersecretion, and impaired mucociliary clearance, initial treatment of cough in active

smokers must include smoking cessation. In most cases, cough due to smoking improves or resolves within four weeks of abstinence from tobacco[9].

Although anti-inflammatory therapy with oral corticosteroids for exacerbations of chronic obstructive pulmonary disease (COPD) is supported by recent clinical trials[69], the effect of therapy specifically on cough has not been evaluated. Universal consensus does not yet exist on the role of inhaled corticosteroids in the treatment of COPD[70]. The antitussive effects of inhaled β_2-agonists and theophylline, agents often used in the management of COPD, have also not been investigated. Ipratropium bromide, however, has been demonstrated in a randomized, controlled trial, to attenuate cough and sputum production[71]. Antibiotic therapy, indicated for presumed acute bacterial infections, likely ameliorates all aspects of a clinical exacerbation, including cough, but the antitussive effect of antibiotics has not specifically been evaluated.

Bronchiectasis, especially during exacerbations, may be associated with copious sputum production. Diagnosis is usually based on clinical and radiographic data. Although several North American studies evaluating the causes of chronic cough have demonstrated bronchiectasis in a very small percentage of referred patients[3–5,12], a recent Brazilian trial reported bronchiectasis to be present in 18% of immunocompetent patients referred to a university outpatient clinic for evaluation of chronic cough[72].

An effective cough is necessary in patients with bronchiectasis to allow mobilization of excessive respiratory secretions. During exacerbations, however, cough may become severe and debilitating, prompting aggressive management. Non-pharmacological therapy for bronchiectasis includes chest physiotherapy and postural drainage. Appropriate antibiotics are likely to improve respiratory symptoms, including cough, during an exacerbation[8]. Two prospective, uncontrolled studies describing a small number of patients with bronchiectasis suggested that β_2-agonists and theophylline are useful in diminishing cough[4,12]. Randomized, double-blind, placebo-controlled studies evaluating beclomethasone[73] and bromhexine[74] added to a regimen of physiotherapy showed neither drug to be effective in decreasing cough frequency and severity.

Non-specific antitussive therapy

Non-specific antitussive therapy is indicated when the etiology of cough is not established, thereby precluding the use of highly effective specific antitussive therapy. Other situations in which non-specific antitussive therapy may be appropriate include short-term usage while awaiting the effect of specific therapy, and in illnesses such as inoperable lung cancer or pulmonary fibrosis, in which specific therapy is not an option.

The goal of non-specific therapy is to suppress cough by inhibiting the cough reflex, regardless of the etiology of cough. Non-specific therapy is often not particularly effective.

Non-specific antitussive agents are most broadly classified as central or peripheral, based on their site of action. Central antitussives act within the central nervous system (CNS) to suppress the responsiveness of one or more components of the central reflex pathway for cough, whereas peripheral agents function outside the CNS, presumably by inhibiting the responsiveness of one or more vagal sensory receptors that produce cough[75]. The sites of action of some non-specific antitussive drugs, however, may not be mutually exclusive[75–77].

Centrally acting agents

Opioids
Drugs such as morphine, which are derived from opium, are generally termed opioids. Those that have sedative properties and may induce dependence are classified as narcotics. Opioid narcotics which are approved as antitussives include codeine, hydrocodone, and hydromorphone. Codeine is the narcotic antitussive of choice because of its lower abuse potential and more favourable side effect profile in terms of sedation and respiratory depression[78].

Codeine, often referred to as the gold-standard antitussive agent, has been demonstrated to be effective against various forms of pathological cough in randomized, double-blind, placebo-controlled trials[79,80]. The recommended antitussive dosage in adults is 10–20 mg every 4–6 hours, not to exceed 120 mg every 24 hours[78]. However, two fairly large, blinded, controlled studies have shown codeine to be ineffective against cough due to acute upper respiratory tract infections[51,81]. These data call into question the validity of the common clinical practice of treating postinfectious cough with codeine or other opioid preparations.

Dextromethorphan is a non-narcotic opioid without significant analgesic or respiratory depressant effects, though it may induce sedation. The drug has been demonstrated to be an effective antitussive in multiple randomized, double-blind, placebo-controlled studies[79,80,82]. It is one of the most widely used antitussives in the United States, with more than 60 dextromethorphan-containing preparations available. The recommended dosage in adults is 10–30 mg every 4–8 hours, not to exceed 120 mg in 24 hours[78].

Diphenhydramine
Diphenhydramine is a first-generation H_1-receptor antagonist that is believed to have antitussive action through a central mechanism[78]. One randomized, double-blind, placebo-controlled trial showed diphenhydramine to be effective in suppressing chronic cough due to bronchitis[83]; however, another study failed to demonstrate an effect against pertussis-induced cough in children[84]. The typical adult antitussive dose is 25 mg every 4 hours, not to exceed 150 mg in 24 hours. As with other drugs of this class, potential side effects include sedation and anticholinergic effects[78].

Caramiphen
Caramiphen is a non-opioid, centrally acting agent with weak anticholinergic properties. Although two randomized, double-blind, placebo-controlled studies have supported the antitussive effect of caramiphen[82,85], this evidence was felt inadequate to gain FDA approval for the drug in the United States

as an over-the-counter antitussive. Caramiphen is available in combination with the decongestant phenylpropanolamine as a prescription preparation (Tuss-Ornade)[78].

Baclofen

γ-aminobutyric acid (GABA) is a central inhibitory neurotransmitter. The GABA-agonist baclofen has been shown, in animal studies, to inhibit cough via a central site of action[86]. Two randomized, double-blind, placebo-controlled studies in healthy human volunteers have demonstrated the ability of oral baclofen to inhibit capsaicin-induced cough.[87,88] A 14-day course of low-dose baclofen achieved a degree of inhibition of capsaicin-induced cough similar to that of a 30 mg dose of codeine.[89] In small studies, baclofen has demonstrated antitussive activity in chronic, idiopathic cough,[90] and in cough due to ACE inhibitors.[65] However, the establishment of a role for baclofen in the treatment of cough awaits further prospective trials.

Peripherally acting agents

Levodropropizine

Levodropropizine, a non-opioid derived from phenylpiperazinopropane, is a peripherally-acting agent whose antitussive effect may be related to the modulation of sensory neuropeptides within the respiratory tract[91]. Levodropropizine has been shown to inhibit induced cough in healthy volunteers[92] and in patients with obstructive lung disease[93], as well as to suppress pathological cough in bronchitic patients in a placebo-controlled trial[94]. In uncontrolled studies, the antitussive effect of levodropropizine was shown to be similar to that of dextromethorphan[95] and dihydrocodeine[96] in patients with pathological cough.

Benzonatate

Benzonatate, a long-chain polyglycol derivative chemically related to procaine, acts peripherally by inhibiting the efferent limb of the cough reflex[78]. The antitussive efficacy of benzonatate in induced cough as well as in subjectively-measured pathological cough was demonstrated in trials performed soon after its release in 1955[78]. A recent report described three patients with advanced cancer and opioid-resistant cough who obtained symptomatic relief with benzonatate[97]. This agent is currently available in a prescription preparation (Tessalon perles). The recommended adult dose is 100 mg (one perle) three times daily, with a maximum of 600 mg daily. The perle should be swallowed intact without chewing to prevent anesthesia of the upper airway.

Inhaled anesthetics

Inhaled lidocaine (lignocaine) is often used during fibreoptic bronchoscopy to suppress cough. Although the antitussive effect of inhaled lidocaine has been demonstrated in studies of capsaicin-induced cough[98], and anecdotally in pathological cough[99,100], prospective, controlled trials are necessary to evaluate the utility of inhaled anesthetic agents in the treatment of cough.

Protussive therapy

The goal of protussive therapy is to improve the effectiveness of cough. Enhancement of cough may be beneficial in situations in which mobilization of copious amounts of respiratory secretions is necessary, such as with bronchiectasis and cystic fibrosis, as well as in postoperative patients, in whom prevention of atelectasis is desired. Protussive therapy may or may not increase cough frequency.

A wide variety of prescription and over-the-counter cough preparations, containing putative protussive agents such as expectorants, mucolytics, and mucokinetic agents, is available. However, most studies evaluating the efficacy of protussive therapy are difficult to interpret, since a patient's subjective response, or an objective measurement of mucus consistency or volume of expectorated sputum, may not correlate with actual improvement of cough effectiveness[8]. As stated in the recent consensus panel report of the American College of Chest Physicians[8], a protussive agent may be presumed to be clinically useful only if it has been shown to significantly increase the clearance of particles from the lower respiratory tract during coughing in adequately performed studies in patients with pathological cough.

By these criteria, randomized, double-blind, placebo-controlled studies have demonstrated the significant protussive effect of hypertonic saline aerosol[101,102] and erdosteine[103] in patients with bronchitis; aerosolized amiloride[104] in subjects with cystic fibrosis; and inhaled terbutaline in conjunction with chest physiotherapy and postural drainage[105] in patients with bronchiectasis. Agents shown to be ineffective in similarly designed trials include bromhexine[106,107], carbocysteine[108], guaifenesin[109], and mercaptoethane sulfonate[101].

REFERENCES

1 French CL, Irwin RS, Curley FJ, Krikorian CJ. Impact of chronic cough on quality of life. *Arch Intern Med* 1998; 158:1657–1661.

2 Schappert SM. Ambulatory care visits to physician offices, hospital outpatient departments, and emergency departments: United States, 1995. *Vital & Health Statistics-Series 13: Data from the National Health Survey.* 1997; 129:1–38.

3 Poe RH, Harder RV, Israel RH, Kallay MC. Chronic persistent cough. Experience in diagnosis and outcome using an anatomic diagnostic protocol. *Chest* 1989; 95:723–728.

4 Irwin RS, Curley FJ, French CL. Chronic cough. The spectrum and frequency of causes, key components of the diagnostic evaluation, and outcome of specific therapy. *Am Rev Respir Dis* 1990; 141:640–647.

5 Pratter MR, Bartter T, Akers S, Dubois J. An algorithmic approach to chronic cough. *Ann Intern Med* 1993; 119:977–983.

6 McGarvey LPA, Heaney LG, Lawson JT et al. Evaluation and outcome of patients with chronic non-productive cough using a comprehensive diagnostic protocol. *Thorax* 1998; 53:738–743.

7 Smyrnios NA, Irwin RS, Curley FJ, French CL. From a prospective study of chronic cough. Diagnostic and therapeutic aspects in older adults. *Arch Intern Med* 1998; 158:1222–1228.

8 Irwin RS, Boulet LP, Cloutier MM et al. Managing cough as a defense mechanism and as a symptom: a consensus panel report of the American College of Chest Physicians. *Chest* 1998; 114(suppl):133S–181S.

9 Wynder EL, Kaufman PK, Lerrer RL. A shortterm follow up study on ex-cigarette smokers: with special emphasis on persistent cough and weight gain. *Am Rev Respir Dis* 1967; 96:645–655.

10 Israili ZH, Hall WD. Cough and angioneurotic edema associated with angiotensin-converting enzyme inhibitor therapy. *Ann Intern Med* 1992; 117:234–242.

11 Marchesani F, Cecarini L, Pela R, Sanguinetti CM. Causes of chronic persistent cough in adult patients: the results of a systematic management protocol. *Monaldi Arch Chest Dis* 1998; 53:510–514.

12 Smyrnios NA, Irwin RS, Curley FJ. Chronic cough with a history of excessive sputum production: the spectrum and frequency of causes and key components of the diagnostic evaluation, and outcome of specific therapy. *Chest* 1995; 108:991–997.

13 Irwin RS, Corrao WM, Pratter MR. Chronic persistent cough in the adult: the spectrum and frequency of causes and successful outcome of specific therapy. *Am Rev Respir Dis* 1981; 123:413–417.

14 Gaffey MJ, Kaiser DL, Hayden FG. Ineffectiveness of oral terfenadine in natural colds: evidence against histamine as a mediator of common cold symptoms. *Pediatr Infect Dis J* 1988; 7:223–228.

15 Berkowitz RB, Tinkelman DG. Evaluation of oral terfenadine for the treatment of the common cold. *Ann Allergy* 1991; 67:593–597.

16 Berkowitz RB, Connell JT, Dietz AJ, Greenstein SM, Tinkelman DG. The effectiveness of the nonsedating antihistamine loratadine plus pseudoephedrine in the symptomatic management of the common cold. *Ann Allergy* 1989; 63:336–339.

17 McLeod RL, Mingo G, O'Reilly S, Ruck L, Bolser DC, Hey JA. Antitussive action of antihistamines is independent of sedative and ventilation activity in the guinea pig. *Pharmacology* 1998; 57:57–64.

18 Corrao WM, Braman SS, Irwin RS. Chronic cough as the sole presenting manifestation of bronchial asthma. *N Engl J Med* 1979; 300:633–637.

19 Johnson D, Osborne LM. Cough variant asthma: a review of the clinical literature. *J Asthma* 1991; 28:85–90.

20 Widdicombe JG. Neurophysiology of the cough reflex. *Eur Respir J* 1995; 8:1193–1202.

21 Advenier C, Lagente V, Boichot E. The role of tachykinin receptor antagonists in the prevention of bronchial hyperresponsiveness, airway inflammation and cough. *Eur Respir J* 1997; 10:1892–1906.

22 Irwin RS, French CL, Smyrnios NA, Curley FJ. Interpretation of positive results of a methacholine inhalation challenge and 1 week of inhaled bronchodilator use in

diagnosing and treating cough-variant asthma. *Arch Intern Med* 1997; 157:1981–1987.

23 Cheriyan S, Greenberger PA, Patterson R. Outcome of cough variant asthma treated with inhaled steroids. *Ann Allergy* 1994; 73:478–480.

24 Shim CS, Williams MH. Cough and wheezing from beclomethasone diproprionate aerosol are absent after triamcinolone acetonide. *Ann Intern Med* 1987; 106:700–703.

25 Doan T, Patterson R, Greenberger PA. Cough variant asthma: usefulness of a diagnostic therapeutic trial with prednisone. *Ann Allergy* 1992; 69:505–509.

26 North American Tilade Study Group. A double-blind multicenter group comparative study of the efficacy and safety of nedocromil sodium in the management of asthma. *Chest* 1990; 97:1299–1306.

27 Shioya T, Ito N, Watanabe A, Kagaya M, Sano M, Shindo T, Miura S, Kimura K, Miura M. Antitussive effect of azelastine hydrochloride in patients with bronchial asthma. *Arzneim-Forsch./Drug Res* 1998; 48:149–153.

28 Tan RA, Spector SL. Chronic cough. *Compr Ther* 1997; 23:467–471.

29 Nishi K, Watanabe K, Ooka T, Fujimura M, Matsuda T. Cough-variant asthma successfully treated with a peptide leukotriene receptor antagonist (Japanese). *Jpn J Thoracic Dis* 1997; 35:117–123.

30 Dicpinigaitis PV, Dobkin JB, Reichel J. Antitussive effect of the leukotriene antagonist zafirlukast in subjects with cough-variant asthma. *J. Asthma* 2002; 39:291–297.

31 Dicpinigaitis PV. Effect of zafirlukast, a leukotriene-receptor antagonist, on cough reflex sensitivity in healthy volunteers: a pilot study. *Curr Ther Res* 1999; 60:15–19.

32 Dicpinigaitis PV, Dobkin JB. Effect of zafirlukast on cough reflex sensitivity in asthmatics. *J Asthma* 1999; 36:265–270.

33 Irwin RS, French CL, Curley FJ, Zawacki JK, Bennett FM. Chronic cough due to gastroesophageal reflux. Clinical, diagnostic and pathogenetic aspects. *Chest* 1993; 104:1511–1517.

34 Ing AJ, Ngu MC, Breslin AB. Pathogenesis of chronic persistent cough associated with gastroesophageal reflux. *Am J Respir Crit Care Med* 1994; 149:160–167.

35 Ferrari M, Olivieri M, Sembenini C et al. Tussive effect of capsaicin in patients with gastroesophageal reflux without cough. *Am J Respir Crit Care Med* 1995; 151:557–561.

36 Ing AJ. Cough and gastroesophageal reflux. *Am J Med* 1997; 103:91S–96S.

37 Ing AJ, Ngu MC, Breslin AB. Chronic persistent cough and clearance of esophageal acid. *Chest* 1992; 102:1668–1671.

38 Irwin RS, Zawacki JK, Curley FJ, French CL, Hoffman PJ. Chronic cough as the sole presenting manifestation of gas-troesophageal reflux. *Am Rev Respir Dis* 1989; 140:1294–1300.

39 Laukka MA, Cameron AJ, Schei AJ. Gastroesophageal reflux and chronic cough: which comes first? *J Clin Gastroenterol* 1994; 19:100–104.

40 Fitzgerald JM, Allen CJ, Craven MA, Newhouse MT. Chronic cough and gastroesophageal reflux. *Can Med Assoc J* 1989; 140:520–524.

41 Waring JP, Lacayo L, Hunter J, Katz E, Suwak B. Chronic cough and hoarseness in patients with severe gastroesophageal reflux disease. Diagnosis and response to therapy. *Dig Dis Sci* 1995; 40:1093–1097.

42 Irwin RS, Zawacki JK, Wilson MM, French CL, Callery MP. Failure of chronic cough due to GERD to resolve despite acid suppression [abstract]. *Am J Respir Crit Care Med* 1999; 159:A830.

43 Allen CJ, Anvari M. Gastro-oesophageal reflux related cough and its response to laparoscopic fundoplication. *Thorax* 1998; 53:963–968.

44 Irwin RS, Zawacki JK, Wilson MM, French CL, Callery MP. Effects at one year of anti-reflux surgery performed for chronic cough due to GERD resistant to medical therapy [abstract]. *Am J Respir Crit Care Med* 1999; 159:A830.

45 Empey DW, Laitinen LA, Jacobs L, Gold WM, Nadel JA. Mechanisms of bronchial hyperreactivity in normal subjects after upper respiratory tract infection. *Am Rev Respir Dis* 1976; 113:131–139.

46 Little JW, Hall WJ, Douglas RG, Mudholker GS, Speers DM, Patel K. Airway hyperreactivity and peripheral airway dysfunction in influenza A infection. *Am Rev Respir Dis* 1978; 118:295–303.

47 Hogg JC. Persistent and latent viral infections in the pathology of asthma. *Am Rev Respir Dis* 1992; 145:S7-S9.

48 O'Connell F, Thomas VE, Studham JM, Pride NB, Fuller RW. Capsaicin cough sensitivity increases during upper respiratory infection. *Respir Med* 1996; 90:279–286.

49 Fujimura M, Myou S, Matsuda M, Amemiya T, Kamio Y, Iwasa K, Ishiura Y, Yasui M, Tagami A, Matsuda T. Cough receptor sensitivity to capsaicin and tartaric acid in patients with Mycoplasma pneumonia. *Lung* 1998; 176:281–288.

50 Eccles R. Codeine, cough and upper respiratory tract infections. *Pulm Pharmacol* 1996; 9:293–297.

51 Freestone C, Eccles R. Assessment of the antitussive efficacy of codeine in cough associated with common cold. *J Pharm Pharmacol* 1997; 49:1045–1049.

52 Holmes PW, Barter CE, Pierce RJ. Chronic persistent cough: use of ipratropium bromide in undiagnosed cases following upper respiratory tract infection. *Respir Med* 1992; 86:425–429.

53 Fujimori K, Suzuki E, Arakawa M. Effects of oxatomide, H_1-antagonist, on postinfectious chronic cough; a comparison of oxatomide combined with dextromethorphan versus dextromethorphan alone (Japanese). *Arerugi-Jap J Allergol* 1998; 47:48–53.

54 Ravid L, Lishner M, Lang R, Ravid M. Angiotensin-converting enzyme inhibitors and cough: a prospective evaluation in hypertension and in congestive heart failure. *J Clin Pharmacol* 1994; 34:1116–1120.

55 Strocchi E, Malini PL, Valtancoli G, Ricci C, Bassein L, Ambrosioni E. Cough during treatment with angiotensin converting enzyme inhibitors. Analysis of predisposing factors. *Drug Invest* 1992; 4:69–72.

56 Woo J, Tan TY. A high incidence of cough associated with combination therapy of hypertension with isradipine and lisinopril in Chinese subjects. *Br J Clin Pract* 1991; 45:178–180.

57 Lacourciere Y, Brunner H, Irwin R et al. and the Losartan Cough Study Group. Effects of modulators of the renin–angiotensin–aldosterone system on cough. *J Hypertens* 1994; 12:1387–1393.

58 Fox AJ, Lalloo UG, Belvisi MG, Bernareggi M, Chung KF, Barnes PJ. Bradykinin-evoked sensitization of airway sensory nerves: a mechanism for ACE-inhibitor cough. *Nat Med* 1996; 2:814–817.

59 Fogari R, Zoppi A, Mugellini A, Preti P, Bauderali A, Salvetti A. Effects of amlodipine, nifedipine GITS, and indomethacin on angiotensin-converting enzyme inhibitor-induced cough: a randomized, placebo-controlled, double-masked, crossover study. *Curr Ther Res* 1999; 60:121–128.

60 Just PM. The positive association of cough with angiotensin-converting enzyme inhibitors. *Pharmacotherapy* 1989; 9:82–87.

61 Tomaki M, Ichinose M, Miura M et al. Angiotensin converting enzyme (ACE) inhibitor-induced cough and substance P. *Thorax* 1996; 51:199–201.

62 Hargreaves MR, Benson MK. Inhaled sodium cromoglycate in angiotensin-converting enzyme inhibitor cough. *Lancet* 1995; 345:13–16.

63 Cazolla M, Matera MG, Liccardi G, De Prisco F, D'Amato G, Rossi F. Theophylline in the inhibition of angiotensin-converting enzyme inhibitor-induced cough. *Respiration* 1993; 60:212-215.

64 Malini PL, Strocchi E, Zanardi M, Milani M, Ambrosioni E. Thromboxane antagonism and cough induced by angiotensin-converting-enzyme inhibitors. *Lancet* 1997; 350:15–18.

65 Dicpinigaitis PV. Use of baclofen to suppress cough induced by angiotensin-converting enzyme inhibitors. *Ann Pharmacother* 1996; 30:1242–1245.

66 Umemura K, Nakashima M, Saruta T. Thromboxane A_2 synthetase inhibitor suppresses cough induced by angiotensin converting enzyme inhibitors. *Life Sci* 1997; 60:1583–1588.

67 American Thoracic Society. Standards for the diagnosis and care of patients with chronic obstructive pulmonary disease. *Am J Respir Crit Care Med* 1995; 152:S77–S121.

68 Nicotra MB, Rivera M, Dale AM, Shepherd R, Carter R. Clinical, pathophysiologic, and microbiologic characterization of bronchiectasis in an aging cohort. *Chest* 1995; 108:955–961.

69 Davies L, Angus RM, Calverley PMA. Oral corticosteroids in patients admitted to hospital with exacerbations of chronic obstructive pulmonary disease: a prospective randomized controlled trial. *Lancet* 1999; 354:456–460.

70 Banner AS. Emerging role of corticosteroids in chronic obstructive pulmonary disease. *Lancet* 1999; 354:440–441.

71 Ghafouri WD, Patil KD, Irving K. Sputum changes associated with the use of ipratropium bromide. *Chest* 1984; 86:387–393.

72 Palombini BC, Villanova CAC, Araujo E et al. A pathogenic triad in chronic cough. Asthma, postnasal drip syndrome, and gastroesophageal reflux disease. *Chest* 1999; 116:279–284.

73 Elborn JS, Johnston B, Allen F, Clarke J, McGarry J, Varghese G. Inhaled steroids in patients with bronchiectasis. *Respir Med* 1992; 86:121–124.

74 Olivieri D, Ciaccia A, Marangio E, Marsico S, Todisco T, Del Vita M. Role of bromhexine in exacerbations of bronchiectasis. *Respiration* 1991; 58:117–121.

75 Bolser DC. Mechanism of action of central and peripheral antitussive drugs. *Pulm Pharmacol* 1996; 9:357–364.

76 Adcock JJ, Smith TW. Inhibitory effects of the opioid peptide BW443C on smaller diameter sensory nerve activity in the vagus. *Br J Pharmacol* 1987; 96:596P.

77 Adcock JJ, Schneider C, Smith TW. Effects of codeine, morphine and a novel pentapeptide BW443C on cough, nociception and ventilation in the unanesthetized guinea pig. *Br J Pharmacol* 1988; 93:93–100.

78 Ziment I. Agents that affect mucus and cough. In: Witek TJ, Schacter EN, eds, *Pharmacology and Therapeutics in Respiratory Care*. Philadelphia: W.B. Saunders; 1994:239–257.

79 Aylward M, Maddock J, Davies DE, Protheroe DA, Leideman T. Dextromethorphan and codeine: comparison of plasma kinetics and antitussive effects. *Eur J Respir Dis* 1984; 65:283–291.

80 Matthys H, Bleicher B, Bleicher U. Dextromethorphan and codeine: objective assessment of antitussive activity in patients with chronic cough. *J Int Med Res* 1983; 11:92–100.

81 Eccles R, Morris S, Jawad M. Lack of effect of codeine in the treatment of cough associated with acute upper respiratory tract infection. *J Clin Pharm Ther* 1992; 17:175–180.

82 Cass LJ, Frederik WS. Quantitative comparison of cough-suppressing effects of Romilar and other antitussives. *J Lab Clin Med* 1956; 48:879–885.

83 Lillienfield LS, Rose JC, Princiotto JV. Antitussive activity of diphenhydramine in chronic cough. *Clin Pharmacol Ther* 1976; 19:421–425.

84 Danzon A, Lacroix J, Infante-Rivard C, Chicoine L. A double-blind clinical trial on diphenhydramine in pertussis. *Acta Pediatr Scand* 1988; 77:614–615.

85 Thomas JT, Henrich AE, Shepherd DA, Sanzari NP. A system for the clinical assessment of the antitussive activity of caramiphen. *Curr Ther Res* 1974; 16:1082–1090.

86 Bolser DC, DeGennaro FC, O'Reilly S et al. Peripheral and central sites of action of GABA-B agonists to inhibit the cough reflex in the cat and guinea pig. *Br J Pharmacol* 1994; 113:1344–1348.

87 Dicpinigaitis PV, Dobkin JB. Antitussive effect of the GABA-agonist baclofen. *Chest* 1997; 111:996–999.

88 Dicpinigaitis PV, Dobkin JB, Rauf K, Aldrich TK. Inhibition of capsaicin-induced cough by the γ-aminobutyric acid agonist baclofen. *J Clin Pharmacol* 1998; 38:364–367.

89 Dicpinigaitis PV, Dobkin JB, Rauf K. Comparison of the antitussive effects of codeine and the GABA-agonist baclofen. *Clin Drug Invest* 1997; 14:326–329.

90 Dicpinigaitis PV, Rauf K. Treatment of chronic, refractory cough with baclofen. *Respiration* 1998; 65:86–88.

91 Lavezzo A, Mellilo G, Clavenna G, Omini C. Peripheral site of action of levodropropizine in experimentally-induced cough: role of sensory neuropeptides. *Pulm Pharmacol* 1992; 5:143–147.

92 Bossi R, Braga PC, Centanni S, Legnani D, Moavero NE, Allegra L. Antitussive activity and respiratory system effects of levodropropizine in man. *Arzneimittel-Forschung* 1998; 38:1159–1162.

93 Bariffi F, Tranfa C, Vatrella A, Ponticiello A. Protective effect of levodropropizine against cough induced by inhalation of nebulized distilled water in patients with obstructive lung disease. *Drugs Under Exp Clin Res* 1992; 18:113–118.

94 Allegra L, Bossi R. Clinical trials with the new antitussive levodropropizine in adult bronchitic patients. *Arzneimittel-Forschung* 1988; 38:1163–1166.

95 Catena E, Daffonchio L. Efficacy and tolerability of levo-dropropizine in adult patients with non-productive cough. Comparison with dextromethorphan. *Pulm Pharmacol* 1997; 10:89–96.

96 Luporini G, Barni S, Marchi E, Daffonchio L. Efficacy and safety of levodropropizine and dihydrocodeine on non-productive cough in primary and metastatic lung cancer. *Eur Respir J* 1998; 12:97–101.

97 Doona M, Walsh D. Benzonatate for opioid-resistant cough in advanced cancer. *Palliative Med* 1997; 12:55–58.

98 Hansson L, Midgren B, Karlsson JA. Effects of inhaled lignocaine and adrenaline on capsaicin-induced cough in humans. *Thorax* 1994; 49:1166–1168.

99 Fuller RW, Jackson DM. Physiology and treatment of cough. *Thorax* 1990; 45:425–430.

100 Trochtenburg S. Nebulized lidocaine in the treatment of refractory cough. *Chest* 1994; 105:1592–1593.

101 Clarke SW, Lopez-Vidriero MT, Pavia D, Thomson ML. The effect of sodium 2-mercaptoethane sulphonate and hypertonic saline aerosols on bronchial clearance in chronic bronchitis. *Br J Clin Pharmacol* 1979; 7:39–44.

102 Pavia D, Thomson ML, Clarke SW. Enhanced clearance of secretions from the human lung after the administration of hypertonic saline aerosol. *Am Rev Respir Dis* 1978; 117:199–203.

103 Olivieri D, Del Donno M, Casalini A, D'Ippolito R, Fregnan GB. Activity of erdosteine on mucociliary transport in patients affected by chronic bronchitis. *Respiration* 1991; 58:91–94.

104 App EM, King M, Helfesrieder R, Kohler D, Matthys H. Acute and long-term amiloride inhalation in cystic fibrosis lung disease: a rational approach to cystic fibrosis therapy. *Am Rev Respir Dis* 1990; 141:605–612.

105 Sutton PP, Gemmell HG, Innes N et al. Use of nebulized saline and nebulized terbutaline as an adjunct to chest physiotherapy. *Thorax* 1988; 43:57–60.

106 Thomson ML, Pavia D, Gregg I, Stark JE. The effect of bromhexine on mucociliary clearance from the human lung in chronic bronchitis. *Scand J Respir Dis* 1974; 90(suppl.):75–79.

107 Mossberg B, Philipson K, Strandberg K, Camner P. Clearance by voluntary coughing and its relationship to subjective assessment and effect of intravenous bromhexine. *Eur J Respir Dis* 1981; 62:173–179.

108 Thomson ML, Pavia D, Jones CJ, McQuiston TAC. No demonstrable effect of S-carboxymethylcysteine on clearance of secretions from the human lung. *Thorax* 1975; 30:669–673.

109 Thomson ML, Pavia D, McNicol MW. A preliminary study of the effect of guaiphenesin on mucociliary clearance from the human lung. *Thorax* 1973; 28:742–747.

Index

THE A. F. OF L.
FROM THE DEATH OF GOMPERS
TO THE MERGER